PRINCIPLES OF ROENTGENOLOGICAL INTERPRETATION

(WITH ADDITION OF A CHAPTER ON RADIATION THERAPY)

By

L. R. SANTE, M.D.

*Professor of Radiology, St. Louis University School of Medicine;
Radiologist-in-chief to the University Hospitals, St. Mary's Hospital, Firmin Desloge Hospital, Mount St. Rose Hospital and
Cardinal Glennon Memorial Hospital for Children; Visiting
Radiologist, St. Louis City Hospital, St. Louis.*

ELEVENTH REVISED EDITION

AN ATLAS OF MINIATURE ROENTGENOGRAMS
has been prepared to supplement
this publication.

EDWARDS BROTHERS, INC.

ANN ARBOR, MICHIGAN

1958

H. K. LEWIS & CO., LTD.
MEDICAL AND SCIENTIFIC BOOKSELLERS
AND STATIONERS
136 GOWER ST., LONDON W.C. 1

PORTUGUESE TRANSLATION
PUBLICACOES PAN-AMERICANAS, LTD.
No. 70-sala 720
RIO DE JANEIRO, BRASIL

Printed in U.S.A.
Lithoprinted by Edwards Bros., Inc., Lithoprinters and Publishers
Ann Arbor, Michigan, 1958

To the Memory

of

My Teachers

WILLIAM H. STEWART

and

WILLIS F. MANGES

PREFACE TO ELEVENTH EDITION

In conformity with our original policy of frequent revisions of this book, to keep its subject matter up to date and consistent with prevailing opinion, it has undergone its eleventh revision.

The entire work has been completely reedited and revised; older concepts have been corrected and newer material supplied. To prevent an unwieldy enlargement of the book, subject matter has had to be condensed into more concise paragraphs in places without interfering with the meaning.

In order to serve this purpose to best advantage, the subject matter has been made very comprehensive— far more than a student could or should attempt to master. The rarer, less important subject matter to the student is, therefore, printed in smaller type in order that it may be readily recognized and omitted by the instructor if desired.

For the student this book will serve primarily as a basic outline for fundamental teaching but in addition as a source of concise radiological information concerning unusual conditions and diseases with which he comes in contact in his clinical work. The present day tendency in medical education to project clinical teaching into the earlier scholastic years has enhanced this need for more detailed clinical information. Confronted with a maze of new medical terms and diseases he must have a comprehensive text to which he can refer for guidance; mere basic essentials are not enough. In a similar manner this concise work will aid the general practitioner in directing x-ray examination for his patient and in evaluation of the radiological findings after they are reported by the radiologist. For the radiological resident it will serve as a guide for the more complete study of the literature, and for the practicing radiologist it may be found helpful in refreshing his memory on points of differential diagnosis encountered in his busy practice.

The illustrations accompanying the text are for the most part line drawings made directly from roentgenograms; there are, in addition, more than 500 half-tone illustrations of the various pathological conditions in order to acquaint the student with the appearance of actual roentgenograms. Subjects marked with an asterisk (*) throughout the text are illustrated in the supplementary half-tone illustrations which accompany each chapter. Lists of questions have been inserted at the end of each chapter to aid the student in review. Ready reference index sheets at the beginning of each section should be found serviceable. References have been removed from the text and concentrated in sections at the end of each chapter of the book.

Material utilized in this book has been gleaned from all available sources; no attempt has been made to give individual credit for old, fully established ideas; to do so would have converted the text into a lexicon of hames, meaningless and confusing to the student; only in unusual instances where further study might be desired are references given.

The method of presentation of bone infections and the scheme of analysis of bone pathology are essentially similar to those utilized by Wm. H. Stewart. The outline for the x-ray analysis of malignancy of bone, obtained from him also, has been further modified to conform to the classification of bone tumors, formulated by the Registry of Bone Sarcoma of the American College of Surgeons, and by other pathologists. The sections on mastoid and sinus pathology, as well as those portions dealing with foreign bodies in the lungs, reflect impressions of the original teaching of Willis F. Manges. Where material or illustrations from other publications have been utilized, direct acknowledgment is made in the text.

The Atlas of Miniature Roentgenograms introduced with the eighth edition as a supplementary means of study has been completed throughout the entire sections on bones, chest, gastrointestinal and biliary tracts and genito-urinary tract. It is hoped that this means of augmenting the illustration of the text may be of added value.

I am deeply indebted to Dr. Ralph Kinsella, Professor Emeritus, and Dr. G. O. Broun, Professor of Medicine and Director of the Department; to Dr. C. R. Hanlon, Professor of Surgery, and Dr. Henry Pinkerton, Professor of Pathology of St. Louis University School of Medicine, for reviewing the medical, surgical and pathological aspects of this book, and to Dr. R. M. O'Brien, Professor of Orthopedic Surgery and Dr. R. E. Funsch, Senior Instructor of St. Louis University School of Medicine, for reviewing the section on bone diseases; Dr. H. H. Kramolowsky, Associate Professor of Clinical Urology, and Dr. W. F. Melick, Assistant Professor of Urology, have kindly revised the section on urology. I am likewise indebted to Dr. Harry Fischer, Associate Professor of Radiology, State University of Iowa College of Medicine, for his assistance in revision of this edition, especially the sections on gastro-intestinal tract, congenital heart disease and radioactive isotopes; to Dr. Mary Lou Thomasson for making the circulation diagrams in congenital heart disease, and to Mr. P. A. Conrath for the new diagrammatic illustrations used in the text.

I wish also to express my appreciation to the personnel of Edwards Brothers, Incorporated for their infinite care and interest in the compilation of this book.

L. R. Sante

TABLE OF CONTENTS

INDEX

TO

BONE PATHOLOGY

OTHER EFFECTS OF TRAUMA
Traum. Osteitis (Kienbock)
Cystic Degen. Scaph. (Preiser)
Spondyl. Traum. Tarda (Kummell)
Radiation Osteitis
Burn Sequestra
Osteochondritis dissecans
Osteochon; Freiberg Infraction
Osseous Changes in leg ulcer
Slipped femoral epiphysis
Caisson Disease
Post-traum. Bone Atrophy. (Sudeck)
Coxa Magna
Scalenus Anticus Muscle Syn.
Fatigue (March) Fractures
Bursitis
Cal. Tendons; (Pelligrini-Stieda)
Phleboliths; Ehlers-Danlos Syn.
Cal. Hematoma
Myositis Ossificans
Infarcts; Caisson Dis.
Semilunar Cartilage Knee
Intervertebral Discs
Vacuum Space Joint
Baker's Cyst
Lipohemoarthrosis

GLANDULAR AND METABOLIC
Thyroid
Gonads
Pituitary: Acromegaly, Adenomata
Thymus:
  Osteogenesis Imperfecta
  Chondrodystrophia Foetalis
  Dyschondroplasia—Ollier's Disease
  Maffucci's Syn.
  Morquio's Dis.
  Stippled Epi.; Thiemann Dis.
Parathyroid: Osteitis Fibrosa
Other Dis. Unknown Etiology
  Polycstotic Fibrous Dyspl.
  Pseudo-fracture-Looser's Zones
  Paget's Disease
  Osteopetrosis
  Xanthomatosis

NUTRITIONAL DISEASES
Osteochrondritis of:
  Femoral head
  Acetabulum
  Tibial Tubercle
  Patella
  Scaphoid Tarsal
  Calcaneal Epiphysis
  Spine
  Sacrum
  Other rarer locations
Constitutional:
  Rickets
  Scurvy
  Osteomalacia
  Calcinosis Interstitialis

BLOOD DYSCRASIAS
Leukemia
Hemolytic Anemias:
  Erythroblastic
  Sickle Cell
  Chr. Hemolytic Icterus
  Marrow Sclerosis
Hemophilia

INFECTIONS
Pyogenic Osteomyelitis
Non-Sup. Osteomyelitis
Tuberculosis
Syphilis
Yaws
Fungus
Actinomycosis
Blastomycosis
Mycetoma (Madura Foot)
Coccidioidal Granuloma
Torula
Parasitic

NERVE CONDITIONS
Neurotrophic:
  Leprosy
  Raynaud's Disease
  Sclerodactylia
  Syringomyelia
  Spinal Cord Tumor
Melorheostosis
Neurofibromatosis

MINERAL POISONING

Lead
Phosphorus
Bismuth
Fluorine
Radium
Renal Rickets:
  Dwarfism
Kaschin-Beck's Disease

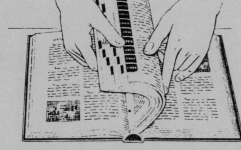

HOW TO USE READY REFERENCE INDEX
Allow the open book to lie flat on the table. Turn to the blue or pink index sheet depending upon the information desired. Select the chapter heading along the margin of the page most likely to contain desired subject. Bend the pages until the thumb mark is found on the margin of the page which corresponds to the chapter heading. The information desired should be in this chapter. If more precise information is desired consult the index at the back of the book.

PART I

BONE PATHOLOGY

(and Associated Pathology of the Adjacent Soft Tissues)

TRAUMA
- A. Fractures (Chapter I)
- B. Dislocations (Chapter II)
- C. Epiphyses and epiphyseal separations (Chapter III)
- D. Other effects of trauma (Chapter IV)
  - 1. from injury to the blood supply
    - a) of cancellous bone structure
      - 1) Traumatic osteitis of carpal bones--Kienböck disease
      - 2) Cystic degeneration of scaphoid (navicular)--Preiser's disease
      - 3) Spondylitis traumatica tarda--Kümmell's disease
      - 4) Radiation osteitis
      - 5) Burns (electrical), sequestration from
    - b) of the subchondral region of a joint
      - 1) Osteochondritis dissecans
      - 2) Deforming osteochondritis of the metatarso-phalangeal joints--Freiberg's infraction
      - 3) Osseus changes in varicose leg ulcer
    - c) of the metaphyseal area
      - 1) Femoral osteochondritis of adolescence--slipped epiphysis--epiphyseolysis
      - 2) Caisson disease--aseptic bone marrow necrosis
  - 2. from injury to nerve supply
    - a) Sympathetic nerve involvement
      - 1) Post-traumatic acute bone atrophy--Sudeck's atrophy
      - 2) Coxa magna
    - b. Nerve Trunks--pressure
      - 1) Scalenus anticus muscle syndrome
  - 3. from deficiency in strength of bone
    - Fatigue fractures
      - 1) March fracture
      - 2) Following roentgen therapy
  - 4. from injury to the adjacent soft parts; with calcareous deposits frequently associated
    - a) Bursae--especially of
      - 1) Subdeltoid
      - 2) Patellar
    - b) Tendons and ligaments
      - 1) Tearing associated with fracture or dislocation
      - 2) Supraspinatus tendon
      - 3) Traumatic calcification of ligaments
      - 4) Collateral tibial ligament--Pellegrini-Stieda disease
    - c) Connective tissue
      - 1) Phleboliths
      - 2) Ehlers-Danlos syndrome
      - 3) Hematoma--especially of thigh
    - d) Muscles
      - 1) Myositis ossificans
    - e) Bone marrow
      - 1) Caisson disease
      - 2) Aseptic infarcts
    - Without associated calcareous deposits
    - a) Cartilaginous structures
      - 1) Separation of semilunar cartilage of knee-- (see dislocations)
      - 2) Displacement of intervertebral disc--(see myelography)
      - 3) Gas or vacuum space within the joint
      - 4) Baker's cyst
    - b) Fat pads of joints
      - 1) Lipohemoarthrosis of knee

Chapter I

FRACTURES

A fracture may be defined as a break in the continuity of the bone. It is manifested in the roentgenogram by a disturbance in the normal texture of the bone and by a break in the periosteal line. Occasionally fractures are not visualized on the initial adequate radiographic examination. This is particularly true in fractures of the carpal scaphoid where upon occasion, the fracture will not be demonstrated until 10 to 14 days have passed, and there has been some absorption at the fracture line. In the fracture zone, the obstruction offered by the bony structure is removed and the x-rays have freer access to the film, producing a darker zone. Roentgenological examination is generally conceded to be the best means at our disposal for the detection of injuries to the bones. While manual examination is sometimes of great value, it subjects the patient to undue trauma and pain and cannot be expected to yield the same information obtainable by roentgenological examination. Since a roentgenogram is really a record of the densities traversed by the x-rays, in one plane only, it is obvious that at least two views at right angles to each other must be made routinely in examination of all fractures. Where two views at right angles to each other are not obtainable, recourse may be had to stereoscopic examination of the part. In many locations it has been found advisable to supplement the ordinary positions with other special examinations. These have been described in detail in the Manual of Roentgenological Technique under Standard Positions.

The detection of a fracture is ordinarily very simple; occasionally, however, a fracture line may be so fine that it requires the keenest perception for its detection; in any event, it is always advisable to make use of a magnifying lens for more detailed examination of the fine bony structure.

Fractures of the long bones may be complete or incomplete. Incomplete fractures are greenstick, or torus in type, or may be stellate, or impacted. Complete fractures may be linear, transverse, oblique, spiral, longitudinal and are further identified by descriptive terms such as angulated, displaced, overriding, etc.

Greenstick fractures are those in which the cortex is ruptured on one side only, the other side remaining intact. They are very rare. Torus fractures are those in which there is folding of the bone but not a definite break. They most frequently occur in cancellous bone of children. In describing any displacement of the bony fragments, the displacement of the distal fragment is always indicated; such displacement may be: anterior, posterior, medial, or lateral. In special locations other terms may be found less ambiguous, as for example, in the forearm or hand, "dorsal" or "palmar"; in the foot "dorsal" or "plantar," etc. Angulation of the fragments is always designated by the direction taken by the apex of the angle, as "dorsal angulation," "medial angulation," etc. Any shortening of the bone indicated by overriding or overlapping of the fragments must be indicated, and its amount estimated. Any statements as to the amount of shortening or the degree of angulation must be merely estimates made with a full understanding of the variations produced by distortion of the image (Klinefelter). Lastly, if the fracture occurs near a joint or other important structure, any involvement of the joint surface by the fracture line must be indicated, since this may influence the method of treatment and the ultimate outcome of the case. Fracture reports therefore should be concise but should always adequately cover the essential points necessary for a clear understanding of the conditions present, as for example: "There is a complete transverse fracture of the right femur in the lower one-third with posterior displacement of the distal fragment and about one-inch overriding. The lower epiphyseal structures are not involved."

Any disturbance in normal relationship, brought about by fracture or deformity from disease, will result in more or less impairment of function of the part. Proper treatment of fractures consists in recognition, reduction, immobilization, and the maintenance of adequate immobilization for a sufficient period of time to allow union to occur.

The normal position of the bones for proper function of the various joints will be designated by systems of lining, under the consideration of fractures of the various parts. Many contributions to this field have been made by Skinner, George, Chamberlain, Boehler and others. Johnson advocates the actual measurement of deviation of these angles from normal and incorporation in the roentgen report. While these systems of lining will determine largely what constitutes good position of a fracture in any given location, still there are certain other fundamental considerations which must be discussed in relationship to fractures in general.

To secure proper growth and union of the fragments, the most important single factor seems to be that relatively large, freshly broken, bony surfaces be maintained in apposition with each other. In certain instances where alignment is maintained by traction, if this is too great, so that there is separation of the broken ends of the bone, union may be delayed or may be entirely inhibited; to be effective therefore, the fractured bony edges should be in close apposition.

As a matter of practical experience it may be assumed that if one third to one half of the broken ends of the shaft of a bone are in close apposition, and the alignment is good, this should be satisfactory for a good functioning result. Where this relationship of the broken fragments is maintained, healing usually takes place with firm union; the greatest quantity of new bone formation is in the location of greatest defect in the alignment; the least new bone formation is on the side of least defect, so that there is a tendency thereby to reestablish the normal alignment of the bone. In time, the medullary canal may be reformed even where the fragments have been grossly displaced.

This is in accordance with Wolff's Law that change in mechanical stress and strain to which a bone is subjected is followed by change in the structure of the bone to conform to the demand made upon it.

As a general rule, the younger the individual, the greater is the likelihood of firm, bony union and the greater the tendency to straighten out deformities and reestablish the normal relationship. In young infants this tendency is so great that if there is side-to-side touching of the fragments, firm bony union will take place, and often the medullary canal will be ultimately reestablished. The younger the individual the more rapidly new bone forms; in young infants new bone formation may be manifested by periosteal proliferation within five days after an injury, whereas in adults it usually requires from two to three weeks before there is any evidence of new bone formation.

The skeleton, both in childhood and adult life is an active dynamic structure as opposed to the previously considered concept that it is an inert structure. Bone activity is constantly occurring. The maintenance of healthy strong viable robust bone depends in large measure upon the continued use and function of the part. It also depends to a certain extent upon metabolic needs and conditions in the body, as for instance, post menopausal osteoporosis. Disuse of a part, either associated first with a fracture or due to some paralytic disorder or other causes, produces bone atrophy in which there is actual diminution in the volume and bulk of a bone due to absorption of bone substance, both calcified and matrix. This is known as osteoporosis. Osteomalacia means a relative demineralization of a normal volume of bone matrix. Clinically the two conditions are indistinguishable, but histologically there is a great difference between them. Osteomalacic or osteoporotic bones heal poorly, as would be expected because of poor vitality of the part.

Nonunions of fractures occur despite the most optimum appearing circumstances. Ordinarily speaking, nonunion is due to one of several factors: failure to obtain reduction; inadequate immobilization (with references to both time and to absolute protection); the presence of soft parts between the bone ends; the presence of infection; circulatory disturbances in one or both of the fractured fragments; finally certain general debilitative conditions wherein the body as a unit does not have adequate vitality or resources to permit or stimulate the healing of the fracture.

Fractures of the long bones heal by two processes. Periosteal and endosteal proliferation. The periosteal union results from proliferation of the cambium layer of the periosteum which is the primitive cellular layer on the underside of the periosteum. Endosteal bone formation occurs by a metamorphosis of the endosteal callus within the medullary cavity of the bone. This process is widely documented in text books of fractures, histology, etc., but in general can be said to consist of the following steps: a) development of a hematoma; b) organization of the hematoma and invasion by fibrous tissue and capillaries; c) phagocytosis of the debris, invasion or appearance of osteoblasts; change in the pH to a more acid media; d) organization of the clot into a pre-bone matrix (osteoid tissue); and e) final calcification and maturation of the osteoid tissue. It will be noted that this is a biochemical phenomenon which occurs in a suitable environment on a previously prepared cellular network. Bone healing occurs fairly rapidly for the most part and most fractures of the long bones have united within several months. Maturation of the callus will then continue over a period of several years, and occasionally with the passage of additional time a previously fractured bone will resume normal alignment and the fracture can no longer be identified.

In the past, fluoroscopic control of reduction played a major role in the treatment of fractures. With the advent of modern orthopaedic surgery, wherein most fractures are handled by a relatively few physicians who are highly skilled in this field, the use of fluoroscopy for this purpose is gradually being abandoned.

A good orthopaedic table, although not essential, is highly desirable, (Figs. A to F). Such a table should provide convenient methods for traction on the extremities without interference with x-ray examination in two planes at right angles to each other. X-ray apparatus best suited to this purpose is two shock-proofed x-ray units, to be operated independently, for securing such views.

Even radiographic examination as a routine measure is not without danger to the operator and patient alike, and before such methods are undertaken, the operator must familiarize himself thoroughly with all aspects of this method, (see chapter on X-ray Protection in the Manual of Roentgenological Technique).

After proper reduction the fragments must be maintained in proper position. Wood is a good splinting material, since it is easily pervious to the passage of x-rays and causes little if any interference with the detail of the fine bony structure. Large amounts of adhesive plaster, especially when wrinkled or rolled, may interfere with bony detail. Salves or ointments with metallic bases sometimes cast very troublesome shadows over the bones. Metal splints--even when constructed of aluminum--may cause considerable obstruction of the rays. Iron bars and bands for reenforcement of plaster casts should be avoided wherever possible. Plaster of Paris, when dry, produces little hindrance to the passage of x-rays. The condition of the fracture and the position of the fragments should be checked up at weekly or biweekly intervals by further x-ray examination to be sure that the fragments have been maintained in proper position. Heavy cotton padding, used in application of plaster cast, packs down after a few days or weeks, and there is also some shrinkage of the soft parts of the extremity from disuse of the part. Both these

conditions result in loosening of the cast and permit spontaneous displacement of the fragments by muscle pull.

Newer methods of fracture care are becoming more widespread. The treatment of fractures emerged from the old school to the present operative aggressive approach with the advent of general surgical refinements and particularly with the introduction of the various antibiotics. The newer methods of treatment are in general well understood. Open reductions, internal fixation using plates, screws, pins, wires, and more recently intramedullary nails. In addition the substitutions of prosthetic appliances for fracture fragments particularly those involving joints, but often to span defects in long bones. In the newer method of treatment the long established fundamentals are not overlooked nor are they changed. Internal

fixation and stability is substituted for external fixation and immobilization in casts, brace, etc. The newer methods offer greater freedom to the patient, permit the introduction of physical therapy much earlier, permitting the restoration of the soft parts, the motion of joint function, early mobilization, etc. The newer methods permit early discharge from the hospital, early return to work, or to family, minimize disuse atrophy by promoting early motion, and in general have radically revised the previous conception of bone and joint lesions.

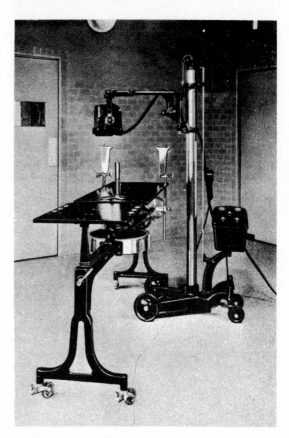

C. General Electric x-ray apparatus in use with table.

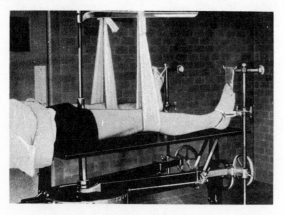

A. Hawley-Scanlan Fracture and Orthopedic Table. A table of more recent design equipped for fracture reductions and orthopedic corrections under biplane radiographic examination. Traction is by screw motion, applied to foot holders which are supported by long adjustable rods which radiate from the center of the table and are capable of almost complete 180° adjustment. Self-contained shockproof x-ray units may be used for radiography in two perpendicular planes.

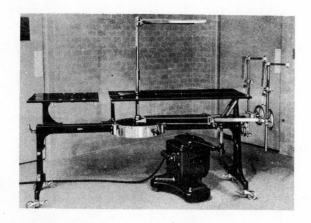

B. Lower extremities under extension, supported by slings suspended from overhead bars.

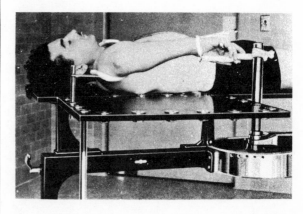

D. Upper extremity under extension in extreme abduction.

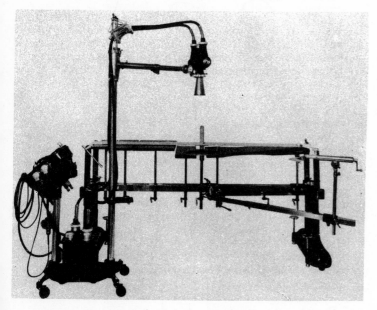

E. Bell Fracture Orthopedic and X-Ray Table. The two table leaves are lowered under the hips and used as a shelf for the x-ray cassette. A canvas strap supports the patient. This is drawn so tightly that there is scarcely any sag when the table leaves are lowered. This facilitates application of plaster or other orthopedic appliance.

F. Bell Table with the tube in position for reduction of long bones. Note that the bulk of the x-ray mechanism is on the opposite side from the working field.

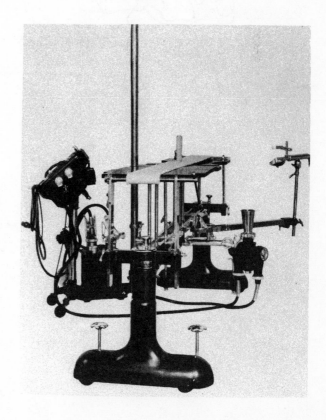

FRACTURES OF THE UPPER EXTREMITY

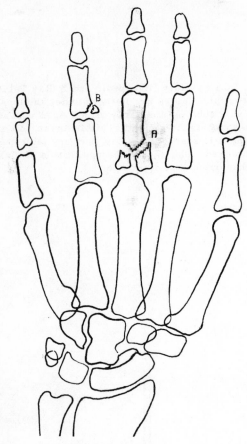

Fig. 1

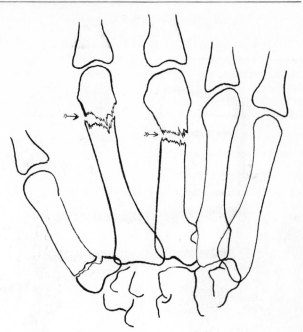

A. Fracture Metacarpals--Palmar View.

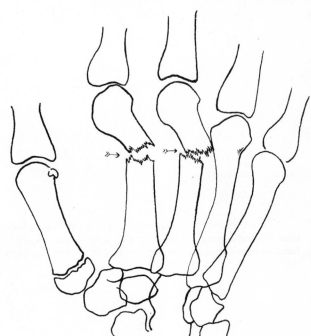

B. Fracture Metacarpals--Oblique View.

Fig. 2

FRACTURES OF THE UPPER EXTREMITY (Continued)

FRACTURES OF HAND PHALANGES. Fractures of the phalanges are usually crushing fractures or chip fractures of the joint margins. Crushing fractures (A) usually require no special treatment other than immobilization and rest for complete recovery. Where there is a tendency to overriding, traction with rubber bands on a board or banjo splint may be necessary. When joint is involved early active motion is necessary.

Chip fractures of the joint margins (B) are most often acquired by a blow on the end of the finger, as in playing baseball. The fact that they involve the joint increases the likelihood of resulting deformity and also of nonunion of the fragments. Early active motion is advisable. These fractures often produce lasting disability, (Gillespie). Fractures of the terminal phalanges usually require attention to soft parts only.

Fractures of the phalanges in general, are relatively slow to show new bone formation.

METACARPAL BONES. Fractures of the metacarpal bones result most frequently from striking a blow with the fist; the force applied to the ends of the metacarpal bones, if sufficiently strong, will cause fracture of one or more of the metacarpal bones with buckling and dorsal angulation. The site of fracture is usually near the distal end of the bone. In some cases bandaging the hand around a ball or bandage roll may serve well to immobilize the fragments; in others a straight board splint will serve the purpose better. In metacarpal fractures the degree of rotation is an important factor. New bone formation occurs early and is prolific unless a joint is involved. Fracture of the proximal end of the metacarpal for the thumb associated with dislocation is known as a Bennett's fracture; it often requires special methods for its successful treatment.

FRACTURE OF SESAMOID BONES. Fractures of sesamoid bones are very rare, but they do occur occasionally. They are of no particular importance but may be painful until the fragments are rounded off, (Jellinger).

FRACTURES OF THE UPPER EXTREMITY (Continued)

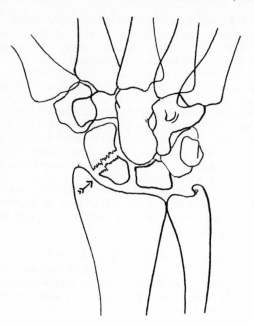

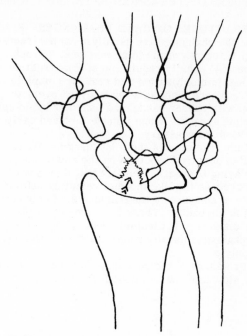

A. Fracture Scaphoid without Displacement.

B. Fracture Scaphoid with Displacement.

Fig. 3

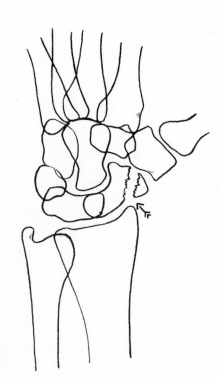

Fig. 3C. Fracture Tuberosity Scaphoid.

FRACTURE CARPAL BONES.* The Scaphoid (navicular) is the bone most frequently fractured in the carpus.

Fracture of the scaphoid is occasionally associated with dislocation of the semilunar bone.   Both the scaphoid and semilunar bones enter into the radiocarpal joint; when the semilunar is dislocated palmarward from the radius, the scaphoid tends to follow, but because of its firm attachment to the distal row of carpal bones it cannot, and fracture of the scaphoid results. Fractures of this bone may be completely through the waist from one joint surface to the other, without displacement of the fragments (A); or this same type of fracture may be through the proximal pole associated with palmar displacement of the medial fragment (B); or there may be simple fracture of the tuberosity of the bone (C).   Where there is no material displacement of fragments, union usually occurs promptly.

Interference with the blood supply of one of the fragments becomes evident by the failure of the fragment to undergo osteoporosis from disuse resulting in a chalky appearance of the avascular fragment. Revascularization, however, takes place after a prolonged period and the bony structure is restored to normal. Where there is displacement of one of the fragments, however, reduction may be impossible and ultimate removal of the displaced fragment may be necessary. Fairly good functional results may result even though a fragment of bone is absent. Since the joint surfaces are involved-- early active motion is the rule in treatment. Fracture of the tuberosity of the bone usually requires no special treatment; it does not involve the joint surface and healing takes place without disability. Fractures of the other carpal bones do occur, but these are usually chip fractures, and present no unusual problem. Nonunion may require fixation of the fragments by a small bone peg. (See relationship to Colles' fracture, p. 10.)

*An asterisk following any title indicates that roentgenographic reproductions illustrating this condition will be found in the pictorial supplement at the end of the chapter.

FRACTURES OF THE UPPER EXTREMITY (Continued)

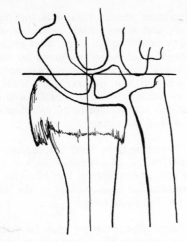

A₁. Impacted Colles' Fracture.

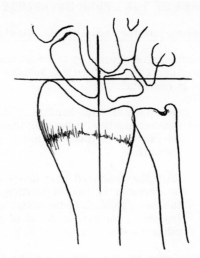

B₁. Colles' Fracture after Reduction.

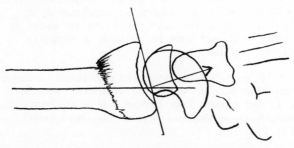

A₂. Lateral View Showing Characteristic Displacement.

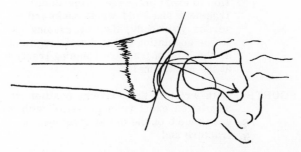

B₂. Lateral View Normal Position.

Fig. 4

FRACTURE--WRIST.* At the wrist joint, the fracture of the lower end of the radius is probably the most frequent fracture of any bone in the body.

A Colles' fracture is a fracture of the distal one and one-half inch of the radius; there is frequently an associated fracture of the tip of the styloid process of the ulna, and the fracture is usually accompanied by a characteristic "silver fork" deformity. The fracture is produced by force applied to the extended hand which results in dorsal displacement of the distal fragment of the fracture and tilting backward of the articular surface of the radius. For proper reduction of a Colles' fracture the normal relationship of the bones must be restored at the wrist joint. If an impaction is present it must be broken up and the deformity corrected. The correction of this disturbed relationship is very necessary for complete recovery of function.

There are three components in the satisfactory reduction:
1. To prevent shortening
2. To avoid displacement
3. To preserve the normal angle of the joint.

The normal relationship of the bones of the wrist joint may be schematically represented by two systems of lining.

First (B₁).

In the palmar view, a line is drawn down the middle of the shaft of the radius to get a clear conception of its normal axis. A second line drawn perpendicular to this, at the level of the tip of the styloid process of the radius should project downward fully one-half to three-quarters of an inch lower than the tip of the styloid of the ulna. Any amount by which this is lacking represents the degree of shortening. (A₁, Impacted Colles' Fracture.)

Second (B₂).

In the lateral view, a line is drawn down the middle of the shaft of the bone to get indication of its true axis. A second line is drawn independently of the first line, across the articular surface of the lower end of the radius; this plane should face palmarward. In impacted Colles' fracture this surface faces dorsalward (A₂). Best results are attained when the normal palmar inclination of the articular surface is attained but if all other relationships are normal and the plane of this articular surface is replaced to at least a perpendicular position with the shaft, then this is permissible for a satisfactory functional result. Greater backward inclination than this will invariably result in a weakening of the grip of the individual after complete healing has taken place.

FRACTURES OF THE UPPER EXTREMITY (Continued)

Surgical procedure for reduction of Colles' fracture:

In order more effectually to assist the surgeon in his reduction of the fracture a knowledge of the procedure is essential.

FIRST: Grasp the affected hand as if you were shaking hands with the individual, and if the fracture is impacted break up the impaction.

SECOND: With the fractured part under the fluoroscope in the lateral position, locate the exact position of the distal radial fragment, placing the thumb of your other hand in contact with it.

THIRD: Grasp the forearm above the fracture firmly with the fingers, thumb in position to exert pressure on the distal fragment and bend wrist backward across your body, thereby causing extreme angulation of the distal fragment at the site of fracture (causing traction at the same time).

FOURTH: With wrist in this extreme position of angulation exert firm pressure with your thumb on the distal fragment of fracture and,

FIFTH: Quickly flex the hand at the wrist. If complete reduction has not been accomplished, repeat the maneuver.

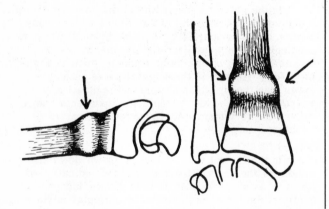

Fig. 4C. Torus fracture of lower end of radius, the most frequent occurrence of this type of fracture is young children.

The fracture should finally be put up with palmar flexion and some ulnar deviation of the hand. Straight board splints are most satisfactory for the maintenance of these fractures in position-- some men prefer only a single dorsal splint, but frequently double splints, palmar and dorsal, will be found most satisfactory. A small notch should be cut out of the dorsal splint to avoid pressure on the lower end of the ulna.

Double board splints lend themselves more readily to application of pressure on the fragments, when this is necessary, and likewise minimize the possibility of constriction of the blood supply from too tight a bandage.

A moulded plaster splint may be found very satisfactory to maintain the fragments in position.

The position of the fragments should be checked up by further roentgenographic examination in about a week or ten days. Four to six weeks is usually sufficient time for healing of ordinary fractures of this type.

In young infants fractures may take on a torous type (Fig. 4C) in which the soft bony structure is folded rather than broken. If an epiphysis is present an epiphyseal separation may result (Fig. 51).

A fracture less commonly encountered at the wrist is a Smith fracture. This is sustained by forcible flexion of the hand on the wrist resulting in a reversal of the deformity with palmar displacement of the distal radial fragment. It is often accompanied by dislocation of the wrist joint, see Fig. 40B.

An interesting observation made on men in the armed forces was that Colles' fracture was commonly encountered when they first entered the service before training had strengthened their muscles and ligaments. Whereas, after this had been accomplished by a period of service, Colles' fracture usually did not result but fracture of scaphoid and dislocation of the semilunar was the most frequent deformity encountered. Similarly, Colles' fracture is more frequent in older individuals who have weaker muscular structures; fracture of the scaphoid occurs more frequently in young adults. Both bones of the forearm is the most frequent fracture site in children.

FRACTURES OF THE UPPER EXTREMITY (Continued)

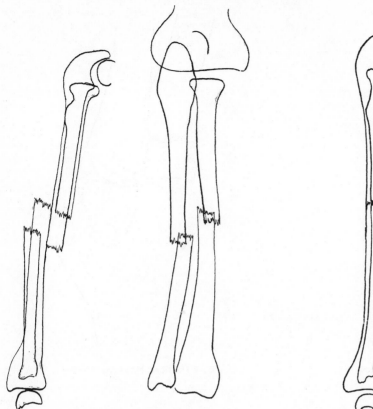

A. Fracture Both Bones Forearm.

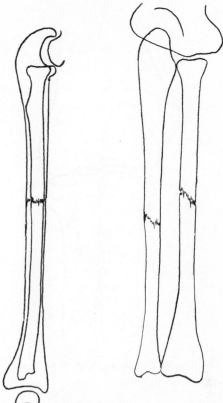

C. After Reduction.

Fig. 5

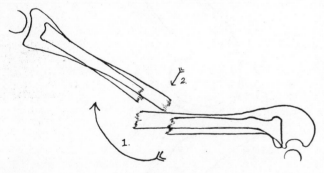

Fig. 5B. Angulated Position for Reduction.

FOREARM FRACTURE. Fractures of the forearm may be either incomplete or complete, of one or both bones. Incomplete fractures occur most frequently in children due to the softer character of the bones. These may be of the "greenstick" type, where the bone is completely fractured through one side and the cortex is still intact on the opposite side. These fractures are undoubtedly much rarer than we formerly supposed. Such fractures often require completion of the fracture before proper replacement of the fragments can be effected. Another type of incomplete fracture which occurs in children is

the "torus" or folding fracture, Fig. 4C, which is due to compression of the soft cancellous bone, and is characterized roentgenologically by a "bulge" in the cortical outline without actual break in the continuity. Obviously recovery from such fractures is prompt with simple immobilization-- they do not need any corrective manipulation unless they result in pronounced disturbance of the normal relationship of the bones. Two to three weeks is ordinarily sufficient time for healing of such fractures.

Complete fractures of both bones of the forearm (A) may be very difficult to replace in proper position. Angulation to increase the deformity with traction is used to reduce the fragture (B). If the bones can be maintained with 1/3 to 1/2 of the fractured surfaces in apposition and the alignment is good this should be satisfactory for a good functional result (C). One precaution which must be observed in fractures of the forearm is that the interosseous space is not encroached upon; encroachment upon this space will result in limitation of pronation and supination. About six to eight weeks is ordinarily required for healing of fractures in this location, in children; longer periods are required for adults.

FRACTURES OF THE UPPER EXTREMITY (Continued)

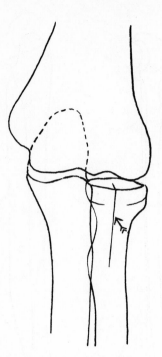

A. Linear Fracture Head of Radius.

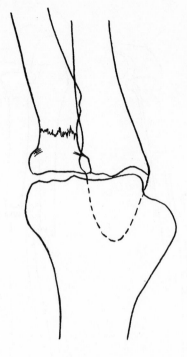

B. Fracture Neck of Radius.

Fig. 6

FRACTURES--ELBOW-RADIUS. Fractures about the elbow most frequently involve the head or neck of the radius, the olecranon or coronoid process of the ulna or the supracondylar region or condyles of the humerus. Fracture of the head of the radius is frequently associated with impacted Colles' fracture; the force applied to the lower end of the radius is transmitted upward through the shaft to the head of the bone which is forced against the capitulum of the humerus. This results in a fine linear fracture of the head of the radius extending into the joint (A). The line of fracture may be so fine that close examination with a lens may be necessary for its detection. Such fractures are of importance only in so far as they involve the joint surface; they may result in limitation of pronation and supination; early active motion (after about a week or ten days) should be instituted to avoid impairment of function. An ordinary sling or right-angle splint should be sufficient for treatment. In every Colles' fracture, palpation should be made over the head of the radius and if pain is elicited, roentgenographic examination of the elbow should be made for the detection of fracture. If the fracture of the head of the radius results in separation of a definite fragment of bone from the head (C), this may require open operation and removal of the fragment before satisfactory function can be restored. Fragments of this sort when widely separated often result in proliferation of large quantities of new bone which may impede function.

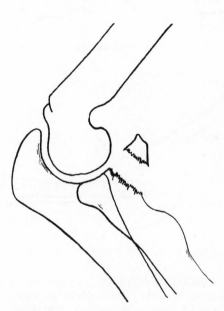

Fig. 6C. Fracture Head of Radius.

Fracture of the neck of the radius (B) rarely gives great difficulty in reduction. Right-angle splint should be sufficient for immediate immobilization. Active motion should be instituted early in the treatment of such fractures to prevent limitation of motion. If the fracture is linear only, without material displacement, many surgeons treat without immobilization merely with a sling.

FRACTURES OF THE UPPER EXTREMITY (Continued)

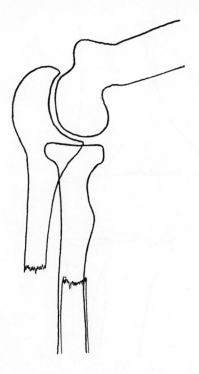

A. Fracture Ulna--Upper Third.

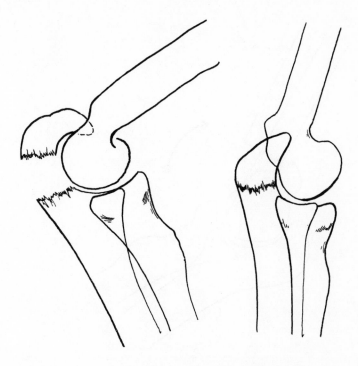

B. Fracture Olecranon Process.

Fig. 7

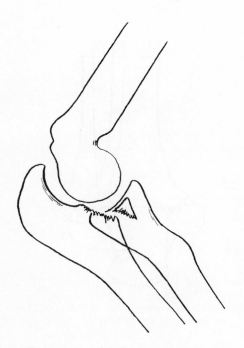

Fig. 7C. Fracture Coronoid Process Ulna.

ELBOW-ULNA FRACTURES. Fracture of the upper third of the ulna may show marked posterior displacement of the upper fragment due to the pull of the extensor muscles (A). Reduction and maintenance of the fragments in position may be impossible without open reduction and internal fixation.

Fracture of the olecranon process of the ulna (B₁ and B₂), may result in wide separation of the upper fragment of the olecranon process due to the pull of the triceps tendon. Relaxation of the muscle by complete extension of the forearm may result in complete replacement of the fragment. If this position alone does not result in replacement of the fragment, open reduction may have to be resorted to for its replacement.

Fractures of the coronoid process of the ulna (C) are usually associated with backward dislocation of the ulna at the elbow joint. Unless the elbow is maintained in an acutely flexed position, spontaneous posterior redislocation of the bones of the forearm is likely to occur at the elbow joint.

Fracture of the upper end of the ulna associated with dislocation of the head of the radius is known as a Monteggia fracture (see Chapter on Dislocations).

FRACTURES OF THE UPPER EXTREMITY (Continued)

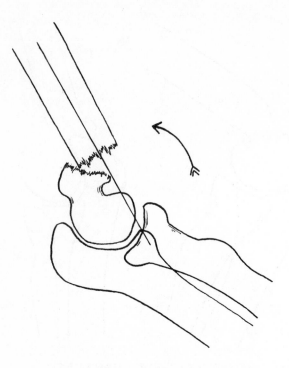

A₁. Supracondylar Fracture of Humerus.

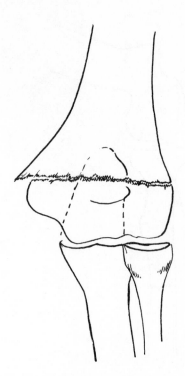

A₂. Supracondylar Fracture of Humerus.

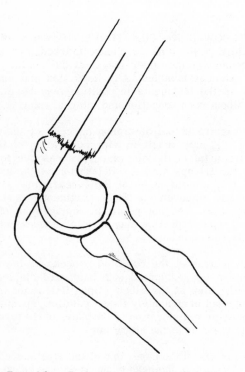

B₁. After Reduction--Normal Position.

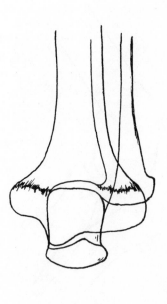

B₂. After Reduction--Elbow Acutely Flexed.

Fig. 8. Fracture of the Lower End of the Humerus.

FRACTURES OF THE UPPER EXTREMITY (Continued)

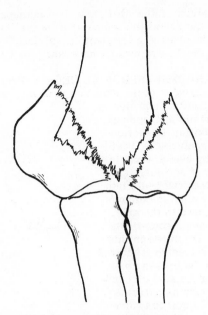

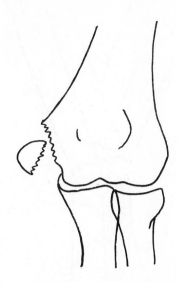

C. Fracture of Both Condyles.   D. Fracture of Inner Condyle.

Fig. 8

ELBOW- -LOWER HUMERUS FRACTURE.*
Supracondylar fracture of the humerus is one of the most common types of injury about the elbow joint. It occurs most frequently in children, during the stage of epiphyseal development. Since there are four centers of ossification for the lower humeral epiphyses, these, together with the deformity from the fracture, give the entire picture a very grave aspect to those who are not thoroughly familiar with the normal structures. The characteristic deformity resulting from supracondylar fracture is caused by posterior displacement of the distal fragment, with or without overriding. $(A_1$ and $A_2)$ This displaces the lower articular surface of the humerus posteriorly. Normally the articular end of the humerus should be anterior to the axis of the shaft. For correction of this deformity manipulative reduction and acute flexion of the elbow in Jones' position is necessary to maintain the fragments in good position, $(B_1$ and $B_2)$, otherwise use Dunlop's traction. Caution should be taken where excessive swelling is present in maintenance of this acutely flexed position that the circulation is not interfered with; it may be impossible at first to secure any more flexion than a right-angle position without interfering with the radial pulse, gradually increasing flexion from day to day.

Fractures of the condyles, either one or both, involving the joint are probably among the most difficult fractures of the elbow to treat (C). Any malposition at all will result in new bone formation filling in the fossa for the olecranon and coronoid processes, which will prevent complete flexion and extension of the joint.

Fractures of the epicondyles, especially of the inner (D), often result in complete detachment of the fragment, which can be palpated as a loose body under the finger. It is often relatively painless. It may be impossible to hold the fragment in good position without operative replacement. If the injury is in a young individual, when subsequent growth is expected of this epiphysis, it should be replaced if possible; if the epicondyle has already completely fulfilled its epiphyseal function, then it may be either left alone if it causes no pain or it may be totally removed if it does. Such fractures in children consistently justify surgical removal.

Occasionally the small fragment of bone, retaining its lower capsular attachment, is slipped through the rent in the capsular ligament to a position inside the joint between the articular surfaces. See epiphyseal separations of inner epicondyle. Figs. 52B and C.

FRACTURES OF THE UPPER EXTREMITY (Continued)

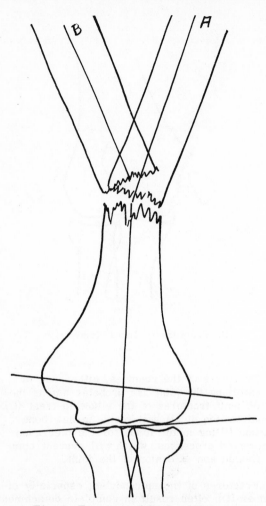

Fig. 9. Fracture of Shaft of Humerus.

middle thirds of the shaft may be accompanied by injury to the radial (musculospiral) nerve. The lower third of the shaft is a frequent site of nonunion. Eight to twelve weeks are usually necessary for firm union.

SHOULDER--SURGICAL NECK.* Fracture of the surgical neck of the humerus is usually accompanied by anterior projection of the distal fragment into the axilla. Reduction of such fractures is best secured by use of a pad in the axilla of sufficient size to bring the fragments into alignment when the elbow is bound down to the side. Since nonunion sometimes occurs in fractures in this location, impacted fractures should not be broken up except under unusual circumstances, such as extreme pain, etc. Eight to twelve weeks is usually necessary for healing of fractures in this location (see combina-

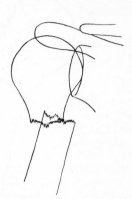

Fig. 10A. Fracture Surgical Neck of Humerus.

tion fractures of surgical neck and greater tuberosity). Early active motion is always advisable in all shoulder injuries.

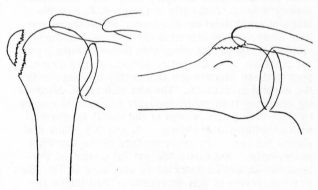

B . Displacement.   B . Reduction by Abduction Position.

Fig. 10B. Fracture of Greater Tuberosity.

HUMERUS--SHAFT FRACTURE.* In fractures of the shaft of the humerus the important fact to be borne in mind about the position of the fragments is to avoid lateral angulation. Normally the carrying angle tends to throw the forearm away from the body film taken palm forward; if angulation of the humerus is medial (A), so as to increase the carrying angle somewhat, this will not interfere with a good functioning result, but if it is lateral (B) the resulting loss of the carrying angle may produce considerable disability. If there is overriding of fragments, traction may be necessary. "Hanging casts" have been found useful for the treatment of these fractures. Under this arrangement a cast is applied to the forearm, elbow and lower humerus with the elbow joint flexed beyond a right angle, immobilizing the fracture, but leaving the shoulder free. Hanging freely, the weight of the cast produces traction. Care should be taken that the cast is not too heavy. Excess traction may pull the fragments apart or even cause subluxation of the shoulder. X-ray examination should be made of the fracture site and of the shoulder from time to time to avoid such a development. This is the only region in which such a hanging cast is of value. Fractures of the upper and

SHOULDER--GREATER TUBEROSITY. The greater tuberosity of the humerus is frequently torn off as a shell of bone and displaced upward. When completely separated it cannot be replaced and held in its normal position except by extreme abduction. The treatment of choice used to be by an abduction or "aeroplane" splint. Open reduction has practically replaced this method of treatment.

After healing in this position, the arm can always be lowered; if allowed to heal with the arm at the side, union of the tuberosity in its high position would prevent proper abduction of the arm by impingement upon the acromion process of the scapula. Union usually requires from six to eight weeks (see combination fractures of the surgical neck and greater tuberosity).

FRACTURES OF THE UPPER EXTREMITY (Continued)

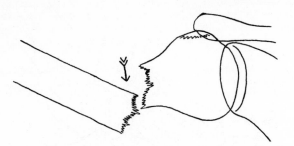

Fig. 10C. Combined Fractures of Surgical Neck and Tuberosity.

FRACTURE--SHOULDER, COMBINED SUR-GICAL NECK HUMERUS AND GREATER TUBER-OSITY. Combined fractures of the surgical neck and greater tuberosity of the humerus present special problems. In order to hold the tuberosity in place an abduction splint is essential, but where there is an associated fracture of the surgical neck of the humer-us an abduction splint acts as a weight pulling down-ward on the distal humeral fragment. This tendency to downward displacement of the distal fragment from the weight of the cast is clearly shown in Fig. 10C. If the displacement of the tuberosity is so great that it must be treated with an abduction splint, then the only alternative to prevent weighing downward of the humeral fragment is to make use of an adjustable splint which can be tightened from day to day or to put the patient to bed until union has occurred. Such fractures may be successfully treated by the hanging cast method, (see p. 16), or open reduction.

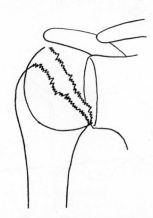

Fig. 10D. Fracture of Anatomical Neck.

SHOULDER--ANATOMICAL NECK HUMERUS. Fractures of the anatomical neck of the humerus often present very trying problems. Such fractures fre-quently are intracapsular and do not unite. The head may be rotated and even slip around entirely to the outer side of the shaft. Under such circumstances surgical intervention is the only alternative.

"Impression" fracture of the head of the hu-merus has been described (Ylwan) from forcibly re-straining patients on a hard wooden bench during electric shock therapy. The fracture is caused by pressure of the posterior edge of the glenoid against the head of the bone during unconsciousness. It ap-pears as a linear depression on the side of the head.

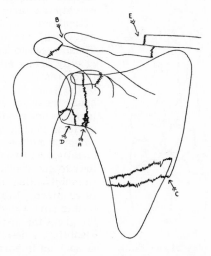

Fig. 11. Fractures of Scapula and Clavicle.

SHOULDER--SCAPULA AND CLAVICLE. The scapula is most frequently fractured through the neck (A), the acromion process (B), the body just above the inferior angle (C), and the glenoid (D). Most fractures of the scapula usually do not require anything more than temporary immobilization, it being almost im-possible to influence the position of the fragments by manipulation, and usually is not necessary, since the functional result is usually satisfactory. Eight to twelve weeks is usually required for firm union. Fracture of the inferior rim of the glenoid, however, is frequently very disabling in spite of all methods of treatment. The lower margin of the rim of the glen-oid serves as attachment for the long head of the tri-ceps muscle and capsular ligament. In lifting heavy weights with arms extended this causes pull on this head of the triceps muscle and the lower rim of the glenoid can actually be fractured in this manner.

The clavicle (E) is one of the most frequently fractured bones in the body; there is usually depres-sion of the outer fragment and some overriding. End to end replacement of the fragments is often difficult and sometimes impossible. Union practically always occurs, however, with good function. Ordinarily a figure of eight bandage about the two shoulders holds the fragments in hyper extension for satisfactory functional result. If badly displaced a large unsight-ly callus may result, which is disfiguring to women patients. Where the cosmetic result is of impor-tance, a figure-of-eight bandage about both shoulders posteriorly, anchored to a hard board "T" splint ap-plied to the back, although uncomfortable, often gives most satisfactory results. Six to eight weeks is usu-ally sufficient to produce satisfactory union.

FRACTURES OF THE LOWER EXTREMITY

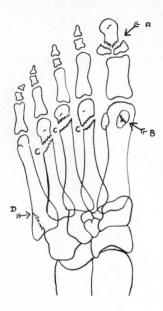

Fig. 12
Fractures of the Foot.

FRACTURES--FOOT PHALANGES. Fractures of the phalanges of the toes (A) are usually crushing fractures, from objects falling on them, or chip fractures of the articular margins, from "stubbing" the toes. These seem to heal more readily than similar fractures of the phalanges of the hand, probably because these joints in the feet are not required to perform such a wide range of motion. Healing usually occurs in from four to six weeks; simple immobilization is all that is required. Fractures of this sort which involve the great toe are most disabling, since this toe is such an important member in locomotion. Manipulation of the fragments into as satisfactory position as possible, and early active motion to prevent stiffening of the joint is the only procedure which can be followed. Very rarely there may be fracture of the sesamoid bones of the great toe (B). Anomalous division of these sesamoid bones is occasionally encountered; care must be taken not to mistake this normal structure for injury. Examination of the opposite foot for comparison will determine the possibility of anomalous division of the bone. Fractures of the inconstant sesamoids of the foot have been described, (Lapidus).

The metatarsal bones are most frequently fractured by the fall of heavy objects (C). If only one or two are broken the others act as splints. Replacement of such fragments in direct apposition is always difficult where any material displacement is present and may at times be impossible. Fortunately, if the normal arches of the foot are maintained, such fractures rarely cause lasting disability. Care must be taken to preserve the normal lateral arch. Downward projection of sharp points should be avoided. A very common fracture of the metatarsal bones is one which occurs through the styloid process at the proximal end of the metatarsal for the little toe (D). Such fractures usually heal merely by immobilization without lasting disability. This is also the site of an anomalous epiphysis which, when it persists into adult life, forms a separate accessory bone known as a Vesalianum. If in doubt, examination of the other foot will settle the question, since anomalies usually occur on both sides. Six to eight weeks is usually required for firm union.

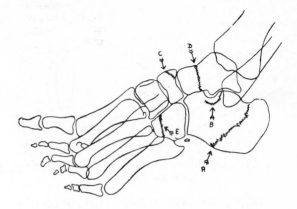

Fig. 13. Fractures of the Tarsal Bones.

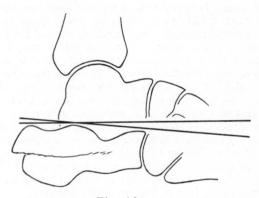

Fig. 13A.

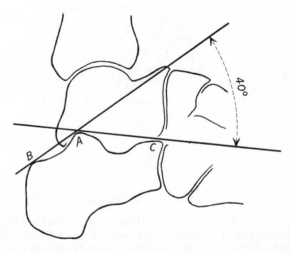

Fig. 13B.

FRACTURES OF FOOT--TARSAL. In fractures of the tarsal bones, the most important factor in securing a satisfactory result is the preservation of

FRACTURES OF THE LOWER EXTREMITY (Continued)

the normal anteroposterior arch of the foot. The most frequent fractures of the tarsal bones are: fracture of the body of the calcaneus (A), of the sustentaculum tali (B), of the navicular (C), talus (D), and nutcracker fracture of cuboid bone (E) by indirect violence, (Hermel and Gershon). The development of "traumatic flat foot" results in disability which is extreme and lasting. The time to correct such defects in the arch is immediately following injury. This can be accomplished by forcibly moulding the foot over a sand bag or some other resisting object and fixing it in plaster in this position until union has taken place. From ten to twelve weeks is usually required for union of such fractures.

A well-defined ossicle is sometimes present at the anterior superior margin of the calcaneus which probably has its origin as a small ununited fracture of the "promontory" of the calcaneus, (Piatt).

IMPACTED FRACTURE OF THE CALCANEUS. The lower portion of the calcaneus is driven upward and forward, resulting in compression of Boehler's salient angle to almost a straight line.

BOEHLER'S ANGLE SHOWING NORMAL STRUCTURAL RELATIONSHIP OF THE CALCAN- EUS. A line drawn from the posterior superior margin of the talo-calcaneal joint (A), through the posterior superior margin of the calcaneus (B), should make an angle with a second line drawn from the same point (A), to the superior articular margin of the calcaneocuboid joint (C), of about 40°. With fracture of the calcaneus this angle may be diminished or reversed. Restoration of this angle is advisable but not essential to a satisfactory result in fractures of the calcaneus. Recently more attention is being given to maintaining a narrow heel and prevention of talocalcaneal arthritis.

FRACTURE OF CALCANEUS. Of these, the fractures of the calcaneus are most disabling, due to the importance played by this bone in the mechanics of walking and weight bearing. Simple moulding of the foot and application of a cast may not be sufficient. Restoration of the normal relationship of the bones is essential. This can be determined from a lateral view of the foot by an estimation of the salient (Boehler's) angle. Normally if two lines are drawn, one from the upper posterior margin of the talo-calcaneal joint to the upper margin of the tuberosity of the calcaneus behind, and the other from this point to the upper articular margin of the calcaneocuboid joint in front, the angle should be about 40°. In fractures of the calcaneus this angle may be greatly reduced due to impaction of the fragments. To restore this angle many methods of manipulation have been devised. Olson has given a very clear description of a modification of Boehler's method which has proven most successful. Two Steinmann pins are inserted through the bones, one through the distal fragment of the calcaneus, the other through the anterior margin of the lower end of the tibia. By turnbuckles attached to pins pressure is exerted. When position

of fragments has been reestablished cast is applied.

A twisting motion of the foot may result in fracture of the sustentaculum tali. This is best shown radiographically by the oblique view of the foot. It is of importance, since the displacement of this process may result in disturbance of the normal arch of the foot, (Wilson).

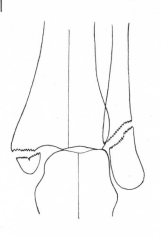 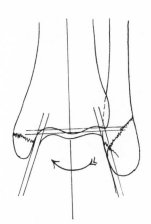

A. Pott's Fracture--   B. After Reduction--
Characteristic Deformity.   Normal Position.

Fig. 14

FRACTURES--ANGLE--POTT'S.* Pott's fracture of the lower end of the fibula is the second most common site of fracture in the body. It frequently is associated with fracture of the inner malleolus (A). There is characteristically lateral displacement of both distal fragments along with the talus and bones of the foot. This causes a disturbance in the normal weight-bearing line which must be corrected to insure a satisfactory functional result. The weight-bearing line extends down the shaft of the tibia, exactly through the middle of the lower tibial articulation and is continued through the exact midportion of the articular surface of the talus. Correction is most effectively carried out by inversion of the foot. A system of lining illustrating the similar spacing on all sides after the joint has been placed in normal position (B) will aid in determining the correct relationship of the bones of the joint; this depends for its accuracy on taking the roentgenogram in true standard position with toes straight forward and foot at right angles to the leg, centering directly over midpoint of the joint. Extensive ligamentum tears may be present which may escape detection unless the full range of joint displacement is explored under anesthesia. Inversion of the foot is the position for reduction of fracture and overcoming characteristic displacement. Care must always be taken to have the foot at right angles to the leg to avoid shortening of the Achilles tendon and other soft tissues. In women accustomed to high-heeled shoes this precaution may not be so essential. Simple fractures of the inner malleolus present no unusual features for reduction or treatment.

FRACTURES OF THE LOWER EXTREMITY (Continued)

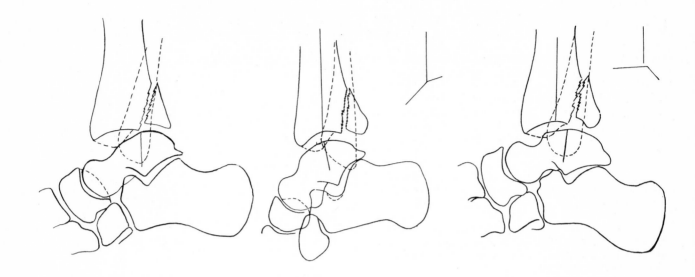

A. Fracture Posterior Articular
Surface of Tibia--Backward
Dislocation.

B. Dislocation Reduced--Foot
Extended.

C. Flexion of Foot--Causing Redislocation
of Foot at Ankle.

Fig. 15

FRACTURE--ANKLE--POSTERIOR ARTICU-
LAR SURFACE OF TIBIA (Trimalleolar Fracture).
Pott's fracture may be accompanied by fracture of
the posterior portion of the articular surface of the
tibia. To the casual observer this third line of fracture, seen only in the lateral view, may be mistaken
for the fracture of the inner malleolus which is seen
clearly only in the anteroposterior position. This
fracture may be associated with backward dislocation of the ankle (A). Since the entire weight of the
body is borne on the tibial articulation it is obvious
that healing with any displacement of this fragment
causing an irregularity of this surface is apt to produce lasting disability. The dislocation is easily reduced by pulling the foot forward (B). The articular
surface of the lower end of the tibia forms an arch
from before backward; flexion of the foot to a right
angle position causes pressure on the posterior
portion of this arch by the talus. If the line of
fracture of the articular surface is too near the
peak of the arch, sufficient shoulder will not be
preserved to withstand the backward pressure
exerted by the talus when the foot is in a flexed
position and backward dislocation of the ankle
joint will again occur (C). It may be necessary
to put the fracture up, with foot in a partial toe
drop position (D) with the full understanding that
this may require tenotomy of the Achilles tendon
from shortening after healing of the fracture has
taken place. In women, an extended position of
the foot is not so disabling since they are accustomed

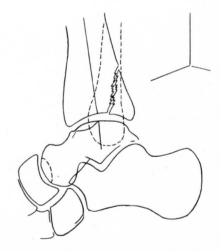

Fig. 15D. Reduction in Optimum Position of Foot.

to high-heeled shoes. Widening of the mortice caused
by fracture of the fibula is necessary before this
fracture can take place.

An excellent roentgenological analysis of the
positions involved in the production of various fractures of the ankle joint and in the method of effective
reduction is presented by T. Hendelberg.

FRACTURES OF THE LOWER EXTREMITY (Continued)

FRACTURE-- BONES OF LEG. Simple transverse fractures of the bones of the leg present no unusual features from fractures of the long bones elsewhere in the body. It must be remembered that the weight-bearing line is transmitted directly down the middle of the tibia and this must be preserved as well as possible. Generally speaking, however, if three fourths of the fractured surfaces are in good apposition and the alignment is good, the position may be considered satisfactory for a good functional result. Reduction and maintenance of this

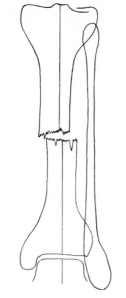

Fig. 15E. Fracture of Leg.

may be accomplished by closed or open means.

If the fragments are overriding or the fracture line is oblique, traction, by extension apparatus and fixation by pins through a cast, or by a constant pull applied to the lower fragment is necessary for maintenance of the fragments in position.

About six to eight weeks is usually necessary for healing. In recent years such fractures of the long bones have been effectively treated by intramedullary nailing. Spot-scanographic examination is an ideal method for determining the length of the intramedullary nail necessary for such surgical procedure. (See Manual of Roentgenological Technique.)

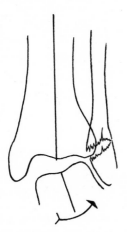

Fig. 16

Evulsion of the internal lateral ligament of the ankle joint, (Fig. 16), is not uncommon in

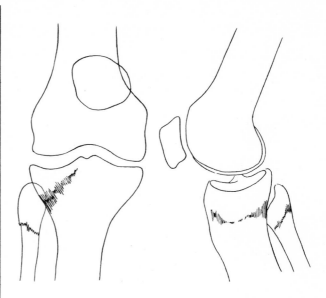

A. Compression Fracture Outer Condyle of Tibia-- Posterior View.

B. Compression Fracture Outer Condyle of Tibia-- Lateral View.

Fig. 17

severe sprains and fractures. Similar evulsion of the external lateral ligament may occur in association with severe sprain without evidence of fracture. Relief of pain and muscular spasm by cocainization will permit a wide range of subluxation of the joint, for substantiation of the diagnosis by further radiographic examination in this position.

KNEE--UPPER TIBIA. Fractures of the condyles of the tibia often result in malalignment of the joint surface. Involvement of the joint surface in fractures of the knee where there is no disturbance in position of the joint surface is not of such grave significance as in other joints, since the intervening semilunar cartilages serve as a buffer to the irregularity of the bone.

Compression fractures of the one or other condyle (A and B), occur from force applied to the inner or outer sides of the knee causing traumatic bow-leg or knock-knee deformity. These are frequently referred to as "bumper fractures" since they usually result from being struck on the side of the knee by the bumper of an automobile. The cartilage is resilient and returns to its natural shape, but the cancellous bone when once compressed retains the deformity. If allowed to heal with the resulting depression of the articular surface, there will be lasting deformity and disability. Operative elevation of the lowered articular surface by inserting a bony wedge often results in restoration of normal position, (Palmer). Early active motion without weight bearing is advisable.

FRACTURES OF THE LOWER EXTREMITY (Continued)

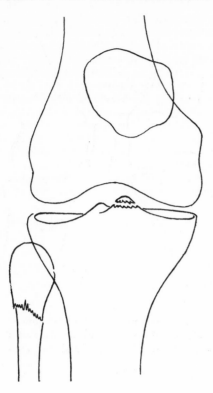

Fig. 18. Fracture of Spine of Tibia.

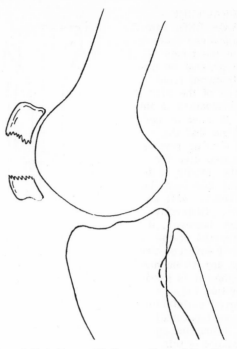

A. Fractured Patella--with Separation of the Fragments.

KNEE--SPINE OF TIBIA. Fractures of the spine of the tibia are comparatively rare; even though they are intracapsular they usually unite sufficiently for good function.

Displaced fractures require replacement; undisplaced fractures are treated as ligamentous injury, usually anterior cruciate ligament.

KNEE--PATELLA* (two figures in next column). Patellar fractures may be longitudinal, transverse or stellate. Longitudinal fractures run in the same direction as the tendon in which the bone lies and consequently the tendon remains intact and there is little if any loss of function. Such fractures may require only a minimum of time before full function is restored.

Complete transverse fractures (A) may result in wide separation of the fragments due to the pull of the quadriceps muscle. Fairly good apposition can usually be attained at the outset by complete extension of the leg (B). If this is not possible open operation may have to be resorted to.

In stellate fractures, excision of the lesser fragments and surgical repair, gives the best hope for satisfactory recovery. Patellar fractures frequently unite only by fibrous union if there is any

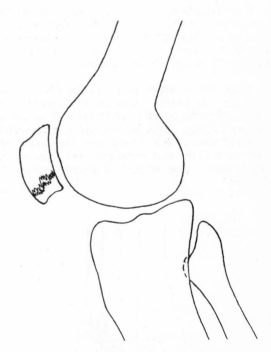

B. Reduction by Extension of Knee.
Fig. 19

material separation of fragments. Separation or stretching of the patellar ligament is indicated roentgenographically by the drawing up of the patella into an unusually high position.

FRACTURES OF THE LOWER EXTREMITY (Continued)

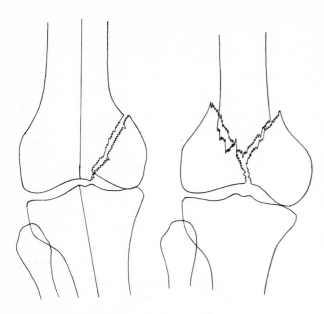

A. Fracture Inner Con-   B. "Y" Fracture of Both
   dyle of Femur.   Condyles of Femur.

Fig. 20

FRACTURE--KNEE CONDYLES. Fractures of the condyles of the femur are likewise very important in so far as their replacement is often very difficult and failure to restore them to their normal position will result in lasting disability. If the fracture line involves the joint directly in the intercondylar space (A), the fact that it involves the joint is not such a serious complication as if it were on a more active portion of the articular surface. Both condyles of the femur may be broken off (B), producing a "Y"-shaped fracture. The fragments in such cases may be very difficult to hold in place--it may be necessary to resort to open operation.

FRACTURE--SHAFT OF FE-MUR (figure 21). Fractures of the lower portion of the shaft of the femur are very frequent; fractures in this location are of especial importance (A). Heavy muscular pull causes backward displacement of the distal fragment with consequent overriding of the fragments and shortening of the extremity. To overcome this muscular pull, heavy traction is necessary.

Extreme traction with the leg in full extension may injure the vessels at the knee, therefore it is better to apply extension with knee in a slightly flexed position. It may be possible under direct fluoroscopic vision to reduce such fractures on a fracture table and to apply a cast; frequently, however, the padding of the cast becomes flattened and the soft parts atrophy from disuse after a time, resulting in sufficient play to permit recurrence of displacement of the distal fragment. Surgical treatment, by the introduction of an intramedullary stainless steel splint down the shaft almost to the lower articular surface of the femur, will serve best to maintain the fragments in good position, (Fig. 21B).

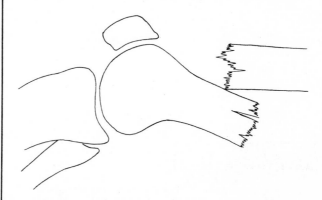

A. Fracture Shaft of Femur--Lower Third with Characteristic Posterior Displacement of the Distal Fragment.

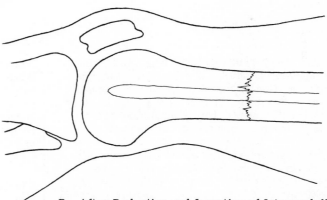

B. After Reduction and Insertion of Intramedullary Nail. Fragments maintained in good position.

Fig. 21

FRACTURES OF THE LOWER EXTREMITY (Continued)

To secure adequate traction it may be found necessary to use a surgical Steinmann pin or Kirschner wire run directly through the condyles of the bone, with application of balanced traction.

If a cast is applied, extension may be maintained by incorporating the pins in the cast.

Time required for complete union of the femur varies a great deal, depending on the age of the individual, degree of separation of the fragments, etc. Ordinarily, however, three months is about the shortest time in which firm bony union can be expected.

In recent years most fractures of the femoral shaft are treated by intramedullary bone splints. This consists of a long, flanged, stainless steel rod which is inserted into the medullary canal, bridging the fractured area and holding the fragments in good apposition and alignment. This form of intramedullary splint has been utilized most successfully in fractures of the femoral shaft in the lower one-third and of the tibia, although it has been used in the shafts of other long bones.

The ultimate results are better under this method of treatment, and the time for healing is usually shortened.

- - - -

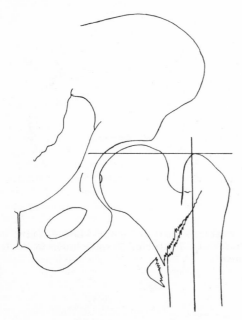 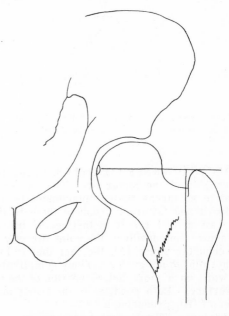

A. Intertrochanteric Fracture of Femur.   B. After Reduction--Normal Position.

Fig. 22

HIP--INTERTROCHANTERIC FRACTURE.* Subtrochanteric fractures and fractures through the upper portion of the shaft present no unusual problems. Fractures in this region may be very troublesome to reduce, but manipulation under traction is the only method at our disposal.

Intertrochanteric fractures (A) extending obliquely between the two trochanters are very frequent. Under certain conditions these may be very difficult to detect; the lining system devised to demonstrate the normal relationship between the neck of the femur and the shaft should aid in detection of such fractures and should give a fair estimate of the amount of shortening. The shaft slips up on the inclined plane of the fracture line, causing the trochanter to be displaced upward. If a line is drawn parallel to the shaft through its midportion, and a second line is drawn perpendicular to it at the level of the great trochanter, this line projected over to the articular surface of the head of the bone should intersect the articular sur-

face at or below the indentation for insertion of the teres ligament. Traction in an abducted position with a Hodgen splint may be used as a method of treatment (B). If there is little displacement or shortening, fixation in plaster may suffice. Fractures of this type usually heal quite readily in three to six months; rarely if ever is nonunion seen in this location.

As a matter of fact very few fractures of this type are treated today by the closed method, the complications of immobilization are too great. Almost all are treated by open operation and nailing; using a flange nail-bone plate of some type such as a Jewett, Key or Neufelt. These consist of a three-flanged nail which is driven through the trochanter into the neck of the femur combined with a bone place which extends down the lateral side of the shaft of the femur and is secured to it.

Isolated fractures of the greater trochanter in adults are very rare; they have been considered by Wilson, Michele, and Jacobson.

FRACTURES OF THE LOWER EXTREMITY (Continued)

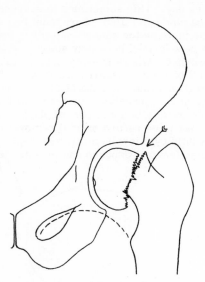

A. Fracture of Neck of Femur.

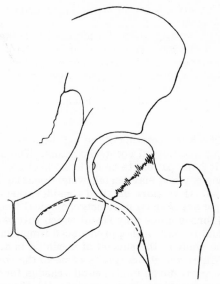

B. After Reduction--Normal Position.

Fig. 23

HIP--NECK OF FEMUR.* Fractures of the neck of the femur are as a rule more serious than any other fracture about the hip (A and B). This is due to the fact that the joint capsule includes almost the entire anterior surface of the neck and at least two thirds of the posterior portion, so that most fractures in this location are really intracapsular fractures. They are sometimes difficult to detect roentgenographically. Shenton's Line (B), the curved line forming the undersurface of the neck of the femur, continued over onto the pelvis, should fall along the upper border of the obturator foramen. This determines the relationship of the neck of the femur with the pelvis. Here, as elsewhere, intracapsular fractures are prone to result in nonunion; whether this is due to deficiency in blood supply of the fragments, interposition of synovial fluid or other cause, the fact remains that a large percentage of such fractures never heal by firm bony union. Fragments may be held in close apposition and in good position by abduction either in a Hodgen splint or by a flanged nail driven into the fragments; in some instances new bone formation and union occur; in others, no vestige of new bone formation ever appears and bony union never takes place. The nearer the fracture is to the anatomical head of the bone, the greater is the likelihood of non-union. Non-union has been attributed by some to lack of blood supply for the broken head of the bone. Studies of the blood supply to the head and neck of the femur would seem to justify this view, (Mussbichler). Certain cases, however, which never unite, years later may still show the head of the bone fully formed and viable in the acetabulum. Still

others attribute non-union to failure of fixation of the fragments. Bone pegs driven into the neck of the the femur to hold the two fragments in position have been used, but only too frequently end in failure. Metallic nails are now used almost exclusively to fix the fragments in position during healing; these have met with more uniform success. The Smith-Petersen nail is the one most frequently used for this purpose. Complete and accurate reduction and impaction of the broken surfaces are great factors in producing union.

SMITH-PETERSEN NAIL

Since the procedure of hip-nailing depends so largely for its success on cooperation with the radiological examination, a brief account of the roentgenological portion of the procedure was thought advisable.

Where fragment of the head of the femur is practically devoid of blood supply and nutrition metallic prostheses may be substituted for artificial replacement of the destroyed structures. Subcapital fractures of the femur result in fair healing; vertical fractures of the neck often show very poor healing while transverse cervical fractures have the greatest tendency for good healing.

Surgical operations using metallic pins and wires have resulted at times after long observation in migration of the metallic objects used for transfixing into vital portions of the body. Burman, et al. have reported migration of surgical pins and wires

FRACTURES OF THE LOWER EXTREMITY (Continued)

used to repair a fracture of the upper humerus, into the mediastinum.

Similar migration of a pin used to transfix a fractured clavicle has been reported by Kremens, et al. Terrafranca, et al. have even described the migration of a Smith-Petersen nail down into the thigh with an immense foreign body cyst of the thigh extending from the groin to the knee.

Check the position of the nail by anteroposterior and lateral roentgenograms. The surgeon may allow the patient to be up in a wheel chair the following day and may permit weight bearing in about 6 months. (For more detailed consideration of the technique see Manual of Roentgenological Technique.)

Fibrous union may result which will permit the individual to walk with a pronounced limp. In an exhaustive study of the subject of nonunion in hip fractures Salner and Pendergrass came to the conclusion that there are three fundamental reasons for failure of healing of fractures in this region: (1) Absence of a cambium layer in the fibrous covering of peripheral callus in the healing process after fracture. This lack of external osteogenic function because of lack of periosteum over the femoral neck is one way in which the process of repair of transcervical femoral fractures differs from ordinary shaft fractures. (2) Angle between neck and shaft because of the shearing force due to the angle of the neck and head, (3) Difficulty in maintaining rigid fixation, and its influence on the blood supply. (A method has been devised for measuring the femoral neck in surgical treatment of fractures of the hip by Van Brunt, q.v.)

Microradiographic studies after injecting the vessels of the upper end of the femur has shown abundant blood supply to the epiphysial margin of the head and the basal layers of cartilage. Truetta and unable to detect any decrease in richness of the arterial tree within the femoral head," so that this does not seem a logical explanation for the high percentage of nonunion associated with advancing age in fractures at this site.

Many things have been used in an attempt to overcome nonunion: diet, administration of calcium salts, etc., all to no avail. Surgeons have recommended and described as beneficial at times, traumatizing the bone on either side by an awl or a chisel or by traumatizing the fracture site by striking the end of the extremity with a rubber mallet repeatedly many times each day. This sometimes is successful where everything else has failed. Care must be taken not to resume function too soon even after union, since often the new-formed bone may soften and again become absorbed. Where nonunion has occurred in spite of all of these measures, recourse may be had to the surgical removal of the head of the bone and its replacement by a prosthesis or artificial femoral head made usually of some sort of plastic material.

A case is on record of total removal of a femur, due to hydatid cyst involvement, with replacement by a cadaveric femur, (Capurro and Pedemonte).

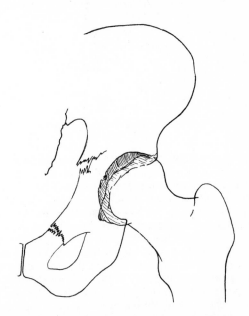

Fig. 24. Central Fracture of Acetabulum.

HIP--ACETABULUM.* Central fracture of the acetabulum, caused by force applied to the greater trochanter, driving the head of the femur through the acetabulum, into the pelvis, is a rather rare but often very painful fracture. Extraction of the head by lateral traction and early passive motion are the chief elements in treatment. The fractured acetabulum always heals, but there is often limitation of motion. Three to six months should usually suffice for repair of the fracture. Rectal manipulation of the fragments may be helpful in moulding them into place, (Jostes).

FRACTURES OF THE SKULL

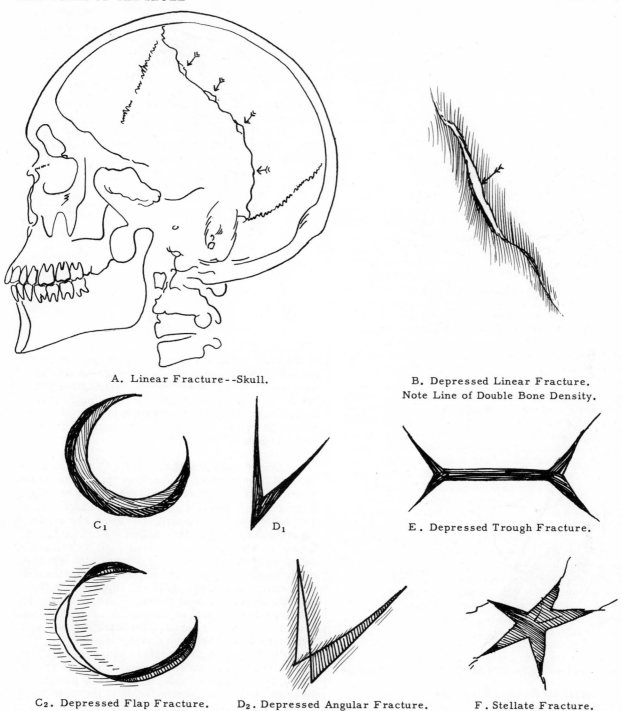

A. Linear Fracture--Skull.

B. Depressed Linear Fracture.
Note Line of Double Bone Density.

C_1

D_1

E. Depressed Trough Fracture.

C_2. Depressed Flap Fracture.

D_2. Depressed Angular Fracture.

F. Stellate Fracture.

Fig. 25

FRACTURES OF THE SKULL.* In fractures of the skull we have an entirely different problem than in fractures of long bones; here we are not concerned so much with the actual injury to the bone, as we are to the possible injury of the underlying brain structures. The injury to the bone itself is secondary; it will heal without much disability to the individual; injury to the brain, however, may cause lasting disability or death.

Interesting observations have been made on the mechanism of skull fractures and prediction of the fracture sites in head injuries by Gurdjian, et al.

Roentgenological examination of the skull is utilized to determine:

FRACTURES OF THE SKULL (Continued)

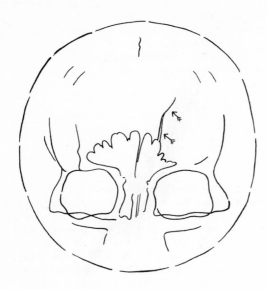

G. Fracture of Skull Involving Frontal Sinus.

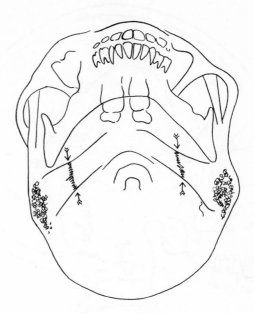

I. Fracture of Skull--Basal.

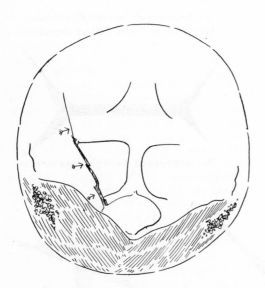

H. Fracture of Skull Involving Foramen Magnum.

1. The actual presence of a fracture,
2. Its character and extent if present,
3. The presence or absence of depression of the fragments,
4. The involvement of any important structures by the line of fracture.

Before it is possible to actually exclude fracture of the skull, five views must be taken; right and left lateral, frontal, occipital and basal. This is necessary since the fracture line may be so fine that unless it is in intimate contact with the film, it often will not show in the roentgenogram; for instance, a right lateral view might not show a fracture of the skull in the left parietal region, nor would a frontal view disclose such a fracture on the left side of the head. Stereoscopic examination cannot be used as a substitute--while often helpful in determining depression or extent of a fracture, it cannot be relied upon to show a fracture on the opposite side of the head.

Linear fractures of the skull (A) must be differentiated from grooves produced by the meningeal arteries, the venous channels and other bony markings. The meningeal arteries spread out fan-shaped from the base of the skull upward; they are tortuous, dividing and subdividing as they extend toward the top of the head. The veins, on the other hand, extend across the sides of the head converging toward the top; they are broader and more shallow than the arteries and often converge into venous lakes, especially in the parietal regions. Linear fractures are blacker in appearance than arterial or venous markings, and usually do not take a course characteristically found with these structures. Arteries divide and subdivide, always diverging and giving rise to branches which become smaller and smaller. Linear fractures rarely divide, but if they do divide, it is only for a short distance; they soon converge again to the main line of fracture, producing a small island of bone; vessels never do this. Other types of fractures of the skull may be flaplike, such as semicircular or circular, troughlike, angular or stellate, depending upon the injury received.

Diastatic fractures of skull or separation of the sutures, is an entity just as important as linear fracture. Care must be taken, however, not to mistake the straight linear inner margin of a suture when superimposed upon the wavy serrated outer margin, as a fracture through the suture, (Danelius).

FRACTURES OF THE SKULL (Continued)

The next thing for consideration is the determination of depression of the fragments. How can depression of a linear fracture be detected in a flat film of the skull? If the fracture line shows a uniform density throughout its entire course, it cannot be depressed, since depression of one or the other fragment, even if ever so slightly, will result in the production of a white line of double bone density at some place in the course of fracture (B). A similar white line of double bone density may be encountered in a flap fracture; whenever it is seen, it is always evidence of depression of the fragment. It is possible, however, for a flap fracture to be depressed without showing a line of double bone density. If you cut a semicircular opening in the top of a fruit can, you will see at once that it is possible to depress the flap without overlapping either side of the opening (C₁). Under such conditions, however, the flap becomes foreshortened and the semicircular opening becomes widened and crescentic in shape. Since we know that the flap originally completely filled the defect, any failure of the shadow of the flap to do so after injury must represent foreshortening of the flap indicating depression. Taken from a slightly different angle, the same flap fracture may show a white line of double bone density (C₂). This is true whether the flap is circular, angular, or irregular, or whether the fragments form multiple flaps as in "gutter" or stellate fractures. (D₁ and D₂, E, F.)

Lastly, the involvement of the adjacent structures is very important. Is the fracture line in close relationship to the motor area of the brain? Does it cross the middle meningeal artery or some other large arterial branch or venous sinus? Does it enter one of the accessory nasal sinuses (G) or the orbit, or one of the foramina such as the foramen magnum (H)?

The detection of the fracture is of prime importance because it indicates the point of maximum trauma to which the underlying structures have been subjected, and also to a certain extent indicates the degree of violence to which the individual has been exposed. Fractures contrecoup must be very rare since we have not encountered any cases in which the maximum injury was not evident at the site of maximum trauma. John Stewart found, in analysis of all skull fractures at the St. Louis City Hospital over a five-year period, that a correct diagnosis was obtained from roentgenographic examination with two lateral views and one view over site of maximum trauma, in 90.5% of all cases. Where fracture of the vault alone was considered, the percentage of correct diagnoses is higher, in basal (I) fractures alone it is much lower.

Failure to find evidence of fracture of the skull should not be allowed to give a sense of false security, since numerous instances have been encountered where fatal intracranial hemorrhage has occurred from brain injury without evidence of fracture of the bone. Voris, Verbrugghen, and Kearne found that 40% of patients dying of head injury have no evidence of fracture of the skull at necropsy.

Traumatic pneumo-cephalus or an intracranial collection of air is a rare complication of fracture of the skull involving the accessory nasal sinuses, (Garland and Mattram). It may undergo spontaneous absorption and healing.

The symptoms which may attend fracture of the skull and intracranial injury may be listed as,

Acute:

1) arterial hemorrhage--often of the middle meningeal artery which must be stopped by operative procedure.

Chronic:

2) subdural hemorrhage from a minimal amount of venous bleeding which does not produce immediate danger but may be treated by dehydration with magnesium sulphate or administration of hypertonic salt solution or glucose,

3) rupture of the arachnoid allowing cerebrospinal fluid to be pumped into the subdural space without provision for its escape--this produces the same symptoms as a hematoma,

4) contusion and laceration of the brain itself with associated edema which of course must be repaired by itself--rest alone can aid in such condition.

Union of fractures of the skull is never attended with large amounts of callus as in fractures of the long bones. Healing of fine linear fractures with partial or complete obliteration of the fracture line may be expected in a fairly large number of instances (Stewart). In children, such fractures may be obliterated in three months; in adults, healing with obliteration of the fracture line takes longer. If there has been any material separation of the fragments the line of fracture may be readily visible years later and indeed may never be completely effaced. Just what governs the union or nonunion of these fragments is not known. It is felt by some that if the pericranium is ruptured, bony union will not take place; others feel that the arachnoid is the prime structure concerned in repair.

After-effects of fracture of the skull depend upon the severity and nature of the injury to the brain structure (Glasser and Shafer; Osmond and Gross). Injuries over the motor area may be followed by epilepsy even years later. Traumatic cysts may develop and subdural hematomas may give rise to intracranial symptoms. Various studies have shown that in an appreciable number of instances, less severe effects such as nervousness, irritability, headaches, change of personality, etc., may develop. Localized thinning of the skull detectable in the roentgenogram may develop within a few months from pressure of a subdural hematoma or an intracranial traumatic cyst or hygroma, (Childe).

Davidoff and Dyke reported a condition known as relapsing juvenile chronic subdural hematoma.

FRACTURES OF THE MANDIBLE AND BONES OF FACE

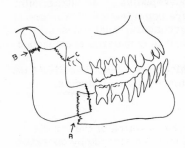

Fig. 26
Fracture of Mandible
A--Angle;
B--Condylar Process;
C--Coronoid Process.

FRACTURES OF THE MANDIBLE.* Fractures of the mandible occur most frequently through the angle or through the body just anterior to the angle (A). The proximal fragment is pulled forcibly upward and medially by the powerful masseter muscle. If wiring of the teeth does not hold the fragments in position, in may be necessary to resort to other methods. Under suitable conditions, the proximal fragment can be forced down and maintained in position by an intradental splint. If necessary Kirschner wires may be placed through the fragments.

Fracture of the condylar process (B) may easily escape detection in the ordinary film; special examination of temporomandibular joint must be made since fracture of this process frequently results from forcible closure of the mouth after dislocation on one or both sides of the jaw. Norgaard has devised a special position for visualization of the condylar process which is, at times, very helpful in visualizing such fractures (Fig. 26C).

Fracture of the condylar process is frequently associated with dislocation of the temperomandibular articulation with the upper fragment medialward (Fig. 26C). The fragment is very difficult to replace and it may be impossible to reduce the dislocation or even to remove the fragment surgically. Strangely enough function is often reestablished with a fairly good result even though the dislocation cannot be reduced.

Fracture of the coronoid process (C) can usually be readily detected and only requires immobilization for its treatment.

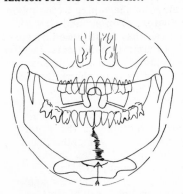

Fig. 27. Fracture of Symphysis of Mandible.

FRACTURE OF THE MANDIBLE NEAR SYMPHYSIS. Fracture of the mandible near the symphysis may completely escape detection in the ordinary lateral view. Frontal view of the mandible is the best method of detecting the presence and extent of such injuries.

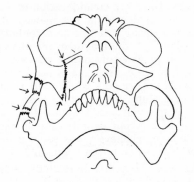

A. Fracture of Zygomatic Arch and Antrum.

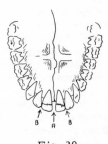

B. Fracture of Zygomatic Arch and Antrum--
Profile View
Fig. 28

FRACTURE OF THE BONES OF THE FACE,* ZYGOMATIC ARCH, and ANTRUM. Fracture of the zygomatic arch is most frequently produced by a direct blow applied to this region. Fracture and depression of the arch is best shown by Titterington's Position (A) or by the tangential view as shown in basal view of the skull (B). Frequently caving in of the antrum is associated with such injuries and the orbit may be involved. Depression of the lateral wall of the antrum and zygomatic arch may be corrected by inserting a hook beneath the depressed bony fragment and pulling outward to normal position.

FRACTURE OF THE MAXILLA AND PALATE. Fracture of the maxilla and palate bone (A) is due to violence applied directly to the upper jaw--such as that received in automobile accidents. Such fractures are best demonstrated by large occlusal films placed in the mouth.

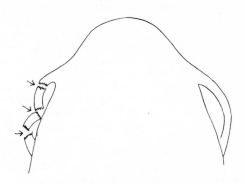

Fig. 29

Immobilization is best secured by wiring of the teeth, or if these are not available, by an intradental splint.

Fractures of the teeth (B) show as linear shadows running across the tooth structure.

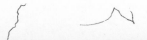

FRACTURES OF THE SPINE--CERVICAL*

Fracture of the spine is of especial importance, not only on account of its function of weight-bearing and motion, but particularly on account of its function of protection to the spinal cord.

The cervical spine is composed of vertebrae, relatively small in size but permitting a wider range of movement than any other portion of the spine. Fractures of this region of the spine must be considered more in the light of restriction of normal motion, than with regard to their weight-bearing function. Owing to the extreme flexibility of this portion of the spine, fractures in this region are very apt to result in displacement and injury to the spinal cord. Injury or compression of the cord above the fourth cervical is very dangerous on account of injury to the segments giving rise to the phrenic nerve; patients suspected of injury to this region should be handled with great care until preliminary examination has definitely excluded gross deformity.

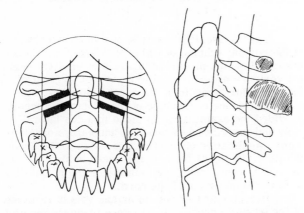

A. Upper Cervical Spine-- B. Upper Cervical Spine--
Normal Lining--A-P   Normal Lining--Lat.

Fig. 30

Fig. 30A shows the scheme of the lining of the normal cervical spine in the antero-posterior view. The atlas and axis articulate by four joints:

1) Anterior ring of the atlas with the odontoid process of the axis permitting rotary motion.

2) Posterior surface of the odontoid process and the transverse ligament of the atlas, which arches across behind, and is the only structure preventing forward luxation of the head.

3 and 4) The two joints between the lateral masses on either side.

The margins of the joints between the lateral masses should be parallel and equidistant. Perpendicular lines drawn through the extreme edges of the joints should be equidistant. The spinous process should be exactly in the midline. If these relationships are present, it may be confidently assumed that the relationship is normal.

Fig. 30B shows the scheme of lining of the normal cervical spine in the lateral view. Lines drawn along the anterior and posterior margins of the upper cervical vertebrae should be parallel; the posterior line, extended upward should fall closely along the posterior surface of the odontoid process. A third line, parallel to the other two lines, drawn through the anterior edge of the posterior tubercle of the axis, shows the posterior tubercle of the axis to be well behind this line. In other words, the posterior tubercle of the first cervical vertebra never extends anterior to the posterior tubercle of the second cervical vertebra in normal relationship.

Deviation of the head from rotation, or flexion with lowering of the chin may cause slight variation in these normal relationships so that one must be on guard against false interpretation of subluxations from such cause.

Coutts in an excellent article on subluxations of this sort has analyzed the various movements of these joints with precise anatomical consideration.

In simple rotation, the transverse ligament is not relaxed and the atlas does not slip forward on the axis. Rotation of the atlas on the axis, however, is limited and requires additional compensatory rotation in the lower cervical vertebrae to bring the head to a full neutral rotary position; tilting and flexion usually accompany rotation. As a result, the spinous processes of the lower cervical vertebrae will deviate from midline in the opposite direction of rotation of the head.

"Subluxation implies relaxation or stretching of the transverse ligament and the slipping forward of the atlas on the axis"; if this is unilateral or predominently on one side, rotation accompanies the deformity.

"When the head becomes fixed in position of rotation through the atlanto-epistropheal joint, with or without subluxation forward, the subject attempts to bring the head to a position of 'eyes front' by rotating through the lower cervical joints in a direction opposite to the rotation deformity. Each of the vertebrae can rotate about eight degrees to either side. The compensatory rotation occurs from the second cervical vertebra down, that is, the second presents the maximum rotation deviation, the lower vertebrae successively approaching the neutral position. The spines of the cervical vertebrae thus rotated deviate to the side of the midline toward which the head is turned, which is the reverse of what occurs when the head is turned on a normal neck.

"A similar mechanism produces lordosis of the lower cervical spine to compensate for the flexion component of the deformity when that is marked."

ROENTGENOLOGICAL OBSERVATIONS

" Lateral view:

1) Increased anterior atlanto-dental interval: This sign is pathognomonic of forward luxation of the atlas.

2) The depth of the shadow of the soft tissues anterior to the first two cervical vertebrae should normally be equal to that. . . of the other cervical bodies.

3) Flexion of the first on the second cervical vertebra: The line joining the inferior borders of the anterior and posterior arches of the atlas, should be

FRACTURES OF THE SPINE (Continued)

parallel or converge posteriorly (to a similar line for the axis), when the head is in a neutral position.

4) Compensatory Lordosis of the Lower Cervical Vertebrae: This sign is present when the flexion of the first on the second cervical vertebra is marked.

5. Failure of the Two Halves of the Posterior Arch of the Atlas to be Superimposed: In a true lateral view the two sides of the posterior arch are superimposed.

6. Evidence of Rotation of the Cervical Vertebrae from the Second Vertebra Downward: The joint spaces of the lateral articulations of the two sides are no longer superimposed, but their shadows are projected, one anterior to the other.

Anteroposterior view:

1) Lateral Deviation of the Epistropheal Spine (Spinous process of the Axis): This is the most important sign to be looked for: Normal cervical spine in rotation shows deviation of spinous processes away from side to which head is rotated: with relaxation of transverse ligament rotation of spinous processes is toward side of rotation of head.

2) Overlapping of the Shadow of the Lateral Masses of the First on the Second Cervical Vertebrae on One or Both Sides: Overlapping is an appearance occurring with flexion and rotation of the first on the second cervical vertebra. It is not pathognomonic of subluxation or of the side on which the forward movement has taken place.

3) Lateral Displacement of the Axis: This sign is subject to many errors of interpretation. In order to give significance to this appearance of lateral displacement the head must be held erect on the spine and both lateral masses must be displaced laterally with respect to the dens. Under these conditions a unilateral displacement represents a pathologic fixation in a position within the normal range of motion. A bilateral displacement of the atlantal lateral masses in opposite directions, however, indicates "fracture of one of the arches of the atlas," (Paul and Moir). A critical analysis of this position have been given by Jacobson and Adler. Attention is called to the diagnostic aid of these lining methods in detection of subluxations of the cervical vertebrae due both to traumatic and regional infections (q.v.).

FRACTURE CERVICAL SPINE--ODONTOID.

Fracture of the odontoid process of the second cervical vertebra is the most dangerous fracture with which we have to deal. The odontoid or toothlike process, projecting upward from the anterior portion of the second cervical vertebra, articulates anteriorly with the inner aspect of the ring of the first cervical vertebra, being held in place posteriorly only by a fibrous ligament extending behind the process from one side of the bony ring to the other. Fractures of this process are very frequent; nothing remains to hold the head upright in its normal position and the upper fragment is carried forward with the head and first cervical vertebra. Forward displacement of

the head and upper fragment is characteristic of this fracture.

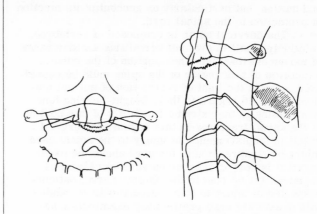

Fig. 31. Fracture of Odontoid Process of Second Cervical.

This is usually clearly shown in a disturbance of the normal scheme of lining of this region. In the lateral view, the posterior tubercle of the first cervical vertebra slips forward to a position in front of the posterior tubercle of the second vertebra; this is always evidence of fracture of the odontoid process, provided the examination is made in a due lateral view and there is no evidence of anomalous development. Application of traction apparatus to the head (Krutchfield tongs) for several weeks holds the parts in normal relationship and minimizes the possibility of fatal compression of the cord.

Blockley and Pruser in an analysis of fracture of the odontoid process in 51 cases found that in children under seven years of age, the injury amounts to a separation at the epiphyseal plate; the displacement is always forward and bony union always results. Whereas in persons over seven years of age there may be no displacement in one-fourth of the cases, in the remainder, forward displacement predominates two to one. Bony union occurs in about one-third of the cases; while absence of bony union is present in the remaining two-thirds.

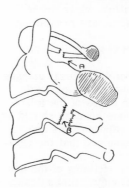

Fig. 32
A. Ring of First
B. Spinous Process

FRACTURE CERVICAL SPINE--RING OF FIRST VERTEBRA. A frequent injury to the first cervical vertebra is fracture of the ring. Unless this is associated with other injury to the upper cervical vertebrae and displacement, it usually does not cause much disability. To demonstrate a fracture of this sort (A), it may be necessary to tilt the head sidewise during examination so as to secure unobstructed

FRACTURES OF THE SPINE (Continued)

unobstructed views of the two sides of the ring. Complete fracture of the ring of the first vertebra can sometimes be detected by a defect in the normal schemes of lining of this region showing wider separation between the two articular processes due to spreading of the ring.

Fractures of the ends of the spinous processes (B) are less dangerous although they may give rise to some pain and disability owing to their ligamentous attachments.

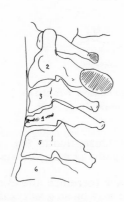

Fig. 33. Compression Fracture of Fourth.

FRACTURE CERVICAL SPINE--COMPRESSION FRACTURE. Another common fracture of the cervical spine is compression of the vertebral bodies; this usually occurs lower down in the region of the fourth, fifth, or sixth cervical vertebra. Sudden forced flexion of the head produced by striking the top of the head on the top of an automobile, results in an undue amount of pressure being brought to bear on the vertebral bodies, producing compression of the cancellous bone. The compression is usually at the anterior margin. Fractures of this sort are best treated by fixation in hyperextension; this takes all undue pressure off the compressed bodies and frequently permits them to resume their normal shape. Ankylosis of the injured segment of the spine by outgrowths of bone bridging across the vertebral spaces results in limitation of motion of this segment of the spine, but accomplishes permanent splinting, relieving pain.

Increase in the thickness of the prevertebral soft tissue space is very suggestive of bone or soft part injury causing hematoma. Loss of the normal lordotic curve may be due to spasm resulting from injury.

WHIPLASH INJURY. Whiplash injury causing fractures of the spinous processes of the lower cervical and upper dorsal spinous processes similar to those seen frequently in clay shovelers, has been reported by Gershon-Cohen.

Taylor has demonstrated a thickening of the ligamentum flavum from injury to the spinal cord in the neck, without fracture of the cervical spine. This occurs from sudden acute forced flexion. Filling of the spinal canal with lipiodol discloses a thickening of the ligamentum flavum on acute backward extension, it is not seen when the neck is held in flexion.

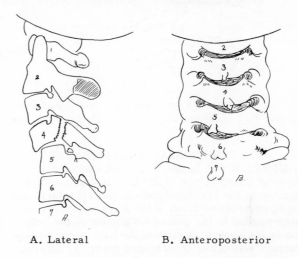

A. Lateral   B. Anteroposterior

Fig. 34. Fracture of Articular Process.

FRACTURE CERVICAL SPINE--ARTICULAR FACETS. Fractures of the articular facets are usually accompanied by dislocation of the vertebrae with consequent danger of pressure on the cord and interference with motion. Wherever malalignment exists, application of traction tends to relieve muscle spasm and reduce the displacement; <u>any manipulation of fractures or dislocations of the cervical spine must be done by an expert surgeon skilled in this procedure.</u>

Injury to the spinal cord without fracture may occur from hyperextension injuries of the neck. (See Other Effects of Trauma.)

FRACTURES OF THE SPINE--DORSAL AND LUMBAR

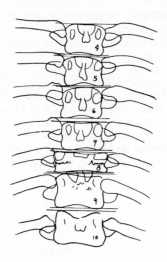

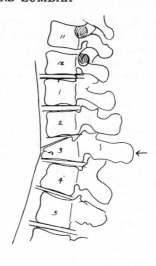

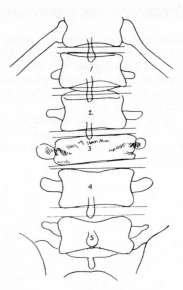

A. Compression Fracture
of 8th D.

B. Compression Fracture
3d Lumbar Vert. Lat.

C. Compression Fracture
3d Lumbar Vert. A-P.

Fig. 35

FRACTURE DORSAL AND LUMBAR SPINE--COMPRESSION.* In the dorsal and lumbar regions the most common type of fracture is compression fracture of the vertebral bodies. Such fractures are due to excessive flexion of the spine with extreme force applied to the cancellous portion of the body; this is the weakest portion of the bone. Compression fracture may occur from violent muscular contraction as seen in metrazol, insulin or electric shock convulsions in treatment of Schizophrenia. Compression fractures of the vertebrae from this cause are most frequently seen in the upper thoracic region, in the 3d to 5th vertebrae.

Roentgenologically, they present a cupping appearance of the upper vertebral margin without anterior compression and are thought therefore to be due to "disc repercussion" rather than hyperflexion as in other compression fractures. Kelly has found that such spinal injuries occur in 1% of the cases.

Posteriorly the vertebra is supported by the heavy articular processes, but anteriorly the spongy cancellous structure of the body is not so resistant to the effects of trauma. The interarticular cartilaginous disc, being elastic, returns to its normal width after compression, while the cancellous body remains wedge-shaped from the effect of the trauma. It is the preservation of the interarticular cartilaginous disc which is a point in differentiation between compression fracture and actual disease processes of the bone, such as tuberculous spondylitis. Tuberculosis destroys the cartilage as well as the adjacent bony structure of the vertebral body; the elastic properties of cartilage are of no avail against the ravages of the disease. It is true that destruction of the vertebral body from secondary malignancy may leave the cartilage intact, but such conditions are usually readily recognizable by the fact that the wedge-shaped deformity follows only after extensive destruction of the bone.

A fine linear groove or channel running from before backward through the body of a vertebra must not be mistaken for a linear fracture; this is the site of nutrient artery and its pathway may remain visible even into adult life.

Compression fractures are therefore attended with kyphotic deformity, which may be so great that the posterior margin of the vertebral body is pressed backward encroaching on the spinal canal; compression or injury to the cord is, of course, the most serious complication which can exist with this fracture. Since the cord proper terminates about the level of the second lumbar vertebra, encroachment on the spinal canal in compression fractures below that level is not of such great importance.

Compression fractures are best treated by fixation in hyperextension. The patient lies prone, supported under the chest and pelvis, allowing the body to sag forward; a plaster-of-Paris jacket is applied in this hyperextended position. Or the patient may lie on his back on a flexible Bradford frame to accomplish the same degree of hyperextension. In many instances this results in almost perfect reestablishment of the normal shape of the body. Fixation must be maintained for at least six to nine months; in severe cases the first three months may well be spent in bed. Roentgenographic examination usually does not show material evidence of healing in less than three months; the first manifestations are usually processes of new bony growth springing from the margins of the vertebral bodies ultimately bridging across from the injured vertebra to the one above and below, Nature's effort to immobilize this segment of the spine. At times, especially where the degree of injury has not been so great, new bone formation is very slow to form, and in certain instances new bone formation may be almost impossible to detect. Baker has pointed out that magnification technique of the finer bony structure may be of great aid in deciding the degree of bone formation.

FRACTURES OF THE SPINE--DORSAL AND LUMBAR (Continued)

Injury to the nucleus pulposus may accompany such fractures of the spine or may occur independently of any evidence of fracture. It may not be manifested at the time of the accident but show up later. The nucleus pulposus has a great deal to do with the normal function of the spine. An analysis of the motion of the lower lumbar vertebrae in normal individuals and in patients with low back pain has been

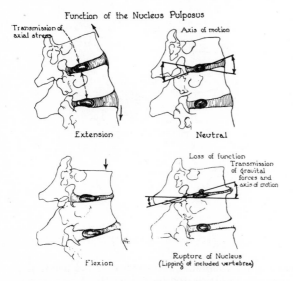

Function of the Nucleus Pulposus

--D.C. Keyes and E.L. Compere

Fig. 35D. Illustrating the Normal Position and Function of the Nucleus Pulposus as a Ball Bearing and Hydraulic Shock Absorber,

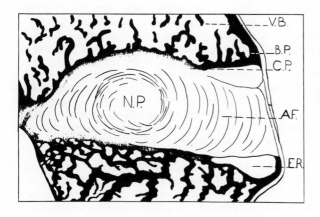

v.b.--vertebral body
b.p.--bone plate
c.p.--cartilage plate
n.p.--nucleus pulposus
a.f.--annulus fibrosus
e.f.--epiphyseal ring

Fig. 35E. Normal Construction of the Intervertebral Disc Showing Relationship of Nucleus Pulposus.

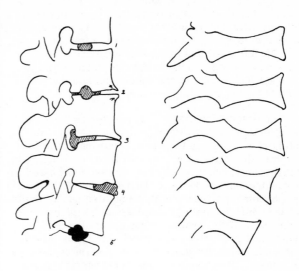

1. Normal Nucleus Pulposus.
2. Herniation Nucleus.
3. Retropulsion.
4. Anterior Displacement.
5. Calcification Nucleus.

Fig. 35F. Illustrating Various Types of Injury to Nucleus Pulposus.

Fig. 35G. Biconcave Vertebrae Due to Pressure of Expanded Intervertebral Nuclei Upon Vertebral Bodies Weakened from Osteoporosis.

made illustrating the fulcrum action of the nucleus pulposus and pointing out the modifying action of the articular facets in extreme motions of the spine, (Gianturco).

The spaces between the bodies of the vertebrae are occupied by semielastic intervertebral discs. These are constructed essentially of three elements: cartilage plates which cover the dense bony plates forming the margins of the adjacent vertebral bodies; a central rounded semifluid body about a centimeter or so in size, the nucleus pulposus and a surrounding bulky fibrous tissue mass the annulus fibrosis which fills the remainder of the space. A delicate cartilaginous ring, thickest in front, serves to buttress the margin of the vertebra and is the site of secondary epiphyseal growth. The nucleus pulposus may be considered as a ball bearing and a hydraulic shock absorber of the spine, (Fig. 35D and E). These nuclei transmit shock from one vertebra to another and are essential to normal function of the spine. With the repeated application of excessive trauma from heavy lifting, etc., the fluid contents of the nucleus pulposus may herniate out through a weak spot in the fibrous capsule. Since constant pressure of soft tissue structure on bone always causes pressure atrophy of the bone, these small hernias pressing against the bony structure of the bodies of the vertebrae give rise to the semicircular pressure defects well posterior on the margins of the vertebral bodies which are quite characteristic of the condition,

FRACTURES OF THE SPINE--DORSAL AND LUMBAR (Continued)

(Fig. 35F, 2 and 5). These semicircular defects seen on radiographic examination caused by Schmorl's nodes usually do not interfere materially with spinal function unless there is associated thinning of the disc.

McRae has pointed out that herniation of the intervertebral disc must be very common, from his investigation of anatomical specimens and that relatively few give disabling symptoms.

SCHMORL NODES.* According to Schmorl, "the affection begins with a diminution of the fluid content of the nucleus pulposus, resulting in the formation in the latter of cracks and fissures running in all directions, which sometimes can be recognized in the roentgenogram owing to their content of air (vacuum phenomenon) whereby it, as pointed out by Knutsson, becomes possible to diagnose an incipient osteochondrosis. If the process progresses, the nucleus shrinks and gradually loses its elasticity and ability to expand; and at the same time the height of the disc diminishes. The degenerative processes are, however, confined to its central part whereas, the fibrous ring remains intact. But as a result of the collapse of the disc and the reduced or entirely lost capacity of the nucleus for expansion, the fibers of the ring become slack and thus a possibility arises for the vertebral bodies to become slightly dislocated in relation to each other. To the continuous small traumata to which their surfaces thereby become exposed they react by sclerosis. The slacking of the fibers of the ring readily explains the possibility for displacement of the vertebral bodies in relation to each other, as a result of which a so-called pseudospondylolisthesis may develop", (Chrom).

No specific symptoms may be produced unless the disc protrudes posteriorly into the spinal canal and causes pressure on the cord, (Fig. 37F 3). This can be demonstrated by Pantopaque injection into the spinal canal or by air injection (see chapter on Myelography), or by direct injection of opaque material into the disc--discography (see Manual of Roentg. Technique). Such protrusions occur most frequently in the lower lumbar region (96%) the site of greatest trauma from weight bearing but they may occur in any location in the spine. Various injuries and diseases of the spine may be complicated by involvement of the nucleus pulposus (see osteoporosis of spine).

Lindbom has stressed injury to the intervertebral discs without immediate evidence of their injury. Subsequent examination months later may show development of fine calcium deposits within any location in the spine. Various injuries and diseases of the spine may be complicated by involvement of the nucleus pulposus (see osteoporosis of spine).

FRACTURE--LUMBAR SPINE--TRANSVERSE PROCESSES. Fractures of the transverse processes of the lumbar vertebrae are usually multiple. They are the result of muscular pull, rather than direct

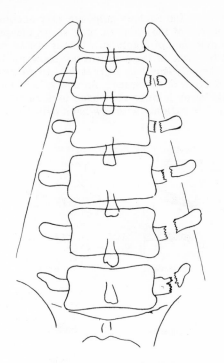

Fig. 36. Fracture Transverse Processes.

trauma to the spine. The shadow of the psoas muscle is often obliterated on the involved side where the injury is severe and the displacement of the fragments may be very great. This is probably due to injury to the muscle and associated hemorrhage from the trauma. If the fragments of the processes show little separation, complete bony union may result after two to three months with relatively slight disability, but if there is wide separation of the fragments, bony union may never take place due to interposition of the muscle. Such a condition results in lasting disability especially in lifting heavy weights. Since these processes which normally give attachment to muscles are not firm, the muscles cannot act with the same effectiveness. Under such conditions there may be pain on attempts at heavy lifting. If nonunion occurs the margins of the fragments become smooth and rounded.

FRACTURE--LUMBAR SPINE--ARTICULAR PROCESSES, "SHEARING FRACTURE." (next page) The articular processes are strong bony structures; an extreme degree of trauma is usually required to produce their fracture. Whenever they are broken, there is usually associated displacement of the vertebra with more or less encroachment on the spinal canal (A). Displacement under such conditions is usually to one side or the other. Traction to reduce the displacement and fixation to promote healing is the usual treatment. Not less than three months and frequently six to nine months or even longer is necessary for complete repair. Rarely slight fractures of the tips of the articular processes occur without spinal

FRACTURES OF THE SPINE--DORSAL AND LUMBAR (Continued)

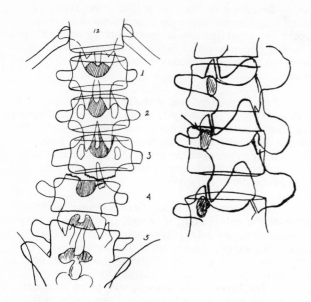

Fig. 37A. Fracture Articular
Processes with Displacement
"Shearing Fracture."

Fig. 37B.
Oblique View.

displacement (B). These may be very small and are
easily overlooked. They may be quite painful and
should always be searched for where there is unexplained pain. Care should be taken not to confuse such
fractures with developmental anomalies which sometimes occur in this region.

Oblique views of the spine (Fig. 37B) taken on
both sides for comparison, should always be made
where there is any suspicion of injury or other
pathology in the articular processes or apophyseal
joints. Fractures in this region may be very easily
overlooked, (Scott). Fractures of such processes
and of the pars interarticularis of the neural arch
may heal even when bilateral, (Roche).

FRACTURE--LUMBAR
SPINE--SPINOUS PROCESS.
Fractures of the spinous
processes are usually due
to direct violence applied
to these projecting bony
prominences. Such frac-
tures are very rare, they
are not usually associated
with other spinal fractures
and consequently are not
as dangerous as other
types. They usually heal
by firm bony union in
about three months without
much disability, but if they
show much separation,
firm bony union may not
take place.

Weinbren has empha-
sized the value of tomog-
raphy for detailed exami-
nation of the spine, for the
detection of small frac-
tures.

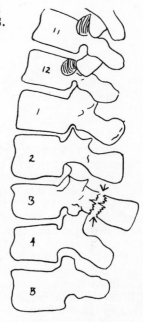

Fig. 38 Fracture
Spinous Process.

FRACTURES OF THE PELVIS

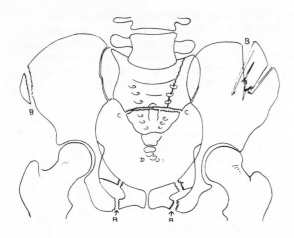

Fig. 39. Fractures of Pelvis.

FRACTURES OF THE PELVIS. The most frequent site of fracture of the pelvis is through the horizontal and descending rami of the pubis (A). Fractures in this location especially if they are near the symphysis or if they show wide displacement are apt to be associated with injury to the bladder or deep urethra. Any injury to these structures is of much greater importance than the fracture of the bones. The rami of the pubis form the boundaries of the obturator foramen, and any disturbance in position may encroach upon this opening. This is of little significance, however, since the obturator foramen transmits only the obturator vessels and nerve. It is covered by a fibrous membrance which gives attachment to three muscles, obturator internus, externus and pyriformis, structures which are not easily damaged. The fracture line may be very near the symphysis or in rare instances the injury may be represented by complete separation of the symphysis pubis.

Such fractures represent a complete break in the bony pelvic ring, and if they are associated with much displacement, sacroiliac separation is likely to become a very distressing complication. Extreme deformities of this sort have been encountered, where one entire side of the pelvis has been displaced upward for several inches.

Treatment of fractures of the pelvis, where there is very little displacement, is best accomplished by fixation either by plaster-of-Paris or strapping. Where there is much displacement, the fragments show a tendency to spread apart; the patient may be suspended in a canvas hammock. If there is also upward displacement of the entire half of the pelvis, traction must likewise be instituted. From three to six months' immobilization is usually required for firm union.

Avulsion of the tuberosity of the ischium, Ischial Apophyseolysis, as a result of muscle pull due to trauma from excessive previous exertion is not too unusual according to Milch. A large cres-

centic fragment of bone is pulled loose from the ischium accompanied by pain, soreness and swelling. Operative investigation, if recent, shows hemorrhage. Recovery occurs with reunion of the fragment. It is most apt to occur in males between 12 and 25 years of age.

Fracture of the rim of the acetabulum may occur with separation of a bony fragment. These are usually associated with dislocation of the femoral head. They usually heal with deformity and disability. Fracture of the body or wing of the ilium (B) is probably next in frequency of pelvic fractures. Such fractures rarely produce much difficulty.

The sacrum is a heavy bone forming the keystone of the pelvic ring; it is well protected by bony prominences and soft tissue pads and is therefore rarely fractured. Fractures of the sacrum do occur (C), however, as a result of sitting down hard, such as accidents occurring while skating. It is quite possible that fractures of the sacrum are more frequent than we suppose, since the natural concavity of the sacrum would favor obscuring of the fracture line when examination is made in the usual way, in a great number of instances. In order to minimize errors of diagnosis in this region, it is well, wherever the sacrum has been subjected to severe trauma, to make the anteroposterior examination from two angles; the first, the usual inclination of the principal ray down the axis of the pelvis, and a second, with the principal ray centered lower and directed more upward towards the head.

The multiple foramina which traverse the sacrum serve to weaken the bone to some extent. Transverse fractures are very apt to extend through these openings, from side to side; whereas longitudinal fractures may occur going through these foramina in a vertical plane parallel to the sacroiliac joint. Since they transmit the sacral nerves, such fractures may be very painful, at least for the first few days or weeks. Repair soon takes place, however, the pain subsides, and there is rarely any material lasting disability. Protection is usually the only treatment necessary and union usually occurs within six to eight weeks.

The coccyx is more subject to trauma (D), from accidents in which extreme force is applied in the sitting position. A definite line of fracture must be demonstrated before a diagnosis of fracture is made, however, since this bone is subject to wide variations in normal individuals. Definite fractures of the coccyx do occur sometimes with considerable displacement of the fragments. After manual reduction of the fragments through rectal palpation, time and protection is all that is required for healing--usually one to two months. At times such fractures are very painful, owing to the coccygeal nerves, which emerge on either side. Sometimes the pain does not subside even with complete healing of the fracture; under such conditions removal of the fragment may have to be resorted to.

QUESTIONS ON FRACTURES

Questions marked with a dagger deal with rare and less-important conditions.

1. Describe briefly points to be considered in the analysis of all fractures.

† 2. Show by diagram the usual site of fracture of the humerus, radius, ulna, scapula, clavicle, femur, pelvis, tibia, fibula.

3. Show by a diagram normal relationship of bones of wrist joint.

4. Show by diagram normal relationship of bones of elbow joint.

5. Show by a diagram the relationship of upper end of humerus to the scapula and clavicle.

6. Show by diagram normal relationship of bones of ankle joint.

7. Show by diagram normal relationship of bones of knee joint.

8. Show by a diagram the method of determining the normal relationship of the femur to the pelvis.

9. What views of the head are necessary to make a definite negative diagnosis of fracture of the skull?

10. How would you determine depression of a fracture from a flat film of the skull?

11. Under what conditions may depression of a fracture be present without showing a double line of bone density?

† 12. What are the most common types of fractures and manner of displacement of fragments in fractures of:

        (a) cervical spine,   (c) lumbar spine (upper),
        (b) dorsal spine,   (d) fifth lumbar vertebra?

13. What are the characteristics of compression fracture of the spine? How would you differentiate compression fracture from tuberculosis of the spine?

14. How long before new bone formation will show in a roentgenogram after a fracture, and upon what does it depend? Do fractures of the skull heal by new bone formation?

15. What is the nucleus pulposus? What is its function?

† 16. What are the roentgenographic manifestations of herniation of the nucleus pulposus?

† 17. How can retropulsion of the nucleus pulposus back into the spinal canal be detected?

18. What dangers are encountered in the fluoroscopic reduction of fractures, and what safeguards are necessary to prevent injury to the patient and operator?

19. Why is the use of a detached head fluoroscope dangerous?

20. Under what circumstances may fluoroscopy be conducted safely at the bedside?

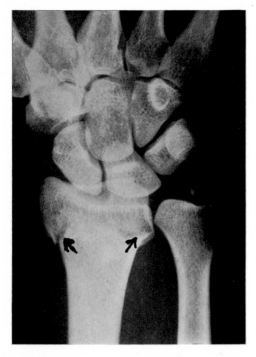

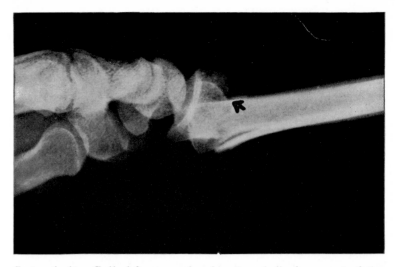

Lateral view Colles' fracture showing dorsal displacement of the distal radial fragment and dorsal inclination of the articular surface of the lower end of the radius.

Impacted Colles' fracture (palmar view), showing disturbance in the normal relationship of the bones of the wrist joint.

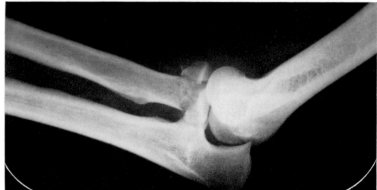

Fracture head of radius into joint with partial dislocation ulna.

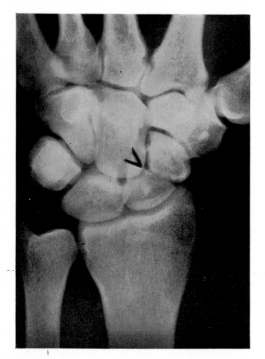

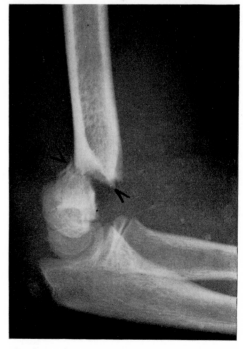

Palmar view of the wrist showing complete fracture of navicular.

Medial view showing supra-condylar fracture of the humerus with characteristic posterior displacement of the distal fragment.

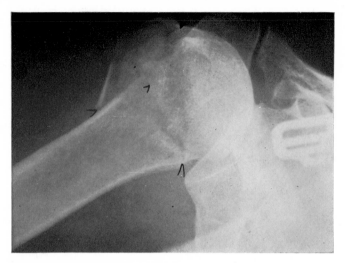

Fracture through the surgical neck of the humerus with associated fracture of the greater tuberosity, in good position.

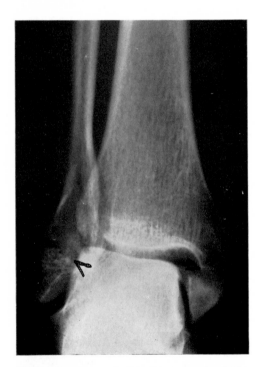

Pott's fracture of the lower end of the fibula with associated fracture of the inner malleolus and characteristic outward displacement of the distal fragments and talus.

$\rightarrow$

Fracture of the shaft of the humerus in the middle third with fragments in good apposition but showing a loss in the carrying angle. Considerable new bone formation is present uniting the fragments. A dark zone between the raised periosteum and the underlying shaft indicates that bone proliferation is still actively going on from the periosteum.

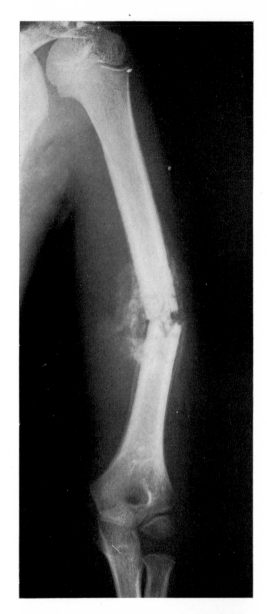

$\rightarrow$

Fracture of the inner-epicondyle of the humerus with wide separation of the fragments.

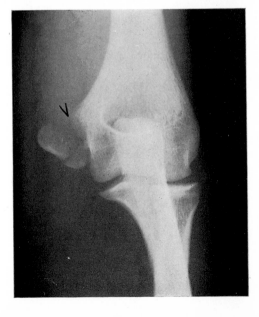

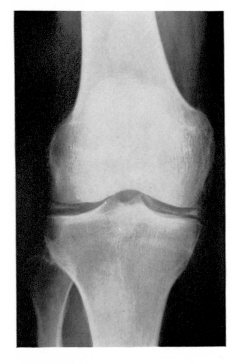

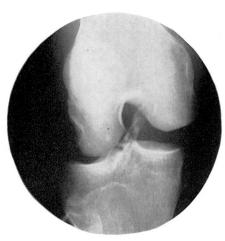

Fracture of tibial spine with tearing of crucial ligaments and dislocation.

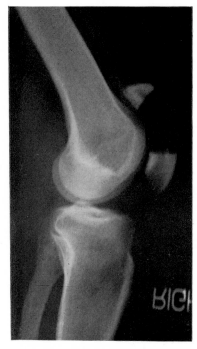

Calcification of interarticular fibro-cartilage following trauma.

Complete transverse fracture of the patella with wide separation of the fragments.

$\longrightarrow$

Avulsion fracture of lower portion of femoral head with associated obturator dislocation.

Reduction of dislocation; perfect function without removal of fragment.

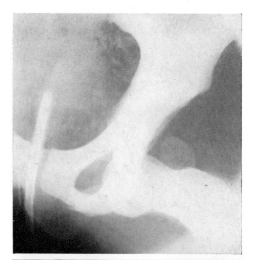

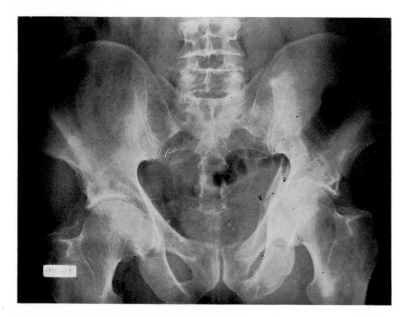

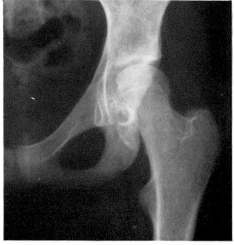

Central fracture of the acetabulum showing the head of the femur driven into the pelvis. Compare with the uninjured opposite side.

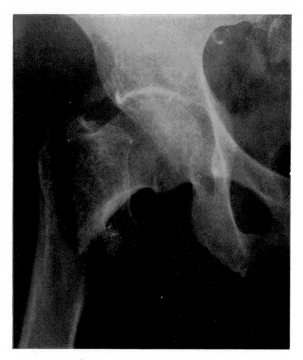

Inter-trochanteric fracture of the femur.

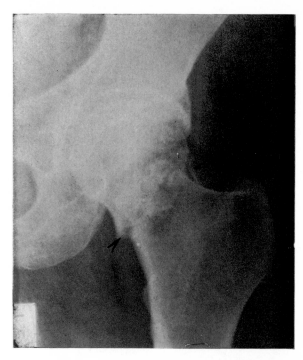

Intracapsular fracture of the neck of the femur.

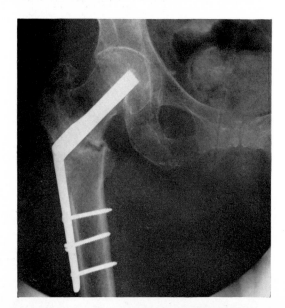

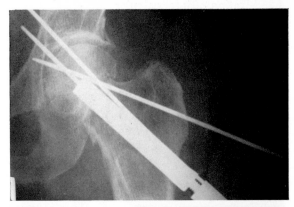

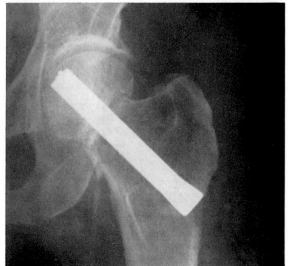

After fixation with flange-nail plate. Antero-posterior and lateral views.

After operative introduction of Smith-Peterson nail. Pins are introduced as guides for directing nail. This operation has reduced mortality as well as non-union from this type of fracture.

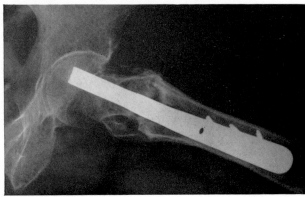

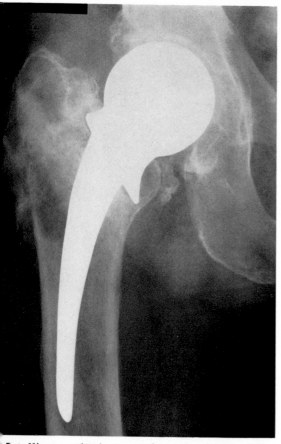

Metallic prosthesis to replace the head of the femur where this structure has become avascular following fracture of the femoral neck.

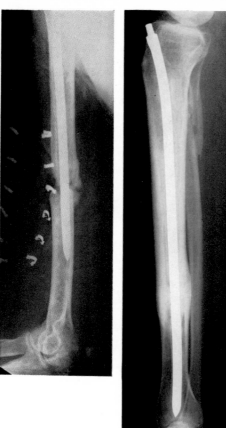
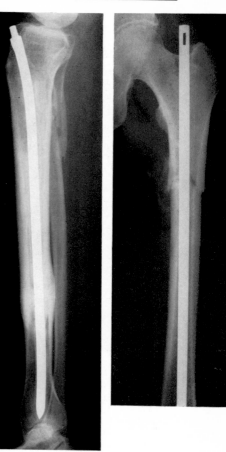

Lottes intramedullary nails for correcting and maintaining position in fractures of the shafts of long bones.

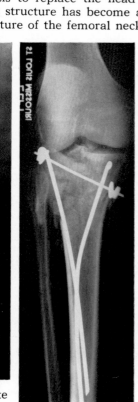
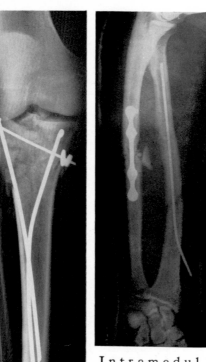

Slotted bone plate for fixation of fracture. Screws extend completely through other side of cortex.

Intercondylar bolt for elevation of plateau fractures upper end tibia, with intramedullary splints.

Intramedullary wire maintaining radial fracture. Lane plate holding ulnar fragments.

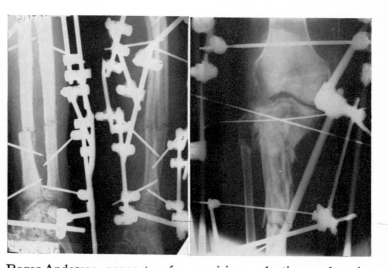

Roger-Anderson apparatus for precision reduction and maintenance of fractured fragments. Metal pins securely fastened in the bony fragment are manipulated by metallic brace outside of the body.—Courtesy Dr. A. H. Diehr.

FRACTURES

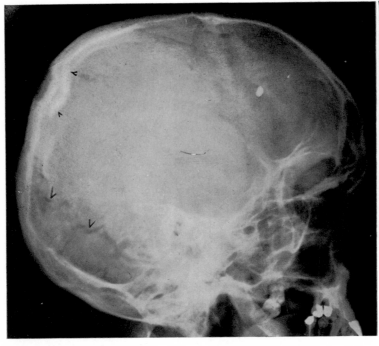

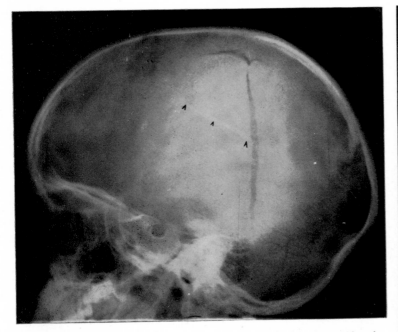

Fracture of the skull showing a small rounded area of depression which is recognized by the zone of double bone density. There is a diastatic fracture of the occipito-parietal suture also.

Frontal view of the same patient showing the depressed and diastatic fractures of the skull.

Flap fracture of the skull showing line of double bone density indicating depression.

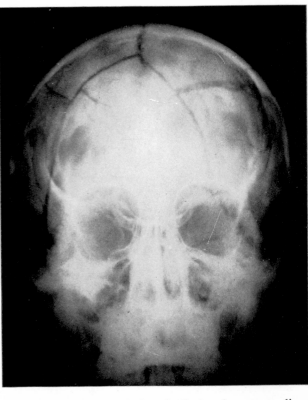

"Eggshell" fracture of the skull showing many lines of fracture. There is no evidence of depression of the fragments.

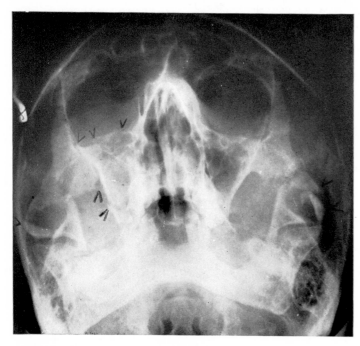

Multiple fractures of bones of face involving antra, rim of orbit, and zygomatic arches.

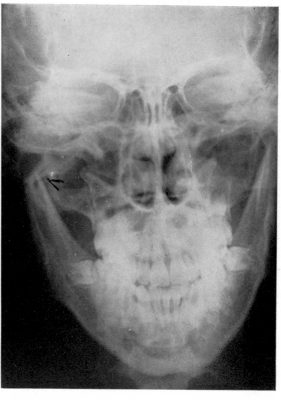

Fracture of the condylar process of the mandible with medial displacement of the upper fragment and medial dislocation of the temperomandibular joint.

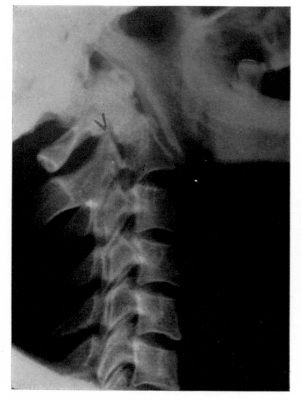

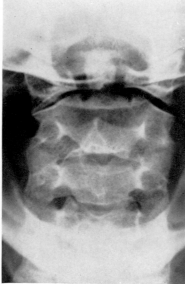

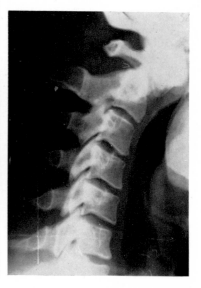

Fracture of the lamina of the second cervical vertebra with an associated dislocation between the second and third.

Fracture of the odontoid process of the 1st cervical vertebra with forward displacement of 1st. on 2d. cervical.

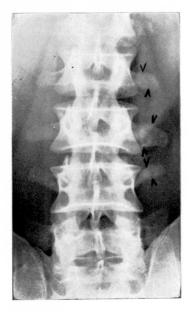

Fractures of the transverse processes of the lumbar vertebrae with only slight separation of the fragments.

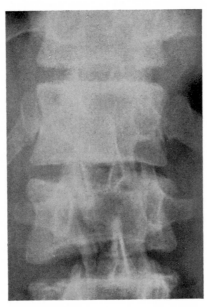 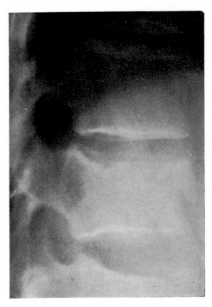

Compession fracture of the body of the first lumbar vertebra with an injury to the upper margin of the second lumbar also. In the antero-posterior view the fracture shows greatest compression on the left side.

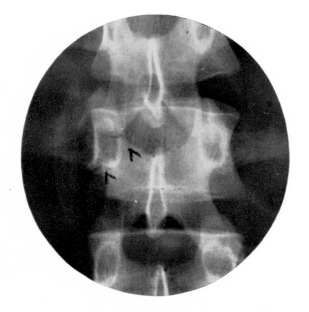 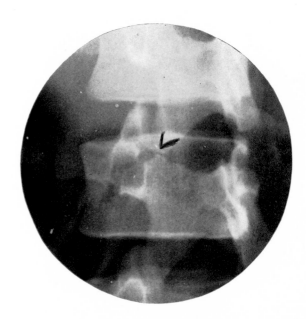

Fractures of the articular processes of lumbar vertebra as seen in anteroposterior and oblique views.

Chapter II

DISLOCATIONS

DISLOCATIONS OF THE UPPER EXTREMITY

Dislocations are usually quite evident clinically, but even in such instances x-ray examination is necessary to be sure that there is no coexisting fracture which might cause excessive damage to the tissues in the attempt to reduce the dislocation.

For the recognition of a dislocation in the radiograph it is necessary that the examination be made in correct standard position, otherwise it will be impossible to properly interpret the relationship which exists between the bones at the joint.

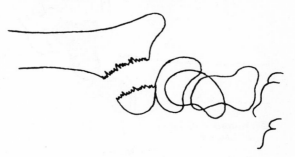

Fig. 40B

DISLOCATION OF RADIAL JOINT AT WRIST.

Uncomplicated dislocations of the wrist joint are rare. When dislocation does occur it is usually associated with fracture of the palmar aspect of the radius and displacement of the carpus and hand palmarward (Smith fracture). Reduction is easily accomplished by pressure but retention in this position requires continued pressure. The fractured fragment often cannot be held in satisfactory apposition for a good functional result.

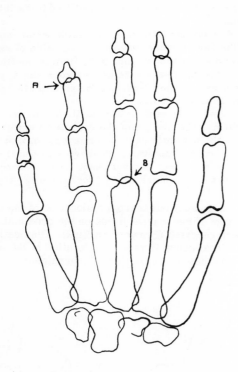

Fig. 40A. Dislocation Phalanges and Metacarpals

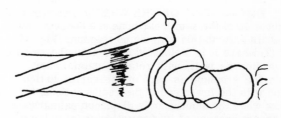

Fig. 40C

DISLOCATION OF THE ULNA AT THE WRIST

JOINT. Spontaneous dislocation of the ulna at the wrist joint occurs whenever the natural length of the radius is lost, either from injury or disease. In any condition which arrests the natural epiphyseal growth of the radial joint, spontaneous dislocation will occur, as in Madelung's Deformity. Rotary dislocation of the ulna at the wrist joint from forcible rolling of the wrist joint under great pressure, occurs in machinery accidents. These may very easily escape detection unless both wrists are examined in the palmar and lateral views. They are sometimes very difficult to reduce.

DISLOCATIONS OF THE HAND.* The phalangeal (A) and the metacarpophalangeal (B) joints are very frequently dislocated. The displacement of the distal portion may be either dorsally or palmarward. They usually are readily reducible by merely exerting traction; occasionally, however, the head of the phalanx may slip through a rent in the capsule, so that it protrudes between the tendons and the displacement cannot be overcome except by open operation.

Fracture-dislocation of the proximal end of the metacarpal for the thumb is known as a Bennett's fracture-dislocation; it often requires special methods of treatment for a satisfactory result.

---

*An asterisk following any title indicates that roentgenographic reproductions illustrating this condition will be found in the pictorial supplement at the end of the chapter.

DISLOCATIONS OF THE UPPER EXTREMITY (Continued)

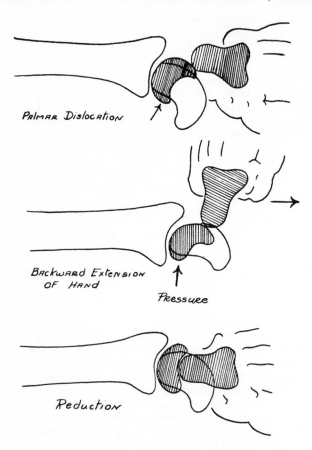

Fig. 41

The following maneuvers have been most successful in reduction of dislocation of the semilunar bone:

1. Grasp the patient's injured hand in a hand clasp, as if you were shaking hands with him (for injuries to the right side, use your right hand; for left-sided injury, shake hands with your left hand).
2. Grasp the patient's forearm above the wrist with your other hand, placing the thumb of this hand on the prominence caused by the edge of the dislocated semilunar bone on the palmar aspect of the wrist.
3. The prominence caused by the edge of this displaced bone can be accurately located by fluoroscopic examination with the injured hand in due lateral position.
4. Exerting firm traction on the wrist joint, bend the hand far backward into a position of extreme hyperextension across your body (in this position, bending the hand backward across your chest, you are in a position to exert your maximum strength for the manipulation).
5. With the hand in this position exert extreme pressure on the margin of the dislocated semilunar bone as the patient's hand is quickly permitted to assume its normal position. Observe with fluoroscope and if the maneuver has not been successful, repeat with more traction and more pressure (Fig. 41).

An unusual intercarpal dislocation of the entire distal row of metacarpal bones on the proximal row has been reported (Brewer and Zink). Dislocation of other carpal bones is rare. Dislocation of the pisiform bone has been reported, (Immermann).

DISLOCATION OF THE WRIST. Two types of dislocation of the semilunar bone are encountered; (1) at its articulation with the os magnum (Fig. 41A), and (2) where it is dislocated at its articulation with the radius as well, with rotation palmarward. Since the scaphoid is part of the carpal articulation with the lower end of the radius it tends to follow when the semilunar is displaced palmarward but cannot because of its firm attachment to the distal row of carpal bones, hence fracture of the scaphoid is commonly encountered when there is dislocation of semilunar at the radial joint. Since the ligaments and tendons shorten quickly to accomodate themselves to the new position, it is urgent to attempt the reduction very soon after injury.
The dislocation is produced with the hand bent far backward, in hyperextension, replacement therefore must be effected with the hand in a similar hyperextended position (Fig. 41B and C).
Since the radiologist is often called upon to assist in the reduction of such dislocations a detailed account of the procedure will be helpful.

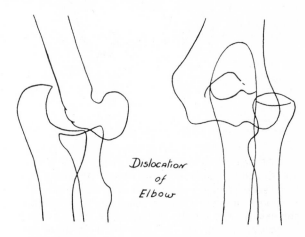

A. Lateral   B. Anteroposterior
Fig. 42

DISLOCATIONS OF THE ELBOW JOINT*
(Fig. 42). Dislocations of the elbow joint are relatively

DISLOCATIONS OF THE UPPER EXTREMITY (Continued)

frequent. The ulna alone may be completely dislocated backward (A and B) so that the lower articular surface of the humerus is in apposition with the anterior surface of the ulna, the coronoid process projecting upward into the position normally occupied by the olecranon process. Such dislocations are frequently accompanied by fractures of the coronoid process of the ulna; if this is the case, the elbow must be held in acute flexion until partial healing has occurred, since any attempt to straighten the elbow may result in spontaneous redislocation. Many stages of partial dislocation due to rotary motion are encountered, but these can easily be recognized from the configuration of the bones. The radius may be dislocated also, (Burman et al).

Such dislocations are produced by extreme extension--consequently they must be reduced by the same mechanism. Using the forearm as a lever, hyperextend at the elbow joint; this presses the tip of the olecranon process against the humerus, thus lifting the coronoid process away from the fossa and

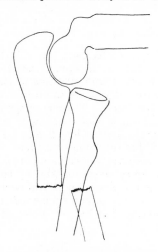

C. Dislocation of Radius

removing the only obstacle to reduction. Flex the elbow and maintain in this position for a few days or a week to permit healing of the torn ligaments.

Dislocation of the radius alone at the elbow joint (C), is usually accompanied by fracture of the upper end of the ulna, (Monleggia fracture-dislocation). The fracture of the ulna may be so severe that the dislocation of the radius is actually overlooked. Since the head of the radius is a plane surface, the reduction of the dislocation itself is usually much easier than replacement of the fracture.

Similar anteromedial dislocation of the head of the radius with paradoxical crossing of the radius producing supination contracture of the forearm may be produced without fracture of the ulna, (Burman). The force of the suddenly contracted biceps muscle, acting upon the radius with the elbow in a position of flexion and supination causes the paradoxical crossing of the radius to the opposite side resulting in supination contracture. This results in a very disabling deformity.

DISLOCATIONS OF THE SHOULDER.[*] The shoulder is probably the most frequent site of dislocation of any joint in the body. The wide range of motion, the rather flail capsular ligament and the extent to which the musculature is depended upon to maintain the

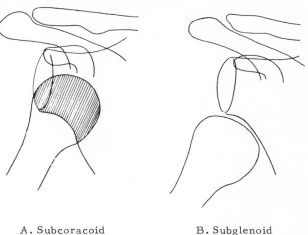

A. Subcoracoid   B. Subglenoid

Fig. 43

joint in place, all motivate to its easy dislocation. In no other location in the body is it so essential that the roentgenographic examination be made in absolutely correct standard position, i.e. with the arm down by the side, palm forward. Rotation of the humerus in the normal joint caused by allowing the palm of the hand to be directed backward, or by flexion of the arm across the chest, will result in a roentgenogram which may readily simulate dislocation of the bones. When taken in standard position at least one third of the articular surface of the humerus should be parallel to and in proper relationship with the glenoid of the scapula, to indicate the joint is in proper place.

Dislocation common at the shoulder joint are subcoracoid (A) and subglenoid (B), both of which are produced in similar fashion by forcible protrusion of the head of the humerus through the weak inferior portion of the capsule. Such dislocations are frequently accompanied by fracture of the lesser tuberosity of the humerus, and even of the anatomical or surgical neck; it is therefore always advisable to secure a roentgenographic examination before reduction of the dislocation is attempted. Reduction is effected by the regular Kocher Method. Posterior dislocations of the head of the humerus are extremely rare in which the head of the humerus is forced backward through the posterior portion of the capsular ligament to a position below the acrmion process or spine of the scapula.

Clinically the fixed position of the head may lead to an indication of the true condition, but it requires a lateral view for definite establishment of the posterior dislocation, (Jacknow and O'Connor). Arden has reported a case of posterior dislocation of both shoulders.

Dislocation of the shoulder may be associated

DISLOCATION OF THE UPPER EXTREMITY (Continued)

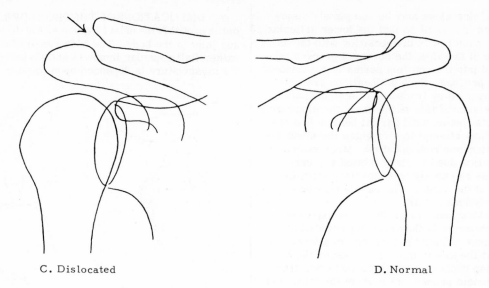

C. Dislocated   D. Normal

with more severe tearing of the ligaments and injury to the soft parts than is evident at roentgenographic examination. The severe damage of the soft parts may ultimately result in calcium deposits in the ligaments and muscles which may be very disabling. If the patient complains of pain after reduction, repeated x-ray examination should be made.

DISLOCATION--ACROMIOCLAVICULAR ARTICULATION.* Separation of the acromioclavicular articulation is occasionally seen as a result of severe downward pull on the arm. Since this joint is so variable in its degree of separation of the bones, even in normal individuals, it is always advisable to make an examination of the opposite shoulder also for comparison (C dislocated; D normal). Examination should be made in the upright position with a weight in the hand. Immobilization to insure proper healing of the torn ligaments is all that is necessary in the way of treatment. Tearing of the coraco-clavicular ligament is a common accompaniment of acromioclavicular separation; it may be followed by calcification of the torn ligament three or four weeks later. In any instance where pain persists weeks after such an injury reexamination by roentgen rays should be made for detection of this possibility. If there is no indication of any such condition within a month, the likelihood of its developing at a later date is very slight.

DISLOCATIONS OF THE LOWER EXTREMITY

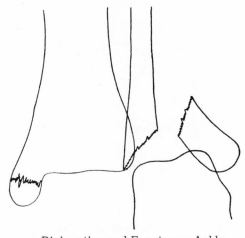

Dislocation and Fracture--Ankle

Fig. 45

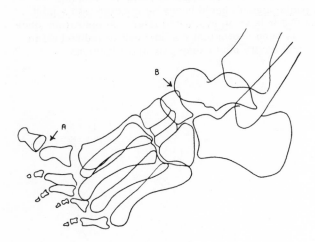

A. Great Toe
B. Talo-navicular Joint

Fig. 44

DISLOCATIONS OF THE FOOT. Dislocation of the toes (A) is rather rare. Usually when it does occur it is readily recognizable in the roentgenogram and is treated by simple traction. The metatarsal bones are rarely dislocated except as a result of severe trauma to the rest of the foot. Their reduction is usually not very difficult.

The most common dislocation in the tarsal region is dislocation of the astragalus (talus) at its joint with the scaphoid (tarsal navicular) (B). The head of the astragalus slips upward overriding the scaphoid, producing an unusual prominence of the head of the bone on the dorsum of the foot. Reduction of such dislocations may be quite easily accomplished if undertaken early, but if reduction is deferred until lapse of considerable time, it may not be possible without severe force applied to the head of the bone to drive it downward into normal position. Open operation may have to be resorted to.

Dislocation of the astragalus (talus) on the os calcis (calcaneus) is very rare; it is usually accompanied by fracture of the sustentaculum tali or other portion of the os calcis. Manipulation of the foot by rotation and pressure over a sand bag under fluoroscopic control is usually the best method of reduction.

DISLOCATION OF THE ANKLE.* The ankle joint is a morticed joint; dislocations of this joint are almost always associated with fracture of some sort. The most common displacement of the bones of this joint is seen in association with Pott's fracture; here the outward displacement of the fractured fibula and the inner malleolus of the tibia carry with them the astragalus causing a luxation of the ankle joint. Correction of the deformity caused by the Pott's fracture results in reduction of the luxation at the ankle joint without difficulty (see Pott's fracture, Fig. 14).

Fahey, et al. have called attention to the fact that fracture-dislocations of the ankle with fixed posterior displacement of the fibula behind the tibia are often difficult to reduce, giving lasting disability.

Backward dislocation of the astragalus (see Fig. 15) is usually accompanied by fracture of the posterior articular margin of the lower end of the tibia; if the fracture line of the tibia is far enough posteriorly so that sufficient "shoulder" is left to hold the ankle joint in position in its flexed position, then no dislocation occurs, but if the fracture line is near the peak of the anteroposterior arch of the lower tibial articulation, then, on assuming a flexed position of the foot, the astragalus is pressed backward on the posterior portion of the articular surface of the tibia and if sufficient "shoulder" is thereby removed, then the astragalus will suffer spontaneous backward re-dislocation. Reduction of the dislocation is simple; with the patient lying on the table under an anaesthetic, grasp the great toe firmly and lift the leg off the table, in this manner the weight of the leg will be sufficient force to effect immediate reduction of the dislocation. To prevent redislocation either the foot must be immobilized in an extended position, running the risk of permanent shortening of the tendo-Achilles from maintenance in this position or forward pressure must be exerted on the heel to prevent backward luxation. At times this becomes a very difficult problem (see fracture of the posterior articular surface of the tibia, Fig. 15).

DISLOCATIONS OF THE LOWER EXTREMITY (Continued)

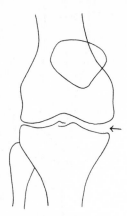

Fig. 46. Dislocation Semilunar Cartilage of Knee with locking of joint. Only under such conditions will there be any widening of the joint space.

DISLOCATIONS OF THE KNEE.* The knee joint is buttressed by strong ligaments and the joint itself is rarely dislocated; when it is, manipulation with traction under fluoroscopic guidance is usually quite effective in causing proper reduction. Certain dislocations of the knee are irreducible due to the complete avulsion of the tibial lateral ligament and interposition of the capsuloligamentous flap within the joint. A characteristic depressed groove on the medial aspect of the knee is a diagnostic sign.

Dislocation of the fibula at its upper articulation with the tibia is rare but should be readily recognized on comparison on the two sides.

Dislocation of the semilunar cartilages of the knee, often is not demonstrable by ordinary roentgenographic examination. Normally the width of the interarticular space is determined by the articular cartilages which cover the ends of the bones; the two semilunar fibrocartilages fit snugly in place acting as buttresses of the joint but not contributing to the interarticular space. The displacement of one of these cartilages then will not permit narrowing of the joint space on one side. With fracture of a cartilage, a fragment may become wedged between the articular surfaces and cause widening of one side of the joint (Fig. 46). Or a "bucket-handle" fracture of the cartilage may occur permitting the cartilage to slip around with the reversed cartilage lying in the intercondylar notch. Unless such displacement is present at the time of examination it may be impossible to detect the condition from the ordinary roentgenogram.

If the joint is stretched immediately by forcible abduction or adduction a partial vacuum will be momentarily produced which may aid in the demonstration of the cartilaginous structures. Or, it may be found worth while to inject oxygen or air for the clearer demonstration of the articular structures,

Bircher's Method, (Oberholzer). (See also Arthrography Manual of Roentgenological Technique). Opaque media should never be injected into a joint unless it is to be evacuated later at operation since it has been shown that confinement of iodized oil in a joint cavity may cause pain and adhesions.

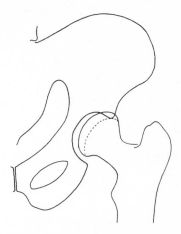

Fig. 47. Posterior Dislocation of Hip

DISLOCATION OF THE HIP.* The hip joint is very rarely dislocated. When dislocation does occur it is almost always in a young, well-built, muscular individual. Sufficient trauma to produce a dislocation of the hip, when applied to an older individual, usually results in fracture of the neck or upper end of the femur. The head of the femur is usually displaced backwardly resting on the posterior rim of the acetabulum, although it may be higher up on the ilium or lower down in the obturator foramen. Roentgenographically the dislocated head of the bone is usually recognized even when it lies directly behind the acetabulum, so that the articular surfaces actually appear to be in proper relationship—the shadow of the femoral head may fall directly over the center of the acetabular cavity. The one telltale point which is always evident, is the fact that the head of the femur, being closer to the film in this abnormal dorsal location, is smaller in size than one would ordinarily expect it to be—a fact which is evident at once if a comparative view is taken of the opposite hip joint. In case of doubt take an oblique view of the hip, (Solovay). Under these abnormal conditions the lining schemes, adapted to show the normal relationship of the bones of the hip joint, do not work out correctly. Reduction under anaesthesia is made by ordinary flexion and rotation manipulation. Even where there is no evidence of bony injury after complete reduction, erosion and cystic destruction of the articular cortex may develop months later due to subchondral necrosis from injury to the blood supply. (Congenital dislocation of the hip is not considered under injuries; it is a congenital malformation considered under developmental anomalies.)

DISLOCATIONS OF THE JAW

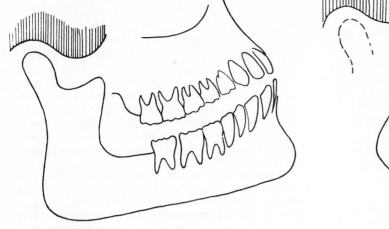

A. Normal Temporomandibular Joint

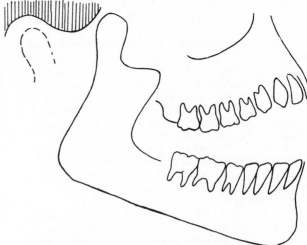

B. Dislocation--Mouth Wide Open

Fig. 48

DISLOCATION OF THE JAW. The temporomandibular articulation is a gliding ginglymus-arthrodial joint; as the mouth is opening, the condyle of the mandible glides forward on its articular surface, its range of forward motion being limited by muscular attachments to the bone and by the eminentia articularis, a bony prominence which forms the anterior portion of the joint. Overdistention of the mouth in eating or from yawning may result in slipping of the condylar process of the mandible forward over the eminentia articularis into such a position that it prevents the closing of the mouth; any attempt to forcibly close the mouth while dislocated may result in fracture of the condylar process. Reduction is usually effected by placing both thumbs in the mouth, exerting firm downward pressure on the molar regions of the mandible, at the same time pressing upward on the chin. Care must be taken by the operator to protect his fingers. If this is not successful, several thicknesses of tongue depressors or the handle of a table knife sufficiently protected, or some similar object, may be placed between the posterior molar teeth of the upper and lower jaws to act as a fulcrum by which the condyle of the mandible may be lifted clear, over the eminentia articularis as upward pressure is exerted on the chin. This maneuver must be carried out carefully without too much force. Very frequently such dislocations of the jaw are associated with fractures of the condylar process of the mandible.

This fracture usually occurs as a result of an upward blow on the chin when the mouth is widely open. In this position the condyles of the jaw slip forward over the eminentia articularis; a sudden blow to the chin does not permit time for the condyle to slip back naturally and a fracture of the condylar

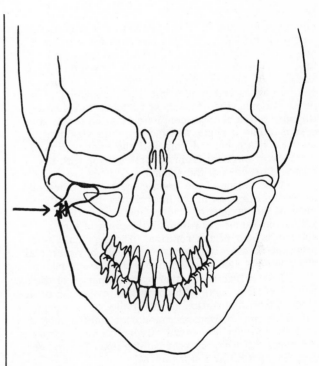

C. Fracture--Dislocation of the Condyle of the Mandible

process results together with a dislocation of the condyle.

Often because of the loose unattached condition of the fragment it cannot be replaced and must be removed. In spite of removal the joint may return to fairly good normal function.

DISLOCATION OF THE SPINE

DISLOCATION OF THE CERVICAL SPINE
(See Fractures of Cervical Spine)

The cervical region permits the widest range of motion of any portion of the spine. It is therefore most susceptible to injuries, both fractures and dislocations. Falling on the head and twisting the neck; a sudden jerk with the head held in some unusual position, may be sufficient to cause dislocation of the cervical spine. The articular facets are so closely applied and so well morticed by each other that simple dislocation without fracture is rather rare. That subluxation does occur under exceptional circumstances, there can be no doubt; the writer has encountered two cases after mastoid operation under anaesthesia.

A very frequent site of such dislocation is between the first and second cervical vertebrae. Very minute changes in position may result in limitation of motion. For the detection of such dislocations the system of lining developed to illustrate the normal relationship of the vertebrae of the upper cervical spine is imperative. The articular surfaces between the first and second vertebrae should be equidistant on both sides and parallel with each other; overlapping of the articular surfaces on both sides indicates luxation of the first forward on the second. In the lateral view dislocation is accompanied by forward displacement of the shadow of the posterior tubercle of the first vertebra in its relationship to the second; complete luxation forward is only possible if rupture of the articular ligament of the first has occurred; this will show separation of the body of the first from its articulation with the odontoid process of the second.

Dislocation of the lower cervical vertebra may be best recognized in the lateral view by malalignment of the various articular facets or in the antero-posterior view by malalignment of the spinous process from rotation. The cervical vertebrae are so closely fitted together that any material displacement can hardly occur without fracture.

Kovács has shown that by examination of the lower cervical spine with downward projection of the x-ray beam, subluxation and deformity of the apophyseal joints may be demonstrated encroaching upon the vertebral artery and nerve. Hypertrophic changes at the vertebral margins encroaching upon the foramen may cause similar impingement.

The atlas and axis articulate by four groups, 1) the anterior ring of the atlas with the odontoid process of the axis; 2) posterior surface of the odontoid process with the transverse ligament; 3 and 4) the joints between the lateral masses on either side. The synovial membranes of all of these joints often communicate freely. These joints are drained by the retropharyngeal lymph nodes into which, by the deep lymphatic channels, the nasopharyngeal, tonsillar areas, middle ears, teeth and nose are also drained, making the spread of infection through these channels readily possible. This may result in <u>spontaneous</u>

<u>forward luxation</u> of the atlas on the axis due to increase in <u>fluid in the joint between the odontoid process of the axis and the ring of the atlas</u>. This is readily detected in the lateral view of the upper cervical spine by increase in width of this articulation, (Coutto).

Rotary luxation of one or the other or both lateral articular masses may result often from apparently trivial injury. Detection is possible only with careful rotational open-mouth views with rotation to either side showing medial or lateral offset of lateral mass on the affected side. Laminagraphy may be of material aid, (Jacobson and Adler).

Manipulation of the cervical spine for the reduction of any such dislocations should only be carried out by an orthopedist or surgeon well informed as to the method and dangers of the procedure. Simple immobilization or traction is imperative to avoid injury pending more complete plans for treatment.

Injury to the cord may occur without dislocation of the cervical spine by hyperextension injuries to the neck (See Pg. 66).

DISLOCATIONS OF DORSAL-LUMBAR SPINE

Dislocation of the vertebrae in the dorsal and lumbar regions rarely, if ever, occurs without associated fracture of the articular facets. The problem here merely becomes one of replacement by traction, manipulation and fixation until healing takes place (see fracture of articular processes of lumbar vertebra).

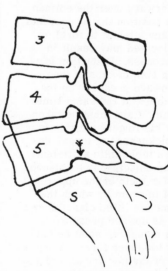

Fig. 49
Spondylolisthesis

SPONDYLOLISTHESIS* (See also Congenital Anomalies) is a condition in which one or more of the lower lumbar vertebrae become displaced on each other or on the sacrum. The condition occurs most frequently between the fifth lumbar vertebra and the sacrum but any other vertebrae may be involved. The upper articular surface of the sacrum forms an inclined plane tilting forward and downward resulting in a tendency to luxation of the fifth lumbar forward on the sacrum.

Ten to fifteen percent of all patients referred for low back pain have this condition; in fully three-fourths of the cases the fifth lumbar vertebra is involved. Usually only one vertebra is involved but occasionally more than one may be involved. Trauma is conceded to be a direct cause of the condition in association with a congenital defect of the neural arch and articular processes of the vertebra which normally support the fifth lumbar in this inclined position and prevent it from slipping forward. This is probably due to nonfusion of the double centers of ossification in the lamina of the lumbar vertebra. This anomaly is rarely seen in infants, but Kleinberg has reported a case in an infant 17 months old. In very few instances does it seem probable that a single intense trauma resulted in the luxation. Usually it can be traced to a series of less severe traumas repeated over a long period of time, such as heavy lifting in patients having a congenital defect of the arch.

Ullmann's lining scheme will aid in detection in cases of slight luxation of the fifth lumbar vertebra (Fig. 49). If a line is erected at right angles to the articular surface of the sacrum at its anterior margin, the fifth lumbar vertebra should remain entirely posterior to this line. If the fourth lumbar vertebra touches this line or projects beyond it, this is evidence of spondylolisthesis. Meyerding has proposed the following classification of spondylolisthesis: Grade I spondylolisthesis showing isthmus defects but without displacement; Grade II showing 1/3 forward displacement on the sacrum; Grade III, 2/3 forward displacement and Grade IV, complete displacement.

This displacement may be between the fourth and fifth or any other lumbar vertebrae. Large outgrowths of bone may result in bridging across between the two bones causing ankylosis of this segment of the spine where displacement is extreme. Fixation by a plaster jacket serves to support the back and decrease the pain. Operative procedure is sometimes resorted to.

The appearance of reverse spondylolisthesis, or posterior displacement of one vertebra upon another, has been generally supposed by most radiologists to be due to a technical error. A study of this condition has led to the conclusion that at times there may be real reverse luxation of the vertebrae (Melamed and Ansfield). These authors divide the true from the false displacements and attribute their cause as follows:

1. True backward displacement of lumbar vertebrae
   A. Due to degenerative processes
   B. Due to disease
   C. Due to trauma
   D. Due to congenital anomalies
2. Apparent backward displacement of lumbar vertebrae
   A. Due to technical factors
   B. Due to anatomical variations

They attribute true retrodisplacement to degeneration of the intervertebral disc and point out that in this condition there is encroachment upon the intervertebral foramen imparting an "hourglass" constriction to this opening. The encroachment of osteophytes growing from the articular margin must not be overlooked as a possible cause of this appearance. Any disease process or other condition which produces tearing or relaxation of the apophyseal joints may give rise to this condition.

Others are also of the opinion that reverse spondylolisthesis may also occur in the other regions of the spine, (Gillespie).

The term "prespondylolisthesis" is sometimes used in cases in which congenital malfusion of the isthmus of the neural arch is present even though luxation has not taken place. Many contend that this is poor practice since it implies that slipping is inevitable, (Garland and Thomas). For description of the arch defects associated with this condition see anomalies of spine.

A new operation, posterior intervertebral fusion of the lumbar spine, has been used by James and Nisbet, for relief of this condition. Failure of fusion of the isthmus on either side permits the posterior segment to rock on the anterior portion, impinging on the 5th lumbar nerve. Removal of posterior Y-shaped segment and posterior fusion of the bodies with an intervertebral graft relieves the condition.

Spondylolisthesis has been reported in the cervical region by Durbin in association with failure of fusion of the lamina. Surgical fusion resulted in relief of symptoms.

DISLOCATION OF THE COCCYX

Dislocation of the coccygeal segments may result from extreme force applied to the coccyx, as in sitting down forcibly upon some hard object. Under such circumstances, it is usually associated with fracture. Manipulation with a finger inserted into the rectum may result in reduction, or it may be necessary to remove the offending fragment. Such fractures may be very painful on account of the coccygeal plexus of nerves which emerge in this region (see fracture of coccyx).

DISLOCATION OF SACRO-ILIAC JOINTS

Actual dislocation of the sacro-iliac joints occurs only as a result of application of extreme degree of trauma to this region, such as falling from a height or being struck by an automobile or railroad train. Such disarticulations are usually accompanied by separation at the symphysis pubis and displacement of the entire side of the pelvis upward. Under such circumstances, lateral fixation in a plaster jacket with extension on one thigh to reduce the displacement is usually sufficient treatment.

SACRO-ILIAC STRAIN

Sacro-iliac strain is another condition in which, often as a result of such trivial trauma as a twisting motion of the trunk, there may be a strain of the ligaments holding the joint in proper firm apposition. Sleeping on a sagging mattress may produce the same result. Such strain permits slight abnormal motion at the joint which results in extreme pain. X-ray examination usually fails to reveal any abnormal relationship at the sacro-iliac articulations; there may be some slight asymmetry of the levels of the two pubic bones at their symphysis, but this sign is sometimes also lacking. This asymmetry may sometimes be elicited by radiographic examination of the patient while standing on one foot.

Firm strapping of the pelvis with pressure pads over the joints on either side should result in relief of pain and reëstablishment of normal function after ten days to two weeks. Manipulation of the joint under anesthesia and fixation may result in relief of the condition. In extreme cases of long standing where all other methods fail, arthrodesis has been recommended.

Many cases of so-called sacro-iliac strain are in truth instances of slipping of an intervertebral disc of the lumbar vertebrae; for detection of such disc displacement see section on myelography.

QUESTIONS ON DISLOCATIONS

Questions marked with a dagger deal with rare and less important conditions.

1. Describe the common sites of dislocations in the hand.

2. Describe the common sites of dislocations in the wrist.

†3. Show by diagram the procedure to be followed in reducing a dislocation of the semilunar (lunate) bone.

4. Name the common types of dislocation about the shoulder joint.

†5. Describe the common sites of dislocation in the foot.

6. Describe the common sites of dislocation in the ankle. Are such dislocations usually associated with fracture?

7. What are the roentgen indications of dislocation of a semilunar cartilage of the knee?

8. Which is the most common type of injury about the hip joint, dislocation or fracture: in a young person? in an older individual?

9. What is the characteristic position in dislocation of the jaw?

10. What are the clinical manifestations of dislocations of the cervical spine? Why are dislocations of the upper four vertebrae so dangerous?

11. How may non-traumatic luxation of the cervical spine be produced?

12. What relationship has infection of the adjacent soft parts to the production of this condition?

†13. What is meant by spondylolisthesis and to what is it usually due? Prespondylolisthesis?

†14. What are the roentgenographic manifestations of spondylolisthesis? Prespondylolisthesis?

15. What is meant by sacro-iliac strain? What is its cause and what are its roentgenographic manifestations?

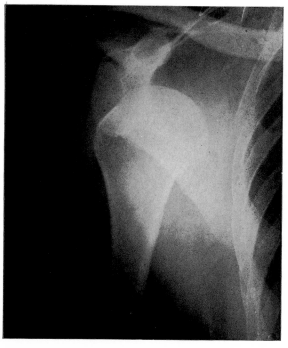

Sub-coracoid dislocation of the humerus.

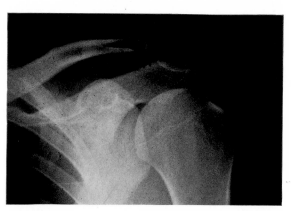

Separation of the acromio-clavicular articulation with elevation of the outer end of the clavicle.

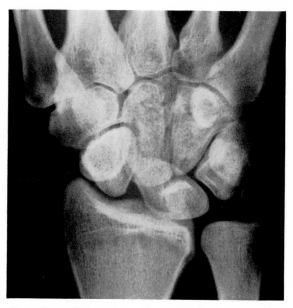

Complete dislocation of scaphoid; partial luxation of semilunar.

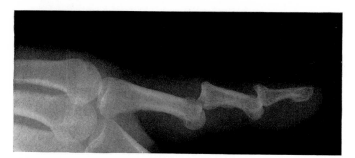

Double dislocation of phalangeal joints of little finger, —courtesy Dr. S. G. Kramer.

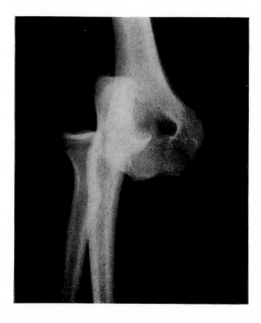

Complete backward and lateral dislocation of both bones of the forearm at the elbow joint in the antero-posterior view (to the left), and the lateral view (to the right).

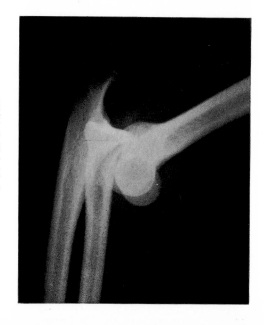

DISLOCATIONS

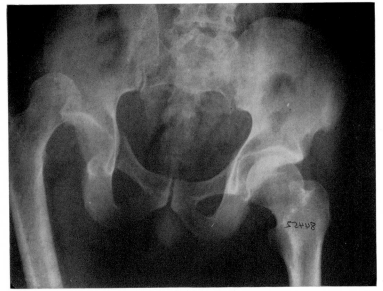

Complete dislocation of the hip showing the head of the femur resting above the acetabulum.

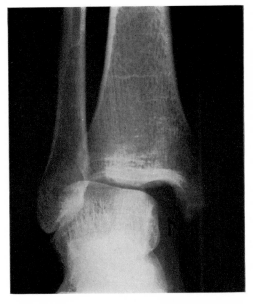

Outward dislocation ankle joint without fracture.

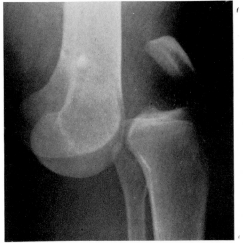

Complete dislocation knee joint without fracture.

→

Lateral view of the lumbo-sacral joint showing spondylolisthesis with forward displacement of the fifth lumbar on the sacrum. Note congenital absence of the articular processes of fifth lumbar and sacrum which normally hold the bones in proper relationship.

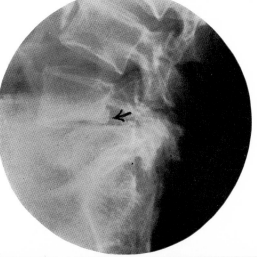

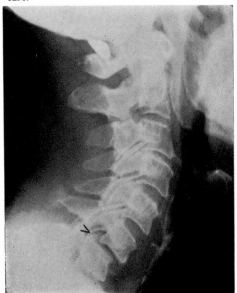

Forward dislocation of the sixth cervical vertebra upon the seventh.

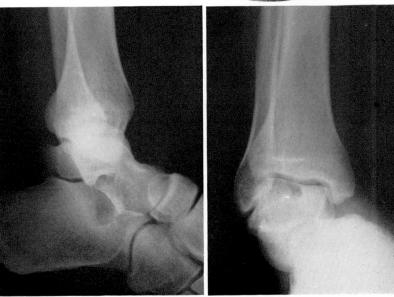

Complete dislocation talo-calcaneal joint without fracture.

Chapter III

EPIPHYSES AND EPIPHYSEAL SEPARATIONS

All bones are preformed in cartilage or membrane. In the natural course of fetal development, a small center of ossification appears in the cartilaginous shaft of the bone and continues to grow until it replaces the entire shaft. At the time of birth complete ossification of the shafts has occurred in all of the long bones. From this point on, the bones must continue their growth, both in thickness and length by other means. The increase in thickness is produced by the osteogenetic layer of the periosteum, and the increase in length is from epiphyseal centers of ossification which develop in the remaining cartilaginous ends of the long bones. These make their appearance in the various localities at different times in the development of the normal individual, and not until full growth is attained does the cartilaginous epiphyseal line unite with the shaft of the bone.

Any interference with the natural development of the bony structure, whether from injury or disease will result in "growth lines" extending perpendicularly across the diaphyseal ends of the long bones. Much can be inferred from the appearance of these lines, (Engeset, et al).

The direction of the nutrient vessels seems to govern in some way the development of the epiphyses. The nutrient artery always runs toward the epiphysis which is last to unite; in bones having only one epiphysis, such as the clavicle, the nutrient artery always runs away from the epiphysis.

The epiphyses are so important that it is imperative that the radiologist be familiar with their location, appearance, and method of development.

The epiphyseal line is naturally weaker than the adjacent bony structure, so that trauma applied at this site may cause separation of the epiphysis rather than a fracture of the bone itself. One characteristic thing which almost always occurs in association with epiphyseal separation is that a small fragment of the diaphysis is usually pulled away with the displaced epiphysis. Since these are the centers upon which future growth of the bone depends, it is essential that they be replaced as accurately as possible and that this operation be undertaken shortly after injury.

Accurate replacement is necessary to promote the most satisfactory conditions for union and subsequent function as a growth-producing structure. The seriousness of failure to resume its growth-producing function is dependent upon the period remaining for function before epiphyseal union; if only a short time of active growth remains the lack of growth will not seriously impair normal development. The most serious deformity which can result is seen in instances in which there is a fracture of the epiphysis across the epiphyseal plate, resulting in loss of function of a part of the epiphysis and continued function of the remainder. This may result in extreme deformity as growth of the bone progresses. It is likewise essential that epiphyseal separation be reduced promptly since bone formation is very rapid--demonstrable, even in three or four days.

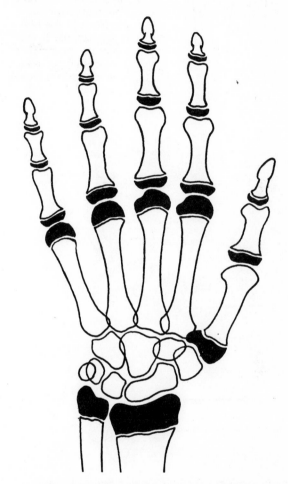

Fig. 50. Epiphyses--Hand and Wrist

EPIPHYSES OF THE HAND. In the hand, the epiphyseal lines are located at the proximal ends of the phalanges, and distal ends of the metacarpal bones, with the exception of the thumb, where the epiphysis for the metacarpal bone is at the proximal end. A good key for remembering the epiphyses of the hand is to draw two fingers of one hand across the knuckles of the other; this indicates the position of the epiphyses of the metacarpal bones at their distal ends, and of all of the phalanges at their proximal extremities (the thumb must be considered as another finger).

EPIPHYSES OF THE UPPER EXTREMITY (Continued)

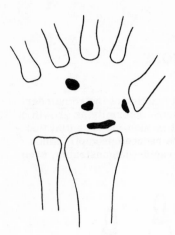

Fig. 50A

OSSIFICATION CENTERS OF CARPAL BONES. There are no epiphyseal lines for the carpal bones. All of these bones are preformed in cartilage and ossify from ossification centers which appear approximately one for each year of life up to the eighth year. The center for the pisiform is the last to appear and it may make its appearance at any time between nine and eleven years of age.

perfect replacement is not absolutely essential to insure continued growth but the best reduction possible is always advisable.

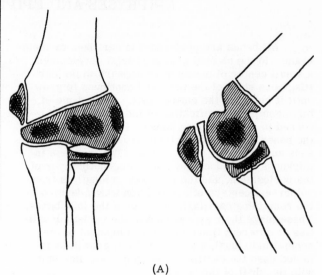

(A)
Ossification Centers and Epiphyses Elbow

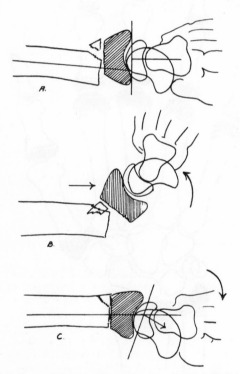

Epiphyseal Separation--Lower Radial Epiphysis
Fig. 51.

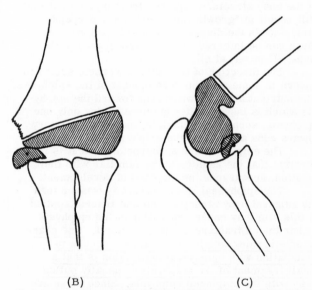

(B)   (C)
Epiphyseal Separation--Inner Epicondyle Humerus
Fig. 52

EPIPHYSES OF WRIST.* Epiphyses for the lower end of the radius and ulna appear as two straight lines across the lower ends of the bones. They have no unusual characteristics. Separation of the lower radial epiphysis is a rather common injury corresponding in a child to Colles' fracture in the adult. The method of reduction and treatment is the same as for Colles' fracture. Replacement should be very accurate so as to insure proper future development; certain studies have been recently made which would indicate that

EPIPHYSES OF ELBOW.* At the elbow joint (A), the epiphysis for the upper end of the radius is merely a straight line across the bone, just beneath the articular cortex. Separation of this epiphysis is somewhat different from similar injuries elsewhere since the capsule of the elbow joint extends far down over the neck of the bone and the articulation of the radio-ulnar joint is on the medial aspect of the epiphysis. This makes the accurate replacement of the displaced epiphysis even more important than similar injuries elsewhere.

*An asterisk following any title indicates that roentgenographic reproductions illustrating this condition will be found in the pictorial supplement at the end of the chapter.

EPIPHYSES OF THE UPPER EXTREMITY (Continued)

The epiphysis for the upper end of the ulna is at the tip of the olecranon process; normally it runs along parallel to the joint, not into it. Occasionally an anomalous division of this epiphysis may be present running across the tip of the epiphysis into the joint. Separation of this epiphysis may be accompanied by upward displacement from the pull of the triceps muscle; under such circumstances the injury must be handled similarly to fractures of the olecranon process with upward displacement of the fragment.

Injury early in life to this epiphysis for the olecranon may result in permanent separation of this structure giving rise to an appearance not unlike that of the patella in the knee. This has been interpreted as a Patella Cubiti, or an anomalous development of a patella for the elbow, (J.E. Habbe).

Ossification centers for the lower end of the humerus are more numerous and somewhat more complicated in arrangement. Four ossification centers, one for each articular surface and one for each epicondyle, appear successively in this region in the following order: first, the center for the capitulum (portion which articulates with radius); second, the center for the inner epicondyle; third, the center for the trochlea (portion which articulates with the sigmoid fossa of the ulna), and fourth, the center for the external epicondyle. As these ossification centers grow, those for the two articular surfaces fuse with each other and with that of the outer epicondyle to form a single epiphyseal line across the lower end of the humerus; that for the inner epicondyle remains separate and forms a second epiphyseal line. Separation of the epiphysis for the lower end of the humerus is rather rare. Accurate replacement is essential, (McLearie and Merson). Usually force of sufficient degree applied in this region results in supracondylar fracture, rather than separation of the epiphysis; when it does result, reduction and treatment are similar to that used for supracondylar fracture.

Separation of the epiphysis for the epicondyle may merely result in a loosening of this bony prominence so that it can be rolled around beneath the finger. Under these circumstances, although it is naturally very difficult to maintain in its proper position, it usually gives little pain or immediate disability. Since the internal epicondyle in its growth aids in the development of the carrying angle, any interference with its function, caused by separation from its normal attachment, may result in failure in development of this very important relationship. If the arrest of epiphyseal growth of the inner epicondyle occurs at an early age when the individual still has a long period of growth to look forward to, then the resulting deformity of the elbow will be great, although it may not appear for several years. If the arrest of growth of this epiphysis occurs at a more advanced age, when only a few years remain before normal union of the epiphysis, then the deformity will not be so great.

Separation of the epiphysis for the inner epicondyle (B & C) sometimes produces a very complicated picture; the separated epiphysis, retaining its capsular attachment from below, may slip through the rent in the capsule into the joint. It becomes wedged between the joint surfaces of the lower end of the humerus and the ulna and is firmly held in this position by the taut capsule. This occurs with the elbow in flexion; if the elbow is extended, the small interposed epiphysis cannot be dislodged and the elbow joint on extension undergoes spontaneous partial or complete dislocation. Under such circumstances surgical removal is the only procedure by which the displaced epiphysis can be dislodged from its position between the joint surfaces. An attempt at fixation of the epiphysis in its normal position may be made, but this is not always successful.

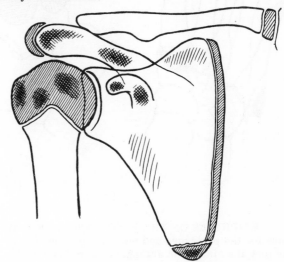

Fig. 53. Ossification Centers and Epiphyses Shoulder

EPIPHYSES OF THE SHOULDER JOINT.* At the shoulder joint, the epiphyses for the upper end of the humerus present a somewhat unusual arrangement. The upper end of the humerus develops by three centers of ossification: one for the head, and one for each of the tuberosities of the bone. These fuse, forming an angular epiphyseal line, apex upward. If during the roentgenographic examination, the central ray is not projected directly across the epiphyseal line, then this angular shape of the epiphysis may appear as a double line, showing not only the anterior, but also the posterior margin of the epiphysis. This must be borne in mind, so as not to mistake this secondary shadow as a fracture of the bone. Separation of the upper epiphysis of the humerus is rather rare owing to its peculiar shape; when it does occur, it presents no unusual features for its reduction and treatment.

The scapula presents seven centers of ossification, two for each process (acromion and

EPIPHYSES OF THE UPPER EXTREMITY (Continued)

coracoid), one for body, one for vertebral margin and one for the inferior angle. Occasionally there is an additional separate epiphysis for the glenoid. The epiphyses for the scapula are rarely injured.

The clavicle shows one epiphysis, appearing as a straight line at its medial extremity. It is one of the latest to appear, and one of the earliest to unite with the shaft. It is rarely injured.

- - - - -

EPIPHYSES OF THE LOWER EXTREMITY

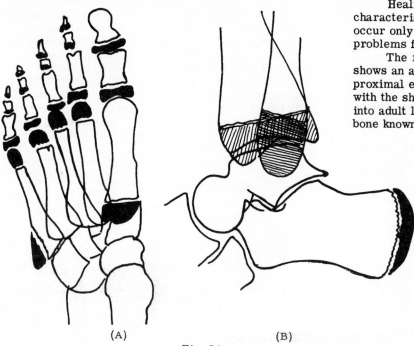

(A)   (B)

Fig. 54

Healing of the bones presents no unusual characteristics. Separations of these epiphyses occur only rarely, and they present no unusual problems for their reduction and treatment.

The fifth metatarsal bone sometimes shows an additional anomalous epiphysis at its proximal end. This epiphysis may not unite with the shaft; under these conditions it persists into adult life as a supernumerary anomalous bone known as a "Vesalianum." Since this is a frequent site of fracture, care must be taken lest a normal epiphyseal line is mistaken for injury; examination of the opposite foot will show any anomalous development, since whenever anomalies occur, they are almost always bilateral. Certain instances have been encountered where the Os Vesalianum was found to be a separate bone, (I. Baastrup).

All of the tarsal bones with the exception of the os calcis (calcaneus) develop by single ossification centers, but they do not appear, as in the wrist, one for each year of life (B). The os calcis is the only tarsal bone to have an epiphyseal line; this is at the extreme posterior portion at the attachment of the Achilles tendon. Complete separation of this epiphysis may show wide displacement, owing to the pull of the Achilles tendon.

In the oblique view of the calcaneus, during the growth period of the epiphysis for the tuberosity, an appearance resembling a tiny chip fracture may be seen on the plantar surface near the epiphyseal line in an otherwise normal individual. This is due to slightly irregular epiphyseal growth, which is not abnormal.

EPIPHYSES OF THE FOOT. The epiphyseal lines for the phalanges and metatarsal bones (A) of the foot are similar in arrangement to those of the hands; namely, at the proximal ends of all of the phalanges, and the distal ends of all of the metatarsal bones with the exception of the great toe. They show as straight lines across the ends of the bones presenting no unusual characteristics. Separations of these epiphyses occur only rarely, and they present no unusual problem for their reduction and treatment.

- - - - -

EPIPHYSES OF THE ANKLE.* At the ankle joint, the epiphyses of the lower ends of the tibia and fibula appear as two straight lines, running across the lower ends of these bones just above the ankle joint. Trauma of a similar nature, which would result in Pott's fracture in an adult, may result in epiphyseal separation of the lower fibular epiphysis. Reduction and treatment are similar to that for Pott's fracture.

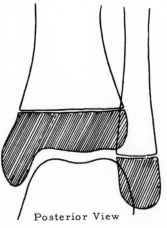

Posterior View

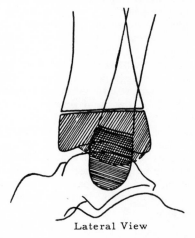

Lateral View

Fig. 55

EPIPHYSES OF THE LOWER EXTREMITY (Continued)

EPIPHYSES OF KNEE. The epiphysis for the upper end of the fibula (Fig. 56) is represented by a straight line running across the upper end of the bone; it presents no unusual features and is rarely injured. The upper tibial epiphysis, however, has certain unusual characteristics worthy of special note; the epiphyseal line runs across the upper end of the bone to provide growth for the shaft of the tibia, then anteriorly it dips down to take in the epiphysis for the tibial tubercle. This tongue-like projection of the tibial tubercle may be separated by trauma from the pull of the patellar tendon or as a result of Osgood-Schlatter's Disease.

The lower femoral epiphysis is indicated merely as a straight line across the end of the bone. This epiphysis is strongly attached and is rarely separated in this generation. In former years this injury was more common. It used to result from catching the leg between the spokes of a wagon and was known as "Wagon-Wheel Fracture." When separation does occur, manipulation under traction is the best method of reduction.

The margins of the lower femoral epiphysis are the most frequent site of irregular bone growth during the developmental period between 4 and 8 years; this irregularity of the articular cortex should not be mistaken for trauma or other bone pathology.

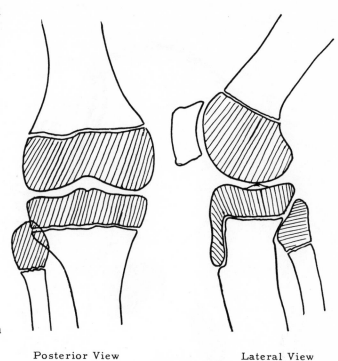

Posterior View   Lateral View

Fig. 56

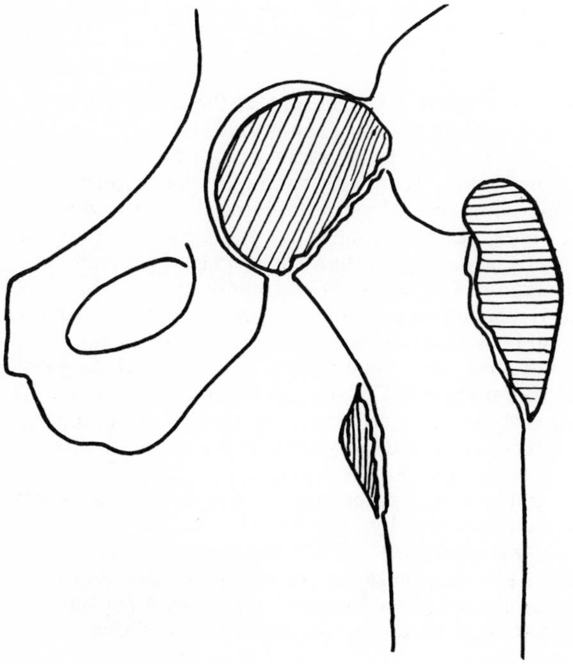

EPIPHYSES AT THE HIP JOINT.* (Fig. 57) There are three epiphyses for the upper end of the femur; one for the head of the bone, and one for each trochanter. Each appears as a straight line across the bone in the respective locations. Separation of any of these epiphyses is rarely seen from acute injury, but slipping of the epiphysis for the femoral head from some nutritional disturbance (juvenile coxa vara) is a well-known disease entity, (see pp. 65,66).

Fig. 57

EPIPHYSES OF THE PELVIS

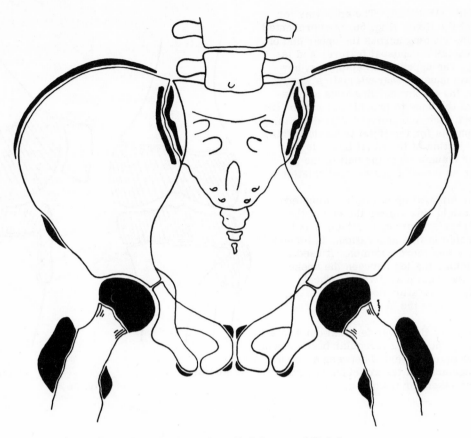

Fig. 58. Secondary Epiphyses of Pelvis

EPIPHYSES OF PELVIS. The innominate bone has three primary and five secondary centers of ossification. The three primary centers are for the ilium, ischium and pubis, seen as the first ossification centers in foetal life. The six secondary centers of ossification which appear at puberty are: one each for the iliac crest, anterior inferior spine of the ilium, pubic bone near its symphysis, tuberosity of the ischium auricular process of ilium, and acetabulum. The epiphyseal center for the crests is a long thin strip of bone which surmounts the rounded upper margin of the ilium; it is always observed roentgenographically without difficulty. The center for the anterior inferior spine is seldom visualized because of its position. The epiphyseal centers for the pubic bones likewise are rarely visualized roentgenographically and their very existence is questioned by some observers. The epiphyseal line between the ischium and descending ramus of the pubis is always well seen—it has rounded margins and should never be mistaken for fracture. The epiphysis for the tuberosity of the ischium is a crescentic structure fitting over the undersurface of this rounded bony prominence, it is readily visualized roentgenographically and should be recognized without difficulty. The

separate epiphyseal structure of the acetabulum may not develop and is rarely visualized.

The sacrum is developed from five vertebral segments which fuse with each other sometimes leaving remnants of not completely eliminated vertebral discs. Each segment has the epiphyseal centers normally present in other vertebral structures but by reason of fusion of the segments may not be clearly recognizable. In addition to these one or two centers of ossification for each wing of the sacrum have been described. These run along parallel to the margins of the sacroiliac joints and are rarely visualized unless by reason of epiphysitis from trauma or other cause they become the site of sclerosis, (E. N. Cleaves).

An ununited epiphysis for the ischial tuberosity has been reported by Slayton.

The epiphyseal center for the articular process of the ilium is rarely recognizable roentgenographically and is not given by many anatomists but has been demonstrated by Rauber-Kopsch and by Shipp and Haggart.

Caffey and Madell have pointed out several variations in the ossification centers of the pelvis at birth.

EPIPHYSES OF THE SPINE

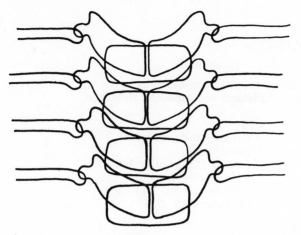

A. Three Primary Ossification Centers for Vertebrae

SPINAL EPIPHYSES (Fig. 59), (Bailey). The vertebrae ossify by three major ossification centers which show roentgenographically as a central and two lateral masses in the spine of an infant (A). These should be fused by six or seven years of age. Five secondary centers of ossification (B & C), appear about the age of puberty:

Two plate-like vertebral rings for the upper and lower margins of the vertebral body, two ossification centers for the tips of the transverse processes and one for the tip of the spinous process. All ossification centers should be firmly united by twenty-five years of age.

The vertebral plates for the upper and lower margins of the bodies appear most clearly in the cervical region. They are continuous rings thinnest posteriorly and in the center, thickest at their anterior margins. The atlas has only the three primary ossification centers; the axis has in addition to the three primary centers common to all vertebrae, two other primary centers for the odontoid process. A secondary center for the tip of the odontoid process develops at about two years which is readily demonstrable roentgenographically and another for the inferior margin of the body about puberty. The seventh cervical has an extra primary center for the costal processes. Secondary ossification centers are observed roentgenographically for the tips of the articular processes; these sometimes persist ununited into adult life, (Wilbur Bailey).

Further investigation more recently undertaken also indicates that many of these secondary centers remain ununited into adult life, (Hadley).

Many question the exact function of these secondary ossification centers indicating that the processes which they represent are merely apophyses and do not function in growth of bone as epiphyses. There is evidence to indicate that the vertebral bodies do not grow in vertical diameter from the vertebral centers which appear at their upper and lower margins, (Bick and Copel). The work of these authors indicates that "in longitudinal development the body of the human vertebra grows as does the diaphysis of a long bone, with true proximal and distal epiphyseal plates. ......enough has been demonstrated to confirm Schmorl's views. The so-called 'epiphyseal

misnamed...... The ring is not an epiphysis and takes no active part in the growth of the vertebral body. It is primarily a cartilaginous ring which ossifies separately. ......It lies outside the metaphyseal area and fuses with the body when longitudinal growth is completed. ......the fibers of the anterior longitudinal ligament insert into its substance."

Large venous sinusoids traverse the mid-zone of the vertebral body. These are supplied by two antero-lateral veins in front and are emptied by two posterior veins which connect with the venous plexus within the neural canal. The transverse horizontal groove traversing the mid-portion of the vertebral body caused by these venous structures should never be mistaken for pathology, (Wagoner and Pendergrass).

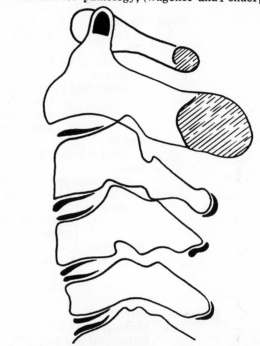

B. Secondary Epiphyseal Centers for Cervical Spine

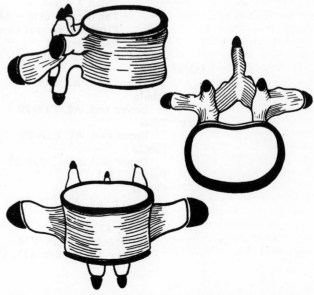

C. Secondary Epiphyseal Centers for Other Vertebrae

Table I

EPIPHYSEAL CENTERS

An anatomical list of the various ossification centers and epiphyses as they appear and unite at the various joints, - Wm. Englebach and Alphonse McMahon.

Upper Extremity:

Hand: Carpus, capitate 1
Hammate - 1-2
Os triangularis 3
Lunate 4

Greater Multangular 5
Navicular 6
Lesser Multangular 7-8
Pisiform 9-11
Metacarpal A3, U14-15
Phalanges A3, U15

Wrist: Radius
    Lower end - A2, U17
Ulna
    Lower end - A7, U18-20

Elbow: Humerus
    Lower end - capitulum A2
              trochlea A10
              outer epicondyle - A11-12   } F and U16
              inner epicondyle - A5-6, U18

Radius
    Head - A-5-6, U16
Ulna
    Olecranon process - A10, U16

Shoulder: Clavicle, A15-17, U22
    Scapula { Acromion A15, U18
            { Coracoid, A1, U15-18
            { Angle and border, A15, U15-18

Humerus:
    Upper end - Head A6-7 mo.
              Greater Tuberosity A2 } F and U
              Lesser Tuberosity A3

Lower Extremity:

Foot: Phalanges A - 3-7, U16
    Metatarsal A - 3-7, U16
    Tarsal: Calcaneus, A6 mo. Epiphysis for A10, U16
            Talus A-7 mo.
            Third cuneiform - A1
            First and second cuneiform A2-4
            Navicular A4
            Cuboid A Birth

Ankle: Tibia
    Lower end, A2, U18
Fibula
    Lower end, A2, U18-20

Knee: Tibia
    Upper end, A1, U18-20
Fibula
    Upper end, A3-4, U18-20
Patella A2-3
Femur
    Lower end, A1, U18-20

Hip: Femur
    Head, A1, U18
    Gt. Trochanter A4-U18
    Lesser Trochanter A13, U17

Innominate: Centers Appear
      3 primary Ilium 8-9 weeks
           Ischium 3 mo. } 7-8 yr. } Well developed at birth U18
           Pubis 4-5 mo. } union }

      5 secondary crest A15-18, U18-20
           Anterior Inf. angle A15-16, U18-20
           Tuberosity Ischium, A15-16, U18
           Symphysis pubis, A16, U18
           "Y" piece Acetabulum U18-20

Spine: Vertebrae,
        3 primary, body 8 weeks
          centers lateral masses 7-18 weeks

        5 secondary
          centers, end of each transverse process, A16, U18
              end of each spinous process A16, U18
              upper and lower surfaces of body, A16, U18

        2 additional centers
        Lumbar vertebra, for mammillary
                 process - A16, U18
        Sacrum: Epiphysis of wing
                near sacro-iliac joints A15-16, U18

A--appear   F--fuse   U--unite

An elaborate report on the appearance and growth of ossification centers in white and negro children has been made. (H. K. Kelly and L. Reynolds, Am. J. Roentg. and Ra. Th., 57:477, 1947.)

Dedick and Caffey have reported the Roentgen Findings in the skull and chest in 1030 new born infants.

Table II

APPEARANCE AND UNION OF BONE CENTERS
ENGELBACH AND McMAHON

Yrs.		Yrs.	
1	Coracoid process scapula	13	Lesser trochanter femur
	Head of humerus (6-7 mos.)	14	U. of head of metacarpals
	Capitate and hamate		(14-15 yrs.)
	Head of femur	15	A. of acromion
	Upper epiphysis tibia (birth)		Inferior angle scapula
	Third cuneiform		U. of centers of scapula
2	Greater tubercle humerus		(15-18 yrs.)
	Capitulum, humerus		A. of sternal end clavicle
	Lower epiphysis radius		(15-17 yrs.)
	Patella (2-3 yrs.)		U. of heads of phalanges, hand
	Lower epiphysis tibia		A. of secondary centers os coxae
	Lower epiphysis fibula		a. Crest of ilium (15-18 yrs.)
	First and second cuneiforms		b. Acetabulum (15-16 yrs.)
	(2-4 yrs.)		U. of primary centers os coxae
3	Os triangularis	16	Union of:-
	Heads of metacarpals		Distal extremity humerus
	Heads of phalanges		Olecranon, ulna
	Heads of metatarsals (3-7 yrs.)		Upper epiphysis radius
4	Lunate		Heads of metatarsals
	Greater trochanter femur		Heads of phalanges, feet
	Upper epiphysis fibula	17	Union of:-
	(3-4 yrs.)		Lower epiphysis radius
	Navicular (tarsal)		Lesser trochanter femur
5-6	U. of head and tubercles	18	Union of:-
	humerus		Head of humerus
	Medial epicondyle humerus		Head of femur
	Upper epiphysis radius		Greater trochanter femur
	Greater multangular		Lower epiphysis tibia
	Lesser multangular (6-8 yrs.)	18-	Union of:-
	Navicular (carpal) (5-6 yrs.)	20	Lower epiphysis ulna
7	Lower epiphysis ulna		Secondary centers os coxae
	U. of ischium and pubis		(20-25 yrs.)
	Epiphysis os calcis (7-9)		Lower epiphysis femur
9	Pisiform (9-11)		Upper epiphysis tibia
10	Olecranon, ulna		Lower epiphysis fibula
	Trochlea, humerus		Upper epiphysis fibula
11	Lateral epicondyle humerus	22	U. of sternal end clavicle
	(11-12 yrs.)	25	

--Wm. Engelbach and Alphonse McMahon

Table II. A chronological list of the various ossification centers with their time of appearance and union as listed by Engelbach and McMahon is reproduced.

A--appear   F--fuse   U--unite

Table III

X-RAY PLATES FOR BONE DEVELOPMENT
ENGELBACH AND McMAHON

Yrs.		Yrs.	
1-5	(1) Full figure, divided on two plates (2) Hands and feet, taken separately (3) Lateral knee for patella	14	Plates listed under ages 13 and 15
		15	(1) Clavicle (2) Scapula (3) Pelvis (half) (4) Lateral foot (5) Hand (6) Lateral elbow
6	(1) Carpals and tarsals (2) Shoulder (3) Pelvis		
7	(1) Pelvis (2) Carpals	16	Elbow (lateral) (Anteroposterior)
8	(1) Carpals (2) Lateral foot	17	Pelvis
9	(1) Carpals (2) Lateral foot	18	(1) Carpals (2) Tarsals (3) Shoulder (4) Pelvis, with hip joint (5) Ankle (anteroposterior)
10	(1) Elbow (lateral) (anteroposterior) (2) Lateral foot		
11	Plates listed under ages 10 and 12	19	Plates listed under ages 18 and 20
12	(1) Elbow (lateral) (anteroposterior) (2) Carpals	20	(1) Carpals, with wrist (2) Knee (anteroposterior) (3) Ankle (anteroposterior)
13	(1) Hip, with half pelvis (2) Anteroposterior elbow	To 25	(1) Clavicle (2) Scapula (3) Pelvis (4) Knee

--From Wm. Engelbach and Alphonse
McMahon (Bull. Assoc. for Study of
Inter. Secretions, Vol. VIII, No. 1,
p. 1045, Jan. 1924)

Table III. For the guidance of the physician in investigation of endocrine disturbance as shown by epiphyseal development, the accompanying table showing parts for examination at different age periods as outlined by Engelbach and McMahon, may be found helpful.

A--appear   F--fuse   U--unite

ENDOCRINE INFLUENCE
on
EPIPHYSEAL DEVELOPMENT

Undoubtedly the time of appearance and union of the various epiphyses is influenced by the endocrine secretions.

The thyroid and anterior lobe of the pituitary are the structures most prominently concerned. According to Zuck's (T.T., J. Pediat., 3:424, 1933) observations, "the thyroid is dominant in growth promotion and anterior lobe of the hypophysis in maturation."

Recent investigation would indicate that the hypophyseal secretion contains many hormones. Experimental work on hypophysectomized puppies has shown that by withholding only the growth hormone (administering all other pituitary secretions), growth of the puppy can be inhibited for years. He will not only fail to grow in size but will still maintain his puppy characteristics, silky hair, awkward incoordination of movements, playful manner, etc. It would seem then, that, at least to some extent, physical growth goes hand in hand with maturation whether the growth hormone of the anterior lobe of the pituitary acts directly or thru its effect on thyroid secretion or whether the thyroid acts upon the pituitary it is difficult to say. At any rate, such puppies did not show other manifestations of thyroid deficiency.

Roentgenographic examination of the various ossification centers should therefore be a key for the detection of possible endocrine disturbances. The time of appearance of the epiphyses is subject to some variation even in normal individuals; there may even be variation in the time of epiphyseal appearance in various regions in the same individual.

At birth, all of the membranous bones are well formed and the shafts of all of the long bones are well ossified. Secondary centers of ossification are present for the head of the tibia and usually for the lower end of the femur; that for the head of the humerus soon appears, usually by the fifth or sixth month, followed soon after, usually the second year by the center for the capitellum. A center of ossification for the capitate carpal bone is the first to appear in the wrist; roughly speaking this is followed for the next seven years by the appearance of one additional ossification center for each year of life in the carpal bones; the pisiform is last to appear— nine to eleven years.

Epiphyseal centers for the metacarpal bones and phalanges of the hand appear in the second and third years. Centers for the proximal phalanges are first to appear, followed almost simultaneously by ossification centers for the corresponding heads of the metacarpals. In the foot the ossification center for the cuboid is present at birth and those for the calcaneus and talus appear at the sixth and seventh months.

In appraising the stage of development of infants and young children then, the bones of the hand and wrist, and the cuboid, calcaneus, and talus of the foot are the most useful.

Todd maintains that epiphyseal development is subject to such great changes due to faulty nutritional states that it can only be relied upon for approximate estimation of maturation. While his method of estimation takes cognizance of epiphyseal development, it is not based primarily upon these structures. Instead, his "Atlas is devoted to stages of maturity decipherable in subepiphyseal surfaces and on the bony contour of ossifying epiphyses." To this end he has formulated "maturation determinators of the skeleton" consisting mainly of contours and characteristics of bone structures of the diaphyseal ends of bones before epiphyseal centers have developed. He utilizes the hand and wrist alone in assaying the stage of bone maturation and his atlas covers growth from three months of age to maturity. Accurate reading of the roentgenograms requires precise observation and practice.

Care must be taken not to mistake incomplete pseudoepiphyseal structures as true epiphyses; they probably represent faulty developmental structures of no pathological significance, (Editorial, Am. J. R. and Ra. Th. 70:149, 1953).

Studies have been made in which, comparison of the actual age in years with the bone age as indicated by skeletal development, was used as a basis for prediction of the ultimate height of the individual at full maturity. Such prediction curves presuppose the continued existence of the same condition which gave rise to increased or decreased velocity of growth in the first place. They are most useful in individuals who show rapid bone growth from endocrine dysfunction.

From Surgical Treatment of the Motor-Skeletal System by F.W. Bancroft and Clay Ray Murray. J.B. Lippincott Co., with permission of authors and publisher:

"It is generally agreed that the femur achieves approximately 3/4 of its growth from the distal metaphysis, and the tibia and fibula approximately 3/5 of their growth from the proximal metaphysis, and that almost 70 per cent of the growth of the lower extremity takes place at the distal femoral and proximal tibial and fibular metaphyses. Therefore, any attempt to arrest growth in the lower extremity will usually be directed at these areas. White has stated that 1/4 to 3/8 of an inch shortening per year during growth will ensue following a destruction of the lower femoral epiphyseal cartilage plate, and that if the upper tibial and fibular epiphyseal plates are similarly destroyed, twice that amount of shortening may be expected.

"The most significant study of this subject of growth of the femur and tibia has been completed by Gill, G.K. and Abbott, L.C. They have removed the computation of bone growth from the realm of guessing to what appears to be scientific accuracy. In a recent presentation, as yet unpublished, "A Practical Method for the Prediction of the Growth of the Femur and Tibia in the Individual Child," these authors have made, I believe, a very significant contribution to the subject of growth arrest. With their permission the method is presented in abstract form:

DETERMINATION OF EXPECTED GROWTH OF NORMAL FEMUR AND TIBIA:

I. Essential Data Required:
  A. Age of Child in years and months.
  B. Skeletal Maturation Age, which may be determined by comparison of antero-posterior x-ray of the hand with the standards in Todd's Atlas for the hand. (Todd, T.W.: Atlas of Skeletal Maturation (Hand), St. Louis, C.V. Mosby Co.)

The skeletal maturation age may also be determined from the knee, but, unfortunately, Todd's standards for the knee are not printed in Atlas form. For this reason it is simpler to determine the skeletal maturation age from the hand.
  C. Total Height. This measurement is taken with the patient standing on a normal leg. Blocks are placed under the short leg until the pelvis is level. The buttocks, shoulders, and head should touch the wall.

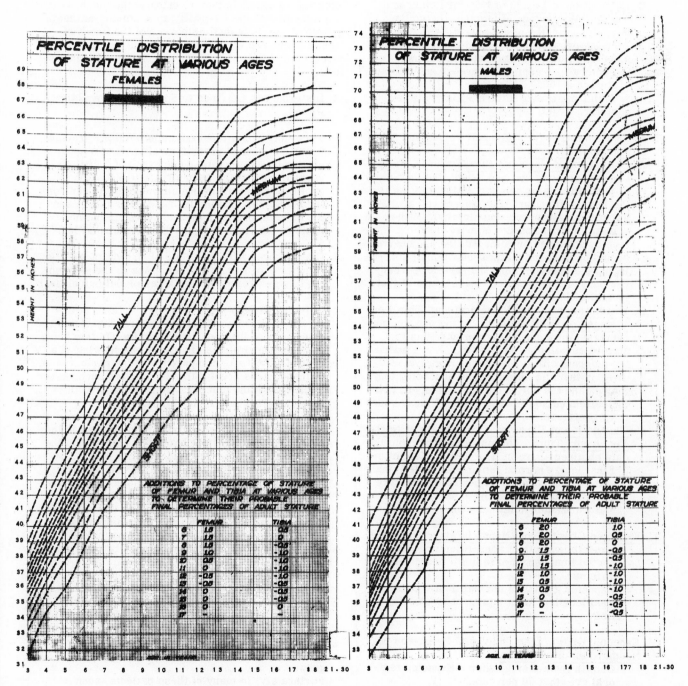

-from GILL, G.K. and ABBOTT, L.C. Arch. Surg. 45:286, 1942, with permission of authors.

D. Lengths of Femur and Tibia. This is to be determined from x-rays of the femur and tibia taken at a distance of six feet, the tube to be centered in the approximate middle of each bone*. From these films the measurements are made as follows:

FEMUR - straight line from tip of femoral head to medial lip of internal femoral condyle at joint line.

TIBIA - straight line from medial lip of internal tibial condyle at the joint line to tip of internal malleolus.

E. Calculation of Length of Normal Femur and Tibia as Percentage of Stature. From the height and lengths of the normal femur and tibia the present femoral and tibial percentages of stature are calculated as follows:

Femoral per cent of stature = Length femur/ stature x 100.

Tibial per cent of stature = Length tibia/ stature x 100.

II. Estimation of Length of Normal Femur and Tibia at Completed Growth.

A. Estimation of Expected Final Stature. From the sex, present age, and height, the individual is placed in his or her percentile position in the Percentile Chart (Fig. 257, Surgical Treatment, Brancroft and Murray). If the skeletal maturation age is more than six months advanced or retarded, the age charted should be the bone maturation age. By following up the chart between the parallel percentile curves, the expected final stature of that individual is obtained.

B. Estimation of Normal Femoral and Tibia Percentages of Adult Stature. To the present percentages of the normal femur and tibia to stature as calculated above in I, E are added the amounts either positive or negative as given in the adjoining subtable according to the sex and the corrected age. This will give the estimated adult percentages of these bones to final stature.

C. Calculation of Expected Final Length of Normal Femur and Tibia. This is calculated from the data obtained above in II, A and B as follows:

Final length normal femur = Expected final stature x adult femoral per cent of stature.

Final length normal tibia = Expected final stature x adult tibial per cent of stature.

III. Expected Growth from Normal Femur and Tibia.

Expected growth of normal femur = Expected final length of femur - present length of femur.

Expected growth of normal tibia = Expected final length of tibia - present length of tibia.

IV. Expected Growth from Individual Epiphyses of Normal Femur and Tibia.

Growth from distal femur = Expected femoral growth x 70 per cent.

Growth from proximal tibia = Expected tibial growth x 55 per cent.

Growth from distal tibia = Expected tibial growth x 45 per cent.

DETERMINATION OF EXPECTED GROWTH OF ABNORMAL FEMUR AND TIBIA:

This method will give only the expected growth of the normal femur and tibia. This information will aid in determining the growth of the shorter leg if in each case a careful study is made of the mechanism of production of the inequality as it relates to the growth of the individual epiphyses of the involved limb. There are three such mechanisms. A brief discussion of the most common example of each follows.

I. Disturbances Confined to Specific Epiphyseal Plates.

This mechanism most commonly follows trauma which has caused premature closure of a specific epiphysis. As the other epiphyses of that limb usually grow at the normal rate, the loss of growth is that amount which would have been contributed by the center damaged. For this reason, the calculations may be made entirely on the basis of the expected growth of the normal leg.

II. Disturbances Affecting Rate of Growth of All Epiphyses of Limb. (This applies to the shortening of an extremity due to anterior poliomyelitis.)

This mechanism most commonly follows poliomyelitis, but may be caused by any long-standing disabling condition of the extremity. In this group the epiphyseal plates are intact but growing at a decreased rate as compared with the normal side. In these cases great difficulty is often encountered in assessing the comparative rates of growth of the normal and abnormal limbs.

In some instances this information may be obtained by placing a small vitallium marked in the shaft of the femur and tibia of the normal and the short leg. We have devised a simple method by which these may be introduced subcutaneously under local anesthesia. Teleroentgenograms are taken immediately after their implantation and then at six-month intervals. In this manner we can measure the growth from each epiphysis of both legs and can determine the comparative rates of growth. From this information the growth of the shorter leg can be calculated quite accurately. Of course, some children are seen so near the end of the growth period that no time is allowed for such studies. In these instances epiphyseal arrest may be safely performed on the basis of the normal rate of growth. Equalization will then result only to the extent to which the corresponding epiphyses of the short leg grow.

Fortunately, in many of these patients, seen at

---

*Spot scanography may also be used for accurate measurement of bone length. See "Manual of Roentgenological Technique."

the age of 11 or 12, in whom the mechanism has been acting since early childhood or infancy, only from two to three inches of shortening is present. Simple analysis of the difference in the length of the bones when compared with the probable growth since the onset of the disease, as may be determined by calculating backward with our method, will show that the actual growth rate of the abnormal leg is so close to that of the normal leg, about 85 per cent, that for all practical purposes the expected growth may be calculated on the basis of growth of the normal leg.

III. Mechanical Loss in Length. (may be associated with mechanisms 1 and 2)

In the third group are placed those cases in which all or the greater part of the inequality is due to a mechanical cause such as loss of substance, overriding, dislocation, or angulation. If study shows that the loss in length has been purely mechanical, then the rate of growth of the epiphyses is normal and the epiphyseal arrest may be carried out on the basis of the normal rate of growth. In many cases there is also a loss of growth due to one of the foregoing mechanisms. In such cases the rate of growth may be determined as above, the epiphyseal arrest performed on the basis of this rate.
The following example will serve to clarify the various steps in predicting the growth of the normal femur and tibia.

Given a girl, age 9 years

Length of femur = 14.8 inches
Height = 53 inches (I,C)
Bone maturation age 10 years (I,B)
Length of tibia = 12.5 inches (I,D)

Femoral per cent of stature = $\dfrac{14.8 \, / \, 100}{53}$ = 28 per

cent. Tibial per cent of stature = $\dfrac{12.5 \, / \, 100}{53}$ = 23.5 per cent (I,E)

The expected total stature = 64 inches (II,A)
Femoral per cent of adult stature = 28 + 0.5 = 28.5 per cent (II,B)
Tibial per cent of adult stature = 23.5 + (-1.0) = 22.5 per cent (II,B)
Final length femur = 28.5 per cent / 64 = 18.2 inches (II,C)
Final length tibia = 22.5 per cent / 64 = 14.4 inches (II,C)
Expected growth femur = 18.2 - 14.8 = 3.4 inches (III)
Expected growth tibia = 14.4 - 12.5 = 1.9 inches (III)
Growth distal femur 3.4 / 70 per cent = 2.4 inches (IV)
Growth proximal tibia = 1.9 / 55 per cent = 1.05 inches (IV)
Growth distal tibia = 1.9 / 45 per cent = 0.85 inches (IV)

Let us suppose that just before the age of eight years this child has suffered an injury which had caused premature closure of the distal epiphysis of one femur, resulting in a shortening of one inch. With no treatment, the final shortening of the femur will be 1 + 2.4 inches or 3.4 inches. Immediate fusion of the distal femoral epiphysis will prevent an increase in inequality, but leave the one-inch discrepancy. To gain complete equality of the upper tibia epiphysis could be blocked at this time. The stature would then be 64 minus 3.4, or 60.6 inches at full growth.

Again let us suppose that this child had poliomyelitis in infancy, which has resulted in 2 1/2 inches shortening of one leg. The short femur is 13.8 inches long or one inch short. The short tibia is 11 inches long, or 1 1/2 inches short. Teleroentgenographic studies with markers for a period of six months have shown that the epiphyses of the short femur were growing at 90 per cent of the rate of the normal femur, and the epiphyses of the short tibia were growing at 80 per cent of the rate of the normal tibia. From this we calculate that the short femur will grow 3.4 / 90 per cent, or 3.1 inches, to a full length of 16.9 inches. The short tibia will grow 1.9 / 80 per cent, or 1.5 inches, to a final length of 12.5 inches. The present discrepancy of 2.5 inches will increase to a final discrepancy of 3.2 inches. As the normal femur will grow 2.4 inches from the distal epiphysis, and the normal tibia will grow 0.8 inch from the distal epiphysis, immediate fusion of these epiphyses will result in equality of length at full growth.

It is also possible to perform epiphyseal arrest so that the knees will be of equal height. For instance, the present length of the normal tibia is now equal to the final expected length of the short tibia, therefore, fusion of the upper and lower tibial epiphyses will place the knees at the same height. Equalization can then be gained by arrest of the distal epiphysis of the normal femur at a later date when the length of the normal femur approaches the final expected length of 16.9 inches of the short femur. This is determined as follows: The normal femur is already 14.9 inches and should grow only 2.1 inches to attain a length of 16.9 inches. Of the 3.4 inches of expected growth of the normal femur, 30 per cent or one inch is contributed by the upper femoral epiphysis, which cannot be fused. Therefore, the growth allowed from the distal femur will be 1.1 inches. During this growth the whole femur will grow 100/70 / 1.1 or 1.6 inches, therefore, the distal epiphysis of the femur should be fused when the normal femur has grown 1.6 inches to a length of 16.4 inches.

Temporary arrest of epiphyseal growth can be obtained by bridging the epiphyseal line with metallic staples. These can be removed later if resumption of growth is desired.

Radiation of epiphyses during active growth in infants can cause marked retardation with ultimate shortening of the extremity, (C. H. Frantz). Growth disturbance appearing as late as ten years after roentgen-ray injury has been reported by A. Langenskiold.

QUESTIONS ON EPIPHYSEAL SEPARATIONS

Questions marked with a dagger deal with rare and less important conditions.

1. Are all bones preformed in cartilage or membrane? Does cartilage show in the roentgenogram? Why? Does bone? Why?

2. What is an epiphysis? Apophysis?

†3. Show by diagrams centers of ossification and epiphyseal lines of:

Upper end of humerus	Ankle joint
Elbow joint	Scapula
Wrist joint	Clavicle
Hand	Pelvis
Knee joint	

4. What is meant by an epiphyseal separation and what are its roentgenographic manifestations?

5. Show by diagram how you would proceed to replace a separated lower radial epiphysis.

†6. Locate the various epiphyses in the hand. What may be used as a key to the epiphyses in the hand?

†7. Locate the centers of ossification and epiphyses of the elbow.

†8. What unusual circumstances frequently attend separations of the epiphysis for the inner epicondyle of the humerus?

†9. Locate centers of ossification and epiphyseal lines for the bones of the shoulder joint.

†10. Locate epiphyseal lines of ossification centers in foot and ankle.

†11. What peculiarity is shown in the epiphyses at the knee?

†12. Locate epiphyses at the hip joint.

†13. Indicate the sites of epiphyseal lines in the pelvis as seen roentgenographically.

†14. Indicate epiphyseal lines of the spine as seen roentgenographically.

15. What influence does endocrine secretion have on bony development?

16. How may the proper bony development for any age be determined?

17. Discuss briefly Todd's method of determination of skeletal maturation.

18. What are growth prediction curves and under what conditions are they of value?

19. How may epiphyseal arrest be permanently secured?

20. How may temporary arrest of epiphyseal growth be established?

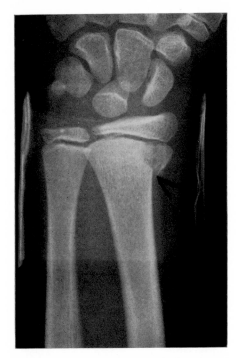

Epiphyseal separation of the lower end of the radius. Note the small fragment of the diaphysis which accompanies the epiphyseal separation.

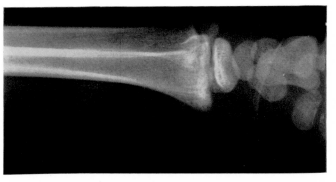

Lateral view showing dorsal displacement of the separated epiphysis of the radius.

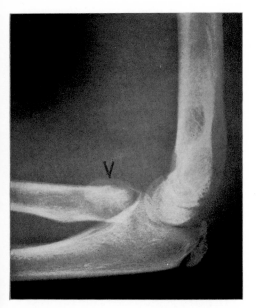

Epiphyseal separation of the head of the radius with forward and downward displacement of the epiphysis so that the articular surface looks forward.

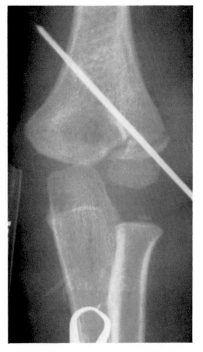

Fixation of epiphyseal fracture of outer condyle of humerus with pin.

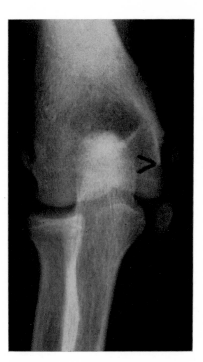

Epiphyseal separation of the epiphysis for the inner epicondyle. The epiphysis often retains its capsular attachment below, and is projected between the joint surfaces of the elbow joint causing locking of the joint and spontaneous dislocation on forcible extension.

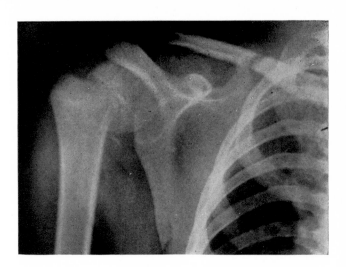

Epiphyseal separation of the head of the humerus with outward displacement of the shaft. There is no dislocation. Note the associated fracture of the clavicle.

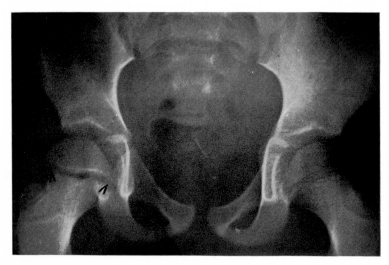

Epiphyseal separation of the head of the femur caused by trauma. The position is good.

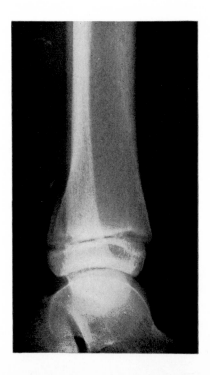

Epiphyseal separation of the lower end of the tibia with slight displacement at the epiphyseal line.

Chapter IV

OTHER EFFECTS OF TRAUMA

Trauma undoubtedly plays a part in the production of other conditions besides actual fracture or dislocation of the bones. Such changes in bony structure seem to be brought about mainly through injury to, 1) the blood supply, 2) the nerve supply, or 3) the adjacent soft part structures.

Effect of Injury to the Blood Supply. Trauma may be insufficient to produce an actual fracture and yet may, especially if repeated many times in the same manner, be sufficient to result in disturbance of the blood supply to the bony structure at some vulnerable part. If the blood supply affected is for the cancellous structure of bone, slow disintegration takes place; roentgenographic examination immediately after injury may show normal bone texture, only after a considerable period of time does the normal bone architecture disintegrate and the bony structure collapse. After a time revascularization takes place and repair is brought about by fibrous tissue replacement of the dead bone, organization and new bone. This is referred to as a process of "creeping replacement" (D.B. Phemister). Sometimes the repair impulse does not continue long enough for complete repair and necrotic areas may remain. If the blood supply that is interfered with is from a small end artery in the subchondral region of a joint, a tiny infarction occurs, depriving a small fragment of the articular cortex of its nutrition. If the blood vessels which are interfered with supply the metaphyseal region of a growing epiphysis, softening occurs and, if the epiphysis is under stress or strain, detachment and slipping of the epiphysis may occur.

Injury to the Blood Supply of Cancellous Bone Examples are:
1) Traumatic Osteitis of the Carpal Bones-- Kienböck's Disease
2) Cystic Degeneration of Scaphoid (Navicular) Bone
3) Spondylitis Traumatica Tarda—Kümmell's Disease
4) Burns
5) After X-Ray Therapy.

The method by which trauma results in these changes is not always entirely clear nor is the traumatic etiology of all the conditions which we will consider under this heading conceded by everyone, but the general consensus of opinion is that trauma is a definite factor in their production.

TRAUMATIC OSTEITIS OF CARPAL BONES-- KIENBÖCK'S DISEASE* (Fig. 60A). Traumatic osteitis of carpal bones is a condition affecting principally the semilunar (lunate) and scaphoid (navicular) bones.

When the condition involves the semilunar, it is known as Kienböck's Disease; when it involves the scaphoid, it is known as Preiser's Disease. The pathologic process, however, is probably similar in both bones. It occurs most frequently in young males, between twenty and thirty years of age.

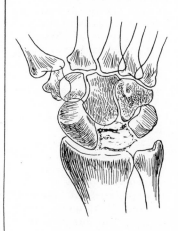

Fig. 60A

The cause of the condition is most frequently ascribed to injury, either a single severe trauma or to repeated less severe injuries, such as striking with the butt of the hand in some manufacturing process.

The ensuing effects are probably the result of interference with the normal blood supply of the bone, not the immediate result of injury. The bone loses its normal shape, becomes irregular in outline and denser in appearance. There is no evidence of infection, merely a condensation of the bone. At times there may be associated cystic degeneration.

Santozki and Kopelmann recognize four stages based on roentgenological and histological findings:
1. roentgenologically normal; histo-pathologically primary subchondral bone necrosis;
2. roentgenologically thickening and rarefaction of the bony structure with maintenance of normal form (no fracture) and occasional sequestrum formation; histopathologically fractures of the necrosed bone trabeculae with intact bony shaft;
3. roentgenologically bone deformity with uneven structure, zones of increased and decreased opacity, and pathological fracture; histo-pathologically layers of granulation tissue with osteoclasts and osteoblasts around the necrotic bone foci, fibrotic bone marrow (resorption of the necrotic bone substance and new bone formation);
4. roentgenologically reappearance of the normal structure leading to complete restitution but with marked deformities; later of the arthritis deformans type; histo-pathologically, restoration of the bone (formation of spongiosa trabeculae with calcium deposits) and changes of the cartilage resulting in arthritis deformans.

Roentgenographically, comparison with the bones of the uninvolved wrist reveals the extent to which the involved bone has been flattened in size and disturbed in contour and density.

---

*An asterisk following any title indicates that roentgenographic reproductions illustrating this condition will be found in the pictorial supplement at the end of the chapter.

Clinically there is pain on motion and swelling over the involved area. The disease is chronically disabling and the bone may have to be removed; even operation may not remove the disability.

SPONDYLITIS TRAUMATICA TARDA (KÜMMELL'S DISEASE) (Fig. 60B). Spondylitis traumatica tarda is a condition in which at some remote period, usually months later, after relatively slight trauma, the spongy vertebral body of the vertebra disintegrates and collapses. At the time of injury there is no roentgenographic evidence of disease and the patient may have no immediate symptoms. Later with collapse of the body of the vertebra, symptoms develop. The posterior portion of the vertebral body is protected from collapse by the stronger more compact articular processes, so that the resulting collapse of the anterior portion of the body produces a wedge-shaped deformity. It may be associated with some thinning of the interarticular disc, but this usually is not a conspicuous characteristic of the disease; this would indicate that the condition has some other etiological factor than injury to the nucleus pulposus.

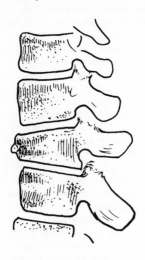

Fig. 60B

The explanation of the condition which seems most plausible is that trauma insufficient to cause actual fracture results in disturbance in the circulation leading to nutritional atrophy. There are some who feel that it may be caused by local hyperemia following traumatic injury to the autonomic nerve control of the capillaries of the bone.

Pathological studies in moderately advanced cases have revealed many small hematomas in the spongiosa of the vertebral bodies with rarefaction of bone; in well-established cases, a complete breakdown of the bony structure was noted. An instance has been reported in which the vertebral disc adjacent to the vertebra also had undergone "a similar process of nutritive starvation through traumatic obliteration of blood vessels and trophic supply."

In any event, the ultimate prognosis is favorable.

HYPEREXTENSION INJURIES TO THE CERVICAL SPINE. It is possible by sudden forcible hyperextension of the cervical spine to cause injury to the spinal cord resulting even in paraplegia and death without any manifestation of fracture or dislocation of the vertebral structures, (Crooks and Birkett). The ligamentum flavum may be torn or the disc ruptured. In a review of this subject Kaplan cites a case in which death occurred from paraplegia following such an hyperextension injury. At autopsy there was complete disintegration of the cord, but no evidence of injury to the bony structures. The findings suggested that, "one cause of the suppression of cord function in such injuries is thrombosis of the spinal arteries and liquefaction necrosis of the cord." Berkin and Hirson have reported a similar case. Taylor suggested and demonstrated that the posterior injury to the cord was caused by forward bulging of the ligamenta flava at the moment of hyperextension. Schneider et al. have illustrated the method by which central cervical spinal cord injury may be sustained from hyperextension injuries of the cervical spine. Forward bulging of the ligamentum flavum impinging on the posterior aspect of the cord at the moment of hyperextension with anterior counter pressure of hypertrophic spurs on the vertebral bodies, causes a simultaneous pinching or squeezing of the cord.

BONE CHANGES IN FROST BITE. Vinson and Schatzki found little if any bone changes in a large percentage of frost bite injuries at any time even if mummification of soft tissue had occurred. Osteoporosis was noted about the fourth to tenth week. Two months after frost bite a sequestrum may form at tip end of terminal phalanx which may separate after another month.

In some cases tiny, rounded punched out areas developed in the bone several months later and there was narrowing of the joint cartilages, similar to the lesions which occur in rheumatoid arthritis.

RADIATION OSTEITIS. Numerous instances of spontaneous fracture following prolonged radiation therapy have been encountered. Such fractures are usually manifested as fine cracks in the cancellous bone structure; they usually heal if given proper immobilization, (Slaughter).

ELECTRICAL BURNS - SEQUESTRATION. Severe electrical or thermal burns may result in complete destruction of the blood supply to a segment of bone which ultimately will result in sequestration of that part. The bone may appear perfectly normal immediately after the accident. Several weeks may elapse before the sequestrum becomes evident in the roentgenogram. This is due to disintegration of the media of the arteries, not the intima.

Grayish white, pearllike globules consisting of calcium phosphate have been found in the edges of such wounds or near the body of the individual. It has been assumed that the high temperature of the electric arc causes melting of calcium salts of the bone, (Pearl; Jellinek; Jaffe).

Injury to Blood Supply of the Subchondral Regions of Joints. Examples are:
1. Osteochondritis dissecans;
2. Osteochondritis deformans metatarsojuvenalis—Freiberg's Infraction.

OSTEOCHONDRITIS DISSECANS* (Fig. 61A). Osteochondritis dissecans is a condition occurring in adolescence or young adult life, characterized by quiet subchondral necrosis, with separation of a small triangular fragment of the articular cortex of the bone. It does not seem to be associated with pyogenic infection, but is most probably caused by interference with the blood supply to the affected area as a result of trauma. The site of most frequent

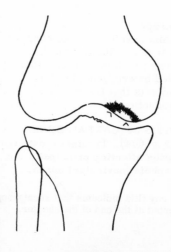

Fig. 61A

involvement is the inner condyle of the femur, although it does occur other locations, such as the head of the femur, the patella, the lower articular surface of the ankle, the head and the capitellum and supratrochlear fossa of the humerus, (Morgan). It may be bilateral and cases have been reported in which it was hereditary.

Roentgenologically the articular cortex of the involved joint shows a small roughly triangular piece of bone separated by a zone of rarefaction from the main bony structure. At the onset the fragment is held in place by the intact articular cartilage, but later on, this may also give way, and the fragment of bone may be extruded into the joint, becoming a joint mouse. If this occurs, or if the involved area is very large, surgical removal may have to be resorted to; if it is small, nature may repair the defect in the bone. Ordinarily it does not produce any marked degree of permanent disability, (Hutchinson).

DEFORMING OSTEOCHONDRITIS OF THE METATARSOPHALANGEAL JOINTS (FREIBERG'S INFRACTION)* (Fig. 61B).

Osteochondritis deformans metatarsojuvenalis is an osteochondritis of the head of the second or third metatarsal bone, occurring most frequently in adolescence but remaining throughout life. Its cause is not definitely known, but it has been most frequently ascribed to trauma applied to the head of the metatarsal bone from abnormal pressure, resulting in some interference with normal blood supply to this portion of the bone. It may be that it is akin to osteochondritis dissecans, but in this instance involves the entire articular end of the bone. It has been seen in tennis players and toe-dancers, but in the majority of instances, no such cause of unusual trauma is present.

Pathologically the process is much the same as in osteochondritis dissecans; there is quiet subchondral necrosis of the bone without evidence of pyogenic infection; ultimately the entire articular surface and head of the bone become destroyed, but there is no periosteal reaction or other manifestation of pyogenic infection. Small loose cartilaginous bodies may be present.

Roentgenographically the head of the involved metatarsal bone shows destruction, losing its normal rounded appearance and acquiring a crescentic in-

dented appearance, the margins of which correspond very closely to the normal extent of the articular cartilage. The margin of the destroyed area is rough and irregular and the end of the bone may be widened and thickened. The articular margin of the adjoining phalanx may be widened to correspond with the widened end of the metatarsal bone, but it ordinarily does not show destruction of bone. There is no periosteal new bone formation.

Clinically this abnormal condition is associated with pain and discomfort, but this is not so severe as to be totally disabling. Once present, the condition tends to persist throughout life. Operations for the removal of the articular end of the bone may be of benefit but removal of the head often only increases the disability.

PANNER'S DISEASE. A somewhat similar disease involving the second metatarao-phalangeal joint and the head of the adjacent metatarsal bone is Panner's disease. Clinically, it is insidious in its onset, begins with pain when walking, showing tenderness to pressure especially over the dorsal aspect. There is soreness on motion especially from side to side but no evidence of infection. It occurs most frequently in girls between 10 and 14 years of age but had been reported in adults.

It runs a protracted course but usually heals spontaneously after a year or so. Application of a plaster cast may be necessary to give relief from pain.

Roentgenographically, the articular surface of the head of the second metatarsal is somewhat flattened and irregular in contour with indentations but it is clearly outlined and never shows the semilunar destruction of the head of the bone seen in Freiberg's Infraction. There is irregular spotty rarefaction and in places more condensed areas; the diaphysis appears normal, the shaft seems slightly thickened. At times small ossicles may develop in the tendons or adjacent fibrous tissue. In severe cases there may be a tremendous overgrowth of the surrounding fibrous tissue and thickening of the tendon sheath. This may be so great that it may give the impression of a neoplasm; if resected it promptly recurs. Calcium salts may be laid down in this newformed fibrous tissue, but this likewise disappears as the condition gets well.

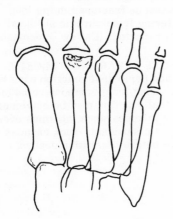

Fig. 61B

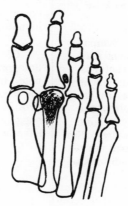

Fig. 61C

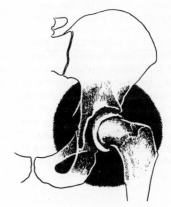

Fig. 61D

Injury to Blood Supply of Metaphyseal Region.
Examples are:
1) Femoral osteochondritis of adolescence
2) Caisson Disease

FEMORAL OSTEOCHONDRITIS OF ADOLES-
CENCE OR SLIPPING OF FEMORAL EPIPHYSIS-
EPIPHYSEOLYSIS (Fig. 61D). The most striking
example of interference with the blood supply to the
metaphyseal area is seen in spontaneous slipping of
the epiphysis for the femoral head. The weakening
brought about by the interference with proper blood
supply permits the epiphysis to slip due to the weight
of the body.

Femoral osteochondritis of adolescence or
spontaneous slipping of the epiphysis for the head of
the femur is a condition occurring in adolescence,
most frequently in males between the ages of twelve
and fifteen years of age. The cause is not definitely
known, but there is evidence to indicate that some
interference with the blood supply to the metaphysis
of the bone, due probably to trauma, may bring about
the condition. The condition is usually unilateral,
but occasionally both sides may be involved.

Clinically the initial symptom is usually limping with stiffness and pain in the joint, followed later
by shortening, limitation of motion and deformity.

Pathological manifestations are sclerosis of
the bone with thickening and oedema of the surrounding soft parts; there is no evidence of infection. The
epiphysis for the head of the bone is displaced downward in relationship to the neck as a result of the
upward pressure of the extremity.

Roentgenographically the epiphysis for the head
may take on a chalky dense appearance, much the
same as the appearance of a piece of sterile dead
bone; the head remains in the acetabulum, but the
diaphyseal fragment of the neck is displaced upward.
Even if the part is put at rest, the process once
started seems to continue to its own conclusion.
Operative replacement of the epiphysis is sometimes
successful but at others it seems to be of little benefit. Best results are obtained in cases where the
condition is discovered early before wide displacement has occurred. A lateral view of the hip may be
of value in appraising the extent of the displacement.
For early diagnosis the epiphysis for the head slips
below a line drawn along the upper edge of the neck
of the femur; normally the upper edge of the head
projects above this line, (Klein).

Effect of Injury to the Nerve Supply. Sympathetic Nerve Involvement. Nerve involvement may
account for pathological defects in bony structures.
This may be from injury to the sympathetic nerves
themselves or actual impingement of nerve trunks
against bony structures. A striking example of the
effect of interference with the nerve supply to bone
is seen in Post Traumatic Acute Bony Atrophy. (For
bone changes following injuries to the central nervous system, see chapter on Neutrophic Conditions of
Bone.)

POSTTRAUMATIC ACUTE BONE ATROPHY—
SUDECK'S ATROPHY*

Posttraumatic acute bone atrophy is a rare condition in which the bones of an extremity, often distal
to the site of trauma, undergo acute bone atrophy after
severe or even slight injury. This condition is most
frequently seen in bones of the hands and feet, but it
occasionally occurs in the diaphyses of long bones. It
may become chronic and run a protracted course.
Plewes reports an instance of about one in 2000 accidents to the hand. There is some close relationship
between Sudeck's atrophy and thickening of the
palmar fascia.

The etiology of this condition is not clear,
but it is believed by some to be due to injury to
the trophic nerves controlling the blood vessels,
thus affecting the blood supply.

Clinically the condition has its onset a few
days after trauma—even slight trauma—with pain,
tenderness and limitation of motion of the joints or
parts distal to the injury. The skin may become
shiny and thin and the joints distal to the injury
may swell and ultimately become ankylosed.

Roentgenologically the bone shows an extreme
degree of bone atrophy or osteoporosis with loss
of lime salts and penciled outline of the bone similar to but much more pronounced than bone atrophy
from disuse. In the cancellous portions of the
bones the atrophic condition assumes a spotty,
motheaten appearance. The transverse diameter
of bone may be especially diminished. There is
associated atrophy of the muscles and subcutaneous
tissue.

One sign by which this condition can be
recognized as differing from ordinary osteoporosis
or atrophy of disuse, is the early atrophy and
thinning of the articular cartilages; ordinary osteoporosis does not affect the cartilaginous structures. Likewise, the pain which is extreme in
this condition seems to become worse with immobilization, a condition contrary to what would be
expected from arthritis. Recovery has been reported following periarterial sympathectomy and
vigorous massage and manipulation, if the bone
and joint changes are not too far advanced. A
somewhat similar condition has been described
following trauma to the large joints, (Jaffe).

Multiple spontaneous fractures in the long
bones of infants suffering from chronic subdural
hematoma have been reported, (Caffey; Jungmann).

OSSEOUS CHANGES IN VARICOSE ULCER.*
Sclerosing osteitis and periosteal reaction have been
noted in patients suffering from varicose veins of
the leg. The periosteal reaction may be extremely
prolific, even shaggy in appearance, at times even
suggestive of osteogenic sarcoma. Such changes
have been noted even before ulceration occurs,
(Gilbert and Voluter).

NERVE TRUNK PRESSURE

SCALENUS ANTICUS, MUSCLE SYNDROME; SCALENUS NEUROCIRCULATORY COMPRESSION

(Fig. 62). Nerve trunks as they go through bony orifices or over bony prominences are apt to become impinged upon the bony structures. Passage of nerves through spinal foramina which have been deformed from injury or disease may give such symptoms. In certain locations the relationship of the vessels and nerves to the bony structure may give rise to the unusual symptoms.

A syndrome occurs consisting of pain along the area supplied by the brachial plexus also occasionally in the deltoid region, supraclavicular fossa, or localized to the seventh cervical spine, due to compression of the brachial plexus or subclavian artery by the scalenus anticus muscle. This muscle arises from the transverse processes of the third, fourth, fifth and sixth cervical vertebrae passing downward and somewhat laterally beneath the clavicle inserting into a tubercle on the first rib. The muscle makes an acute angle with the portion of the first rib lateral to it due to the downward slope of the rib. In patients having an anomalous cervical rib or prominent trans-

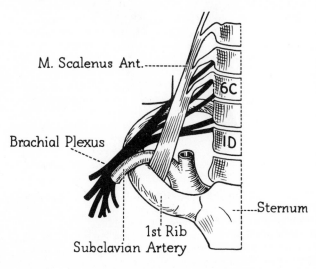

M. Scalenus Ant.

6C

ID

Brachial Plexus

Sternum

1st Rib

Subclavian Artery

Fig. 62

verse process of the seventh cervical vertebra, this angle is most pronounced. The subclavian artery and brachial plexus lie behind the scalenus anticus muscle passing over the rib along the outer margin of the muscle. Pressure of the muscle, on either the nerve plexus or the artery or both, gives rise to a characteristic syndrome.

This consists of: 1) pain over the area supplied by the brachial plexus, occasionally over the deltoid area, supraclavicular fossa or localized to the seventh cervical vertebra; 2) numbness and hyperaesthesia usually along the ulnar distribution; 3) muscular weakness; 4) the pulse may be diminished on the affected side, and, 5) there may be tenderness over the scalenus muscle.

The condition may occur as a result of muscular activity by some unusual movement of the shoul-

der; or it may occur without reference to muscular activity especially in slender-necked individuals. The explanation for the development of this condition in later life, or following extreme exhaustion, is found in the relaxation of the muscles allowing the shoulder to droop. Elevation of the shoulder and immobilization usually gives relief; otherwise surgical cutting of the scalenus anticus muscle or removal of a projecting cervical rib (Spurling and Bradford) must be resorted to.

DEFICIENCY IN BONE STRENGTH; FATIGUE FRACTURES OR MARCH FRACTURE; STRESS FRACTURE.

MARCH FRACTURE (PIED FORCE) (Fig. 63). This is a condition which involved the distal portion of the shaft of one or more metatarsal bones, although any other of the weight-bearing bones may be involved. It is characterized by a localized prolific overgrowth of periosteal new bone. Usually no history of direct trauma can be obtained and no actual line of fracture may be visible in the roentgenogram. In one instance where the involved bone resected because of suspicion of malignancy, microscopic evidence of fracture was detected. The periosteal thickening is often related to the insertion of the interosseous muscle. It is most frequently seen in soldiers, nurses and others whose duties require them to be on their feet for long periods of time.

Experiments conducted by the U.S. Army indicate that the condition becomes more prevalent as the weight of the soldier's pack is increased and his training becomes more strenuous. It is also believed from these experiments that

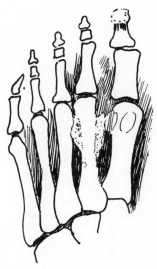

Fig. 63

such microscopic fractures occur as a result of tiring out of the muscles causing unusual strain on the ligaments which permits microscopic movement in the cancellous structures of the bone. This abnormal movement stimulates new bone formation which may appear as a linear area of bone sclerosis when the fracture involves cancellous bone, or as pronounced periosteal new bone formation if it involves the compact shaft of a bone. These fractures are therefore referred to as "fatigue fractures." They occur most frequently in the metatarsal bones, os calcis, tibia, hip, and bones of the pelvis. Recovery is prompt on relief from the abnormal activity. Similar fractures of the fibula occur in skaters (C. F. Ingersoll), and fractures of the first rib have been reported from carrying heavy weights, (barracks bag fractures).

Burrows has reported the occurrence of fatigue

infractions of this type in the middle of the tibial
shaft of ballet dancers. The chief symptom was localized pain on leaping; roentgenologically there was
a soft tissue swelling over the skin and a horizontal
fissure with infraction. Devas and Sweetnam have
reported 50 cases of stress fracture of the fibula in
athletes especially in runners, some with abrupt and
some with insidious onset. All heal after prolonged
rest.

ROENTGEN (THERAPY) FRACTURES

Somewhat similar spontaneous fractures have
resulted after prolonged roentgen therapy for other
cause. These are probably due to endarteritis which
tends to produce aseptic necrosis. In radiation
therapy of carcinoma of the cervix the dose of radiation received by the hip joint is usually below
that necessary to produce complete devitalization of
the bony structures. The subcapital zone of the femur
is rendered more susceptible to a "stress" or "insufficiency" type of fracture however. These fractures usually heal well if not displaced after a prolonged period and complete aseptic necrosis rarely
develops, (Bontiglio). Stephenson and Cohen in reviewing 21 fractures of the hip following radiation
therapy conclude that damage to the bone cells themselves must be a contributing cause since microscopic examination of the blood vessels did not seem
to show such serious damage.

Effect of Injury to the Adjacent Soft Tissue
Structures. Injury to soft tissue structures adjacent to bones and joints may result in pathology
detectable in the roentgenogram. In order for
such lesions to be detectable there must be some
change in density of the pathological area and the
surrounding soft structures. For instance, air in
the tissue, associated with compound fractures or
infection with gas-forming organisms would be
readily detectable. Gas or vacuum spaces produced
by sudden forcible separation of joint surface are
readily visualized as dark streaks within the joint
outlining its articular cartilage. Calcium deposit in
the soft tissues likewise serves to demonstrate certain pathological states within the soft tissues. Calcification in the soft tissues may result from chronic
irritation of the bursae or tendinous attachments or
from large unabsorbed hemorrhage into the interstitial or intermuscular tissue.

Gondos has suggested the term periarthritis
calcarea for what is commonly called bursitis, manifesting itself as calcium deposits in tendons, bursae,
etc. Such lesions occur in association with practically all of the joints of the body.

CALCIUM DEPOSIT IN SOFT TISSUES; LIGAMENTS, TENDONS, BURSAE AND CARTILAGE. (Fig. 64A & B).

Calcareous deposits in bursae as a result of
trauma or chronic irritation is very common. The
sites of most frequent involvement are in the sub-
deltoid bursa or as occurs more frequently in the
supraspinatus tendon near the shoulder joint (Fig.
64A), and in the prepatellar bursa in the knee (Fig.
64B). Such calcareous deposits may be due to exces-

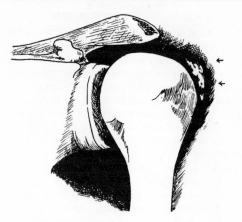

Fig. 64A

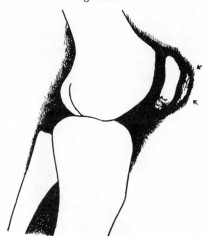

Fig. 64B

sive calcium in the synovial fluid or calcium deposit
in the tendon itself, in which case it can form very
rapidly, even within three or four days. Or it may
be a deposit in the wall of the bursa, in which case
it is a much more chronic process. Excess calcium in
the bursal fluid may give rise to the appearance in
the roentgenogram. Roentgenographically, this condition presents the appearance of a dense calcium deposit in the region of the bursa. Roentgen therapy
has proven successful in most cases, giving prompt
relief especially in very acute cases. Chronic cases
may also be favorably affected. Obstinate cases may
require surgery. Howes and Alicandri have described
five views of the shoulder to detect such calcified deposits about the shoulder.

Whitcomb has pointed out the development of
pressure erosions from such calcified deposits by
pressure on the bone.

Tearing of ligaments associated with fractures
or dislocations may lead to excessive calcification.

Prominent locations in which this occurs is in
acromio-clavicular separation and in tearing of the
interosseous ligament of the forearm.

Excessive pressure upon a ligament or bursa
over bony prominence by a cast, if continued for a
long period of time, may result in calcification in the
ligament or bursa.

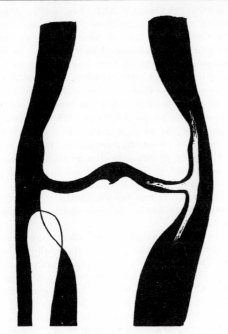

Fig. 64C

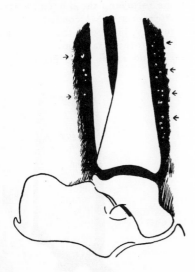

Fig. 64D

Calcification of the intervertebral discs in children has been observed (Peacher and Storrs) possibly as a result of infection or trauma, with subsequent absorption even after a three year period.

MILK DRINKER'S SYNDROME

Extreme calcinosis with large amounts of calcium deposited in the soft tissues of the body, occurring in individuals who for some reason have been required to drink large quantities of milk such as in the treatment of peptic ulcer, in the presence of renal insufficiency constitute "milk-drinker's syndrome." Pointed out first by Burnett, et al. as a syndrome following the prolonged intake of milk and alkali, it is evident that the essential diagnostic findings are calcinosis with large calcium deposits throughout the soft parts, in an individual with renal insufficiency. Poppel et al. have reported two additional cases with striking findings.

Dworetsky has reported the complete disappearance of the calcium deposit after restriction of the intake of milk.

Calcification of interarticular fibrocartilage especially of the knee (Fig. 64C) is not an uncommon finding with few if any symptoms. Calcified deposit in hyalin articular cartilage is a rather rare occurrence. Bunje and Cole have reported such a case with multiple joint involvement with mild arthritic symptoms but nothing to indicate its etiology.

TRAUMATIC CALCIFICATION OF COLLATERAL TIBIAL LIGAMENT OF THE KNEE--PELLIGRINI-STIEDA'S DISEASE (Fig. 64C). As its name implies, this is a calcium deposit in the collateral tibial ligament or bursa which follows trauma. It may result from pressure of a cast. At the onset the injury may not seem very severe, but the patient complains of pain, in spite of negative roentgen findings. Several weeks or months later, calcium deposits in the soft tissues overlying the medial condyle of the femur will be seen to develop. This may be due to calcium deposit in the ligament or in the long slender bursa which is in close relationship to the ligament.

Other bursae of the knee may, likewise, show calcium deposit, (Norley and Bick).

Roentgenographically this appears as a dense calcareous band running along the inner side of the knee joint, from one-half to eight centimeters long and two or three millimeters thick, bridging across between the bones of the knee joint. Often the calcareous deposit can be seen to extend for a short distance into the interarticular cartilage at its attachment. A similar condition may occur in the Achilles tendon.

The prognosis as to ultimate complete recovery must be very guarded. It would seem that roentgen therapy might be of some avail since it is of value in the treatment of bursitis elsewhere. Too early surgical interference may result in recalcification.

Heat and diathermy rarely restore proper function. Since x-ray therapy is of value in bursitis elsewhere, it may be of value in this location. Surgical removal may be necessary.

Osteosis Cutis is a condition in which small rounded bone deposits develop within the skin, near tendons or joints. According to Riebel and Praver it probably represents repair of traumatic or infectious origin with calcification and subsequent heterotopic bone formation.

PHLEBOLITHS.* Calcareous deposits occur in the walls of the veins, especially where they are subjected to trauma or constant irritation. They are frequently observed as rounded white deposits in the soft tissues anterior to the tibia. They should not be confused with calcium deposits in the soft tissues from other causes.

EHLERS-DANLOS SYNDROME (Fig. 64D). Numerous rounded shotlike nodules, showing calcium incrustation resembling phleboliths occurring in the subcutaneous tissues of the extremities have been described as part of Ehlers-Danlos Syndrome, (J.F. Holt). Microscopically, they appear to be degenerated fat globules encrusted with calcium salts. The other factors constituting the syndrome are:

1. hyperplasticity of the skin
2. fragility of the skin and blood vessels
3. hypermobility of the joints
4. pseudotumors over the bony prominence.

It is probably due to a developmental anomaly since it is frequently associated with other variations. They differ in appearance from phleboliths in that they have a clear center appearing ringlike in place of solid structures. Katz and Steiner have emphasized the microscopic appearance by special staining methods to show hypertrophic elasticity of the tissues. They have called attention to large masses of ectopic bone which occasionally develop in muscles about the hip; which occur in paroplegia.

A classical case has been reported by Katz and Steiner in which there were large masses of mature bone in the lower extremities, especially in the hip muscles.

CALCIFIED HEMATOMA* (Fig. 64E). A large hematoma of the soft parts may not absorb but may undergo calcification. In order for blood to undergo calcification in the tissues it seems that it must be in interstitial or intermuscular tissue.

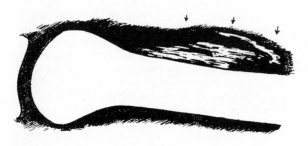

Fig. 64E

The irregular blood clot undergoes calcification or even ossification instead of absorption and becomes visible in the roentgenogram. Because calcium deposit is present does not mean that the condition is permanent; many cases have been observed in which such calcium deposits, if treated early, disappear upon application of heat. Otherwise surgical removal may be necessary. Too early surgical removal may result in recurrence. Such calcified deposits are within the interstitial tissues and cannot be considered as true examples of myositis ossificans.

A condition known as Werner's Syndrome has been described in which widespread calcium deposits occur in the soft tissues, tendons, ligaments and bursae. There is associated arteriosclerosis of all arteries, with exception of cerebral vessels involving the media of the vessel, (Herstone and Bower). Subperiosteal extravasation of blood, especially in the region of the pericranium, cepholhematoma results in a rounded elevation which may within a few weeks present a circular calcium incrustation visible in the roentgenogram.

MYOSITIS OSSIFICANS (Fig. 64F). Myositis Ossificans is a condition in which calcification occurs in the striated muscles. It usually follows trauma resulting in intermuscular hemorrhage. In place of physiological absorption with restoration of function, the blood undergoes calcification and ossification, resulting in replacement of the muscle with bone causing more or less impairment of function, depending upon the degree of involvement. The brachialis anticus muscle in the arm, and the vasti muscles of the thigh are most frequently involved. It may occur to a marked degree in hemiplegics or in paralytics from spinal cord injury. It may be hereditary and progressive, involving all of the muscular structures of the body; the cause is not known, (Miller and O'Neill). An unusual case has been described by Singleton and Holt.

Roentgenologically, the calcareous deposits may be recognized arranging themselves along the muscle fibers. The calcification does not extend into the tendon, consequently in the roentgenogram a space free from calcification can be seen in the immediate vicinity of the bony attachment. In this regard, it differs from ordinary exostosis formation which springs from the bone, and grows outward into the soft tissue as a result of chronic irritation or infection. The linear striations following the muscular structure will usually differentiate this condition from sarcoma of bone. Frequently, however, the bone may not be laid down in such orderly fashion. Once deposited in muscle it rarely undergoes resorption.

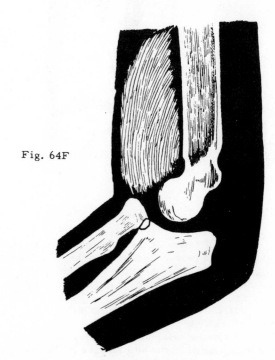

Fig. 64F

GAS OR VACUUM SPACES WITHIN JOINTS; (Phantom Nucleus Pulposus) (Gershon-Cohen, et al.) (Fig. 64H). Gas or vacuum spaces may occur within the joints as a result of forcible separation of the joint surfaces. This produces dark streaks of decreased density outlining the cartilaginous margins of the joint which are readily visualized (Fig. 64G). It has been suggested that the phenomenon is probably due to, "gas from surrounding fluids which have been vaporized as the result of a partial vacuum," (Marr).

The development of the same phenomenon at the symphysis pubis in women with relaxation of this joint from pregnancy (Camiel and Aaron) suggests that the loss of normal tight maintenance of the joint surfaces may be a decisive factor in development of the condition.

The fact that this may be produced at will, by forcibly stretching, in many of the less stable joints of the body such as the knee and shoulder, would indicate that it probably does not in itself depend upon any pathological state for its development. This method is used for roentgenological demonstration of the interarticular cartilages of the knee (see Manual of Roentgenological Technique).

A similar appearance occurs, however, in the intervertebral joints of the spine without manipulation or injury, unassociated with herniation of the disc which would indicate that some other mechanism may be present. Raines suggests that "the radiolucencies are due to disc degeneration which produces a cracking or fissuring of the disc substances."

CAISSON DISEASE - BONE MANIFESTATIONS, (Fig. 64I). Gases go into solution in ever-increasing amounts as the gas pressure is increased; if the gas pressure is then released the supercharged solution will rapidly give off its excess charge of gas in the form of bubbles. A common example of this reaction is seen in the bubbles of gas which form in soda water when the cap of the bottle is removed. Similarly, in individuals who work under increased air pressure such as divers, the blood becomes supercharged with air. If the individual is transferred too quickly to ordinary atmospheric pressure, the excess air in the blood will form bubbles of gas free in the circulating blood. It has long been known that such individuals experience severe pains and muscular contractions known as the "bends."

The cause of the "bends" has been shown to be due to air emboli in the vessels in and about the joints. Aseptic infarcts of this type occur in the bone marrow. These are not detectable at the time but later heal with calcification showing in the roentgenogram as irregular calcium deposits within the medullary canal.

Roentgenographically, in the acute stage, these bubbles of air can be demonstrated in the periarticular regions as radiotransparent areas. They may be demonstrable only for a short time but when they first occur they can be readily recognized.

It seems that fatty tissue is most likely to be attacked and undergo necrosis from such emboli possibly because of its greater absorbability of nitrogen. The mechanism by which the bone changes

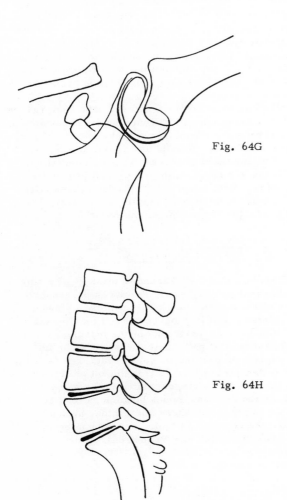

Fig. 64G

Fig. 64H

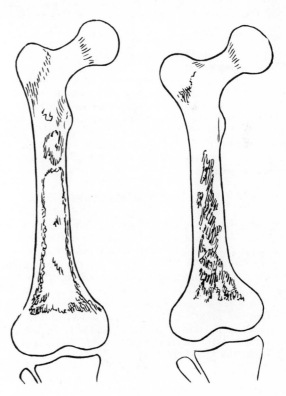

Fig. 64I

found in the roentgenogram are produced is not fully understood in so far as experimental air embolism is not followed by such changes. Perhaps pressure from gas liberated within the medullary canal may play a part in the death of the bone marrow. At any rate large areas of aseptic marrow necrosis may result. These may not be demonstrable at the time but later the necrotic tissue is replaced by irregular calcification within the medullary canal which is readily demonstrable in the roentgenogram. Calcification occurs at first at the edges of the area of fat necrosis but as time goes on the entire area may be replaced by an irregular area of calcium deposit. Similar changes may be seen about the joints with areas of aseptic necrosis, fibrocystic changes and exostosis formation. Oddly enough, many instances have been reported of similar bone changes in individuals who have never been subjected to air pressure. These probably represent marrow infarction from other causes. Experimental infarction of bone in animals produces similar results (Foster).

A similar appearing lesion has been reported in which microscopic examination revealed, "bone and cartilage imbedded in blood clot. The bone trabeculae were in general well preserved. Only small areas of cartilage appeared normal; the rest showed degenerative changes of varying degree, and small areas of calcification," (Laurence and Franklin). No mention was made of infarction and there was no history of trauma.

Strangely enough, small infarcted areas near the joint margins may give rise to cystlike areas of destruction resembling malum coxae senilis. This is probably one of the most common manifestations of Caisson Disease.

It is believed by some that small calcified islands of cancellous bone may be due to small bone infarcts during development, (Steel).

Poppel and Robinson point out that the lesions encountered in Caisson Disease may at least at the onstart be more like snow caps in the bony structures over the ends of the bone before destruction has taken place. The location of the lesions are most frequently in the humerus in the head and about the knee. Infarcts in the medullary canal may not be detectable for several months.

BAKER'S CYST OF THE KNEE (Fig. 64J).
This is a herniation of the capsule of the knee joint posteriorly into the popliteal space. It presents a palpable tumor mass which is attached to the capsule of the joint and can be clearly demonstrated by removal of fluid and injection of air into the knee joint. It probably is originally caused by trauma. Complete resection and repair is essential for cure.

The knee joint is subject to many variations in its extent and location. A large plica may divide the suprapatellar portion of the joint, and it is possible for similar cystic swellings to occur in many locations about the joint, (Pipkin).

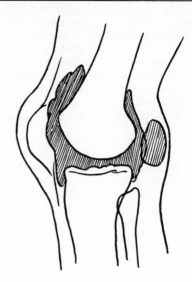

Fig. 64J

SKELETAL TRAUMA IN INFANTS

Attention has been called to the amazing roentgen manifestations of unrecognized skeletal trauma in infants, (Silverman). For the most part, these represent calcification of hemorrhage from ligamentous and periosteal tears resulting usually from strain on various joints. They may not be immediately detectable, but within a short time calcification begins to take place.

Multiple spontaneous fractures have been reported in association with chronic subdural hematoma.

Fat pads are normally present about the elbow, over the olecranon, coronoid and radial fossae, which serve to buffer these processes in their normal motion. These are most commonly viewed best in the lateral view. With effusion into the joint these fatty deposits will be displaced dossally or ventrally depending upon the degree of distension, (Norell).

ROENTGEN MANIFESTATIONS OF MUSCULAR DYSTROPHY

This is a disease of unknown etiology affecting the myoneural junction which results in progressive wasting of the musculature. It is usually a disease of early childhood and is progressive. It may be associated with pseudohypertrophy of the muscles.

The essential pathological change is due to gross replacement of the muscle by fat. The fat being of lesser density appears as translucent shadows within the muscle fascia, deposited in the same direction as the muscle. Bones become as long as usual but suffer in thickness and contour because they lack the stimulus in their growth by normal muscle pull, (Lewitan and Nathanson).

LIPOHEMOARTHROSIS (Fig. 64K). This is a condition in which the fat pads of a joint are ruptured as a result of fracture into the joint. Oil is liberated by the fatty tissue which, being lighter than blood and other fluid in the joint, layers itself on top. Roentgenograms made in the lateral view with horizontal projection of the X-ray beam will demonstrate this apparent fluid level.

Injuries to other soft part structures may be recognized by the effect which they produce on adjacent bony parts; displacement of the intervertebral disc may result in its protrusion into the spinal canal producing pressure symptoms.

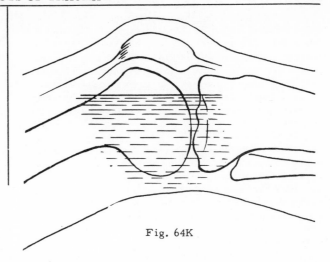

Fig. 64K

QUESTIONS ON OTHER EFFECTS OF TRAUMA

Questions marked with a dagger deal with rare and less important conditions.

†1. What is Kümmell's disease and describe its X-ray appearance?

2. What is Kienböck's disease and what is its etiology?

3. Describe briefly the structure of the Intervertebral Disc and the X-ray findings resulting from its displacement.

4. How may protrusion of the intervertebral disc into the spinal canal be detected?

5. What is Osteochondritis Dissecans and how is it manifested in the roentgenogram? In what location is it most frequently found?

6. What are the X-ray manifestations of Osteochondritis Deformans Metatarsojuvenilis (Freiberg's Infraction) and to what is it due?

†7. What is meant by Femoral Osteochondritis of Adolescence or Slipping Femoral Epiphysis and what is its cause? At what age does it usually occur?

8. What is the etiology of Pelligrini-Stieda's Disease?

†9. What is Sudeck's posttraumatic atrophy and to what is it due?

†10. What is meant by the condition known as Multiple Spontaneous Idiopathic Symmetrical Fractures and to what is it attributable?

†11. What are the clinical and roentgenological manifestations of March Fracture? What evidence is there to indicate that it is of traumatic origin?

12. Describe roentgen findings in myositis ossificans and how may it be differentiated from exostosis formation?

13. Under what conditions do calcified deposits appear in the soft tissues?

†14. What bone lesions are found in Caisson disease, in the acute and in the chronic stages and to what are they due? Aseptic infarcts?

15. What structures are involved in Baker's cyst and how may the diagnosis be established roentgenologically?

16. What is lipohemoarthrosis and how may it be detected?

17. How may vacuum or gas shadows be produced in joints and to what are they due?

Chapter V

ANALYSIS OF BONE PATHOLOGY

In considering the roentgenographic evidence of disease, one must be impressed from the outstart that roentgenological diagnosis is made, not upon any hit-or-miss basis, from recollection of some similar appearing roentgenogram seen at some previous time, but only after systematic analysis of the manifestations of disease found on careful examination. Various diseases by virtue of specific chemical action of their toxins, produce varying reactions in the normal elements of bone structure. Certain added physiological processes, such as bone atrophy, serve also to complicate the picture.

On account of this response of various elements of bone structure to different disease processes it has become possible to formulate a systematic scheme of analysis to assist in their diagnosis.

One must bear in mind that roentgen diagnosis consists of:

(1) detection of pathology in the roentgenogram,

(2) its proper evaluation,

(3) correlation of the roentgen manifestations with other elements of the history and clinical findings, and,

(4) an exercise of judgment as to the greatest degree of probability under the circumstances.

The detection of pathology in a roentgenogram presupposes a thorough and complete acquaintance with the normal; the evaluation of the nature of the pathologic process, once detected, requires a full knowledge of the modes of response of various structures to disease; correlation of the roentgen manifestations with the history and clinical findings demands a broad knowledge of the symptomatology of disease and finally the exercise of judgment as to the greatest degree of probability under the circumstances requires analytical consideration which develops as experience is acquired.

Radiographic detection of any changes in bone depends upon variation in the contour or density of its structure. These may be due to decreased density of the bone as in physiologic bone atrophy or pathologic bone destruction, or they may be due to increase in density due to bone production. It is upon these principles that the entire system of bone analysis is based.

POINTS IN THE ANALYSIS OF BONE LESIONS

A. Point of Origin
B. Bone Production or Destruction
C. Expansion or Non-Expansion
D. Condition of the Cortex
E. Invasion or Non-Invasion
F. Bone Atrophy

A. <u>Point of Origin</u>. By point of origin is meant the actual point from which the pathology arises in the bone. There are five possible points of origin of a disease process in the long bones:

1. Periosteum—example, periosteal sarcoma.

2. Cortex—example, osteoma.

3. Medullary canal (central or endosteal)—example, osteomyelitis.

4. Epiphysis—example, tuberculosis.

5. Articular surface--example, pyogenic arthritis.

B. <u>Bone Production or Destruction</u>. By bone production we mean evidence of activity of bone-forming elements. Since the periosteum is the chief bone-forming structure, any evidence of periosteal reaction must be considered as evidence of new bone formation. Three main types of periosteal reaction are recognized, (Fig. 65A):

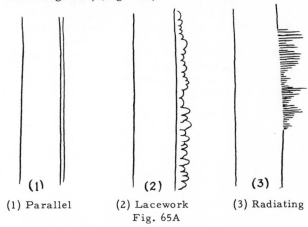

(1) Parallel   (2) Lacework   (3) Radiating
Fig. 65A

1. The parallel type in which the periosteal new bone is laid down in parallel layers along the shaft of the bone; this occurs as a result of trauma, pyogenic infection or lues; a similar appearance is sometimes encountered, especially in premature or new born infants where the shafts of the long bones may have a "duplicated" appearance due to incomplete ossification, which gives the impression of an active periosteal reaction.

2. The lacework type, in which small lines of periosteal new bone radiate outward from the shaft, looping back to form irregular rounded bumps on the bone; this may be considered as almost characteristic of syphilis. A somewhat similar lacework type of periostitis occurs in hypertrophic osteoarthropathy from anoxia, and occasionally in association with pyogenic osteomyelitis. Any irritation of the periosteum in syphilitic patients, be it from trauma, pyogenic infection or other cause, may initiate the lacework type of reaction.

3. The radiating type, in which fine spicules of bone radiate outward perpendicular to the shaft, like a sunburst, ending free on the soft tissues; this is almost always indication of a malignant tumor. Very rarely a similar radiating appearance may occur during healing of a fracture; or a shaggy appearance of periosteal reaction may accompany varicose leg ulcer due to chronic passive congestion or pressure on bone of a soft tissue mass such as an aneurysm.

Another form of bone production is bone sclerosis indicated in the roentgenogram by a thickening of the cortical bone and a condensation of its structure.

This occurs most frequently as a result of syphilitic osteitis, or long-standing pyogenic infection. Destruction of a joint cartilage allowing direct apposition of bony surfaces results in dense sclerosis or "eburnation" of the bone.

By bone destruction we mean actual destruction of the bone cells, resulting in a defect in the bony structure. An example of a disease in which bone destruction alone plays a prominent part is tuberculosis. An example of a disease in which bone production is most evident is syphilis. One in which both destruction and production are going on at the same time is osteomyelitis.

C. Expansion or Nonexpansion. By expansion is meant the symmetrical enlargement of the shaft of a bone as the result of a central new growth (Fig. 65B). It is always indication of a slow-growing tumor of central origin such as a bone cyst. Mere local bulging on one side of the shaft does not constitute true expansion; it may be described as local enlargement.

An example of such asymmetrical bulging is the cyst-like structures seen within the cortex of long bones in fibrous dysplasia.

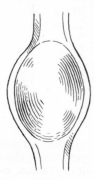 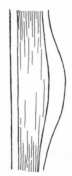

Expansion   Not True Expansion
Fig. 65B

D. Condition of the Cortex. The cortex may be thickened from proliferation of cortical bone, as in syphilitic osteitis; or it may be thinned as a result of pressure atrophy, from a central new growth. It may remain intact, as it usually does in benign lesions, or it may be broken through early in the course of the disease as it usually is in malignant conditions. Not all diseases which break through the cortex are malignant; osteomyelitis, for instance, shows erosion through the cortex to permit egress of pus from the medullary canal; in this instance, however, the cortex is broken through in many places, leaving good bone structure in between. Malignant tumors, on the other hand, never do this; they invade and destroy by a multiplication of cells along an unbroken front, sweeping the cortex before them.

Is the bone straight or deformed? Certain diseases, by weakening the bony structures, result in bowing of the bones, with thickening of the cortex on the convex side and thinning on the concave side. In generalized Osteitis Fibrosa Cystica (Von Reckinghausen) and in Polyostotic Fibrous Dysplasia a gnarled appearance of the bony outline develops from the bulging of cyst-like areas throughout the bone.

E. Invasion or Noninvasion. By invasion is meant the extension of a new growth originating in bone out into the surrounding soft tissues. If the growth originates within the medullary canal, invasion presupposes the rupture of the cortex; if it originates in the periosteum, invasion may occur directly without disturbance of the cortical structure.

F. Bone Atrophy, (Osteoporosis; halisteresis). This is a normal physiological process, which results from disuse of any bone, either voluntary, from immobilization of a part, or enforced from pain due to some disease process.

According to prevailing opinion bone tissue normally undergoes a continuous process of bone destruction and repair. Large osteoclastic cells are continuously engaged in destruction of bone cells and osteoblasts continuously repair the damage. The purpose of this seemingly futile process is however, very logical on more mature consideration. According to Wolff's Law, bone trabeculae develop the greatest strength along the lines of greatest stress and strain. As an individual grows his changing configuration and posture develop changes in the stress and strain put upon the bone. Increase in strain stimulates osteoblastic activity, while decrease in strain favors increase in activity of the osteoclastic cells. So in this manner the osteoclastic cells are encouraged to remove the useless bony structures and osteoblasts are stimulated to replace them with stronger bone in the regions in which greater strength is required. It is by this process of bone destruction, where the bone is not needed, and bone production where it is necessary for repair that fractured fragments are again brought into line and satisfactory function redeveloped. The influence of the endocrine secretions on calcium metabolism and osteoporosis is seen in menopausal and senile osteoporosis.

The blood supply is an important element in maintaining this function. Normal bone structure is rich in calcium salts, 58% as calcium phosphate, and 7% calcium carbonate. These calcium salts are present as an intercellular deposit, within their cell structure.

Opinion is still divided as to the exact means by which calcium salts reach the bone and are deposited in its cellular structures; it is quite probable, however, that they are carried by the blood in the form of soluble phosphates which are precipitated in insoluble form by some action of the bone cells. Of one thing, however, we are quite sure, that there is continuous calcium metabolism, both constitutional and local, with constantly changing calcium deposit in bones. The constitutional calcium metabolism is probably regulated by activity of the endocrines, principally the parathyroid glands; evidence of this is seen in tumors of the parathyroid where hypersecretion of these glands is associated with an extreme degree of loss of calcium salts of all of the bones of the body. Loss of calcium salts under these conditions constitutes a definite pathological process. The calcium metabolism of any particular extremity is vitally dependent upon the degree of activity of the extremity and upon an intact blood supply. If an extremity of a normal individual is immobilized on a splint for six to eight weeks, it will be found on roentgenological examination that the bones have lost much of their calcium salts; this physiological process is known as atrophy of disuse.

Authorities maintain that the decrease in density suffered by bone on disuse is due to an actual suspension of the normal reparative process of the bone which is stimulated by activity, thus permitting the natural destructive process to predominate. They have found that the actual calcium content per bone cell is the same as in normal cells—only the cells are fewer in number.

Roentgenographically in bone atrophy the bony structure loses its normal density, becoming darker in appearance and acquiring a penciled outline. The trabecular structure of the bone can still be made

Summary of Chemical Findings in Neoplastic Diseases of the Bone
Woodward, Arch. Surg. 47:368, 1943.

Disease	Serum Acid Phosphatase	Serum Alkaline Phosphatase	Serum Phosphorus	Total Serum Calcium	Sulkowitch Reaction Urine	Urine Bence Jones Protein	Total Serum Protein
Chondroma, Osteochondroma osteoma, exostosis	. . . . . .	Normal	Normal	Normal	. . . . . .	. . . . . .	. . . . . .
Solitary bone cyst	. . . . . .	Normal	Normal	Normal	. . . . . .	. . . . . .	. . . . . .
Giant cell tumor	Normal	Normal, slightly raised	Normal	Normal	. . . . . .	. . . . . .	. . . . . .
Osteogenic sarcoma	Normal	Usually high	Normal	Normal	. . . . . .	. . . . . .	. . . . . .
Endothelioma of bone	. . . . . .	Normal, slightly raised	Normal	Normal	. . . . . .	. . . . . .	. . . . . .
Reticulum cell lymphosarcoma of bone	. . . . . .	Normal, slightly raised	Normal	Normal	. . . . . .	. . . . . .	. . . . . .
Rickets	. . . . . .	High	Normal or low	Normal or low	. . . . . .	. . . . . .	. . . . . .
Inflammatory disease of bone	. . . . . .	Usually normal	Normal	Normal	. . . . . .	. . . . . .	. . . . . .
Osteolytic metastic disease	Normal	Normal, moderately high	Normal or High	Normal or High	Pronounced	Negative	Normal
Osteoplastic metastatic not from prostate	Normal	High	Normal	Normal	Normal	Negative	Normal
Carcinoma prostate metastatic to bone	High in 70%	High	Normal	Normal	Normal	Negative	Normal
Plasma cell myeloma	Normal	Normal slightly raised	Normal or High	Normal or High	. . . . . .	Positive in 60%	Normal to very high
Senile osteoporosis	Normal	Normal	Normal	Normal	Normal	. . . . . .	Normal
Hyperparathyroidism	. . . . . .	High	Low	High	Pronounced	. . . . . .	. . . . . .
Osteitis deformans	Normal	High	Normal	Normal	Normal	. . . . . .	Normal
Osteomalacia	Normal	Moderately raised	Normal or low	Usually low	Usually slight	. . . . . .	Normal or low

It will be noted that in general all benign tumors of bone show normal values; malignant or potentially malignant bone growths show normal or slightly raised serum alkaline phosphatase with other determinations normal.

Osteolyticbone metastases show high blood calcium and phosphorus determinations, a condition which is shared only with plasma cell myeloma, (certain urinary findings serve to differentiate these two conditions).

Osteoblastic bone metastases all show high serum alkaline phosphatase but that those originating from carcinoma of the prostate have in addition high acid phosphatase (a distinguishing characteristic in the differential diagnosis of this condition if it is present).

In nutritional diseases such as rickets, the alkaline phosphatase is high; while hyperparathyroidism is practically the only condition in which there is a consistent change in the calcium-phosphorus ratio.

Further consideration of the blood chemistry values in various bone diseases is given by E. B. Flink.

In hypoparathyroidism the chemical findings are practically the reverse of hyperparathyroidism.

out, in fact it may be accentuated in appearance. In other words, the bone cells themselves are still quite intact; they have not been destroyed, and all that is required for restoration of calcium salts and return to a normal state is the resumption of function of the part. This is known as bone atrophy of quality or osteoporosis; it is a physiological process and not a pathologic state. Such reaction is dependent upon an intact, unobstructed circulation.

Loss of 30% of the calcium is necessary before atrophy is evident roentgenologically.

Atrophy of quantity is the expression used to indicate a reduction in the size of any bone or portion thereof, as compared to its fellow of the opposite side. Such a condition is seen following infantile paralysis. It develops usually from the lack of stimulation of normal muscular activity.

Pressure atrophy of bone is seen where tumors of the soft parts cause undue pressure on normal bone structure; for example, pressure of an aneurysm or tumor against the spine will in short time cause a pressure defect with erosion and destruction of the bony structures. Pressure from an aneurysm of the interosseous artery in the forearm or popliteal in the knee will produce gross erosion of the knee. Herniation of the nucleus pulposus producing undue pressure of the herniated nucleus on the vertebral bodies will cause a rounded pressure defect on the adjacent margin of the vertebra; excessive pressure of the brain substance against the inner wall of the cranium, from chronic increased intracranial pressure associated with brain tumor, will give rise to an accentuation of the convolutional markings on the skull, known as convolutional atrophy. Pressure from soft part tumor, such as synovioma or reticulum cell sarcoma, will produce pressure defects on bone. This may be due in part to stasis of venous flow since anything which causes stasis may result in periosteal spicule formation. Due consideration must be given to these physiological conditions in any analysis of bone pathology.

Correlation of the roentgen with the clinical and laboratory findings is essential.

CLINICAL HISTORY. The clinical history may be of utmost importance and may prove the deciding factor in the diagnosis.

The age of the patient may be of importance, since certain diseases predominate in certain age periods.

Congenital conditions are, of course, manifested at birth or shortly thereafter, when restriction of proper function draws attention to the abnormal development.

Certain diseases are apt to occur in certain age periods; from birth to three years of age, rickets, scurvy and congenital syphilis are the most common diseases of bone.

Acute pyogenic epiphysitis and epiphysitis of the nonsuppurating variety occur during the growth period of the various epiphyses. With normal fusion of the epiphyses these conditions disappear.

Between five and fifteen years of age, tuberculosis and osteomyelitic infection are most common; while both diseases do occur in adult life, they are most commonly encountered during this age period.

Bone tumors of congenital origin may not manifest themselves until many years after birth when by their growth they cause limitation of function; this is naturally a variable period dependent upon the size and character of the growth. Bone cysts are most common in early life—under twenty-one years of age—probably because they tend to heal spontaneously thereafter. Giant-cell tumor on the other hand is most apt to occur in adults. Sarcoma of bone may occur at any time, but secondary carcinoma is a disease predominating in adult life.

Pyogenic infective arthritis can occur during any period. Arthritis of the atrophic type is a disease most frequently encountered in early adult life, while hypertrophic arthritis is common to the later years of life, past forty.

Likewise, sex may be of importance since certain diseases are more apt to occur in one sex than the other; for instance, in females carcinomatous bony metastases are more apt to be of the osteoclastic type, whereas in males the osteoblastic type predominates.

The past history may provide the clue to a satisfactory understanding of the case; osteomyelitis or some other bone disease in childhood may explain the appearance of the bone in adult life.

The history of the present illness is above all the most important. Was there a history of trauma? If so was there indication of a pathological process before the trauma? A fracture of a bone resulting from trauma may be due to a weakened condition from a previous disease process such as a bone tumor.

What was the duration of the illness? On this point alone may depend the differential diagnosis; for example, certain stages of tuberculous epiphysitis closely resemble epiphysitis from pyogenic origin; only a knowledge of the duration of the illness would serve to differentiate the conditions.

Is there fever or other manifestation of infection? This may serve to differentiate between infection and other processes such as bone tumor.

Finally, due consideration of laboratory findings, such as urinalysis, bacterial examination, blood counts, and blood chemistry, must be considered (see table on preceding page).

QUESTIONS ON BONE ANALYSIS

1. What method of analysis would you use in the determination of the character of a bone lesion?

2. Of what advantage is the clinical history in the differential diagnosis of bone diseases?

3. What is meant by:

> Point of Origin,
> Production or Destruction,
> Expansion or Nonexpansion,
> Condition of the Cortex,
> Invasion or Noninvasion,
> Bone Atrophy?

4. What types of atrophy of bone are recognized and give their roentgen characteristics? What is atrophy of quality? of quantity? pressure atrophy?

5. What is meant by osteoporosis and what is the physiological explanation of its development?

6. In what disease is blood chemistry of special advantage in differential diagnosis?

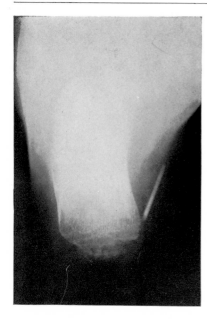
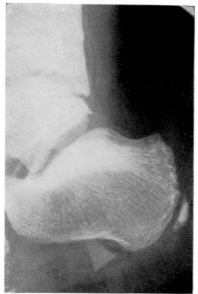

← Triangular fragment of glass seen in the soft tissues of the heel. Glass shows in the radiograph in direct proportion to the mineral content.

Knife blade protruding into the skull; in place for several years. Metallic objects cast dense shadows in the radiograph. →

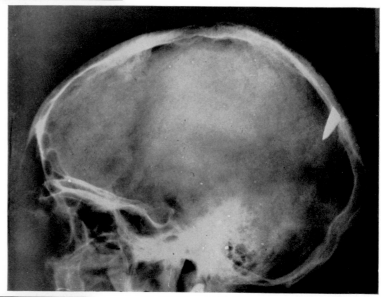

Lateral view of the skull showing a large defect in the parietal bone following previous operative procedure.
↓

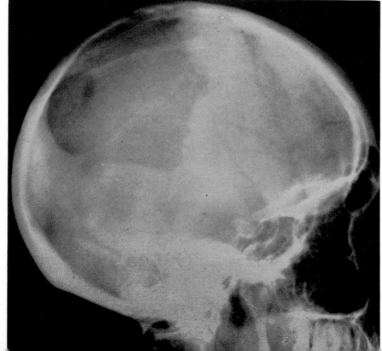

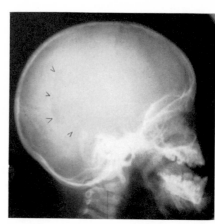

Pressure erosion of traumatic intra-cranial cyst which developed several months after injury to skull without evident fracture,—courtesy Dr. E. C. Funsch.

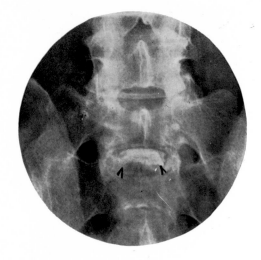

← Antero-posterior view of the lumbo-sacral joint showing calcification of the nucleus pulposus in this region.

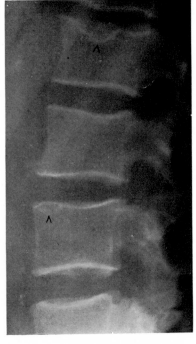

Areas of semilunar deformity at the vertebral margins due to pressure absorption from herniation of the nucleus pulposus. →

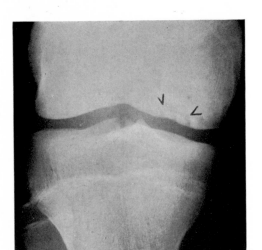

Osteochondritis dissecans, showing a small fragment of the articular cortex of the lower end of the femur separated by aseptic necrosis probably due to trauma, a condition which usually involves the inner condyle.

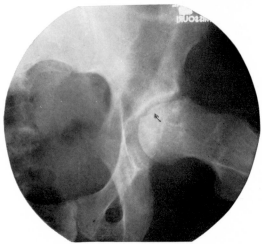

Osteochondritis of hip showing fragment off superior articular cortex of femoral head.

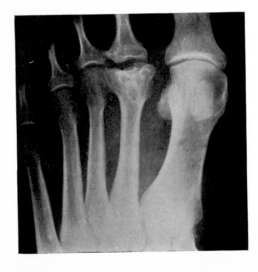

← Freiberg's Infraction of the head of the second metatarsal, probably due to aseptic necrosis from long continued trauma.

Kienböck's disease showing irregular destruction of the lunate, probably the result of disturbance in the blood supply to the bone from trauma. →

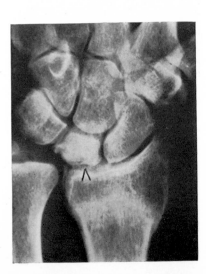

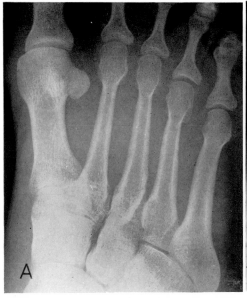 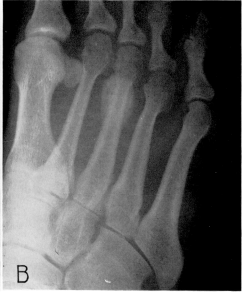 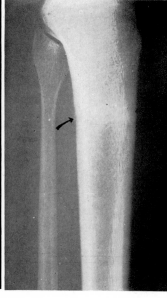

MARCH FRACTURE. Excessive strain from tiring of muscles by unusual activity such as forced marches under heavy loads, causes spontaneous fracture from disintegration of bone structure.

A. At time patient first complained of pain no fracture could be seen.

B. One month later definite overgrowth of new bone is seen on the middle metatarsal from constant irritation of the insidious fracture.

MARCH FRACTURE OF THE TIBIA after prolonged strenuous maneuvers.

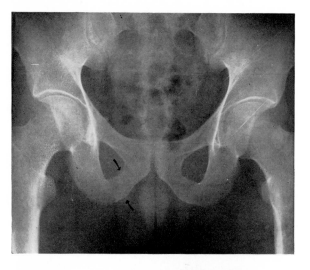

March Fracture of the pelvis. Note fracture of pubic bone.

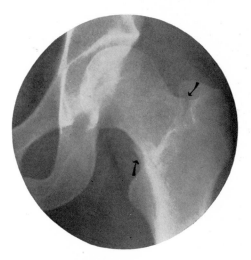

MARCH FRACTURE OF THE HIP

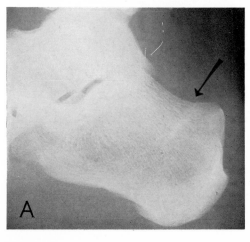 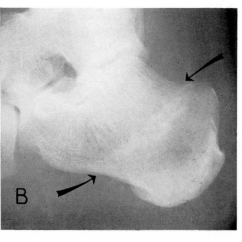

←

MARCH FRACTURE OF THE CALCANEUS.

Such fractures seem to occur most frequently at the site of greatest strain.

A. Slight condensation of the bone structure at site of fracture.

B. Eighteen days later.

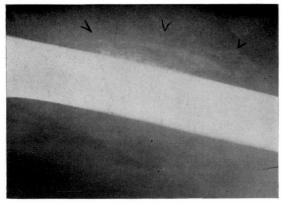

Irregular area of calcification in the soft tissues on the anterior aspect of the femur due to calcifying hematoma.

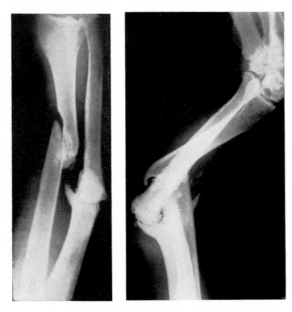

PSEUDARTHROSIS, or false joint following ununited fractures of both bones of the forearm.

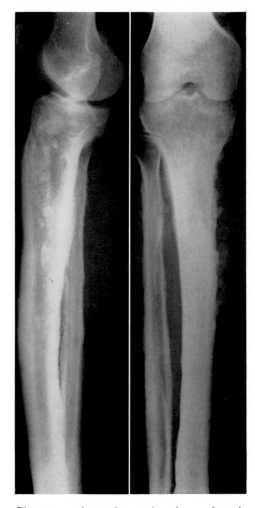

Shaggy periosteal reaction from chronic irritation and passive congestion of varicose leg ulcer.

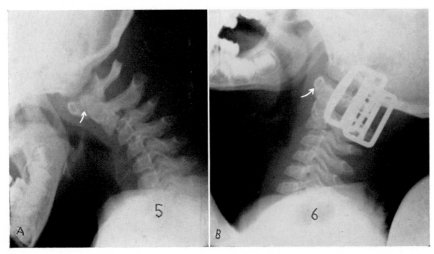

Spontaneous forward luxation of 1st on 2d cervical vertebra from relaxation of supporting ligament due to infection. A. Head held in extreme flexion, note separation of odontoid process from articulation with ring of 2d. B. Head held in full extension by traction; joint space closed.

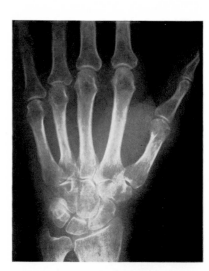

SUDECK'S ATROPHY. A condition in which extreme bone atrophy follows trivial trauma.

DISEASES OF BONE

(and adjacent soft parts)

NUTRITIONAL DISEASES (Chapter VI)

A. Regional, Aseptic Necrosis of Epiphysis; (affecting bone structure, only in isolated locations; these may be influenced by glandular or metabolic malfunction).

  1. Osteochondritis deformans juvenalis; aseptic necrosis of epiphysis epiphysis.

   (a) Femoral head—LEGG-CALVÉ-PERTHES' DISEASE

   (b) Acetabulum—Intrapelvic protrusion—(OTTO PELVIS)

   (c) Tibial tubercle—(OSGOOD-SCHLATTER'S DISEASE)
       Medial tibial condyle—(BLOUNT'S DISEASE)

   (d) Patella—primary center (KÖHLER'S SECOND DISEASE)—
       secondary center (SINDING-LARSEN'S DISEASE)

   (e) Tarsal Scaphoid—(KÖHLER'S DISEASE)

   (f) Calcaneal Epiphysis—(SEVER'S DISEASE)

   (g) Osteochondritis of secondary epiphyseal centers of Spine—
       subchondral necrosis of vertebral bodies—(SCHEUERMANN'S
       DISEASE). VERTEBRA PLANA—(CALVÉ).

   (h) Sacrum—epiphysitis of wing of sacrum

   (i) Other rarer locations of osteochondritis of the epiphyses

  2. Multiple Epiphyseal Dysplasia

B. Constitutional;

From deficiency in diet

  1. Rickets—infantile, foetal and late

  2. Osteomalacia

  3. Scurvy (BARLOW'S DISEASE)

  4. Calcinosis Interstitialis

From excess in diet

  1. Hypervitaminosis A

  2. Hypervitaminosis D.

Chapter VI

NUTRITIONAL DISEASES OF BONE

A. REGIONAL NUTRITIONAL DISTURBANCE; OSTEOCHONDRITIS DEFORMANS JUVENALIS; ASEPTIC NECROSIS OF EPIPHYSIS

During the stage of active growth, usually during the adolescent period, certain changes may appear within the epiphyseal structures of the body, the exact cause of which is not fully understood. The initial lesion is due to avascularization of the epiphyseal structure, resulting in a localized nutritional disturbance. The epiphysis becomes softened and undergoes quiet necrosis. Fragmentation and disintegration of the epiphysis may occur, but bacterial infection with suppuration does not result. The condition may not progress beyond the point of softening of the epiphyseal structure. A similar process sometimes involves ossification centers of tarsal bones. In general it may be said that during the first decade the primary ossification centers are involved and during the second decade the secondary centers are affected. Different changes occur in epiphyses in various locations depending upon the peculiarities of function of the various regions involved.

The common sites of aseptic necrosis are:

1. Epiphysis for femoral head (Legg-Calvé-Perthes' Disease)

2. Acetabulum, resulting in intrapelvic protrusion of the acetabulum (Otto Pelvis)

3. Tibial tubercle (Osgood-Schlatter's Disease)

4. Tarsal Scaphoid (Navicular) (Köhler's Disease)

5. Calcaneal Epiphysis (Sever's Disease)

6. Osteochondritis of spine—subchondral necrosis of epiphyses for vertebral bodies—(Scheuermann's Disease)

7. Sacrum—Osteochondritis of epiphyses for wing of sacrum near sacroiliac joints.

The exact cause of this phenomenon is not fully understood; the underlying pathology represents a local nutritional disturbance of the epiphysis, interfering with its normal development from disturbance of its blood supply. The fundamental pathological process is the same in all locations in which it is found in the body; the findings are modified in various locations, depending upon the stresses and strains upon the particular epiphyseal structure involved.

Roentgenological investigations made by P. G. K. Bentzon on the epiphysis of freshly amputated limbs after injection with cinnabon and red lead disclosed that in the epiphyses most frequently involved the location of the arteries was such that they could easily be traumatized. He found that, "arteries to the epiphyseal nuclei must pass through or along the epiphyseal cartilage first. From the radio-clinical observations compared with the results of anatomical studies and experiments on animals, it lies nearest to conclude that the lesion to the wall of the artery does not result in the closing of the vessel, but in an interruption of the vasomotoric nerves in the adventitia, with a consequent condition of arterial hyperemia and that it is a condition connected with this arterial hyperemia of the osseous tissue that causes the reaction to set in."

Certain published cases of occurrence of the condition in individuals who had received large doses of thyroid extract over a considerable period of time lend support to the possibility of endocrine influence in the development of the condition. However, Brailsford doubts the influence of endocrine disturbance as an etiological factor.

It will be noted that this condition is confined largely to epiphyses of the spine and lower extremities; only isolated instances have been reported of involvement of the epiphyses of the upper extremities and elsewhere; in these there is almost always some question of associated trauma. Likewise, even in the epiphyses most frequently involved of the lower extremities it is only those in which there is some unusual strain on the epiphyseal line either by reason of angular attachment of the epiphysis, or by strong muscular pull that the condition develops. The epiphysis for the head of the femur, for instance, attaches obliquely to the shaft so that the epiphyseal attachment is strained by the transmission of the body weight to the shaft. It probably requires the added stress and strain of weight bearing or heavy muscular pull for the ultimate interference with the blood supply leading to disturbance in local nutrition. At the knee, for instance, it is not the lower femoral epiphysis or the upper tibial epiphysis in which this condition develops, but in the epiphyseal prolongation for the tibial tubercle, a location which is subjected to strong muscular pull from the quadruceps muscle. Likewise, the lower tibial epiphysis which transmits the body weight directly does not become involved whereas the epiphysis for the calcaneus, which is subjected to heavy muscular pull, from the Tendo Achilles, develops the disease. The tarsal scaphoid, the keystone for the arch of the foot, is likewise subjected to indirect strain. It would seem therefore that the subjection of the epiphyseal line to unusual strain must play a definite part in its final necrosis and destruction through damage to the nutrient arteries and interference with local nutrition.

Whatever the immediate cause may be, there is always found on microscopic examination a disturbance in chondral ossification with aseptic necrosis of the epiphysis. At a later stage the necrotic tissue is broken down and replaced by new-formed osteoid bone. The microscopic picture is one which would be expected with disturbance of the local nutrition from interference with the blood supply.

In the active stage it responds to protective treatment; only rarely does it persist into adult life causing failure of union of the epiphysis.

OSTEOCHONDRITIS OF EPIPHYSIS FOR FEMORAL HEAD (LEGG-CALVÉ-PERTHES' DISEASE)* (Fig. 66). When the condition involves the epiphysis for the head of the femur, it is known as Legg-Calvé-Perthes' Disease.

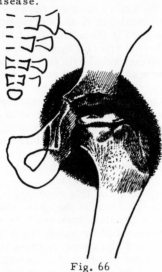

Fig. 66

Clinically the disease is manifested by pain in the region of the hip, limitation of motion, muscle spasm and rigidity--all symptoms common to beginning tuberculosis of the hip. The first roentgen manifestation of epiphysitis is flattening of the top of the femoral head, (coxa plana). This is followed by widening of the epiphyseal structure and broadening of the neck of the bone. The epiphyseal line becomes more horizontal. The articular cartilage is preserved and the acetabulum is not involved. The process is not in any sense an arthritis nor do joint complications ever arise. At the onset the joint cartilage may even appear to be widened. Due to the weight-bearing function of the hip, fragmentation of the epiphysis may result if the patient is allowed to continue to use the part.

The changes are probably initiated by the interruption of epiphyseal nutrition after which the epiphysis undergoes varying degrees of necrosis. The blood supply of the epiphysis is derived mainly from the periosteum of the diaphysis. Almost complete disintegration and fragmentation of the epiphysis may occur, but the articular cartilage remains intact, probably deriving its nourishment from the synovial membrane.

Attention has been called to an hereditary factor in Perthe's Disease by observation of 54 cases in one family, (Jequier and Fredenhagen).

Roentgenographically, in the very early stage, changes may not be demonstrable. After the condition is fully established, there is:

1. Avascularization of the epiphyseal structure manifested by a chalky appearance of the epiphysis, which becomes discernible as osteoporosis, develops in the remainder of the bony structures.

2. Softening of the epiphysis, with flattening of the head due to pressure from weight-bearing, with consequent widening of the femoral neck.

3. Fragmentation of the epiphysis and cystlike degeneration of the subepiphyseal structures.

4. Later, revascularization takes place with gradual loss of chalky appearance and resumption of normal bone architecture.

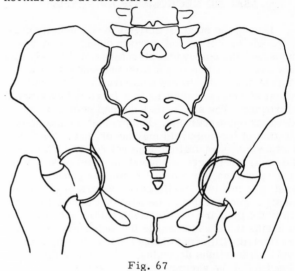

Fig. 67

5. The joint cartilage is always preserved.

6. The process never extends across the joint space to involve the acetabulum.

Hyperplasia of the involved side of the pelvis has been observed by Martin.

If function is eliminated, the patient can be assured of ultimate recovery without ankylosis, much shortening or material loss of function. In this region involvement is frequently bilateral. After recovery epiphyseal growth continues in a normal manner and shortening never takes place, if proper treatment is instituted early in the disease. Delayed epiphyseal union may occur at the site of any of the epiphyseal structures. Holsti has reported involvement at the ischiopubic junction. Occurrence in this location is difficult to explain, except on the basis of associated trauma. He has pointed out that it is impossible to differentiate this condition from physiologically irregular mineralization upon the roentgen findings alone.

INTRAPELVIC PROTRUSION OF THE ACETABULUM; OSTEOCHONDRITIS JUVENALIS ACETABULI; JUVENILE OSTEO-ASTHENIC PROTRUSION.* (Fig. 67). Intrapelvic protrusion of the acetabulum is a condition in which, by reason of a softening of the bony structure of the acetabulum or some other pathological process, the femoral heads cause an intrapelvic protrusion of these structures. Not unless the floor of the socket crosses or touches the linea

*An asterisk following any title indicates that roentgenographic reproductions illustrating this condition will be found in the pictorial supplement at the end of the chapter.

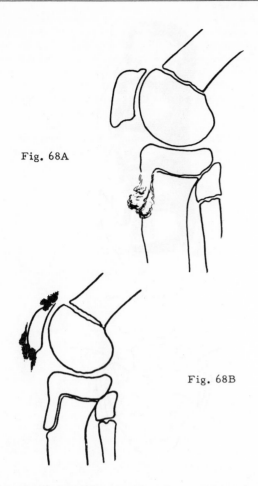

Fig. 68A

Fig. 68B

terminalis can it be considered a condition of this type. It is almost always bilateral showing in the roentgenogram as rounded protrusions encroaching upon the pelvic cavity.

Kristiaan Overgaard has listed three groups:

1. Secondary protrusion following a focal disease process having a definite history of previous illness or trauma.

2. Primary osteoarthritic protrusion, arthritis deformans where the osteophytes build a shelf about the head of the femur producing a ball and socket joint and even cause a hole in the center of the acetabulum.

3. Juvenile osteo-asthenic protrusion due to weakness of the bone tissue. (See p. 206.)

It seems highly probable that at least in one form this condition may result from epiphysitis of the "Y"-shaped epiphyseal lines of the acetabulum due to a process essentially similar to the other epiphyseal lesions here described. Depending upon the degree of intrusion, there is more or less limitation of abduction at the hip joint. In adult female patients, extreme deformity may result in possible difficult delivery during subsequent pregnancy. It is twice as frequent in women as in men.

OSTEOCHONDRITIS OF EPIPHYSIS FOR TIBIAL TUBERCLE (Osgood-Schlatter's Disease)* (Fig. 68A). The epiphysis for the upper end of the tibia dips down in a tonguelike process to take in the epiphysis for the

tubercle of the tibia. When the tubercle of the tibia is involved by this epiphyseal disease, it becomes softened and is easily detached by the pull of the patellar tendon for which it serves as attachment. This condition is known as Osgood-Schlatter's Disease.

Clinically the condition is usually not suspected until, from some slight trauma, the epiphysis for the tubercle pulls away from the upper end of the tibia, the patella rising to a high position. This results in inability to extend the leg at the knee. The condition is usually bilateral. Fixation in intended position results in recovery and complete restoration of function.

Osteochondritis confined to the region of the medial tibial condyle has been reported, giving rise to nonrachitic bow legs, BLOUNT'S DISEASE (see anomalies).

OSTEOCHONDRITIS OF OSSIFICATION CENTERS OF PATELLA. Osteochondritis of the primary ossification center has been reported by Köhler.

Occasionally the patella may have additional secondary centers of ossification. These occur most frequently on the lateral side giving rise to longitudinal division of the patella; they may appear however as small secondary centers at the upper or lower patellar margin. Epiphysitis of these secondary centers (Sinding-Larsen's Disease) (Fig. 68B) results in aseptic necrosis very similar to that seen involving other epiphyses in the body. It is an exceedingly rare condition however; very few cases have been reported. Spontaneous recovery results without disability as the result of rest (Wolf).

RETARDATION OF OSSEUS DEVELOPMENT OF TARSAL NAVICULAR (KÖHLER'S DISEASE)* (Fig. 69). The ossification center of the tarsal scaphoid (navicular) bone sometimes is affected by this condition, resulting in retardation of osseus development of the bone. This condition is known as Köhler's Disease. There is evidence to indicate that the retardation of development of the navicular may be due to interference with normal blood supply.

In certain instances when the foot has been put in a cast the failure of atrophy of the navicular with its resulting chalky appearance is evidence of avascularity of the bone. As revascularization takes place, the normal bone architecture is re-established and recovery occurs.

Roentgenographically the center of ossification for the tarsal scaphoid remains small and irregular in outline, much retarded in its development in comparison with the other normally developed tarsal bones. Since it may be regarded as the keystone in the development of the normal arch of the foot, it becomes very important, wherever this condition is found, to maintain the normal arch during the development period. When this is done, ultimate complete recovery should result without disability. The disease is usually bilateral and is self-limited.

Sometimes the tuberosity of the navicular may alone be involved; under these circumstances there is a separate center of ossification for the tubercle which ultimately results in an accessory anomalous bone to which is attached the tendon of the tibialis posticus muscle.

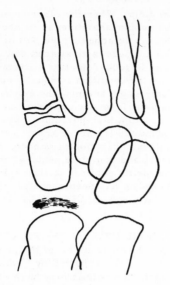

Fig. 69

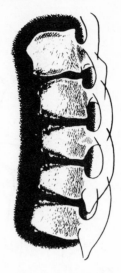

Fig. 71

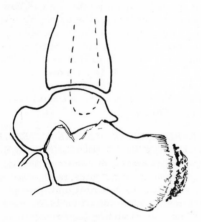

Fig. 70

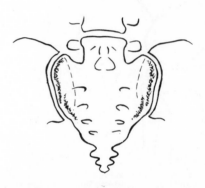

Fig. 72

OSTEOCHONDRITIS OF EPIPHYSES FOR
CALCANEUS (SEVER'S DISEASE) (Fig. 70). Osteochondritis of the epiphysis for the calcaneus is rather
rare. Roentgenographically it results in a fluffy,
worm-eaten fragmented appearance of the epiphysis,
with irregularity of the adjacent posterior portion of
the body of the bone.

OSTEOCHONDRITIS OF SECONDARY EPIPHYS-
EAL CENTERS OF SPINE--SUBCHONDRAL NECRO-
SIS (SCHEUERMANN'S DISEASE) (Fig. 71). Osteochondritis of the spine or subchondral necrosis of the
epiphyses for the vertebral bodies is a similar process occurring most commonly in the dorsal region.
In this location also it apparently is a self-limited
process. It is characterized by development of kyphosis of the spine in otherwise normal healthy adolescent children.

The tendency of children to imitate the posture
of others has been cited as a possible factor in the
development of several instances in the same family
or community, (F. H. Kemp and D. C. Wilson).

The same underlying pathological process as
seen in epiphysitis elsewhere involves the epiphyseal
rings for the margins of the vertebral bodies.

These secondary centers for the upper and
lower surfaces of the vertebral bodies are ringlike in
character skirting the margins of the vertebral bodies;
they appear normally about the twelfth year and unite
with the bodies in the early twenties. In adolescence
these may be delayed in appearing; if present they
become rarefied and irregular; these changes are
usually more marked anteriorly; wedging of the vertebral bodies may result, giving rise to kyphotic deformity. Occasionally the disease may be limited to
the vertebral rings of a few or even a single vertebra
causing malunion and persistence into adult life. It
may develop as a result of carrying heavy weights by
young individuals during this stage of development.
Recent microscopic studies have thrown some doubt
on the true epiphyseal character of these vertebral
rings. At any rate, the vertebral margins from which
the vertebral bodies grow in height behave in the
same way as epiphyseal structures.

If proper fixation and support of the spine is
instituted, complete recovery without deformity may
result, but if untreated, permanent spinal deformity
will most likely be the ultimate outcome.

Williams has made a detailed study on the differential diagnosis and sequelae of juvenile vertebral osteo-chondrosis with observations on the ultimate results of this type of involvement.

EPIPHYSITIS OF WING OF SACRUM (Fig. 72). Epiphysitis of the epiphyses for the wings of the sacrum may, on account of its close proximity to the sacroiliac joint, result in symptoms of sacro-iliac strain or arthritis of this joint. The lateral epiphyses for the wing of the sacrum are elongated structures, two on either side, running along the outer margins of the wing of the sacrum. They usually appear between the fifteenth to eighteenth year and unite in the nineteenth year or early twenties, (Cleaves).

Roentgenographically these epiphyses are rarely seen and unless they become the site of disease they may be entirely overlooked. With the development of epiphysitis, however, there is a haziness of the sacroiliac joint along the sacral margin, and an associated irregular sclerotic appearance of the adjacent bone. If much time has elapsed before the condition is detected it may be difficult to differentiate from sacro-iliac arthritis, (Cleaves). If the time of onset can be established at eighteen or nineteen years of age, this is very suggestive of sacral epiphysitis.

Proper treatment with rest and immobilization should result in recovery, but failure to provide proper treatment may result in permanent disability, owing to the close proximation of the sacro-iliac joint.

A sclerotic appearance confined to the iliac side of the sacro-iliac joint is often a forerunner of spinal arthritis or Marie-Strumpell's Disease.

OSTEITIS CONDENSANS ILII. A somewhat similar appearing lesion is seen in osteitis condensans ilii. There is a similar sclerotic appearance in the sacro-iliac regions, but this seems to be confined to the iliac side of the joint. The joint cartilage does not seem to be involved in this instance and the joint space is well preserved. It usually occurs at the lower margin of the joint and rarely shows associated arthritic changes. The symphysis may also be involved. It must always be remembered that Marie-Strumpell's disease always starts with sacro-iliac joint involvement on the iliac side of the joint. However, Marie-Strumpell's disease almost always occurs in men, and osteitis condensans ilii predominates in women; likewise, the former disease is associated with other spinal involvement, whereas the latter disease is confined to the iliac bone adjacent to the sacroiliac joint. It has been shown (Rauber-Kopsch quoted by Ude) that epiphyseal growth centers occur on the articular processes of the ilia and it would seem possible that epiphysitis in this location would offer a satisfactory explanation of this disease, (Gillespie and Lloyd-Roberts; Hutton).

Wells, after a study of 67 cases found that 80% had previous pregnancy. Since the commonest cause of low back pain in women studied was muscular imbalance occurring post partum osteitis condensans therefore occurs in a group particularly prone to low back pain for other reasons.

OTHER RARER LOCATIONS OF EPIPHYSITIS

This form of epiphyseal disease may occasionally involve many other regions in the body. Other ossification centers which have been reported as involved are:

Coracoid process of scapula, epiphysis for,
Clavicular epiphyses—(Friedrich)
Humeral head—(Lewin)
Humerus, epiphysis for capitellum—(Panner)
Radial, head—(Brailsford)
Ulnar distal epiphysis (Burns)
Ulnar proximal epiphysis for olecranon
Metacarpals, heads—(Mauclaire)
Carpal pisiform
Iliac crests—(Buchman)
Pubic Symphysis—(Van Neck)
Ischio pubic junction—(Voltancoli)
Femoral neck (Gutig and Hertzog)
Femoral trochanter—(Monde Felix)
Tibial head (Ritter)
First metatarsal, proximal (Wagner)
Patellar primary center (Köhler)
Vertebral body, Primary center (Calvé)

Astragalus (Mouchet) (Smyth)
Cuneiform, Medial (Buschke)
Sesamoid bones of great toe

Fairbank has described a condition of irregular ossification of several epiphyses which did not conform to any of the osteochondritis conditions commonly met with during the adolescent period. The epiphyses become fragmented with areas of irregular density, and consequent shortening. In the knee the femoral condyles become flattened and angular with the lateral condyle showing a shallow depression. In the shoulder the epiphysitis ultimately results in flattening of the humeral head. Whereas in the foot the phalangeal epiphyses may even exhibit small apparently loose fragments. All epiphyses ultimately unite but there may be resulting deformity.

B. Constitutional Nutritional Disturbances

RICKETS—INFANTILE * (Fig. 73). Rickets is a nutritional disturbance, due to Vitamin D deficiency, occurring chiefly in infancy during the first three years of life, characterized by profound changes in the calcium content and epiphyseal structures of the bones.

The bones are the great reservoirs for calcium. Approximately 85 to 90% of the calcium salts of bone are phosphates, which are convertible into soluble salts by the body tissues and thrown into the general circulation. When, from any cause, the concentration of soluble calcium salts in the blood diminishes, then these storehouses of calcium in the bones are drawn upon to maintain the calcium content of the bones. Vitamin D is the element which prepares the calcium salts in the diet for absorption from the intestines and maintains proper calcium concentration in the blood,

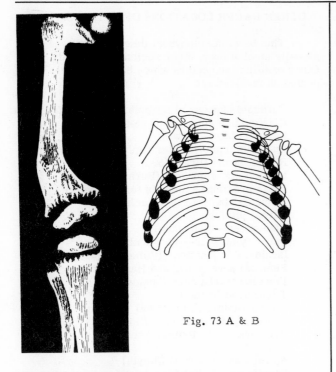

Fig. 73 A & B

adult life the zone narrows down to a white line running transversely across the bone. These dense zones of phosphosclerosis, due to arrested growth, are referred to as, "growth lines." They may be due to any severe interference with growth.

Roentgenographical analysis then of the picture of fully developed rickets shows:

1. Enlargement of the ends of long bones.
2. Rachitic rosary from involvement of costo-chondral junction of ribs.
3. Haziness and cupping of the diaphyseal ends of the bones.
4. Widening of the zone of osteoid formation between the epiphyseal center and the diaphysis.
5. Osteoporosis but no actual bone destruction.
6. Bowing of the shaft of the bone with thickening of the cortex on the concave and thinning on the convex side.
7. Occasionally spontaneous fractures may occur, but the cortex is never broken through except by trauma.
8. Periosteal proliferation is present only rarely. Serum alkaline phosphatase is high in rickets, but the serum phosphorus and calcium are low. In a rare condition known as osteoblastic dysplasia, the lesions of the long bones closely resemble rickets but the alkaline phosphatase is low, (Schlesinger, et al.).

FOETAL RICKETS. Cases have been reported in which the foetus on birth already presented the characteristic evidences of rickets. Thus it is evident that Vitamin D deficiency, if extreme, may be passed on to the foetus in utero, (Terrafranca and Zellis).

LATE RICKETS.* It has been amply proven also that rickets may again become manifest in the growing bones at a later period as a result of extreme Vitamin D deficiency. When it occurs at a later age it presents all of the epiphyseal changes and other characteristics of the infantile type. Both the foetal and late types are rarely seen in this country.

Vitamin D - Resistant Rickets. Some cases of rickets require larger doses of Vitamin D to affect a cure of the condition, in some cases even as high as 500,000 units daily for a time. These have been spoken of as Vitamin D resistant. They are often present in older children, four to five years of age. Their epiphyseal growth is often retarded. The condition is rare, (Holt).

Dent and Harris have presented forms of rickets and osteomalacia which appear to be hereditary in nature. While they seem to present the picture both roentgenologically and clinically of these Vitamin D deficient diseases they do not respond to such treatment. It is possible that these are the type of Vitamin D resistant type reported elsewhere.

RENAL RICKETS (Renal Osteo-dystrophy). Renal rickets is a condition due to chronic severe impairment of kidney function in which the bone

thereby conserving the normal calcium content of the bones. Rickets develops from a lack of vitamin D in the diet; therefore, in order to maintain the blood calcium the bones lose their calcium salts. With the loss of calcium salts the bone loses its strength, so that from weight bearing or muscle pull, bowing of the bones is apt to occur. Rickets is the most common cause of knock-knee and bow-leg deformities. Spontaneous fractures may occur from weakening of the bones. Rickets is a disturbance of calcium metabolism, not of bone growth; consequently the cortex of the bone, continuing its growth (according to Wolff's Law) as a response to greatest stress and strain, becomes thickest on the concave side and thinnest on the convex side; at the epiphyseal line the continually forming osteoid tissue fails to calcify, resulting in enlargement of the ends of the bone, widening of the zone of preliminary osteoid formation and cupping of the epiphyseal line. This enlargement of the ends of the bones is very evident at the costo-chondral junctions of the ribs giving rise to the so-called Rachitic Rosary (Fig. 73B). This also occurs in scurvy. When it does occur it may be considered as a response to trauma from strain on the weakened cortex of the bone. The centers of ossification in the epiphysis rarely show any apparent change. Only very rarely is slight periosteal reaction present.

Administration of vitamin D, either as cod-liver oil or by exposure of the skin surface to ultra-violet rays, results in rapid deposit of calcium salts in the new-formed osteoid tissue with the formation of an extremely wide and dense preliminary zone of calcification at the diaphyseal side of the epiphyseal line. Even after recovery some remnant of this zone of calcification remains to indicate the period of malnutrition experienced by the individual; in manifestations resemble true rickets very closely. It is more an intoxication than a disease of nutrition and owes its name only to the resemblance of the bone lesions to those of rickets. There is hyperplasia of the parathyroid glands and hyperfunction of these structures resulting in an extreme degree of osteoporosis (see Hyperparathyroidism and Renal Dwarfism).

OSTEOMALACIA. Osteomalacia is a disease due to defect in the calcification of the bony matrix; osteoid bone fails to calcify. This may be due to lack of Vitamin D. It is rarely encountered in this country; China, India and portions of Europe are the most frequent regions of occurrence. It occurs most frequently in pregnant or lactating women; due to the increased calcium demands of pregnancy and lactation, the calcium and phosphorus of the blood are disturbed and there is an increase in calcium excretion. The alkaline phosphatase is usually high, which serves to differentiate this condition from osteoporosis of other cause.

Clinically the disease manifests itself by pain, ranging from dull backache to intense pain on slightest motion. The patient walks with a characteristic waddle.

The process is one in which bone that has once been well calcified loses its calcium salts. The physiological destruction of old bone and its replacement by new osteoid tissue goes on in a normal way, but for some unknown reason the calcium liberated from the old bones is not utilized by the organism to calcify the new osteoid tissue, but instead is lost principally in the feces.

ROENTGENOLOGICAL CONSIDERATION. There is often marked deformity of the pelvis and long bones. Compression deformity of the pelvis occurs due to the weight bearing. Fractures are common with poor callus formation. There may be bending of the long bones.

The medullary canal is widened and the cortex becomes extremely thin, even as thin as paper. Periostitis may be present. The bone presents an indistinct hazy appearance with lack of contrast between it and the soft tissues. The trabeculae range from a faint to a coarse and uneven network, and may give the appearance of crumbling. The long bones appear widened at the diaphysis. They may resemble osteitis fibrosa cystica, but the cystic formation is not so definite and the softening is more pronounced. The late or healed stage shows distortion of the pelvis with recalcification.

Baker has described two cases in which he was able to demonstrate defects in the fibre system of the bone matrix by means of polarized light and various tissue stains. There was no evidence of involvement of the collagen connective tissue of other structures. Roentgenographically the picture presented by both patients was similar in appearance to osteomalacia occurring at advanced age, but the reactions to chemical tests were at variance with this condition. He has designated this condition as Fibrogenesis Imperfecta Ossium.

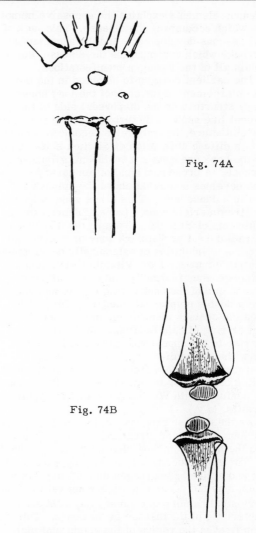

Fig. 74A

Fig. 74B

SCURVY*—(Barlow's Disease) (Fig. 74). Scurvy is a nutritional disease due to deficiency of Vitamin C in the diet; characterized by hemorrhages throughout the body which result in certain characteristic bone changes. It is a disease of ossification occurring most frequently between six and ten months of age. It never occurs in breast-fed infants and rarely if ever is it present in new born infants. Vitamin C is contained in fresh fruits and vegetables such as oranges, lemons, grapefruit, tomato juice, etc., and is present in fresh milk. Boiling or pasteurization destroys this vitamin in milk.

The effect of Vitamin C deficiency is on the cells of mesenchymal origin producing an inability of the supporting tissues to produce and maintain intercellular substances. These substances are the collagen of all fibrous tissue, matrix of bone, dentine and cartilage, including non-epithelial cement substance of vascular epithelium, and are essential to all normal osteoblastic and chondroblastic development. Without proper collagenous material, osteoblastic proliferation all but ceases, and cartilaginous growth, although still possible, results in formation of imperfect cartilage structure. Being an essential element of vascular structure,   the lack of these collagenous elements explains the excessive hemorrhages which accompany the disease. This lack of normal osseous development, and the associated hemorrhage which accompanies the disease, serve to explain all of the roentgen manifestations.

The earliest changes to be noted in the bones are an enlargement of the ends of the long bones. The bony structure on the diaphyseal side of the epiphyseal line shows a disturbance in the normal bone architecture, the trabeculae become fragmented, there is a diffuse absorption of calcium salts and the end of the bone presents a translucent, ground-glass appearance. A broadened band of temporary calcification develops somewhat above the epiphyseal plate with a dense zone. This dense zone is known as the "trümmerfeld zone," (zone of debris) or as the white line of Fraenkel. Toward the diaphyseal side a radiolucent gerüstmark zone or scurvy line is seen due to inhibition of osteoblastic development and matrix formation from Vitamin C deficiency. It is homogeneous in density and runs uniformly across the end of the bone giving rise to an appearance of a double epiphyseal line, (Fig. 74B). The ossification centers themselves may present a dense deposit or ring of calcification about their edges, giving rise to the appearance of an ossification center within an ossification center known as Wimberger's Sign, very frequently seen in the ossification centers for the tarsal bones. This should not be confused with Wimberger's sign in syphilitic epiphysitis, (q.v.).

As the disease progresses, hemorrhages into the various organs and structures of the body give rise to the most prominent characteristics of the disease. The gums become soft and spongy; the teeth loosen and active hemorrhages may occur; this manifestation may not occur if teeth are not yet present. Subperiosteal hemorrhage causes the most striking characteristic of the disease in the bones. This may be seen first in the region of the epiphyseal plate where the periosteum is firmly attached. Injury from pressure on the weakened bone causes a small subperiosteal hemorrhage closely limited to the periosteal attachment is followed by spicules of periosteal new bone formation along the stripped-up periosteum which project almost perpendicularly outward from the region of the epiphyseal line. This is known as Pelkan's Sign (Fig. 74A). Later on, more extensive subperiosteal hemorrhage may strip the periosteum from the entire shaft, giving rise to a boggy mass intimately connected with the shaft of the bone (Fig. 74C). This is the most acute stage of the disease, giving rise to extreme pain and disability which may even resemble paralysis. The presence of a hard, painful tumor mass intimately connected with the bone, without fever, may clinically simulate sarcoma. The femur is frequently involved. Extensive subperiosteal hemorrhage may cause spontaneous dislocation of the epiphysis.

Separation takes place through the weakened translucent zone; the epiphyseal plate with its periosteal attachments intact is literally floated off of its diaphyseal attachment by the extensive subperiosteal hemorrhage.

Even at this stage, the therapeutic test is most decisive in its action; the results of the administration of orange juice for twenty-four hours is almost miraculous; the pain is relieved; the patient feels better, and even uses the involved extremities. On resuming proper diet, the subperiosteal blood clot becomes ossified, the displaced epiphysis undergoes spontaneous correction due to the retained periosteal attachment to the epiphyseal plate and calcium salts again become deposited normally. The periosteal attachment to the epiphyseal bone plate explains the spontaneous restoration of the epiphyses as healing takes place. The irregular thickening of the shaft is restored to normal after a few months or a year.

The characteristics of this disease (Bromer) may be outlined as:

Early:
1. Loss of calcium salts in diaphyseal ends of bones and ground-glass appearance; (not specific).
2. Formation of dense zone of temporary calcification (trümmerfeld zone, with adjacent band-like zone of decreased density, gerüstmark or scurvy zone) above giving rise to the appearance of a double epiphyseal line. At the onset the zone of decreased density may be present only at the edges, referred to as the "corner sign."
3. Ring of calcification about ossification centers resembling an ossification center within an ossification center, (Wimberger's Sign).

Fully Established:
4. Spicules of new periosteal bone formation extending outward from epiphyseal line (Pelkan's Sign).
5. Large subperiosteal hemorrhages stripping up periosteum of shaft with subsequent calcification.
6. Spontaneous displacement of epiphysis.

Repair:
7. Absorption of hemorrhage and ossification by periosteum.
8. Spontaneous correction of displaced epiphysis.
9. Redeposit of calcium salts and resumption of normal bone growth.

The presence of a rosary in both rickets and scurvy serve to differentiate these conditions from congenital syphilis in which no rosary occurs. Many points serve to differentiate scurvy from rickets; in scurvy there is no bowing such as is seen in rickets; in scurvy the gerüstmark zone of decreased density is narrow, of even density and extends clear across the diaphyseal end of the bone whereas, in rickets no such zone exists; in scurvy there is no delay in calcification of new formed bone and a wide trümmerfeld zone of provisional calcification is present whereas, in rickets unossified bone forms a wide zone at the metaphyseal end; in scurvy there are large subperiosteal hemorrhages.

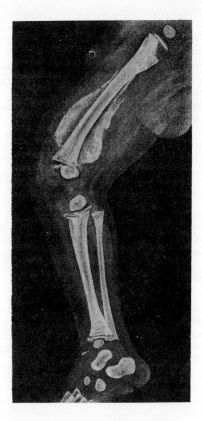

Fig. 74C

Dennis and Mercado have reported the development of scurvy after the prolonged use of folic acid antagonists as therapeutic agents for other conditions. The bone changes are typical as a result of long standing aminopterin therapy.

CALCINOSIS INTERSTITIALIS * (Fig. 74D) is a condition in which calcium salts are deposited in the subcutaneous tissues throughout the body. This is probably due to some fault of calcium metabolism rather than trauma and might perhaps be better considered under that heading. It may remain local (Circumscripta) or it may progress to an extreme degree involving practically the entire body (Universalis). Calcium deposits may have a tendency to occur about joints; the frequent association of calcinosis with scleroderma, dermatositis or vasomotor disturbances when there is vascular derangement or a degenerative condition of the connective tissue or fat suggests dystrophic calcification, (Cole).

Administration of a ketogenic diet over a considerable period has resulted in a complete disappearance of the calcium deposits in some cases; others do not seem to be influenced by any therapeutic measure. Sausa and Chaves have reported a case showing development of the condition in a previously healthy child at three years. Adults may also be involved.

TUMORAL CALCINOSIS (Calcinosis Circumscripta) (Thomson and Tanner). Tumoral calcinosis seems to be a distinct entity of the general condition,

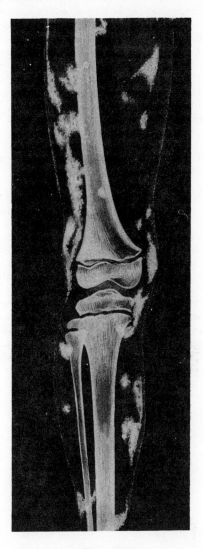

Fig. 74D

calcinosis. Three brothers were described with large calcium tumor about the shoulder which appeared and enlarged for one year. Operative removal was followed by recurrence elsewhere. The cause could not be determined.

CHALKY "GOUT". This is another form of calcinosis circumscripta. It is characterized by small rounded chalk deposits in the subcutaneous tissues about the smaller phalangeal joints. Roentgenologically the dense chalky content of these nodules is readily discernible, differentiating them from the tophi associated with gout. It is the clinical appearance which so closely resembles gouty deposits. A type of Lipo-calcino-granulomatosis has been described by Oosthuizen, et al.

HYPERVITAMINOSIS A (Rothman and Leon). Administration of excessive quantities of Vitamin A over a long time results in striking constitutional manifestations and pathological findings in bone structure: severe emaciation, hemorrhagic rhinitis, loss of hair, softening of bones, with spontaneous fracture and even death in two to four weeks.

Daily dosage of 200,000 to 300,000 units of Vitamin A (usually taken as oleum percomorphum) for several months is usually necessary to produce the condition, (J. Caffey). It may be safely assumed that no case of hypervitaminosis A will occur with 75,000 units daily or less.

A parallel type of periosteal reaction is present over the long bones and clavicles especially in the midportion of the shafts with swelling of the overlying soft tissues and muscles. Calcified rings appear about the epiphyses.

The appearance is strikingly similar to infantile cortical hyperostosis. This similarity has been commented upon by E. B. Shaw, in discussion of an article by Toomey and Morissette. There are certain variations; the periosteal reaction is more massive and laminated in an infantile cortical hyperostosis but it is present in both; hypervitaminosis A occurs in first year of life, whereas infantile cortical hyperostosis has its onset in early infancy within the first two years; infantile cortical hyperostosis shows mandible most apt to be involved whereas, in hypervitaminosis it is not; hypervitaminosis A recovers rapidly within a few days or weeks after withdrawal of excessive dosage of Vitamin A, whereas infantile cortical hyperostosis continues for months along its natural course before recovering.

HYPERVITAMINOSIS D (Jeans; Caffey). Vitamin D is used primarily in infants in the treatment of rickets. In adults it has been found of value in the treatment of some forms of arthritis. The U.S.P. dosage recommended for children is 300 to 400 units daily; adults require proportionately less, approximately 400 units.

Numerous cases have been reported where these doses have been greatly exceeded, especially in the treatment of chronic arthritis. Large doses for a short time produce symptoms of intoxication, nausea, vomiting, diarrhea and abdominal discomfort. Continued over a long period of time, this leads to weight loss, debility and damage to cells of various organs, arteries and arterioles which become the repository of calcium salts. If continued, it may lead to death. These changes usually accompany hypercalcemia and hyperphosphatemia. Metastatic calcium deposits occur in various organs and in and about joints. In the bones of growing children there is a dense deposit of mineral in the zone of provisional calcification in the metaphyses of long bones.

It has been pointed out that all signs and radiograph findings of hypercalcemia have been found in children in whom history of hypervitaminosis D cannot be proved; these are designated as idiopathic hypercalcemia, (Shiers, et al.).

QUESTIONS ON NUTRITIONAL DISEASES OF BONE

Questions marked with a dagger deal with rare and less important conditions.

1. Give characteristics of: Legg-Calvé-Perthes' Disease; state probable cause and differential diagnosis from tuberculous arthritis.

†2. Intrapelvic protrusion of the acetabulum; what is its cause and ultimate result?

†3. Osgood-Schlatter's Disease.

†4. Köhler's Disease of tarsal scaphoid and how does it differ from the other forms of epiphysitis mentioned above?

†5. Subchondral necrosis of spine.

6. Describe the bone changes of rickets and their roentgenographic appearance. What pathological changes are present and how can they be explained? What is meant by foetal rickets and late rickets? What is renal rickets and in what way is it related to ordinary rickets?

†7. What is osteomalacia and what are its characteristics? What relationship does it seem to have to endocrine secretion? to vitamin deficiency?

8. To what is scurvy due and how does it manifest itself in bones, in the early stages? When well advanced? When healed? How do the X-ray findings vary from congenital syphilis?

†9. What is calcinosis interstitalis and describe its roentgen appearance?

10. Describe the roentgen characteristics of Hypervitaminosis A.
What dosage of Vitamin A is necessary to produce this effect, and how is it treated?

11. Describe the roentgen appearance of Hypervitaminosis D. What other conditions does it most resemble?

12. In what way does Hypervitaminosis A resemble Infantile Cortical Hyperostosis and how may they be differentiated?

13. What is meant by "chalky gout"? Does it have any relationship to true gout?

QUESTIONS ON NUTRITIONAL DISEASES OF BONE.

INFECTIONS OF BONE (Chapter VII)

BACTERIAL

A. Pyogenic Infection

  1. Acute Osteomyelitis

    a. Hematogenous Origin
      In Adults
        Medullary or deep type
        Subperiosteal type
      In Infants and Children
        Metaphysial involvement
        Epiphyseal Type (non-tuberculous epiphysitis)
    b. Direct Extension (localized) origin
      Osteitis Pubis

  2. Chronic Osteomyelitis

    a. Following acute osteomyelitis
    b. Brucella osteomyelitis
    c. Chronic bone abscess, (BRODIE'S ABSCESS)
    d. Osteoid osteoma

B. Nonsuppurating Osteomyelitis of GARRÉ

C. Infantile Cortical Hyperostosis

D. Tuberculosis of Bone

  1. Short and Long Bones,

    a. Diaphysis
    b. Metaphysis
    c. Epiphysis (cancellous end of bone)
    d. Joint (arthritis)

  2. Irregular Bones especially

    a. Spine (vertebral bodies)
    b. Carpal bones, especially os magnum
    c. Tarsal bones, especially os calcis

  3. Flat Bones, especially cranial bones

    a. Cystic type of tuberculous involvement

SPIROCHETAL INFECTION

E. Syphilis, (LUES)

  1. Congenital syphilis
  2. Epiphysitis
  3. Syphilitic lesions of later life

    a. Periostitis
    b. Osteitis
    c. Osteomyelitis

F. Yaws

G. Fungous Infection

  1. Actinomycosis
  2. Blastomycosis
  3. Mycetoma, (Madura Foot)
  4. Coccidioidal Granuloma
  5. Torula

H. Parasitic Infection

  1. Ecchinococcus Cyst

Chapter VII

INFECTIONS OF BONE

A. PYOGENIC BACTERIAL INFECTION

1. ACUTE OSTEOMYELITIS
   a. Hematogenous Origin:
      In children and young adults
         Medullary or deep type, which results
         from involvement of the medullary
         canal by infection gaining entrance by
         way of the nutrient artery.
         Subperiosteal type, which occurs when
         the pyogenic organisms gain entrance
         by way of the blood stream to the sub-
         periosteal region.
      In Infants
         Metaphyseal Involvement
         Epiphyseal type--(non-tuberculous epi-
         physitis)
   b. Direct Extension (Localized) Origin
      Spread from soft part infection
      Spread from an infected joint.
      Direct Inoculation—Foreign body piercing
      bone.

Approximately 90 per cent of hematogenous osteomyelitis cases occur in children 5 to 15 years of age.
Staphylococcus aureus is the most common etiological agent.

Acute pyogenic osteomyelitis is an infection of
bone by pyogenic organisms. The long bones are
most frequently involved; only very rarely is the
spine or skull the site of osteomyelitic involvement.
Spinal involvement is usually as a direct extension
from pyogenic pulmonary infection and involvement
of the skull usually follows spread of infection from
the sinuses or scalp. Its outstanding roentgenological
characteristic is the co-existence of bone production
and bone destruction.
There are two general forms of the disease; the
Hematogenous and Direct Extension Type.

ACUTE PYOGENIC OSTEOMYELITIS OF HEMATOGENOUS ORIGIN: MEDULLARY OR DEEP TYPE*

CLINICAL MANIFESTATIONS

1. Age—5-15 years, although it can occur at any
   age; in recent years infantile involvement is
   becoming more prevalent.
2. Sex—No predominance.
3. Race—No predominance.
4. Site of Inoculation—medullary canal by way of
   the nutrient artery.
5. History and course of disease—The onset may

be sudden with chills followed by high fever and leucocytosis. Even though the infection is deep in the
medullary canal, the manifestations of localized infection, pain, heat, redness, swelling, loss of function
may be present. Pain is usually severe, but may not
be clearly confined to the area of involvement; for instance, involvement of the upper end of the femur may
have pain referred to the knee. There may be a pre-
existing suppurating lesion such as an abscess or
other type of pyogenic infection in the body, but frequently no such history can be obtained. The disease
may be more insidious and gradual in onset.

During the first seven to ten days pus accu-
mulates in the medullary canal, but actual bone
destruction or production may not be evident. The
pus, being of similar density to the bone marrow, may give no evidence of its presence in the
roentgenogram. However, even at this early stage,
evidence of minute bone destruction may be seen
in the metaphyseal region by careful examination
and comparison with the same region of the opposite side. This is probably due to the fact that
the small veins draining the infected medullary
canal offer avenues for extension of the infection.
Therefore, if all other manifestations of osteomyelitis are present, do not wait for roentgen
evidence of bone destruction, but proceed with
treatment.

The advent of chemotherapy has revolutionized
the treatment; sulpha drugs, penicillin and other
antibiotics, will abort the infection if administered
early. Even when given after the condition is well
established they may exert a very favorable influence, check the advance of the infection and has-
ten recovery. At any rate as soon as the condition
is suspected clinically, chemotherapy should be instituted. In the light of our present knowledge
simple aspiration of subperiosteal or soft part
abscess often serves well to restrain the harmful
effect of stripping up of the periosteum. If the
disease has advanced so far that surgical treatment
is thought advisable, simple drilling into the shaft
for detection of the infection is not sufficient for
drainage; nothing short of resection of a gutter of
bone (saucerization) will suffice.

Early administration of chemotherapy will materially modify the picture usually produced by unchecked osteomyelitis or may even abort the disease.
As a result, the typically described form is now
seldom seen.

---

*An asterisk following any title indicates that roentgenographic reproductions illustrating this condition will be
found in the pictorial supplement at the end of the chapter.

PATHOLOGICAL INVOLVEMENT AND ROENTGENOLOGICAL FINDINGS. Bacteria entering through the nutrient artery are deposited in its smaller branches in the medullary canal. The end arteries are arranged in loops in the metaphyseal ends of the bones; therefore, the initial effect of the infection may be in the metaphyseal region. This portion of the bone, being soft and cancellous, may be the site of most extensive destruction. With the proliferation of organisms the infection tends to extend if unchecked along the line of least resistance up and down the medullary canal (Fig. 75A). Even as this extension occurs there are multiple areas of localized erosion of bone due to the bacterial toxins which finally result in complete perforation of the cortex of the bone in widely separated localities, leaving good bone structure between

sufficient so that there is no manifestation of toxic absorption, then there is no need for hasty operative procedure; if there _is_ evidence of toxic absorption any surgical procedure should be limited to securing adequate drainage.

When the involucrum has assumed sufficient strength to take on the function of the destroyed bone then operative procedure may be undertaken for the removal of necrotic material. In children under three years of age simple drainage of the infection or aspiration without exploration of the bone; and immobilization in a cast often gives better results than extensive operative drainage of the medullary cavity.

Chemotherapy if instituted sufficiently early in the course of the disease may not only influence the

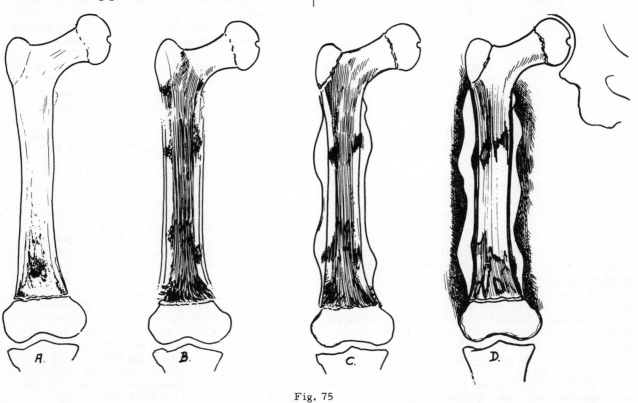

Fig. 75

(Fig. 75B). With the perforation of the cortex the pus reaches the subperiosteal region and the periosteum is stripped up from its bony attachment by the burrowing of the pus. Finally, however, from a process of distension and erosion, the periosteum itself is broken through, thus allowing the escape of pus through the soft parts to the outside (Fig. 75C). If sufficient drainage is thus established the toxic manifestations will disappear.

With the involvement of the periosteum, this structure is stimulated to new bone formation as a part of the reparative process. Large amounts of periosteal new bone may surround and practically reestablish the destroyed bone. The new-formed periosteal bone is called the involucrum. If drainage is

clinical course of the disease but may so modify the roentgen manifestations that they may be at great variance with those ordinarily encountered. In place of large areas of stripped-up periosteum with resulting extensive sequestra formation (Fig. 75), the periosteal reaction is often at a minimum. The intact periosteum likewise offers adequate blood supply to the underlying bone and consequently bone destruction is limited and repair a simpler and more rapid process. The destroyed bone fills in and is replaced by sclerotic proliferation of the bone cells themselves giving a denser appearance to the trabeculae. It is more rapid and stronger following the natural physiological method of bone repair. The entire process may be over in 30 to 60 days, whereas without chemotherapy the disease may be prolonged for many years.

SEQUESTRUM FORMATION (Fig. 75C). If the infection is unchecked extending up and down the shaft, stripping up the periosteum, sequestration will occur. The blood supply of bone comes from two main sources: the nutrient artery and the osteogenic layer of the periosteum. With the involvement of the medullary canal by infection the source of blood supply to the bone normally furnished by the nutrient artery is cut off. As the pus which erodes through the cortex to the subperiosteal region undermines and strips up the periosteum in its effort to gain drainage, it thereby removes from the bony cortex the only other adequate blood supply for the nutrition of the bone. When any tissue is deprived of adequate blood supply, it dies; so it is that with the elimination of the blood supply to certain portions of the bone they die and are ultimately sloughed off. This is due to the action of osteoclasts on the infarcted area. When separated, such a piece of dead bone is known as a sequestrum. Since sequestra are the usual sources of persistent drainage in osteomyelitis, and since the sinuses caused by them will not close until they are completely absorbed by the body secretions (sequestra are not removed by osteoclastic action), discharged spontaneously or removed by surgical procedure, their recognition in the roentgenogram is an all-important point. Such sinuses sometimes persist for years; or they may close only to be reestablished when the pressure of underlying pus becomes sufficiently great.

ROENTGEN MANIFESTATION OF SEQUESTRUM FORMATION (Fig. 75D). There are two rather distinct characteristics by which sequestra can be recognized; first, a sequestrum usually presents a more chalky white appearance than the surrounding bone, and second, sequestra never show active proliferation of periosteal new bone. If any normal bone is placed at rest for four to six weeks, it undergoes absorption of the calcium salts; this condition is known as bone atrophy, or osteoporosis. This normal absorption is dependent upon an intact blood supply; in the case of sequestrum formation the blood supply to the sequestrum is destroyed and physiological absorption cannot take place. The piece of dead bone, therefore, retains its calcium salts and does not undergo the normal physiological atrophy. In contrast with the surrounding atrophied bone the sequestrum presents a chalky white appearance. This is an outstanding feature of sequestrum formation.

The second characteristic of sequestrum formation is the failure of periosteal proliferation in contact with the sequestrated bone. By definition, a sequestrum is a piece of bone that dies because it is deprived of its blood supply, due to the stripping up of the periosteum; therefore no periosteal reaction can be present springing from the dead bone. Sequestration may involve the entire shaft or may be limited to small areas in the cortex of the bone. In either event the sequestrum is usually surrounded by an area of liquefaction or destruction of the bone, which,

in turn, is surrounded by an area of bone sclerosis In this state the disease becomes chronic and in its well-walled-off state will rarely show any benefit from chemotherapy.

With the removal of all sequestra, healing rapidly takes place. The primary infection is usually limited to the medullary canal, and rarely spreads beyond the epiphyseal line, although in exceptional cases it may spread to the epiphysis and even involve the joint. A hole completely through a bone is known as a cloaca.

Frequently the primary infection is followed by numerous metastatic infections in the other bones in far removed localities (Fig. 76). These metastatic infections may be subperiosteal and are often not suspected until the drainage of the primarily infected bone has been established. Not until the pain of the primary infection is relieved does the patient notice the less painful secondary site of involvement. Subperiosteal infection of this sort rarely goes on to extensive suppuration and sequestrum formation.

ROENTGENOLOGICAL CHARACTERISTICS— MEDULLARY TYPE OSTEOMYELITIS

1. Point of Origin.

From the widespread manifestations of the disease seen in the roentgenogram, the point of origin is obviously the medullary canal.

2. Bone Production or Bone Destruction.

In pyogenic infection of bone of all sorts, there are manifestations of bone destruction and bone production going on at the same time. This simultaneous occurrence is a differential point in the diagnosis of this disease. New bone formation is manifested principally by periosteal reaction, usually of the parallel type. It is possible in a person suffering from lues for pyogenic infection to activate the luetic involvement, giving rise to the lace-work type of periosteal reaction. In certain localities, especially phalanges, new bone production may be very slow in formation and may not appear until there is considerable destruction. Later on in the course of the disease, bone production may manifest itself as a sclerosing osteitis, especially bordering small areas of confined suppuration and necrosis. Bone production may be so pronounced that under certain circumstances the condition may resemble bone sarcoma.

3. Expansion or Nonexpansion.

No expansion of bone is present, since the process starting in the medullary canal spreads up and down the shaft and erodes through the cortex. The acute character makes expansion impossible.

4. Condition of the Cortex.

The cortex is broken through in numerous

places leaving areas of good bone structure in between. This is a characteristic of infection and is a differential point between osteomyelitis and malignancy. One of the characteristics of malignant tumors arising in medullary canal is their early erosion through the cortex, but in this instance there are not multiple areas of erosion with good bone in between as in osteomyelitis.

5. Invasion or Noninvasion.

There is no true invasion of soft parts by the tumor mass. Sinuses pierce the soft parts and discharge pus from the medullary canal, but no true invasion occurs as by tumor formation. In the case of tumor growth the invasion is by multiplication of cells which literally sweep the cortex away before it.

SUBPERIOSTEAL TYPE OF OSTEOMYELITIS*

This type of osteomyelitis is most frequently seen in association with the extensive medullary type at some remote location as a metastatic involvement. The pyogenic organisms which produce the original medullary involvement, circulating in the blood stream, find lodgment in the subperiosteal tissue of some other bone by way of the periosteal blood supply. The development of such foci may be influenced by slight trauma such as that incident to the heel resting on the bed, or the rubbing of the bed clothes on the big toe. Pyogenic infection of this type usually tends to remain more localized in the subperiosteal tissues and often does not spread far from the original site of inoculation, being limited by cortical bone on the one side and periosteal new bone formation on the other. The confinement of the infection under the stripped-up periosteum leads to layer upon layer of newly-formed periosteal bone. Only very rarely is the cortex eroded; rarely if ever does this erosion from such foci extend into the medullary canal.

Clinically the manifestations are not painful to the same degree as those of the primary medullary involvement and often their presence may not be suspected until adequate drainage of the primary infection relieves the pain in that region.

Roentgenological Characteristics Subperiosteal Type Osteomyelitis (Fig. 76).

1. Point of Origin.

Subperiosteal region causing stripping-up of periosteum with extreme degree of periosteal reaction. These areas may be from a few centimeters in length to areas involving one-half of the shaft.

2. Bone Production or Bone Destruction.

There are large amounts of new periosteal bone production, usually layer upon layer of bone of parallel type of reaction. Bone destruction is limited to slight erosion of the cortex or it may not be detected at all. Sequestrum formation is rarely present and if it does occur, is usually very small.

3. Expansion or Non-expansion.

No true expansion; any enlargement of bone is due to periosteal reaction. The shaft still retains its normal configuration.

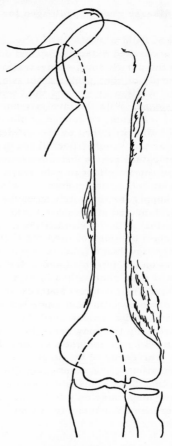

Fig. 76

4. Condition of Cortex.

Ordinarily cortex remains intact, but there may be erosion and destruction.

5. No true invasion of the soft parts.

In recent years, the condition seems more prevalent taking on the appearance of dense sclerosis with a central area of bone destruction confined to one end of a long bone, (Neligan and Warrick).

OSTEOMYELITIS IN INFANTS

Osteomyelitic infection in young infants may show marked variation from the manifestations described in adults. The source of infection in most instances is thought to be infection from diaper rash or other skin diseases but many cases are seen in which no source of the infection can be found. Any of the pyogenic organisms may be the cause but the streptococcus and staphylococcus are the most common offenders.

It is blood borne as in adults and seems to have a predilection for the metaphysial regions. It has a tendency to spread to the epiphysis and may cause spontaneous epiphyseal separation as in scurvy. The epiphyseal structure is often involved and may be destroyed. The infection may spread to involve the joint giving an impression of a primary joint infection. The amount of fluid may be increased so much as to cause spontaneous dislocation of the joint.

Clinically, the process may seem more insidious, with relatively low fever, relatively slight pain and disability.

Roentgenographically there is localized rarefaction of the diaphysial end of the bone. Often rounded areas of bone destruction occur in diaphyses and epiphysis but sequestration is not common. There is an epiphyseal reaction in the region of bone involvement. The epiphysis may be separated or the joint dislocated.

The prognosis in very young infants is much less favorable than in older individuals but chemotherapy gives a great advantage in treatment. Subperiosteal collection of pus may be successfully aspirated without operative drainage. A type of low-grade infection occurring in infants, known as spondylarthritis (q.v.) is characterized by narrowing of the intervertebral discs and some sclerosis of the vertebra, developing insidiously and lasting several months. Complete recovery is the usual outcome; it resembles most tuberculous spondylitis from which it must be differentiated.

Acute bacterial osteomyelitis most commonly affects the long bones, but it may involve any bone in the body. Although a rare occurrence, it may affect the spine. Pneumococcus osteomyelitis of the spine has been reported as a complication of pneumonia, and typhoid involvement of the spine was a not too uncommon occurrence in the days when typhoid was a prolific disease. The Friedlander bacillus has been reported as a cause in South African individuals.

Osteomyelitis variolosa or osteomyelitis resulting from small pox infection or vaccinia usually occurs in children of other countries where small pox is prevalent presenting similar findings, (Bertcher).

ACUTE PYOGENIC EPIPHYSITIS (NONTUBERCULOUS) Fig. 77

Acute pyogenic epiphysitis is a rather rare condition in which the blood-borne infection primarily attacks the epiphysis of older children. The process usually spreads to involve the adjacent diaphyseal structure, but rarely progresses for any great distance down the medullary canal. The articular car-

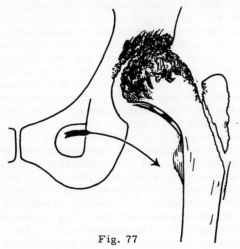

Fig. 77

tilage forms a barrier to the spread of the infection of the joint, although complete destruction of the joint may result.

This type of pyogenic infection of bone is most frequent in relatively young children, usually between the ages of three and seven years, but it may occur at any age up to the age of complete union of the epiphyses. The upper end of the femur and upper end of the tibia are the most frequent sites of involvement.

Clinical Characteristics of Acute Pyogenic Epiphysitis. The onset is sudden with fever, pain, muscle spasm and other signs of local inflammation. There is periarticular swelling and sometimes the development of effusion in the joint. As the disease progresses there is bone destruction, and sequestrum formation. Sinuses may form to the outside, discharging the pus. The disease may become chronic, similar to osteomyelitic infection elsewhere in the bone. Chemotherapy in this condition also may prove very beneficial if given early.

Pathological and Roentgenological Characteristics of Acute Pyogenic Epiphysitis. Pyogenic infection involving the cancellous bone of the epiphysis results in bone destruction, which varies in amount with the severity of the infection. This is very rapid, often being quite pronounced by the end of the third or fourth week. The destruction may be carried to the point of fragmentation or complete destruction of the epiphysis. The destructive process is so rapid that it is evident in the roentgenogram before sufficient time has elapsed to permit absorption of lime salts from atrophy of disuse. The pyogenic infection may or may not form fistulous tracts to the outside; frequently the end of the extremity becomes large and swollen with the pyogenic process remaining confined to the tissues. The destroyed bone and cartilage is replaced by new bone formation from proliferation of the adjacent periosteum. The end result may be destruction of the function of the epiphysis and failure of future growth or limitation of motion of the joint.

These pathological manifestations result in the following roentgenological characteristics:

1. Point of Origin: epiphysis.
2. Bone Production or Destruction: both occur at the same time in the involved area.
3. No true Expansion.
4. Cortex although broken through in numerous places shows areas of good bone between.
5. No true Invasion of soft parts.

The only condition in which the roentgenographic picture may resemble this condition is tuberculous epiphysitis. The main difference between the manifestations of these two conditions is that acute pyogenic epiphysitis is much more rapid, requiring only days and weeks for the same degree of bone changes that would require months and years from tuberculous involvement. As a result, bone atrophy which is a physiological result of disuse of any bone does not have time to occur before bone destruction in acute pyogenic epiphysitis, whereas in tuberculous epiphysitis, bone atrophy is evident long before bone destruction occurs. Also bone destruction by pyogenic processes is repaired by new bone formation, periosteal and cortical, while purely tuberculous destruction is repaired primarily by fibrous tissue only; when actual bone production is present with tuberculous disease it is usually a manifestation of associated pyogenic infection.

Infection of epiphyses especially of the metacarpals and metatarsals from osteomyelitis or other systemic infection may result in loss of function of the epiphysis and stunting of its growth. Attention has been called to the tendency of smallpox to cause this deformity. There may be no such demonstrable etiology however; the condition may be symmetrical, affecting the same toe or finger on each side.

DIRECT EXTENSION TYPE OF OSTEOMYELITIS
Fig. 78

The bone may become involved by spread of pyogenic infection:
    From the soft parts
    From infection of an adjacent joint
    From direct inoculation by a foreign body
In all these types the area of infection tends to remain local, rarely, if ever, extending to involve the entire medullary canal. Actual involvement is first manifested by hazy appearance of the outline of the bone from erosion of the cortex. This process takes longer and is not as severe as that seen where pus is confined to the medullary canal under pressure and is seeking an outlet. Periosteal new bone pro-

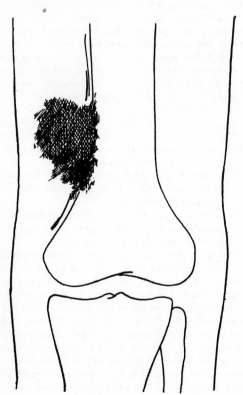

Fig. 78

duction is not as extensive, but usually manifests itself as a thin white line running along the shaft of bone adjacent to the area of erosion.

When the process spreads from an infected joint the cancellous portion of the bone offers a ready medium for extension of the disease. In the cancellous portion actual bone destruction may be difficult to differentiate from bone atrophy, but the disintegration of the trabecular bone from actual destruction of the bone cells can usually be made out.

If the infection is directly inoculated by a penetrating foreign body or as in a compound fracture, the manifestations of infection begin at the point of inoculation and spread to the adjacent bony structure. Incision and evacuation of the infection to the outside materially lessen the danger of extension to the bone.

Roentgenological Characteristics of Localized Type Osteomyelitis.

1. Point of Origin.
    At the periphery of the bone, with variations, depending upon the type.

2. Bone Production or Bone Destruction.
    Both bone production and bone destruction are present, but the reaction is usually more localized. Destruction is usually confined to a local erosion. Sequestra, if present, are usually small.

3. Expansion or Nonexpansion. None.

4. Condition of the Cortex.
    Eroded near site of infection; there may be associated sequestrum formation.

5. Invasion or Noninvasion.
    No true invasion of the soft parts.

OSTEITIS PUBIS AND ISCHII. This is a condition which develops in the pubic bones at their symphysis and in the ramii of the ischia shortly after operative procedures on the prostate and bladder neck, (Cohen). It is probably due to some low-grade type of infection, although the causative organism cannot ordinarily be isolated. Batson has demonstrated a wealth of venous supply to the bones of pelvis and hip which might explain extension of infection to these areas after bladder and prostate operations. We have encountered a case in which an acute destructive arthritis of the hip joint followed such an involvement of the symphysis some weeks after recovery of the primary lesion. It is attendant with considerable pain. Similar extension of infection to the spine following prostatectomy has been reported by Liming and Youngs.

Roentgenologically, the bony structures of the pubic and ischial regions undergo osteoporosis and erosion later followed by dense sclerosis with shaggy periosteal reaction; and occasionally small, cystlike areas of destruction are present. The condition is favorably influenced by x-ray therapy, (Goldstein and Rubin). All other supportive and biological methods may have to be used. The process may involve months and years before complete restoration to health. Ultimate cure frequently results in fusion of the symphysis pubis, (Lame and Chang).

CHRONIC OSTEOMYELITIS

Not until every vestige of destroyed bone is removed does the osteomyelitis process heal. The involucrum may become sufficiently strong to take on the function of the part, and the individual may be up and about, carrying on his normal activities, but numerous small isolated areas of bone destruction, usually with associated tiny sequestra, will still keep the discharging cutaneous sinuses active for years. Such sinuses may close temporarily, only to be followed by accumulation of infectious material, reopening with reestablishment of the sinus.

Such remaining foci are usually represented by small destroyed areas of the bone, or by dependent pockets formed by the infection in the cancellous bone which do not favor normal drainage. In either case surgical correction is essential to avoid a long period of invalidism. Being well walled off, chemotherapy has little influence on lesions of this sort. Osteomyelitis from brucella infection is usually very chronic giving rise to localized areas of bone destruction with sinuses which persist over a long period of time. Such foci usually cannot be differentiated roentgenographically from osteomyelitis from other cause. Streptomycin may be effective in the cure of such infections, (Lowe and Lipscomb).

Other unusual types of osteomyelitis are those produced by typhoid and paratyphoid organisms.

Where typhoid fever still exists bone infection involving almost any region of the body occurs. The bone reaction is very similar to other types of pyogenic infection with sclerosis, periosteal reaction, and even necrosis with sequestration.

Paratyphoid infection, although very rarely encountered, produces a much different, almost characteristic appearance. Rounded punched-out areas of destruction appear in the diaphyses of the bones (usually of the knee), bordering upon the epiphyseal line. These are surrounded by areas of sclerosis of the bone and periosteal reaction. The process is similar in some respects to that produced by the cystic type of metaphyseal tuberculosis or sarcoid involvement of bone but is much more rapid, all cases being healed in from two to three months, (Forssman). Friedlander bacilli may cause infection in many other tissues besides the lung. It may be the etiological organism in osteomyelitis, and in this role may be associated with formation of gas in the soft tissues.

CHRONIC ABSCESS OF BONE
BRODIE'S ABSCESS

Brodie's abscess (Fig. 79A) may be defined as a small solitary area of destruction in the cancellous bone, caused by chronic attenuated pyogenic infection, usually staphylococcus. The condition does not provoke severe constitutional or local reaction. There is nothing to indicate a tuberculous etiology. It usu-

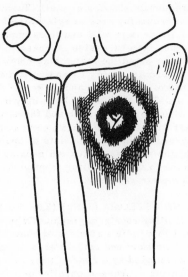

Fig. 79A

ally occurs in young adults, most frequently in males, in a proportion of five to one.

The condition occurs in the tibia in a majority of all cases. The lower end of radius, femur and humerus are the other common sites; but it may occur in any location.

Clinically, this condition occasionally follows an acute infectious process or trauma, but most often occurs without any definite known etiology. The onset is slow, characterized by a rheumatic boring pain, which may be worse at night. The course is chronic, seldom producing any febrile reaction. Chemotherapy has proven of little value.

Pathology and Roentgenological Characteristics, Brodie's Abscess. Pathologically there is a central area of bone destruction located near the end of a long bone, usually without any external fistula or periosteal reaction. This is manifested in the roentgenogram by an area of translucency one to two centimeters in

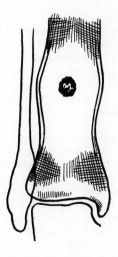

Fig. 79B

diameter, frequently showing a small central sequestrum and a surrounding area of sclerosis of the bone.
The reaction process is mild and finds expression as
sclerosis rather than excessive increase in volume;
the cortical bone about the lesion may show increased
density. If sclerosis is very extensive it may obscure the area of rarefaction and make the diagnosis
more difficult. The shaft of the bone may be normal
in contour or fusiform in outline and there may be
some proliferation of the overlying periosteum.

The treatment usually consists of opening and
curretting of the abscess cavity and packing with
iodoform gauze to insure healing from below, which
results in complete recovery.

OSTEOID OSTEOMA (Jaffe) (Fig. 79B). This is
a condition similar roentgenographically in practically
every respect to Brodie's abscess of bone. It presents a small well defined central area of bone destruction, surrounded by a zone of bone sclerosis
often with varying degrees of parallel periosteal reaction. A small area of increased density within the
destroyed area may be readily interpreted as a tiny
sequestrum. From the roentgen standpoint the two
conditions cannot be differentiated, (J. F. Hamilton).
These usually occur in the ends of long bones, but
they may occur in other locations. Fagerberg and
Rudström have described an instance in which the
arch of a vertebra was involved.

Microscopically, Jaffe has found within the area
of destroyed bone a nidus or nest of osteoid tissue,
with varying degrees of newly formed bone. This latter gives the roentgen impression of a sequestrum
whereas it may really be an evidence of repair by
newly formed bone. At any rate excision of the area
always results in cure. Flaherty et al. have recently
reported on 54 cases of proved osteoid osteoma with
analysis of findings. Knutsson has stressed the not
infrequent occurrence of this condition in children;
because of the excessive production of periosteal reaction its nature may be obscured.

Another rare condition which may give rise to
confusion in diagnosis is nonsuppurative osteomyelitis of Garré.

NONSUPPURATIVE OSTEOMYELITIS (Garré)
This is a more insidious type of osteomyelitis characterized by bone production and sclerosis, with a
limited amount of bone destruction and osteoporosis,
which does not suppurate.

Clinical Manifestation. The disease occurs in
youth and middle age.

A frequent site of involvement is the femur. In
a majority of instances only a single bone is involved.

The disease may have an acute onset with fever
and leucocytosis which rapidly subsides into a clinical course extending over a period of months or
years, or the onset may be insidious and the symptoms appear latent. Some give a history of previous
illness, such as typhoid, influenza, or focal infections, but in the majority of cases no history of previous infection is obtainable.

After the acute onset the patient usually experiences pain of a dull character, with swelling and
tenderness, but only slight constitutional disturbances.

The fever when present is only slight (98.6°-100° F)
and the leucocytosis is mild (8,000-12,000). The patient presents himself for one of the following symptoms: pain, swelling, deformity, limitation of motion
or even fracture.

Pathological and Roentgenological Findings.
The condition is probably due to a low-grade infection in the lymphatics of the bone.

The roentgenogram may present any or all of
the following reactions.
1. Sclerosis.
2. Periosteal Reaction.
3. Bone Destruction.
4. Osteoporosis.

The most outstanding characteristic of the condition is the osteosclerosis either confined to a
small localized area, or involving the entire shaft of
the bone. This may be so pronounced that it even obliterates the medullary canal. This may be homogenous or spotted with areas of destruction. The
areas of destruction produce a moth-eaten appearance and often suggest small cyst formations, but
sequestrum formation does not occur. Destruction
of bone is usually not a prominent feature.

The degree of ossification may vary from an
area beneath the periosteum, producing subperiosteal
localized ossification, to a large irregular mass of
new bone attachment to a normal shaft throughout its
entire length. The periosteum varies in its reaction
from a smooth, rounded deposit to a shaggy bone
production with spicules standing out from the shaft.
This type is often confused with osteogenic sarcoma.

Upon operation a straw-colored fluid is freed
from the marrow cavity, but no evidence of pus is
found. The medullary canal is filled with necrotic
and hemorrhagic material. On culture the staphylococcus aureus is usually found. Suppuration soon
develops following surgical intervention, however.

Differential diagnosis is difficult; in its purely
sclerotic form it resembles the sclerotic osteitis of
lues from which it can hardly be distinguished by
roentgen examination alone. When associated with
periosteal reaction it may resemble Ewing's Sarcoma, or if bone destruction is a prominent feature
it may be confused with osteolytic sarcoma. Due to
its confusion with the various types of sarcoma of
the bone, correct diagnosis is vital. If in doubt, a
biopsy should be taken before any extensive or deforming operation is undertaken.

INFANTILE CORTICAL HYPEROSTOSIS
(Figs. 80A, B, C) (Caffey and Silverman). This is a
condition appearing in infants within the first three
months of life in which local painful swellings appear
in the soft parts over the long bones, ribs, cheeks,
jaws, scapulas, and clavicles. The patient becomes
irritable and feverish with loss of appetite and sensi-
tiveness on handling. Some patients have pseudo-
paralysis, dysphagia, pleurisy, anemia, leucocytosis,
monocytosis, increased sedementation rate and increased serum phosphatase.

The condition is usually self-limited running
its course in a few months and terminating in recovery with restoration of the bones to normal.

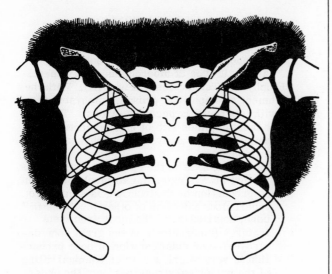

Fig. 80A

Occasionally, however, resolution is not complete and late crippling effects remain, (Caffey). The bone retains its enlarged size, with absorption of the bulky shaft from within causing enlargement of the marrow cavity. Bridges of cortical bone to adjacent bony structures, such as the bones of the forearm, may result causing interference with function. The enlarged shaft tends to cause corresponding enlargement of the adjacent epiphysis.

Some doubt as to its infectious nature has developed because of the report of an instance, (Nelson) of prenatal development of the disease in a woman who had received massive dose estrogen therapy.

An instance has been reported where the condition followed vaccination, (Delano and Butler).

Roentgenographically there is boggy periosteal reaction and diffuse sclerosis of the bone in the region beneath the superficial swelling.

The periosteal reaction may be very thick giving the appearance of subperiosteal infiltration, the sclerosis varies depending upon the degree of periosteal involvement. The cause has not been determined but it is believed that the condition may be due to some unusual type of infection the exact nature of which is not understood.

Some cases of leukemia have been reported in children which produce a very similar periosteal reaction and some degree of bone destruction and sclerosis but these are attended with other confirmatory blood changes. Acute leukemia in children runs a rapid and fatal course; whereas this condition clears up within a few months with restoration of the bony structure to normal. Engelmann's disease (q.v.) produces a similar sclerotic appearance, but this is probably not due to infection. Allen et al. have recently surveyed the 34 cases reported in the literature with discussion.

TUBERCULOSIS OF BONE*

Tuberculous infection may attack any structure of bone in any location giving rise to widely varying

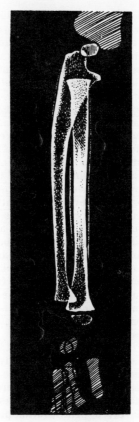

Fig. 80B

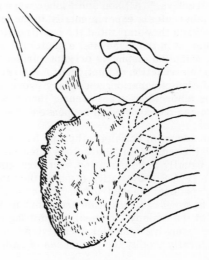

Fig. 80C

manifestations. It may be primary in the bony structure or it may be secondary from some other focus in the body such as tuberculous synovitis, arthritis or rarely pulmonary tuberculosis. Formerly the bovine type of tuberculosis was responsible for a large majority of skeletal involvement; today with almost universal pasteurization of milk and inspection of cattle, this source of infection has almost disappeared. Human type still remains a dangerous source; and all cases of bone tuberculosis should have chest roentgenograms in search of active foci.

In order to understand more readily the roentgen manifestations of the disease in its various forms the essential underlying pathology must be borne in mind. By and large, tuberculosis must be considered as the great bone destroyer. It is one of the diseases characterized by formation of granulomatous masses; when these invade bone, they destroy not only by liberation of bacterial toxins but by pressure of their invading granulomatous deposits. The process is rather slow and insidious, lasting for months and years, rather than days and weeks. If tuberculous granulations develop beneath the periosteum, it will be stripped from its underlying bony attachment and periosteal reaction will occur from its mechanical stimulation. This occurs very rarely and usually to a very limited degree, but it must be borne in mind that it is possible. The roentgen appearance is very similar to that caused by subperiosteal invasion of leukemic infiltration. If the pressure from these tuberculous granulations is great and the cortical structures soft, as in children, expansion of the bone may occur; if the bony cortex is unyielding, as in adults, necrosis occurs.

Ultimate repair of the destroyed bone is largely by fibrous tissue formation, only rarely and usually to a very limited degree does new bone formation occur as a reparative process after tuberculous infection. Allison states that, "In all my cases when compact bone was involved, proliferation predominated; when cancellous bone was affected, the lesions proved to be destructive." Allison and Fisher were able to produce tuberculosis experimentally in the long bones of dogs. When they implanted the bacilli under the periosteum or in the diaphysis, a proliferative process resulted; when the epiphysis or joint surface was inoculated, this reaction did not occur. If however, by reason of sinus formation, secondary pyogenic infection of the tuberculous tract occurs, then new bone formation can be expected in response to the pyogenic organisms.

The advent of antibiotic therapy has done much to change the outlook in tuberculous infections. Streptomycin, usually in combination with para-amino-salicylate (P.A.S.), by static action on the tubercle bacillus, "retards the destructive process of the disease, hastens reossification and shortens the duration of the malady", (Jones), permitting earlier and more extensive remedial operative procedures. These naturally modify the processes of natural healing.

SITES OF BONE INVOLVEMENT

The principal sites of tuberculous bone involvement are:
Short and Long Bones,
    a) epiphysis—(cancellous end of bone)
    b) joint— (arthritis)
    c) diaphysis
    d) metaphysis—(cystic involvement)
Irregular bones, especially,

    a) spine—(vertebral bodies)
    b) carpal bones, especially os magnum
    c) tarsal bones, especially os calcis
Flat Bones, especially cranial bones
    a) Cystic type of tuberculous involvement.

Epiphyseal Tuberculosis (Fig. 81A). With the establishment of epiphyseal growth, epiphyseal infection with tuberculosis becomes evident. This is by far the most common site of involvement.

Roentgenological analysis of epiphyseal tuberculosis indicates,

Point of origin, is in the epiphyseal structures, almost always extending to involve the joint,

Bone production or destruction, is similar to tuberculous infection of other locations in bone; destruction is the most prominent feature—(tuberculosis is the great bone destroyer)—any manifestation of bone production is very slight, due to mechanical lifting of the periosteal structures from the underlying cortex by invasion of granulations.

Expansion or Non-Expansion: No true expansion of the bone.

Condition of Cortex: Broken through in many places from erosion with sinus formation to give exit to the products of infection.

Invasion of Soft Parts: There is no true invasion since the process is not of neoplastic origin.

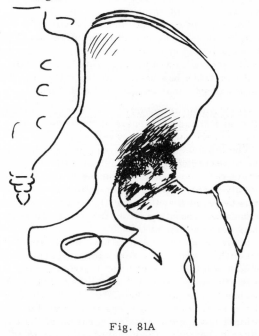

Fig. 81A

Since in a great many instances the epiphysis is intimately connected with the articular cortex of a joint, any involvement of this structure therefore is apt to result in an involvement of the joint. In a great majority of instances the areas of tuberculous destruction start in the epiphysis and spread to involve the joint. Tuberculous infection of bone is a slow insidious process, requiring months and years for its development rather than days and weeks as compared to pyogenic infections. In the beginning stage of tuberculous involvement, especially in this location, there may be no detectable evidence of pathology in the roentgenogram, and yet, there may be extreme pain causing limitation of use of the part. This in turn results in physiological absorption of lime salts —osteoporosis; not until later on is bone destruction from the tuberculous process evident in the roentgenogram. As a result osteoporosis may be present in this condition before bone destruction is evident, a condition which is just the reverse of pyogenic infection.

The first evidence of cortical involvement may be a hazy appearance of the articular cortex in the subchondral area caused by invasion by tuberculous infection. Since this always leads to spread of the infection to the joint it may be considered as a forerunner of tuberculous arthritis. With involvement of the subchondral region, the cartilage becomes affected; tuberculous granulations extend into the joint covering the cartilage like a pannus destroying it. The erosion is greatest in the noncontacting parts of the joint.

Ultimate repair of the destroyed bone is by fibrous tissue formation, rarely by new bone formation unless secondary infection has occurred with pyogenic organisms.

It may be said then that in epiphyseal tuberculosis there is:
1. Haziness of articular cortex, in subchondral region.
2. Osteoporosis of the bone from limited use due to pain, occurring before destruction.
3. Bone destruction as manifested by irregular areas of disintegration in the cancellous tissue.
4. Ultimate repair months or years later by fibrous tissue; very little if any manifestation of new bone formation.

TUBERCULOUS ARTHRITIS: While tuberculous arthritis occurs by extension from epiphyseal involvement in a large majority of instances, there are undoubtedly instances of tuberculous infection of joints which are primarily synovial. The manifestations of tuberculous arthritis is taken up in greater detail in the chapter on arthritis.

DIAPHYSEAL TUBERCULOSIS (Fig. 81B and C). In infants and very young children, before the epiphyseal centers are well established, tuberculosis often attacks the diaphyseal structures or shafts of the bones. The short bones of the hands and feet are most frequently involved giving rise to tuberculous dactylitis or spina ventosa tuberculosa. It may take on a multiple cystic appearance as described by Jungling.

In this location the picture is quite characteristic. When the disease involves the diaphysis of the long bones it presents a more varied appearance. In the long bones of infants it has a tendency not to remain confined to the medullary canal (as in dactylitis), but to involve the subperiosteal layer of the perios-

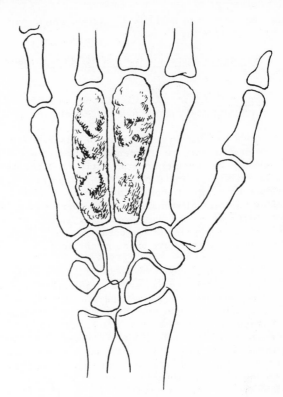

Fig. 81B

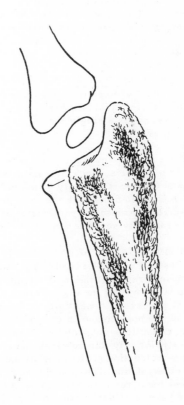

Fig. 81C

teum, giving rise to periosteal reaction which may
serve to confuse the picture.

Roentgenological analysis of diaphyseal tuberculosis.

Point of Origin: Medullary canal as indicated
by the symmetrical central destruction of bone.

Bone Production or Destruction: there is extensive destruction, usually central but only rarely
is there any evidence of bone production. Occasionally tuberculous granulations may develop in the subperiosteal region, stripping the periosteum up and
causing mechanical stimulation of the periosteum. At
times this may be the most prominent feature of the
bone lesion giving rise to an appearance as if there
were a bag-like structure encasing the bone.

Expansion or Non-expansion: The relentless
slow growth of tuberculous granulations in the medullary canal destroys the cancellous bony structures
and soon exerts pressure on the cortex of the bone.
In children the bony structures are less firm, yielding
to pressure, with resulting thinning of the cortex and
expansion of the bone. The shaft changes its normal
slender appearance to that of a thin-walled fusiform
expansion. This is thought by some to be due to a
histamine-induced hyperaemia which in turn causes
decalcification causing the bone to become soft permitting it to accommodate itself to its central granulomatous mass. The appearance is similar to that of
a slow-growing central neoplasm with the exception
that usually the entire shaft is involved and frequently
there is multiple bone involvement.

Condition of the Cortex: The cortex is thinned
from central pressure and may even after a prolonged
period be broken through, but this is usually in numerous places, not in a single location as it is in
malignant tumors.

Invasion or Non-invasion: There is no true invasion of the soft parts, since it is not a neoplastic
growth; the soft tissues are only involved by fistulous
tracts which form to discharge the infectious material. These alone are so characteristic of the condition that they usually serve to establish the diagnosis.

METAPHYSEAL TUBERCULOSIS (Fig. 81D)
(Multiple Cystic Type) (Alexander and Mansuy). In
the metaphyseal regions, the mode of infection is
believed to be by way of the end arteries and the
pathological process is essentially different; the
character of the bony tissue in this region gives rise
to different cancellous character of the bony structure and the relatively thin cortical structure permits easier destruction of the bony tissue and less
likelihood of expansion. The character of the circulation makes local occlusion possible. As a result
cone-shaped areas of destruction occur, finally becoming rounded and cystlike with occasionally tiny
sequestra, but these are usually quickly destroyed

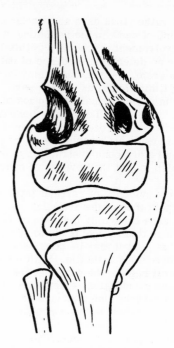

Fig. 81D

leaving only the punched-out appearance. Any of the
other elements of bone reaction may also be present
depending upon the circumstances and degree of involvement of the various bone elements.

The process may spread to involve the entire
length of the bone. Vastine and Bacon describe it
as follows:

"Cystic tuberculosis of bones in children is due
to dissemination of tubercle bacilli through the blood
stream. Large cystlike formations involve the
bones. In the roentgenogram rarefaction originates
in the marrow which may be single or multiple. The
process may appear diffusely through the entire bone
or may appear as circumscribed rarefactions in
certain sites of predilection. In the diffuse type the
cortex and medulla cannot be differentiated. The entire bone is characterized by weblike structure of
increased density. This is the initial stage and represents the more acute process."

Where no secondary infection is present, there
is only moderate sclerosis of the bone. The circumscribed type is characterized by a round rather
smoothly outlined, punched-out area of decreased
density. The cortex is a paper-thin shell. There may
be a faint ring of sclerosis about these cystic areas
or a clear-cut margin with no alteration in the density
of the surrounding bone. This type represents a healing stage and these cysts may proceed without appreciable change "for a long time or may progress to
abscess formation with eventual sinus formation." In
rare instances, such cystic areas of destruction may
appear throughout the entire shaft of a bone (F. Ziady
and G. Selzer).

"SPONDYLARTHRITIS." (Osteomyelitis of Spine) (Saenger). This condition, occurring in infants and young children, is characterized by insidious onset, slowly progressive over a one or two months' period, finally healing in from two to eight months, with restoration to normal in most cases. It gives the impression of a low-grade type of infection.

Roentgenographically it is characterized by marrowing of the intervertebral discs and some sclerosis of the adjacent margins of the vertebral bodies. It may closely resemble tuberculous spondylitis from which it must be differentiated; in this condition, however, the dissolution of the cartilage and sclerosis develop much more rapidly (Guri).

PERIOSTITIS DEFORMANS. Periostitis Deformans is a condition described by Sorians, as a hyperostosing disease characterized by superimposed periosteal layers of periosteal involving chiefly the phalanges. The appearance is not unlike syphilitic or tuberculous dactylitis. The condition appears to run a definite course subsiding after a period of months or a year. The roentgenographic findings four appearances:

 a) periosteal thickening covering the bone with exhuberant bony growth through which the shaft can usually be visualized,
 b) osteophytes or osseous nodules,
 c) periarticular osteophytes,
 d) alterations in the osseous tissue with diffuse bony condensation, followed by osteoporotic zones invading the entire bone.

There may be some connection of this condition with toxiallergic action of tuberculosis, affecting only susceptible individuals.

TUBERCULOSIS IN SPECIAL LOCATIONS; SPONDYLITIS

Tuberculous spondylitis (Fig. 81E). The most frequent site of involvement with bone tuberculosis is the spine. The infection attacks the vertebral body in very much the same manner as it does cancellous bone structure elsewhere. Tuberculous infection invades the cancellous structure causing necrosis of bone with spread to the intervertebral cartilaginous disc and causes its ultimate destruction also. The articular processes are composed of denser more compact bone; they are rarely involved, remaining as buttresses in supporting the spinal column. The weight of the body exerted upon the diseased vertebra causes collapse with resulting wedge-shaped deformity; compression of the vertebra may cause a greater compactness of the unabsorbed lime salts giving a roentgenographic picture simulating bone sclerosis. The angulation produced by the collapse of the vertebral body results in kyphotic deformity and prominence of the spinous process of the involved vertebra. The two other conditions most likely to be confused with tuberculous infection of the spine are compression fracture of the vertebral body, and metastatic malignant involvement. Tuberculosis destroys the intervertebral disc while in both of these other conditions, the disc is preserved; in com-

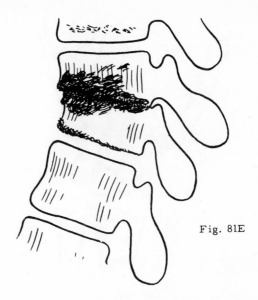

Fig. 81E

pression fracture the disc is elastic and returns to normal after trauma, while metastatic malignant involvement destroys the cancellous bone but does not affect the cartilage. Large venous sinusoids traverse the middle of the vertebral body, the decrease in density which marks their passage must not be confused with actual bone destruction, (Wagoner and Pendergrass).

Modern methods of examination with the tomograph may lead to earlier diagnosis of the tuberculous involvement and thereby shorten the course and severity of the disease as pointed out by Perroy and Mestre.

The tuberculous infection is confined by strong ligaments and heavy muscles and the bulging shadow of a paravertebral abscess can be seen clearly in the roentgenogram. If the involved area is below the 10th thoracic vertebra bulging of the psoas muscle may be present indicating a psoas abscess. By this means the infection may be spread to adjacent vertebrae, or distant vertebrae may be involved by blood stream inoculation. With fixation by plaster jacket or fusing operation, the process may heal and the patient recover.

Certain unusual cases of tuberculous spondylitis have been reported without destruction of the disc with "sclerosis" of the vertebra. It is possible that this might be of the type of metaphyseal involvement seen in the long bones with cystic involvement (Auerbach and Stemmerman; and Poppel, et al.).

Rare cases of psoas abscess have been reported due to pure staphylococcus infection without tuberculous involvement, (Zadek).

Tuberculosis of the Carpal Bones (Fig. 81F). Involvement of the bones of the wrist is very rare but the bone which is occasionally involved is the os magnum. The process is essentially similar to that seen in other bones except that being almost entirely surrounded by articulating surfaces, the involvement

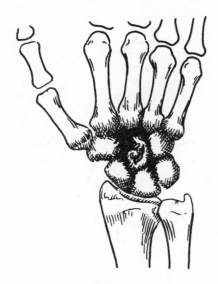

Fig. 81F

is almost complete. The outline of the entire bone becomes hazy, this is followed by osteoporosis which further serves to obliterate the bony outline. Finally destruction occurs, sinuses may develop and a long-drawn-out process ensues. If recovery occurs without operative procedure, ankylosis may be expected.

Tuberculosis of the Tarsal Bones (Fig. 81G). Any of the tarsal bones may become involved, but the most common site of the disease is in the cancellous structures of the os calcis. Although the articular surface may become involved, the disease may remain confined to the body or tuberosity of the bone assuming more the cystic type similar to that seen in metaphyseal involvement. In this region especially, compression of the partially destroyed bone may, through a greater compactness of the unabsorbed lime salts, give an impression in the roentgenogram of sclerosis of the bone surrounding the destructive area.

Cystic Tuberculosis of Flat Bones: The cranial bones are most frequently involved. The condition is extremely rare, being confined almost entirely to in-

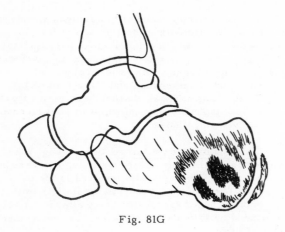

Fig. 81G

fants and young children. Tuberculous involvement of these bones takes on a much different picture from that seen in long bones. The infection starts in the middle table in the diploetic structure (Erdheim). It spreads to the adjacent portions of the inner and outer tables producing rounded areas of destruction. The hole in the inner table is usually somewhat larger than that in the outer table so that on roentgen examination the margins of the destroyed areas present a fringelike appearance of lessened density. Immediately beyond this the bone may present a sclerotic appearance. New areas of involvement may extend out from the margins of the destroyed areas.

In differentiation from other diseases the condition resembles luetic osteitis from which it may be most difficult to differentiate roentgenographically. The punched-out areas of Schüller-Christian's disease are clear cut and smooth without the ragged edges or sclerotic margins. At times, after roentgen therapy to Schüller-Christian lesions they may fill in at the margins giving a somewhat similar appearance. Metastatic carcinoma produces a worm-eaten appearance of destruction which is not at all similar to this condition; other elements such as age of the patient, primary carcinomatous involvement, etc., serve to aid in the diagnosis. An interesting survey of the modern concept of tuberculous diseases has been made by Poppel, et al.

SPIROCHAETAL INFECTIONS
SYPHILIS (Lues) OF BONE

In general it may be stated that syphilis is the great bone producer. In every condition in which syphilis occurs, there is almost always some manifestation of bone production. Syphilis may be congenital or acquired. Either form may give rise to any of the lesions of bone encountered in the disease. Naturally the greatest number of cases of congenital involvement are in infants or young children. Syphillis, like other infections, produces different reactions during the growth period in children and in adults.

CONGENITAL SYPHILIS* (Fig. 82) usually manifests itself at or immediately after birth; it may disclose itself in two ways, either as,
1. parallel periosteal reaction involving multiple long bones, or
2. syphilitic epiphysitis and metaphysitis, showing bone destruction.

Either one or the other of these two lesions seems to predominate in any given case; where multiple periosteal involvement occurs, destructive lesions of the epiphysis appear to be absent or less prominent; on the other hand, when epiphyseal lesions are most pronounced, any periosteal reaction will usually be confined to the regions immediately adjacent to the destroyed areas. Attention has been called to the presence of the parallel type of periosteal elevation in the long bones of apparently healthy new born infants. This is especially likely to occur in premature infants. It has been suggested that it may be a manifestation of a local exaggeration of the normal appositional growth of bone. Hancox does not feel that it has any relationship to disease. Ordinarily, it

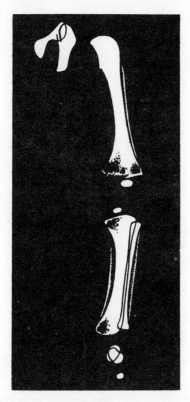

Fig. 82

disappears rapidly; if it remains or shows its first appearance sometime after birth, it would seem that the presence of such a reaction in the bones of a young infant should be considered as suspicious of congenital lues until proven otherwise. In our experience either of these manifestations is more reliable than the Wasserman test in the diagnosis of congenital syphilis in young infants within the first few weeks of life. The lacework type of periosteal syphilis is rarely, if ever encountered in the newborn infant.

If untreated, however, the infantile lesions may subside with apparent healing, only to break out again in a few months or years later with new bone manifestations. At this time the lace-work type of periostitis may become very evident, and heavy deposits of periosteal new bone may even give an impression of scurvy.

The picture may be very readily confused with scurvy, rickets, or even heavy metal poisoning; confirmatory clinical signs therefore must always be present. In scurvy the zone of destruction is uniform going completely across the bone, with a zone of increased density below giving the appearance of a double epiphyseal line. The administration of antiluetic treatment such as penicillin causes almost immediate regression of the pathological lesions with apparent restoration to normal within a few weeks. Continued observation over many months fails to reveal evidence of recurrence of the disease. During this healing stage differentiation from scurvy may be

most difficult; in scurvy, however, periosteal reaction is bulky. In luetic involvement at any stage there is no evidence of rosary formation. In rickets, the expanded enlargement of the end of the bone, the widened zone of epiphyseal bone growth, the extreme degree of osteoporosis and the lack of pronounced periosteal reaction all serve to differentiate the condition. Heavy metal poisons produce a much more intense zone of calcium deposit at the epiphyseal line, usually however without destruction, periosteal reaction or the other manifestations of luetic involvement.

SYPHILITIC EPIPHYSITIS

The lesions of the epiphyseal region are characterized by:

1. Irregular serration of the epiphyseal line— caused by saw-toothed areas of destruction in the diaphysis which usually does not go completely across the entire width of the bone. These may occur most pronouncedly in the diaphyseal regions of the inner condyles of the tibias and femurs and in the upper humeral epiphyses giving rise to Wimberger's Sign (not to be confused with Wimberger's Sign in scurvy, q.v.). In this location this finding is almost diagnostic in itself.
2. A very small amount of parallel periosteal reaction may arise over the diaphyseal region immediately above the epiphyseal line.
3. A light zone of increased calcium deposit may be present just beyond the epiphyseal line.

Syphilitic epiphysitis in older children takes on a similar appearance with irregular bone destruction at the epiphyseal line often with Wimberger's Sign, some adjacent bone sclerosis and periosteal reaction on the adjacent diaphyseal side. Engeset, Ekk and Gilje recognize five zones in the repair of syphilitic epiphysitis depicting the various structural changes and signs.

SYPHILITIC LESIONS OF LATER LIFE*

Clinical Manifestations. In later life individuals of any age may be attacked by syphilitic bone disease without respect to sex or mode of life. It may involve one or several bones. The tibia is the most common site in long bones. Frontal eminences and parietal bosses are the most frequently involved bones of the skull. The destruction of the bridge of the nose is a common manifestation of involvement in the facial bones. Spirochete pallida multiply in great numbers in areas of active bone growth; they may even be observed within osteoblasts.

Syphilis may attack any structure of bone causing any combination of the following manifestations:

A. Periostitis
B. Osteitis
C. Osteomyelitis
D. Arthritis

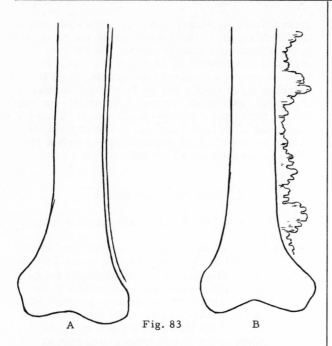

Fig. 83

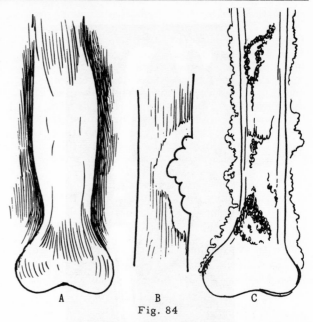

Fig. 84

Pathological Characteristics and Their Radiological Manifestations

A. SYPHILITIS PERIOSTITIS (Fig. 83A and B). Occurs in two forms:
1. The parallel type, and
2. The lace-work type of periosteal reaction. The parallel type is represented roentgenologically by a white line running along parallel to the shaft of the bone (Fig. 83A). This type is usually found on many of the long bones in young infants suffering with congenital syphilis. The parallel type is not characteristic of syphilis; it occurs also from trauma and infection. In older individuals the parallel type of periosteal reaction is not so frequently encountered from syphilis but is more apt to be the result of trauma or infection.

The lace-work type of periosteal reaction at any age is characteristic of syphilis (Fig. 83B). This type of periosteal reaction consists of short spicules of newly formed bone radiating outward perpendicular to the shaft and bending backward in loops, producing a "lacework" appearance. None of the other structures of bone are involved. Periostitis is most commonly seen on the anterior surface of the tibia, and lateral surface of the distal end of the ulna. This is probably due to the fact that in these locations the periosteum is most subject to repeated trauma. Syphilitic periostitis of the metacarpals and phalanges is known as dactylitis (spine ventosa syphilitica).

It differs from tuberculous dactylitis in that the periosteum is merely raised by bulky subperiosteal granulations covering the shaft like a cloak with little if any bone destruction; the intact shaft can be clearly seen through the bulky periosteal reaction.

(B) OSTEITIS, as the name implies, has its origin in the cortex (Fig. 84A). It is a condition in which the bone structure becomes dense and sclerotic showing an ivorylike appearance from the excessive calcium deposit. In any instance in which there is osteitis without accompanying bone destruction, syphilis must be suspected. Osteitis is shown in the roentgenogram as a thickening of the bone structure. It probably is akin to fibrosis and scar tissue formation as seen in chronic infections of the soft parts. Osteitis may be the forerunner of gumma formation in the bone. Gumma formation may occur in the center of a large area of bone sclerosis as a result of a reduction in the blood supply from the sclerotic process itself (Fig. 84B), or it may occur without previous sclerosis of the bone. When gumma formation does occur, it has similar roentgenographic characteristics in bone to which a syphilitic lesion has in the skin or soft parts, namely, a scalloped circinate lesion with indurated margins. Gumma in the long bones is seen most often in the humerus and tibia; in the skull, it often involves the parietal and frontal eminences.

In uncomplicated syphilitic osteitis, there is bone production only, in the form of sclerosis. If this leads to gumma formation, then bone destruction occurs as well. There is some thickening of the bone, which often becomes fusiform, but no true expansion of the shaft occurs. The cortex is sclerotic and eburnated, but is not broken through except where destruction occurs from gumma and this appearance is quite characteristic. There is no true invasion of soft parts. Syphilitic gumma however may occur without much bone sclerosis; merely representing a destroyed area in the bone. It may be difficult under these circumstances to differentiate from metastatic carcinoma.

(C) SYPHILITIC OSTEOMYELITIS. Syphilitic osteomyelitis is a condition similar in all respects to pyogenic osteomyelitis with the exception that the roentgenographic appearance is out of all proportions to the clinical manifestations of the disease (Fig. 84C). Upon this point alone the differential diagnosis may rest. Clinically the patient may not seem very sick but roentgenographically his condition may seem very severe. There is usually a greater amount of bone production and less actual bone destruction than in pyogenic osteomyelitis. The roentgen characteristics, therefore, are similar to osteomyelitis of pyogenic origin:

1. Central or medullary origin.
2. Bone production and destruction occurring at the same time.
3. No true expansion of shaft.
4. Breaking through cortex with good bone in between.
5. No invasion of soft parts as by a tumor mass.

(D) SYPHILITIS EPIPHYSITIS is a congenital manifestation of the disease and has been fully discussed under that heading.

(E) SYPHILITIC ARTHRITIS will be taken up in detail in the chapter on Arthritis.

YAWS

Yaws is a tropical disease caused by the Treponema pertenue, rarely seen in the United States.

It may affect any or all of the bones of the body. It shows itself roentgenographically as a low-grade osteomyelitis usually originating in the medullary canal. The cortex is thickened and the periosteum may be stripped up from the bone. Two types are described:

1. The more active type in which there is destruction of cortex with or without periosteal repair due to the fact that the periosteum may be destroyed, resulting in cavities within the cortex, often just beneath the periosteum.

2. A more chronic form in which rounded vacuoles appear in the bone. These vary in size from 1 mm. to 2 or 3 cm. in diameter. There may be considerable deformity of the shaft.

The process may attack articular surfaces, causing erosion of the bone beneath the cartilage. Roentgenographically the diagnosis can rarely be made except in regions where the disease is prevalent.

FUNGUS INFECTIONS OF BONE
ACTINOMYCOSIS

Actinomycosis is a disease caused by the streptothrix actinomyces or ray fungus, occurring in the United States, especially in the upper Mississippi Valley. Infection with this organism causes "lumpy-jaw" in cattle. It is believed that the organism may be frequently harbored about the teeth and tonsils and that it need not be contracted by chewing grass or straw. It is a chronic infectious disease characterized by suppurative lesions in the soft parts; when the infection spreads to involve the bone it produces a localized osteomyelitis

similar to that caused by pyogenic infection. "Sulphur granules" occurring in the discharge are almost pure colonies of the organism; final diagnosis must be made by their detection.

Clinical Manifestations and Roentgenological Characteristics. This disease occurs most frequently in young adults--males predominate. It may involve the mandible, long bones or spine although any of the bones of the body may be involved.

The clinical manifestations vary according to location of involvement.

When it involves the jaw, there is enlargement from brawny edema and fibrosis of the tissues of the mouth and tongue (wooden tongue). Pain may be slight, especially at the onset, or may become very severe when the disease is well advanced.

The mandible is usually involved by spread of the soft-part infection, causing a localized osteomyelitis. The roentgenographic appearance may be indistinguishable from pyogenic osteomyelitis or other types of mycotic infection. There is destruction of the bone often with rounded circinate border, with sclerosis and increased deposit of lime salts near the margin of the destroyed area. Periosteal reaction is usually not very pronounced when the mandible is involved unless secondary infection by pyogenic organisms is present. When the long bones are involved periosteal reaction may be prolific even resembling sarcoma. A rather characteristic "lumpy" appearance of the adjacent soft parts may lead to the suspicion of the type of infection but differential diagnosis is usually dependent upon finding the characteristic organisms in the pus.

When the spine is attacked, two patterns of reaction are recognized, (Bayling and Wear). If primary in the vertebrae, a "soap-bubble-like appearance develops showing multiple small areas of rarefaction surrounded by zones of normal or dense bone. Paravertebral soft tissue swelling is present along the involved segments or beyond. Or, if spinal involvement is secondary due to spread from abdominal infection a totally different picture is produced; intense sclerosis develops with long spur-like projections running longitudinally along the spine bridging across the vertebrae. Eburnated bone, changes the lateral margins of the vertebrae into a bridge replacing the fine trabecullar pattern into sclerotic bone. Any destruction which may be present is overshadowed by bone production. Collapse of the vertebral bodies and narrowing of the discs is only slight. At operation granulomatous masses not unlike tumors are found which may be difficult to differentiate from new growth. Sinus tracts may be present.

BLASTOMYCOSIS OF BONE

Primary bone lesions of blastomycosis are almost certainly hematogenous in origin with unknown portal of entry. Bone involvement occurs most frequently as part of a systemic infection. Clinically and roentgenologically it resembles tuberculosis.

Clinical Manifestations. Sudden onset with pain, worse at night, is a constant early symptom. There is little or no elevation of temperature unless the bone involvement is a part of a systemic infection. At the onset involvement of the long bones resembles ordinary acute pyogenic osteomyelitis except for the mild febrile reaction and absence of leukocytosis. Without cutaneous lesion there is no hint as to the type of infection. Later the persistent sinuses following spontaneous or surgical drainage, together with X-ray findings and identification of the organism, clinch the diagnosis. Coccidioidal granuloma can only be differentiated by laboratory methods. Due to the chronic course, it may resemble tuberculosis with associated pyogenic infection.

Pathological and Radiological Characteristics. Early lesions in the long bones may show periostitis or central necrosis alone or in combination. Multiple adjacent foci usually coalesce.

The one more or less constant feature of the roentgenologic findings is the presence of a sharp line of demarkation between the involved areas and the adjacent normal-appearing bone. In the short bones, single or multiple areas of complete destruction may be seen involving chiefly the central portions of the bones. If close to the articular surface, a thin shell of bone may remain beneath the cartilage or the joint may be completely destroyed.

When the spine is involved it resembles tuberculosis most effectively. There is destruction and collapse of one or more vertebral body, with narrowing of the disc with little if any bone production. There is paravertebral abscess formation which dissects under the spinal ligaments, (Reeves and Pedersen).

MADUROMYCOSIS
MYCETOMA - (MADURA FOOT)

A chronic diffuse infiltration of tissues (usually of a foot) by one of several varieties of the ray fungus. In the characteristic advanced form, the foot is tremendously swollen and has many sinuses. The universal permeation of tissues may leave the foot diffusely destroyed and the bones barely visible in the roentgenogram. The roentgenographic appearance resembles that of actinomycosis.

There are areas of bone destruction and large areas of shaggy new bone formation. The roentgenographic appearance is not characteristic, and the final diagnosis can only be made by microscopic examination, (Carroll).

COCCIDIOIDAL GRANULOMA—OF BONE

Coccidioidal granuloma is due to an infection with Oidium Coccidioides normally found in the soil, (Carter). The disease is most prevalent in the San Joaquin Valley, California, but in recent years

it has spread to Southern Texas and adjacent areas. Clinically it is usually present in the skin and soft parts and when bone involvement occurs it is usually due to spread of the soft part infection or to inoculation through the blood stream. Clinically it is thought that the condition presents two phases; a primary phase of lung involvement characterized by a mild "influenzal" attack possibly associated with "erythema nodosum" which goes on to recovery within a few weeks. This is followed by a secondary granulomatous stage which may come on at an irregular interval, involving various bones of the body. Only a small percent develop the secondary stage, (Benninghoven and Miller).

Involvement of all of the bones of the body, with the exception of the facial bones, has been described. When the long bones are involved, the infection has a predilection for bony prominence. When the spine is involved, the disease affects bodies, arches, processes alike, showing no preference. Depending upon the manner of spread of the infection, the point of origin when the bone is involved is either peripheral, in the case of direct extension from infection of the soft parts, or central, as occurs when inoculation is into the bone by way of the blood stream. The reaction in bone is predominantly destructive; the margins of destroyed area may be punched out or may appear rather diffuse. They are usually multiple and have a tendency to involve bony prominences about the joints, although they may be either epiphyseal or diaphyseal in location. Except in the bones of the hands and feet, they seem to prefer cancellous bone. Areas of bone destruction in skull involvement may show their greatest diameter at the periphery in the outer table. When the lesion is near a joint, a plate of bone often remains between the destroyed area and the joint; the cartilage is not destroyed as consistently as in tuberculosis.

The degree and character of bone production is variable; in many instances no bone production is present at all, even after long chronic involvement. Bone production may occur, however, as periosteal new bone formation or bone sclerosis about the lesion; this is most marked after operative interference or secondary infection. In any event it is slow in formation and unlike osteomyelitis only occurs late in the disease; it may be shaggy in type, showing spicules radiating into the tissue.

Joints are usually involved from adjacent infection of bone or soft parts. Under exceptional circumstances infection may be primarily in the joint itself. The earliest manifestation may be merely increase in synovial fluid in the joint. The clinical findings may precede any roentgen manifestation; in any event the roentgen findings are not characteristic of the disease. Owing to its chronicity, the condition with which it is most frequently confused is tuberculous arthritis. In this regard it must be said that joint involvement is exceptional. There is no evidence in this disease of selective destruction of noncontacting cartilages, or selective preservation of weight-bearing cartilages; there is no tendency to erosion of the articular cortex beneath a preserved cartilage with formation of so-called "Kissing Sequestra" as described in tuberculous arthritis.

The diagnosis must be ultimately made by microscopic examination.

Disseminated Granuloma Inguinale has been reported, (Rhinehart and Bauer) throughout the long and short bones of the body without evidence of sclerotic reaction. The changes resemble those seen in metastatic malignancy and are not specific for the condition. In association with a genital lesion, such multiple osseus lesions should be suspicious of spread of the disease. Biopsy with demonstration of DONOVAN bodies is necessary to establish the diagnosis.

TORULA (Cryptococcus), (Carter). Torula infection seems to have a great predilection for skin, meninges, and the lung structures. Very rarely does it affect bone; when it does it is usually due to direct extension from some other pre-existing lesion elsewhere in the body.

A granulomatous mass develops in the cancellous tissue at the end of a long bone, and spreads to involve the joint, causing bone destruction with or without bone sclerosis. Its extremely invasive character is a characteristic of all fungus infections. One rather striking characteristic is its extension to the skin presenting numerous ulcerations and sinuses. When the skull is involved it produces punched out areas of destruction. Potassium Iodide therapy usually cures the disease unless meningeal infection develops. Healing of the local lesion may be accompanied by ankylosis if the joint cartilage is destroyed.

PARASITIC INFECTIONS
Ecchinococcus Cyst of Bone

Bone involvement occurs in less than 1% of the cases of ecchinococcus disease. The condition is very uncommon in the United States.

Clinical Manifestations. The development in bones is slow, insidious, and latent. Pain occurs only late in the disease and usually follows some complication, usually a fracture or infection; it is usually of an intermittent character. Pathological fracture may occur. There is usually a large palpable fluctuating tumefaction in the region of the bone involvement.

Pathological and Roentgenological Findings.

1. Early in the disease there are one or many small cystic areas of destruction like bunches of grapes--rounded, punched out, sharply outlined.

2. But without periosteal reaction or condensing osteitis at the periphery--no new bone formation.

3. Later the bony enlargement may become perceptible or palpable, with fusiform expansion. The bony swelling has a typical areolar appearance infiltrated by large cavities of more or less irregular contour but discrete.

4. The cortex is reduced to a shell under the periosteum which may be broken through spontaneously.

The picture resembles cystic osteitis from an anatomical standpoint. Diagnosis from the roentgenogram alone is difficult and frequently impossible.

QUESTIONS ON INFECTIONS OF BONE

Questions marked with a dagger deal with rare and less-important conditions.

1. What two general types of osteomyelitis are recognized?

2. How does infection gain access to the bone in the medullary type? In the localized type?

3. What are the clinical manifestations of osteomyelitis?

4. How long an interval of time may elapse before osteomyelitis gives evidence in the roentgenogram? Where are the first manifestations of infection most frequently found?

5. Show by diagram how the infection spreads and how it gives rise to the roentgenological manifestation of the disease.

6. Using the scheme of bone analysis, indicate the roentgenological manifestations of osteomyelitis when untreated by drugs. After use of chemotherapy.

7. What is meant by involucrum? By sequestrum? By cloaca formation?

8. Describe the roentgen findings in the subperiosteal type of osteomyelitis. To what are they due?

9. What are the roentgen manifestations of acute (nontuberculous) epiphysitis?

10. How does the localized, direct-extension type of osteomyelitis differ from the deep medullary type?

†11. What is meant by Brodie's abscess and what are its clinical and roentgen manifestations?

12. How does tuberculous infection manifest itself in the diaphysis? Is diaphyseal tuberculosis a common or rare occurrence? Describe epiphyseal involvement.

†13. What is spina ventosa tuberculosa? How does it differ from spina ventosa syphilitica?

14. What predominating characteristic is present in all types of syphilitic bone involvement?

15. Describe roentgen appearance of syphilitic: periostitis, osteitis, osteomyelitis, epiphysitis, gumma, and arthritis.

†16. What are the roentgen manifestations of Garré's nonsuppurating osteomyelitis?

†17. What is infantile cortical hyperostosis and what bones does it usually involve?

†18. What are the roentgen manifestations of chronic fungus infections? Can they be differentiated from other types of chronic pyogenic infection roentgenologically? How can the diagnosis be made?

†19. What are the roentgen manifestations of coccidioidal granuloma? What geographical locality is the source of such infections?

†20. What are the roentgen manifestations of torula infection in bone?

†21. How is infection with ecchinococcus cysts manifested?

†22. What are the roentgen manifestations of yaws?

GLANDULAR AND METABOLIC DISTURBANCE (Chapter VIII)

Influencing Bone Growth

- A. Thyroid
    1. Hypothyroidism—Cretinism
    2. Hyperthyroidism

- B. Gonads
    1. Hypogonadism
        Post menopausal osteoporosis
    2. Hypergonadism

- C. Pituitary
    1. Anterior Lobe
        a. Deficiency
        b. Hyperfunction—Acromegaly
    2. Pituitary Disease—Adenomata
        a. Chromophobic
        b. Eosinophilic
        c. Basophilic

Influencing Bone Structure

- D. Thymus
    Defects in mesenchymal development
    1. Osteogenesis Imperfecta, (Fragilitas Ossium; Periosteal Aplasia)
        a. Congenita
        b. Tarda
        c. Idiopathic Osteopsathyrosis
    Defects in chondro-osteal development
    1. Achondroplasia, (Chondrodystrophia Foetalis)
    2. Dyschondroplasia (Ollier's Disease)
    3. Diaphyseal Aclasia, (Multiple exostoses)
    4. Dyschondroplasia with hemangiomata, (Maffucci's Syndrome)
    5. Chondroosteodystrophy, (Morquio-Brailsford Disease)
    6. Chondrodystrophic Calcificans Congenita; (Punctate Epiphyseal Dysplasia; Stippled Epiphyses)
    7. Thiemann's Disease

- E. Parathyroid
    1. Hyperparathyroidism (Von Recklinghausen's Disease)
    2. Osteitis Fibrosa (Cystica)
        Generalized
        Localized

- F. Other Diseases of Unknown Etiology
    1. Fibrous Dysplasia of Bone
        Polyostotic
        Monostotic
    2. Looser's Transformation Zones, (Pseudo Fractures), Vascular Erosion
    3. Osteitis Deformans, (Paget's Disease)
        Ivory Vertebra
    4. Leontiasis Ossea
    5. Osteopetrosis, (Marble Bones—Albers-Schonberg's Disease)
    6. Osteopathica Hyperostotica Sclerotisans Multiplex Infantilis, (Engelmann's Disease),
        Progressive Diaphyseal Dysplasia
    7. Osteopoikilosis
    8. Tubular Sclerosis of Bone
    9. Familial Metaphyseal Dysplasia

- G. Lipoid Granulomatosis of Bone - Xanthomatosis
    1. HAND-SCHÜLLER-CHRISTIAN'S DISEASE
    2. LETTERER-SIEWE'S DISEASE
    3. EOSINOPHILIC GRANULOMA
    4. GAUCHER'S DISEASE
    5. NIEMANN-PICK'S DISEASE
    6. GARGOYLISM (HUNTER-HURLER DISEASE)

Chapter VIII

GLANDULAR AND METABOLIC DISTURBANCES

There can be no doubt of the influence of the endocrine secretions on certain features of bone growth and metabolism. The functions of the various endocrine glands are so complexly interrelated, however, that it is difficult to determine the specific effect of any particular secretion on bone metabolism or growth. Certain outstanding examples, however, serve as a guide to the effect of various endocrine secretions on bone, (Clark).

The various disturbances in bone growth have been considered as definite disease entities in order to more clearly elucidate the subject; that these conditions overlap in many respects will be evident as the subject is pursued. Sears has correlated and discussed the various bone dystrophies in a very interesting manner.

THYROID. "The thyroid has little or no primary action on the rate of growth but profound influence on differentiation of bone tissue." Growth may proceed for a time in absence of the hormone, but tissue differentiation is delayed and osseous nuclei are late in appearing. Such retardation in epiphyseal development is seen in cretinism; generalized retardation may lead to dwarfism.

When they do appear they may be irregular and fragmented. The best method for determining the cause of their delay in development is to observe their response to the administration of thyroid medication.

Conversely, under the influence of increased thyroid secretion, there is an increase in differentiation of bone tissue, and an increase in the ossification of epiphyses and osseous tissue differentiation. A number of bone dyscrasias have been attributed to malfunction of the thyroid gland, especially chondrodystrophia foetalis.

Extreme hypothyroidism may result in decalcification of the bones. Ordinarily this is merely of osteoporotic variety but if the decalcification is rapid, all of the changes of osteitis fibrosa cystica may be present and the condition may resemble hyperparathyroidism. Under these conditions the differential diagnosis will depend upon the blood analysis; in hyperthyroidism the calcium-phosphorus ratio is normal, whereas in hyperparathyroidism there are high calcium and low phosphorus values.

GONADS. "The effect of the gonads on skeletal development is said to be due to the elaboration of sex hormone, a product of interstitial cells. No one fully understands the exact mechanism controlling epiphyseal closure, but there is reason to believe the gonads are deeply concerned in the process. In case of sexual precocity, the epiphyses unite long before the normal time. Conversely, if the gonadal function is impaired or lost during childhood or adolescence, the epiphyses remain open, growth continues beyond

the normal time and eunuchoid gigantism results. The pituitary-gonad-thyroid interrelation introduces many ramifications of thought relating to epiphyseal closure, and a diversity of opinion exists. Until further evidence is offered, it will simplify matters to regard epiphyseal closure as predominantly a function of sex hormone."

Post-menopausal osteoporosis is a condition in which an extreme degree of osteoporosis develops after the menopause, presumably from lack of gonadal secretion. There is a deficiency in the organic matrix of bone from lack of osteoblasts or deficiency of protein to lay down in the matrix. It does not differ from osteoporosis from other cause, except that it involves all of the bony structures and attains a severe degree. In osteomalacia the alkaline phosphatase is usually high; in ordinary senile osteoporosis it is usually normal, never elevated. It is usually impossible to cause redeposition of calcium salts in the weakened bony structures by any means.

Hypergonadism is very rare. It results in sexual precocity and rapid growth. It is characterized by early appearance of the epiphyses (due to the thyroid influence), rapid bone growth (due to the influence of the pituitary), and early closure of the epiphyses (due to excess sex hormone).

Though there is rapid early growth, early closure of epiphyses results in a shorter stature.

ADRENAL. "Adrenal cortex tumors result in the same clinical picture as basophilic adenomas of the pituitary (Cushing's Syndrome), and certain tumors of gonadal origin; pseudohermaphroditism (hypertrophy of the clitoris and stenosis of the vagina), pubic hair and deep voice. There is early appearance of increase in development of all ossification centers, but these do not show premature closure.

"In the absence of tumor, the effect of the adrenal, if any, on skeletal growth, remains unknown."

Precocity of bone growth also occurs in adrenal hyperplasia.

THYMUS. No known definite effect on skeletal growth; it is thought by some that it has an inherent effect upon the development of mesenchymal tissue as indicated in the number and function of the osteoblasts.

PARATHYROID. Parathyroid hormone has no direct effect on bone growth except its influence on fixation and mobilization of calcium.

PINEAL. Has no known effect.

PITUITARY. The pituitary is considered as the pacemaker for the other endocrine glands. Many hormones are elaborated in the pituitary; there are three most concerned with bone growth.

1. Growth hormone of the pituitary gland, which probably is elaborated by the acidophilic cells of the anterior lobe, plays a major role in controlling rate of bone growth. Decreased pituitary secretion produces dwarfism (asexual ateleiosis; Lorain type of infantilism). Increased pituitary secretion produces increase in bone growth, especially the long bones; if this occurs before epiphyseal closure, gigantism results, whereas if it occurs after epiphyseal union, acromegaly occurs. It has little effect on the rate of appearance or closure of epiphyseal centers.

2. Thyrotropic principle (of the pituitary gland) is presumably derived from the alkaline fraction of the anterior lobe. "It is closely allied to the growth hormone and serves as a connecting link between pituitary and thyroid. Pure excess or deficiency would theoretically have the same effect on skeletal development of hyperthyroidism and hypothyroidism respectively."

3. "Gonadotropic principle (of the pituitary gland) is probably elaborated by the basophilic cells of the anterior lobe and serves as a connecting link between pituitary and gonad. While it probably has no direct action on skeletal development, it has an important secondary effect through its influence on development and function of the gonads."

ACROMEGALY*(Fig. 86B). Acromegaly is a disease which is due to the hyperfunction of the anterior lobe of the pituitary gland. It is characterized by a general overgrowth of the skeletal system in individuals past adolescence. If increased function occurs before closure of the epiphyses, there is stimulation of their growth, and gigantism results. The epiphyseal structures appear at their normal time and unite at their normal time; there is merely excessive growth due to stimulation of growth hormone; it may result from an eosinophilic tumor of the pituitary or merely from hyperplasia of eosinophilic cells.

CLINICAL AND ROENTGEN FINDINGS. This condition usually develops in adult life, but occasionally occurs at an earlier period. It is seen with about equal frequency in both sexes. There is a general increase in size of the entire skeleton; the texture of the bone becomes coarse and thick. The head becomes larger, and is elongated in the anteroposterior diameter; the frontal bone becomes prominent and the sinuses become large. The sella turcica is usually enlarged. The most prominent bony enlargement is seen in the lower jaw; the mandible protrudes far beyond the upper jaw so that normal dental occlusion is interfered with. The extremities become thickened and enlarged; this is especially noticeable in the bones of the hands, which become broad and thick, with tufting of the terminal phalanges and clubbing of the fingers, giving rise to the so-called "spade hand". Moore has observed a series of acromegalic patients having thyroid toxicity and hyperostosis of the skull for which he proposes the name, Troell-Junet Syndrome.

PITUITARY TUMORS—ADENOMATA—(See Intracranial Neoplasms)

The pituitary cells are classified according to their staining qualities as follows:

(A) The chromophobe or chief cells which take the stain poorly   (52% of the cells).

(B) The eosinophil cells which have an affinity for the acid eosin   (37% of the cells).

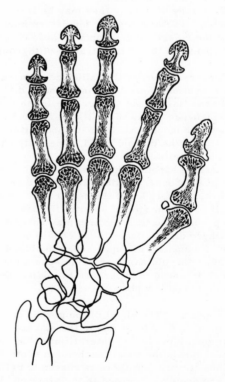

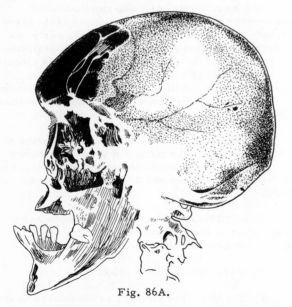

Fig. 86A.

Fig. 86B.

*An asterisk following any title indicates that roentgenographic reproductions illustrating this condition will be found in the pictorial supplement at the end of the chapter.

(C) The basophil cells which have an affinity for the basic stain   (10% of the cells).

Development of adenoma in these cells produces different clinical and roentgenological manifestations depending upon the cell structure involved.

(1) The Chromophobe Cell Adenoma is characized by formation of a bulky tumor of the pituitary which in turn causes both enlargement of the sella turcica and hypofunction of the gland from pressure. The tumor usually reaches a large size before its pressure is manifested. The earliest symptoms may be those arising from local pressure of the enlarged gland, such as visual defects, headaches, etc. The condition of the cells may be likened to the thyroid cells in colloid goitre, with myxedema. The chromophobe seems to be the resting stage of the pituitary cell. With the development of hypofunction, other clinical manifestations make their appearance. In the male there is impotency with testicular atrophy and loss of secondary sex characteristics; not infrequently there may even be reversion to female characteristics. In the female there is amenorrhea from lack of stimulation of the ovary and consequent failure of the follicle to ripen. There may be other findings such as increased sugar tolerance, low blood pressure, secondary anemia, obesity and polyuria.

(2) The Eosinophilic Cell Adenoma makes its presence known by the well-known syndrome of acromegaly. The sella turcica may be somewhat enlarged, but this is part of a generalized enlargement of the entire skeletal system; it never attains a size sufficient to produce pressure as chromophobic adenoma. Kyphosis due to osteoporosis of the spine is usually present. A decreased sugar tolerance with glycosuria and hyperglycemia is found in a large percentage of cases. Masculinization of the female with hypertrichosis of the face, deep bass voice and amenorrhea are usually present. Hypertension and atherosclerosis are a part of the picture. Polycythemia may be present, connective tissue and fatty tumors are not infrequent.

(3) The Basophilic Type of Adenoma results in the syndrome called "basophilism" (Cushing syndrome). The tumor itself is extremely small, never exceeding a few millimeters in size and never causing pressure enlargement of the sella turcica. This type of tumor is characterized by a rapidly acquired, usually painful adiposity, confined to the face, neck, and trunk, the extremities being spared. There is a tendency to become round shouldered, even to the point of becoming shorter in stature; this may be associated with lumbosacral pains. There is sexual dystrophy shown by early amenorrhea in the female and ultimate impotence in the male. There is an alteration in the normal distribution of hair shown by tendency to hypertrichosis of the face and trunk in females, a dusky plethoric appearance of the skin

with purplish lineae atrophicae, vascular hypertension, variable backache, abdominal pains, fatiguability and ultimate extreme weakness.

It is now known that similar symptoms may be produced by hypoadrenalism from tumor of the adrenal or thymus.

Roentgen ray examination does not usually show any enlargement of the sella turcica, since the tumor is never more than a few millimeters in size. In severe cases, however, there is a peculiar softening of all the bones, due to calcium salt absorption, most pronounced in the spine, pelvis and skull. In the spine this may be sufficiently pronounced to cause impaction of the vertebral bodies and decrease in height. There may be spontaneous fractures. The bone changes may suggest hyperparathyroidism.

Wang and Rubbins have discussed the findings in 38 cases of this disease stressing their similarity to hyperparathyroidism. Sissons in a study of 4 such cases has concluded that the osteoporosis in this condition is due largely to interference with the proliferation of osteoblasts and cartilage cells and with their formation of new bone in the presence of a normal amount of osteoclastic bone resorption. The bone changes are comparable with those produced in experimental animals by the administration of A.C.T.H. or cortisone.

Roentgen therapy is the only method of value up to the present time.

Progeria is a condition of premature aging. It usually commences in early infancy progressing to senility within a few years; the individual having the short immature stature of a child develops the facial and bodily appearance of a senile individual. Arteriosclerosis is a prominent feature; arthritis is often present. Although dwarfism results, epiphyseal development is said to correspond with the age of the individual. It may be associated with a craniopharyngioma causing multiple glandular deficiencies.

DEFECTS IN MESENCHYMAL DEVELOPMENT

OSTEOGENESIS IMPERFECTA,* (FRAGILITAS OSSIUM; IDIOPATHIC OSTEOPSATHYROSIS; PERIOSTEAL APLASIA) (Figs. 87A and B). Osteogenesis imperfecta is a disease of the bony structures due to an inherent defect in mesenchymal development resulting in a deficiency in the number and the function of the osteoblasts. Key maintains that the inherent defect is not in the decrease of osteoblasts but in their inability to form new bone. There must be many degrees of involvement, some showing greater amounts of osteoporosis and deformity, others less change in lime salts but still showing the feature of multiple fractures to a marked degree.

Clinically the disease is manifested by:
1. Multiple fractures resulting from trivial traumas which ordinarily do not cause fracture. Such fractures are usually attended

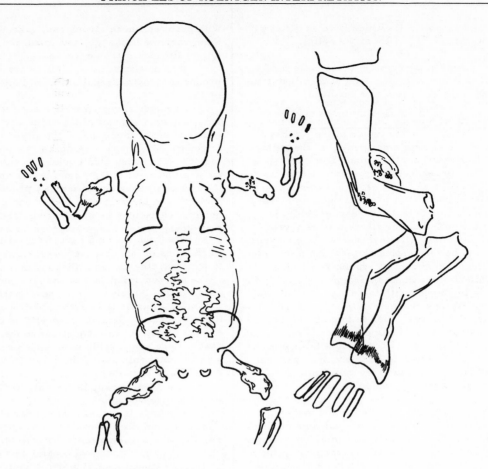

Fig. 87A

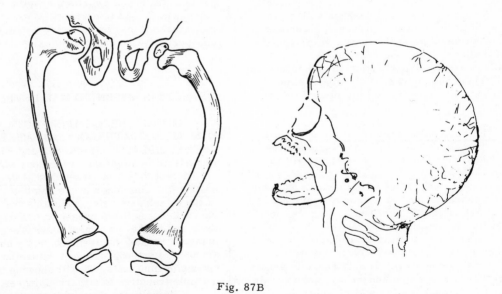

Fig. 87B

with little pain and heal readily.

2. Deformity due to multiple fractures and bowing of the weakened bony structures.
3. Enlarged, soft, "rubber ball" skull.
4. Blue sclera in the congenital types.
5. Profuse sweating which develops early with-

in the first few weeks and persists through-out life.

The classification and nomenclature of this condition varies greatly. Some use the above names interchangeably, while others use them to describe different entities. The term Osteogenesis Imperfecta is used when the condition is of congenital origin. This type is further subdivided into Osteogenesis Imperfecta Congenita and Osteogenesis Imperfecta Tarda, depending upon the time elapsing before the condition makes itself evident. Both these types have blue sclera which most writers depend upon for establishing a definite congenital origin.

The term Idiopathic Osteopsathyrosis, however, is to be confined to that type of the disease occurring in childhood which usually shows the same manifestations as Osteogenesis Imperfecta with the exception of the blue appearance of the sclera, thus differentiating it from the disease of congenital origin.

While the etiology is unknown, many believe it to be due to some sort of an endocrine disturbance, possibly of the thymus gland. There is no indication of vitamin deficiency or disturbance in calcium-phosphorus content of blood.

Clinically the skull and long bones show the greatest manifestations; the femur and humerus are the long bones most frequently involved. Fractures frequently present in both types, heal readily; they may even heal with hyperplastic callus as in cases reported by Baker, and Vandemark and Page, which was of sufficient amount to suggest osteogenic sarcoma. Microscopically the rapidly multiplying bone cells give a picture not unlike that of osteogenic sarcoma which makes the condition even more difficult to evaluate (Strach). A familial element in the occurrence of hyperplastic callus formation has been reported by Hilton.

OSTEOGENESIS IMPERFECTA—CONGENITA* (Fig. 87A). The patient shows evidence of the disease at birth, the majority being born with numerous fractures. The extremities are usually deformed presenting curvatures and nodular prominences from previous fractures (Fig. 87A). The skull may be as thin as parchment and is a membranous bag showing only a few small isolated areas of ossification; many Wormian bones producing a reticulated appearance which is quite characteristic; it is often spoken of as a "rubber ball head." Due to the soft condition of the cranial bones, the skull may sag over the spine, showing broadening on either side and flattening on top, (Tam-o'Shanter skull). In other instances it may show no change. These children usually die early as a result of intercurrent infection. If the patient lives, profuse and continued sweating, beginning usually during the second week, becomes a prominent feature. The patient remains a chronic invalid for life.

Pronounced honey combing at the ends of the bones occasionally occurs; it is designated as osteogenesis imperfecta cystica.

OSTEOGENESIS IMPERFECTA—TARDA*(Fig. 87B). This is an infantile type not manifest at birth, appearing only when the child begins to walk. Occasionally the disease may not manifest itself until early adolescence or adult life. There is often little, if any, pain associated with these fractures; this is thought to be due to the fact that they are often subperiosteal. The skull bones may appear thin and reticulated. In this type we have the blue discoloration of the sclera

(leptoscleria-thin membrane), also. Deafness may be an associated symptom. When the disease appears later in life the probability of survival is greater; as time goes on there is a tendency toward recovery.

Microscopic examination indicates that the process is due to failure of fibroblasts to differentiate into normal osteoblasts. There are fractured spicules and regional hemorrhages; healing takes place readily but with bone which has been arrested in the chondroblastic stage; normal bone marrow becomes converted into a fibrous type.

ROENTGENOLOGICAL MANIFESTATIONS

Congenital Form, (Congenita), (Fig. 87A). When the condition is present at birth the bones of the extremities may have a gnarled, stubby and thickened appearance. They are bowed and misshapen, and multiple fractures are usually present. The cortex is thin but there may be no osteoporosis at this time. The tables of the skull may appear normal or they may be extremely thin, and often calcification and ossification seem to be entirely lacking in some areas; there is wide separation of the sutures and fontanelles. Achondroplasia gives an almost identical picture at birth, minus the fractures.

Late Form, (Tarda), (Fig. 87B). There is marked thinning of the cortex, and bowing of the long bones. Generalized osteoporosis is usually present; when extreme there may even be cystic changes. Marked atrophy or constriction of the shaft produces an appearance of widening of the metaphysis and epiphysis. An irregular appearance of the epiphysis is often present. This form does not usually show the gnarled, stubby appearance of the bones seen in the congenital form and fractures may be of the subperiosteal folding type. The cortex may be as thin as paper and there is marked bowing of all of the bones. The skull bones may be thin and checkered.

IDIOPATHIC OSTEOPSATHYROSIS.* This type of the disease is not distinguishable from the other forms except that there is not the same tendency to extreme osteoporosis and consequent bowing deformities; brittleness of the bones is present, however, resulting in multiple fractures. Deformity is due to multiple fractures, not to weakening from osteoporosis. It is not associated with blue sclera and is to some extent self-limiting, subsiding at about the age of puberty. The onset is usually in the third year of life. In this type there is extreme deformity of the extremities resulting from the occurrence of multiple fractures. The slightest exertion may cause fracture; such fractures are comparatively painless; union is unusually rapid. They may heal with large hyperplastic callus formation having bony spicules radiating outward from the shaft of the bone even resembling sarcoma, (Baker). The skull shows bilateral increase in its diameters with unusual prominence of the frontal and occipital bones. The femur and humerus are the long bones most often involved (KEY).

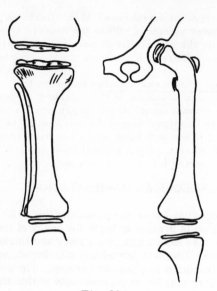

Fig. 88A

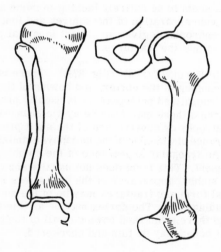

Fig. 88B

The pathology is similar in all forms of the disease. There is a decrease in osteoblasts which results in deficient ossification of bone. On chemical analysis there is no lack of the inorganic constituents of bone, and fragility cannot, therefore, be dependent upon this factor. The bone shows scanty cancellous structure and an increase in medullary elements.

Roentgenological Manifestations. In this type there may be a greater disproportion in the size of the epiphysis with the diaphysis of the long bones. The diaphysis may be slender and often irregular. The cortex is very thin but general decrease in density of the bone is not as pronounced as in the other form. There is marked deformity due to numerous fractures. The more pronounced epiphyseal changes distinguish this type—otherwise the roentgen picture is very similar.

DEFECTS IN CHONDRO-OSTEAL DEVELOPMENT

ACHONDROPLASIA,* (CHONDRODYSTROPHIA FOETALIS), (Fig. 88). This disease is a cartilaginous dystrophy, presenting many different forms, either unilateral or symmetrical in distribution and usually congenital in origin. It usually begins in the fetus, but may not manifest itself until the second or third year of life. In a great many instances such individuals are stillborn. The condition is more frequent in males. It has been traced through five generations (Bangson).

The etiology is not definitely known, but cases have been reported in which cellular reaction in the thymus and thyroid glands were prominent, suggesting an interference with endocrine function. Also only one ossification center is present for the basilar process of the skull in place of the three normally found, suggesting some pituitary dysfunction.

Clinically the condition may present itself in four forms:

1. As true dwarfs (Achondroplastic Dwarf).
2. As very short limbs with normal trunks.
3. Large heads and peculiar faces.
4. Involvement of single members.

The most typical picture is a normal-sized body, with exceedingly shortened extremities; a large head with a characteristic depression at the root of the nose. The head is round and globular and the face is small. Often prognathism accompanies the other changes of the head. This deformity is due to the fact that the basilar structures of the skull develop by one small center of ossification only, rather than the three centers usually present. The lack of development of this portion of the skull leaves all subsequent enlargement of the head to expanding of the vault in order to accommodate the increasing brain structure.

The spine is shortened and may show either lordosis or kyphosis; giving rise to a prominence of the buttocks.

The extremities are much shortened, usually most evident in their proximal segments. The hands are often short and broad and the fingers are of equal length. The ring and little fingers may diverge from the others producing the trident hand. Any of the bones of the extremities may be curved, but this is more common in the femurs and the arms. Either genu valgum or varum may be present or there may be no bowing at all—the disease presents wide variations in different cases.

ROENTGENOLOGICAL CHARACTERISTICS. Since this is a condition affecting primarily the growth of the long bones, due to disturbed epiphyseal growth, from failure of normal bony replacement of cartilage, it is evident that these changes produced in this location would give rise to the most important roentgenological findings in the disease. Failure of the normal epiphyseal growth leaves the affected bones shorter than normal. The shortness of the extremities is often referred to as micromelia.

Periosteal proliferation continues without interference, often in excessive amounts, causing the

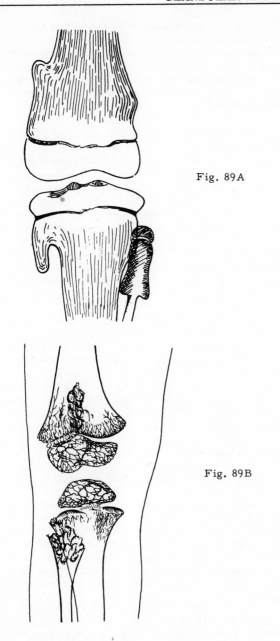

Fig. 89A

Fig. 89B

dral laying down of bone, resulting in bowing of the bone and subsequent changes in the epiphyseal structures (Snoke).

Hyperplastic Type. In other instances the bones may be perfectly straight. They are short and thick, showing abnormal width of the diaphyseal ends without corresponding epiphyseal enlargement—overhanging diaphysis. In these cases the epiphysis itself is broad and flat and denser than usual, without widening of the zone of temporary calcification, and there is marked thickening of the cartilage plate.

Malacic Type. In the malacic type the long bones may show relatively little involvement; the greatest variation may be seen in the spine, chest and pelvis. The vertebrae are often wedge-shaped and the secondary ossifying nuclei are reduced in size; this results in a ragged, irregular, beaklike projection of the anterior margins of the vertebral bodies, resulting in kyphosis. In these cases the laying down of endochondral bone, although inadequate, is none the less uniform.

The pelvis is narrow and flat. Often the lower half of the acetabula are absent, affording articulation for only one-third of each femoral head. Coxa vara is a frequent deformity.

The skull, when involved, shows disproportion between the vault and the face. The base of the cranium is short; the clivus is deep and the sella turcica is smaller than normal; the nose is retracted.

The condition is of benign character. It has been observed that patients suffering from this disease show bone formation if thyroid extract and the growth hormone of pituitary are administered (Ketcham). This lends further support to the belief that this condition may be of endocrine origin.

Some indication of an hereditary origin must be considered due to the case reported by Lenk as hereditary metaphyseal dysostosis in which this condition was traced through three generations.

Rare cases have been reported of associated hypertrophy of the long bones and skin defects (Touraine-Dolente-Gole Syndrome). The condition is manifested by shaggy periosteal reaction over the long bones similar to that seen in association with leg ulcer, and a thickening of the folds of skin of the face, extremities, ankles, and hands. The presence of excessive amounts of estrogens in the male suggests that this may have some bearing on the etiology (Linwold and Duryee).

DIAPHYSEAL ACLASIA (Ellis and Taylor). Diaphyseal aclasia, (multiple osteomata or exostoses; hereditary deforming chondrodysplasia) (Fig. 89A) may occur as an hereditary manifestation at various epiphyseal lines all over the body; often such growths occur in families for many successive generations. They are often very irregular in shape and originate by broad bases from the shaft. They are in no sense malignant and need not be removed unless they interfere with normal function; they stop growing at maturity. If removed surgically they do not tend to recur. Very rarely such tumors may undergo malignant degeneration—chondromyxo sarcoma.

bone to attain even greater thickness than normal. This may result in overhanging the diaphysis at the epiphyseal line.

During the growth period the bones may present widely differing appearances. Kaufmann recognized three different types of involvement histologically: a) hypoplastic, b) hyperplastic, and c) malacic. Hypoplastic. The long bones may be bowed, showing marked changes, with irregularity and widening of the zone of temporary calcification, thickening of the cartilaginous plate, especially on the concave side of the bone, in response to Wolff's law of bone formation. This is considered as the roentgen manifestation of the hypoplastic type; it is believed to be due to weakness and irregularity in the original endochon-

DYSCHONDROPLASIA* (OLLIER'S DISEASE)

(Fig. 89B). Dyschondroplasia is recognized as a distinct disease entity, differing from chondrodysplasia foetalis and diaphyseal aclasia which it may resemble. It is characterized by failure of portions of the epiphyseal cartilage, which ordinarily contributes to increase in the length of the bone, to ossify, maintaining its cartilaginous structure and persisting as nodules and masses within the bone at its diaphyseal end. These irregularly expanded cartilaginous areas with absence of overlying cortical bone inhibit the normal epiphyseal growth in the areas which they occupy; the intervening areas of normal bone continue to grow resulting in gross deformity and shortening of the bone. This results in widening of the diaphysis with linear striations of bone spreading out fanlike toward the epiphyseal line with the cartilaginous structures in between. These bony striations correspond closely to the pattern produced by the nutrient arteries at the ends of the bones, leading to the assumption that they may have something to do with the development of the condition. In later life irregular calcareous deposits occur throughout the cartilaginous masses. It may be confined to a single extremity or to a solitary bone, (Bromer and John).

The bone marrow itself is not impaired; it is the existence of this normal bone marrow in the presence of cartilaginous rests which distinguishes this condition from other forms of chondrodysplasia.

While this condition is commonly referred to as Ollier's Disease, it seems most probable from his own original description that he was really dealing with diaphyseal aclasia.

DYSCHONDROPLASIA WITH HEMANGIOMATA—(MAFFUCCI'S SYNDROME) (Krause; Carleton, et al.).

This is a condition in which dyschondroplasia is associated with multiple hemangiomas about the ends of the bones with clusters of phleboliths and calcifications. The deformity becomes so grotesque at times especially in the hands and feet that they are no longer recognizable, and amputation may become necessary. The bony structures may appear normal at birth, the disease showing its first manifestations in prepubertal years. Small nodules one to two centimeters in size appear in the long bones. They may show unilateral or asymmetrical distribution. Soft bluish veins forming tumorlike masses appear in the extremities and trunk. The bones become fragile and fractures follow trivial injuries. Asymmetrical development of the two sides of the body may result in secondary deformities such as pes planus, genu valgum, scoliosis, etc. The disease becomes stationary after full growth, but most are short and have poor muscular development. Occasionally malignant tumors develop in the bone lesions.

On roentgenographic examination, the small bones of the hands and feet, but not the carpus or tarsus, show multiple small cystlike areas, (enchondromata); these may affect the long bones, ribs, scapulae, and vertebrae also.

Microscopic examination shows that the dyschondroplasia results from failure of absorption of the cartilaginous growth plate of the epiphysis. The changes may be congenital or they may be brought about by endocrine dysfunction. It is possible that the association of dyschondroplasia and multiple hemangiomata may be coincidental.

CHONDROOSTEODYSTROPHY—(MORQUIO-BRAILSFORD'S DISEASE) (Pohl; Fairbanks).

In this condition there is fragmentation and distortion of the epiphyses of long bones. There is primarily a disturbance in the change of cartilage into bone; the condition is more a dysplasia rather than an aplasia, but there is little, if any, shortening of the bones. Wedge-shaped deformity and narrowing of the vertebrae result in kyphosis which may not be suspected until the child sits up. Other deformities of the large joints, knock knees, misshaped heads, depression of the chest, etc., accompany the condition. The disturbance may result in dwarfism due mainly to the spinal maldevelopment.

Other bodily structures may also be involved, clouding of the cornea, thickening of the skin and coarsening of the hair. There is often premature closing of the sutures and atrophy of the optic nerve. The condition is often familial, but it is not necessarily so. A patient having this disease has been observed during pregnancy, with birth of a child having normal skeletal structure. The etiology is not definitely known, but it is believed that the condition is due to mucoid degeneration of cartilage in place of normal calcification (Russo). Hunter-Hurler Syndrome or Gargoylism may produce almost identical deformity (see Xanthomatosis), but differentiation can usually be made.

A very rare condition resembling Morquios' Disease, Dysplasia epiphysialis multiplex characterized by a fragmented appearance of all of the epiphyseal structures of the body has been reported, (Fairbank, et al.). The epiphysis seems to ossify from numerous discrete centers, but normal trabeculation occurs after union. It lacks other characteristics.

CHONDRODYSTROPHIA CALCIFICANS CONGENITA (CHONDRO-DYSPLASIA, STIPPLED EPIPHYSES).

Stippled calcifications appear in the epiphyseal cartilages before ossification. There is some flaring in the epiphyseal ends of the bones and an increase in the zone of temporary calcification at the epiphyseal lines. The condition is congenital and has been reported in numerous children in the same family (Gerard). The calcifications disappear by the age of three years (Rapp) if the patient survives, and there does not seem to be any permanent ill effect (Fairbanks). They frequently die under one year of age from infection. In a case reported by Coughlin et al, there was definite shortening of the long bones, resembling achondroplasia. Thickening of the skin and cataract may be associated findings. The subject may be of low mentality. A case has been reported in utero by Frank and Denny.

Sheach and Middlemiss have reported a case with complete radiological and pathological findings from which they conclude that the condition is one of delayed differentiation and development of the cartilaginous elements with myxoid areas and fibroblastic colonisation; absence of secondary ossification centers and defective formation of the peripheral endochondral component of the terminal metaphyseal cortex. They have been unable to find a single report of this condition in an adult.

Dysplasia epiphysialis hemimelica (tarso-aclasis) (Fairbank) is a rare fault in epiphyseal growth in which portions of the epiphyseal cartilage are enlarged with numerous centers of ossification producing abnormality of form and function in the various epiphyses at which they may be located. The cartilaginous mass may remain attached giving much the appearance of osteochondromata or may become separated forming loose cartilaginous masses in the joint or soft tissues. They never involve more than one extremity and always show unilateral involvement. Their etiology is not known. Treatment consists in removal or correction of deformity.

THIEMANN'S DISEASE.* This is a very rare disease characterized by fissuring and fragmentation of the epiphyses especially of the hands and feet, the proximal joint of the great toe and the 1st tarso-metatarsal joint. These defects recover and union of the epiphyses occurs at the proper time (Schinz, et al.).

PARATHYROID

The part played by the parathyroid glands in the various bone dyscrasias is not fully understood. The principal function of the parathyroid glands appears to be the regulation of the calcium-phosphorus content of the blood. In general the calcium content of the blood bears an inverse ratio to the phosphorus. Neuromuscular tone and irritability are affected by the blood calcium so that the parathyroids also indirectly influence these functions. They have no influence on the absorption of calcium salts by the intestines—this is a function of Vitamin D. Calcium salts, absorbed from the intestinal tract, are deposited in the bones; these become the great storehouses for calcium salts which may be called upon if need be to supply deficiency of calcium which may occur in the blood stream from any cause. It has even been shown that if the calcium intake in the diet is sufficient, Vitamin D can maintain the normal calcium level in the blood even after removal of the parathyroids; it is possible therefore for the bony structure to retain its normal appearance even in the presence of parathyroid disease.

HYPOPARATHYROIDISM

Deficiency of secretion of the parathyroid glands usually follows interference with their blood supply or accidental injury or removal during operative procedures of the neck. The principal function of the parathyroid glands is calcium regulation, so that hypocalcemia resulting from decreased secretion results clinically in tetany. Cataracts may also occur from the low serum-calcium level. The serum phosphorus is proportionally high, and in practically all other respects the chemical findings are just the reverse of hyperparathyroidism, (See p. 79).

The roentgen findings may be lacking in well established cases there may be some increased density of the bones and difficulty in dental development. The appearance of calcium deposits in the basal ganglia may be the main clue to the diagnosis. The administration of parathormone raises the calcium level with amelioration of the symptoms.

PSEUDOHYPOPARATHYROIDISM

Under this term Albright et al. described a familial disease of metabolism in which parathyroid glands seemed to be normal in structure and function, "The chief feature distinguishing it from other forms of chronic hypoparathyroid tetary is the lack of response to parathormone," (Cusumano, et al.). Changes in the hand and skull may be a clue to the diagnosis.

1. Tetany without evidence of renal disease, steatorrhosa or generalized osteomalacia without response to administration of parathormone.

2. Shortening of one or more metacarpal or metatarsal bones.

3. Clinical picture of shortness of stature, thickset appearance, round facies, mental retardation and short stubby fingers.

4. Soft tissue calcification involving the basal ganglia and subcutaneous tissues.

HYPERPARATHYROIDISM,* GENERALIZED OSTEITIS FIBROSA CYSTICA—(von RECKLINGHAUSEN'S DISEASE). Hyperparathyroidism from increased secretion of parathormone from whatever cause, either glandular hyperfunction or tumor formation, results in increase in blood calcium. To maintain this unusual concentration of calcium in the blood the great storehouses of calcium salts in the long bones are called upon to give up their calcium deposits. As a result osteoporosis and various fibrocystic lesions develop in the long bones (Fig. 90A) and pathological fractures may result from their weakened condition. Along with the increase in blood calcium there is a corresponding decrease in blood phosphorus. The neuromuscular irritability is decreased and the patient develops an extreme degree of myotonia. Extensive skeletal deformity may result from softening, bending and fracture of the bones.

Clinically, the onset is usually with pain of the rheumatic type in the bones and joints; this is often referred to the hip, radiating down the leg. Muscular weakness and fatigue develop and there is often loss of weight.

Renal calculus, or other unusual calcium deposit, may result from hypercalcemia. Such deposits are referred to as "calcium metastases."

Roentgenologically, the loss of calcium content produces an extreme degree of osteoporosis, of the bony structures; some portions of the bones give up their calcium salts more readily than others so that the bones may have an irregular spotty appearance.

1. Subperiosteal resorption of cortical bone, usually seen most pronounced in the phalanges and tufts of the fingers and in the proximal ends of the tibiae on their medial aspects, is a most important diagnostic sign (Ginyler, and Jaffe). The margins of the involved bone present a lacy appearance of trabeculae, denuded of periosteum and cortical bone. This is a manifestation of primary Hyperparathyroidism and Renal Osteodystrophy (Renal Rickets), (Fig. 90A).

2. Pugh has pointed out that,
"The loss of the lamina dura which is seen in dental roentgenograms is another manifestation of subperiosteal resorption of bone. . . the periodontal membrane is a specialized form of periosteum."

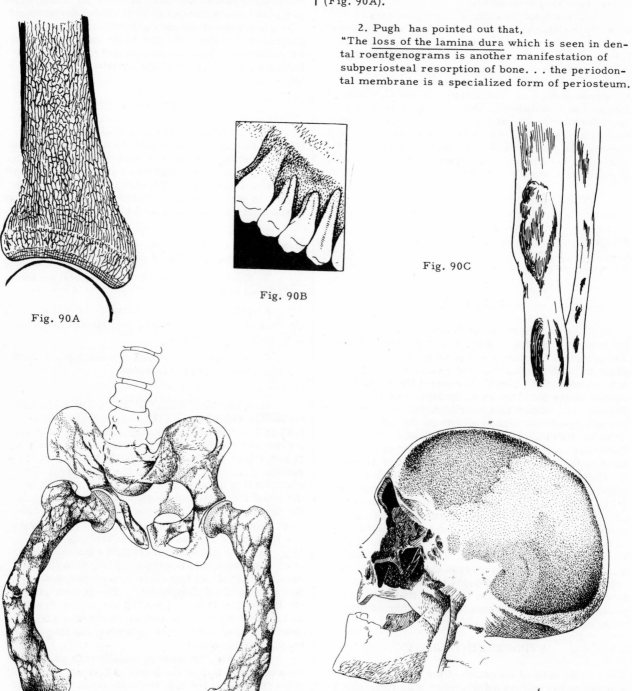

Fig. 90A

Fig. 90B

Fig. 90C

Fig. 90D

Fig. 90E

The lamina dura is actually the cortical portion of bone around the teeth. . . the loss of the lamina dura has been reported as occurring in other conditions besides hyperparathyroidism and renal osteodystrophy. There is no lamina dura in edentulous patients, and therefore, in many elderly persons the loss of the lamina dura cannot be depended upon as a diagnostic criterion." (Fig. 90B).

3. The trabeculae become coarse and may break down to form areas of cystic degeneration. (Fig. 90C). These cystic areas are most obvious near the ends of the diaphyses of the long bones, especially the tibia, and on the superior and inferior margins of the ribs. These small cysts are filled with clear straw-colored fluid. Being caused by degeneration and resorption of bone structure, they never cause true expansion of the shaft of a bone no matter how large they become.

4. In extreme cases the bones become softened and weak from the loss of lime salts so that they may become bowed and curved into grotesque shapes; the lower extremities show coxa vara deformity and similar deformities may develop in the ribs (Fig. 90D).

5. Similar osteoporotic changes occur in the skull with loss of normal bone architecture and assuming of a granular appearance (Fig. 90E). This irregular, matted, stippled appearance is associated with osteoporosis of the skull which is rather distinctive of the condition; the bony structures seem thickened even resembling Paget's disease.

6. Besides the granular osteoporosis common to other bones, there is usually visible in the vertebrae a coarse perpendicularly striated fibrocystic appearance. Kyphosis and Scoliosis may occur; or the vertebrae may develop biconcave deformity (Fig. 90F) due to pressure of the expanding nucleus pulposus on the bodies weakened by osteoporosis. Similar biconcave deformity of the vertebral bodies occurs in old age in hyperparathyroidism and in other osteomalacic diseases, due to pressure of expanded nucleus pulposus on the softened vertebral bodies. In its advanced stage it may be indistinguishable from Polyostotic Fibrous Dysplasia; in this condition, however,

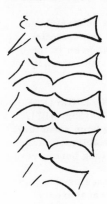

Fig. 90F

the cyst-like areas are not true cysts but are filled with fibrous tissue. Differentiation is imperative since polyostotic fibrous dysplasia is in no way associated with parathyroid tumor.

The diagnosis is made then: 1) on the roentgen evidence of irregular subperiosteal bone resorption most frequently observed in the middle phalanges of the hands, the edges of the tibiae and the skull, 2) on the high calcium-phosphorus ratio in the blood stream, and 3) on the detection of renal calculi from the increase in calcium excreted in the urine.

Surgical removal of a parathyroid tumor, or in certain instances its destruction by roentgen therapy, has led to recovery from the disease with reestablish-

ment of the normal bone structure. Operation may be relied upon to stop the progress of the disease and relieve the pain but in some instances the bone structure does not return to normal.

PSEUDOHYPOPARATHYROIDISM. Albright, et al. in 1950 described the following features of the disease: 1) Clinical and laboratory evidence of chronic parathyroid insufficiency; tetany without evidence of renal disease, steatorrhea or generalized osteomalacia. Despite these findings patients show little or any response to parathormone. 2) Shortening of metacarpal and metatarsal bones. 3) Clinical picture of shortness of stature, thickset appearance, round facies, mental retardation and short stubby fingers. 4) Soft-tissue calcification involving the basal ganglia and subcutaneous tissues. Cusmano has added six similar cases to the literature.

OTHER BONE DISEASES OF UNKNOWN ETIOLOGY. Localized OSTEITIS FIBROSA; (Hartley)(Fig. 91A). It has now been generally accepted that this is a condition which develops as a result of generalized decalcification from systemic cause. It develops as a response of bone tissue to extreme decalcification of bone structure, occurring in many widely different bone conditions where extreme osteoporosis is a prominent feature. It should be considered therefore as a condition, not a disease entity. It occurs in hyperparathyroidism caused by a parathyroid tumor; but it is also present in Paget's disease where parathyroid tumors cannot be found.

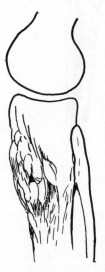

Fig. 91A

In osteitis fibrosa, multiple areas in the bones undergo absorption and decalcification with fibrous tissue replacement and cystlike formations. Isolated areas may show greatest involvement or there may be rather uniform involvement throughout all of the long bones. The cortex is thinned and may or may not show expansion. It remains intact unless pathological fracture occurs from weakening of the bony structures; when such fractures occur they tend to heal readily. There is no periosteal reaction and no soft tissue tumor.

There is a current belief among a number of pathologists that osteitis fibrosa is essentially the same pathological process as that seen in bone cyst, and even in giant cell tumor the defect in development merely occurring at different times and in different locations in respect to bone growth (McWirter).

FIBROUS DYSPLASIA OF BONE*—POLYOSTOTIC OR MONOSTOTIC, (WEIL) (ALBRIGHT'S SYNDROME) (Fig. 91B). This is a peculiar type of bone dysplasia characterized by 1) destructive lesions of bone, 2) pigmented areas in the skin, 3) in the female a precocious sexual development without loss of fertility, and 4) at times multiple arteriovenous aneurysms, (Albright, et al.).

Roentgenologically cystlike lesions develop in the bones; they are usually multiple, showing a tendency to unilateral distribution. They have their point of origin within the cortical layer, not in the medullary canal; an important differential point. This is indicated by the eccentric character of the cystlike area; viewed at right angles this area may give the impression of central (medullary) origin. Such cystlike areas may show greatest expansion in toward

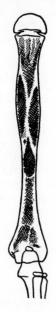 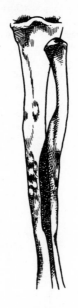

Fig. 91B$_1$ Fig. 91B$_2$

the medullary canal or outward toward the edge of the shaft, depending upon the location of the lesions. Enlargement takes place toward the side of least resistance; if the site of involvement is immediately beneath the cortical margin, the cystlike area may give the appearance of a bleb on the surface of the shaft.

There is fibrous tissue replacement within the cystlike area of involvement but no fluid; in this respect it differs from generalized osteitis fibrosa cystica, in which similar areas of destruction are due to true cysts containing fluid.

The earliest manifestation of this disease is seen as a tiny, cystlike area of destruction occurring within the cortex of an otherwise normal appearing bone. There is localized bulging of the cortex but no true expansion of the shaft since expansion is defined as symmetrical enlargement of the shaft of a bone. Even later on when the areas of involvement become large and coalesce true expansion is not a prominent feature of the disease.

When far advanced the eccentric location of the bulging areas produces a knarled appearance rather than one of uniform expansion. In the ultimate stages where irregular bone involvement has progressed to an extreme degree this characteristic is lost. The cortex remains intact; it is at first thinned on the side of greatest involvement but later (as a result of stimulation of bone growth—Wolff's Law) becomes

much thicker on this side indicating that the destructive process in the bone is within the cortical layer. In this tendency to involve the cortical layer it differs from ordinary (solitary) bone cyst. The skull is frequently involved, showing cystlike areas of destruction of the vault and dense, more homogeneous sclerosis of the basilar structures and face, resembling Leontiasis Ossea.

In a study of 39 cases of Fibrous Dysplasia involving the skull and facial bones, Fries has described the roentgen involvement as: 1) pagetoid, resembling Paget's disease; 2) sclerotic, manifested by dense sclerosis; 3) cyst-like, showing cystic areas within the sclerotic bone.

Fibrous dysplasia may rarely involve one or more vertebral structures (Ledoux-Lebard, and Soulquin), producing fine vertical striations with horizontal lines of condensed bone or even resembling the irregular appearance of angiomatous involvement. Occasionally, a picture resembling fibrous dysplasia of the skull is encountered in Pyle's disease in which there is lack of normal tubular development of the bones (Neuhauser). Unusual cases associated with lipoid granulomatosis of the bone have been reported (Harriman, and Millar).

In this condition osteoporosis is not a prominent feature and the calcium-phosphorus ratio remains unchanged, thus differing from hyperparathyroidism in generalized osteitis fibrosa cystica—von Recklinghausen's Disease. This lack of osteoporosis maintains the strength of the bone in polyostotic fibrous dysplasia so that the bones although extensively involved, never become soft; they may fracture from thinning of the cortex but they never develop the gross deformities from bending of the bones seen in generalized von Recklinghausen's Disease.

The condition is progressive; no form of treatment has been found to be effective; x-ray therapy is of no value.

We have observed a case in which a solitary cystlike lesion was removed surgically with healing of the local lesion, only to be followed by occurrence of similar lesions elsewhere in the skeleton. An unusual case has been recorded of occurrence of a massive hemorrhage with absorption of a large section of the tibia (Schlesinger, et al.).

There may be involvement of a solitary bone, but the same characteristics prevail (monostotic form). Many solitary cystlike lesions seen in the bones, although filled with fibrous tissue, are not necessarily of this type (Wells).

LOOSER'S TRANSFORMATION ZONES (PSEUDO FRACTURES) (VASCULAR EROSIONS) (Fig. 91C). This is a peculiar condition affecting bone structure. Linear zones appear transversely or obliquely across the longitudinal axis of the shafts of long bones, resembling fractures.

The lesions present an appearance as if a thin section of the bone has been erased transversely across the shaft. The bone architecture on either side of the defect is somewhat sclerotic but otherwise not disturbed, however, and the bone at the edges of the defect is in perfect alignment. This perfect alignment will serve to distinguish this condition from true fracture. At the onset they may appear only as

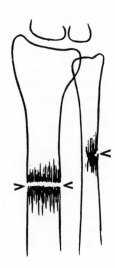

notches in the bone, but they soon extend to traverse the entire width of the bone. Why these defects should arrange themselves in straight lines directly across the long axis of the bone is at first difficult to understand. Observations made by LeMay and Blunt probably explain the etiology of this unusual condition. These investigations have found that Looser's Transformation Zones are invariably associated with arteries closely applied to the bone in these locations; it is then believed that these zones of decreased density are due to pressure absorption caused by the arteries as they traverse the bone in its weakened state.

Fig. 91C

These lesions may occur in a wide variety of pathological conditions such as Rickets, Late Rickets, Paget's Disease and Osteomalacic conditions. It has formerly been observed that in most instances they seem to be associated with insufficiency states in which the vitality is lowered and the bone is subjected to unusual strain (Camp and McCullough).

The bone may be so weakened in these regions that actual fractures may occur. The multiple spontaneous symmetrical fractures reported by Milkman (known as Osteoporosis Melolytica or Milkman's Syndrome) are undoubtedly of the same origin, the symmetrical character of the lesions being explained by the symmetry of anatomical structures on the two sides of the body.

OSTEITIS DEFORMANS (PAGET'S DISEASE)*
(Fig. 92). Osteitis Deformans is a chronic deforming disease of bone. It occurs most frequently in adults over forty years of age, males are more frequently affected. The cause of the disease is not definitely known. While its pathological picture suggests its relationship to parathyroid hyperfunction, actual tumors of this gland have not been found in connection with the disease.

The disease is usually solitary in its occurrence but has been reported in the father and two daughters of the same family, (Irvine). The first manifestation of the disease may be enlargement of the head; the individual notices that he requires a larger-sized hat or his friends may notice the increase in the size of the skull.

Involvement of the spine causes the patient to become stooped, and round shouldered. The clavicles are bowed forward, the femurs outward and the tibiae forward. The entire skeleton may be involved or the disease may be confined to a single bone. The disease is always associated with pronounced arteriosclerosis. Except for slight pain, usually of a rheu-

matic type, and weakness there are no subjective symptoms.

Roentgenologically the skull presents a typical appearance (Fig. 92A). The bones are thickened from two to five times the normal thickness. The increase in thickness is confined entirely to the diploe and outer table, so that there is no encroachment on the cranial cavity and consequently no symptoms of increased intracranial pressure. The process is one of bone rarefaction and condensation going on at the same time, causing a mottled "wooly" appearance of the thickened bone. The bones of the face are usually not involved; occasionally, however, the process involves the bones of the base of the skull, causing encroachment on the various foramina with development of symptoms depending upon the cranial nerve or structure involved; involvement of the petrous bone, for instance, may result in deafness.

Softening of the bones of the skull may result in invagination of the upper cervical spine, through the foramen magnum into the cranium (platybasia, Fig. 111), giving rise to various nervous manifestations.

In certain instances the bones of the skull may merely show circumscribed areas of rarefaction. The condition is known as Osteoporosis Circumscripta (Fig. 92A); it is not a disease entity but merely the transitional stage of Paget's Disease from normal to Paget bone (Kasabach and Gutman).

Bossi and Pisani have questioned the relationship between osteoporosis circumscripta and Paget's disease in many cases, feeling that it is still a definite entity rather than a transitional stage of Paget's disease and that the name Schuller Disease II be still retained.

The long bones show an increase in bulk which is due to an overgrowth of bone, not to expansion. The cortex is thickened on both sides and bowing occurs on the side opposite to the greatest muscular bulk. Texturally, the bone presents a wide-meshed

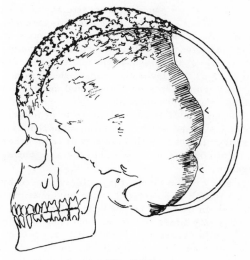

Fig. 92A

coarsely reticulated structure, in the interstices of which is a softer tissue relatively deficient in calcium. The outline of the bone is smooth, but there is irregular encroachment on the medullary canal. The trabeculae show strandlike accentuation and rearrangement running longitudinally up to the joint cortex. This serves to differentiate this condition from osteoblastic type of metastatic carcinomatous involvement and lues (Fig. 92B). Looser's transformation zones may develop transversely across the shaft of a bone. In rare instances Paget's disease may be associated with calcareous deposits in the soft tissues of the legs. As the disease progresses, bone sclerosis and condensation become more evident until the entire

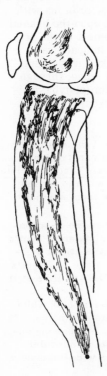

bone may become white and chalky in appearance, devoid of any evidence of normal structure. The appearance is like that encountered with syphilitic sclerosis, or even sclerotic osteogenic sarcoma. Periositis is rarely if ever present. The chronicity of the condition and the multiple sites of involvement usually is sufficient for differentiation from these conditions. When there is generalized bony involvement the resemblance to polyostotic fibrous dysplasia may be striking.

When the spine is involved the cancellous portion of the vertebral bodies is replaced by a dense calcareous deposit which produces a chalky appearance in the roentgenogram. There is no change in size or contour and the discs are well preserved. A similar picture is produced by metastatic osteoblastic carcinoma; unless other bones are involved, the two conditions cannot be differentiated.

Fig. 92B

Microscopically the bone shows fibrocystic changes similar to other bone diseases in which there is rapid decalcification of the bone but in addition there are other findings which are considered characteristic of the disease. In place of the thin curved lines of the Haversean canals there is a mosaic pattern of hematoxylin-stained cement lines producing islands of new bone.

The failure of Paget's disease to produce evident changes in the normal calcium-phosphorus ratio serves further to differentiate it from other diseases of bone. The serum phosphatase, however, is increased.

A study of the circulatory effects caused by Paget's Disease has resulted in the observation that it produces an extreme increase in volume flow, as much as twenty times the amount present in normal bone. Paget's disease is chronic and progressive; nothing has been found to modify its course. In an appreciable number of instances the bone lesions may undergo malignant change (Editorial Lancet).

IVORY VERTEBRAE (VERTEBRAE NOIRE; VERTEBRAE OPAQUE). A number of instances have been reported in the literature in which an isolated vertebra was involved. To these the term "ivory vertebra" has been applied in the literature. They probably represent isolated involvement of Paget's disease.

In his original communication, Paget did not describe involvement of the bones of the face; cases have been encountered, however, in which the facial bones were involved. A strikingly similar condition which has its origin and shows its greatest involvement in the facial bones is known as Leonitiasis Ossea.

LEONITIASIS OSSEA (HYPEROSTOSIS CRANII; CARNIOSCLEROSIS) (Fig. 93). This is a rare disease of unknown etiology found most often in individuals in early decades of life. It produces enormous, diffuse hyperostosis, beginning usually in the bones of the face and extending to those of the skull. This localized overgrowth of bone may become stationary or may be slowly progressive.

Leontiasis Ossea gets its name from the leonine or lionlike expression given to tne face by the thickened facial bones. The condition may give an appearance suggestive of swelling of the soft parts.

It is usually confined to the bones of the face and skull but cases of generalized involvement of the other bony structures have been described (Garland; Knaggs, Evans, and Pygott, et al.).

Two types are recognized: the creeping periosteal and the diffuse osteitic but in practice both types may be seen occurring simultaneously in the same patient.

Clinically the disease usually begins in the sinuses or nasal fossae, spreading slowly with involvement of the nasal bones, zygomata, lower orbits

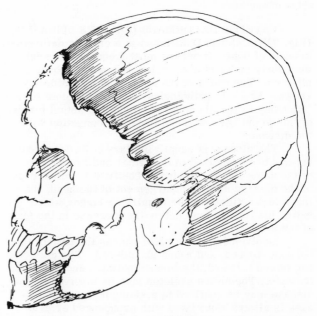

Fig. 93

and rami of the mandible. The alveolar processes of the lower and upper jaws are involved. Of the skull bones, the frontal and temporal bones are the most often affected.

The diseased areas, which are painless, show no evidence of inflammation. The condition is either slowly progressive with constant enlargement of the bones, or it may undergo a stationary phase. Neuralgic pains due to obliteration of the supra- and infraorbital foramina are common. Speech and mastication may be disturbed. Narrowing of the orbital cavity may occur with protrusion of the eyeball and subsequent disturbance in vision, amblyopia, and finally blindness. The base of the skull when involved causes disturbances of smell, taste, and hearing. Even paralysis of the extremities may occur. There is no thickening of the soft parts as occurs in acromegaly.

The most striking pathologic feature of the condition is a marked thickening and later a pronounced increase in the density of the bones of the face and skull. The cranial bones often attain a thickness of 3 cm. or more. On cross section, the inner and outer tables of the skull cannot be differentiated. The homogeneous aspect may be interrupted by scattered patches of soft fibrous-looking material and in rare cases cystic degeneration of such fibrous patches may be seen. The bone is soft and vascular, the surface being smooth.

From a histological standpoint, leontiasis ossea presents a picture somewhat similar to either Paget's or Recklinghausen's disease (if cystic degeneration is present). The localized lesions of Polyostotic Fibrous Dysplasia give a similar appearance when they involve the skull.

The disease is progressive; nothing has been found consistently beneficial in arresting its growth. Plastic surgery may be used for cosmetic effect. In a single case in which we have given X-ray therapy, the growth has not progressed in 25 years.

This condition has been considered with Paget's disease because of its close resemblance to that disease. Some pathologists consider it a variant of this condition. It does not possess any of its osteomalacic qualities.

Roentgenographic examination reveals a deforming enlargement of the bones of the face and skull with localized narrowing of the medullary portions. All bone architecture is lost and the bones assume a chalky white appearance. There is secondary narrowing of the foramina, orbits and sinuses. The detail of the bone varies from a pagetoid lamellation, to multiple cysts corresponding to Recklinghausen's disease.

OSTEOPETROSIS,* (Marble Bones; Albers-Schönberg Disease) (Fig. 94) (Kummell).

Osteosclerosis
Osteopathia hyperostotica (sclerotisans) multiplex infantilis
Chalky bone

This is a rare disease of bone growth of unknown etiology, characterized by excessive osteoblastic activity of the osteoblastic cells, without sufficient activity of the osteoclasts normally present in healthy bone. There is, in addition, excessive calcium deposit, imparting an abnormal brittleness and hardness to the bones. This excessive bone growth encroaches upon the bone marrow, gradually replacing the bone marrow structures, giving rise to extreme anemia. Microscopic examination of the bone lesions in the earliest stages, before overgrowth of bone has caused complete sclerosis of the medullary structures, would indicate a "perivascular inflammatory tissue reaction with lymphocytic infiltration and some giant cells," which would suggest the possibility of some primary inflammatory lesion as the basis of development of the disease.

CLINICAL CONSIDERATIONS. Ages range from new born to forty-eight years. It may be present at birth; or it may even be diagnosed in utero (Jenkinson); the new-born child may show no evidence of the disease, yet may develop the condition within the first few months of life. The condition is usually first suspected following a relatively painless pathological fracture. Or the first manifestation may be an enlarged skull, giving the impression of hydrocephalus (Kneal and Sante). There may be progressive narrowing of the visual fields and retardation of development.

Consanguinity seems to play a part; it occurs even generations later in children of cousins. Eight instances have been reported in three generations in one family (McPeak), and a mother and three children have been reported by Pirie. It may or may not terminate fatally. Kelly and Lawlah found four cases in the third generation.

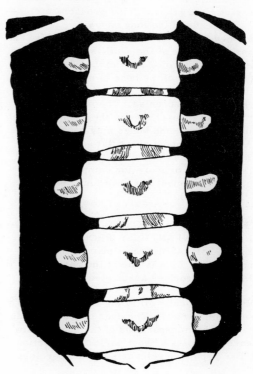

Fig. 94

FAMILIAL METAPHYSEAL DYSPLASIA; This is a similar condition, at least, the cranial manifestations are practically the same as leontiasis ossea. There is a chalky white thickening of the bones of the face and jaw; gradual obliteration of the nasal sinuses, orbits, auditory canals and cranial foramina. The eyes set unusually widely apart, and the thickened prominent cheek bones give a leonine expression. Faulty dentition is due to the involvement of the alveolar structures. Mori and Holt have pointed out that the diagnosis of familial metaphyseal dysplasia is dependent upon the roentgen observation of splayed long bones. Indeed they may be one and the same condition. Piatt et al. have recently reported nine cases stressing the benign character of the disease in some people.

PATHOLOGICAL AND ROENTGENOLOGICAL CONSIDERATIONS. Diagnosis of the disease is dependent upon the roentgen manifestations. The bony structures may appear normal at birth and not until a few months, or even a year has passed, do the characteristics of the disease become evident. At this time the growing bones in the diaphyseal regions begin to show an unusual increase in density which progresses to involvement of the entire shaft. Parallel longitudinal striations in the cancellous ends of the long bones fading out as they approach the compact portion of the shaft are due to long columns of remaining unchanged cartilaginous cells. These have been described as osteopathia striata by Voorhoeve, but we have observed this phenomenon in association with developing osteopetrosis and are convinced of the common identity of these conditions. Hurt has described a similar case in which the identity seemed evident.

White transverse lines of increased density may also be distinguished in the diaphyseal ends of bones due to excessive bone growth. This produces a clubbing effect of the ends of the long bones.

In fully developed cases the bones are white and structureless. The base of the skull is thickened and the depth of the sella turcica is diminished. Wherever the spongy portion of the bone is not sclerosed, it exhibits bone atrophy or osteoporosis with a well-defined meshwork of trabeculae. The bones appear chalky, but there is little change in the shape although at the shoulder and knee the bones may become club-shaped. The bone is almost avascular and any fractures which may occur in this stage are slow to heal, often requiring a year or more for complete union.

No form of treatment has been found to arrest or relieve the condition.

OSTEOPATHIA HYPEROSTOTICA SCLEROTISANS MULTIPLEX INFANTILIS; PROGRESSIVE DIAPHYSEAL DYSPLASIA; (Engelmann's Disease) (Engelmann; Sears). This is one of the very rare congenital bone dystrophies associated with osteosclerosis. The condition becomes evident in childhood, involving practically all of the long bones being bilateral and symmetrical. The ends of the bones appear normal but the mid-portions of the shafts show uniform dense sclerosis without periosteal reaction, very much like syphilitic sclerosis but the serology is negative. There is some lengthening of the bones with slight bowing. The bones of the skull show patches of sclerosis in the bone; the hands and feet appear normal. The sclerosis appears to be due to overgrowth of cortical bone, (Singleton, et al.).

Laboratory examinations are all essentially negative. Bone biopsy fails to show any abnormality in the structure of the bone.

This condition can be differentiated from marble bones by the confinement of the sclerosing portion to the mid-portion of the shaft, whereas, in marble bones the sclerosis advances from either end to involve the entire shaft. It can be differentiated from infantile cortical hyperostoses described by Caffey and Silvermann by its lack of periosteal or soft tissue reaction, and by its failure to produce fever and other symptoms of infection. Likewise this condition is persistant, whereas, infantile cortical hyperostosis recovers and disappears in a few months.

Neuhauser has described a similar closely related condition with bone changes and wasting anomalous neuromuscular signs, under the title Progressive Diaphyseal Dysplasia.

An hereditary type occurring in siblings has been reported by Ribbing and by Paul; and Van Buchan et al. Van Bucham et al. have reported a twin brother and sister with a similar condition under the title, Hyperostosis Corticolis Generalisata Familiaris.

Singleton et al. have reported a case in which they call attention to "the presence of thickening of the vessel walls in the biopsy specimen ... suggests that the disease may be on a vascular basis."

Griffiths has reported a case with widespread involvement with a complete analysis of the 17 reported cases with sufficient detail to justify the diagrams.

OSTEOPOIKILOSIS (Spotted Bones; Osteopoecilia; Osteopathia Condensans Disseminata) (Fig. 95). Osteopoikilosis is a condition in which there are numerous small areas of condensation in the bones throughout the skeleton without clinical symptoms. The condition is usually discovered by accident.

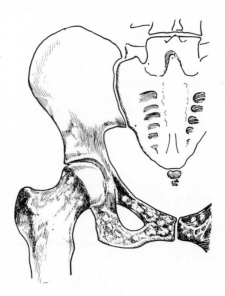

Fig. 95

These islands of condensation occur most abundantly in the cancellous portions of the bones. The trabeculae are thicker than normal, giving the impression of compact bone; they vary from 2 mm. to 2 cm. in size. The fully formed epiphyseal structures are usually free from involvement. They are of three types: spherical or spotty form, striated or elongated form, and a mixed type in which both forms of lesions occur. All bones may be involved except ribs and spine. The skull is rarely involved.

The condition is hereditary, possibly developing from a congenital cartilage defect; some authors consider the condition as a manifestation of dyschondroplasia. There is no change in blood calcium or phosphorus (Wilcox).

TUBULAR SCLEROSIS OF BONE. (Baumann-Schenker and Uehlinger). This is a condition in which the trabeculae of cancellous bone structure appear to be markedly thickened and accentuated. Microscopic examination of the bone structure gives the impression of sclerosis of the bone trabeculae with tunneling. Viewed on end these give the appearance of spotted bones. It is apparently of no pathological significance.

Familial Metaphyseal Dysplasia (Pyle; Hermel, et al.). This is a peculiar type of deformity of the shafts of the long bones in which there is irregular constriction of the shafts in their midportions with relative thickening of the cortex and encroachment upon the medullary canal. The ends of the bones are unusually enlarged and club-shaped; the cortex is thin and the trabecular structure fine. There is no pain or disability other than that occasioned by the deformity. Two instances have been reported in which the disease occurred in brother and sister.

METAPHYSIAL DYSOSTOSIS

This is an exceedingly rare condition in which the cartilaginous metaphysis does not ossify, resulting in dwarfism. The ends of the shaft are bulky and densely calcified. It differs in appearance from dyschondroplasia.

LIPOID GRANULOMATOSIS OF BONE

XANTHOMATOSIS*—RETICULO-ENDOTHE-LIOSIS; (HAND-SCHÜLLER-CHRISTIAN'S SYNDROME; EOSINOPHILIC GRANULOMA; LETTERER-SIEWE'S DISEASE; HUNTER-HURLER SYNDROME; GAUCHER'S DISEASE: NIEMANN-PICK'S DISEASE) (Fig. 96). At least the first three of these conditions are thought to be somewhat different aspects of the same disease. Fraser and Strong have pointed out their relationship to the reticulo-endothelial system. Xanthomatosis is a disturbance of fat metabolism. In the Hand-Schüller-Christian type, lipoid masses, particularly cholesterol and its esters, are deposited in the reticuloendothelial system, leading to definite roentgenological lesions in the skull, long bones and lungs.

In Gaucher's disease the stored substance is lipoprotein; in Niemann-Pick's disease the deposits are a phosphated lipoid. In these conditions the lipoids are stored in the phagocytic cells of the reticuloendothelial system.

The etiology is unknown, but endocrine disturbances are seen with retardation of physical-mental development. There is also adiposogenital dystrophy probably from pituitary insufficiency. This may be the cause or may be the result of faulty fat metabolism.

Clinically, Hand-Schüller-Christian's Disease occurs most frequently in young children, although an increasing number of cases are being reported in adults; 50% of cases are in children under six years of age.

Three prominent features of the syndrome are:
1. Rounded punched-out bony defects in the skull and other bones
2. Exophthalmos
3. Diabetes insipidus

The bony defects are due to deposits of fat, hyperplasia of the reticuloendothelial elements increasing the size of the small areas of lipoid deposit until they form large tumors of yellow fat. Pressure atrophy probably accounts for the bony defects. Exophthalmos is dependent upon destruction of the roof of the orbit and replacement by fatty tumor. Diabetes insipidus is present only if the cholesterol and fatty deposits occur around the region of the sella turcica causing destruction of the bony support for the pituitary. Any of the bones of the body may be involved, but the most common sites of involvement are the wings of the ilia, upper portion of the femurs and ribs. The bones may be so weakened that pathological fractures occur.

Vertebra Plana - Calvé's Disease. The vertebrae may be involved by the destructive lesions even to the point of complete collapse of the body giving an appearance of vertebra plana (Calvé's Disease), (Torgersen). Observation during the development of the condition reveals a progressive osteolytic process in which the vertebral body becomes narrower and narrower to the point of only a fine remaining plate of bone due to eosinophilic granuloma. Compere, E.L. et al. have observed coincidental widening of the cartilaginous discs above and below the involved vertebra. Subsequent examination may reveal recovery with regaining of almost the entire original height of the vertebra.

Fatty deposits are frequently seen in the lungs differing in size from minute miliary lesions to large blotchy areas of consolidation. They are not of especial importance except to strengthen the view that this is a constitutional disease. Physiological studies do not indicate that the lungs play an essential role in fat metabolism (Markowitz and Mahn).

Gingivitis is an early symptom, and xanthomatous lesions of the skin are common. Enlargement of the liver may be present with jaundice.

Roentgenologically, the most characteristic lesions by which the disease may be recognized are seen in the skull and other flat bones. The defects in the bone appear as punched-out areas with smooth, often circinate borders, with clear-cut edges involving the entire thickness of the bone. The areas may be single or multiple and may show a button of sequestrated bone (Wells). In the skull the calvarium is most frequently involved, but there may be involvement of the base, sinuses, orbits, mastoids or facial bones. There is ordinarily no sclerosis of the surrounding bone or other indication of bone production; in this respect it differs from syphilitic involvement. Schüller has reported, however, some evidence of bone sclerosis about the lesions in the occipital region of the skull as a manifestation of healing.

Hand-Schüller-Christian's disease is a very fatal disease; treatment recommended is
1. Fat-restricted diet.
2. Insulin.
3. X-ray therapy.

None of these are as a rule very effective. X-ray therapy has, in our experience, been most disappointing.

EOSINOPHILIC GRANULOMA*

This is a condition which seems to be closely related to Hand-Schüller-Christian's disease producing similar punched-out areas in the skull and other flat bones, especially the ilia and ribs (Fig. 96C).

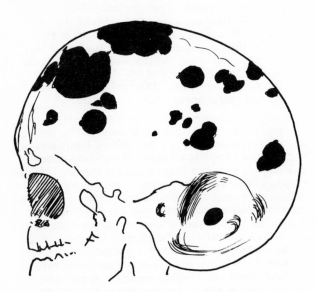

Fig. 96A

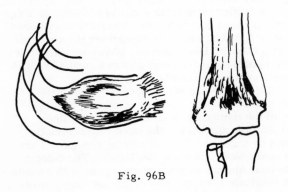

Fig. 96B

The long bones and bodies of the vertebra may also be involved. Vertebral destruction may be so great that there is complete collapse of the body giving rise to the appearance of vertebra plana. Bone involvement may be limited to a single punched-out area in the skull or one of the long bones. We have observed one case in which there was separation of the sutures without convolutional atrophy, probably due to a deposit of granulomatous material over the cerebral cortex.

On exploration these areas of bone destruction are filled with greyish-brown granulomatous masses which reveal on microscopic examination large numbers of reticulo-endothelial and other blood cells with a large number of eosinophile cells. These are sometimes so predominant that they impart a red color to the entire section.

These tumors vary markedly in one respect however from Hand-Schüller-Christian's disease in that they are usually very amenable to small doses of x-ray therapy, usually undergoing complete recovery. This is so small in amount that the quantity of x-radiation delivered in radiography may be sufficient to cause regression, (Platt and Eisenberg). The amount and character of the x-ray therapy administered with successful results is similar to that used in the control of infection. Spontaneous regression of a solitary lesion may occur. Curettment of a solitary lesion may cause healing, (Hunter). Nitter has reported 3 cases occurring with a localized lesion in the pelvis, 2 of which healed after x-ray therapy, one in which surgery was unsuccessful.

An instance has been reported in which there was both lung and diaphragmatic involvement in addition to the involvement of the bony structure, thus further indicating its similarity to Schüller-Christian's Disease, (Ackerman).

An unusual case has been reported in which the terminal phalanx was involved (Loehr).

LETTERER-SIEWE'S Disease. This is a closely related condition similar roentgenologically in many respects to Hand-Schüller-Christian's Disease and to eosinophilic granuloma. It differs in that it is a non-lipoid reticulo-endotheliosis. Histologically

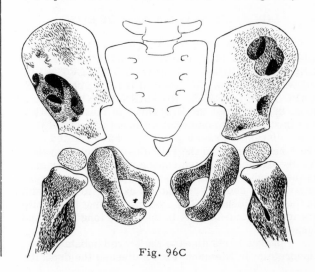

Fig. 96C

the lesions are devoid of lipoid. It is considered by some to be a different stage of the disease. It occurs only in infants less than two years of age and is almost always fatal.

Letterer-Siewe's Disease is thought to be a variant of the other xanthomatous diseases. It often shows rounded, punched-out areas of destruction in the skull similar to Hand-Schüller-Christian's Disease, but these are never as extensive. The long bones may be involved in the metaphyseal regions and there may be such extensive blood vessel changes as to suggest multiple hemangiomata on microscopic examination. There may be heavy periosteal reaction and the process may resemble acute leukemia. It may involve the spine and spread to the adjacent soft parts like an abscess. In certain instances it has healed with merely curettement where it was in an accessible location; recurrence even years later is not uncommon. The lungs are almost always involved, with miliary infiltration or larger areas of consolidation and there is usually generalized lymph node enlargement with eosinophilic infiltration. There may also be visceral involvement of the liver and spleen. Instances are reported where it resembled osteoid osteoma. The name Histocytoma has been proposed to designate these conditions since the tumor masses are composed of histiocytes filled with fat, foam cells, eosinophiles, and macrophages.

GAUCHER'S DISEASE (Fig. 97). A rare, familial, chronic, constitutional, nonhereditary disease of metabolism characterized by the deposition of cerebroside kerasin in certain cells of the reticuloendothelial system.

CLINICAL CHARACTERISTICS. The most outstanding characteristics of the disease are splenohepatomegaly, which occurs without ascites; occasionally lymph-adenopathy, subicteric pigmentation of the exposed parts of the skin, pingueculalike thickness of the ocular conjunctiva, hemorrhagic diathesis, and unique changes in the bones. A hypochromic type of anemia may develop with slight but early leucopenia. Frequently thrombocytopenia and spastic irritative contractions and tremors of the central type occur. The femur usually shows the most typical changes, but all of the bones may become involved.

PATHOLOGY. Large so-called Gaucher cells containing complex substances in their cytoplasm with eccentrically placed nuclei and wrinkled protoplasm are traversed by a fine fibrillar network. These cells are considered as characteristic of the disease. They are found in all organs where elements of the recticulo-endothelial system are present.

ROENTGENOLOGICAL MANIFESTATIONS. Any of the long bones may be involved but the femur shows the most extensive changes; it may be the only bone showing manifestation of involvement. The bone lesions are produced by permeation of the interstitial tissue with gaucher cells and the roentgenographic appearance produced depends upon the degree of involvement and the characteristics of the bone archi-

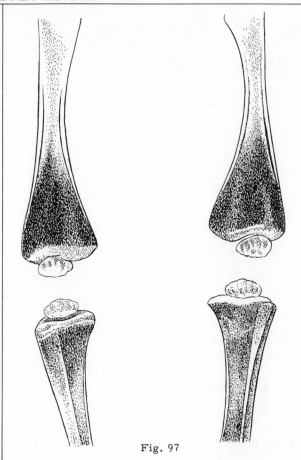

Fig. 97

tecture in the region of the bone involved. In the long bones the fine trabeculae are the first to be eliminated by pressure atrophy from gaucher cells giving rise to the appearance of coarsening of the trabecular structure. In the ends of the long bones the more delicate trabecular structure results in more extensive absorption with development of a fine, almost fibrillar network of remaining trabeculae. The cortex is thinned and the shaft itself becomes widened giving rise to the "club-shaped" lower end of the femur so characteristic of the disease.

Tennent has stressed symmetrical enlargement of the lower ends of the femurs, with cortical thinning, loss of the normal medial concavity and central patchy rarefaction as being the essential elements of bone involvement.

Pathological fracture may occur in the region of the neck of the femur or elsewhere where the bone is under stress. Numerous small rounded spots of bone sclerosis are encountered—these are probably due to multiple minute areas of trauma applied to the weakened trabeculae which give way and are either compressed or give rise to stimulation of new bone in an effort of repair (Reed and Susman; Windholz and S. Foster; and Tennent).

The most effective treatment is splenectomy.

NIEMANN-PICK'S DISEASE. In Niemann-Pick's disease the findings are very similar to those found in Gaucher's Disease. Examination of the fatty deposits shows that they consist of phosphated lipoids.

GARGOYLISM, (HUNTER-HURLER DISEASE). This is a congenital condition characterized by multiple symmetrical skeletal deformities with a superimposed disturbance of lipoid metabolism (Harvey).

It is now agreed that this condition must be classified with the lipoidoses with superimposed endocrine disorder, probably the effect of lipoid disturbance on the hypothalamus causing pituitary and thyroid dysfunction.

Hypothalamic disturbances are probably connected with changes seen in the pituitary and thyroid glands, and these in turn with some clinical features of the disease such as chondrodystrophy and dwarfism.

The hypophyseal dysfunction is attributed to "blebs caused by escape of cerebrospinal fluid into adjacent tissues in early embryonal life." The clinical picture is given as:

a) kyphotic disproportionate dwarfs from "beaking" of the anterior inferior margins of the twelfth thoracic or first lumbar vertebra

b) large head, grotesque face resembling gargoyles and any type of skull deformity without erosion or enlargement of sella or evidence of increased intracranial pressure

c) bilateral corneal opacities

d) hepato splenomegaly

e) mental deficiency

A condition described in Morquio-Brailsford Disease shows essentially similar bone lesions without other features of the syndrome. The vertebral bodies are biconvex and rounded, and the discs biconcave; in Morquio-Brailsford Disease the bodies are flat. In both conditions kyphosis is due to deformity of the twelfth thoracic or first or second lumbar vertebrae, with increased motion at this point. In gargoylism one body is smaller than the other and is displaced backward: there is beaking of the lower anterior edge of vertebra while in Morquio-Brailsford Disease there is usually symmetrical pointing in the middle of the anterior vertebral body; other conditions may destroy the vertebra (eosinophilic granuloma). There is no mental deficiency in Morquio-Brailsford Disease, while this condition is regarded as "one of the best defined types of mental retardation," (Caffey).

The roof of the acetabulum is usually sloping (shelving); there is coxa valga but no gross enlargement. The ends of the radius and ulna usually slope towards each other showing delay in growth. The hands are spadelike and the bases of the metatarsals are pointed, short, thick and honeycombed.

QUESTIONS ON GLANDULAR AND METABOLIC DISTURBANCES

Questions marked with a dagger deal with rare and less-important conditions.

1. What influence does thyroid dysfunction have on bone growth?

2. Describe the skeletal changes in acromegaly and to what are they due?

3. What three types of pituitary adenomata are recognized and what are their chief clinical and roentgenological manifestations?

4. What is osteogenesis imperfecta and describe the roentgen manifestations in its various types?

†5. Describe the roentgen appearance of chondrodystrophia foetalis (achondroplasia). To what is it due?

†6. Describe the roentgenographic appearance of generalized osteitis fibrosa cystica (von Recklinghausen's Disease).

7. What are the clinical and roentgenological manifestations of fibrous dysplasia of bone, monostotic and polyostotic?

8. How may Polyostotic Fibrous Dysplasia be differentiated from von Recklinghausen's Disease roentgenographically and pathologically?

9. What are the clinical and roentgenological manifestations of osteitis deformans (Paget's disease)?

†10. What is meant by osteoporosis circumscripta and with what disease is it intimately associated?

11. In what locations does Paget's disease occur as a localized manifestation?

12. Could you differentiate roentgenologically between localized Paget's disease of the vertebral bodies and osteoblastic carcinoma? How could the differential diagnosis be made?

†13. Describe the clinical and roentgenological manifestations of leontiasis ossea.

14. What is meant by "Marble Bones"? How does the condition develop and what are its roentgenological characteristics?

†15. Describe the roentgen findings in Osteopathia Hyperostotica Sclerotisans Multiplex Infantilis (Engelmann's Disease) and how may it be differentiated from Marble Bones and Infantile Cortical Hyperostosis of Caffey and Silvermann?

16. What is meant by Osteopoikylosis? Punctate Epiphyseal Dysplasia? Tubular Sclerosis of Bone? Of what pathological significance are they?

17. What is xanthomatosis and for what type of bone changes is it responsible? What is Hand-Schüller-Christian's syndrome? What is meant by Eosinophilic Granuloma and what relationship does it bear to Hand-Schüller-Christian's disease? To Letterer Siewe's Disease?

†18. What are Gaucher's and Niemann-Pick's diseases and how do they differ from xanthomatoses of other types, clinically and roentgenographically?

†19. Describe HURLER-PFAUNDLER'S SYNDROME.

BLOOD DYSCRASIAS (Chapter IX)

Bone Changes in

    A. LEUKEMIA

        1. Lymphatic

        2. Splenomyelogenous

    B. HEMOLYTIC ANEMIAS

        1. Erythroblastic or Mediterranean Anemia (COOLEY)

        2. Sickle Cell Anemia

        3. Chronic Hemolytic Icterus

        4. Myelosclerosis (Marrow Sclerosis)

    C. HEMOPHILIA

Chapter IX

BLOOD DYSCRASIAS

BONE CHANGES IN LEUKEMIA; LYMPHATIC; SPLENOMYELOGENOUS LEUKOCYTHEMIA

Lymphatic leukemia is a fatal disease, characterized by hyperplasia of the white-blood-cell-forming tissues throughout the body. Usually there is a striking increase in white blood cells with many abnormal cell forms.

Clinically the outstanding characteristic of the disease is the painless enlargement of the lymph glands and lymphoid tissues all over the body. Hyperplasia of smaller lymphoid deposits results in the appearance of lymphoid masses in locations in which they normally are not encountered; the spleen is also enlarged. There is a rapidly increasing anemia followed by the symptoms which ordinarily develop from any secondary anemia; weakness, general malaise, loss of weight, dyspnea and palpitation. Spontaneous subcutaneous hemorrhage occurs. In the terminal stages or with peritoneal involvement hyperpyrexia may develop.

Ordinarily at the onset in either lymphatic or splenomyelogenous leukemia there is no roentgenographic evidence of the disease; occasionally, however, bony involvement may develop in either. Generalized osteoporosis may develop; this is most pronounced just adjacent to the epiphyseal line. In children, narrow bands of increased density 2 to 5 mm. in width may traverse this dark zone at the ends of the long bones due to calcium deposits during remissions in the disease. Epstein has found that the vertebral bodies go through similar changes. In certain instances there may be small areas of actual bone erosion, in the diaphyseal regions. The periosteum may be elevated from subperiosteal infiltration, giving rise to an appearance spoken of as "cloaking of the periosteum," or it may be raised in laminated layers. The picture may resemble scurvy or even neuroblastoma, (Silverman). Monocytic leukemia may also produce similar changes in the bones. In adults especially, diffuse osteosclerosis may develop due to increased production of cancellous bone.

The disease is invariably fatal; roentgen therapy offers amelioration of symptoms and some prolongation of life. In extremely acute cases, especially in infants, X-ray therapy is contraindicated. Amelioration of symptoms with filling in of the zones of decreased density with dense new bone occurs following treatment with folic acid antagonists-aminop-terin, but this at best is only a temporary measure.

Chloroma. This is an unusual form of myeloid leukemia characterized by deposits of tumor-like material in the skeleton, especially in the subperiosteal tissues. Involvement of the skull and orbit predominates producing "chloromatous facies". The masses are greenish yellow on section but appear slaty-blue in color when viewed through the skin.

The lesions are not characteristic but when they are encountered in a case having blood findings of leukemia they are significant. Without knowledge of the blood findings the picture may suggest scurvy, neuroblastoma, suprarenal disfunction, (Kemp and Williams).

BONE MANIFESTATIONS IN HEMOLYTIC ANEMIAS.

The anemias may be divided into two main groups: a) hemolytic anemia, in which the anemia is due to destruction of previously well-formed blood cells; b) the deficiency anemias, in which there is defective blood formation, (Teall).

ERYTHROBLASTIC ANEMIA.* Erythroblastic or Mediterranean anemia (Cooley) Fig. 98, is an anemia usually affecting children descended from nationalities bordering on the Mediterranean, especially Italian and Greek. The condition seems to be congenital, but the cause is not known. In most cases, the disease is well advanced before the end of the first year. The skin shows a peculiar muddy or icteric tinge, but the sclera remains clear. Many have been described as mongoloid in appearance. The head is usually greatly enlarged, especially in the parietal regions. Both the liver and spleen are increased in size.

The blood picture is characteristic: large numbers of erythroblasts and immature cell forms are found especially after splenectomy; leukocytosis is present; and there is evidence of increased fragility. The icteric tinge is probably due to hemolysis. Characteristic bone changes occur in the anemias of children which are probably not primary but secondary to the anemia. In all types of this disease, due to the profound anemia, hyperplasia of the bone marrow develops to which may be traced all of the manifestations of bone involvement.

PATHOLOGICAL AND RADIOLOGICAL MANIFESTATIONS. The cranial vault in the early stages shows an increased porosity of the medullary portion; the diploetic structures are more pronounced but both

---

*An asterisk following any title indicates that roentgenographic reproductions illustrating this condition will be found in the pictorial supplement at the end of the chapter.

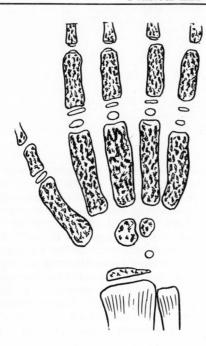

Fig. 98

the outer and inner tables of the skull are thin.

The earliest manifestations of bone involvement may be seen within the first year as transverse lines of increased density adjacent to the epiphyseal cartilages, either along or associated with similar zones of decreased density. These are symmetrically distributed in multiple bones throughout the body.

Microscopically, the opaque lines are due to dense trabeculae with increased calcium matrix. These findings are caused by a transient disturbance of endochondral bone formation (Janus and Dietz).

When fully developed the trabeculae become accentuated and thickened, producing a lattice-work appearance of the medullary portion (Fig. 98). The bones lose their slender curved appearance becoming thicker and squared at the ends. There is rarely any periosteal reaction. The entire picture is the result of pressure from hyperplasia of the bone marrow. In the later stages, there is even greater thickening of the diplöe which may even become four times its normal thickness due to hyperplastic changes of the bone marrow. The outer table may become so thin that it cannot be distinguished in the roentgenogram; the parietal bones are the sites of greatest thickening. There may be spicules of bone radiating outward like hair standing on end. Or, as usually occurs in this form of anemia, there may be no skull involvement at all.

In the long bones, there is a widening because of an increase in the medullary portion. Rarefaction of the medulla results in a translucent appearance in the roentgenogram. There is enlargement and accentuation of the trabeculae of the medulla which is more marked at the metaphyseal end. Thinning of the cortex may lead to pathological fracture. Periosteal elevation is rarely observed. Joint changes have been

recorded. The changes are similar to those seen in the short bones but are not so pronounced. There may be involvement of the pelvis, vertebrae, ribs, clavicles and scapulae as well as the long bones. Erythroblastic anemia has been reported in adults showing essentially similar reactions. The long bones may develop a sclerosis however causing filling in of the medullary canal.

SICKLE-CELL ANEMIA
Fig. 99

Sickle-cell anemia is a chronic hemolytic anemia associated with abnormalities of the hemoglobin molecule characterized by peculiar sickle-shaped red blood cells. Contact with air affects the sickle cells so that special laboratory procedure is essential for their proper demonstration.

It occurs primarily in the negro race or from countries bordering on African territory; a few instances have been reported of its occurrence in white individuals. Sickle cells are encountered in 7% of all negros without abnormal manifestations.

Clinically it is characterized by anemia, abdominal crises, joint pains, leg ulcers and other manifestations depending on the organ involved. These conditions result from the underlying basic pathologic processes of excessive blood destruction and abnormal erythropoiesis with resulting bone marrow hyperplasia; thrombosis and infarction. These pathological processes are the basis for development of all of the unusual bone manifestations which occur.

Roentgenologically the skull especially in children presents a similar but more striking appearance to that of the other anemias, with thickening of the bones of the cranium, especially in the parietal regions, thinning of the outer table, allowing the active diploe to produce spicules of new bone radiating out-

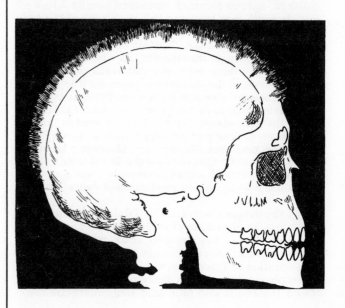

Fig. 99

ward from the skull margin, described as "hair stand-ing on end," (Fig. 99). In adults this appearance is not usually encountered. There is instead a thickened granular appearance of the skull bones.

In sickle-cell anemia the long bones may be involved also, although this is very rare. We have, however, seen instances in which destructive areas have been present in the lower end of the humerus, with hyperplastic periositis. Widespread infarction and marrow hyperplasia produce many bizarre roent-gen manifestations (Hamburg). Mosley and Manley have stressed the joint manifestations which are probably due to infarctions, not unlike those produced in caisson disease from nitrogen embolism. There is asceptic necrosis (especially of the femoral and humeral heads of the hip and shoulder joints), with flattening or disintegration of the weight-bearing portion, and secondary sclerotic and hypertrophic arthritic changes about the joint.

Extensive bone infarction of the shafts of long bones is stressed by Rowe and Haggard with seques-tration of almost the entire shafts and involucrum pro-duced by the proliferating periosteum, very similar to that produced in osteomyelitis by infection.

The spine, especially in adults may show bal-looning of the vertebrae and even osteosclerosis, (Kraft and Bertel).

Persons suffering with this condition frequent-ly are afflicted with leg ulcers, gall stones, and epistaxis (Weil and Lerner).

No form of treatment is definitely satisfactory. Splenectomy is of doubtful value. In some instances of early involvement X-ray treatment has been found beneficial.

Chronic Hemolytic Icterus. In this disease, bone changes are not so apt to be present but when they do occur they present essentially similar le-sions to those seen in erythroblastic anemia.

BONE CHANGES IN DEFICIENCY ANEMIA

Myelosclerosis, (Marrow Sclerosis). This is a condition in which, from some unknown cause the bone marrow undergoes progressive degeneration with replacement by a gelatinous material and fibro-sis. With the continuous loss of blood-forming struc-tures there is an attempt made by the rest of the hemopoietic system to compensate for the loss re-sulting in splenomegaly and hepatomegaly. There is a profound change in the blood picture; anemia with nucleated red cells and other young forms and changes in the white cells similar to aleukemic luekemia. This gives rise to extreme weakness with aches and pains in the bones and joints.

Secondary myelosclerosis, where the condition follows extensive involvement of the red bone mar-row, such as osteopetrosis, Paget's disease, and ex-tensive invasion of the bone by tumor, may produce similar changes (Bersack and Feinstein).

It would seem from this that the blood changes may be incidental to the bone marrow destruction from whatever cause and that the fibrosis and sclerosis which follow are reparative processes. It may be considered then as a dyscrasia of the reticu-loendothelial system of unknown etiology having a de-pressing action on normal bone-forming elements of the bone marrow.

ROENTGENOGRAPHICALLY. The bones show a dense sclerotic appearance due to thickening of the trabecular structure, fibrosis of the marrow spaces with some calcification. In its extreme degree it may present an appearance almost as dense as fluorine deposits or even of marble bones. In the flat bones of the pelvis and in the bodies of the vertebrae the appearance may resemble that of metastatic osteo-blastic carcinoma (Sussman).

HEMOPHILIA—JOINT INVOLVEMENT (Gohrmley, et al.)

In hemophilia there is difficulty in the coagu-lating elements of the blood, not in its cytology. The marked tendency to spontaneous hemorrhage which is characteristic of this disease may result in bone changes in and about the joints which are at times difficult to differentiate from other types of arthritis. Spontaneous hemorrhages into the joint may at first produce haziness of the joint similar to effusion of any other type. Early lesions may be rounded, well-defined areas of cortical erosion beneath the carti-lage. Large hemorrhages beneath the cartilage may strip up this structure, depriving it of blood supply so that it becomes destroyed and leaves the articular cortex bare and eroded. New bone production may result in irregular osteophite formation, or the blood clots may become organized with fibrosis and calci-fication; producing a picture not unlike cystic degen-eration of bone seen in mallum coxae senilis; anky-losis may result. At times the extensive destruction of bony tissue caused by this condition may even re-semble osteogenic tumor (Echternacht).

Most hemorrhagic manifestations occur near the epiphyseal line during the stage of active bone development; as a result the epiphysis enlarges to conform to the increased size of the bone-forming area. The expanded and enlarged epiphysis which re-sults, therefore, will be a clue to the underlying cause in future years. This is especially noteworthy in the head of the radius and in the knee. (See chapter on arthritis.)

QUESTIONS ON BLOOD DYSCRASIAS

Questions marked with a dagger deal with rare and less-important conditions.

1. What bone changes are noted in lymphatic leukemia?

2. To what are they attributable and do they differ materially from secondary malignant involvement from other cause?

3. What manifestations in the cranial bones are more or less common to all hemolytic anemias of childhood?

4. Describe the characteristic appearance of the skull in erythroblastic anemia. What manifestations occur in the long bones?

5. What bone manifestations are present in sickle-cell anemia?

6. What racial characteristics are always present in sickle-cell anemia? Are sickle cells found in the blood of normal negroes?

†7. What bone manifestations are present in chronic hemolytic icterus?

†8. What is meant by bone marrow sclerosis and what are its roentgen manifestations?

†9. What roentgen manifestations have we of hemophilia and where do they occur?

DISEASES OF BONE (Continued)

NEUROPATHIC LESIONS OF BONE (Chapter X)

Neuropathic Disturbances

1. Without other manifestations of abnormality

2. Leprosy

3. Raynaud's Disease

4. Sclerodactylia

5. Injuries and Tumors of the Spinal Cord

6. Melorheostosis

7. Neurofibromatosis; Bone changes in (VON RECKLINGHAUSEN'S DISEASE)

8. Arthropathy - Syringomyelia; Charcot

NEUROPATHIC LESIONS OF BONE

NEUROPATHIC DISTURBANCES*
Fig. 100

Even though there may be doubt of the actual existence of "trophic" nerves, (Delano), there can be no doubt as to the trophic effects produced in bone by nerve disturbances. The effects are most pronounced in the metacarpal and metatarsal bones and phalanges of the hands and feet. The distal ends of the bones become smaller in calibre and the terminal phalanges become atrophied to fine points. This process of bone resorption may continue until the heads of the metacarpal and metatarsal bones are completely separated from the distal ends of the shafts of the bones. Such pronounced bone lesions are usually accompanied by punched-out trophic ulcers of the soft parts. Whether the condition is due to the direct influence of the nerves on bony growth or indirectly to the effect of the nerves on the blood vessels cannot be definitely asserted. Cutting down of the blood supply alone does not always result in these bone changes; they do not occur in arteriosclerosis or diabetic gangrene.

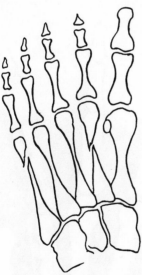

Fig. 100

In by far the greatest number of instances there may be no manifestation of the cause of the condition and the patient may appear otherwise normal. Numerous conditions in which other manifestations of neurotrophic disturbances are present show similar changes. Notable examples are:

Leprosy
Raynaud's
Sclerodactylia
Endarteritis-Obliterans (Buerger's Disease)

Syringomyelia
Certain types of Spinal Lues
Tumors and Injuries to the central nervous system

BONE AND JOINT LESIONS IN LEPROSY (Esguerra-Gomez and Acosta). According to the specifications of the International Congress of Leprosy at Cairo, 1938, there are two types of leprosy: 1) the nerve or neural type including all cases of benign leprosy with polyneuritic manifestations (disorder of sensation, trophic changes, paralysis, mutilations) or macules of non-leprous nature "leprides" or both; 2) lepromatous type formerly called cutaneous in which are grouped all cases of malignant leprosy with poor resistance and unfavorable prognosis with lesions especially of the skin.

Cutaneous leprosy rarely is attendant with bone lesions whereas the neurological type is most frequently associated with neurotrophic atrophy of the bones (Faget and Mayoral). Bone changes therefore are not pathognomonic: similar roentgenological changes are seen in congenital anomalies, and in other neurotrophic disturbances. The neurotrophic process is very slow requiring ten to twenty years for the digits to become atrophied. Generally speaking there is progressive atrophy of quantity, the terminal phalanges and other short bones of the hands and feet become pointed and spindle shaped, progressing proximally until all of the bones are involved. Marked contractures occur especially in the hands in the neurotrophic form of the disease; in the lepromatous type contractures and pointing of the bones is not a usual finding. In leprosy the added element of anesthesia permits the ready association of injury and secondary infection, with the characteristic reaction which these conditions produce. Periostitis does not usually accompany the atrophic lesions, unless secondary pyogenic infection occurs. Suppurative lesions of the soft parts may show shaggy periosteal reaction of the bone underlying the region of the superficial ulcer.

It has been pointed out, (Cooney and Crosby) that "the phalanges in the feet are often preserved intact even when there is marked destruction of the metatarsal and tarsal bones. In contrast the absorption of the phalanges of the hands always occurs before involvement of the metacarpal bones, beginning at the distal phalanx." It is felt that this is due to the fact that in the feet it is the heads of the metatarsal bones and in the hands the tips of the carpal phalanges that are subject to the maximum trauma and pressure in ordinary function and use. Ainhum has been recorded as an occasional lesion in leprosy.

Occasionally in association with lepromatous leprosy a type of cystic degeneration has been de-

---

*An asterisk following any title indicates that roentgenographic reproductions illustrating this condition will be found in the pictorial supplement at the end of the chapter.

scribed which is called osteitis multiplex cystica; this condition is due to absorption of lime salts giving rise to a honeycombed appearance from numerous punched-out cystlike areas of radiolucency. Such vacuoles do not determine any peripheral reaction but when they approach the cortical covering they distend and sometimes destroy it. Various abnormalities of the bone structure due to perivascular injury may occur; enlargement of the canal for the nutrient artery has been observed.

Zones of hypercalcification and widening of the proximal ends of one or more phalanges covering adjoining phalanx like a cap, called "hooded" appearance, may occur.

Phalangeal, two forms, 1) resorption, 2) resorption after atrophy, gives picture designated as "collar button," "hooded," or "hour-glass" form.

RAYNAUD'S DISEASE. Raynaud's disease is an obscure condition characterized by spasm of the terminal blood vessels to symmetrical parts of the body often resulting in symmetrical gangrene of the distal phalanges. This condition occurs mainly between the ages of 18 and 30, especially in women. It is probably the result of a neuro-vascular disturbance. As a symptom, symmetrical gangrene may occur in the course of syringomyelia, tumors of the cord, leprosy and tabes.

CLINICAL CHARACTERISTICS. The patient suffers from periodic attacks of spasm of the terminal blood vessels. Attacks generally begin with dysesthesia and a dead feeling in the fingers or other symmetrically situated parts of the body: toes, lobes of ears, nose. The affected members look pale and waxy, and feel cold. This is the stage of asphyxia. It may be of short or long duration and pain may be very intense. The involved parts become hyperesthetic. This stage is replaced by cyanosis, the skin becoming bluish or livid, and the pain becoming more intense. Insomnia, anorexia, and psychic upsets are the rule. Fever is absent. In the severe cases where the cyanosis is prolonged, gangrene supervenes.

ROENTGENOGRAPHIC APPEARANCE. Only after repeated attacks over a long period of time do bone changes develop. There is a marked atrophy of quantity of the bones; the phalanges of the hands and feet become spindle-shaped and pointed, giving rise to a spearlike appearance. There is absorption of the distal phalanges even to complete disappearance; rarefied areas appear in the heads of the metacarpals but rarely do they undergo such spindle-shaped atrophy as seen in other atrophic conditions.

INJURIES AND TUMORS OF THE SPINAL CORD. Spinal cord injury with paralysis may result in the development of large hyperostoses, frequently bridging a joint. These form rapidly and may attain huge proportions, often 6 to 8 centimeters in thickness. When the lower extremities are involved they may be associated with the development of bladder stone. An instance has been reported, (Larsen and

Wright) in which a similar type of massive bony outgrowth has developed bridging the hip joint, following paralysis from poliomyelitis. They may develop within muscles (myositis ossificans) or in the existing ligaments. Surgical removal may be carried out only to be followed by recurrence, (Miller and O'Neill).

Lodge has pointed out that extreme degree of osteoporosis and spontaneous fractures are also common accompaniments of paraplegia but this is probably due to prolonged disuse.

MELORHEOSTOSIS;
MONOMELIC FLOWING HYPEROSTOSIS
Fig. 101

Melorheostosis (Kraft) is a flowing hyperostosis of bone usually involving multiple bones of a single extremity; bilateral involvement has been reported (Carpender, et al.). The X-ray appearance of the bone has been likened to that of a molten stream of wax running down the side of a candle. Definite diagnosis of the condition can be made only by roentgenographic examination.

The etiology is unknown, but the distribution of the hyperostosis is usually along the distribution of a nerve suggesting some nerve influence in its development. In unusual cases the skull, jaw, spine and ribs may be involved.

Microscopically there is concentric perivascular ossification but this is hardly sufficient to characterize the disease.

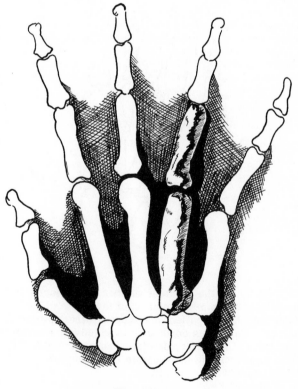

Fig. 101

CLINICAL MANIFESTATIONS. The first signs of the condition are usually noted during childhood or adolescence; but the condition may not be noticed until adult life.

The onset is insidious and the progress extremely slow. There may be no symptoms at all and the condition may be discovered quite by accident. Low-grade intermittent rheumatic pains may be present which may disappear for months or years. The symptoms even in severe cases may be very vague. The condition may be slowly progressive or remain quiescent for years.

In advanced cases deformities occur which result in shortening of the extremity. The muscles of the involved extremity tend to become atrophic.

Roentgenologically, the involved bone shows a dense cortical hyperostosis, resembling sclerotic bone extending longitudinally along one side of a long bone. The bone shows an irregular wavy contour with thickening of the shaft.

A case has been reported in which a previous skull injury was thought to have some bearing on the development of melorheostosis in the arm, (Fejer).

The process extends to the very margin of the articular cortex and may be present in the adjacent bones, but the joint itself usually remains free from involvement. Only in very advanced cases is there interference with joint function. The hyperostosis cannot have its origin from periosteal proliferation, since it extends beyond the normal location of this structure. Several of the bones of an extremity may be involved, usually showing a distribution along the course of a nerve. The medullary cavity is encroached upon by the overgrowth of bone.

When the shoulder or hip is affected, bony masses appear frequently in the soft parts, lodging usually in the muscles or under the skin. These formations may be confluent, presenting a bizarre appearance. Sympathectomy has been performed for the relief of pain (Hess and Street).

No other form of treatment has been found to influence the disease.

NEUROFIBROMATOSIS OF VON RECKLINGHAUSEN*

This is a condition which manifests itself primarily by multiple small neurofibromatous nodules arising from the peripheral nerves. It is now thought by some to be an hereditary condition.

Other associated conditions which have been described are "coffee-colored splotches" of the skin, mental deficiency, other congenital developmental defects, involvement of the central nervous system and rarely involvement of the bony structures.

Involvement of bone structures is primarily due to atrophy or destruction from pressure of the nerve tissue nodules. Holt and Wright list six groups of bone changes:

1. Erosive defects due to the presence of neurofibromas contiguous to bone.
2. Scoliosis.
3. Disorders of growth, including both over- and under-development.
4. Bowing and pseudarthrosis of the lower leg.
5. Intra-osseous cystic lesions.
6. Congenital anomalies.

The most characteristic roentgen findings are small cystlike areas of absorption in the bony structures caused by pressure of neurofibromatous nodules forming within the bony tissue (Brooks and Lehman). Microscopic examination fails to disclose any infiltration of the bone by the nerve tissue.

There is often pronounced osteoporosis and softening of the bone which frequently leads to extreme degrees of kyphosis. Malignant degeneration is not uncommon; it leads to pronounced bone destruction. Notching of the undersides of the ribs may occur when intercostal nerves are involved, giving an x-ray picture similar in all respects to that found in coarctation of the aorta. Abnormalities of bone growth such as hyperplastic periostitis associated with elephantiasis of the extremity is probably a manifestation of circulatory stasis (Friedman).

NEUROPATHIC ARTHROPATHY. Notable examples of nerve influence on the development of certain types of arthritis is seen in Charcot joint and Syringomyelia. The extreme disintegration of the joint structures seen in these conditions is probably due largely to unrestrained trauma in an anaesthetic joint (see chapter on arthritis).

QUESTIONS ON NERVE CONDITIONS AFFECTING BONE

Questions marked with a dagger deal with rare and less-important conditions.

1. Describe the influence of long-standing neurotrophic disturbances on the bones of the hands and feet.

†2. What is the roentgenographic appearance of leprosy?

†3. What is the ultimate effect of Raynaud's disease on the terminal bony structure?

†4. What is melorheostosis and what indication have we that it may have some relationship with nerve distribution?

†5. Is it ever progressive? Does the hyperosteal new bone spring from the periosteum? If not, why not? Is it ever associated with pain? How may it be treated?

6. What bone manifestations may be associated with paraplegia?

7. Describe the bone lesions most commonly encountered in neurofibroma.

MINERAL POISONS AND OTHER INTOXICATIONS AFFECTING BONE (Chapter XI)

A. Metallic Poisoning

From Ingestion or Inhalation of Metallic Salts
1. Lead
2. Phosphorus
3. Bismuth
4. Fluorine
5. Radium

From Lodgment of a Lead Bullet in Bony Structure

B. Vitamins

Hypervitaminosis A
Hypervitaminosis D

C. KASCHIN-BECK'S Disease

Chapter XI

MINERAL POISONS AND OTHER INTOXICATIONS AFFECTING BONE

From Ingestion and Inhalation*

In growing children the continued intake of heavy metallic substances into the body in sufficient quantity and over sufficient period of time leads to certain roentgenographic changes in the bones. Often the cause of the intoxication is not suspected until bone changes seen at roentgenographic examination indicate the true nature of the condition.

Metallic salts, such as lead, phosphorus and bismuth are deposited in the bones along with normal calcium. Observations on rachitic patients with lead intoxication indicate that the lead is mobilized with the calcium since the zone of increased density did not form as long as the rickets remained untreated, but that as soon as the rickets was treated, heavy deposits of calcium and lead became evident in the zone of previous osteoid bone.

The most frequent source of intoxication in lead poisoning is from inhalation from burning of old storage battery boxes or in infants from ingestion of lead paint chewed from toys, (Cooper).

In children these deposits are most pronounced on the diaphyseal side of the epiphyseal line at the

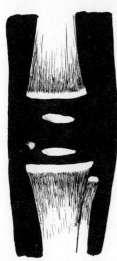

Fig. 102

zone of temporary calcification, showing in the roentgenogram as zones of increased density (Fig. 102). Any of the heavy metals may cause such deposits and one cannot be distinguished from the other. The condition has been observed in new-born infants as a result of bismuth given to the mother as antiluetic medication. The longer the duration, the wider this zone of calcification becomes. A line of increased density can be present in perfectly normal infants from Vitamin D administration either as cod liver oil or ultraviolet ray exposure; in lead poisoning this zone is denser.

Chemical analysis of the bone in the region of these dense zones showed that "lead was deposited in inverse ratio to calcium. The zones of greatest density in the roentgenogram showed less calcium, but four times as much lead as the cortex," (Vogt). Microscopically this line of increased density appears to be due to enormous increase in radiopaque cancellous tissue and decrease in marrow space.

After relinquishing the intake of metallic salts, these dense zones gradually diminish in width but may not disappear completely for years. They do not remain across the ends of long bones as permanent manifestations of former growth disturbance such as the "growth lines" seen persisting after rickets but merely continue to show a zone of increased density within the newly-formed metaphyseal bone. This would indicate that the abnormal processes occurring in these conditions are radically different, the one produced in rickets being a structural defect in the bone resulting in a scar-like alteration of the bony architecture which remains as a permanent defect moving farther and farther from the epiphyseal line as bony growth progresses, the other, zones of metallic deposit, resorbing by the blood stream only to be redeposited at the epiphyseal line in the natural process of bone growth. Such chronic intoxication may be sufficient for the development of lead encephalitis months or even years after all outside contact has been eliminated.

In severe lead poisoning there may be associated encephalitis, which may result in increased intracranial pressure with convolutional atrophy and separation of the sutures. Encephalography discloses hydrocephalus with excessive amount of cerebrospinal fluid. This may not develop until years later; once established it may be permanent. Epileptic convulsions may develop.

In adults metallic deposit is so uniform that it cannot be detected in the roentgenogram.

Phosphorus poisoning presents, in addition to the usual findings of metallic poisoning, other manifestations in the mandible. Irregular areas of bone destruction appear, especially along the alveolar margins; the teeth may become loose and fall out. The picture is similar to osteomyelitis caused by pyogenic infection and cannot be distinguished from it roentgenographically.

Fluoride osteosclerosis has been described in miners working in rock having a high fluorine content (2 to 5%). Recently fluorosis has been reported from fluorine in the drinking water in some parts of Texas, ranging from 4.6 to 12 parts per million; concentrations in excess of 1.5 parts per million are said to produce occasional fluorosis. Long residence in such areas is necessary before such a condition develops.

Roentgenographically there is an increase in density of all the bones of the skeleton, due to thickening of the trabeculae and increased calcium deposit producing a chalky appearance of the vertebrae. This occurs even in adult fully developed bone. This is the only condition in which metallic salts, deposited in adult bone structure, causes demonstrable increase in density. In severe cases spinal ligaments may show deposit as well, (Stevenson and Watson). Etch-

---

*An asterisk following any title indicates that roentgenographic reproductions illustrating this condition will be found in the pictorial supplement at the end of the chapter.

ing of the teeth may be a point in differential diagnosis of fluorine poisoning.

Other types of metallic poisons, because of their great toxicity, do not result in demonstrable bony deposits since they cannot be tolerated in sufficient quantities for a sufficient length of time.

RADIUM POISONING. When salts of radium element are taken into the body, even in extremely small quantities, they become stored in the bones, similar to other metallic substances. The greatest danger from radium poisoning is due to the fact that the bone marrow is constantly bombarded by radiation from the radium with which it is in such close contact. Even in infinitesimal quantities, the biological effect of radium in such intimate contact with blood-forming structures of the bone marrow produces a profound effect. A notable example is that of the watch dial painters of New Jersey, who, by repeatedly pointing their paint brushes in the corners of their mouths swallowed infinitesimal quantities of radium element. The effect is especially great on account of the alpha particles which have 10,000 times the biological effect of gamma rays. The result is a profound anemia with reduction of red blood cells and marked reduction in the number of white blood cells of the blood. Once present, the effect of the radium is continuous.

Roentgenographically, the radium poisoning produces areas of worm-eaten destruction in the bones. These are often evident in the skull near the suture lines. After the disease has been established for some time, shaggy periosteal reaction may result. As a result of the long-continued exposure of the bone to this radiation, a number of instances have been observed in which osteosarcoma developed. Osteogenic sarcoma has been developed experimentally in animals from radium poisoning (Harris and Bunker).

LEAD POISONING FROM BULLET. Lead poisoning from lodgment of a lead bullet in bony structure, although rare, has been definitely proved in a number of recorded cases (Senturia). Just why so few cases have developed from the large number of gun shot wounds which occur is difficult to understand.

Lodgment of the bullet in bone in close relationship to a joint seems to be an important factor in the subsequent development of systemic lead intoxication. Roentgenograms taken years later in such cases reveal marked changes from the original appearance of the bullet, and in the distribution of metallic fragments. Numerous lead deposits seem to be within the joint capsule or are encapsulated in the surrounding soft tissue.

RENAL (RICKETS) (Fig. 103) OSTEITIS—RENAL DWARFISM. Renal rickets is a form of rachitic involvement of bone, which occurs as a result of chronic interference with the kidney function. It occurs as a result of long-continued gross retention of waste products in the blood stream associated with chronic interstitial nephritis or nephrosclerosis from pyelonephritis and has even been encountered with polycys-

tic and other forms of defective kidney. It also may be due to obstruction of the lower urinary tract. It is not primarily due to a faulty metabolism from lack of vitamin D, but is the result of a disturbance in the normal calcium-phosphorus ratio in the blood from the deficiency in kidney function.

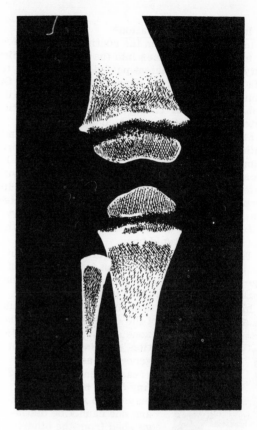

Fig. 103

Albright gives the sequence of events as:
a) renal insufficiency
b) phosphate retention
c) tendency toward a low level of serum calcium
d) hyperplasia of the parathyroid glands to meet this tendency

In rare instances in which the condition is of long duration it may become accompanied by osteitis fibrosa generalisata and may be confused with primary hyperparathyroidism.

The bone changes produced are in many respects similar to those of true rickets: there is loss of lime salts, with accentuation of bone markings, enlargement of the diaphyseal ends of the bones, haziness and irregularity of the epiphyseal lines, but rarely is the zone of active osteoid formation as wide as in true rickets. There may be bowing of the bones and stunting of the growth, giving rise to a form of renal dwarfism in contradistinction to true rickets. Periosteal bone formation is sometimes a prominent feature. The skull may be enlarged and the bones thickened; in extreme cases they may take on a fuzzy appearance. The vertebrae may show marked loss of lime salts with biconcave deformity and relative increase in the width of the interarticular discs. Calcium metastases to other organs may occur.

The radiological changes which occur in renal osteitis have been summarized concisely by Sussman and Poppel.

This condition is differentiated from true rickets by:

1. The presence of a chronic renal disorder, resulting in the damming back of waste products in the blood,
2. By high phosphorus and low calcium in the blood,
3. By the failure of Vitamin D in the diet to correct the condition.
4. By the appearance of dense arteriosclerotic changes usually of the Monckeberg type if present.

Weens and Marin have pointed out that calcification and sclerosis of the arteries may be encountered in infants in clinical conditions, renal rickets in hyperparathyroidism; Vitamin D intoxication; in progeria associated with growth disturbance and profound metabolic changes. They point out that many cases of arteriosclerosis have been reported in infants which have no evident etiology.

At times it may resemble other dysostoses of bone, producing dwarfism (Muller and Sissons).

Individuals suffering with this disorder rarely attain adult life; they usually succumb to uremia.

Celiac disease, due to lack of normal absorption from the diseased intestinal mucosa, also produces osteoporosis of the bone, but this in no way resembles renal rickets.

OXALOSIS. This is a rare condition encountered in children in which calcium oxalate deposits were found in tissues throughout the body, especially in the urinary tract and bones. Death occurred from renal failure. Dunn describes the unusual bone lesions occurring throughout the body in association with this condition; the skull and mandible show a moderate granular osteoporosis; the vertebrae show similar "soft-wally" osteoporosis but no evidence of compression; there was severe osteoporosis in the diaphyseal ends of the long bones sharply delineated by the epiphyseal lines without gross evidence of epiphyseal involvement; sharply defined transverse lines at the margins of the involved areas which are symmetrical in all areas of involvement and may indicate the time of onset of the condition. Unlike renal rickets which it somewhat resembles, the epiphyseal line itself is not widened nor irregular. The parathyroid glands were investigated and appeared normal. It is assumed therefore that the condition is due to a primary disturbance of oxalate metabolism.

KASCHIN-BECK'S DISEASE. This is a disease affecting the bones and joints, which has been observed only in a small area of Siberia. The etiology is not definitely known, but it is thought to be due to pollution of the drinking water with manure.

The changes usually appear during the growing period, between nine and sixteen years of age; males predominate.

Clinically there is irregular swelling and enlargement of the joints with acute rheumatic pain. There is shortening of the bones and atrophy of the muscles.

Roentgenologically, the epiphyseal cartilages are primarily involved. There are areas of destruction in the bones and development of the long bones is checked, causing shortening. The process is most pronounced in the phalanges where the epiphyses become unrecognizable and sink into the deepened and widened metaphyses.

QUESTIONS ON MINERAL POISONS AND OTHER INTOXICATIONS

Questions marked with a dagger deal with rare and less-important conditions.

1. What are the roentgen manifestations of lead poisoning in the long bones in children? In adults?

2. Is lead deposited in the bone marrow in adults and does it cause any perceptible increase in density of the bone?

3. Does excessive bismuth administration cause any manifestation in the bones of children? Of adults?

4. Is there any metallic poison which produces increase in density of bones in adults?

†5. How is fluorine taken into the body in cases of poisoning and under what conditions does this occur in industry?

6. What are the dangers of radium poisoning and what manifestation does it present in the long bones?

7. Why is the ingestion of radium element even in extremely small doses so dangerous?

8. What is Renal Rickets and how does it manifest itself in the roentgenogram?

†9. What is KASCHIN-BECK'S disease; where does it occur and how does it manifest itself roentgeno-graphically?

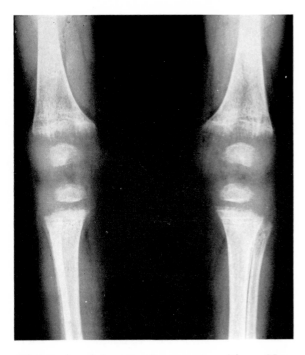

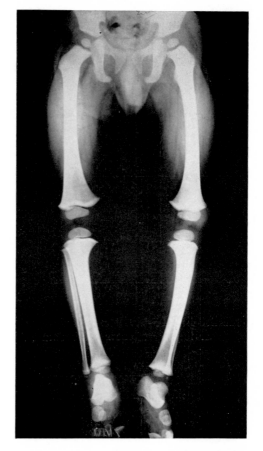

Rickets involving the lower extremities. Note the loss of lime salts; the flaring of the ends of the long bones; the saucer-shaped hazy epiphyseal lines due to continuous widening of zone of active growth. There is most bowing where the bones are subjected to weight-bearing.

Healed rickets showing bowing of the bones, thickening of the cortex on the concave side and thinning on the convex side.

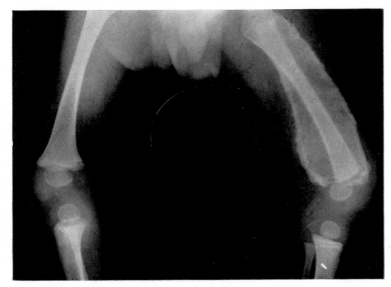

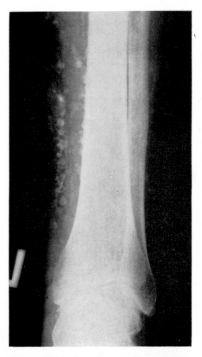

Scurvy showing spontaneous separation of the epiphysis and large sub-periosteal hemorrhage stripping up the periosteum. Compare with opposite unaffected structure.

Phleboliths in the walls of the veins of the leg.

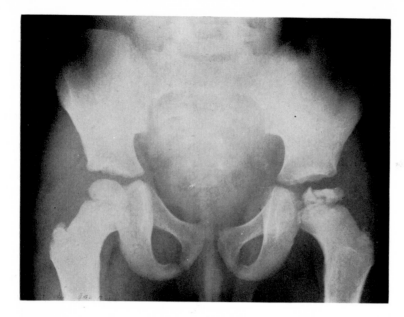

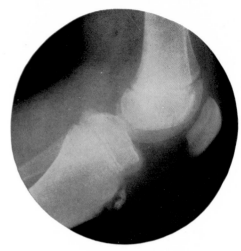

Osgood - Schlatter's Disease showing the softened epiphysis for the tibial tuberosity separated by the pull of the patellar tendon.

Perthe's Disease, involving the epiphysis for the head of the femur. Note the flattening and fragmentation of the head, the widening of the neck and the lack of involvement of the articular cartilage and acetabulum.

Bilateral intra-pelvic protrusion of the acetabula, a condition of unknown etiology but probably associated with epiphysitis of the acetabular epiphyseal lines. Of no significance other than the pelvic deformity produced. The deformity causes some limitation of motion and may interfere with delivery in the female.

↓

Koehler's Disease of the tarsal navicular bones due to epiphysitis affecting these centers of ossification. Usually bilateral but not interfering with the ultimate complete growth of the bone.

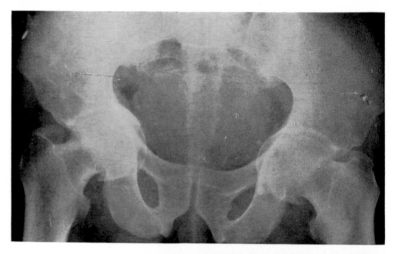

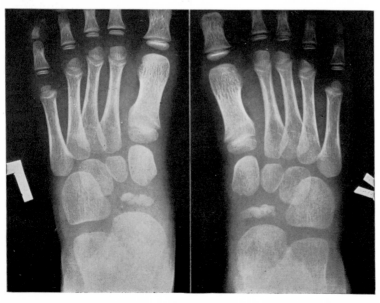

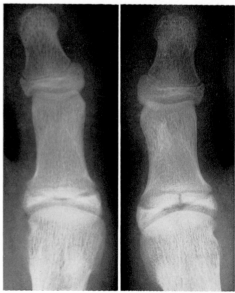

Thiemann's Disease, split epiphyseal centers of phalanges. Spontaneous healing with union of epithsyses.

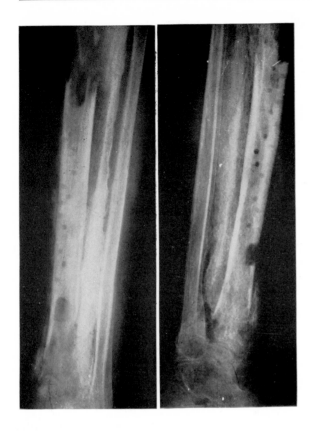

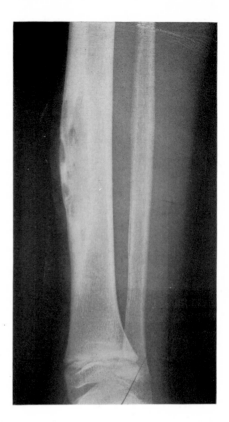

Osteomyelitis involving the entire shaft of the tibia. Note the large sequestrum of the shaft with the numerous drill holes. The sequestrum is chalky in appearance and is surrounded by a heavy involucrum of new bone formation. Before the advent of chemotherapy this was the usual result of osteomyelitis.

Localized osteomyelitis of the anterior margin of the tibia from introduction of infection through a puncture wound in this region.

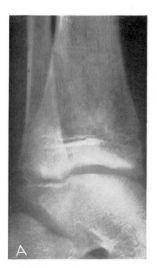
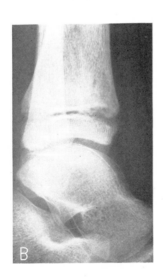
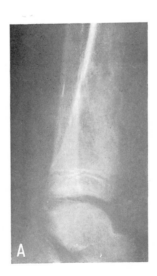
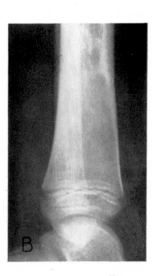

OSTEOMYELITIS UNDER THE INFLUENCE OF CHEMOTHERAPY

A. Although the fever and pain had subsided roentgen examination on August 14th showed definite destruction of the diaphysis at the lower end of the tibia. There was only slight periosteal reaction.

B. By September 15th (one month later) the destructive process had completely healed and was replaced by normal bone architecture. All symptoms had subsided and the patient was up and about.

A. Extensive bone destruction with subperiosteal infection one month after onset.

B. One year later under chemotherapy complete healing has taken place with minimum deformity and without sequestrum formation.

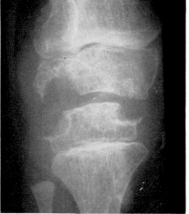

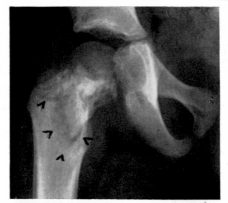

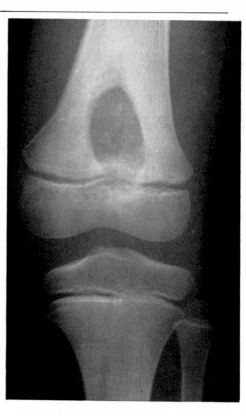

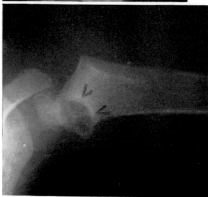

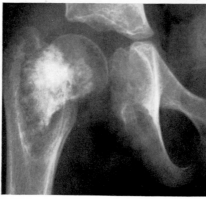

Cystic Tuberculosis showing cystic areas of destruction; upper, involving epiphysis; lower, diaphyseal region. Joint not involved.

Diaphyseal Tuberculosis acute stage involving neck of femur, showing bone destruction and periosteal reaction. One year later sequestration and fibrous tissue repair.

Cystic Tuberculosis, cyst-like area of destruction confined to diaphyseal region. Epiphysis and joint not involved.

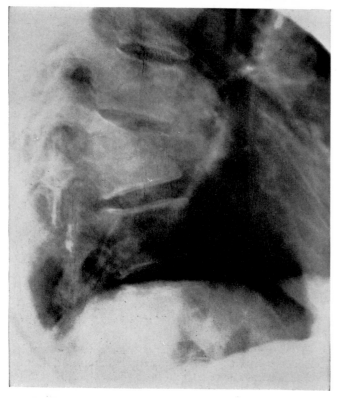

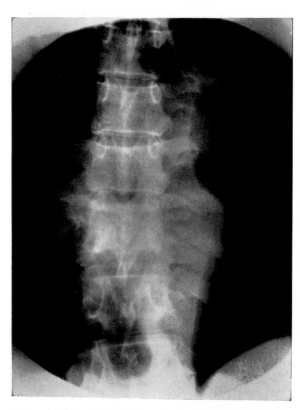

Tuberculosis of the spine in the lateral view showing complete destruction of the inter-articular disc and fusion of the bodies of the two vertebrae.

Tuberculosis of the spine, same patient, seen in the antero-posterior view, showing the development of a tuberculous abscess around the area of bony involvement.

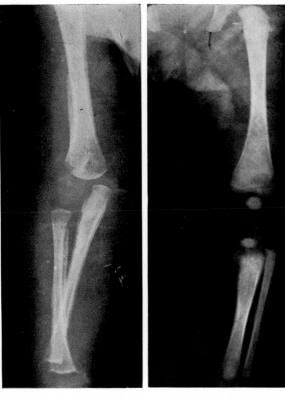

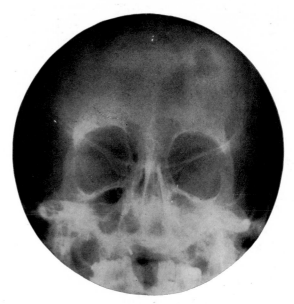

Gumma of the frontal bone showing irregular areas of destruction surrounded by areas of sclerotic bone.

Multiple periosteal reaction is a frequent finding of congenital syphilis in new-born infants. Epiphysitis of luetic origin showing destructive areas in the diaphysis, serration of the epiphyseal lines and some periosteal reaction.

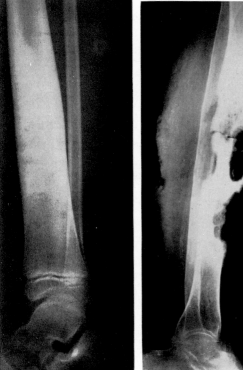

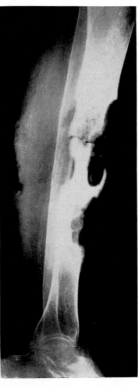

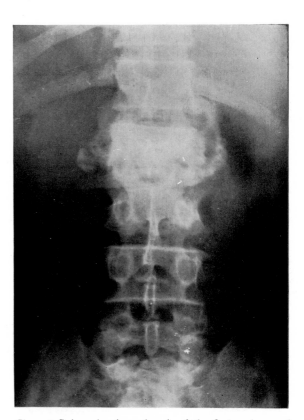

Syphilitic ostitis. Note the uniform thickening of the cortex without periosteal reaction.

Gumma of the tibia developing within an area of osteosclerosis. Osteosclerosis may precede gumma formation.

Charcot Spine, showing sclerosis of the first and second lumbar vertebrae with extensive destruction of the vertebral bodies and cartilages and a large amount of surrounding debris and detritus.

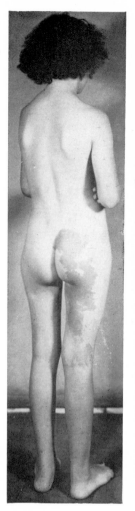
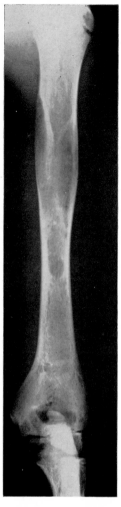
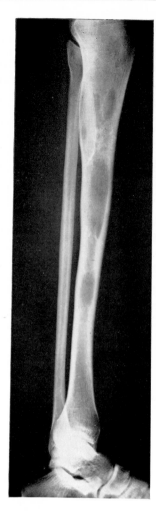
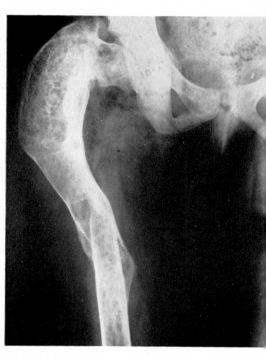

Site of original involvement, note eccentric appearance of expanded "cyst"-like area in the greater trochanter; also, fracture through another area of involvement in the shaft.

EARLY LESIONS OF POLYOSTATIC FIBROUS DYSPLASIA
Twelve year old girl
Showing Albright's Syndrome:

1. Early Menstruation; (8 years of age);
2. Large pigmented area on back of thigh;
3. Multiple "cyst"-like areas of bone involvement. Note crescentic appearance of *intracortical* lesions.

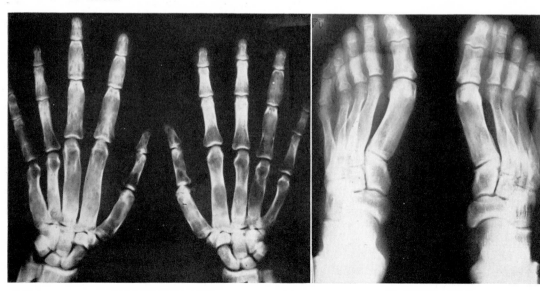

Hands and feet of advanced case of polyostatic fibrous dysplasia; note, enlargement and elongation of involved bones and loss of bone architecture.

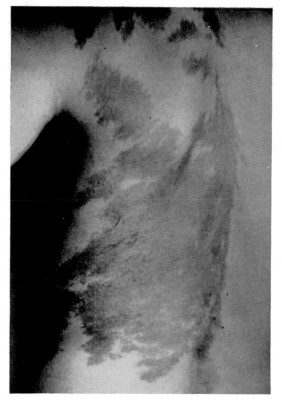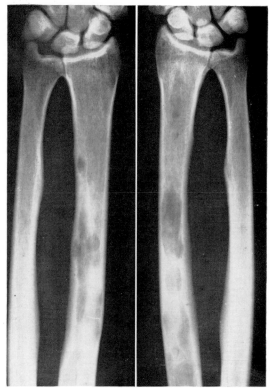

ADULT POLYOSTOTIC FIBROUS DYSPLASIA — OF LONG STANDING

Large pigmented areas covering the greater portion of the back, side, and chest of an adult male, with generalized polyostotic fibrous dysplasia (Albright's syndrome).

Tiny lesion starting in cortex of radius, evidence of "earliest" involvement. Almost all of the other bones showed extensive involvement by polyostotic fibrous dysplasia.

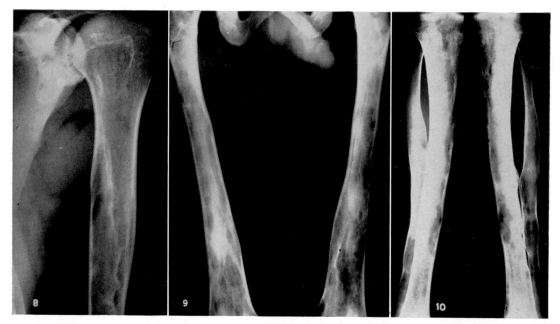

8. Crescentic lesions in shaft of humerus, most characteristic of polyostotic fibrous dysplasia.

9. Extensive involvement of both femurs, causing thick, knobby appearance, with thinning of the shafts but no bending deformity.

10. Bones of both legs similarly involved; somewhat elongated because of hyperplastic process.

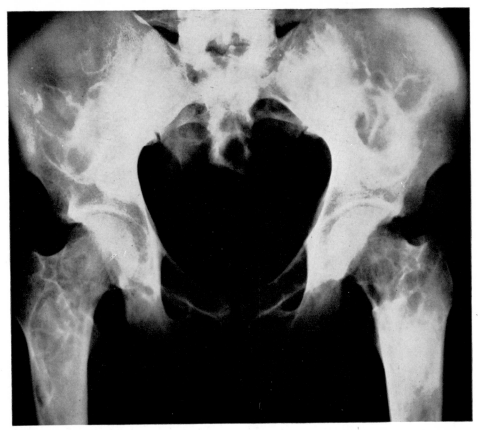

Pelvis showing ring-like structures surrounding areas of sclerotic appearing bone, characteristic of polyostotic fibrous dysplasia.

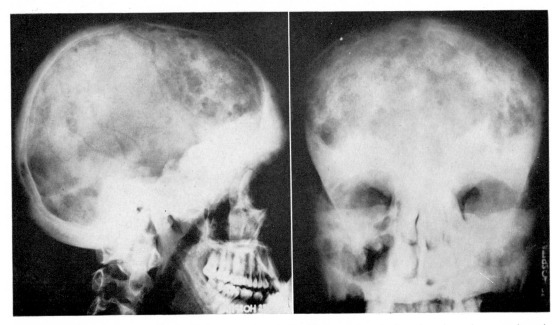

Extensive involvement of skull from polyostotic fibrous dysplasia, showing dense sclerosis of compact bony structures at base and tendency to cystic formation over the calvarium.

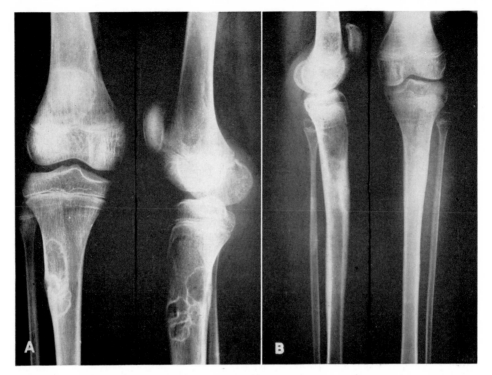

A. Two "cyst"-like areas in shaft of tibia and smaller area in femur from fibrous dysplasia of bone. No other involvement was found at this time. Areas were excised.

B. Complete healing and filling in of resected area with new bone formation. No recurrence.

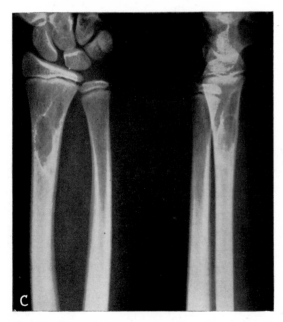

C. Further development of polyostotic fibrous dysplasia in opposite radius a number of months later.

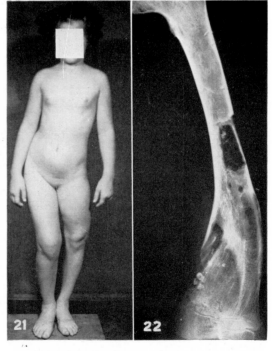

21. Dyschondroplasia (Ollier's disease). Note deformity and shortening of femur.

22. Characteristic appearance of bone lesions at diaphyseal end of bone with areas of intervening decrease in density due to remnants of cartilage.

Irregular growth results in deformity and shortening of the bone.

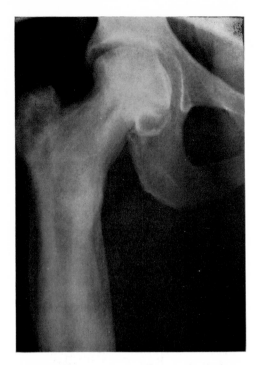

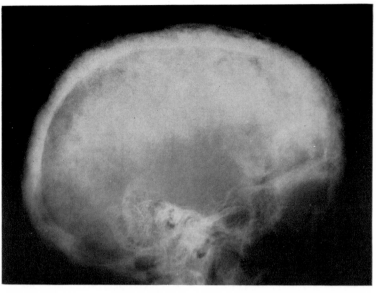

Paget's Disease of the skull. Note the extreme thickening of the outer table of the skull with moth-eaten appearing bone.

Paget's Disease may affect a single bone without disturbing any of the other bones in the skeleton. Bone condensation and bone rarefaction going on at the same time. The femur is a frequent site of involvement.

Acromegalic enlargement of skull and overgrowth of the sinuses and jaw from increased anterior pituitary secretion. The sella is not unusually enlarged. →

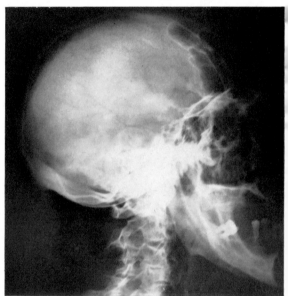

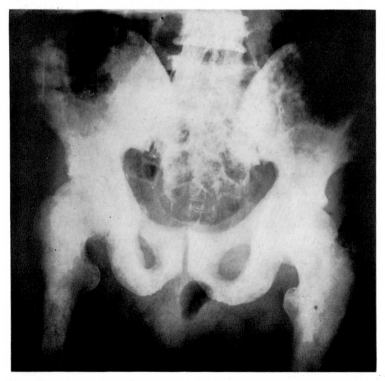

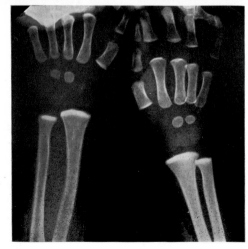

Paget's Disease involving the pelvis showing the characteristic spotty moth-eaten appearance of the bony structure.

Lead poisoning in a child from swallowing paint off of toys. Note the dense zone of calcification at the epiphyseal lines.

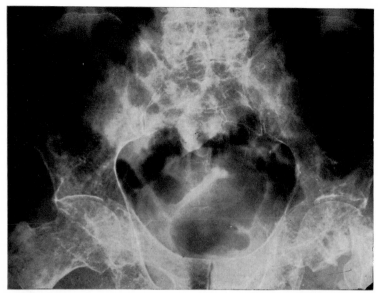

Osteoporosis of the bones of the pelvis from hyperparathyroidism. Numerous spontaneous fractures occur owing to the weakening of the bones.

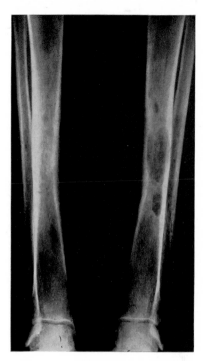

Multiple cystic areas in the bones due to hyperparathyroidism.

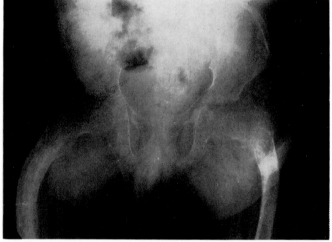

Osteogenesis Imperfecta Tarda. Note the lack of lime salts and the extreme bowing of the bones. Spontaneous fractures are frequent.

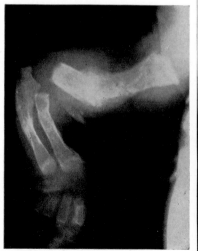

Osteogenesis Imperfecta Congenita showing multiple fractures.

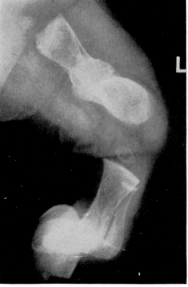

Osteogenesis Imperfecta Congenita showing multiple fractures.

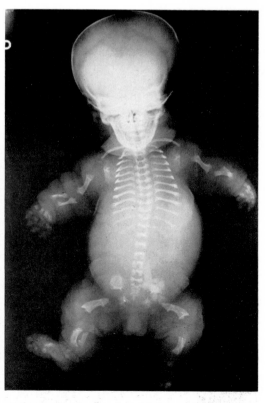

Achondroplastic dwarf at birth; resembles osteogenesis imperfecta but there are no fractures.

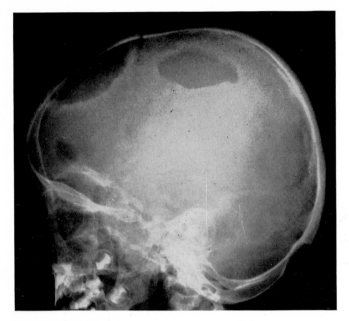

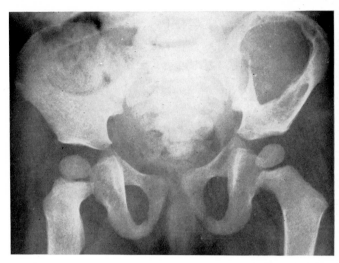

Hand-Schüller-Christian's Disease involving the flat bones of the skull. Note the rounded, punched-out areas in the bone.

Hand-Schüller-Christian's Disease involving flat bones of pelvis.

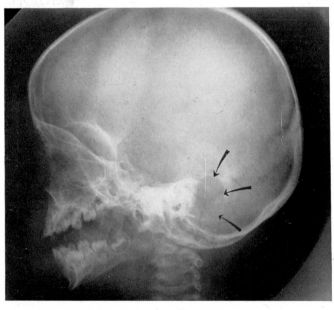

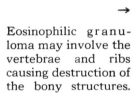

Eosinophilic granuloma may involve the vertebrae and ribs causing destruction of the bony structures.

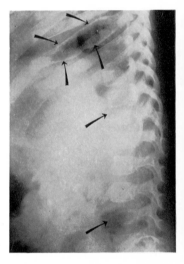

EOSINOPHILIC GRANULOMA

A disease of bone closely resembling Hand-Schüller-Christian's Disease characterized by large rounded sharply-defined defects in flat and irregular bones. Separation of the sutures may occur from increased intracranial pressure *without* convolutional atrophy.

Eosinophilic Granuloma involving the flat bones of the pelvis. The appearance is in every respect similar to Hand-Schüller-Christian's Disease. Microscopic examination however shows abundant eosinophiles the distinguishing characteristic. Radiation therapy is very effective in the treatment of the disease.

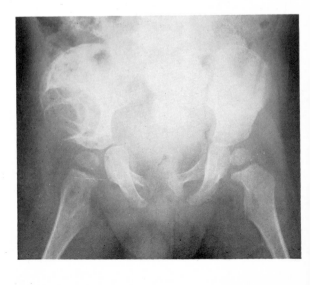

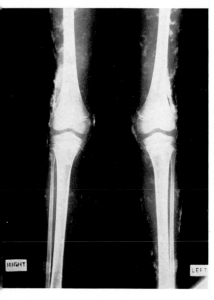

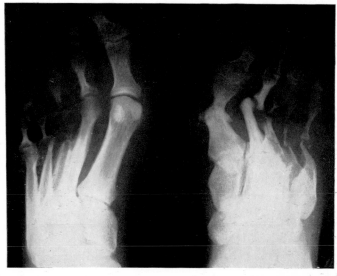

← Calcinosis Inter-stitialis, a condition in which irregular calcium deposits are laid down in the interstitial tissues.

Neurotrophic disturbance causing spindle-shaped deformity of the metatarsal bones and phalanges.

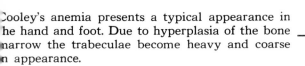

Cooley's anemia presents a typical appearance in the hand and foot. Due to hyperplasia of the bone marrow the trabeculae become heavy and coarse in appearance. →

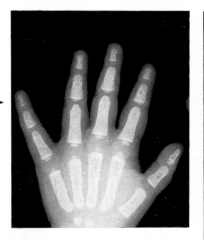

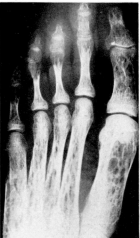

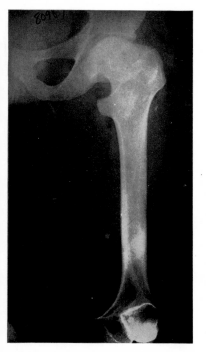

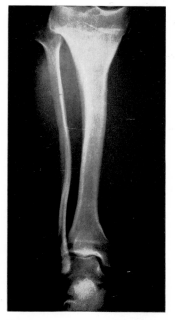

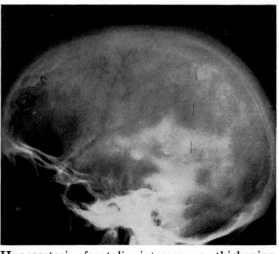

Achondroplasia showing the short thick appearance of the long bones. This condition accounts for many of our dwarfs.

Hyperostosis frontalis internus, a thickening of the inner table of the skull in the frontal region which is thought to be due to some type of endocrine pathology.

DISEASES OF BONE

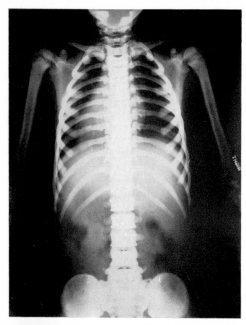

Osteopetrosis, or marble bones is a condition in which all of the bones of the body become chalky in appearance obliterating the normal bone structure.

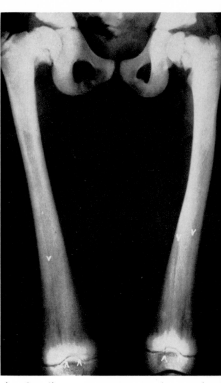

Osteopetrosis. As the disease progresses, a dense scleroti[c] zone appears along the diaphysial side of the epiphysial lin[e] which gradually extends to involve the entire shaft. Dar[k] longitudinal lines appear within the calcifying bone whic[h] probably represent columns of uncalcified cartilaginous cell[s]

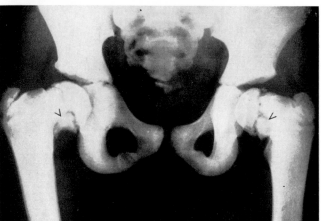

Osteopetrosis. Spontaneous infractions of the lower margins of the necks of both femurs due to stress and strain on bone at this point. Upper part remains intact and continues its normal growth while the lower part does not grow. This gives rise to extreme coxa vara and knock knee deformity.

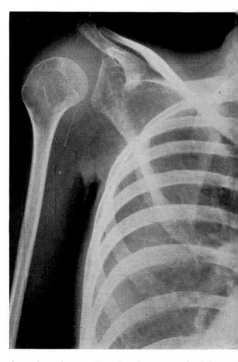

Atrophy of quantity showing a marked loss o[f] substance in the bony structures of th[e] shoulder from infantile paralysis.

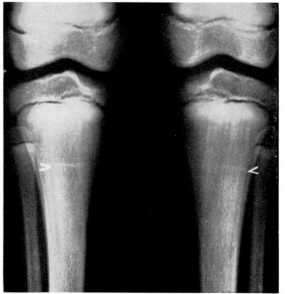

Osteopetrosis. In some instances dense transverse lines appear across the diaphysial ends of the bones, indicating short periods of remission of the disease. Such remissions have been reported.

CONGENITAL ANOMALIES AND ANATOMICAL VARIATIONS (Chapter XII)

General Defects - considered under "glandular and metabolic."

    A. Achondroplasia; Chondrodystrophia Fetalis

    B. Dyschondroplasia

    C. Osteogenesis Imperfecta—congenital type

    D. Osteopetrosis, Osteosclerosis Fragilis Generalisata—Marble Bones (ALBERS-SCHÖNBERG'S Disease)

    E. Osteopoikilosis

    F. Chondrodystrophy Calcificans Congenita

    G. EHLERS-DANLOS Syndrome

Local Anatomical Variations

    A. Skull

        1. Acrania-anencephaly

        2. Macrocephaly, (megalocephaly)

        3. Hydrocephalus

    Craniostenosis

        1. Microcephaly

        2. Oxycephaly, Turricephaly, (tower skull)

        3. Dolichocephaly, (long skull)

        4. Brachycephaly, (short skull)

        5. Plagiocephaly, (slanting skull)

        6. Scaphocephaly, (scaphoid skull)

    Ocular hypertelorism

    Cranial Dysostoses

        1. Cleidocranial dysostosis

        2. Lacunae skull (luechenschaedel)

        3. Localized thinning of cranial bones

        4. Platybasia, (Basilar Impression, Basilar Invagination)

        5. Persistence of parietal foramina

        6. Sinus pericranii

    B. Spine

        1. Spina bifida

            a. Vera

            b. Occulta

        2. Supernumerary and malformation of vertebrae

        3. Absence of, or fusion of cervical spine—(KLIPPEL-FEIL SYNDROME)

        4. Block Vertebra

        5. Occipitalization of the Axis

        6. Sacralization

        7. Elongation transverse process

        8. Spondylolisthesis from congenital absence of articular processes

C. Chest

    1. Supernumerary or absence of ribs
       Cervical and lumbar ribs

D. Pelvis

    1. Congenital dislocation of hip

    2. Pelvic Deformity associated with:
       Extrophy of bladder
       Bifurcation of coccyx

E. Extremities

    1. General Involvement

      a. Hemihypertrophy—hemiatrophy

      b. Intrauterine amputations and fractures

    2. Local Involvement

      a. Upper extremity

          SPRENGEL'S DEFORMITY

          Elevated Scapula

          MADELUNG'S DEFORMITY—Radius Curvus

          Absence of or fusion of bones—deformities

          Supernumerary bones

      b. Lower extremity

          Congenital dislocation of hip (see pelvis)

          Deformity lower tibial epiphysis from irregular development

          Tibia Vara—upper epiphyseal deformity

          Tibia Recurvatum

          Absence of or fusion of bones—deformities

          Bipartite patella

          Talipes equinovarus

          Talipes calcaneovalgus

          Arthrogryposis multiplex congenita

          Genu Recurvatum

          Lipomatosis involving bone

          Talo-navicular synostosis

          Supernumerary bones

Chapter XII

CONGENITAL ANOMALIES AND ANATOMICAL VARIATIONS

GENERAL DEFECTS

"The sequences of growth and differentiation together will lead to normal development." Interference with either may result in wide physical and physiological variations. Neuhauser in an article on "Growth, Differentiation and Disease," points out the hereditary and environmental influences in production of developmental defects. Two factors are responsible for development: genetic and environmental. Certain disease may be due to abnormality in a single gene locus, such as achondroplasia, marble bones, possibly osteogenesis imperfecta and many other simple hereditary defects. "It has been postulated that once in ten thousand births there is a gene mutation that will produce achondroplasia, which in turn, will be expressed in subsequent offspring as a mendelian dominant." Environmental factors, harmonal and nutritional, are much more varied and complicated in their action. "Likewise, environmental abnormalities may react on the development of the organism in such a way that genetic abnormalities are simulated and the two may be indistinguishable clinically." Some such responsible agents are: infection of the pregnant woman with rubella, Vitamin deficiencies, exposure to roentgen-rays and other harmful agents such as nitrogen mustard.

In achondroplasia, dyschondroplasia and osteogenesis imperfecta there is an inherent deficiency. Because of the influence of harmonal imbalance, this group of diseases has been considered in greater detail under "Glandular and Metabolic Diseases".

LOCAL ANATOMICAL VARIATIONS

Anomalies of development involving only localized regions or single bones, which do not interfere with natural function, are often referred to as anatomical variations, and are considered in most instances as being normal for the individual. Such variations may be congenital in origin or may be the result of injury or disease during the developmental period.

ANOMALIES OF SKULL—ACRANIA* (Fig. 103) Acrania, or complete absence of the cranium, is a congenital anomaly recognizable roentgenographically before birth. The condition may be suspected clinically from hydramnios which frequently accompanies the condition, but definite diagnosis must be made by roentgenographic examination. There is partial or complete absence of the cranial structure; the bones of the face are small and drawn, giving an apelike appearance. The condition is frequently associated with anencephaly—complete or partial failure of development of the brain.

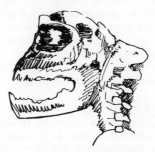

Fig. 103

MEGALOCEPHALY—MACROCEPHALUS. Any condition in which the head attains an unusually large size. Any skull in which the brain and contents weigh 1639 to 1650 gm. (Welcker).

HYDROCEPHALUS (Fig. 104). This is a condition of megalocephaly in which the size of the skull is due to the dilatation of the ventricular structures. The sutures are widely separated and the fontanelles remain large and extend well down

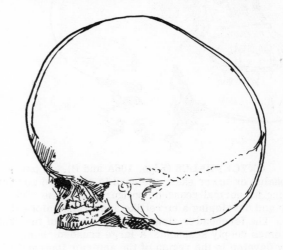

Fig. 104

---

*An asterisk following any title indicates that roentgenographic reproductions illustrating this condition will be found in the pictorial supplement at the end of the chapter.

into the suture lines. The condition is usually due to chronic increase in intracranial pressure from some interference in cerebrospinal circulation. The chronic increase in intracranial pressure results in thinning of the cranial bones and an increase in the convolutional markings and bulging of the frontal portion. There is an extreme degree of brain atrophy. The sella turcica may be flattened out from pressure. Such individuals usually die in infancy; if they do survive they usually remain idiots.

CRANIOSTENOSIS; (CRANIOSYNOSTOSIS). Premature closure of certain sutures may give rise to various peculiar shapes of the skull. Contraction is perpendicular across the long axis of the suture. This results in serious restriction to brain development. The brain increases almost three times during the first year, and the circumference of the skull increases to within approximately one inch of its adult size by five years of age. Closure of sutures after cerebral development is completed does not lead to abnormal cranial shapes. Hope, et al., have called attention to the need for prompt diagnosis since operation to be effective must be in the early months of life.

MICROCEPHALUS (Fig. 105). Microcephalus is, as its name implies, a condition in which the skull is smaller than normal. This is because of a deficiency in brain development, not to craniostenosis. It is usually recognizable at birth or even in utero. The bones of the face develop, but the size of the skull does not increase; the sutures may be closed at or soon after birth. Such individuals are usually idiots. They may die at an early age, but frequently live well into adult life.

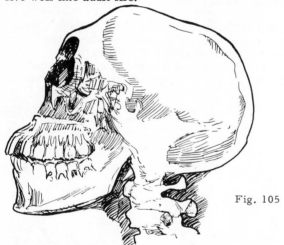

Fig. 105

OXYCEPHALUS (Figs. 106A and B). In oxycephalus or tower skull, the head is elongated upward, losing its normal rounded configuration in the midline and developing a turretlike appearance along the top. The forehead is slanting and the base of the skull becomes deeply scaphoid. A large rounded "bump" may develop in the region of the anterior fontanelle; the bony covering in this region is very thin and the brain substance may herniate out into this pocket.

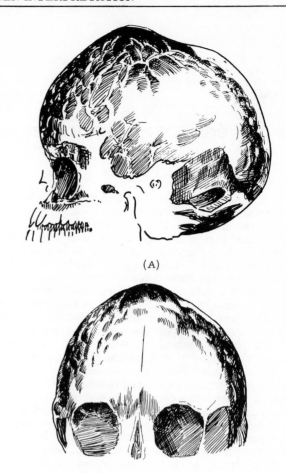

(A)

(B)

Fig. 106

There is marked convolutional atrophy due to increase in intracranial pressure; and damage may result to the brain substance.

Many other types of deformity occur, usually with less serious consequences:

Dolicocephaly - long skull, Fig. 107.
Brachycephaly - short skull, Fig. 108.
Scaphocephaly - scaphoid skull - front of skull coming to a peak like the prow of ship.
Trigonocephaly - triangular skull, pointed forehead.

OCULAR HYPERTELORISM. A peculiar deformity of the skull, in which the orbits are widely separated, producing a flattening of the bridge of the nose and shortening of the skull. The lesser wing of the sphenoid is retarded in its development; this condition is not resultant from malfusion of sutures but is a distinct entity.

Cleidocranial Dysostosis. A condition in which there is defective closure of the sutures associated with complete or partial absence of the clavicles. In extreme instances the shoulders may be brought to-

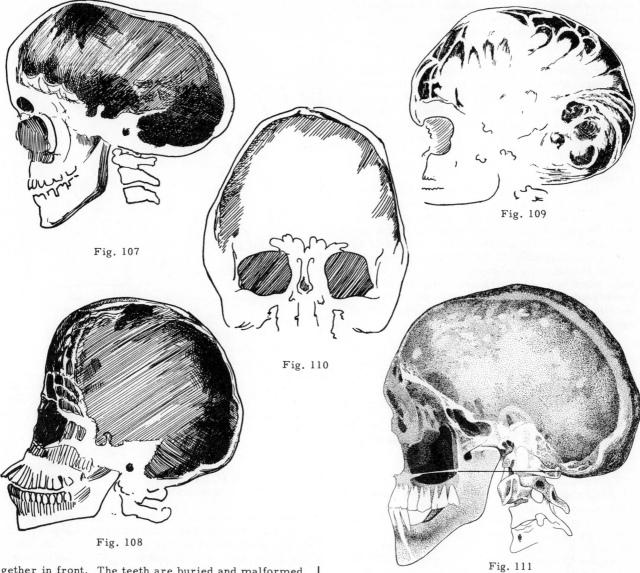

Fig. 107

Fig. 109

Fig. 110

Fig. 108

Fig. 111

gether in front. The teeth are buried and malformed, and there is dysostosis of the phalanges of the hand, (Ingram; Eisen).

Eltorm, (H., Acta. Radiol., 26:69, 1945) has summarized the roentgen findings as follows:
1. defects in the calcium of the skull
2. Wormian bones in the occipital bone
3. sclerosis of the petrous portion
4. aplasia of the pneumatic spaces in the temporal and frontal bones
5. small upper and lower jaws
6. total retention of the permanent teeth
7. spina bifida in the cervical and thoracic columns
8. excessively developed transverse processes of the seventh cervical
9. markedly defective clavicles
10. defective development of the scapulae with defective coronoid process and glenoid cavity
11. aplasia of the medial epicondyle and capitellum of the humerus
12. brachyphalangia
13. defective development of the iliac bones with poor development of the acetabulum on both sides
14. split pelvis
15. bilateral congenital coxa vara

Acrocephalosyndactyly is an unusual type of congenital deformity consisting of: 1. A very high skull, flat posteriorly with the vertex in the superofrontal region; 2. syndactylism of the four extremities, (Cooper).

Lacunae Skull (Leuchenschaedel)* (Fig. 109). This condition presents an appearance of rounded pits or depressions in the skull, especially in the parietal regions. There is usually an associated increase in intracranial pressure as indicated by separation of sutures and distended fontanelle. Spina bifida almost always accompanies the condition. On palpation the skull gives a parchmentlike impression. Cases have been reported of multiple occurrences of this and other anomalies in the same family. The condition is congenital and the cause is unknown.

THINNING OF AREAS IN CRANIAL BONES (Fig. 110). These are rather rare anomalies seen most frequently bilaterally in the parietal or occipital regions; they may occur in any location but are usually symmetrical. Studied in profile the bone is seen to consist of thin layers of compact bone, devoid of diploetic structure. There is no encroachment on the cranial cavity and no interference with cerebral function.

Most roentgenologists accept the view that this condition is due to a dysplasia of the diploetic layer, that for some unknown reason the diploetic structure does not develop properly between the two compact layers just as in certain instances mastoids do not undergo pneumatization. No instance has been recorded in which cranial bones of normal structure were found to undergo atrophy. Examples of this deformity have been found in Egyptian mummies and the writer has observed it in the skull of an Indian removed from an Indian mound.

PLATYBASIA (Basal Impression; Basilar Invagination (Fig. 111). This is a condition in which softening of the cranial bones from congenital deformity or acquired disease, leads to invagination of the upper portion of the cervical spine, upward through the foramen magnum into the cranial cavity. Because of the weakened condition, the bone structure is not sufficiently strong to maintain the weight of the head; it is frequently seen in association with Paget's disease, (Poppel, et al.).

Pressure on the medulla and pons may give rise to many untoward neurological symptoms even resembling multiple sclerosis.

Chamberlain has devised a line from the posterior margin of the palate to the posterior edge of the foramen magnum, above which the odontoid process of the second cervical vertebra should not extend; projection above this line constitutes Platybasia. McGregor has developed an angle, between two lines drawn from the center of the sella turcica, one to the nasion or root of the nose, the other to the anterior margin of the foramen magnum; this angle should not exceed 140°. In both instances the roentgenogram must be made with the patient in a due lateral position.

PERSISTENT ENLARGEMENT OF PARIETAL FORAMINA (Fig. 112). Very rarely the parietal foramina remain enlarged and persist into adult life. They appear in the roentgenogram as two symmetrically placed rounded openings on either side of the midline in the parietal bones. They are in about the same location and appear very similar to the trephine openings made preparatory to ventricular puncture. Their margins are somewhat beveled. They can be palpated as two depressions on the head, but cause no pain or disability.

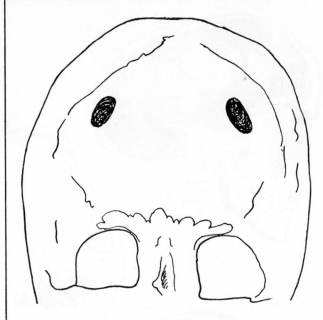

Fig. 112

SINUS PERICRANII. This is a congenital vascular anomaly in which an emissary vessel connects with an intracranial blood sinus through an abnormal foramen in the skull. Ritvo, M. (Roentgen Diagnosis of Diseases of the Skull, Paul Hoeber, N.Y. 1949) cites a case in which the engorged structure formed a visible lump on the forehead while in the recumbent position but disappeared when erect.

ANOMALIES OF SPINE

CORONAL CLEFT VERTEBRA. A rather rare anomaly in the appearance of the bodies of the vertebrae of new born or still born infants as seen in the lateral view, produced by delayed fusion of the anterior and posterior ossification centers for vertebral body. A number of vertebrae may be involved giving the appearance of a coronal cleft. These later fuse into normal structures.

SPINA BIFIDA * (Fig. 113A). The spine, with its many segments, is subject to numerous anomalies and anatomical variations. Perhaps the most common anomaly of the spine is the failure of the neural arch to close—spina bifida; this is indicated in the roentgenogram by a defect in the laminae and usually by an absence of the spinous process. If the defect is confined to the bony structure, the condition is spoken of as Spina Bifida Occulta; if it is accompanied by a meningocele or myelocele it is known as Spina Bifida Vera. The former is of no significance, causing no symptoms; the latter is serious in direct proportion to the degree of soft-part involvement. This defect is most commonly countered in the region of the fifth lumbar vertebra and upper portion of the sacrum, although it may occur at any level. In addition to these defects of the laminae, there may be congenital absence or

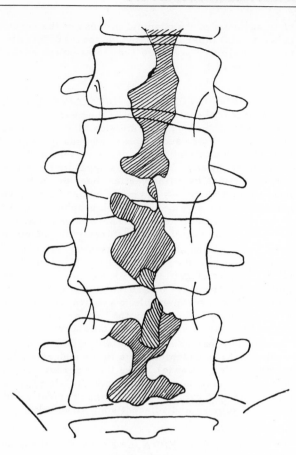

Fig. 113A

rudimentary development of the pedicles or articular processes.

Fullenlove, and Williams question the role of congenital defects and anatomical variations as independently a cause of backache.

SUPERNUMERARY AND MALFORMATION OF THE VERTEBRAE* (Fig. 113B). Supernumerary and hemivertebrae are rather common; they occur in any portion of the spine, but the most frequent location is in the lumbar region. The existence of only eleven ribs may give the impression of a supernumerary lumbar vertebra, whereas only the normal number may be present. Usually, such supernumerary segments are normal in size and shape, causing no pathological symptoms or deformity. Occasionally malformed vertebral segments are encountered which cause deformity and disability. These usually take on the form of wedge-shaped bodies with malformed lateral masses; they may be supernumerary or may represent malformation of a natural segment. They are due to imperfect segmentation of ossification centers during development. Their differentiation from vertebral injuries may at times be difficult.

Scoliosis or other spinal deformity, when congenital, may result from malformation of vertebrae (structural) or may result from muscular imbalance during the developmental period (postural) (Fig. 113C).

By detection of primary curve by roentgen methods, (See Manual of Roentgenolical Technique), correction can be accomplished by wedging casts, followed by fusion. Much can be accomplished in rectifying the condition.

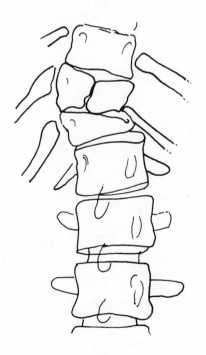

Fig. 113B

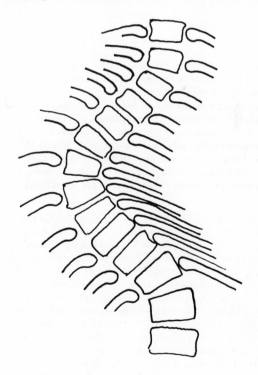

Fig. 113C

CONGENITAL ABSENCE, FUSION OR DEFORM-
ITY OF CERVICAL SPINE (KLIPPEL-FEIL SYN-
DROME) (Fig. 114A). A rather striking anomaly
which has been encountered in absence of the entire or
a portion of the cervical spine. The remaining bony
structure representing the cervical portion of the
spine may be fused into an irregular bony mass.

Clinically there is:
1. Absence of, or shortening of the neck.
2. Lowering of the hair line.
3. Limitation of motion.

This constitutes what is known as Klippel-Feil
Syndrome.

Other anomalies may be present, such as Spina
Bifida. A wide variety of neurological symptoms may

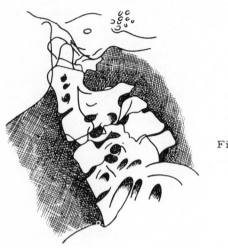

Fig. 114A

be present, such as paralysis, torticollis, and other
contractures and even mental impairment. The prognosis as to life is good.

In recent years it has been found that many
such individuals have had symptoms of rheumatoid
arthritis in infancy and there is a growing feeling
that the deformity may be in some way due to this
disease during early years. Bonola had devised a
plastic operation for the correction of this deformity
which promises some relief from this condition.

OCCIPITALIZATION OF THE ATLAS. (McRae
and Barnum). This is a specific congenital bony deformity in the region of the foramen magnum due to
some degree of bony union between the atlas and the
adjacent skull. There is usually bony continuity between the anterior arch of the atlas and anterior lip
of the foramen magnum. Laminography may be necessary to demonstrate this assimilation. Impingement
of the posterior portion of the odontoid on the cord is
responsible in large measure for the many varied
neurological symptoms, which frequently simulate
multiple sclerosis. Fusion of the upper cervical
vertebrae serves to alleviate this. Apparently platybasia is not a common accompanying cause. Com-

plete agenesis of the odontoid process of the second
cervical with other associated vertebral deformity
may give similar pressure symptoms on the cord,
(Schultz, et al.).

DIASTEMATOMYELIA, (DIPLOMYELIA). This
is a "congenital malformation of the neural axis
characterized by a sagittal division of a segment of
the spinal cord or cauda equina and usually associated
with anomalous development of the vertebrae,"
(Neuhauser, et al.). The cord is separated into two
lateral portions by a fine vertical bony or cartilaginous septum which may be visible on ordinary roentgen
examination or may require myelographic examination
to show the dividing septum. There is associated
widening of the vertebral structures in the involved
area with malformation of the vertebra, failure or
bizarre fusion of the neural arches. Many unusual
neural defects of gait, locomotion and development of
the lower extremities are associated with this condition which may be amenable to surgical correction.
It occurs most frequently in the lumbar and sacral
region but may be encountered elsewhere in the spine.
Tomography may be a valuable aid in diagnosis;
myelography is essential for a fuller understanding of
the cord defect, (Cowie). Like the hyperostosis which
develops in association with paraplegia, there is, in
some cases, an overgrowth of shaggy periostitis of
the upper femurs and adjacent bony structures.

BLOCK VERTEBRA, or FAILURE OF SEG-
MENTATION (Fig. 114B). Due to faulty segmentation
of the centra of the vertebra, the vertebral bodies
may be fused into a single bony block. This is usually of little significance. It can usually be readily differentiated from injury or disease since there is almost always some trace of the intervertebral disc
remaining. This is most frequently seen in the cervical region, occasionally in the dorsal but very
rarely in the lumbar spine.

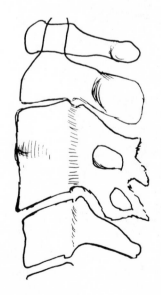

Fig. 114B

SACRALIZATION* (Fig. 114C). The lower portion of the lumbar spine and the upper sacral segment is the site of a large number of anatomical variations. The most frequently encountered variation in this region is enlargement of one or both transverse processes of the fifth lumbar vertebra. The processes may be broad and expanded, giving the appearance of a butterfly; they may encroach upon and even form false joints with the sacrum. Such a condition is known as sacralization. In itself it is of no clinical significance, and does not give rise to any symptoms. When it is present on one side only it does produce a potential weakness which may render the sacroiliac joints more susceptible to strain or injury.

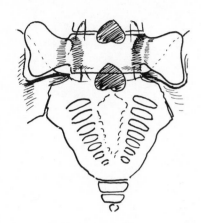

Fig. 114C

ELONGATION OF THE TRANSVERSE PROCESSES (Fig. 114D). Elongation of the transverse processes of the fifth lumbar vertebra with impingement on the ilium has been described as a cause of low back pain but the consensus of opinion is that actual impingement rarely occurs.

BIFURCATION OF THE COCCYX is a rare anomaly, occasionally seen with development of two complete coccygeal structures. Other variations in development are common.

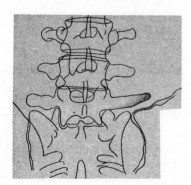

Fig. 114D

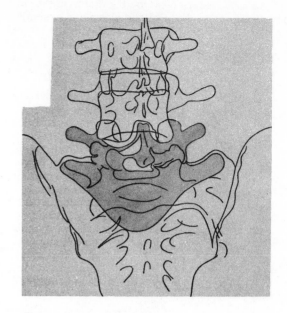

Fig. 115A

SPONDYLOLISTHESIS. (Figs. 115A & B). Congenital or acquired defects of the pars interarticularis or isthmus often associated with rudimentary development of the articular processes may result in lack of proper support of the vertebra, with consequent slipping of the vertebra downward and forward, a condition known as spondylolisthesis. In most instances, trauma, usually of a continuous repeated

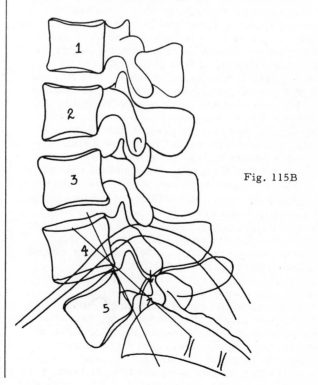

Fig. 115B

type, is a necessary contributing factor in the presence of this anomaly. Oblique views are essential to demonstrate such anomalous defects; the lateral view is essential for estimating the degree of forward luxation. Any of the lumbar vertebrae may be involved but the condition is most frequently seen in the fifth lumbar.

Spondylolisthesis of the fifth lumbar vertebra forward and downward on the sacrum presents a characteristic picture in the anteroposterior view, (Fig. 115A).

Roentgenologically the condition may be suspected from examination of the anterior roentgenogram from the following findings, (Garland and Thomas):

1. Overlapping transverse processes of the 5th lumbar on the sacrum.

2. Obscuring of the outline of the fifth lumbar vertebra.

3. Apparent increase in density of body of fifth lumbar vertebra.

4. Angulation and crowding of laminae and spinous processes.

Spondylolisthesis of the fifth lumbar forward and downward on the sacrum is best seen in the lateral view. The degree of luxation can best be estimated from the lateral view. Ullmann's line for estimating the degree of luxation is very helpful (Fig. 49).

Meschan's lining method (Fig. 115B) of stability determination although more complicated is a more exact method. This consists of drawing two lines (lateral view) one connecting the posterior-superior and posterior-inferior margins of the fifth lumbar, and other connecting the posterior-inferior margin of the fourth lumbar and the posterior-superior margin of the sacrum. These lines when prolonged may intersect above or below; may be parallel or may coincide in a single line. Normally these lines should intersect at or below the fifth lumbar vertebra, or if the lines are parallel they should not be more than 3 mm. apart. In true spondylolisthesis the lines intersect above the fifth lumbar and the degree of angle determines the severity of the spondylolisthesis as follows: Up to 10 degrees indicates slight, 11 to 20 degrees is moderate and greater than 20 is severe. When the lines are parallel more than 3 mm. distance is abnormal. Any variation of these measurements found in films taken in recumbent and upright position or in position of hyperextension of the body indicates the degree of instability of the back. True spondylolisthesis is usually indication of a painful, weak back but Bistrom has directed attention to the fact that at times complete luxation of the lumbosacral joint and other congenital anomalies may be present without pain or disability.

The isthmus defect of the fifth lumbar vertebra is best seen in the oblique views (Fig. 115C). Both oblique views should be taken for comparison. In this view an anomalous defect in the pars interarticularis or isthmus between the articular processes can be readily seen. The defect is most frequently bilateral (Garland and Thomas).

Horizontal sacrum in which the articular surface of the sacrum is rendered almost perpendicular

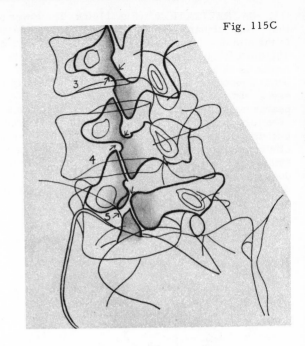

Fig. 115C

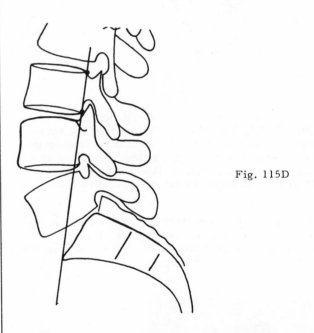

Fig. 115D

thereby producing an excessive strain upon the apophyseal joints. If a line drawn through the posterior margins of the lower three lumbar vertebrae projected downward passes in front of the sacrum it is considered to be sufficiently displaced to give rise to symptoms.

ILIAC HORNS. (Thompson, Walker, and Weens). Iliac Horns are bilateral osseous processes arising from the posterior surface of the iliac bones. Occur in association with deformity of joints and faulty development of fingernails. They are not necessarily isolated bony (anomalies) malformations but are manifestations of hereditary arthrodysplasia and fingernail dystrophy.

Bates has pointed out that posterior iliac horns occur in arthrodysplasia in association with dysplasia of the fingernails.

SUPERNUMERARY OR ABSENCE OF RIBS*
(Figs. 116A & B). Extra ribs, either above, attached to the cervical spine (cervical ribs) (Fig. 116A) or below, attached to the upper lumbar vertebra (lumbar ribs) (Fig. 116B) are frequently encountered. Cervical ribs vary in size from extremely prominent transverse processes of the seventh cervical vertebra to large fully developed rib structure. They may, under exceptional circumstances, cause pressure on the brachial plexus with consequent neuralgic symptoms. As a result of contraction of

the scalenus anticus muscle the subclavian artery and brachial plexus may be impinged against such a cervical rib, giving rise to scalenus anticus muscle syndrome.

Weston has determined their hereditary nature; "It is of interest to note that the anomalies are more pronounced in the third generation than in the second generation."

Lumbar ribs are usually quite rudimentary and cause no untoward symptoms; they merely represent elongated processes of bone, projecting outward from the transverse processes of the first lumbar vertebra, articulating with them by definite articular surfaces. Similarly one or more ribs may be congenitally absent. (Gershon-Cohen and Delbridge; Bowie and Jacobson).

ANOMALY OF STERNUM. The lower segment of the sternum is very frequently deformed with remnants of remaining cartilage so as to give the impression of abnormal destruction.

SYNOSTOSIS OF RIBS (Fig. 116C). Synostosis, or fusion of the anterior free ends of 2 ribs is not uncommonly met with. It usually involves the fourth or fifth ribs anteriorly. Division or bifurcation of a rib occurs less frequently.

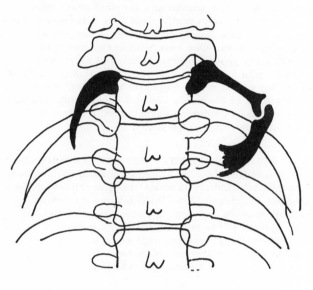

Fig. 116A

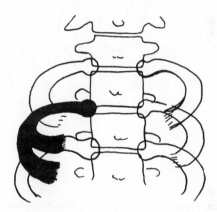

Fig. 116C

RHOMBOID IMPRESSION (Fig. 116D). Pronounced impressions on the under surfaces of the inner ends of the clavicles are made by heavy rhomboid ligaments. They are of no pathological significance.

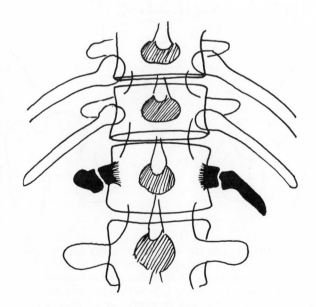

Fig. 116B

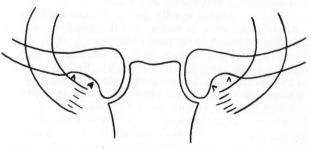

Fig. 116D

ANOMALIES OF THE PELVIS; CONGENITAL DISLOCATION OF HIP* (Fig. 117). One of the most common anomalies encountered in the pelvis is congenital dislocation of the hip. The condition is probably due to a malposition of the fetal parts. The head of the femur not being in its normal position, the acetabulum remains shallow and does not assume its normal cup-shaped appearance. Since it does not function properly, growth is interfered with and the bones of the entire lower extremity remain small in comparison with those of the other normal member. The head and neck of the femur remain in an abnormal position disturbing the normal relationship with the pelvis, as indicated by Shenton's Line. There is no bone erosion or destruction, but the head of the bone may be small or the capital epiphysis smaller than its fellow of the opposite side, A system of lining has been devised, (Martin), for the proper evaluation of the normal and detection of true dislocations of the hip joint, (See Manual of Roentgenolical Technique).

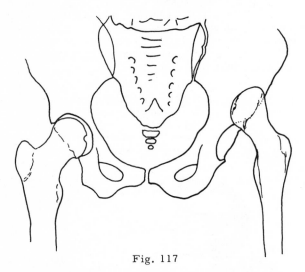

Fig. 117

Two types are recognized; the endogenous type resulting from developmental arrest of the roof of the acetabulum with shallow acetabular cavity and the dynamic type produced by the presence of abnormal forces which are responsible for the dislocation of the femoral head from the acetabulum such as relaxation of ligaments about the hip and muscular imbalance. This may serve to explain the occasional coexistence of spina bifida and congenital dislocation of the hip.

The condition usually goes unnoticed until the child tries to walk, at which time the waddling gait attracts attention to the true condition. A system of lining is helpful in evaluation of the deformity, (See Manual of Ronetgenolical Technique). Reduction of the dislocation, if attempted early, may be successful. In young infants skeletal traction in abduction has given most satisfactory results (Crego). If reduction is maintained the pressure of the femoral head, in its normal position during the developmental period, may produce an acetabular socket sufficiently deep for a satisfactory functional result.

CONGENITAL COXA VARA. Congenital coxa vara is an unusual condition characterized by deformity of the head and neck of the femur which develops within the first few years of life. There is fragmentation of the neck at the lower epiphyseal line forming a triangular fragment of bone which interferes with growth of the lower portion of the neck producing coxa vara. During adolescence the epiphysis may give way, entirely, resulting in upward displacement of the shaft. At this stage it cannot be differentiated from the condition known as "slipped epiphysis" of adolescence. The etiology is not known, but there is some indication that this condition may be due to Vitamin A or D deficiency early in life. Finby, et al. suggest the tentative hypothesis that deficient osteogenesis in the femoral neck region with development of pseudoarthrosis may be the cause. The only treatment is early recognition and surgical correction.

Almond has recently cited four instances occurring in the same family indicating the congenital aspect of this condition. One case with serial radiographic examination shows clearly the normal epiphyseal growth up to 5 months, with fragmentation of the neck at the lower end of the epiphyseal line by 2 years, persistence of Shenton's line and consequent shortening and finally beginning ossification of defect with coxa vara deformity at 4 years.

PELVIC DEFORMITY WITH EXSTROPHY OF THE BLADDER (Fig. 118). Exstrophy of the bladder, a congenital anomaly in which there is failure of the anterior bladder wall to close, leaving the entire bladder mucosa exposed, is associated with certain bony defects in the pelvis. The pubic bones are small and rudimentary, showing wide separation at their symphysis, often five or six inches. This produces surprisingly little difficulty in walking.

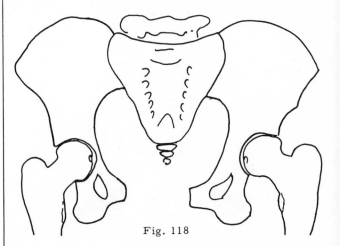

Fig. 118

ANOMALIES OF THE EXTREMITIES, HEMIHYPERTROPHY; LOCAL GIGANTISM: HEMIATROPHY. Certain forms of anomalous development affect the entire extremity. Hemihypertrophy or local gigantism is a condition in which one extremity or member develops to greater size than the other. The cause of this excessive growth is not known; it may be caused by an abberation of tissue differentiation. The structures themselves are larger and often the same influence on growth can be seen on the bones of the pelvis or shoulder. The condition may not be noticeable until the child starts to walk. Nothing has been found to influence the condition during growth; after growth is fully established corrective operations can be undertaken. Hemiatrophy may also occur without apparent cause.

INTRA-UTERINE AMPUTATIONS AND FRACTURES.* Intra-uterine amputations from accidents

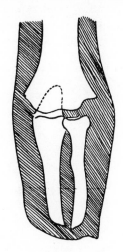

Fig. 119

to the fetus in utero are occasionally observed (Fig. 119). These may be due to constrictions produced by the umbilical cord, amnionic adhesions, etc. Such constrictions may so interfere with the blood supply to the part that failure to develop results; this may be so great that the extremity is amputated in utero. Recent conception of the method of development of such anomalies is that they merely represent cessation of differentiation at some time in the process of limb development. They may not go on to full amputation but merely persist as constriction bands about the extremity.

Intra-uterine fractures from osteogenesis imperfecta usually present a knarled appearance at the sites of fracture of the long bones from callus. Other instances of isolated, localized, curving deformity of long bones have been noted which have been attributed to healed intra-uterine fractures (Dawson). The pathological process may develop from a somewhat similar process to that of Ainhum in which a constricting, fibrous band develops in the soft parts about the great or little toe (usually in negroes), causing constriction of the parts and gradual interference with the circulation. We have observed such deformity in a newborn child about the forearm. It may be that by some such process, amputation is produced in utero (See Lipomatosis of bone).

VARIATIONS OF UPPER EXTREMITY— SPRENGEL'S DEFORMITY (Fig. 120). Sprengel's deformity of the scapula is characterized by decrease in size of the body of the scapula and prominent overgrowth of the spine and acromion processes (Fig. 120A). It is of no pathological significance. It is associated with an unusually high position of the scapula.

Elevated scapula, somewhat akin to Sprengel's Deformity, is a condition in which the scapulae are found in an extremely high position. This causes some deformity, but is of no other significance. In-

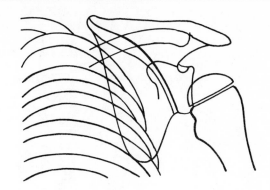

Fig. 120A

stances in which the glenoid cavity is congenitally shallow (glenoid hypoplasia) result in easy dislocation of the shoulder joint and are often spoken of as "habitual dislocation" (Fig. 120B), (Owen). Bilateral humerus varus deformity of the upper ends of the humeri has been reported by Davies. Rudimentary supernumerary duplication of the clavicle has been reported by Golthamer, but this seems to be of little if any pathological significance.

The supracondyloid process of the humerus (Kriss) is a spur-like projection of bone, varying from a small outgrowth to one more than a centimeter in length, projecting outward and downward from the ulnar side of the humerus several centimeters above the elbow joint. Investigation of the inmates of the St. Louis City Sanitarium by Robert J. Terry disclosed 25 instances of this anomaly. This was considered a vestigeal remnant from lower animal development. It may cause nerve pressure.

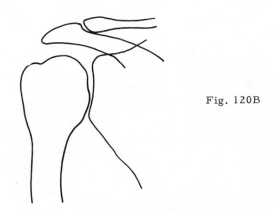

Fig. 120B

MADELUNG'S DEFORMITY—(RADIUS CURVUS) (Fig. 121A). This is a deformity affecting the forearms due to arrest of growth of a portion of the lower radial epiphysis. It is more common in females than in males in ratio of four to one. It occurs with surprising uniformity at twelve to fourteen years of age. The first manifestation of the condition may be an unusual prominence caused by the spontaneous dorsal dislocation of the ulna at the wrist, due to the fact that the arrest in epiphyseal growth of the radius

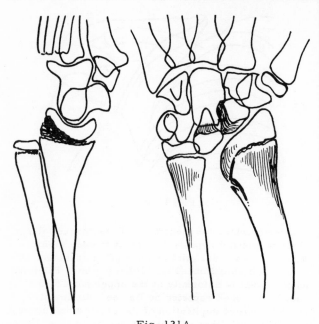

Fig. 121A

makes this bone shorter than the ulna which grows at
a normal rate and, therefore, becomes longer. If
there is arrest of only one portion of the radial epiphysis the radius becomes curved—Radius Curvus.
Union of the epiphyses causes arrest of the condition,
but the deformity persists. Casts and restraining
splints are of no avail; destruction of the epiphysis
leaves the member shorter; permitting the condition
to go on until union of the epiphyses has occurred results in such adaptation of the tissues to this new position that osteotomy or other orthopedic operations
are difficult and ineffective. A similar condition occurs in the tibia at the ankle and at its upper end,
Tibia Vara, (Fig. 123D).

ROENTGENOLOGICAL MANIFESTATIONS.
There is a thinned appearance of lower radial epiphysis on the inner side with only a very fine line of
epiphyseal growth; on the outer side the epiphysis is
of normal thickness.
    A rarefied area on the diaphysis often develops
beneath the area of inactivity of the epiphyseal growth.
If the condition has persisted for a long time, the
radius will be curved with the lower radial articulation directed inward, and the ulna will have undergone
spontaneous dorsal dislocation, protruding downward
over the carpus for several centimeters.

PATELLA CUBITI (Fig. 121B). Either as a result of an inherent developmental defect or because of
an injury to the epiphyseal structure for the olecranon
process of the ulna early in its development, this epiphysis becomes divided forming a separate structure,
much like the patella at the knee joint. Hence the name
patella cubiti. It is of no pathological significance,
(Habbe; Kjelland).

ABSENCE OF OR FUSION OF BONES OF UP-
PER EXTREMITY (Fig. 121C).* Any of the bones of
the upper extremity may be entirely absent. The
humerus may be missing with the forearm articulating
at the shoulder joint. Either of the bones of the forearm may be absent; when this anomaly exists there is
usually associated absence of the corresponding portion of the carpal and metacarpal bones. Many types
of fusion of the carpal bones occur.

STUNTING OF GROWTH OF METACARPAL OR
METATARSAL BONES, (Fig. 121D). Strictly speaking, this may not be a developmental anomaly but
rather an acquired deformity resulting from interruption of growth of epiphysis for a metacarpal or meta-

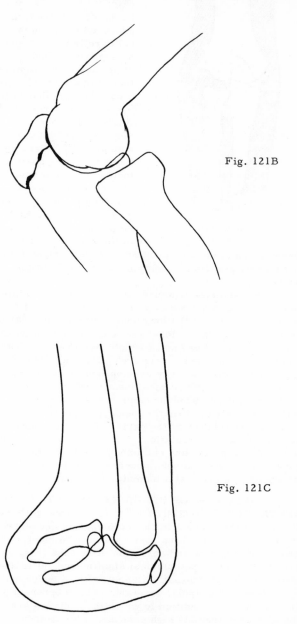

Fig. 121B

Fig. 121C

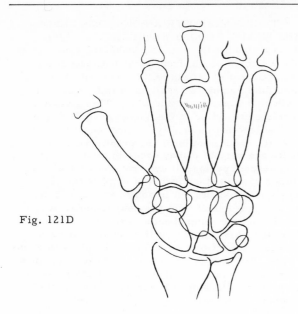

Fig. 121D

3) often a cardiac defect—usually an interatrial septal defect
4) increase in glucose tolerance "like that seen in pituitary cachexia or severe hypopituitarism."

There is no anatomical evidence to indicate endocrine gland disturbance except possibly the pituitary.

The etiology factor of arachnodactyly may be a primary inherent pituitary disturbance with a secondary mesodermal tissue defect. Later in life no manifestation of the previous infection may be discernible, the deformity alone remaining.

SUPERNUMERARY BONES OF THE UPPER EXTREMITY (Fig. 122). Numerous supernumerary bones are recognized in the upper extremity. These are especially numerous in the wrist and hand.

POLY AND SYNDACTYLISM. Many forms of polydactylism and syndactylism may occur. An unusual form of chondroectodermal dysplasia—Ellis van Creveld Disease, (Caffey), consists of hypoplasia of the teeth and nails; progressive shortening of bones of the extremities from the trunk to the periphery. Many types of variation in bones of hands and wrists; interference with normal maturation of epiphyseal centers, as seen especially in knees and elbows. The upper tibial epiphysis is small and located medialward, the proximal end of the tibial shaft is widened and pointed; this and similar changes at the proximal end of the ulna and distal end of the radius seem to be pathognomanic.

An unusual type of syndactyly associated with a

tarsal bone. This may be due to epiphysitis either of unknown etiology or from some pyogenic infection elsewhere in the body, such as osteomyelitis. It has been reported as a complication of small pox. It is rather remarkable to note, however, that occasionally, without apparent cause, similar bones may be involved on both sides.

ARACHNODACTYLY—MARFAN'S SYNDROME (Moehlig). This syndrome consists of:
1) long, slender spider fingers
2) highly arched palate

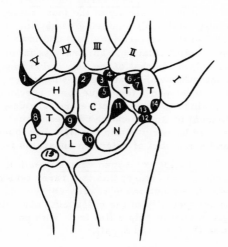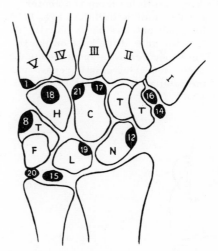

—Bogart, from Dwight's "Anatomical Variations"

1. Os Vesalius	8. Ulnare externum	15. Triangulare
2. Secondary capitate	9. Epipyramis	16. Practrapezium
3. Styloid	10. Epilunatum	17. Subcapitatum
4. Parastyloid	11. Centrale	18. Hypolunatum
5. Metastyloid	12. Radial externum	19. Humular
6. Secondary trapezoid	13. Epitrapezium	20. Secondary pisiform
7. Secondary trapezium	14. Paratrapezium	21. Os of Gruber

Fig. 122

tower-like short skull and prominent jaw is known as Acrocephalo-Syndactyly.

VARIATIONS IN LOWER EXTREMITY—ABSENCE OF OR FUSION OF BONES.

In the lower extremity as in the upper, any of the bones may be absent. The femur may be missing with articulation of the bones of the leg at the hip. Either of the bones of the leg may be missing; when they are missing there is usually a deficiency in the corresponding bones of the foot. Fusion of the calcaneus and cuboid (calcaneo-cuboid coalition) or of the talus and navicular (talonavicular synostosis) is sometimes encountered. There may be associated congenital ankylosis of the phalangeal joints. Malformation of tarsal bones and other structures occur with deformities such as talipes equinovarus and valgus. Fusion of the metatarsal bones may occur in varying degrees.

CONGENITAL PSEUDOARTHROSIS, usually of the bones of the leg, is an anomalous condition in which a false joint is produced, probably from trauma to the fetus, causing fracture in utero. Nonunion of the fracture results and the bones become spindly in appearance. Such conditions may be cured and union effected by delayed autogenous bone graft (Moore).

FABELLA. An anomalous sesamoid bone, the fabella, is a frequent finding in the lateral head of the gastrocnemius muscle, behind the knee, (Hessen). It is of no pathological significance but must merely be recognized as an anatomical variation.

Bifid patella is a deformity occasionally encountered. The bone, ossifying from two centers, shows a permanent longitudinal division, Fig. 123A.

Congenitally small patellas occur usually displaced well to the outer side of the knee on the lateral condyle. These may result in spontaneous dislocation of the patella requiring plastic repair and replacement of the patellar insertion to avoid dislocation, (Nickerson).

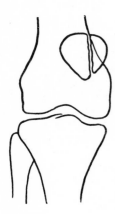

Fig. 123A

TIBIA VARA; OSTEOCHONDROSIS DEFORMANS TIBIAE; BLOUNT'S DISEASE (Fig. 123B).

This is a condition, much like Madelung's deformity of the wrist, in which, from some unknown cause, there is arrest of growth of the medial portion of the upper tibial epiphysis resulting in failure of normal growth of this portion of the tibia. This gives rise to a beaklike projection of the medial condyle of the tibia and bow-leg deformity. It may be unilateral or bilateral. It does not have any predilection for any definite age period; it may occur in infancy or during the adolescent period. It does not show the characteristics seen in other forms of epiphysitis. Its etiology is not known but in some instances it may have been associated with previous trauma. It has been shown to develop about a year after osteomyelitis of the tibia, (Morris). If it occurs during the formative stage it may be influenced and the deformity even corrected by application of braces and other orthopedic appliances, but if it occurs after the bone growth is well developed it can only be corrected by osteotomy, (Barber).

TIBIA RECURVATUM (Lubschitz) (Fig. 123C). This is an anomalous deformity in which the tibia bows backward in place of forward due probably to uneven growth of the upper tibial epiphysis. In this case the anterior portion of the epiphysis is deficient in growth. In most cases the cause is not apparent.

IRREGULAR GROWTH LOWER TIBIAL EPIPHYSES (Fig. 123D). This results in forward or medial bowing of the tibia similar to the other conditions which are due to irregular epiphyseal growth.

Talipes equino varus (clubfoot)* (Fig. 123E). A congenital anomaly of the foot caused possibly by faulty fetal position during gestation. The foot is held in a downward (equinus) and inward (varus) position with rotation. This results in the axis of the os calcis and that of the astragalus impinging upon each other which interferes with correction. Kite has developed a technique for correcting the deformity which is very effective and is widely used (see Manual of Roentgenological Technique). Treatment should be early within the first few months of life and some sort of retention apparatus is necessary.

Talipes calcaneo valgus constitutes a deformity opposite in nature; this is a rarer type of deformity which is much more readily corrected. Tarsal coalition especially of the calcaneus, navicular and talus gives rise to "rigid flat foot" with pain and dysfunction (Vaughn and Segal).

Arthrogryposis multiplex congenita (Fig. 123F) (Lewin) is a condition of unknown etiology characterized by persistent flexure or contracture of a joint due to thickening of the articular and periarticular structures only. Muscle bundle atrophy, osteoporosis, flexion and extension deformities are invariable

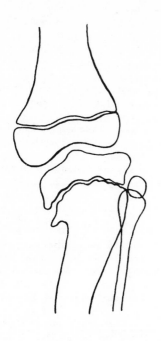

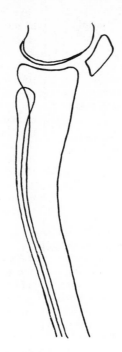

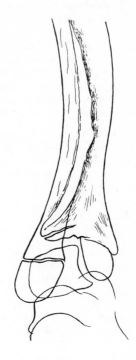

Fig. 123B   Fig. 123C   Fig. 123D

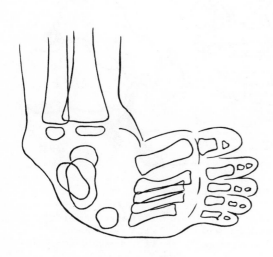

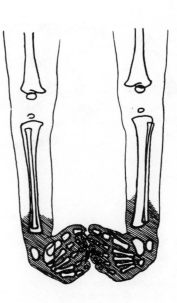

Fig. 123E   Fig. 123F

findings. The extremities are usually held in a stiff extended position and there is limitation of motion. When the lower extremity is involved there is marked clubfoot deformity. When the knee is involved it must be differentiated from genu recurvatum, a condition in which there is abnormal mobility in extension but limited flexion, (Jacobson, et al.). Hypoplasia of the acetabulum and congenital dislocation of the hip are frequent findings.

Congenital Vertical Talus. A very rare cause of congenital flat foot, from a vertical position of the talus and low articulation with the navicular. Most instances of flat foot are due to club foot deformity, (Osmond-Clarke).

Ainhum (Spinzig) is a condition occurring almost exclusively in negroes in which a fibrous band develops in the soft tissues, usually of the great toe, encircling the member, interfering with the circulation from its contraction. This condition has also been observed in the little toe, (Stack). The author has observed a similar condition in a white child with a fibrous constriction band about the forearm which interfered with proper muscular development but caused no demonstrable variation in bone formation.

Lipomatosis involving bone. A peculiar congenital condition reported only in the legs and feet in which there is fat replacement of the muscles, tendons, and ligaments of the leg and foot with invasion of the cancellous bony structures causing cross-fusion of the bones and gross deformity of the struc-

tures. The foot becomes a misshaped mass which is hardly recognizable. Contraction rings of fibrous tissue are present about the ankle somewhat similar to those seen in Ainhum, (Barnetson).

Congenital interference with growth differentiation may produce similar constriction rings or so-called "intrauterine amputation," (q.v.).

Generalized lipomatosis may involve bone, causing macrodactylia and localized hypertrophy of the tissues, (Fainsinger and Harris).

An extremely unusual case suggesting Lipoid Reticulosis of Bone has been described by Burkitt, (Fairbank).

In addition to these, instances of hyperphalangism and supernumerary epiphyses have been reported, (O'Rahilly).

SUPERNUMERARY BONES OF LOWER EXTREMITY. The recognized supernumerary bones of the lower extremity are illustrated in Fig. 123G. In addition, March, et al. have reported the os sustentaculi a supernumerary bone associated with the sustentaculum tali. Certain bones also become fused.

Talo-navicular Synostosis in which there is congenital fusion of these two bones is occasionally encountered. It does not seem to produce much disability.

Calcaneo-navicular coalition has also been noted as a developmental variation (Chambers), often without unusual symptoms.

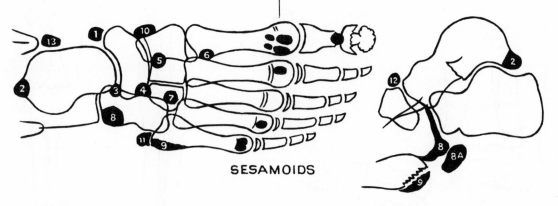

SESAMOIDS

—Brailsford "Radiology of Bones and Joints"

1. Os tibiale externum (accessory scaphoid)
2. Trigonum
3. Secondary os calcis
4. Secondary cuboid
5. Intercuneiform
6. Intermetatarsum
7. Uncinatum
8. Peroneal sesamoid (articulating with inferior surface of cuboid)
8a. Peroneal sesamoid
9. Epiphysis of fifth metatarsal
10. Paracuneiform
11. Vesalianum
12. Astragalo-scaphoid ossicle
13. Os subtibiale (Fairbank)

Fig. 123G

QUESTIONS ON CONGENITAL ANOMALIES AND ANATOMICAL VARIATIONS

Questions marked with a dagger deal with rare and less-important conditions.

1. Name five conditions in which there seems to be some congenital disturbance in normal bone development.

2. To what are Achondroplasia, Dyschondroplasia, and Osteogenesis Imperfecta attributed? Why?

3. What is meant by Osteopetrosis (Marble Bones) and describe briefly its characteristic roentgen appearance.

4. What is Osteopoikilosis and how does it manifest itself roentgenographically? Does it have any influence on the health of the individual?

5. Describe briefly the meaning of the following conditions:
   Acrania
   Microcephaly
   Megalocephaly
   Oxycephaly
   Dolichocephaly
   Brachycephaly
   Scaphocephaly
   Ocular hypertelorism
   Cleidocranial dysostosis
   Lacunnae skull
   Localized thinning of cranial bones
   Persistent enlargement of parietal foramina

6. Describe the following anomalies in spinal development:
   Spina Bifida Occulta
   Spina Bifida Vera
   Supernumerary and malformed vertebrae
   Klippel-Feil Syndrome
   Sacralization
   Spondylolisthesis from congenital defects

7. In what two locations are supernumerary ribs most often found? Are they of any pathological significance? What is synostosis of a rib?

8. What are the roentgen manifestations of congenital dislocation of the hip? What is meant by congenital Coxa Vara?

†9. What bony deformity of the pelvis usually accompanies extrophy of bladder? Does it cause serious disability in walking?

†10. What is hemihypertrophy and what is its cause?

†11. What are the cause and roentgen appearance of intrauterine amputations?

12. What is meant by Sprengel's Deformity of the Scapula? Is it of any significance?

†13. Describe Madelung's deformity and indicate the method by which it is brought about.

†14. To what may the stunting of growth of the metacarpal or metatarsal bones be due?

†15. Name and locate the supernumerary bones of the hands and wrist.

†16. Name and locate the supernumerary bones of the foot.

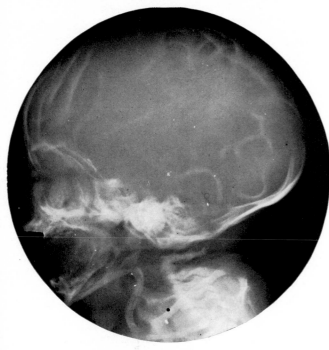

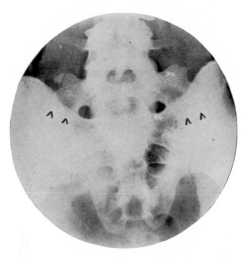

Luechenschaedel or Lacunae Skull giving the appearance of rounded areas of thinning of cranial bones. Congenital. Usually associated with spina bifida.

Sacralization of the expanded transverse processes of the fifth lumbar vertebra. This is a developmental anomaly of little pathological significance.

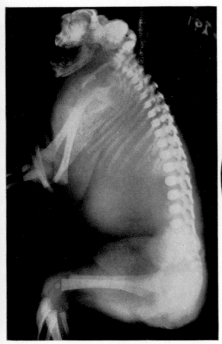

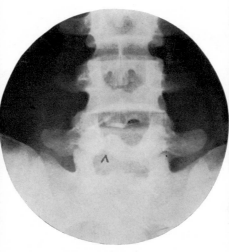

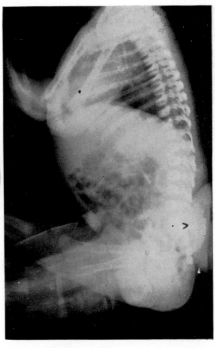

Anencephaly, showing the lack of development of the cranial structures.

Spina bifida occulta, a lack of fusion of the laminae of the fifth lumbar vertebra, a developmental anomaly of no pathological significance. Not to be confused with true spina bifida.

Spina bifida, showing a defect in the vertebral structure in the lower lumbar region with a protruding sac.

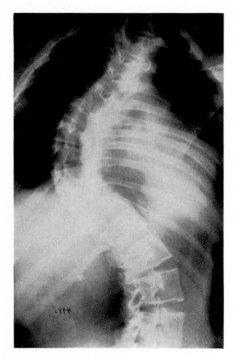

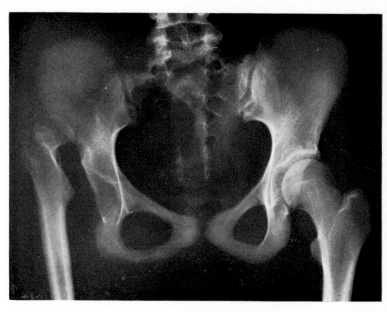

Congenital dislocation of the hip showing the lack of development of the head and shaft of the involved femur. The acetabulum is shallow compared with the opposite side.

Scoliosis of the spine with rotation of the bodies of the vertebrae.

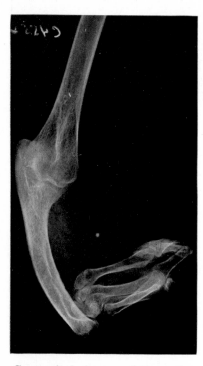

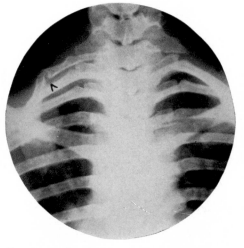

Cervical rib showing an accessory cervical rib on one side with a joint.

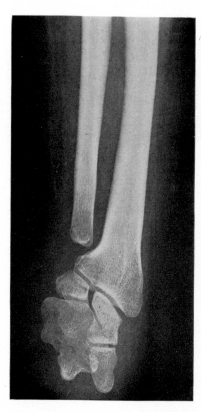

Congenital absence of the radius and bones of the thumb.

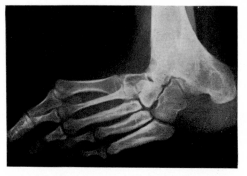

Congenital absence of the hand from an intra-uterine amputation at the wrist.

Talipes Equino-Varus, congenital club-foot deformity; Tibio-Talo-Calcaneal Coalition.

TUMORS OF BONE (Chapter XIII)

A. Benign, Arising from:

  1. Cortex

    a. Osteoma

    b. Osteochondroma—single

    c. Chondroma—ecchondroma

  2. Medullary Canal (Central)

    a. Cyst—osteitis fibrosa cystica

    b. Giant-Cell Tumor

    c. Chondroma—Enchondroma (Central Chondroma), multiple in phalanges, single in long bones

    d. Chondroblastoma—solitary ends of long bones

    e. Non-osteogenic Fibroma

    f. Angioma

B. Malignant

  1. Primary Tumors (Types of Osteogenic Sarcoma), arising from:

    a. Periosteum

      Ossifying Periosteal Sarcoma

      Nonossifying (Fibro-) Periosteal Sarcoma

      Chondromyxo- (Periosteal) Sarcoma

    b. Medullary Canal (Endosteal)

      Osteolytic types of Sarcoma

        Osteolytic sarcoma—rapidly growing and slow growing

        Giant-cell sarcoma—malignant degeneration of giant-cell tumor

        Myeloma-

          Plasma cell

          Myelocytoma

          Erythroblastoma

          Lymphocytoma

        Chondroblastic Sarcoma

     c. Cortex

        Ewing's Sarcoma (Endothelial myeloma)

     d. Extraosseus Osteogenic Sarcoma

     e. Adamantinoma (Ameloblastoma) of long bones

  2. Metastatic Tumors of Bone

     a. Sarcoma

     b. Carcinoma

        Osteoblastic (osteoplastic)

        Osteoclastic

     c. Lymphoblastoma—

        Reticulum Cell Sarcoma
        Lymphosarcoma
        Hodgkin's Granuloma
        Hodgkin's Sarcoma
        Giant Follicular Lymphoma

     d. Neuroblastoma

C. Tumors in Special Locations

  1. Skull

  2. Jaw

  3. Soft Part Tumors Causing Bone Pressure

Chapter XIII

TUMORS OF BONE

Many tumors originate from bony structures; some are benign, many are malignant. It is the chief purpose of the roentgenological examination to detect those characteristics which help to differentiate benign from malignant lesions. In order to concentrate the material on this important subject for study, the American College of Surgeons maintains a Bone Tumor Registry in which physicians are invited to register their cases.

BENIGN TUMORS OF BONE

There is general accord as to the characteristics of benign tumors as described by the Registry, (James Ewing).

1. Osteogenic series,
    Exostosis
    Osteoma
2. Chondroma series
    Chondroma
3. Giant-Cell Series
    Epiphyseal giant cell tumors
4. Angioma Series
    Cavernous Angioma
    Plexiform Angioma

This classification is based on histogenesis; for the purpose of differential roentgen diagnosis however, these tumors may better be considered from the standpoint of the structures from which they arise and the physical characteristics which they produce in the bony structures.

All tumors arising from the periosteum without exception are malignant, so that under the heading of benign tumors we have only those for consideration which arise from the cortex and medullary canal.

Benign bone tumors arising from the cortex are of three types:

1. Osteoma
2. Osteochondroma
3. Multiple Exostoses

OSTEOMA* (Fig. 124A). An osteoma is a new growth composed of bony tissue springing from the cortex and extending out into the soft tissues. They usually arise from the bone near the diaphyseal side of the epiphyseal line and are always directed away from the joint. As the bone lengthens by the natural process of growth they get farther and farther away from the end of the bone, but obviously they can never reach its midportion. They may arise by a narrow pedicle or by a broad sessile base. In a pure osteoma

the free margin is rounded and smooth. One characteristic point by which they can always be identified and differentiated from inflammatory outgrowths (or exostoses) is the fact that in osteomas the architecture of the bone extends from the shaft directly out into the bony growth; this is not the case in exostosis formation. When they occur in the skull they arise from the cortex without cartilaginous element, being hard and ivory-like, and are known as ivory osteomata.

OSTEOCHONDROMA (Fig. 124B). An osteochondroma is similar to an osteoma with the exception that there are also cartilaginous elements in the growth. These tumors originate in a similar manner to osteomas and roentgenographically the appearance is very similar; the terminal free end of the growth, however, in place of having a rounded smooth surface presents scalloped calcareous deposits in the soft tissues just beyond the end of the bony pedicle. The intervening cartilaginous portion of the tumor, of course, does

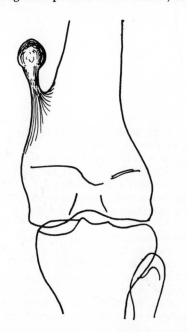

Fig. 124A

not show in the roentgenogram and as a result these rounded deposits of bone seem to be free in the soft tissues. Wherever this appearance exists it is a definite indication of the existence of cartilaginous elements in the tumor.

---

*An asterisk following any title indicates that roentgenographic reproductions illustrating this condition will be found in the pictorial supplement at the end of the chapter.

Rare instances have been reported where such tumors which retain their cartilaginous elements into later life have undergone malignant degeneration.

Pure chondromatous exostoses (ECCHONDROMA) must-be rather rare. Theoretically they should represent cartilaginous outgrowths of bone similar to osteochondromas but without osseous elements. Indeed many observers feel that all three of these tumors represent the same process at different stages; that they all originate as chondromas, changing into osteochondromas and finally into pure osteomas as the cartilage is replaced by bone. Extraskeletal deposits of bone and cartilage occasionally occur. Purser has described one in the soft tissues of the foot adjacent to the great toe.

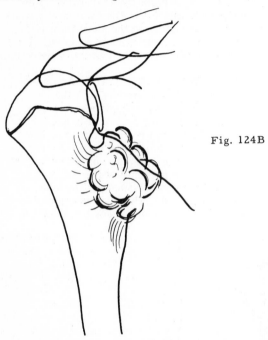

Fig. 124B

Such tumors need not be disturbed unless by their position they interfere with function. If they do, simple local removal will suffice; they never tend to recur. They are tumors arising from normal cartilaginous structures (ecchondroma) in contradistinction to enchondroma, cartilaginous tumors occurring where cartilage does not normally occur.

Small periosteal (or subperiosteal) cartilage tumors have been reported by Lichtenstein and Hall, showing surrounding zone of sclerosis; benign without recurrence after local removal. Kimmelstiel and Rapp, have designated radiologically similar lesions, "apparently benign tumurous but destructive and infiltrative hyperplasia of connective tissue", as "periosteal desmoids".

BENIGN MEDULLARY TUMORS. The most common types of benign tumors arising from the medullary canal are:
  a. Bone Cyst
  b. Benign Giant-Cell Tumor

c. Chondroma
d. Fibroma—Osteitis fibrosa cystica
e. Angioma

All of these have certain similar roentgenographic characteristics. All originate from the medullary canal; they are all slow-growing tumors so that the cortex is expanded by the gradual pressure of their growth. Although often expanded to paper thinness, the cortex is not broken through by invasion of the growth; if breaking of the cortex does occur it is due to fracture resulting from the frail condition of the bone. Periosteal reaction or any other form of new bone formation is never present except as an instrument of repair after fracture. There are, however, certain other characteristics which serve to differentiate these lesions.

Geschickter and Copeland feel that bone cyst, giant-cell tumor and osteitis fibrosa are manifestations of a similar process as it occurs in different localities of the bone. Giant-cell tumor occurring most frequently in the cancellous end of the bone is permitted more unrestrained growth since the thin cortex offers little resistance; bone cyst, occurring in the metaphyseal region meets stiffer resistance in the form of stronger cortical structures causing greater pressure to be exerted on the tumor structures, and finally osteitis fibrosa occurring in the diaphysis of the bone is subjected to greatest pressure from thick cortical bone resulting in abundant fibrous tissue with small cysts.

BONE CYST* (Fig. 125). While not truly neoplastic in origin they produce lesions similar to true tumors and must be considered in differential diagnosis. They almost always occur in children under twenty years of age and probably represent a localized disorder of bone growth.

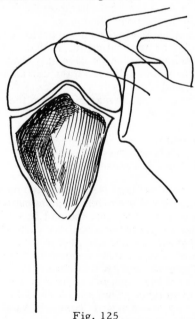

Fig. 125

They are central in origin causing uniform expansion of the bone. The cortex is thinned but not broken through except from trauma and there is no periosteal reaction. Occasionally true cysts occur which are asymmetrical and show true lateral expansion, (Hutter).

Unicameral (single cavity) bone cysts occur in the shafts at the diaphyseal ends of the long bones. They usually abutt directly on the cartilage plate of the epiphysis, but never extend into the epiphyseal structure. Bone cysts tend to undergo spontaneous healing as a layer of spongiosa bone is deposited over the cartilage at the epiphyseal end of the bone during the regular process of bone growth; so that by adult life they should be filled in. Surgical attempts to heal a cyst by implantation of bone chips before the cyst has moved away from the metaphyseal region may end in absorption of the bone chips and reestablishment of the cyst.

Cysts usually contain clear fluid with scant lining membrane. At times they may contain large quantities of blood which oozes in through capillaries lining the cyst wall; these are known as "aneurysmal bone cysts." Sherman and Soong have recently emphasized the characteristics of this tumor. They present a varied picture and are the only types of bone cysts which may occur in adults. They occur in either the diaphyseal or metaphysial regions of long bones; they usually are excentric with indication of origin in one side of the cortex, or periosteum or endosteum although they may in their stage of full-blown development appear to be central in origin; and they may be traversed by bony septa giving the impression of giant cell tumor variants which some still hold them to be. Curettement and packing will heal the lesions or they may be filled with bone chips taken from the crest of the ilium.

Bone cysts during their stage of healing are known as "latent" or healing bone cysts. They may be recognized roentgenographically by the fact that they are usually somewhat removed from the epiphyseal end of the bone; the degree of expansion is less and the cortical walls are thicker. They are usually found in early adult life. These fill in with fibrous tissue and ultimately with bone. If operated in the healing stage theymmay be designated as non osteogenic fibromata, (Maudsley and Stansfeld).

Observations by Ponseti and Friedman would indicate that such lesions can arise from other causes also. They have observed such a case for thirteen years. During this time such a defect appeared in the upper metaphyseal region of the humerus, regressed, and finally disappeared as it traveled downward into the shaft, with growth of the bone. This complete cycle was repeated for three separate times, the site of first appearance of the bony defect being always in the same place in the metaphyseal region. The essayists conclude that since the lesions arose in the same location in each instance that this would indicate some internal difficulty in the ossification process of the bone at this point. Such lesions are similar to those described as cystlike, nonosteogenic fibroma, metaphyseal fibrous defects, monostotic fibrous dysplasia.

GIANT-CELL TUMOR*, (OSTEOCLASTOMA), (Fig. 126). Benign giant-cell tumor, although it also occurs as a single lesion in the ends of long bones, is most prone to occur in adults. In this case the age of the patient may be a determining factor in the diagnosis.

It is central in origin, causing a large area of destruction with expansion of the bone, looking very much like a cyst except that it occurs almost exclusively in individuals over 20 years of age whereas bone cyst occurs in individuals below that age. It must be considered only as locally malignant, since it usually does not tend to metastasize. By its continuous growth it causes breaking through the cortex. Being slow growing the periosteum has an opportunity to throw out barrier after barrier of bone in front of successive breaks in the cortex. This is known as trabeculation and is almost characteristic of tumors of this type. It is the only tumor of medullary origin which produces new bone. It usually responds to radiotherapy.

Ordinarily giant-cell tumor may be considered as a benign growth, without metastases or local recurrence after operation. Very rarely, however, tumors of this sort appear to undergo malignant degeneration and instances have been recorded of actual metastasis of giant-cell tumor cells.

Development of an irregular infiltrative margin in a previously well defined giant cell tumor is presumptive evidence of malignant degeneration.

Haas and Ritter have reported a case of "benign" giant-cell tumor with embolic metastasis in prepuce of the penis 2 1/2 years later.

The typical picture of benign giant-cell tumors as described occurs in the cancellous ends of the long bones well into the epiphysis. Other atypical variants occur, however, in which spindle cells predominate with relatively fewer giant cells. This is considered as a healing form of giant-cell tumor. They frequently occur in the small and irregular bones especially the vertebrae; and a case has been reported in which the patella was involved, (Shorvon). They have been reported in the skull and nasal sinuses.

NON-OSTEOGENIC FIBROMA (Fig. 127). Fibromas of bone of this type (Jaffe and Lichtenstein) are relatively rare. They form tumors similar to enchondromas involving the ends of the long bones, (often the fibula) but differ in that they usually occur as single tumors. Osteitis fibrosa is a fibrous tissue replacement of bone. It is possible that isolated fibromas may be in some way related. Some contend that these are really not neoplastic.

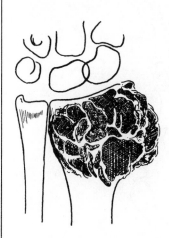

Fig. 126

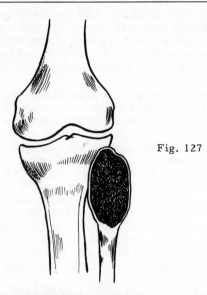

Fig. 127

SUBPERIOSTEAL LIPOMA. A benign subperiosteal lipoma has been described by Hummel and Truong-Thi-Danh presenting the appearance of a large smooth radiolucent subperiosteal mass raising the periostrum over one-third of the femoral shaft.

BENIGN CHONDROMA—ENCHONDROMA* (Fig. 128). Chondromas, on the other hand, are usually multiple, occurring in the smaller bones of the hands and feet. While the roentgen characteristics of the individual lesions are the same, the site and manner of involvement is the determining factor.

BENIGN CHONDROBLASTOMA. Very rarely (Geschickter and Copeland give the incidence as 5 in 2000 cases), benign chondromas affect the end of the shaft of a long bone, producing a picture similar to bone cyst, or giant-cell tumor. Occurring most frequently in, or in close relationship to the epiphysis, they are spoken of as chondroblastomas (Codman). In this location they may expand the bone and may be

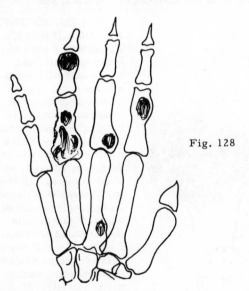

Fig. 128

associated with some sclerosis. The few cases which we have treated have responded well after x-ray therapy, with filling in of the destroyed areas of newly formed dense bone.

Eleven verified cases have recently been reported by Sherman and Uzel, who give the important points in roentgen diagnosis as 1) age—usually occurring during adolescence as the epiphyseal line is closing; 2) location—all tumors were medullary, usually occurring in the epiphyseal region even though closed, but encroaching into the metaphyseal area. It was always found to be at least touching the epiphyseal line; 3) areas of osteolysis which were universally found with 4) fine thread-like strands of bone and occasional peristeal reaction. An instance has been reported (Gramiak et al.) in which multiple rounded well defined hemangiomatous lesions have been present in the skull and long bones throughout the body.

ANGIOMA OF BONE (Fig. 129). Angiomatous growths usually involve the cancellous structure of bone. They are most commonly encountered in the vertebral bodies and skull, but may occur in the long bones.

Roentgenographically this condition may be recognized in the vertebral type by enlargement of the cancellous channels of the bone, thinning of the septa and a consequent reduction in density of the entire bone (Fig. 129A). Cranial bone involvement causes a peculiar stellate arrangement of the dilated channels in the bone; when present in this location they frequently are associated with angiomas of the scalp and brain (Fig. 129B). These are the types most commonly encountered. Clusters of rounded defects, frequently in the occipital or parietal bones, may be due to large venous lakes of blood vessels. Very rarely the shaft of a long bone is involved with thin-walled, multiple, expanded lesions due to angioma; these are frequently referred to as bone aneurysms when they involve the shaft or end of a long bone they usually show irregular asymmetrical expansion and when they involve the vertebrae they cause extensive destruction. Because of its appearance it has been described as "soap bubbly," resembling giant-cell tumor. Lesions which resemble multiple hemangiomata have been encountered in the metaphyseal regions of the long bones, associated with Letterer-Siewe's Disease in infants under two years of age.

Ewing recognizes both benign cavernous and plexiform antiomas and malignant angioendothelioma. Expansion of such angiomas may encroach on adjacent structures such as the spinal cord causing secondary symptoms from pressure, (Foster and Heublein.).

Large cavernous areas filled with blood have been reported as hemorrhagic bone cysts, bone aneurysms or hemorrhagic giant-cell tumors.

Rare cases of multiple angiomatous involvement of long bones have been reported, (Ackerman and S. Hart).

At their onset they cause no clinical symptoms; by the time attention is drawn to them they have produced large vacuolated areas in the expanded ends of

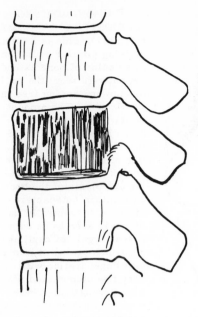

Fig. 129A

the long bones. As time goes on heavy trabeculae form, traversing the cavernous spaces; originating in the regions of the nutrient vessels they radiate in all directions like a "sunburst." Still later solid fibrous tissue fills in the blood spaces causing eventual removal of the blood sinuses. These processes may recede under the influence of roentgen therapy.

The main classification is based on histogenesis indicating the type of cells of which the tumor is composed and in this respect is excellent but designation of the subvarieties seems very confusing; it certainly does not "lend itself to the practical needs of the radiologist." This is because tumors of the same cell type may occur in many locations in the bone, and often, present marked variations in their appearance depending upon their location and the structures which they involve. For this reason it still seems desirable to classify the subvarieties of tumors according to their roentgenological manifestations (see attached chart, "Roentgen Analysis of Bone Malignancy"; pp. 191-2 under Type of Tumor and Cells).

Since there is no epithelial structure in bone there can be no primary growth of carcinomatous type arising from the bone; any primary malignancy must be sarcomatous or endotheliomatous in nature. Any malignant tumor therefore arising from bone structures may be designated as Osteogenic Sarcoma.

PERIOSTEUM. OSSIFYING OSTEOGENIC SARCOMA;*(designated by Registry of Bone Sarcoma as, "Medullary and Subperiosteal") (Fig. 130A, not to be confused with Periosteal Sarcoma of the Registry). Ossifying periosteal sarcoma is a rapidly growing, very malignant tumor. Microscopically it is of the small round-cell type springing from the osteogenetic layer of the periosteum. It occurs in especially healthy individuals and in many instances follows trauma usually of a bruising nature. It is usually attendant with pain and disability. It grows rapidly and within a few weeks may attain considerable size. Metastases develop soon, especially to the lungs; in many instances by the time the diagnosis is made, metastases to the lungs or brain have already occurred.

Roentgenographically the picture is quite characteristic. Heavy radiations of new bone project outward at right angles to the shaft of the bone ending free in the soft tissues. There is little if any erosion

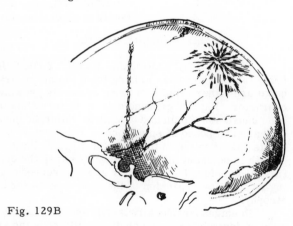

Fig. 129B

PRIMARY MALIGNANT TUMORS OF BONE

The classification of malignant tumors of bone adapted by the Registry of Bone Sarcoma of the American College of Surgeons, (Ewing), 1939 revised edition is as follows:

MALIGNANT BONE TUMORS

1. Osteogenic Series
   a) medullary and subperiosteal
   b) telangectatic
   c) sclerosing
   d) periosteal
   e) fibrosarcoma, medullary, subperiosteal
2. Chondroma Series
   a) chondrosarcoma
   b) myxosarcoma
3. Giant-Cell Tumors
   a) benign, malignant
7. Liposarcoma

4. Angioma Series
   a) angio-endothelioma
   b) diffuse endothelioma
5. Myeloma Series
   a) plasma cell
   b) myelocytoma
   c) erythroblastoma
   d) lymphocytoma
6. Reticulum-cell Sarcoma

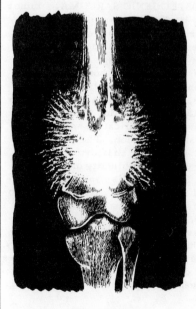

Fig. 130A

of the shaft and an appearance of dense sclerosis of the bone may develop. There is, of course, no expansion of bone since the growth is from the inner osteogenetic layer of the periosteum. The growth extends out into and invades the soft parts making a palpable tumor mass; it is not medullary in origin, but may extend through the cortex to invade the medullary canal. For that reason it has been designated as "medullary and subperiosteal" by the Bone Registry. At times the tumor is so bulky and large that it seems to spring from the cortex itself. Grunow cites various types of bone tumor with radiating spicules. The shaggy periosteal reaction associated with varicose ulcerations of the leg may at times resemble an actual new growth; usually however both bones show similar periosteal reaction--a condition which would not be likely to occur in primary osteogenic sarcoma. Bone changes associated with tropical ulcer and largely confined to the cortex and periosteum and are much smoother in appearance, their occurrence is confined to the tropics, (Brown and Middlemiss).

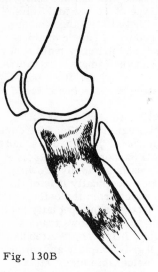

Fig. 130B

SCLEROSING OSTEO SARCOMA (Fig. 130B). This is a form of osteogenic sarcoma in which the ends of long bones are involved by a slowly progressive sclerotic process, which "converts the bone into a solid mass of very dense ossified tissue--as dense as ivory." This is not due to periosteal proliferation and indeed no periosteal bone production can be recognized in the roentgenogram.

The process is usually relatively slow, the symptoms such as pain and disability may be mild. The natural progress may require several years but even after a prolonged period metastases may develop. Few are saved even with early amputation. Roentgen therapy usually does not have very much effect.

PAROSTEAL OSTEOGENIC SARCOMA, a tumor recognized originally by Geschickter and Copeland has recently been verified by Stevens, et al., after a study of 19 such cases. Parosteal osteogenic sarcoma is described as "an unusual type of primary malignant densely ossified tumor of bone arising and proliferating roentgenographic characteristics are the encircling, dense, lobular and juxtacortical nature of the growth, the failure of the lesion to destroy the cortex, the heterogeneity of ossification and the failure to produce periosteal elevation. The presence of a thin free space between tumor and cortex is often seen with the proper degree of obliquity of the view."

Differentiation from myositis ossificans, osteochondroma parosteal ivory osteoma, sclerosing osteogenic sarcoma, ossifying hematoma and exhuberant callus must be made.

A few cases have been reported of multiple osteogenic tumors of this sort occurring simultaneously. It is possible that they may represent bone metastases by secondary spread of such tumors to bone. This is likewise very infrequent, (Ackerman).

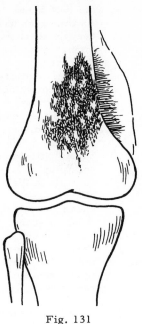

Fig. 131

CHONDROMYXO (PERIOSTEAL) SARCOMA (Fig. 131). This is a tumor showing similar radiation of spicules of bone extending outward from the periosteum and ending free in the tissues. The amount of new bone produced is much less, however, and there is greater infiltration of the tumor into the cortex and medulla causing osteolysis of the bone rather than osteosclerosis. Microscopically the tumor is seen to be composed largely of cartilage cells undergoing myxomatous degeneration with very few elements of new bone production. These tumors likewise are very rapidly growing and very fatal, metastasizing freely to other structures.

MEDULLARY CANAL

OSTEOLYTIC SARCOMA—RAPIDLY GROWING* (Fig. 132A). Sarcomas arising from the medullary canal are either rapidly growing or slowly growing in character. Rapidly growing osteolytic sarcomas of bone cause some pain and disability. Microscopically they are composed of spindle cells and abortive osteoblasts. Originating in the medullary canal, their growth is so rapid that they literally sweep the cortical bone before them as their growth proceeds, giving no time for expansion of the bone or even for bone atrophy.

Roentgenographically they present a central area of destruction in the shaft, usually near the end of a long bone, with one side of the cortex swept away as the tumor advances to invade the soft parts. There is no periosteal reaction or other indication of new bone formation.

These tumors are very malignant and few individuals suffering from them are ever saved by amputation or any other procedure.

The Bone Registry does not recognize this type of osteolytic lesion as a separate bone tumor entity but feels that the cell type is essentially the same as in bone producing types of sarcoma and that the osteolytic characteristics are produced by conditions of growth and environment. What ever the reason it certainly gives different roentgen characteristics.

OSTEOLYTIC SARCOMA—SLOW-GROWING* (Fig. 132B). Slower-growing osteolytic sarcoma originating centrally produces much the same picture as the rapidly growing type with the following exceptions:

1. that the slow-growing character of the tumor permits expansion of the cortex, and

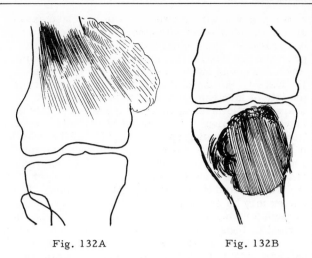

Fig. 132A   Fig. 132B

2. the cortex is not broken through until later in the course of the disease and then never in such a sweeping manner. There is little if any periosteal reaction.

Microscopically these tumors are of abortive osteoblasts and spindle cells. Their appearance is similar to other slow-growing benign lesions of bone such as cyst, chondroma, giant-cell tumor, and great difficulty may be experienced in their differentiation. Precious time may therefore be lost; in any doubtful case a biopsy should be taken.

GIANT-CELL SARCOMA—MALIGNANT DEGENERATION. Some authors have experienced malignant changes and metastatic involvement in giant-cell growths which they ascribe to a malignant development in these growths. Geschickter and Copeland feel that this is apt to occur in a giant-cell tumor after improper treatment with the development of true osteogenic sarcoma.

CHONDROBLASTIC SARCOMA. This is a tumor of medullary origin characterized by a rounded area of bone destruction occurring in the cancellous end of the bone near the site of former epiphyseal line. Expansion of the bone may or may not be present indicating the rapidity of growth of the tumor. If the cortex is eroded through there may be some periosteal bone formation.

Microscopically these tumors are composed of young cartilage cells although some giant cells are found near the margin.

Of this group giant-cell tumor, chondroblastic sarcoma and myeloma are the only ones showing any evidence of benefit by X-ray treatment. In most instances the growth can be checked, in some instances actual regression occurs. Radical surgery is not ordinarily necessary for relief of giant-cell tumor. X-ray treatment is ordinarily all that is necessary for giant-cell tumor, but for chondroblastic sarcoma surgery should be the method of choice.

MYELOMA* (Fig. 132C). A myeloma is a tumor arising from the various cellular elements of the bone marrow; large and small lymphocytes, granular leuko-

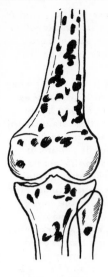

Fig. 132C

cytes and nucleated red cells. The recognized types of myeloma (Ewing) are:

1. Plasma cell myeloma;
2. Myelocytoma, derived from granular leukocytes;
3. Lymphocytoma, derived from lymphocytes;
4. Erythroblastoma, derived from nucleated red cells.

This condition may be present for a long time without manifestation of tumor masses in the bone, indeed recent work would indicate that only a small percentage of these cases (10 to 15 per cent) ever show roentgen evidence of bone destruction from tumors. In such cases reliance must be placed therefore upon sternal puncture for diagnosis. The presence of Bence-Jones protein in the urine confirms the diagnosis when found but unfortunately these bodies are present in only a small percentage of cases; hyperglobulinemia is frequently present. Bence-Jones protein is only present in 65% of all instances.

Tumor masses, when present, may appear simultaneously over widespread areas throughout the bony structures suggesting the possibility of multiple origin "multiple myeloma" or a single larger tumor may be the only indication of initial involvement, (Blum).

Roentgenographically the multiple type of myeloma presents numerous rounded areas of destruction in the bone, varying from a few millimeters to a centimeter in diameter having a smooth almost punched-out appearance. There is ordinarily no periosteal reaction and the bone is rarely weakened enough to cause spontaneous fracture. They usually cause widespread involvement of the skull, spine, ribs, pelvis and long bones. The bones of the hands may also be involved. The multiple small punched-out areas produced in the skull produce an appearance which is almost characteristic. In the spine especially the cancellous bone structure may take on an appearance of coarse accentuation of trabeculae. An unusual case has been reported, (Krainin, et al.) showing radiating type of bone formation throughout the entire shaft.

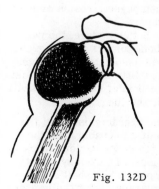

The disease usually occurs in young adults but rare cases have been reported in children. The roentgenological manifestations are very similar in the long bone lesions but in the vertebrae the destructive process is so great that the vertebral bodies become almost completely flattened, (Jansson). Atypical forms

Fig. 132D

of myeloma may occur in which larger solitary tumor masses appear in one or more bones; these cannot be differentiated by roentgen examination alone from other types of solitary osteolytic tumor such as that shown in Fig. 132D.

RETICULUM CELL SARCOMA (Fig. 132D) when fully developed may give the picture of a solitary expanding central growth near the end of a long bone; the roentgen picture does not differ at this stage from any other type of slow growing central tumor. It is rounded or ovoid in the beginning when it occurs in the ends, and fusiform when it occurs in the shafts of long bones. As it progresses it grows between the trabecular structure up and down the shafts producing a mottled irregular shaggy appearance of the bone; there is only slight periosteal reaction. It may involve the soft parts; the tumor may be bulky and there may be great pain. This form of tumor has proved very sensitive to radiation therapy, (Sherman and Snyder). Instances in which this type of tumor originated in the skull have been reported by Strange and de Lorimier. A study of 33 cases has been undertaken by Wilson and Pugh.

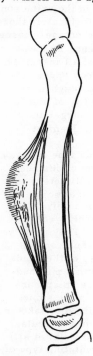

Fig. 133

EWING'S ENDOTHELIOMA;
(Diffuse Endothelioma of Bone; endothelial myeloma) (Fig. 133). It is now recognized by most observers that Ewing's tumor is a definite entity. There are still some who maintain that histologically it cannot be differentiated from reticulo-sarcoma of bone, (Magnus and Wood). Clinical signs and behavior however serve to differentiate between the growths.

This is essentially a disease of childhood, over half of the cases occurring before twenty years of age. In a series of 111 cases only 5 occurred beyond 30 years of age, (Sherman and Soong).

The long bones are most frequently involved, approximately 50%, but the small bones of the foot and flat bones of the pelvis and skull are also frequently involved. The midportion of the shaft is most frequently involved although there may be involvement of the metaphyseal resion or even the epiphysis.

Clinically the onset is not as severe, the pain is not as great as in other bone tumors and the growth is not as rapid. There may be associated fever giving the impression of an osteomyelitic involvement. Metastases may occur to distant points, such as the skull or other bony structures, or the lungs.

Roentgenologically, the characteristics of the tumor vary somewhat depending probably upon the influence of the bony structure of the various locations in which the tumor arises. There may be diffuse involvement of a large part of the shaft of the bone. The marrow space enlarges giving the impres-

sion more of a diffuse swelling than localized expansion of the shaft seen with other slow-growing tumors of endosteal origin. Bone absorption from central pressure and destruction may progress to the point where barely an outline remains of the bony cortex. Periosteal reaction of the parallel type occurs over the site of involvement and often shows a rather characteristic layer upon layer appearance "like the layers of an onion". The amount of periosteal reaction varies depending upon the rapidity of the growth; it is especially pronounced after radiation therapy and may give an appearance suggestive of sclerosis of the shaft. Periosteal bone formation is never of the trabeculated type seen in giant-cell tumor. The cortex may be perforated and the tumor may break through forming a bulky mass in the soft tissues; the periosteal bone may appear to end free in the tissues.

A few instances have been recorded where patients with tumors have survived a five-year period after radiation therapy alone or in combination with amputation or other treatment. Winham has reported a case of primary rib involvement with metastases to the lung with ten-year survival.

NON-OSSIFYING PERIOSTEAL FIBROSARCOMA. A well recognized type of osteogenic tumor arising from the outer fibrous layer of the periosteum. Since this periosteal layer is not concerned with bone formation these tumors do not show periosteal new bone. The designation of these tumors by the Registry as Periosteal Sarcoma (1d) is apt to cause confusion among radiologists who reserve this unqualified term for tumors associated with radiating periosteal new bone formation. The bony structure remains intact and does not show destruction. The tumor mass closely connected with the bone can be palpated in soft parts; it may, by pressure, leave its imprint upon the bone or may even displace adjacent bones by its growth. It may metastasize to other bones or to the lungs; very few individuals suffering with this condition are ever saved even by radical amputation.

Ewing, describes these tumors as being, " of spindle cell structure, showing varying grades of malignancy, absence of bone production, peculiar metastatic tendencies, presenting such notable specific features as to require recognition as a separate type of bone sarcoma. The origin from the outer layer of the periosteum and preservation of the shaft, serve to distinguish it roentgenographically from the distructive forms of bone tumors."

There is a remarkable predelection of the tumor to produce multiple metastases in the periosteum of many other bones, a feature rather exclusively enjoyed by this process and suggesting peculiar physiological properties.

EXTRAOSSEOUS OSTEOGENIC SARCOMA. A very rare type of osteogenic tumor which arises in the soft parts from remnants of bone-forming tissues remaining from the developmental period. They are characterized by dense, irregular masses of bony tissue occurring in the soft parts well apart from the normal bony structure; they appear to start from numerous foci simultaneously. They are very rapidly growing, metastasizing to the regional lymph nodes and to the liver and spleen. About 60% of osteoid extraosseous deposits are malignant. X-ray therapy has only palliative effect.

ADAMANTINOMA (AMELOBLASTOMA). Adamantinomata occur principally in the mandible. Occasionally however such tumors are found in the shafts of long bones especially the tibia. Here, as in the mandible, they tend to remain localized showing indication of their malignancy only in their tendency to recur if not completely removed. Morgan and Mackenzie have reported a case in which metastasis to a rib occurred 22 years after amputation of the leg for the primary growth in the tibia.

Five-Year Survivals after Treatment of Malignant Bone Tumors. It is generally accepted that high amputation is the treatment of choice. Even this method holds scant hope of survival. Coley and Harrold have analyzed 59 cases of osteogenic sarcoma with five-year survival, principally after amputation. X-ray therapy does not seem to be curative; however, there can be no doubt of its palliative value in relief of pain by checking growth, and prolongation of life. There are indications that intensive preoperative x-ray therapy to produce a stage of quiescence in tumor growth, followed by amputation, holds greater hope of ultimate cure than immediate operation without x-ray therapy. Some instances of survival have occurred following local resection only. Tudway has concluded therefore that:

1. Deep x-ray therapy in high dosage followed by local resection should be given serious trial especially;
   a) in the upper limb
   b) in the group with atypical clinical or radiographic signs or histology; resembling that of inflammatory lesions
   c) with grade I histology
   d) in the young
2. Deep x-ray therapy followed by amputation should be used for osteogenic sarcoma if;
   a) local resection would leave a lower limb more unsuitable than an artificial leg,
   b) response to x-ray therapy is poor
3. Deep x-ray therapy alone should be used:
   a) if the patient is unsuitable for or refuses operation, and,
   b) palliatively if, metastases are present or the tumor is too advanced or the patient is not fit for radical treatment
4. Amputation alone should be used, palliatively for pain or fungation, when x-ray therapy has failed to relieve or is not obtainable,
5. Biopsy and histological grading must be performed in every case. A histological diagnosis is most important
6. Records of every case should be sent and discussed by a group with special experience in tumors.

EXPLORATION OF MALIGNANT GROWTHS. Such a large percentage of malignant tumors of bone are fatal, no matter what type of therapy is instituted, that there can be little likelihood of rendering this prognosis less favorable by exploration and biopsy. This should be done in every case before radical operation is undertaken; if little can be accomplished toward cure of malignancy, surely no harm should be done by unnecessary mutilating operations.

Numerous instances have been pointed out where bone lesions, thought to be malignant, might have been needlessly subjected to amputation, (Brailsford). If amputation is decided upon, it will have a greater opportunity for success if it is performed in the quiescent period after x-ray therapy during the stage of suspension of active growth.

Furthermore, reliance upon a single roentgenogram or upon the opinion of a single radiologist is hazardous in any instance. The same may be said concerning the interpretation of the microscopic section; only pathologists well trained in bone pathology are competent to make the final decision. Holt assembled a group of unusual tumors in infants and children which illustrate the difficulty in roentgen diagnosis in many cases.

METASTATIC TUMORS OF BONE

METASTATIC SARCOMA. Secondary sarcomatous growths, metastatic in bone usually take on the characteristics of the primary growth. They usually produce destructive lesions without bone reaction or repair.

METASTATIC CARCINOMA IN BONE. Carcinomatous metastases in bone are of two varieties: osteoblastic and osteoclastic.

OSTEOBLASTIC CARCINOMATOUS METASTASES* (Fig. 134A) show definite rounded cotton-ball-like areas of bone condensation throughout the bony structure especially in the cancellous areas. These may become confluent producing a chalky white sclerotic appearance of the bone. In the vertebral bodies and bones of the pelvis this appearance often cannot be differentiated from Paget's Disease.

They are most frequently found as secondary

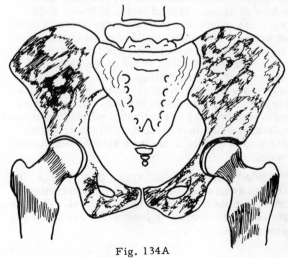

Fig. 134A

growths from the denser types of cancer, such as scirrhus carcinoma, especially carcinoma of the prostate.

OSTEOCLASTIC CARCINOMATOUS METASTASES* (Fig. 134B), as its name implies, shows multiple destructive lesions throughout the bones without expansion or periosteal reaction. They usually follow the softer adenomatous types of carcinoma especially carcinoma of the breast, and therefore occur more frequently in women.

Rare cases have been noted where heterotopic ossification occurred in an area of metastatic carcinoma of the rectum. Ossification of such soft part metastases for ordinarily soft or osteoclastic types of carcinoma is difficult to understand. (Senturia, et al).

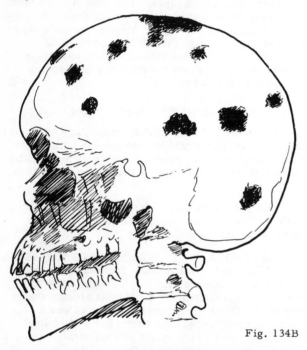

Fig. 134B

BONE METASTASES FROM HYPERNEPHROMA. Metastatic lesions from hypernephroma may produce an unusual type of lesion in bone. Such tumors are osteolytic, forming large areas of bone destruction within the medullary canal of a long bone, and osteoblastic as well, due to thickening of the bone trabeculae. The edges of the destroyed areas are not sharply defined but show irregular margins due to infiltration of the trabeculae which extends to the very edge of the bony cortex. Thickened septa give rise to an internal pattern made up of loculations which may pulsate. The tumor grows rapidly so that little if any bone atrophy has time to develop.

BONE METASTASES FROM HEPATOMA. Primary hepatomas are very rare; bone metastases from such tumors are even more unusual. They form bulky osteolytic tumors in bone which are in no way characteristic.

Roentgen study of 33 patients with histologically proved melanoma metastasizing to bone were found to have the following characteristics, (Selby, et al.):

The roentgen appearance of bone metastases from melanoma is not specific, but they are usually osteolytic, oval in shape, medullary in location and show cortical destruction. A few of the metastases in this series presented unusual features of sclerosis and a bulky soft tissue mass.

Melanoma metastases are more likely to occur in flat bones. In somewhat less than half of the cases observed there was a soft tissue component.

BONE METASTASES FROM NEUROBLASTOMA (SYMPATHETICOBLASTOMA). These rather rare tumors may arise wherever sympathetic nerve tissue exists; they are most frequently encountered in the adrenal medulla in children under five years of age. As a rule the primary growth is suspected only after metastases are found. These have a predilection for the liver and for the skull and long bones, but they may occur in the chest and other locations also.

Metastatic bone lesions from neuroblastoma produce small, ill-defined areas of cortical destruction in the ends of the long bones, in the diaphysis usually without periosteal reaction, which have as a distinguishing feature their symmetrical distribution, for instance, the lower ends of both femurs, and upper ends of the humeri which are the most common site of involvement. If the periosteum is stripped up by tumor growth of either the parallel or radiating type may develop. If this disease is widespread then this symmetrical distribution is not such a striking feature; spine or pelvis may be involved. Skull involvement shows a granular blotchy appearance with cyst-like bumps in the cranial bones; there is usually an increase in intracranial pressure from a layer of tumor tissue between the brain and the skull bones; this causes wide separation of the sutures without convolutional atrophy, a point in differentiation of this type of tumor. This is not a point of absolute differentiation, however, since certain granulomatous lesions, such as eosinophilic granuloma, may produce the same lesion. Spinal involvement, destruction of vertebral body with collapse, widening of the disc, paravertebral extension of the process resembling paraspinal abscess such as that seen in connection with tuberculosis of the spine, are the principal manifestations of the disease.

An abdominal tumor may be present from involvement of the adrenal or liver; such tumors may be associated with calcification.

Study of forty cases at the Boston Children's Hospital has shown that the hopeless prognosis usually given is not justified; roentgen therapy may result in regression or even cure, (Wyatt and Farber). A more recent study by Sherman and Leaming based on 34 cases reveals a wide variety of bone involvement.

BONE CHANGES IN MALIGNANT LYMPHOMA (Coles and Schulz). The following classification of Malignant Lymphomata is offered by Jackson and Parker:

Reticulum cell sarcoma
Lymphosarcoma
Hodgkin's granuloma
Hodgkin's sarcoma
Giant follicular lymphoma
Thirteen percent of these conditions show bone involvement.

Reticulum Cell Sarcoma may be primary in bone or it may present secondary lesions (see Primary Tumors of Bone for characteristics of Reticulum Cell Sarcoma).

The secondary lymphomatous lesions of the others may show similar lesions.

Bone Lesions of Hodgkin's Disease. There is certain similarity between the bone manifestations of Hodgkin's Disease and those of metastatic malignancy. Thus in the manner of spread to the bones either condition may be by direct lymphatic extension or by the blood stream. The commonest sites in either condition are in bones having a rich blood supply. The bones most frequently involved are the vertebrae, pelvis, femur and sternum. Any of the other bones may be involved, however.

Only rarely are the bones involved in Hodgkin's Disease. Pain may or may not precede bone involvement; it may be of dull aching or severe lancinating type. It is produced either by invasion of nerve trunk or direct invasion of the bone. Bone involvement occurs late in the disease and usually indicates terminal stage.

PATHOLOGICAL AND RADIOLOGICAL MANIFESTATIONS. There is nothing characteristic roentgenographically in the bone lesions which might be considered as pathognomonic of malignant lymphoma. The lesions are either destructive or productive or both; cartilage is not involved and the joint is not invaded. In the long bones, the involved portion is usually near the proximal end. The condition may progress to involve the entire bone. Skull roentgenograms reveal both osteoblastic and osteoclastic reactions, the latter predominating with the areas of destruction surrounded by zones of increased density of varying degrees.

The lesions have been classified into four groups:
1. Osteoclastic
2. Osteoblastic
3. Combined
4. Indifferent

The changes represented by the first three types are self-evident; the fourth type is discerned only with the nicroscope. In the indifferent type the bone marrow is replaced by lymphogranulomatous material without sufficient change to produce roentgen findings.

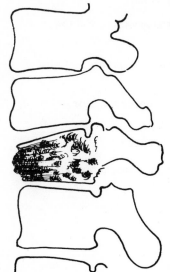

Fig. 135

It will be noted that these exclude leukemias and the disease which is termed paragranuloma by Jackson and Parker.

TUMORS IN SPECIAL LOCATIONS

EFFECT OF SOFT PART TUMORS ON BONE.
Soft part tumors, regardless of their nature, may cause pressure atrophy or destruction if in close proximity to the bone. This is especially true if the tumor mass pulsates, such as an aneurysm.

Aortic aneurysms produce pressure destruction of the anterior vertebral margins, eroding first the less dense cancellous bone, followed later by the dense plates of cortical bone which form the upper and lower margins of the vertebrae. Aneurysm of the interosseous vessels in the leg causes pressure erosion and shaggy periosteal proliferation which may even be mistaken for periosteal new growth; usually both bones bear evidence of the reaction.

Pressure of a soft part sarcoma or a nonossifying periosteal sarcoma arising from the nonosteogenetic layer of the periosteum may cause similar erosion of the adjacent bone. Slight periosteal reaction within the area of involvement from vascular and lymphatic stasis may serve to confuse the picture.

Nerve tissue nodules which occur in neurofibromatosis cause pressure erosion wherever they come into close proximity with the bone, such as the notching of ribs caused by development of such nodules along the intercostal nerves.

Glomus tumor of the neurovascular organs at the ends of the fingers give rise, through constant pressure, to scalloped-out pressure defects on the sides of the terminal phalanges, (Schulz).

TUMORS OF THE SKULL. Tumors arising in the skull both benign and malignant are very rare. The most frquent benign tumor arising from the cranial bones is the osteoma. These present dense rounded bony structures from 1/2 cm. to 9 or 10 cm. in diameter. These may spring from the bone at any place, either growing outward producing unsightly deformity of the skull, or inward into the cranial cavity. It is surprising what size these intracranial osteomata can attain with relatively little symptom. The most frequent location is within an accessory nasal sinus, usually the frontal sinus. When they occur in this location unless they interfere with drainage, they cause little trouble, (see nasal sinuses). Other rarer tumors are osteochondroma, giant-cell tumor, fibroma, angioma, dermoid cyst and teratoma.

Malignant tumors arising in the skull may be of any type found in long bones and present similar roentgen findings. Those having special characteristics are considered in relationship with the most important structures which they involve or are associated with; such as meningioma, osteogenic sarcoma, fibrosarcoma and chloroma.

CHORDOMA; DUMBBELL TUMOR. By reason of its origin in the spinal cord, and tumors which originate within the spine finding egress through the vertebral foramina, so called dumbbell tumors affect the bony structure merely by pressure erosion and will be considered under spinal lesions (q.v.).

Tumors of the Jaw

The most important tumors of this region are taken up in connection with the teeth.

QUESTIONS ON TUMORS OF BONE

Questions marked with a dagger deal with rare and less-important conditions.

1. Do any benign tumors arise from the periosteum?

2. Do any malignant tumors arise from the cortex?

3. What is the nature of tumors arising from the medullary canal, malignant or benign?

4. Name three common benign tumors arising from the cortex and give the roentgen characteristics of each.

†5. What is meant by diaphyseal aclasia (multiple exostoses) and in what respect do these tumors differ from ordinary osteoma?

6. Name five types of benign tumors arising from the medullary canal and give their roentgen characteristics.

7. What are the characteristics of bone cyst, giant-cell tumor and enchondroma chondroblastoma and how may they be differentiated?

†8. What are the characteristics of angioma of bone? Where do such lesions occur most commonly?

9. Of what types must all primary osteogenic tumors be? Can carcinoma be primary in bone? What is meant by a bone aneurysm?

10. What are the roentgen characteristics of ossifying periosteal sarcoma? Of chondromyxo-sarcoma of the periosteum? Can the nonossifying variety be detected roentgenographically?

11. What are the roentgen manifestations of Ewing's endothelial myeloma of bone? Is it a radiosensitive tumor?

12. Describe briefly the roentgen findings in (medullary) osteolytic sarcoma; chondroblastic sarcoma. How do the rapidly growing and slow-growing varieties differ roentgenographically?

†13. What are the characteristics of multiple myeloma? Are Bence-Jones bodies always found in the urine in association with such tumors?

14. What are the usual characteristics of secondary tumors in bone? What are neuroblastoma and what is peculiarly characteristic of their metastatic lesions in bone?

15. What two types of secondary carcinomatous lesions are recognized in bone and describe their characteristic appearances?

16. What bone changes sometimes occur with lymphatic leukemia and Hodgkin's disease?

17. What procedure would you always carry out before undertaking or recommending radical operation in any questionable tumor of bone?

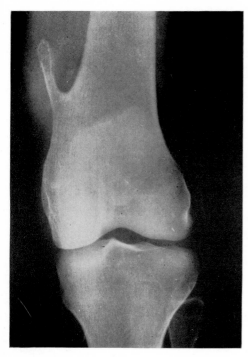

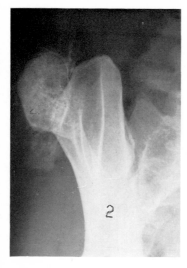

Osteoma of crest of ilium, an unusual location.

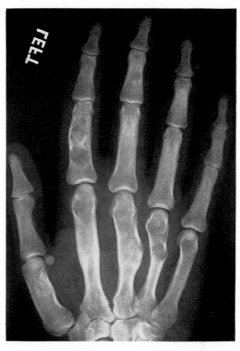

Osteoma of the lower end of the femur showing rounded peg-like upward projection of the growth. Osteomas are characterized by continuation of the bony texture out into the new growth. A cauliflower-like end of the growth is indication of associated cartilaginous content.

Multiple enchondromata involving the smaller bones of the hand. Note the areas of destruction and expansion of the shafts of the bones.

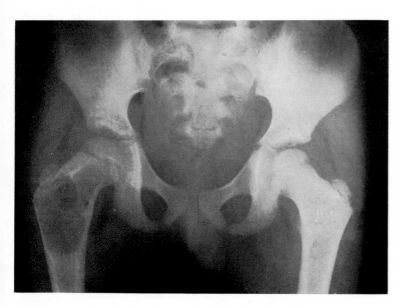

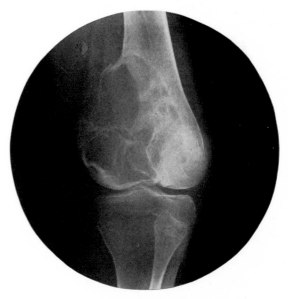

Benign cyst involving the neck of the femur. Note the area of destruction and the symmetrical expansion of the shaft of the bone.

Giant cell tumor of the lower end of the femur showing a large rarefied area in the bone with partitions of bony structure known as trabeculation.

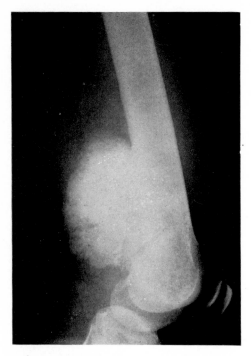

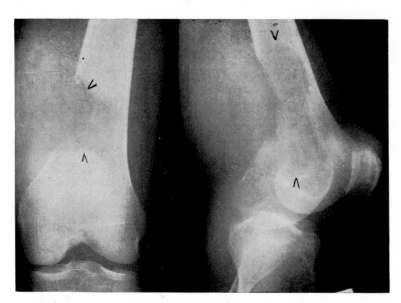

Rapidly growing endosteal sarcoma causing rapid destruction of the cortex without bone expansion.

Osteogenic sarcoma showing the finger-like projections of bone extending outward from the cortex and sub-periosteal layer. This radiating type of bone proliferation is almost always due to malignant new growth.

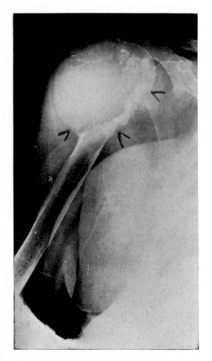

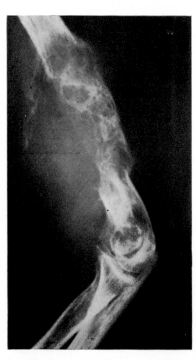

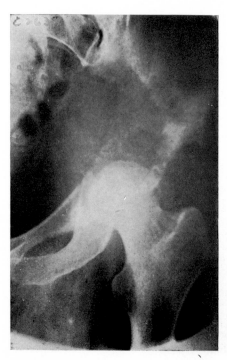

Slow-growing endosteal sarcoma showing expansion of the bone as the tumor increases in size.

Small round cell sarcoma showing the laying down of new bone formation after X-ray treatment.

Rapidly growing endosteal sarcoma practically destroying the acetabulum.

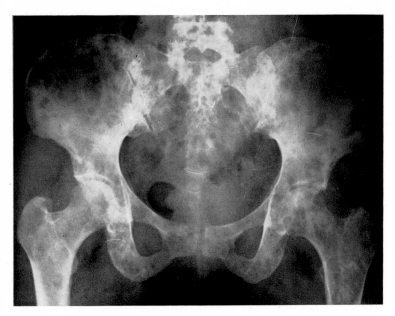

Osteoclastic carcinoma, secondary to a carcinoma of the breast, showing multiple areas of destruction throughout the bones of the pelvis.

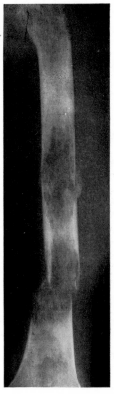

→ Metastatic carcinomatous involvement of the femur showing multiple irregular areas of bone destruction with a pathological fracture. Malignant tumors rarely metastasize below the elbows and knees.

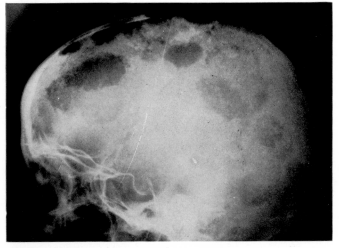

Numerous areas of bone destruction from secondary carcinomatous involvement.

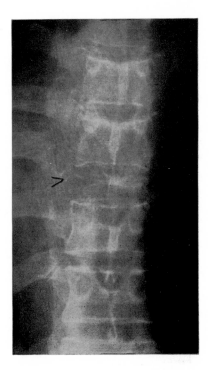

→ Metastatic carcinoma of the spine showing complete destruction of the body of a vertebra without attacking the adjacent cartilaginous structures. Only a small plate of bone remains.

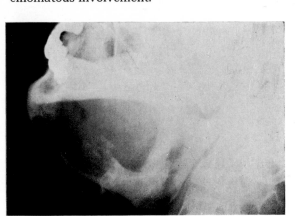

Carcinoma of the mandible from extension of a carcinoma of the tongue. Note the areas of bone destruction and lack of periosteal reaction.

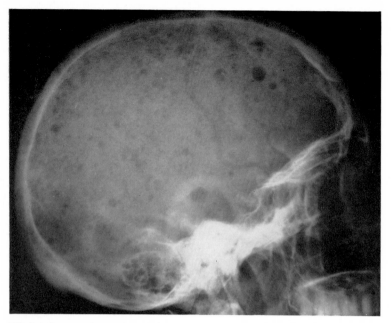

Multiple myeloma involving skull, showing numerous punched-out areas of destruction characteristic of the condition.

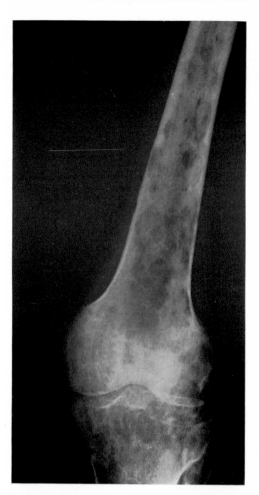

Multiple myeloma involving the femur and structures below the knee. Numerous rounded well-defined areas of destruction are seen in the cancellous structures without expansion of the bone or periosteal reaction. The areas involved extend to all of the bones in the body even below the elbows and knees.

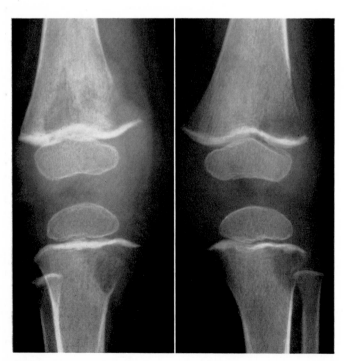

Sympathetic neuroblastoma showing symmetrical metastases in lower ends of both femurs. This is the only tumor of childhood which metastasizes in this manner.

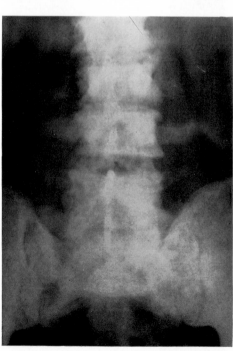

Osteoblastic carcinoma involving the spine and adjacent pelvic structure secondary to carcinoma of the prostate. Note similarity in appearance to Paget's Disease.

ARTHRITIS

ARTHRITIS AND PERIARTICULAR CONDITIONS (Chapter XIV)

ACUTE ARTHRITIS
ACUTE SYNOVITIS
TRANSIENT SYNOVITIS OF HIP JOINT IN CHILDREN

A. Acute Infectious Arthritis of Proved Etiology.

    1. Acute Polyarticular Rheumatism.

    2. Acute Syphilitic Arthritis

    3. Acute Pyogenic Infective Arthritis

        a. Staphylococcus

        b. Streptococcus

        c. Gonococcus

        d. Pneumococcus, etc.

    4. Tuberculous Arthritis

B. Traumatic Arthritis

C. Gouty Arthritis

    1. Differentiation from:

        a. Rheumatoid Arthritis

        b. Calcinosis circumscripta - chalk "gout"

        c. Sarcoid

CHRONIC ARTHRITIS

(Any of the forms described under acute arthritis may be prolonged into a chronic state)

D. Rheumatoid (Atrophic) arthritis, (Probably infectious arthritis, etiology unknown)

    Synonyms: (Proliferative)
                (Infective)
                (Arthritis Deformans)

    1. Still's Disease

    2. Felty's Disease

    3. Psoriasis

    4. Arthritis Mutilans

    5. Ankylosing Spondylitis - Marie Strumpell, etc.

E. Degenerative (Hypertrophic) Osteoarthritis (Metabolic Arthritis)

    1. Malum Coxae Senilis

F. Hypertrophic Pulmonary Osteoarthropathy
   Chronic Idiopathic Hypertrophic Osteoarthopathy

G. Neurotrophic Arthritis - Charcot

H. Arthritis Associated with other Constitutional Conditions

   1. Sarcoid

   2. Hemopoietic Arthritis

   3. Ochronotic Arthritis

   4. Caission Disease - Fibrocystic Arthritis

I. Unusual Types of Arthritis associated with local lesions.

   1. Arthritis Sicca

   2. Arthritis associated with Intrapelvic Protrusion of the Acetabulum—Otto Pelvis.

   3. Osteochondromatosis

   4. Coxa magna following synovitis of hip

   5. Primary Neoplasms of the joint (cyst xanthoma; hemangioma; giant cell tumor; synovioma; synovial sarcoma; pigmented villonodular synovitis)

Chapter XIV

ARTHRITIS

ACUTE SYNOVITIS

TRANSIENT SYNOVITIS OF THE HIP JOINT IN CHILDREN. This condition is characterized by sudden onset with pain in hip usually without cause or x-ray findings in the bony structures, (Edwards). Close observation will usually disclose the swollen appearance of the muscles surrounding the hip joint, the ileopsoas, obturator internus and gluteus minimus muscles, forming an enlarged baggy mass about the joint. There is no disturbance of the joint itself or of the bony structures and the condition soon subsides and returns to normal. It is probably due to oedema and swelling from allergic reaction, exposure to cold or possibly trauma.

ACUTE ARTHRITIS

Through the efforts of a Committee of the American Rheumatism Association the subject of arthritis has been reviewed and considerably clarified, (Primer of Arthritis, revised edition, 1942, published by the American Medical Association). The report points out that, "roughly speaking the great majority of the cases of arthritis fall into one or another of five groups:

1. the frankly infectious cases, caused by specific micro-organisms,

2. cases that are probably infectious but of unproved etiology,

3. the degenerative forms of joint disease, which are often spoken of as arthroses,

4. arthritis resulting from physical injury to the joint by trauma,

5. gouty arthritis."

For purposes of roentgen consideration they have been rearranged somewhat; acute rheumatic fever has been included under Infectious Arthritis of known etiology, and Traumatic Arthritis has been advanced to a position before Degenerative Arthritis. In so doing it has been found that the entire classification of Arthritis can readily be separated into Acute and Chronic types without further alteration. While such a change does not interfere with the clinical classification, it aids materially in the roentgen consideration of these conditions.

A. INFECTIOUS ARTHRITIS OF PROVED ETIOLOGY. This includes all cases of arthritis caused by specific organisms. Different types of infection result in various manifestations depending upon the type of organism.

1. ACUTE POLYARTICULAR RHEUMATISM. From the clinical manifestations of the disease its infectious character has been partially established. It is pretty well accepted that it is due to constitutional infection with some strain of streptococcus or virus infection. Strictly speaking, it should not be considered in this classification until the actual etiological agent has been identified but it is such a distinct entity that it was thought best to include it in this group.

In acute polyarticular rheumatism the site of involvement is almost entirely periarticular, the joint surface itself being relatively uninvolved. Clinically the disease is attended by pronounced constitutional reaction—chills, fever, prostration and evidence of severe local involvement of the joints. There is redness, swelling and extreme pain. Numerous joints are involved and there is a tendency to jump from one joint to another.

Roentgenographically there is no demonstrable change in the structures of the joint. The articular cortex is smooth, the cartilage still remains intact as indicated by the space between the ends of the bones, and there is no evidence of periosteal reaction on either side of the joint. The joint itself is not damaged and when the disease process subsides it

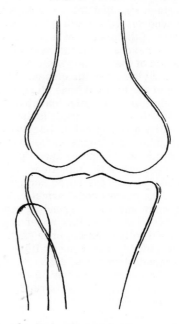

Fig. 136

returns to normal without impairment of function.

2. ACUTE SYPHILITIC ARTHRITIS (Fig. 136).

Acute syphilitic arthritis, for instance, resembles acute polyarticular rheumatism so closely that they often cannot be differentiated without roentgeno-graphic examination. Acute syphilitic arthritis, likewise, has its greatest evidence of involvement in the periarticular structures; the joint surface itself is not involved. The one distinguishing feature is periosteal reaction, usually of the paral-lel type, seen running along the shaft of the bone on either side of the joint. Syphilis is the great bone producer; periosteal new bone formation is the type of bone production present in this syphi-litic lesion. In this case also the joint itself is relatively free from involvement and when the process subsides there is no permanent damage. This is now a rare type of arthritic involvement, seen more frequently in the days when syphilis was at its unrestrained height. Prompt recognition and cure of syphilis by antibiotics has almost completely eliminated this form of the disease.

3. ACUTE PYOGENIC INFECTIVE ARTHRITIS*

(Fig. 137). Arthritis caused by pus-producing or-ganisms presents much the same picture regardless of the type of organism producing the infection. Three, more or less distinct, stages can be recog-nized through which the process of joint infection passes if the infection is unchecked.

1. Swelling of the joint from periarticular ede-ma and increase in fluid. This is often a very tran-sitory stage, showing no change in the bony struc-ture. If the amount of fluid is extreme this can be recognized roentgenographically by the bulging of the joint capsule and even in certain locations such as the knee joint, by the separation of the joint sur-faces. This stage may last for a few days or weeks, or the clear synovial fluid may rapidly change to pus. Distention of the joint may be so extreme that it results in spontaneous dislocation of the joint.

2. Erosion of the cartilage followed by destruc-tion of the underlying articular cortex. This process of destruction of the cortical bone often makes its initial appearance near the joint margins, at the site of tendinous attachments, as small isolated areas of decreased density and cortical disintegration. Or, the entire articular cortex may undergo simultaneous complete destruction, depending upon the site of in-oculation and severity of the infection.

3. Replacement of destroyed portions of the cartilage and bone by new bone formation with varying degrees of ankylosis depending upon the amount of destruction. Cartilage never regenerates except to a very limited degree; once destroyed it can only be replaced by new bone or fibrous tis-sue. In all pyogenic infections, destroyed cartilage is replaced by new bone formation; in contradis-tinction, tuberculous destruction is repaired by fi-brous tissue formation.

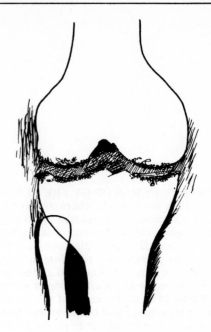

Fig. 137

Young infants, within the first few years of life, are subject to an extremely virulent involve-ment by pyogenic arthritis of the hip joints. The disease may be so rapid and the swelling so severe that spontaneous dislocation of the hip joints may result.

Pyogenic arthritis may present varying de-grees of virulence common to the organism pro-ducing the infection. For instance, staphylococcus infection tends to remain localized to the joint while streptococcus arthritis may spread to the ad-jacent bones, producing osteomyelitis, depending upon the severity of the infection. The gonococcus is notorious for its rapid destruction of cartilage and subsequent ankylosing deformities. Gonorrheal infections seem to have a predilection for certain locations: the under surface of the patella, for instance, causing destruction of the cartilage in this location; the plantar surface of the calcaneous at the attachment of the plantar fascia, causing spur formation, etc.

Gonorrheal arthritis does not always cause such extreme destruction, however; it may be that the toxic condition gives rise to arthritis in some cases without actual local infection with gonorrheal organisms.

Pneumococcus arthritis is usually part of a general systemic infection with this organism.

Typhoid fever occasionally produces an ar-thritic condition usually limited to one or two vertebrae with narrowing of the disc and sclerosis of the vertebral body and pronounced hypertrophic outgrowths of bone.

The advent of chemotherapy has vastly changed the outlook in acute types of pyogenic

---

*An asterisk following any title indicates that roentgenographic reproductions illustrating this condition will be found in the pictorial supplement at the end of the chapter.

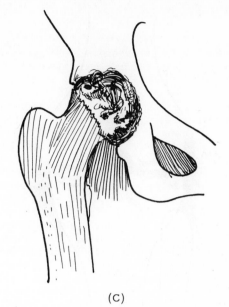

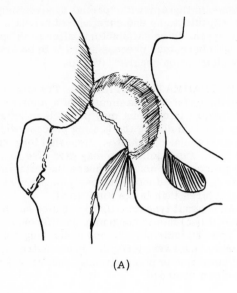

(A)

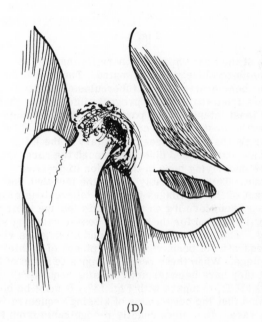

(C)

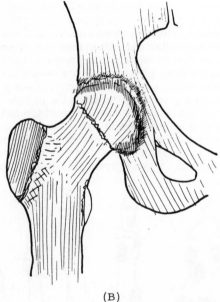

(B)

(D)

Fig. 138

arthritis. In many instances, injection of Penicillin directly into the joint after aspiration of pus changes the course of the disease.

TUBERCULOUS ARTHRITIS* (Fig. 138A, B, C, D). Tuberculous arthritis, on the other hand, is a much more protracted process. Whereas pyogenic arthritis requires days and weeks, tuberculous arthritis lasts for months and years. In this case also the progress of the infection may be followed through a number of stages.

1. (Fig. 138A) First there is a stage of hyperaemia of the joint, causing a hazy appearance of the joint structures. During this period there is pain, muscle spasm and interference with nor-

mal function. This stage may continue for many weeks providing a basis upon which the next stage develops.

2. (Fig. 138B) Bone atrophy, with loss of lime salts, develops from disuse. The pathologic process is so slow and insidious that bone atrophy results before bone destruction develops. This is one of the characteristic differences between the tuberculous and pyogenic types of arthritis.

3. (Fig. 138C) Finally, after months, there is the stage of destruction of cartilage and bone. Destruction of the cartilage is indicated by the gradual narrowing of the space between the ends of the bones; the destruction of cartilage removes the natural structures which normally hold the

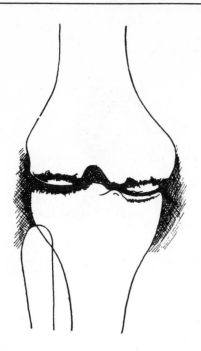

Fig. 138E

ends of the bones apart and permits them to become more closely approximated. The character of the bone destruction in tuberculous arthritis differs from that seen in pyogenic infection in that it is least intense in the portions of the joint subjected to most intimate contact. In pyogenic arthritis the process seems to start at the joint surface and proceed directly through the cartilage to the underlying bone in the region of greatest contact. This is probably due to the fact that the contact of the cartilages prevents tuberculous granulations from forming on these parts leaving their destructive action for the adjacent less-contacting surfaces. The bone is undermined and often gives rise to sequestra of bone, covered by pieces of viable cartilage. When these occur on opposite sides of the joint they have been termed "Kissing Sequestra" (Fig. 138E), compare with Fig. 137. It must be borne in mind that the occurrence of kissing sequestra is very rare, often more readily recognizable from the pathological specimen than in the roentgenogram.

4. (Fig. 138D) Lastly, there is the stage of repair which always requires years for its completion. Bone and cartilage destroyed by tuberculous infection are replaced largely by fibrous tissue formation. This, of course, is invisible in the roentgenogram, leaving only the shaggy irregular appearance of the injured bone.

Any of these forms of arthritis involvement may occur at any age period. Tuberculous arthritis, however, is more prone to occur in childhood, although it is sometimes seen in adult life. Pyogenic involvement is most common in late childhood and early adult life.

In recent years, antibiotic therapy has permitted operative procedures otherwise not possible.

Streptomycin therapy with "partial synovectomy, partial capsulectomy and curettage of necrotic foci in bone appear to be satisfactory; after such operations the tuberculous process appears to be arrested and recalcification occurs", (Wilkinson).

B. TRAUMATIC ARTHRITIS. Trauma alone may be the cause of inflammation of a joint. A fracture extending into a joint may produce an inflammatory reaction during the healing process which is known as traumatic arthritis. Repeated long-continued trauma to a joint also may give rise to an arthritic process. In many instances the inflammatory process is centered more intensely in the periarticular structures than in the joint itself.

An unusual type of arthritic change has been reported (Rose) due to congenital indifference to pain. The articular surface and underlying cortex of an ankle underwent irregular bone destruction from lack of sensation to pain. Gradual recovery occurred as sensation returned.

C. GOUTY ARTHRITIS* (Fig. 139). Gout primarily affects the periarticular tissues, usually involving the smaller joints, such as the toes. In the early stages it is rarely diagnosable roentgenologically. Later, after repeated attacks, urate deposits in the periarticular and subcutaneous structures and joints give rise to an arthritic process. Gout comes on in paroxysms, with intermittent periods of relief during which there is clinical return of the joint to normal. In any instance in which the pain is of this character, especially where the great toe is the site of involvement, gout should be seriously considered. After repeated attacks the sodium urate deposits may produce such trauma to the joint that hypertrophic changes result. When fully established the roentgen

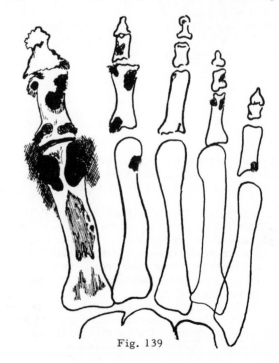

Fig. 139

picture is quite characteristic; the transparent urate deposits appear as well-defined, rounded, punched-out areas of erosion near the joint margins. The rounded punched-out areas which occur near the phalangeal joints in rheumatoid arthritis may resemble gouty deposits.

The phalangeal lesions of sarcoid often resemble gout. They appear as rounded, punched-out areas at the joint margins but usually extend into the cancellous bone, showing pressure absorption and coarsening of the trabecular structures.

Hypercholesteremic xanthomata of the tendons occur in the extremities presenting rounded masses often more than a centimeter in diameter, which by pressure causes notch-like resorption of the bone especially of the phalanges, (March, et al.). The bony lesions may resemble gout.

Lyford and Shapiro have reported a case in which gout caused a similar area of bone replacement in the patella.

When large, especially when present on the articular margins of the knee joint they may be due to pressure from meniscus ganglia, (Albert).

CHALKY "GOUT". This is a condition in which rounded subcutaneous nodules appear near the terminal phalangeal joints of the fingers, causing redness, swelling and intense pain. The redness and swelling may so strongly suggest infection that surgical incision is carried out. In reality this condition is not related in any way to gout; the close resemblance of the cutaneous nodules to tophi is undoubtedly the cause of this mistake. Roentgen examination at once discloses the heavy calcium content of these nodules, differentiating them from tophi which are deposits of urate crystals which are radiolucent.

CHRONIC ARTHRITIS

Any of the acute types of arthritis may be prolonged into the chronic stage. Excluding these types where the etiology is fairly well understood, there still remains a large number, the origin of which is rather obscure. These fall into two large groups, the Rheumatoid (Atrophic) and Degenerative (Hypertrophic) Osteoarthrosis. Description of these under many other names has given rise to much confusion. A Committee of the American Rheumatism Association, after due consideration, decided upon the above-named classification; the recommendations outlined in their "Primer on Arthritis" will be briefly referred to with pertinent quotations:

"Nichols and Richardson showed that all chronic joint disease is due either to proliferative changes beginning in the synovial membrane or to degenerative changes originating in the joint cartilage." These changes are most manifest in the two great divisions of chronic arthritis.

D. RHEUMATOID (ATROPHIC) ARTHRITIS* (Figs. 140 and 141) has been described under many titles:

Proliferative,
Infective,
Arthritis Deformans.

Regardless of the name, the pathology is the same.

In Rheumatoid (Atrophic) Arthritis (Figs. 140 and 141) the most characteristic pathological changes are found in:

1. The synovial membrane.

"Early in the disease, excessive proliferation of the synovial cells causes thickening of the synovial lining. It appears edematous and is grayish or pinkish red. The number and size of the villi are greatly increased. At this stage of the disease the synovial fluid content is increased."

These being soft tissue changes are not demonstrable in the roentgenogram. At this stage no change can be detected.

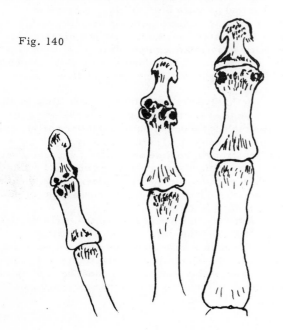

Fig. 140

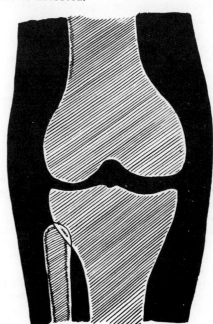

Fig. 141

2. The articular cartilage.

The articular cartilage does not show appreciable changes early in the course of the disease. "As the disease progresses, the changes in the articular cartilage become more obvious. It appears grayish white, is softer and may contain larger ulcerations. If the proliferation of the synovial lining tissue continues, it will eventually extend on to the articular cartilage and may envelop it completely. When the opposing articular cartilages are both enveloped with such inflammatory granulation tissue (pannus), fibrous tissue ankylosis is apt to occur. The advancing pannus not only smothers the underlying cartilage, it actually invades it. Such invasion may be so extensive as to destroy completely the articular cartilage and bony ankylosis may follow."

"Small areas of atrophic bone destruction often referred to as punched-out areas, are a prominent feature of rheumatoid arthritis and must be considered in the differential diagnosis with gouty arthritis."

Destruction of the joint cartilage is manifested roentgenographically by the narrowing of the inter-articular space; the two ends of the bones seem to get closer together.

Osteoporosis is an early manifestation of the disease, probably due to loss of function from pain; there is no periosteal reaction, but irregular proliferation of bone may occur in connection with the punched-out areas of bone destruction as a reparative process, giving the appearance of associated hypertrophic arthritis. Indeed, mixed types of arthritis are possible.

3. The articular ends of the bones.

"The proliferative connective tissue seen in the subchondral marrow spaces is the result of the invading pannus penetrating from the articular surface. Late in the disease the bony cortex of the adjoining bones is reduced in thickness, the trabeculae are fewer in number and the bone marrow is more vascular."

There is some periarticular swelling and increase in synovial fluid but these are not distinctive features. Roentgenographically this manifests itself as bone atrophy. The lesions seen at roentgenographic examination are essentially atrophic in character, atrophy of cartilage and bone—without any manifestation of bone production, other than the proliferative changes which occur in association with the punched-out areas of bone absorption.

When this disease occurs in young adults, it usually affects the larger joints; it may involve only a single joint or, it may affect almost all of the joints of the body—progressing from one to another. Its etiology is not known; focal infection may play a part.

"Fewer than one fourth of the patients 'recover', one half 'improve', or the disease becomes 'quiescent', and the remaining one fourth become progressively worse." When it affects adults, it is usually more chronic and is more likely to be confined to the small joints, especially of the hands. The clinical manifes-

tation and x-ray findings are so different in the two types of the disease that it seems possible that they may be due to different etiologies; yet the pathological picture is the same. The disease progresses, with acute exacerbations and long periods of quiescence. Roentgen therapy is of great aid in these acute stages of exacerbation. In recent years instances have been recorded where function was restored by operative insertion of a vitallum metal cup over the head of the femur, or a plastic prosthesis.

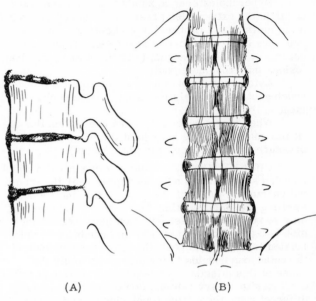

(A)   (B)

Fig. 142

MARIE STRUMPEL'S DISEASE (SPONDYLOSE RHIZOMELIQUE)—SPONDYLITIS OSSIFICANS LIGAMENTOSA (Fig. 142B). The Committee of the American Rheumatism Association has classified Marie-Strumpel's and Von Bechterew's Spondylitis as rheumatoid because of their close resemblance. Still's disease is due to similar arthritic manifestations in children. In addition Felty's disease and arthritis associated with psoriasis have been classified as atrophic. These forms of ankylosing spondylitis are thought by some observers to be separate entities.

In this type of arthritis the sacro-iliac joints are the site of first involvement. In the spine the disease is first manifested in the lower portion and progresses upward. There is usually rapid onset with prostration, confinement to bed, generally severe pain. The stiffness progresses rapidly and pathological changes involve the entire spine. In some cases, however, the onset may be insidious with local pain, the first manifestation.

Attention has been called to the early roentgen signs of sacro-iliac involvement, (Rolleston).

The adult sacro-iliac joint shows a dense margin of cortical bone; whereas, the adolescent joint does not show this dense margin and the joint space is wider. As the disease develops the margins of the joint become hazy and sclerotic. This is best seen at the upper margin of the sacrum.

Roentgenographically, the vertebrae show change in form with "squaring" of the anterior margin and there is generalized demineralization. The intervertebral discs are normal in size and remain intact and the paraspinal ligaments become ossified. In the antero-posterior view the appearance is that of a molten or "bamboo spine."

The costotransverse joints of the ribs and the apophyseal joints of the vertebrae become involved.

Marie-Strumpell's Disease differs from Bechterew's Disease in that in the former the onset is sudden and the course rapid, and the intervertebral spaces or discs remain normal in all cases; in the latter the condition is slowly progressive and the intervertebral discs are atrophied and there are calcified deposits.

The etiology of both diseases is unknown.

Roentgen therapy may be of great palliative value. Through its relief of pain it enables the individual to engage in greater freedom of motion and thus aids combating the ankylosing process (Baker, et al.).

A somewhat similar appearing vertebral ligamentous calcification bridging across segments of the vertebrae is probably due to a more or less physiological aging process; in this condition the sacroiliac joints appear free, in true Marie-Strumpell's disease the sacroiliac joints are the earliest portion to be involved, (Smith, et al.).

Rheumatoid (atrophic) arthritis of the apophyseal articulations of the spine has been described. Clinically the disease manifests itself by pain and progressive stiffening of the back very much like ankylosing spondylitis; in fact, it probably is a form of Marie-Strümpel's disease although at the outstart it may not have the same roentgen characteristics. It occurs in younger individuals and is very insidious but may progress very rapidly to involve the entire spine. Roentgenologically there is osteoporosis of the articular processes with thinning of the articular cartilages but the interarticular discs remain intact. There is no evidence of bone production. In the active stage roentgen therapy has been of some value.

ARTHRITIS MUTILANS. An unusual type of chronic arthritis has been described in which there is wasting of the heads of the metacarpal bones and phalanges with tapering and narrowing of the distal ends, together with widening of the bony structures at their bases. The joint spaces may be obliterated. As a result the bony structures become shortened and the fingers retract within a normal-sized skin, producing wrinkling of the skin. The fingers assume a "main en lorgnette" deformity. The reason for this unusual type of arthritic involvement is not clear, (Nielson and Snorrason).

ANKYLOSING SPONDYLITIS—VON BECHTEREW; MARIE STRUMPEL (Fig. 142A and B). Under this heading two conditions must be considered having somewhat similar characteristics and X-ray findings; Von Bechterew's spondylitis (A), and Marie-Strumpell disease (B).

VON BECHTEREW'S SPONDYLITIS (SPONDYLITIS DEFORMANS)—SPONDYLITIS MUSCULARIS—(Fig. 142A). In this condition there is a slowly progressive stiffing of the spinal column beginning in the cervical and thoracic regions and extending downward, associated with kyphosis. Accompanying signs of nerve involvement may occur such as hypotonia and atrophy of muscles of the back, and paralysis; diminished cutaneous sensations or psychic phenomena. Stiffness and pain preceding the joint ankylosis; other joints may be involved.

Roentgenologically there occurs dorsal kyphosis and narrowing of the vertebral bodies, atrophy of the intervertebral discs, with much deposit of calcium in the cartilages and ossification of the paraspinal ligaments. Knaggs feels that this type of spondylitis has its origin in muscularatony; that atrophy of the vertebral discs results, followed by ankylosis of the vertebral bodies from the resulting contact of the bony structures.

E. DEGENERATIVE (HYPERTROPHIC) OSTEOARTHROSIS.* (Fig. 143).

In Degenerative Hypertrophic Arthrosis the chief underlying pathological changes are found in:

1. The articular cartilage.

The articular cartilage becomes softened, undergoes fibrillation and splitting which is first evident at the margins. The process is extremely slow and insidious so that repair of the fibrillated cartilage by new bone formation takes place almost simultaneously. This is indicated in the roentgenogram by small spicules of new bone growing out from the joint margins; these are spoken of as exostoses (or osteophytes). As the disease progresses, the cartilage becomes somewhat thinner but it rarely completely disappears.

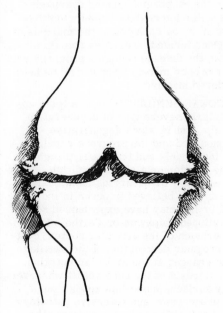

Fig. 143

2. The articular ends of the bones.

The bones retain their normal lime-salt content and bone atrophy does not occur. If there is much thinning of the cartilage, as is sometimes seen in the advanced stages, bone becomes closely applied to bone; whenever this occurs, eburnation results; eburnation of the ends of the bones produces ivorylike density of the bony structures. The articular cortex may become irregularly shaped and notched; exostosis formation may become so pronounced that ankylosis occurs from bridging of the joint by the bony outgrowths. If broken off from trauma they become loose bodies within the joint known as "joint mice." Occasionally, especially in well-advanced cases, small nodular areas are seen at the joint margins. Such fibrous nodules occurring near the small joints of the fingers are known as Heberden's nodes.

Little if any periarticular swelling occurs and the synovial membrane shows little change.

This condition is very common in late adult life. It rarely occurs before forty years of age, but is present to some degree in most people after fifty years of age. The spine is a favorite site of hypertrophic spondylitis and exostosis formation can be well seen at the joint margins of all of the vertebrae.

The cause is not definitely known but it seems most likely that it is a manifestation of the general wear and tear of life rather than a specific focal infection. Obesity, causing excessive trauma to the weight-bearing joints, or faulty posture may be a contributory cause. Heredity is probably also a factor. Lack of certain elements in the diet may be a cause.

Faulty elimination of waste products—constipation—may permit the harboring in the body of excessive amounts of toxic material. The regions most frequently involved are the spine, hips and knees, although all joints may be involved. When it involves the spine such exostoses usually cause little or no symptoms but they may attain considerable size, even encroaching upon and causing pressure on the spinal canal, or pressing upon the esophagus causing dysphasia.

Small triangular intercalary bone formations may occur between the osteophytes at the margins of the vertebrae. Once formed, exostoses remain forever; if untreated, the disease becomes progressively worse, but under proper management it may be held in check or rendered inactive.

MALUM COXAE SENILIS. This is a term applied to a particularly severe type of degenerative arthritis of the hip joint in which degenerative changes are pronounced and the progress rapid. It occurs in older individuals and trauma is thought to be a factor in the development of the condition, either immediately after injury or occurring insidiously many years after. It is believed to occur in individuals who in earlier life may have experienced some trauma such as slipped epiphysis or Perthe's Disease. There is erosion of the articular cortex, cystlike areas and irregular destruction of the cartilage and hypertrophic changes at the articular margins. Eburnation and sclerosis of the bone result wherever the denuded bony surfaces come into apposition. From the rapid progression and extensive pathology it is quite evident that there is some process other than ordinary hypertrophic arthritis; this is probably a loss of adequate nutrition from interference with the blood supply from trauma or senility. As the head of the bone undergoes destruction, it elongates causing deepening of the acetabulum which in turn causes restriction of abduction and adduction at the hip joint.

F. NEUROPATHIC ARTHROPATHY—CHARCOT (Fig. 144). Neurogenic conditions may give rise to rather grave arthritic disorders. Perhaps the best example of such a type of arthropathy is Charcot joint. This is a manifestation of trauma applied to an anesthetic joint. Syphilitic destruction of the sensory nerves is the greatest cause of development of this condition. It has been shown experimentally that resection of the posterior nerve roots in cats, followed by traumatization of a joint with thermocautery resulted in the prompt development of Charcot joint (Eloesser). Similar joint reaction has been described with diabetes mellitus, (Cozen; Bolen).

Bolen has pointed out that more recent investigation indicates their occurrence also in leprosy, peripheral nerve injury, pyogenic soft tissue infections following puncture wounds and other infections subject to trauma. The etiology of charcot joints from diabetes still remains controversial.

There are two general types of involvement, the hypertrophic or sclerotic, and the other, atrophic. In the hypertrophic type the primary process in the joint destruction is the development of a pannus of connective tissues and blood vessels which spreads over the joint surface, resulting in fibrous tissue invasion and destruction of the cartilage. Cortical bone becomes in contact with cortical bone resulting in dense sclerosis and eburnation. Efforts at repair only make the picture more confused; heavy outgrowths of bone from the joint margins form large osteophytes which may become broken off and add to the debris which surrounds the joint. In the atrophic form there is marked bone destruction without visible new bone production, and little if any actual osteophyte formation; the ends of the bones may be merely worn away, giving rise to a "drum stick" appearance. When it involves the spine the vertebral body may collapse and there may be calcium scattered in the immediate neighborhood. There may be a spindle-shaped appearance in the soft tissues, and it may be difficult to differentiate from tuberculosis of the spine.

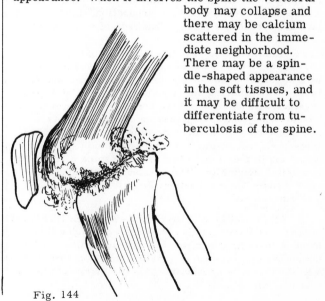

Fig. 144

Brittleness of the bones is an outstanding feature to which much of the debris about the joint can be ascribed, (Moller).

Clinically Charcot joint is characterized by an enlarged painless joint, waxy and spindle-shaped in appearance. Once the process starts, it progresses rapidly to an extreme degree of tissue destruction; often within a few months.

Roentgenologically the condition is manifested by:
1. Extreme disintegration of the joint, practically all identity of the joint structures being lost.
2. Deposit of a large amount of debris about the joint due to tissue destruction.
3. An ivorylike eburnation of the bone.

SYRINGOMYELIA. Similar involvement of the joints of the upper extremities occur in this condition; there is extensive fragmentation of the articular margins with gross disintegration of the joint; large amounts of periosteal new bone formation and dense sclerosis beneath the articular cortex. There is lack of osteoporosis since the joint is anaesthetic. The shoulder joint is by far the most frequent site of involvement. A case of this type has been reported, (Meyer, et al.) in which complete disruption and disintegration of the shoulder joint occurred in less than two and one-half months.

G. ARTHRITIS ASSOCIATED WITH OTHER CONSTITUTIONAL CONDITIONS.

1. BOECK'S SARCOID INVOLVING BONE (Fig. 145), (Holt and Owens). In patients suffering from sarcoid disease elsewhere in the body, deposits of sarcoid material in the tissue adjacent to the joint may result in deformity of the joint and replacement of the underlying bone by sarcoid material. Only about ten to fifteen per cent of patients with sarcoidosis show bone lesions.

Microscopically this material shows tubercles with epitheloid and giant cells much resembling tuberculosis; but guinea pig inoculation with sarcoid material fails to produce tuberculous disease. For this reason, cases have undoubtedly occurred in which sarcoid was mistaken for tuberculosis or even giant-cell tumor of bone on the basis of a false pathological report. This is a granulomatous process which invades the medullary cavity, causing lacunar absorption from pressure. Such pressure absorption leads finally to fragmentation and destruction of the finer trabeculae, causing apparent osteoporosis. Lacunar coalescence results in small localized cavities in the bone, rounded, ovoid, pear-shaped; either solitary or multiple.

Roentgenographically the lesions appear as rounded, clear-cut, punched-out areas near the joint margins, especially of the smaller joints of the hands and feet. They resemble the lesions produced by gout but show a smoother border. Sometimes they arise near the middle of the joint surface, extending by fingerlike projections into the joint. The bones may become deformed on account of disturbance in articular relationship from loss of bony structure and they may attain a reticular appearance from the coarsened trabecular structure. There is no evidence of bone production. There may be associated lung involvement, (p. 281).

The disease is rather insidious and should, because it occurs at, or in close relationship to joints, (Crissey and Day), be more properly considered as an unusual type of chronic arthritis.

2. CONSTITUTIONAL HEMATOPOIETIC ARTHRITIS. Certain constitutional and hematopoietic diseases may be associated with arthritic manifestations. For instance, in hemophilia, leukemia, etc., there is a pronounced tendency to spontaneous hemorrhage into joints and periarticular tissues. This may give rise to arthritic symptoms and signs. The roentgen picture varies greatly.
1) thinning of cartilage, subchondral cyst formation and spurs,
2) or gross deformity of ends of bones if hemorrhage occurs in growing stage of bone,
3) or a diffuse periarticular density corresponding to the synovial capsule probably from fibrosis. (See Blood Dyscrasias).

Large defects have been reported in the adjacent bony structures such as the wing of the ilium with irregular ossification in the fascia and connective tissue, (Petersen).

3. OCHRONOTIC ARTHRITIS—(ALKAPTONURIA). Alkaptonuria is an hereditary fault probably in phenol metabolism which may be associated with all grades of discoloration of the urine from brown to black. The urine may be discolored when passed or may turn dark on standing due to the alkaptone (hemogentisic acid) one of the products of deranged metabolism in the urine. About one-half of the cases of alkaptonuria are associated with ochronosis—the staining of skin (ears), sclera, articular cartilages, intervertebral discs, tendons, valves of heart and even of the bones with deep bluish-brown pigment.

An appreciable number of these cases develop pain, swelling and deformity of the joints, usually one or more large joints, or spine and numerous smaller

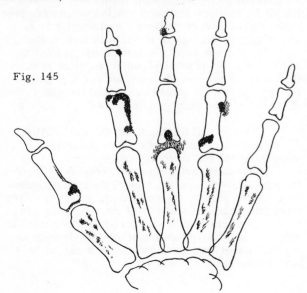

Fig. 145

joints of hands or feet; this is known as ochronotic arthritis.

Roentgenographically ochronotic arthritis shows as its most striking characteristic irregular calcified deposits in the bursae, tendons and cartilages of joints. When the spine is involved there is often universal calcification of all interarticular discs and spinal ligaments giving an appearance somewhat similar to Bechterew's spondylitis. There is pronounced osteoporosis giving rise to the appearance of large exostoses extending out from the joint margin, (Hertzberg),(Pomeranz, et al.), (Thompson).

4. FIBROCYSTIC DESTRUCTIVE ARTHRITIS FROM CAISSON DISEASE. Air emboli from Caisson disease occurring about the joint result in rounded fibrocystic areas of asceptic necrosis in the articular cortex of the bone with areas of sclerotic bone repair and erosion and destruction of the joint cartilage. The condition may not be distinctive in its joint manifestations at the outstart and the joint pains may be attributed to "rheumatism." Roentgenographic examination however, discloses the changes resulting from asceptic fibrocystic necrosis. A similar picture is produced by Malum Coxae Senilis.

H. UNUSUAL TYPES OF ARTHRITIS OR PERIARTHRITIS.

1. ARTHRITIS SICCA. Arthritis sicca is a peculiar type of dry arthritis which usually attacks the shoulder joint causing progressive erosions and destruction of the head of the humerus. It attacks young adults and its cause is not known although it has been attributed to tuberculosis.

2. ARTHRITIS associated with INTRAPELVIC PROTRUSION OF THE ACETABULUM (OTTO PELVIS). This is a condition in which the acetabular sockets of the hip joints protrude into the pelvis, giving rise to an arthritic condition. Only those cases in which the floor of the acetabulum touches or crosses the linea terminalis should be considered as intrapelvic protrusion. When the condition is encountered in young individuals it seems highly probable that it may be due to epiphysitis but this has never been absolutely proven. It occurs twice as often in females as in males and is frequently bilateral. Otto's original description of the condition was in an adult. Development of the condition in an adult is believed to be due to softening of the floor of the acetabulum from trauma or low-grade infection.

Three groups are recognized (Overgaard).
1) Secondary protrusion following a focal disease process—those in whom there is a definite history of previous illness.
2) Primary osteoarthritic protrusion associated with Arthritis Deformans, in which there is no focal disease, where the disease is limited to the acetabulum.
3) Juvenile osteo-asthenic protrusion in which there is a weakness of the bony tissue permitting protrusion possibly due to epiphysitis but this has never been proven.

3. OSTEOCHONDROMATOSIS. Cartilaginous fragments, broken off in early life, may remain in the joint giving rise in later life to multiple large calcified rosettelike structures floating loosely in the joint; this condition is known as chondromatosis. If such loose bodies interfere with function or produce pain, they must be removed (Mussey and Henderson).

4. COXA MAGNA (Ferguson,and Howorth). This is a condition which has been observed following a short period of synovitis of the hip. Clinically the condition starts with slight fever and enlargement of the inguinal nodes. The first symptom is limping and the extremity is held in a flexed, adducted position. With rest the symptoms subside promptly. Immobilization is continued for periods of 6 to 10 months and complete recovery occurs.

Roentgenologically the epiphysis for the femoral head enlarges during this period; there is no erosion or bone destruction, no periosteal reaction, merely enlargement of the femoral head. It is possible that the prolonged immobilization may have something to do with the condition.

5. ARTHRITIS OF LUSCHKA'S JOINTS OF THE CERVICAL SPINE may be considered as a definite entity not because of the type of arthritic involvement but primarily because of the location of the joints involved. Luschka's joints are small synovial structures in the cervical spine called hemiarthroses intervertebrales. They are located between the posterior and lateral aspects of the lower five cervical vertebrae. They are quite small measuring only a few millimeters in size but are so located that hypertrophic spurs at their joint margins intrude upon the spinal foramina causing pressure on the spinal nerves. They are best visualized in the lateral and oblique views of the cervical spine.

6. XANTHOGRANULOMATOUS DISEASE OF BONE WITH POLYARTHRITIS. This is a type of rheumatoid polyarthritis described by Golden and Richards, in which advanced cystic changes are present in the long bones showing histologically a xanthogranulomatous type of lesion with foam cells.

Roentgenologically enormous cystic swellings of the limbs are present resembling cystic areas in the bones. These may be confined to the periarticular regions or may extend throughout the entire shaft of the bone. The etiology is unknown.

7. PRIMARY NEOPLASMS OF THE JOINT. These may be of many types; Cyst; Xanthoma; Hemangioma; giant cell tumor synovioma.

Fortunately arthritis due to neoplasms involving the joint is very rare. In such cases the characteristics of the growth, its location and extent of involvement determine the severity of the symptoms and roentgenographic picture produced. If the growth itself does not destroy surrounding bony tissues, as primary synovioma, it is doubtful if it can be detected roentgenographically.

Differentiation of synovial sarcoma from benign pigmented villonodular synovitis as indicated by Lewis, is as follows:

1) If the nodular soft tissue masses are in part or wholly outside the joint capsule, the lesion is not villonodular synovitis but may be synovial sarcoma, fibrosarcoma or some other condition.

2) If the lobulated soft tissue masses in or near the joint contain scattered and irregular deposits of amorphous lime, the lesion is almost certainly a sarcoma. If the lesion of the soft tissues of the joint has invaded bone, the condition is probably synovial sarcoma.

Synovial sarcomas do not tend to metastasize (Knutsson). The most important differences between synovialoma and synovial fibrosarcoma according to Jonsson.

1) Synovialoma contain endothelium-lined cavities, formations which are lacking in synovial sarcoma (Bloom and Pattinson).

2) Synovialoma metastasize often, not to say regularly to the regional lymph glands. Synovial lymphosarcoma do not. Both types of tumor, on the other hand, metastasize to the lungs and other distant organs.

3) Synovialomas are often highly radiosensitive, synovial fibrosarcoma insignificantly so.

8. HYPERTROPHIC PULMONARY OSTEOARTHROPATHY—OSTEOPHYTOSIS—BAMBERGER-MARIE'S DISEASE (Fig. 146). This is a condition involving the bones and tissues of the hands and feet, which develops in association with chronic lung pathology such as suppuration, bronchiectasis or chronic lung abscess, or in association with carcinoma of the lung. This is thought to be due to anoxemia from impairment of normal lung function. Liver damage associated with chronic pulmonary disease is thought to be the cause.

ROENTGENOLOGICAL MANIFESTATIONS. The first manifestation of the process is in the enlargement of the soft parts at the ends of the fingers, resulting in so-called "club-fingers." On roentgenographic examination, the bones appear normal at this stage. As the condition becomes prolonged, the terminal phalanges become expanded at their tips and a generalized periostitis particularly along the shafts of the metacarpals and phalanges develops, which may be difficult to distinguish from that of lues. The little finger and thumb often show the first and greatest involvement. The shafts of the bones may not show any change until later, when they also show delicate lacy periosteal reaction much like the lacework type of periosteal reaction from syphilis. In very severe cases the process may cause heavy shaggy periostitis involving the shafts of all the long bones. Joints frequently are swollen, but the cartilage remains intact. The pulmonary lesion which gives rise to the periosteal reaction may be present for a long time without any manifestation of bone involvement when suddenly, without any apparent change in the pulmonary conditions the periosteal reaction develops. Once it starts it progresses rapidly.

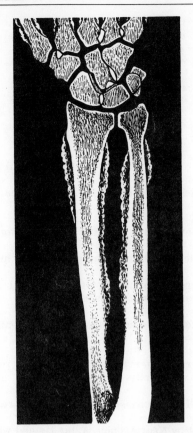

Fig. 146

An idiopathic form of this condition is recognized which is in no way related to the pulmonary hypertrophic osteoarthropathy associated with chronic lung suppuration and malignant lung involvement. It is an extremely rare condition in which no such etiological factors are present. Three of the twenty-five reported cases are in females.

It has its onset at puberty with pain which shows seasonal variations. There is enlargement of the extremities and clubbing of the fingers.

The long bones show uniform dense sclerosis and lacelike periosteal reaction very much like the ordinary variety of pulmonary osteoarthropathy. The skull is also involved. The face shows a leonine appearance and there is increased vascularity of the bones. The epiphyses are also involved. The phalanges are small and pointed. There is hyperchromic anemia, probably due to bone marrow encroachment. A number of unusually severe cases with pronounced periosteal proliferation and sclerosis of the shafts of the long bones have been reported (Temple and Jaspin). Wiles et al. have recently called attention to a rare but definite malacia of the joint cartilage of the patella which may be the precurser of osteoarthritis; it affects the soft parts first and during this stage does not show roentgen manifestations.

NERVE PRESSURE FROM SPINAL IMPINGEMENT. Luschka joints (Boreadis and Gershon-Cohen) are two small joint spaces on either side of the lower five cervical vertebrae, located between the lateral aspects of the lower five vertebral bodies adjacent to the annulus fibrosus of the intervertebral disc. Their importance has been stressed by many writers because of their close relationship to nerve and vascular structures.

The male process projects upward from the vertebra below into the female impressions of the vertebra above, anteromedially to the mixed nerve root and posteromedially to the vertebral artery vein and sympothetics as they pass through the vertebral foramen. Pressure on these structures by degenerative processes of the joints or hypertrophic exostoses may give very distressing symptoms from pressure of these structures.

QUESTIONS ON ARTHRITIS

Questions marked with a dagger deal with rare and less-important conditions.

1. Does trauma ever cause arthritic manifestation? Under what circumstance?

2. Does Polyarticular Rheumatism produce any manifestations in the roentgenogram? Why?

3. What are the roentgen manifestations of Acute Syphilitic Arthritis and how do they differ from those of Acute Polyarticular Rheumatism?

4. What are the clinical manifestations of Pyogenic Infective Arthritis and what roentgen signs does it produce?

5. What are the roentgen manifestations of Tuberculous Arthritis? Through what stages does it progress? What is arthritis sicca?

6. Describe briefly the changes seen in Gouty Arthritis and discuss their causes.

7. What is meant by Neurotrophic Arthritis and what are its roentgen characteristics?

†8. Describe involvement of bone by Sacroid. What joints does it usually involve?

†9. To what is arthritis, associated with hematopoietic diseases, due?

10. What two general forms of chronic arthritis are recognized by the American Committee for the Control of Rheumatism?

11. What are the roentgen characteristics of Atrophic Arthritis? Of spinal apophyseal joints?

12. What are the roentgen characteristics of Hypertrophic Arthritis?

13. Describe the roentgen characteristics of Ochronotic Arthritis and to what are they due?

14. What is meant by Malum coxae senilis and where does it usually occur? Arthritis from Caisson disease?

†15. Describe briefly the clinical manifestations and roentgen findings in Bechterew's spondylitis and Marie-Strumpell's disease.

†16. What arthritic changes occur as a result of Intrapelvic Protrusion of the Acetabulum (OTTO PELVIS)?

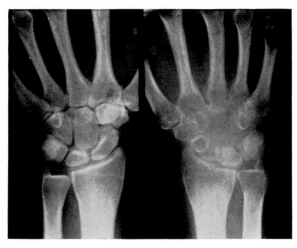

Infective arthritis showing complete disintegration of the joint cartilages of the right wrist joint. Compare with the clear-cut bony margins of the left wrist.

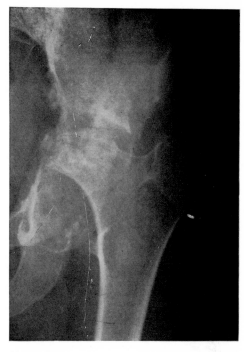

Tuberculous arthritis of the hip showing complete destruction of the head of the bone and of the adjacent acetabulum. Healing takes place by fibrous tissue production and not by new bone formation. There is several inches shortening.

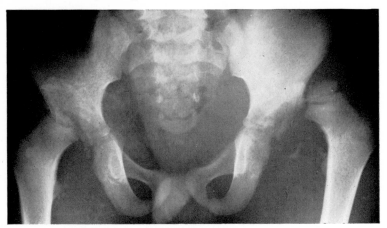

Bilateral spontaneous dislocation of hips from acute pyogenic arthritis.

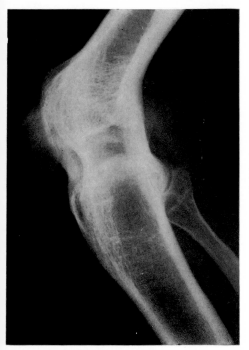

← Ankylosis of the knee joint from infective arthritis. The joint is bridged by solid bone formation.

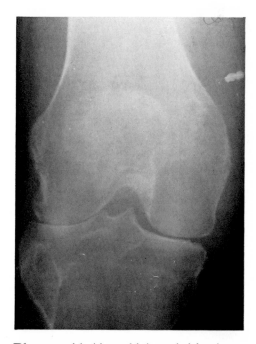

Rheumatoid (Atrophic) arthritis showing loss of lime salts, pencilled outline of bone, atrophy without bone production. There is destruction of articular cartilage as well.

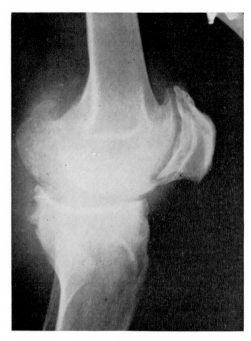

Hypertrophic arthritis of the knee show-ing heavy outgrowths of bone from the joint margins and tendinous attachments with some thinning of the cartilage. There is no loss of lime salts.

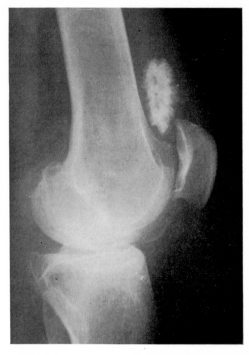

Osteochondromatosis; joint mouse due to calcification of a loose cartilaginous body within the joint usually occurring from injury during the developmental period of an individual.

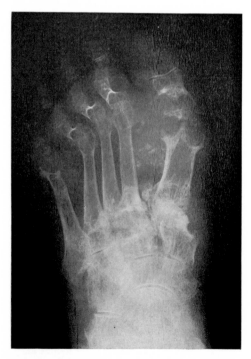

Gout, showing the characteristic punched-out areas of bone destruction at the joint margins produced by urate deposits.

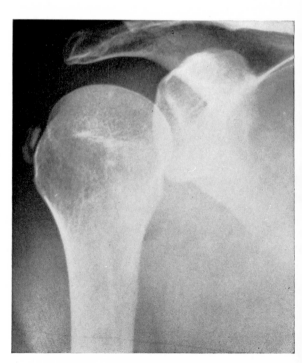

Calcareous deposit in the wall of the sub-deltoid bursa or supra-spinatus tendon.

REFERENCES FOR BONE PATHOLOGY

Fractures

Klinefelter, E. W., "The Influence of Position on the Measurement of the Projected Bone Angle," Am. J. Roentgenol., 55:722, June 1946.

Johnson, C. R., "The Measurement of the Deformity Alignment Accompanying Fracture," Radiol., 36:100, 1941.

National Bureau of Standards, Medical X-Ray Protection up to Two Million Volts, Ch. 11, Section 6, 1-d, 1949.

Gillespie, H. W., "The Significance of Minor Bone Injuries," Brit. J. Radiol., 19:173, 1946.

Jellinger, D. L., "Fracture of a Sesamoid Bone of the Thumb," Am. J. Roentgenol., 57:619, 1947.

Burman, M. S., Sinberg, S. E., Gersh, W., and Schmier, A. A., "Fractures of the Radial and Ulnar Axes," Am. J. Roentgenol., 51:455, 1944.

Sylwan, T., "Impression Fractures in the Caput Humeri in Connection with Electroshock," Acta Radiol., 32:455, 1949.

Lapidus, P. W., "Sesamoids Beneath All the Metatarsal Heads of Both Feet," J. Bone and Joint Surg., 22:1059, 1940.

Boehler, L., "Diagnosis, Pathology and Treatment of Fractures of the Os Calcis," J. Bone and Joint Surg., 13:75, 1931.

Piatt, A. D., "Fracture of the Promontory of the Calceneus," Radiol. 67:386, 1956.

Olson, Paul F., "The Treatment of Fractures of the Os Calcis," J. Bone and Joint Surg., 21:747, July 1939.

Wilson, G. E., "Fractures of the Calcaneus," J. Bone and Joint Surg., 32A:59, 1950.

Warrick, C. K., and Bremner, A. E., "Fractures of the Calcaneus," Brit. J. Radiol., 35B:33, 1953.

Hendelberg, T., "The Roentgenographic Examination of the Ankle Joint in Malleolar Fractures," Acta Radiol., 27:23, 1946.

Palmer, I., "Compression Fractures of the Lateral Tibial Condyle and Their Treatment," J. Bone and Joint Surg., 21:674, 1939.

Wilson, M., Michele, A. A., and Jacobson, E. W., "Isolated Fractures of the Lesser Trochanter," J. Bone and Joint Surg., 21:776, 1939.

Mussbichler, H., "Arterial Supply to the Head of the Femur," Acta Radiol., 46:532, 1956.

Burman, M., Grossman, S., Rosenak, S., "The Migration of a Fracture-transfixing pin from the Humerus into the Mediastinum," Am. J. Roentgenol., 76:1061, 1956.

Kremens, V., and Glauser, F., "Unusual Sequela Following Pinning of Medial Clavicular Fracture," Am. J. Roentgenol., 76:1066, 1956.

Terrafranca, R. J., Zellis, A., and Babyn, R., "Large Foreign Body Cyst with Migration of Smith-Peterson Nail," Am. J. Roentgenol., 76:1070, 1956.

Van Brunt, E. V., "A Method of Measuring the Femoral Neck in Surgical Treatment of Fractures of the Hip," Am. J. Roentgenol., 76:1163, 1956.

Davidson, W. D., "Determine of Alignment in Hip-Nailing Procedure," J. Indiana M. A., 35:461, 1942.

Capurro, R. G., and Pedemonte, P. V., "Hydatic Cysts of the Femur," J. Bone and Joint Surg., 35B:84, 1953.

Trueta, J., and Harrison, M. H. M., "The Normal Vascular Anatomy of the Femoral Head in Adult Man," J. Bone and Joint Surg., 35B:442, 1953.

Blockley, N. J., and Pruser, D. W., "Fractures of the Odontoid Process of the Axis," J. Bone and Joint Surg., 36B:794, 1956.

Jostes, F. A., "Fracture of the Acetabulum with Central Dislocation of the Head of the Femur," J. Bone and Joint Surg., 18:483, April 1936.

Roche, M. B., "Healing of Bilateral Fracture of the Parainterarticularis of a Lumbar Neural Arch.," J. Bone and Joint Surg., 32A:428, 1950.

Weinbren, M., "Value of Tomography in Examination of Fractured Vertebrae," Acta Radiol., Supp. 116:184, 1954.

McRae, D., "Asymptomatic Intervertebral Disc Protrusions," Acta Radiol., 46:9, 1956.

Lindbom, A., "The Roentgenographic Appearance of Injuries to the Intervertebral Disc," Acta Radiol., 45:129, 1956.

Milch, H., "Ischial Apophysiolysis: New Syndrome," Bull. Hosp. Joint Dis., 14:188, 1953.

Sv. A. Chrom., "On the Incidence of Osteochondrosis," Acta Radiol., 26:49, 1945.

Scott, W. G., "Low Back Pain Resulting from Arthritis and Subluxations of the Apophyseal Joints and Fractures of the Articular Facets of the Lumbar Spine," Am. J. Roentgenol., 48:491, 1942.

Gurdjian, E. S., Webster, J. E., and Lissner, H. R., "Observations on Prediction of Fracture Site in Head Injury," Radiol., 54:313, 1950; 60:226, 1953.

Danelius, G., "The Occasional Appearance of Both Inner and Outer Suture Lines in Roentgenograms of the Skull Simulating Fissure Fracture," Am. J. Roentgenol., 55:315, 1946.

Stewart, John, "Fractures of the Skull," J.A.M.A., 77:2030, Dec. 24, 1921.

Voris, H. C., Verbrugghen, A., and Hearns, J. J., "Head Injuries," J.A.M.A., 115:1765, 1940.

Garland, L. H., and Mattram, M. E., "Traumatic Pneumocephalus," Radiol., 44:237, Mar. 1945.

Stewart, Wm. H., Skull Fractures, Paul Hoeber, Pub., N. Y., 1925.

Ritvo, M., Roentgen Diagnosis of Diseases of the Skull, Paul Hoeber, Pub.

Glasser, M. A., and Shafer, F. P., "Skull and Brain Traumas; Their Sequelae," J.A.M.A., 98:271; Jan. 23, 1932.

Osmond, L. H., "Correlation of Disability with Roentgen Findings Head Injuries," Radiol., 41:1, July 1943.

Gross, R. J., "Roentgenological Aspects of Head Trauma," Am. J. Roentgenol., 64:399, 1950.

Childe, A. E., "Localized Thinning and Enlargement of the Cranium," Am. J. Roentgenol., 70:1, 1953.

Davidoff, L. M., and Dyke, C. G., "Relapsing Juvenile Chronic Subdural Hematoma," Bull. Neurol. Inst. of New York, 7:95, 1938.

Kelly, J. P., "Fractures Complicating Electro-convulsive Therapy and Chronic Epilepsy," J. Bone and Joint Surg., 36B:70, 1954.

Baker, C. D., Frank E. Lane, R.T., Everett L. Pirkey, "Roentgen Examination of Old and New Trauma of the Spine with the Ultrafine Focus Roentgen Tube," Am. J. Roentgenol., 75:144, 1956.

Keyes, D. C., and Compere, E. L., "The Normal and Pathological Physiology of the Nucleus Pulposus of the Intervertebral Disc," Am. J. Roentgenol., 31:568, 1934.

Gershon-Cohen, J., Budin, E., and Glauser, F., "Whiplash Fractures of the Cervicodorsal Spinous Processes: Resembling Shoveler's Fracture," J.A.M.A., 155:560, 1954.

Dislocations

Brewer, A. A., and Zink, A. C., "Unusual Intercarpal Dislocation," Radiol., 41:185, 1943.

Immermann, E. W., "Dislocation of the Pisiform," J. Bone and Joint Surg., 30A:489, 1948.

Burman, M., "Paradoxical Crossing of the Radius in Antero-Medial Dislocation of the Head of the Radius to Give Supination Contracture of the Forearm," Am. J. Roentgenol., 70:422, 1953.

Jacknow, A. S., and O'Connor, L. J., "Posterior Dislocation Humerus," A.M.A. Arch. Surg., 72:479.

Arden, G. P., "Posterior Dislocation of Both Shoulders," J. Bone and Joint Surg., 36B:558, 1956.

Solovay, J., "Posterior Oblique View in Dislocation of Hip," Am. J. Roentgenol., 72:1045, 1954.

Kovacs, A., "Subluxation and Deformation of the Cervical Apophyseal Joints," Acta Radiologica., 43:1, 1955.

O'Connor, Sylvester J., and Jacknow, A. S., "Posterior Dislocation of the Shoulder," A.M.A. Arch. Surg., 72:479, 1956.

Coutts, M. B., "Atlanto-epistropheal Subluxations," Arch. Surg., 29:297, 1934.

Fahey, J. J., Schlenker, L. T., and Stauffer, R., "Fracture Dislocation of the Ankle with Fixed Displacement of the Fibula Behind the Tibia," Am. J. Roentgenol., 76:1102, 1956.

Jacobson, G., and Adler, D. C., "Examination of the Atlanto-Axial Joint Following Injury," Am. J. Roentgenol., 76:1081, 1956.

Paul, L. W., and Moir, W. W., "Non-Pathologic Variations in Relationship of the Upper Cervical Vertebrae," Am. J. Roentgenol., 62:519, 1949.

Jacobson, G., and Adler, D. C., "An Evaluation of Lateral Atlanto-Axial Displacement in Injuries of the Cervical Spine," Radiol., 61:355, 1953.

Gianturco, C., "A Roentgen Analysis of the Motion of the Lower Lumbar Vertebrae in Normal Individuals and in Patients with Low Back Pain," Am. J. Roentgenol., 52:261, 1944.

Oberholze, R. J., "Arthropneumoroentgenograph (Bircher's Method)," Am. J. Roentgenol., 38:524, 1937.

Kleinberg, S., "Spondylolisthesis," J. Bone and Joint Surg., 16:441, 1934.

Ullmann, H. J., "A Diagnostic Line for Determining Subluxation of the Fifth Lumbar Vertebra," Radiol., 2:305, 1924.

Melamed, A., and Ansfield, D. J., "Posterior Displacement of the Lumbar Vertebrae," Am. J. Roentgenol., 58:307, 1947.

Gillespie, H. W., "Vertebral Retroposition (Reversed Spondylolisthesis)," Brit. J. Radiol., 24:193, 1951.

Garland, L. H., and Thomas, S. F., "Spondylolisthesis," Am. J. Roentgenol., 55:275, March 1946.

James, A., and Nisbet, N. W., "Posterior Intervertebral Fusion of the Lumbar Spine," J. Bone and Joint Surg., 35B:181, 1953.

Meyerding, H. W., "Low Backache and Sciatic Pain Associated with Spondylolisthesis and Protruded Intervertebral Disc," J. Bone and Joint Surg., 23:461, 1957.

Durbin, F. C., "Spondylolisthesis of the Cervical Spine," J. Bone and Joint Surg., 36B:734, 1956.

Epiphyses and Epiphyseal Separation

Habbe, J. E., "Patella Cubiti," Am. J. Roentgenol., 48:513, 1942.

McLearie, M., and Merson, R. D., "Injuries to the Lateral Condyle Epiphysis of the Humerus in Children," J. Bone and Joint Surg., 36B:84, 1954.

Baastrup, C. I., "Os Vesalianum Tarsi and Fracture of Tuberositas ossis Metatarsi V," Am. J. Roentgenol., 9:695, 1922.

Cleaves, E. N., "Adolescent Sacro-iliac Joint," Am. J. Roentgenol., 38:450, 1937.

Caffey, J., and Madell, S. H., "Ossification of the Pubic Bones at Birth," Radiol., 67:346, 1956.

Slayton, C. A., "Ischial Epiphysiolysis," Am. J. Roentgenol., 76:1161, 1956.

Rauber, A., and Kopsch (Kopsch, Dr. Fr.): Lehrbuch und Atlas der Anatomie des Menschen, Abteilung 2 Knochen-Baender, Vierzehnte Auflage, George Thieme Vertag. Leipzig, 1932.

Shipp, F. L., and Haggart, G. E., "Further Experience in the Management of Osteitis Condensans Ilii," J. Bone and Joint Surg., 32A:841, Oct. 1950.

Bailey, D. K., "The Normal Cervical Spine in Infants and Children," Radiol., 59:712, 1952.

Bailey, Wilbur, "Persistent Vertebral Process Epiphyses," Am. J. Roentgenol., 42:85, 1939.

Hadley, L. A., "Secondary Ossification Centers and the Intraarticular Ossicle," Am. J. Roentgenol., 76:1095, 1956.

Bick, E. M., and Copel, J. W., "Longitudinal Growth of the Human Vertebra," J. Bone and Joint Surg., 32A:803, Oct. 1950.

Wagoner, G., and Pendergrass, E. P., "Intrinsic Circulation of the Vertebral Body," Am. J. Roentgenol., 27:818, 1932.

Kelly, H. K., and Reynolds, L., "Appearance and Growth of Ossification Centers and Increases in the Body Dimensions of White and Negro Infants," Am. J. Roentgenol., 57:477, 1947.

Dedick, A. P., and Caffey, J., "Roentgen Findings on the Skull and Chest in 1030 Infants," Radiol., 61:13, 1953.

Engelbach, Wm., and McMahon, Alphonse, "Epiphyses," Bull. Assoc. for Study of Inter. Secretions, Vol. VIII, No. 1, P. 1045, Jan. 1924.

Todd, T. W., Atlas of Skeletal Maturation, C. V. Mosby, Co., Pub., St. Louis, 1937.

Editorial, "Pseudo-Epiphyses in Hand and Foot," Am. J. Roentgenol., 70:149, 1953.

Bancroft, F. W., and Murray, Clay Ray, Surgical Treatment of the Motor-Skeletal System," J. B. Lippincott Co., Pub.

Gill, G. G., and Abbott, L. C., "Practical Method of Predicting the Growth of the Femur and Tibia in the Child," Arch. Surg., 45:286, 1942.

Frantz, C. H., "Extreme Retardation of Epiphyseal Growth from Roentgen Irradiation," Radiol., 55:720, 1950.

Langenskiold, A., "Growth Disturbance Appearing 10 Years after Roentgen Ray Injuries," Acta Chir. Scandinav., 105:350, 1953.

Phemister, D. B., "Fractures of the Neck of the Femur, Dislocations of the Hip, and Obscure Vascular Disturbances Producing Aseptic Necrosis of the Head of the Femur," Surg., Gynec. and Obst., 59:415, 1934.

Other Effects of Trauma

Santozki, M., and Kopelmann, S. A., "A Contribution to the So-Called Malacia of the Os Lunatum and Os Naviculare," Abstract, Am. J. Roentgenol., 22:383, 1929.

Crooks, F., and Birkett, A. N., "Fractures and Dislocations of the Cervical Spine," Brit. J. Surg., 31:252, 1944.

Kaplan, C. J., "Cervical Hyperextension Injuries with Paraplegia," J. Bone and Joint Surg., 35B:97, 1953.

Berkin, C. R., and Hirson, C., "Hyperextension Injury of the Neck with Paraplegia," J. Bone and Joint Surg., 36B:57, 1954.

Taylor, A. R., "The Mechanism of Injury to the Spinal Cord in the Neck Without Damage to the Vertebral Column," J. Bone and Joint Surg., 33B:543, 1951.

Vinson, H. A., and Schatzki, R., "Roentgenologic Bone Changes Encountered in Frostbite, Korea, 1950-51," Radiology, 63:685, 1954.

Schneider, R. C., Cherry, G. and Pantek, H., "Syndrome of Acute Central Cervical Spinal Cord Injury," J. Neurosurg., 11:546, 1954.

Slaughter, D. P., "Radiation Osteitis and Fractures Following Irradiation," Am. J. Roentgenol., 48:201, 1942.

Pearl, F. L., "Electric Shock," Arch. Surg., 27:227, 1933.

Jellinek, S., "Changes in Electrically Injured Bones," Brit. J. Radiol., 31:23, 1926.

Editorial, "Bone Changes in Electric Current Injuries," Am. J. Roentgenol., 54:525, 1945.

Jaffe, R. H., "Electropathology," Arch. Path., 5:837, 1928.

Morgan, P. W., "Osteochondritis Dissecans of the Supratrochlar Septum," Radiol., 60:241, 1953.

Hutchinson, R. G., "Osteochondritis Dissecans—Unusual Cases," Brit. J. Radiol., 16:147, 1943.

Panner, H. J., "A Peculiar Characteristic Metatarsal Disease," Acta Radiol., 1:319, 1922.

Klein, A., Joplin, R. J., Reidy, J. A. and Hanelin, J., "Roentgenological Features of Slipped Capital Femoral Epiphysis," Am. J. Roentgenol., 66:361, 1951.

Plewes, J. W., "Sudeck's Atrophy in the Hand," J. Bone and Joint Surg., 36B:195, 1956.

Jaffe, H. L., "Bone Rarefaction After Trauma to Large Joint Regions Without Fracture," Radiol., 33:305, 1939.

Caffey, J., "Multiple Fractures in the Long Bones of Infants Suffering from Chronic Subdural Hematoma," Am. J. Roentgenol., 56:162, 1946.

Jungman, A., "Spontaneous Fracture of the Femur in an Infant with a Large Occipital Meningocele," Radiol., 61:231, 1953.

Gilbert, R., and Voluter, G., "Contribution a L'Etude Radiologique des Modifications Osseuses et cutanées concomitantes dans la Region des Jambes," Acta Radiol., 29:403, 1948.

Spurling, R. G.,and Bradford, F. K., "Scalenus Neurocirculatory Compression," Ann. Surg., 107:708, 1938.

Ingersoll, C. F., "Ice Skater's Fracture," Am. J. Roentgenol., 50:469, 1943.

Burrows, H. J., "Fatigue Infraction of the Middle of the Tibia in Ballet Dancers," J. Bone and Joint Surg., 36B:83, 1956.

Devas, M. B., and Sweetnam, R., "Stress Fractures of the Fibula," J. Bone and Joint Surg., 36B:818, 1956.

Bontiglio, M., "The Pathology of Fracture of the Femoral Neck Following Irradiation," Am. J. Roentgenol., 70:449, 1953.

Stephenson, W. H., and Cohen, B., "Post-Irradiation Fractures of the Neck of the Femur," J. Bone and Joint Surg., 36B:830, 1956.

Gondos, B., "Observations on Periarthritis Calcarea," Am. J. Roentgenol., 77:93, 1957.

Howes, W. E., and Alicandri, B. B., "A Method of Radiologic Examination of the Shoulder," Radiol., 50:569, 1948.

Whitcomb, W. P., "Bones-Excavation of Humeral Head by Calcareous Deposits of Supraspinatus Tendinitis," Radiol., 66:237, 1956.

Peacher, W. G., and Storrs, R. P., "Cervical Disc Calcifications in Childhood," Radiol., 67:396, 1956.

Bunje, H., and Cole, W. R., "Calcification of Articular Cartilage," J. Bone and Joint Surg., 36B:874, 1956.

Burnett, C. H., Commons, R. R., Albright, F. and Howard, J. E., "Hypercalcemia Without Hypercalcuria or Hypophosphatemia, Calcinosis and Renal Insufficiency; Syndrome Following Prolonged Intake of Milk and Alkali," New England J. Med., 240:787, 1949.

Poppel, M. H., and Zeitel, B. E., "Roentgen Manifestations of Milk Drinker's Syndrome," Radiol., 67:195, 1956.

Norley, T., and Bick, W. H., "Calcification of the Bursae of the Knee," J. Bone and Joint Surg., 31A:417, 1949.

Riebel, F. A., and Praver, L. L., "Osteoma Cutis," Am. J. Roentgenol., 78:73, 1957.

Holt, J. F., "The Ehlers-Danlos Syndrome," Am. J. Roentgenol., 55:420, 1946.

Katz, I., and Steiner, K., "Ehlers-Danlos Syndrome with Ectopic Bone Formation," Radiol., 65:352, 1955.

Herstone, S. T., and Bower, J., "Werner's Syndrome," Am. J. Roentgenol., 51:639, 1944.

Miller, L. F., and O'Neill, C. J., "Myositis Ossificans in Paraplegics," J. Bone and Joint Surg., 31A:283, 1949.

Dworetzky, M., "Reversible Metastatic Calcification (Milk Drinker's Syndrome)," J.A.M.A., 155:830, 1954.

Singleton, E. B., and Holt, J. F., "Myositis Ossificans Progressiva," Radiol., 62:47, 1954.

Foster, L. N., et. al, "Experimental Infarction of Bone and Bone Marrow," J. Bone and Joint Surg., 33A:396, 1951.

Laurence, W., and Franklin, E. L., "Calcifying Enchondroma of Long Bones," J. Bone and Joint Surg., 35B:224, 1953.

Steel, H. H., "Calcified Islands in Medullary Bone," J. Bone and Joint Surg., 32A:405, 1950.

Gershon-Cohen, J., Schraer, H., Sklaroff, D. M., and Blumberg, N., "Dissolution of the Intervertebral Disk in the Aged Normal," Radiol., 62, 383, 1954.

Marr, J. T., "Gas in Intervertebral Discs," Am. J. Roentgenol., 70:804, 1953.

Camiel, M. R., and Aaron, J. B., "The Gas or Vacuum Phenomenon in the Pubic Symphysis During Pregnancy," Radiol., 66:548, 1956.

Raines, J. R., "Intervertebral Disc Fissures (Vacuum Intervertebral Disc)," Am. J. Roentgenol., 70:964, 1953.

Poppel, M. H., and Robinson, W. T., "The Roentgen Manifestations of Caisson Disease," Am. J. Roentgenol., 76:74, 1956.

Pipkin, G., "Lesions of the Suprapatellar Plica," J. Bone and Joint Surg., 32A:363, 1950.

Silverman, F. N., "The Roentgen Manifestations of Unrecognized Skeletal Trauma in Infants," Am. J. Roentgenol., 69:413, 1953.

Norell, H. G., "Roentgenologic Visualization of Extracapsular Fat: Its Importance in Diagnosis of Traumatic Injuries to Elbow," Acta Radiol., 42:205, 1954.

Lewitan, A., and Nathanson, L., "Roentgen Features of Muscular Dystrophy," Am. J. Roentgenol., 73:226, 1955.

Woodward, H. Q., "Role of the Chemical Laboratory in Diagnosis of Neoplastic Disease of Bone," Arch. Surg., 47:368, 1943.

Flink, E. B., "Calcium, Phosphorus and Phosphatase as Aids in the Diagnosis of Bone Lesions," Radiol., 50:72, 1948.

Nutritional Diseases

Bentzon, P. G. K., "Roentgenological Investigations Concerning the Arterial Supply of the Epiphyses," Acta Radiol., 8-618, 1927.

Jequier, M., and Fredenhagen, H., "L'heredite de la dystrophic epiphysaise des hanches," Radiol. Clin., 17:92, 1948.

Martin, H. E., "Germetrical-Anatomical Factors and Their Significance in the Early X-Ray Diagnosis of Hip-Joint Disease in Children," Radiol., 56:842, 1951.

Holsti, L. R., "Osteochondritis Ischiopubica," Acta Radiol., 45:178, 1956.

Overgaard, Kristiaan, "Otto's Disease and Other Forms of Protruscio Acetabuli," Acta Radiol., 16:390, 1935.

Wolf, J., "Larsen-Johansson Disease of the Patella," Brit. J. Radiol., 23:335, 1950.

Kemp, F. H., and Wilson, D. C., "Some Factors in the Aetiology of Osteochondritis of the Spine," Brit. J. Radiol., 20:410, 1947.

Williams, E. R., "Observations on Differential Diagnosis and Sequelae of Juvenile Vertebral Osteochondrosis," Acta Radiol. Supp., 116:293, 1954.

Cleaves, E. N., "Adolescent Sacro-iliac Joints," Am. J. Roentgenol., 38:450, 1937.

Gillespie, H. W., and Lloyd-Roberts, G., "Osteitis Condensans," Brit. J. Radiol., 26:16, 1953.

Hutton, C. F., "Osteitis Condensans Ilii," Brit. J. Radiol., 26:490, 1953.

Wells, J., "Osteitis Condensans Ilii," Am. J. Roentgenol., 76:1141, 1956.

Terrafranca, R. J., and Zellis, A., "A Case of Congenital Rickets," Radiol., 60:192, 1953.

Smyth, I., "Bilateral Osteochondritis of the Middle Cuneiform Bone," Radiol., 68:575, 1957.

Shepard, E., "Multiple Epiphyseal Dysplasia," J. Bone and Joint Surg., 36B:458, 1956.

Schlesinger, B., "Rickets with Alkaline Phosphatase Deficiency; An Osteoblastic Dysplasia," Arch. Dis. Childhood, 30:265, 1955.

Holt, J. F., "Vitamin D Resistant Rickets," Am. J. Roentgenol., 64:590, 1950.

Dent, C. E., and Harris, H. H., "Hereditary Forms of Rickets and Osteomalacia," J. Bone and Joint Surg., 36B:204, 1956.

Baker, S. L., "Fibrogenesis Imperfecta Ossium," J. Bone and Joint Surg., 36B:378, 1956.

Bromer, R. S., "Roentgenray Diagnosis of Infantile Scurvy," Am. J. Roentgenol., 19:112, 1928.

Dennis, J. M., and Mercado, R., "Scurvy Following Folic Acid Antagonist Therapy," Radiol., 67:412, 1956.

Cole, W. R., "Calcinosis," Guy's Hosp. Rep., 102:56, 1953.

Sausa, A., and Chaves, J. P., "Calcinosis," J. Bone and Joint Surg., 35B:423, 1953.

Thomson, J. E. M., and Tanner, F. H., "Tumoral Calcinosis," J. Bone and Joint Surg., 31A:132, Jan. 1949.

Oosthuizen, S. F., LaRoux, P., and de Wet, A. S., "Calcino-Universalis: Type Lipo-Calcino-Granulomatosis," Brit. J. Radiol., 23:598, 1950.

Rothman, P. E., and Leon, E. E., "Hypervitaminosis A ," Radiol., 51:368, 1948.

Caffey, J., "Chronic Poisoning Due Excess of Vitamin A," Pediatrics, 5:672, 1950.

Toomey, J., and Morisette, R. A., "Hypervitaminosis," Am. J. Dis. Child., 73:473, 1947.

Jeans, P. C., "Vitamin D," J.A.M.A., 143:177, 1950.

Caffey, J., "Vitamin A Poisoning," Editorial, Am. J. Roentgenol., 67:818, 1952.

Shiers, J. A., Neuhauser, E. B. D., and Bowman, J. R., "Idiopathic Hypercalcemia," Am. J. Roentgenol., 78:19, 1955.

Infections of Bone

Neligan, G. A., and Warrick, C. K., "The Value of Radiology in the Diagnosis and Management of Pyogenic Osteitis in Childhood," J. Faculty of Radiol., 5:112, 1953.

Liming, R. W., and Youngs, F. J., "Metastatic Vertebral Osteomyelitis Following Prostatic Surgery," Radiol., 67:92, 1956.

Cohen, H. H., "Osteitis Pubis," J. Urol., 55:84, 1942.

Flaherty, R. A., Puch, D. G., and Dockerty, M. B., "Osteoid Osteoma," Am. J. Roentgenol., 76:576, 1956.

Knutsson, F., "The Roentgenographic Appearance of Osteoid Osteoma in Children," Acta Radiol., 45:125, 1956.

Allen, D. H., Browne, F. S., and Pierce, A. W., "Infantile Hyperostosis," Am. J. Roentgenol., 76:576, 1956.

Batson, O. V., Ann. Int. Med., 16:38, 1942.

Goldstein, A. E., and Rubin, S. W., "Osteitis Pubis Following Subrapubic Prostatectomy," Am. J. Surg., 74:480, 1947.

Lame, E. L., and Chang, H. C., "Pubic and Ischial Necrosis Following Cystostomy and Prostatectomy (Osteitis Pubis)," Am. J. Roentgenol., 71:193, 1954.

Lowe, G. H., and Lipscomb, P. R., "Brucellosis Osteomyelitis," Surg., 22:525, 1947.

Forssman, G., "Three Cases of Skeletal Changes Round the Knee Joint in Paratyphoid Fever in Infants," Acta Radiol., 27:294, 1946.

Fagerberg, S., and Rudström, P., "Osteoid Osteoma of a Vertebral Arch," Acta Radiol., 40:383, 1953.

Hamilton, J. F., "Osteoid Osteoma," Surg., Gynec. and Obst., 81:465, 1945.

Caffey, J., and Silverman, W. A., "Infantile Cortical Hyperostoses," Am. J. Roentgenol., 54:1, 1945.

Caffey, J., "On Some Late Skeletal Changes in Chronic Infantile Cortical Hyperostoses," Radiol., 59:651, 1952.

Bennett, H. S., and Nelson, T. R., "Prenatal Cortical Hyperostosis," Brit. J. Radiol., 26:47, 1953.

Delano, P. J., and Butler, C. D., "The Etiology of Infantile Cortical Hyperostoses," Am. J. Roentgenol., 58:633, 1947.

Jones, A. R., "The Influence of Hugh Owen Thomas on the Evolution of the Treatment of Skeletal Tuberculosis," J. Bone and Joint Surg., 35B:309, 1953.

Girwood, W., "Multiple Cystic Tuberculosis of Bone (Jungling's Disease)," J. Bone and Joint Surg., 35B:285, 1953.

Soriano, M., "Periostitis Deformans," Ann. Rheumat. Dis., 11:154, 1952.

Alexander, G. H., and Mansuy, M. M., "Disseminated Bone Tuberculosis (so-called Multiple Cystic Tuberculosis)," Radiol., 55:839, 1950.

Saenger, E. L., "Spondylarthritis in Children," Am. J. Roentgenol., 64:20, 1950.

Ziady, F., and Selzer, G., "Multiple Cystic Tuberculosis of Bone," Clin. Pract. Cape Town, South Africa, 1:346, 1942.

Guri, J. P., "Pyogenic Osteomyelitis of the Spine," J. Bone and Joint Surg., 28:29, 1946.

Wagoner, G., and Pendergrass, E. P., "Intrinsic Circulation of the Vertebral Body," Am. J. Roentgenol., 27:818, 1932.

Auerbach, O., and Stemmerman, M., "Roentgen Interpretation of the Pathology in Pott's Disease," Am. J. Roentgenol., 52:47, July 1944.

Poppel, M. H., Lawrence, L. R., Jacobson, H. G., and Stein, J., "Skeletal Tuberculosis," Am. J. Roentgenol., 70:936, 1953.

Zadek, I., "Acute Non-Tuberculosis Psoas Abscess," J. Bone and Joint Surg., 32A:433, 1950.

Hancox, N. M., and others, "Radiological 'Double Contour' Effect of Long Bones of Newly Born Infants," Arch. Dis. Childhood, 26:543, 1951.

Engeset, A., Eek, S., and Gilje, O., "On the Significance of Growth in the Roentgenological Skeletal Changes in Early Congenital Syphilis," Am. J. Roentgenol., 69:542, 1953.

Bayling, J., and Wear, J. M., "Blastomycosis and Actinomycosis of the Spine," Am. J. Roentgenol., 69:395, 1953.

Reeves, R. J., and Pedersen, R., "Fungous Infection of Bone," Radiol., 62:55, 1954.

Carter, R. A., "Coccidiodal Granuloma: Roentgen Diagnosis," Am. J. Roentgenol., 25:715, 1931.

Benninghoven, C., and Miller, E. R., "Coccidioidal Infection in Bone," Radiol., 38:663, June 1942.

Rhinehart, W. J., and Bauer, J. T., "Disseminated Granuloma Inguinale of Bones," Am. J. Roentgenol., 57:562, 1947.

Carter, R. A., "Infectious Granulomas of Bones and Joints with Special Reference to Coccidiodal Granuloma," Radiol., 23:1, 1934.

Glandular and Metabolic Disturbances

Ellis, V. A., and Taylor, J. G., "Diaphyseal Aclasis," Brit. J. B. and Jt. Surg., 33B: 110, 1951.

Clark, D. M., "The Practical Value of Roentgenography of the Epiphyses in the Diagnosis of Endocrine Disorders," Am. J. Roentgenol., 35:752, 1936.

Sear, H. R., "The Congenital Bone Dystrophies and Their Co-Relation," J. Faculty Radiol., 4:221, 1953.

Moore, S., "The Troell-Junet Syndrome," Acta Radiol., 39:485, 1953.

Wang, C. C., and Rubbins, L. L., "Cushing's Disease: Its Roentgenographic Findings," Radiol., 67:17, 1956.

Sissons, H. A., "Osteoporosis of Cushing's Syndrome," J. Bone and Joint Surg., 36B:418, 1956.

Strach, E. H., "Hyperplastic Callus Formation in Osteogenesis Imperfecta," J. Bone and Joint Surg., 35B:417, 1953.

Hilton, G., "Familial Hyperplastic Callus Formation," J. Bone and Joint Surg., 35B:411, 1953.

Baker, S. L., "Hyperplastic Callus Simulating Sarcoma in Two Cases of Fragilitas Ossium," J. Path. and Bact., 58:609, 1946.

Vandermark, W. E., and Page, M. A., "Massive Hyperplasia of Bone Following Fractures of Osteogenesis Imperfecta," J. Bone and Joint Surg., 30A:1015, 1948.

Key, J. A., "Brittle Bones and Blue Sclera; Hereditary Hypoplasia of the Mesenchyme," Arch. Surg., 13:523, 1926.

Bangson, J. S., "Several Generations of Achondrotlasia," J. Hered., 17:393, 1926.

Snoke, P. O., "Chondrodystrophia Fetalis," Am. J. Roentgenol., 29:31, 1933.

Lenk, R., "Hereditory Metaphyseal Dysostosis," Am. J. Roentgenol., 76:569, 1956.

Bromer, R. S., and John, R. L., "Ollier's Disease, Unilateral Chondrodysplasia," Am. J. Roentgenol., 26:428, 1931.

Krause, G. R., "Dyschondroplasia with Hemangiomata (Maffuccis Syndrome)," Am. J. Roentgenol., 52:620, 1944.

Carleton, Alice, "Maffucci's Syndrome," Quart. J. Med., 11:203, 1942.

Phol, J., "Chondro-Osteodystrophy, (Marquios' Disease)," J. Bone and Joint Surg., 21:187, 1939.

Fairbank, H. A. T., "Chondro-Osteo-Dystrophy," J. Bone and Joint Surg., 31B:291, 1949.

Russo, P. F., "Chondroosteodrystrophy: Marquios' Disease; Case Observed during Pregnancy," Radiol., 41:42, 1943.

Christensen, W. R., Rukan, Lin, and Berghoot, J., "Dysplasia Epiphysalis Multiplex," Am. J. Roentgenol., 74:1059, 1955.

Rapp, G., "Chondrodystrophia Calcificans Congenita," Am. J. Roentgenol., 49:77, 1943.

Fairbank, H. A., "Dysplasia Epiphysialis Punctata," J. Bone and Joint Surg., 31B:114, 1949.

Coughlin, E. J., "Chondrodystrophia Calcificans Congenita," J. Bone and Joint Surg., 32A:938, 1950.

Frank, W. W., and Denny, M. B., "Dysplasia Epiphysialis Punctata," J. Bone and Joint Surg., 36B:118, 1954.

Sheach, J. M., and Middlemiss, J. H., "Dysplasia Epiphysialis Punctata," Brit. J. Radiol., 29:111, 1956.

Fairbank, T. J., "Dysplasia Epiphysialis Hemimelica (Tarso-apiphysial aclasis)," J. Bone and Joint Surg.,

Cusmano, J. V., Baker, D. H., and Finby, N., "Pseudohypoparathyroidism," Radiol., 67:845, 1956.

Schinz, A. R. et al., Roentgen. Diagnostic, Grune and Stratton, 4 Vols., New York, 1951-54.

Ginyler, A. M., and Jaffe, N. L., "Osseous Findings in Chronic Renal Insufficiency in Adults," Am. J. Path., 17:293, 1941.

Pugh, D. G., "Subperiosteal Resorption of Bone," Am. J. Roentgenol., 66:577, 1951.

Hartley, J. N. J., "Giant-Cell Tumors, Osteitis Fibrosa, and Bone Cysts. A Study of Their Aetiological Relation," J. Faculty Radiol., 4:10, 1952.

McWhirter, R. J., "Giant Cell Tumours, Osteitis Fibrosa, and Bone Cysts," J. Faculty Radiol., 4:1, 1952.

Harriman, D. G. F., and Miller, J. H. D., "Fibrous Dysplasia of Bone with Skeletal Lipoid Granulomatosis," J. Bone and Joint Surg., 36B:95, 1954.

Albright, F., Butler, A. M., Hampton, A. O., and Smith, P., "Syndrome Characterized by Osteitis Fibrosa Disseminata, Areas of Pigmentation and Endocrine Dysfunction, with Precocious Puberty in Females," New Eng. J. Med., 216:727, 1937.

Fries, J. W., "The Roentgen Features of Fibrous Dysplasia of the Skull and Facial Bones," Am. J. Roentgenol., 77:71, 1957.

Schlesinger, P. J., et al., "Fibrous Dysplasia," J. Bone and Joint Surg., 31A:187, 1949.

Wells, P. O., "Fibrous Dysplasia of Bone (Monostotic)," Radiol., 52:642, 1949.

LeMay, M., and Blunt, J. W., Jr., "A Factor Determining the Location of Pseudo-Fractures in Osteomalacia," J. Clin. Invest., 28:521, 1949.

Camp, J. D., and McCullough, J. A., "Pseudofractures in Diseases Affecting the Skeletal System," Radiol, 36:651, 1941.

Irvine, R. E., "Famial Paget's Disease with Early Onset," J. Bone and Joint Surg., 35B:106, 1953.

Kasabach, H. H., and Gutman, A. B., "Osteoporosis Circumscripta of the Skull and Paget's Disease," Am. J. Roentgenol., 37:577, 1937.

Bossi, R., and Pisani, G., "Osteoporosis Circumscripta Cranii, (Schuller Disease)," Brit. J. Radiol., 29:445, 1956.

Editorial, "Circulatory Effects of Osteitis Deformans," Lancet, 2:568, 1946.

Garland, L. H., "Generalized Leontiasis Ossea," Am. J. Roentgenol., 55:37, 1946.

Knaggs, R. L., Inflammatory and Toxic Disease of Bone, William Wood and Co., 1926.

Evans, J., "Leontiasis Ossea," J. Bone and Joint Surg., 35B:229, 1953.

Pygott, F., and Scott, M. G., "Leontiasis Ossea (Virchow Type)," Brit. J. Radiol., 27:31, 1954.

Kummell, H., "Aerytlicher Verein in Hamburg," Munchen Med Wchnschr., 51:365, 1904.

Jenkinson, E. L., Pfisterer, W. H., Latteier, K. K., and Martin, M., "A Prenatal Diagnosis of Osteopetrosis," Am. J. Roentgenol., 49:455, 1943.

Kneal, E., and Sante, L. R., "Osteopetrosis (Marble Bones)," Am. J. Dis. Child., 81:693, 1951.

McPeak, C. H., "Osteopetrosis," Am. J. Roentgenol., 36:816, 1936.

Pirie, A. H., "The Development of Marble Bones," Am. J. Roentgenol., 24:147, 1930; 30:618, 1933.

Mori, P., and Holt, J. F., "Cranial Manifestations of Familial Metaphyseal Dysplasia," Radiol., 66:335, 1956.

Voorhoeve, N., "L'image Radiologique Non Encore Decrite d'une Anomalie du Squelette," Acta Radiol., 3:407, 1924.

Hurt, R. L., "Osteopathia Striata—Voorhoeve's Disease," J. Bone and Joint Surg., 35B:89, 1953.

Engelmann, G., "A Case of Osteopathia Hyperostotica (Sclerotisans) Multiplex Infantilis," abs., Am. J. Roentgenol., 22:377, 1929.

Sears, H. R., "Engelmann's Disease," Brit. J. Radiol., 21:236, 1948.

Ribbing, S., "Hereditary Multiple Diaphyseal Sclerosis," Acta Radiol., 31:522, 1949.

Paul, L. W., "Hereditary Multiple Diaphyseal Sclerosis (Ribbing)," Radiol., 60:412, 1953.

Neuhauser, E. G. D., Schwachman, H., Wittenborg, M., and Cohen, J., "Progressive Diaphyseal Dysplasia," Radiol., 51:11, 1948.

Van Buchan, F. S. P., Hadders, H. N., and Ubbens, R., "The Unknown Familial Disease of the Skeleton: Hyperostosis Corticalis Generalista Familiaris," Acta Radiol., 44:109, 1955.

Griffiths, D. L., "Engelmann's Disease," J. Bone and Joint Surg., 36B:312, 1956.

Harmston, G. J., "Osteopathia Condensans Disseminata," Radiol., 66:556, 1956.

Holly, L. E., "Osteopoikilosis," Am. J. Roentgenol., 36:512, 1936.

Wilcox, L. F., "Osteopoikilosis," Am. J. Roentgenol., 27:580, 1932.

Baumann-Schenker, R., and Uehlinger, E., "Ucher Tubulare Sklerose des Skeletts," Radiol. Clin., 16:221, 1947.

Pyle, E., "A Case of Unusual Bone Development," J. Bone and Joint Surg., 13:874, 1931.

Hermel, M. B., et al., "Familial Metaphyseal Dysplasia," Am. J. Roentgenol., 70:413, 1953.

Fraser, J., "Skeletal Lipoid Granulomatosis (Hand-Schuller-Christian's Disease)," Brit. J. Surg., 22:800, 1935.

Torgersen, J., "Vertebra Plana in Lipoidosis (Hand-Schuller-Christian's)," Acta Radiol., 27:638, 1946.

Compere, E. L., Johnson, W. E., and Coventry, M. B., "Vertebra Plana (Calvé's Disease) Due to Eosinophilic Granuloma," J. Bone and Joint Surg., 36A:969, 1954.

Rosselet, E., and Rosselet, P. J., "Vertebra Plana Osteonecrotica (Maladie de Calvé) a propos d'une localisation rare," Radiol. Clin., 24:746, 1956.

Markowitz, C. A., and Mahn, F. C., "Role of Lung in Metabolism of Fat," Am. J. Physiol., 93:521, June 1930.

Wells, Col. P. O., "The Button Sequestrum of Eosinophilic Granuloma of the Skull," Radiol., 67:746, 1956.

Platt, J. L., and Eisenberg, R. B., "Eosinophilic Granuloma of Bone," J. Bone and Joint Surg., 30A:761, 1948.

Hunter, T., "Solitary Eosinophilic Granuloma of Bone," J. Bone and Joint Surg., 36B:545, 1956.

Ackerman, A. J., "Eosinophilic Granuloma of Bones Associated with Involvement of the Lungs and Diaphragm," Am. J. Roentgenol., 58:733, 1947.

Nitter, L., "Three Cases of Eosinophilic Granuloma of the Pelvis in Children," Acta Radiol., 46:731, 1956.

Loehr, W. H., Eosinophic Granuloma of Bone in the Hand," Am. J. Roentgenol., 57:568, 1947.

Mercer, W., and Duthie, R. B., "Histiocytic Granulomatosis," J. Bone and Joint Surg., 36B:279, 1956.

Tennent, W., "Gaucher's Disease—The Early Radiological Diagnosis," Brit. J. Radiol., 18:356, 1945.

Reed, J., and Sosman, M. C., "Gaucher's Disease," Radiol., 38:579, 1942.

Tennent, W., "Gaucher's Disease—The Early Radiological Diagnosis," Brit. J. Radiol., 18:356, 1945.

Harvey, R. M., "Hurler-Pfundler Syndrome (Gargoylism)," Am. J. Roentgenol., 48:732, 1942.

Caffey, J., "Gargoylism (Hunter-Hurler Disease, Dysostosis Multiplex, Liposhondrodystrophy," Am. J. Roentgenol., 67:715, 1952.

Singleton, E. B., Thomas, J. R., Worthington, W. W., and Hild, J. R., "Progressive Diaphyseal Dysplasia (Engelmann's Disease)," Radiol., 67:233, 1957.

Blood Dyscrasias

Epstein, B. S., "Vertebral Changes in Childhood Leukemia," Radiol., 68:65, 1957.

Silverman, F. N., "The Skeletal Lesions in Leukemia," Am. J. Roentgenol., 59:819, 1948.

Kemp, T. A., and Williams, E. R., "Chloroma," Brit. J. Radiol., 15:157, 1941.

Teall, C. G., "A Radiological Study of the Bone Changes Hemolitic Anemia and Leukemia in Children," Brit. J. Radiol., 12:601, Nov. 1939.

Janus, W. L., and Dietz, M. W., "Osseous Changes in Erythroblastosis Fetalis," Radiol., 53:59, 1949.

Hamburg, A. E., "Skeletal Changes in Sickle-Cell Anemia," J. Bone and Joint Surg., 32A:893, 1950.

Rowe, C. W., and Haggard, M. E., "Bone Infarcts in Sickle-Cell Anemia," Radiol., 68:66, 1957.

Bromer, R., "Rickets and Infantile Scurvy Occurring in a Case of Osteogenesis Imperfecta," Am. J. Roentgenol., 55:30, 1946.

Weil, I. F., and Lerner, H. H., "A Case of Long-Standing Sickle Cell Anemia with Marked Bone Changes," Am. J. Roentgenol., 60:251, 1946.

Mosley, J. E., and Manley, J. B., "Aseptic Necrosis of Bone in Sickle-Cell Disease," Radiol., 60:656, 1953.

Bersack, S. R., and Feinstein, H. R., "Secondary Myelofibrosis with Progressive Generalized Osseous Eburnation," Am. J. Roentgenol., 56:470, 1946.

Sussman, M. L., "Myelosclerosis with Leukerythroblastic Anemia," Am. J. Roentgenol., 57:313, 1947.

Gohrmley, R. K., et al., "Bone and Joint Changes in Hemophilia," J. Bone and Joint Surg., 30A:589, 1948.

Neuropathic Lesions of Bone

Delano, P. J., "The Pathogenesis of Charcot's Joint," Am. J. Roentgenol., 56:189, 1946.

Esguerra-Gomez, G., and Acosta, E., "Bone and Joint Lesions in Leprosy," Radiol., 50:619, 1948.

Faget, G. H., and Mayoral, A., "Bone Changes in Leprosy," Radiol., 42:1, Jan. 1944.

Cooney, J. P., and Crosby, E. H., "Absorptive Bone Changes in Leprosy," Radiol., 42:14, Jan., 1944.

Larsen, L. L., and Wright, H. H., "Para-Ossification, A Complication of Anterior Poliomyelitis," Radiol., 69:103, 1957.

Miller, L. F., and O'Neill, C. J., "Myositis Ossificans in Paraplegics," J. Bone and Joint Surg., 31A:283, 1949.

Lodge, T., "Bone, Joint and Soft Tissue Changes Following Paraplegia," Acta Radiol., 46:435, 1956.

Kraft, E., "The Pathology of Monomelic Flowing Hyperostosis or Melorheostosis," Radiol., 20:47, 1933.

Carpender, J., Baker, D. R., Perry, S. P., and Outland, T., "Melorheostosis," Am. J. Roentgenol., 49:398, 1943.

Fejer, E., "Uber einen Interessanten Fall von Mëlorheostosis," Acta Radiol., 29:112, 1948.

Hess, W. E., and Street, D. M., "Melorheostosis," J. Bone and Joint Surg., 32A:422, 1950.

Holt, J. F., and Wright, E. M., "The Radiologic Features of Neurofibromatosis," Radiol., 51:647, 1948.

Brooks, R., Lehman, E. P., "The Bone Changes in Recklinghausen's Neurofibromatosis," Surg., Gynec. and Obst., 38:587, 1924.

Friedman, M., "Neurofibromatosis of Bone," Am. J. Roentgenol., 51:623, 1944.

Mineral Poisons and Other Intoxications

Cooper, G., "An Epidemic of Inhalation Lead Poisoning with Characteristic Skeletal Changes in the Children Involved," Am. J. Roentgenol., 58:129, 1947.

Vogt, E. C., "A Roentgen Sign of Plumbism," Am. J. Roentgenol., 24:550, 1930.

Stevenson, C. A., and Watson, A. R., "Fluoride Osteosclerosis," Am. J. Roentgenol., 78:13, 1957.

Evans, R. D., Harris, R. S., and Bunker, J. W. M., "Radium Metabolism in Rats and the Production of Osteogenic Sarcoma by Experimental Radium Poisoning," Am. J. Roentgenol., 52:353, Oct. 1944.

Senturia, H. R., "The Roentgen Findings in Increased Lead Absorption due to Retained Projectiles," Am. J. Roentgenol., 47:381, 1942.

Sussman, M. L., and Poppel, M. H., "Renal Osteitis," Am. J. Roentgenol., 48:726, 1952.

Müller, G. M., and Sissons, H. A., "Rickets Simulating 'Metaphysical Dysostosis,' " J. Bone and Joint Surg., 33B:231, 1951.

Weens, H. S., and Marin, C. A., "Infantile Arteriosclerosis," Radiol., 67:168, 1956.

Dunn, H. G., "Oxalosis," Am. J. Dis. Child., 90:58, 1955.

Congenital Anomalies and Anatomical Variations

Neuhauser, E. B. D., "Growth, Differentiation and Disease," Am. J. Roentgenol., 69:723, 1953.

Ingram, F. L., "Cranio-cleido-dysostosis," Brit. J. Radiol., 20:332, 1947.

Eisen, D., "Cleidocranial Dysostosis," Radiol., 61:21, 1953.

Poppel, M., Jacobson, H. G., Duff, B. K., and Gottlieb, C., "Basilar Impression and Platybasia in Paget's Disease," Radiol., 61:639, 1953.

Cooper, R., "Acrocephalosyndactyly," Brit. J. Radiol., 26:533, 1953.

Chamberlain, E., "Basilar Impression, (Platybasia)," Yale J. Biol. Med., 11:487, 1939.

McGregor, M., "The Significance of Certain Measurements of the Skull in the Diagnosis of Basilar Impression," Brit. J. Radiol., 21:171, 1948.

Fullenlove, T. M., and Williams, A. J., "Comparative Roentgen Findings in Symptomatic and Asymptomatic Backs," Radiol., 68:572, 1957.

Neuhauser, E. B. D., Wittenborg, M. H., and Dehlinger, K., "Diastematomyelia," Radiol., 54:659, 1950.

Bonola, A., "Surgical Tretament of Klippel-Feil Syndrome," J. Bone and Joint Surg., 36B:440, 1956.

Rowley, K. A., "Coronal Cleft Vertebra," J. Fac. Radiologists, 6:267, 1955.

McRae, D. L., and Barnum, A. S., "Occipitalization of the Atlas," Am. J. Roentgenol., 70:23, 1953.

Schultz, E. H., Levy, R. W., and Russo, P. E., "Agenesis of the Odontoid Process, " Radiol., 67:102, 1956.

Cowie, J. N., "Diastametamyelia," Brit. J. Radiol., 24:156, 1951; 25:263, 1952.

Biström, O., "Congenital Anomalies of Lumbar Spine of Persons with Painless Backs," Ann. Chir. et Gynaec. Fenniae, 43:102, 1954.

Garland, L. H., and Thomas, S. F., "Spondylolisthesis," Am. J. Roentgenol., 55:275, 1946.

Meschan, I., "Spondylolisthesis," Am. J. Roentgenol., 53:230, March 1945.

Thompson, E. A., Walker, E. T., and Weens, H. S., "Iliac Horns," Radiol., 53:88, 1949.

Gershon-Cohen, J., and Delbridge, R. E., "Pseudarthrosis, Synchondrosis and Other Anomalies of the First Ribs," Am. J. Roentgenol., 53:49, 1945.

Bowie, E. R., and Jacobson, H. G., "Spondylolisthesis," Am. J. Roentgenol., 54:161, 1945.

Weston, W. J., "Genetically Determined Cervical Ribs," Brit. J. Radiol., 29:455, 1956.

Bates, J. C., U.S. Armed Forces M. J., 5:865, 1954.

Martin, H. E., "Geometrical-Anatomical Factors and Their Significance in the Early X-Ray Diagnosis of Hip-Joint Disease in Children," Radiol., 56:842, 1951.

Finby, N. F., Jacobson, H. G., and Poppel, M. H., "Idiopathic Coxa Vara in Childhood," Radiol., 67:10, 1956.

Almond, H. G., "Familial Infanite Coxa Vara," J. Bone and Joint Surg., 36B:539, 1956.

Dawson, G. R., "Intra-Uterine Fractures of the Tibia and Fibula," J. Bone and Joint Surg., 31A:406, 1949.

Owen, R., "Bilateral Glenoid Hypoplasia," J. Bone and Joint Surg., 35B:262, 1953.

Davies, A. G. M., "Bilateral Humerus Varus," Brit. J. Radiol., 29:295, 1956.

Golthamer, C. R., "Duplication of the Clavicle; (Os Subclaviculare)," Radiol., 68:576, 1957.

Kriss, N., "Clinical Significance of the Supracondyloid Process of the Humerus," Am. J. Roentgenol., 76:1154, 1956.

Habbe, J. E., "Patella Cubiti," Am. J. Roentgenol., 48:513, 1942.

Kjelland, P. M., "A Rare Anomaly in the Elbow—Patella Cubite," Acta Radiol., 26:491, 1945.

Moehlig, R. C., "Arachnodactyly (Marfan's Syndrome)," Am. J. Roentgenol., 61:797, 1949.

Bogart, F. B., "Variations of the Bones of the Wrist," Am. J. Roentgenol., 28:638, 1932.

Dwight, T., A Clinical Atlas: Variations of the Bones of the Hands and Feet, J. B. Lippincott, Phil., 1907.

Caffey, J., "Chondroectodermal Dysplasia (Ellis-van Creveld Disease)," Am. J. Roentgenol., 68:875, 1952.

Moore, J. R., "Delayed Autogenic Bone Graft in the Treatment of Congenital Pseudarthrosis," J. Bone and Joint Surg., 31A:23, 1949.

Hessen, I., "Fabella (Sesamum Genu Superius Laterale)," Acta Radiol., 27:177, 1946.

Nickerson, S. H., "Pathology of the Anomalies Found in Knee Joints," Am. J. Roentgenol., 53:213, 1945.

Morris, H., "Tibia Vara," Brit. J. Radiol., 21:242, 1948.

Barber, C. G., "Osteochondrosis Deformas Tibiae," Am. J. Dis. Child., 64:831, 1942.

Lubschitz, K., "Case of Tibia Recurvate," Acta Radiol., 27:81, 1946.

Lewin, P., "Arthrogryposis Multiplex Congenita," J. Bone and Joint Surg., 7:630, 1925.

Osmond-Clarke, H., "Congenital Vertical Talus," J. Bone and Joint Surg., 36B:334, 1956.

Jacobson, H. G., Herbert, E. A., and Poppel, M. H., "Arthrogryposis Multiplex Congenita," Radiol., 65:8, 1955.

Spinzig, E., "Ainhum: Its Occurrence in the United States," Am. J. Roentgenol., 43:246, 1939.

Stack, J. K., "Ainhum," J. Bone and Joint Surg., 32A:444, 1950.

Barnetson, J., "Two Cases of Lipomatosis Involving Bone," Brit. J. Radiol., 20:426, 1947.

Fainsinger, M. H., and Harris, L. C., "Generalized Lipomatosis Involving Bone," Brit. J. Radiol., 23:274, 1950.

Vaughn, W. H., and Segal, G., " Talipes Calcanea Valgus," Radiol., 60:855, 1953.

O'Rahilly, R., "Radiological Investigation of a Case of Pedal Hyperphalangism and Supernumerary Phalangeal Epiphysis," Brit. J. Radiol., 19:432, 1946.

Burkitt, D., and Fairbank, H. A. T., "An Unusual Lipoid Reticulosis of Bone," J. Bone and Joint Surg., 36B:109. 1954.

Brailsford, J. F., The Radiology of Bones and Joints, J. A. Churchill, Ltd., London.

March, H. C., and London, R. I., "The Os Sustentaculi," Am. J. Roentgenol., 76:1114, 1956.

Chambers, C. H., "Congenital Anomalies of the Tarsal Navicular with Particular Reference to Calcaneo-Navicular Coalition," Brit. J. Radiol., 23:580, 1950.

Hope, J. W., Spitz, E. B., and Spade, H. W., "The Early Recognition of Premature Cranial Synostosis," Radiol., 65:183, 1955.

de Marchi, E., J. Radiol. et electrol., 36:665, 1955.

Tumors of Bone

Ewing, James, Registry, Neoplastic Disease (revised edition), W. B. Saunders Co., 1939.

Hutter, C. G., "Unicameral Bone Cyst," J. Bone and Joint Surg., 32A:430, 1950.

Purser, D. W., "Extraskeletal Osteochondromata," J. Bone and Joint Surg., 36B:871, 1956.

Sherman, R. S., and Soong, K. Y., "Aneurysmal Bone Cyst: Its Roentgen Diagnosis," Radiol., 68:54, 1957.

Maudsley, R. H., and Stansfeld, A. G., "Non-Osteogenic Fibroma of Bone," J. Bone and Joint Surg., 36B:714, 1956.

Lichtenstein, L., and Hall, J. E., "Periosteal Chondroma," J. Bone and Joint Surg., 34A:691, 1952.

Sherman, R. S., and Uzel, A. R., "Benign Chondroblastoma of Bone," Am. J. Roentgenol., 76:1132, 1956.

Taylor, F. W., "Aneurysmal Bone Cyst," J. Bone and Joint Surg., 36B:293, 1956.

Barnes, R., "Aneurysmal Bone Cyst," J. Bone and Joint Surg., 36B:301, 1956.

Gramiak, R., Ruiz, G., and Campeti, F. L., "Cystic Angiomatosis of Bone," Radiol., 69:347, 1957.

Kimmelstiel, P., and Rapp, I., "Cortical Defect Due to Periosteal Dismoids," Bull. Hosp. Joint Dis., 12:286, 1951.

Peimer, R., "Giant Cell Tumor of Skull and Nasal Sinuses," A.M.A. Arch. Otolaryng., 60:186, 1954.

Brown, J. S., and Middlemiss, J. H., Brit. J. Radiol., 29:212, 1956.

Shorvon, L. M., "Giant Cell Tumors (Osteoclastomata)," Brit. J. Radiol., 19:474, 1946.

Geschickter, C. F., and Copeland, M. M., Tumors of Bone, J. B. Lippincott Co., Phil., 1949.

Haas, A., and Ritter, S. A., "Benign Giant Cell Tumor of Femur with Embolic Metastasis in Prepuce of Penis," Am. J. Surg., 89:573, 1955.

Stevens, G. M., Pugh, D. G., and Dahlin, D. C., "Roentgenographic Recognition and Differentiation of Parosteal Osteogenic Sarcoma," Am. J. Roentgenol., 78:1, 1957.

Jaffe, H., and Lichtenstein, L., "Non-Osteogenic Fibroma of Bone," Am. J. Path., 18:205, 1942.

Hummel, J. A., and Truong-Thi-Danh, "Case of Periosteal Lipoma," J. Radiol. et electrol., 35:737, 1954.

Foster, D. B., and Heublein, G. W., "Hemangioma of Vertebra Associated with Spinal Cord Compression," Am. J. Roentgenol., 57:556, 1947.

Ackerman, A. J., and Hart, M. S., "Multiple Primary Hemangioma of the Bones of the Extremity," Am. J. Roentgenol., 48:47, 1942.

Ewing, James, Neoplastic Diseases, W. B. Saunders Co., 1939, Revised Edition.

Ackerman, A. J., "Multiple Osteogenic Sarcoma," Am. J. Roentgenol., 60:623, 1948.

Blum, S. D., "Solitary Myeloma of Bone," Am. J. Roentgenol., 57:239, 1947.

Krainin, P., et al., "Multiple Myeloma with New Bone Formation," Arch. Int. Med., 84:976, 1949.

Jansson, G., "Roentgenologic Skeletal Changes in Myeloma in Childhood (Platyspondylis Generalisata Myelomatosa)," Acta Radiol., 27:73, 1946.

Sherman, R. S., and Snyder, R. E., "The Roentgen Appearance of Primary Reticulum Cell Sarcoma of Bone," Am. J. Roentgenol., 58:291, 1947.

Magnus, H. A., and Wood, H. L. C., "Primary Reticulo-sarcoma of Bone," J. Bone and Joint Surg., 36B:258, 1956.

Sherman, R. S., and Soong, K. Y., "Ewing's Sarcoma: Its Roentgen Classification and Diagnosis," Radiol., 66:529, 1956.

Morgan, A. D., and Mackenzie, D. H., "A Metastasizing Adamantinoma of the Tibia," J. Bone and Joint Surg., 36B:892, 1956.

Strange, V. M., and de Lorimier, A. A., "Reticulum Cell Sarcoma Primary in the Skull," Am. J. Roentgenol., 71:40, 1954.

Winham, A. J., "Ewing's Tumor of a Rib with Pulmonary Metastases," Am. J. Roentgenol., 71:445, 1954.

Coley, B. L., and Harrold, C. C., "An Analysis of 59 Cases of Osteogenic Sarcoma with Survival for 5 Years or More," J. Bone and Joint Surg., 32A:307, 1950.

Tudway, R. C., "The Place of External Irradiation in the Treatment of Osteogenic Sarcoma," J. Bone and Joint Surg., 35B:9, 1953.

Brailsford, J. F., "Some Experiences with Bone Tumours," Brit. J. Radiol., 20:129, 1947.

Holt, J. F., "Unusual 'Bone Tumors' in Infants and Children," Radiol., 61:749, 1953.

Senturia, H. R., Schechter, S. E., and Hulbert, B., "Heterotopic Ossification in an Area of Metastasis from Rectal Carcinoma," Am. J. Roentgenol., 60:507, 1948.

Selby, H. M., Sherman, R. S., and Pack, G. T., "A Roentgen Study of Bone Metastases from Melanoma," Radiol., 67:224, 1956.

Wyatt, G. M., and Farber, S., "Neuroblastoma Sympatheticum," Am. J. Roentgenol., 46:485, 1941.

Sherman, R. S., and Leaming, R., "Roentgen Findings in Neuroblastoma," Radiol., 60:837, 1953.

Jackson, H., and Parker, F., Hodgkins Disease, New England J. Med., 234:103, 1946.

Mathis, W. H., and Schulz, M. D., "Roentgen Diagnosis of Glomus Tumors," Radiol., 51:71, 1948.

Coles, W. C., and Schulz, M. D., "Bone Involvement in Malignant Lymphoma," Radiol., 50:458, 1948.

Grunow, O. H., "Radiating Spicules, a Non-specific Sign of Bone Disease," Radiol., 65:200, 1955.

Wilson, T. W., and Pugh, D. G., "Primary Reticulum-cell Sarcoma of Bone with Emphasis on Roentgen Aspects," Radiol., 65:343, 1955.

Arthritis

Edwards, E. G., "Transient Synovitis of the Hip Joint in Children," J.A.M.A., 148:30, 1952.

Wilkinson, M. C., "Synovectomy and Curettage in the Treatment of Tuberculosis of Joints," J. Bone and Joint Surg., 35B:209, 1953.

Rose, G. K., "Arthropathy of the Ankle in Congenital Indifference to Pain," J. Bone and Joint Surg., 35B:408, 1953.

March, H. C., "Hypercholesteremic Xanthomata of the Tendons," Am. J. Roentgenol., 77:109, 1955.

Lyford, J., and Shapiro, D., "Gout as a Cause of Isolated Circumscribed Cyst of the Patella," Radiol., 66:380, 1956.

Smith, C. F., Am. J. Roentgenol., 74:1049, 1955.

Nielson, B., and Snorrason, E., "Arthritis Multilans ('Main et Doigt en Lorgnette')," Acta Radiol., 27:607, 1946.

Eloesser, L., "Of the Nature of Neuropathic Affections of the Joints," Ann. of Surg., 66:201, 1936.

Rolleston, G. L., "The Early Radiological Diagnosis of Ankylosing Spondylitis," Brit. J. Radiol., 20:288, 1947.

Cozen, L., "Charcot Joints Secondary to Diabetes Mellitus," Am. J. Roentgenol., 64:277, 1950.

Meyer, G. A., Stein, J., and Poppel, M. H., "Rapid Osseus Changes in Syringomyelia," Radiol., 69:415, 1957.

Bolen, J. G., "Diabetic Charcot Joints," Radiol., 67:95, 1956.

Moller, P. F., "Roentgen Picture of Tabetic Arthropathies and Affections of Bones," Acta Radiol., 26:535, 1945.

Baker, L. D., et. al., "Marie Strumpell's Arthritis," J. Bone and Joint Surg., 32A:848, 1950.

Holt, J. F., and Owens, W. I., "The Osseous Lesions of Sarcodosis," Radiol., 53:11, 1949.

Riley, E. A., "Boeck's Sarcoid," Am. Rev. Tubercu., 62:231, 1950.

Michael, M., Jr., et al., "Scardosis," Am. Rev. Tubercu., 62:403, 1950.

Crissey, R. E., and Day, A. J., "Ochronosis," J. Bone and Joint Surg., 32A:688, 1950.

Petersen, J., "Case of Osseous Changes in Patient with Hemophilia," Acta Radiol., 28:323, 1947.

Hertzberg, J., "On Osteoarthrosis Alkaptonuria (Ochronosis Acetabuli) with Description of One Case," Acta Radiol., 26:484, 1945.

Pomeranz, M. M., Friedman, L. J., and Tunick, I. S., "Roentgen Findings in Alkaptonuric Ochronosis," Radiol., 37:295, 1941.

Thompson, M. M., Jr., "Ochronosis," Am. J. Roentgenol., 78:46, 1957.

Boreadis, A. G., and Gershon-Cohen, J., "Luschka's Joints of the Cervical Spine," Radiol., 66:181, 1956.

Overgaard, K., "Otto's Disease and Other Forms of Protrusis Acetabuli," Acta Radiol., 16:390, 1935.

Mussey, R. D., and Henderson, J. S., "Osteochondromatosis," J. Bone and Joint Surg., 31A:619, 1949.

Ferguson, A. B., and Howorth, M. B., "Coxa Plana and Related Conditions at the Hip," J. Bone and Joint Surg., 16:781, 1934.

Golden, G. N., and Richards, H. G. H., "Xanthogranulomatous Disease of Bone with Polyarthritis," J. Bone and Joint Surg., 35B:275, 1953.

Lewis, W., "Roentgen Diagnosis of Pigmented Villonodular Synovitis and Synovial Sarcoma of the Knee Joint," Radiol., 49:26, 1947.

Knutsson, F., "Two Synovial Fibrosarcomas (Jonsson)," Acta Radiol., 29:4, 1948.

Jonsson, G., "Points Regarding Synovial Fibrosarcoma," Acta Radiol., 29:356, 1948.

Bloom, R., and Pattinson, J. N., "Osteochondromatosis of the Hip Joint," J. Bone and Joint Surg., 33B:80, 1951.

Temple, H. L., and Jaspin, G., "Hypertrophic Osteoarthropathy," Am. J. Roentgenol., 60:232, 1948.

Wiles, P., Andrews, P. S., and Devas, M. B., "Chondromalacia of the Patella," J. Bone and Joint Surg., 36B:95, 1956.

INDEX
FOR
THE CHEST

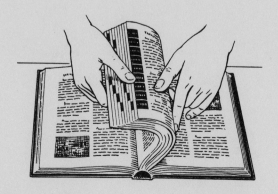

PART II

CHEST

NORMAL RESPIRATORY SYSTEM (Chapter XV)
  I. Roentgen Anatomy
    A. Topography of Lung
      1. Position of interlobar septa
      2. Bronchial tree and segments of lung
    B. Roentgen Examination of Lung Fields
      1. Hilum
      2. Peribronchial markings
      3. Parenchyma
      4. Pleura
      5. Diaphragm
    C. Microscopic Structure of Lung
      1. Primary lobule
    D. Anomalies
      1. Agenesis
      2. Anomalous lobes
          Azygos lobe
          Accessory inferior lobe
      3. Atresia bronchi
      4. Diaphragm
  II. Physiology of Respiration
  III. Respiratory Function

PATHOLOGY OF RESPIRATORY ORGANS (Chapter XVI)
  I. Larynx and Trachea
    A. Foreign Bodies
    B. Tracheal Displacement
    C. Tracheal Compression
    D. Anomalies
    E. Tumors of Trachea and Larynx
  II. Bronchi
    A. Bronchial Irritation
      1. Inhalation gases
      2. Beryllium and other irritating chemicals
    B. Acute Respiratory Infection
      1. Bronchitis—Bronchiolitis
      2. Influenza (LaGrippe); Virus Bronchitis
      3. Active acute congestion— rheumatic fever
    C. Asthma
    D. Emphysema (See section on emphysema and cystic disease of lungs)
    E. Bronchostenosis or Occlusion
      1. Causes
          a. Foreign body
          b. Bronchiogenic tumor
          c. Bronchial tuberculosis
          d. Secretions
          e. Developmental anomalies
      2. Results of
          a. Atelectasis from complete occlusion (see section on atelectasis)
          b. Obstructive emphysema from partial occlusion (see other types of emphysema)
    F. Bronchial Dilatation
      1. Bronchiectasis
      2. Anomalies—congenital cystic disease
      3. Agenesis
      4. Middle Lobe Syndrome
    G. Broncholithiasis

219

H. Broncho-esophageal Fistula
   1. Congenital— with atresia of esophagus
   2. Acquired— from new growth of esophagus
III. Lungs
   A. Circulatory Disturbances of Lungs
      1. Passive pulmonary congestion— haemosiderosis
      2. Pulmonary edema—hypostatic "pneumonia"—azotemic edema (allergic)
      3. Eosinophilic Infiltration— Loeffler's Syndrome
      4. Embolism; thrombosis; infarction—annular shadows of unusual type
      5. Thrombosis of pulmonary artery— Pulmonary Ischemia
      6. Polycthemia
   B. Infections—Bacteria and Virus
      1. Pneumonia
         a. Lobar Pneumonia
         b. Bronchopneumonia
               Infiltrative
               Purulent
               Friedlander Bacillus Pneumonia
         c. Septicemic (streptococcus) Pneumonia
         d. "Glandular" Pneumonia
               Tularemia
               Measles
               Whooping Cough
         e. Interstitial Pneumonia—Virus
               Hamman—Rich Type
               Influenza, Types A and B (epidemic)
               Psiticosis
               Varicellar Pneumonia
               Rickettseal Pneumonias
               Q Fever
               Toxoplasmosis
               Jaagsiekte—alveolar adenomatosis
         f. Spirochetal Infections
               Syphilis (spirocheta pallidum)
               Leptospirosis (Weil's Disease)
         g. Aspiration Pneumonitis
               1. Water— drowning
               2. Foods
               3. Lipoid Pneumonitis
               4. Kerosene Intoxication from aspiration
               5. Other irritating fluids
         h. Collagen Diseases
      2. Lung Abscess
      3. Pulmonary Tuberculosis
         a. Childhood first infection
         b. Adult type of reinfection
               Infiltrative—exudative types
               Acute lobar pneumonic type
                  caseous
                  "epituberculosis"
               Chronic diffuse interstitial fibrosis (tuberculous)
               Bronchial tuberculosis
               Miliary tuberculosis
               American Tuberculosis Association Classification
               Surgical treatment—artificial pneumothorax, phrenicotomy
               Artificial pneumoperitoneum
               Thoracoplasty; Pneumolysis
               Pneumonectomy
      4. Mycotic Infections
         a. Actinomycosis
         b. Blastomycosis
         c. Coccidioidomycosis
         d. Moniliasis
         e. Cryptococcosis (Torula)
         f. Histoplasmosis

        g. Maduromycosis
        h. Aspergillosis
        i. Penicillosis
        j. Spores of maple bark fungus
        k. Bagasse Disease

C. Collagen Diseases
D. Aspiration Irritant and Harmful materials into the lungs
    1. Lipoid Pneumonitis
    2. Kerosene Intoxication from Aspiration
    3. Gases
    4. Water—drowning
    5. Foods
E. Pneumoconiosis
    1. Silicosis
    2. Asbestosis
    3. Anthracosis
    4. Tremolite Talc
    5. Calicosis
    6. Siderosis—Arc-welder's lung
    7. Beryllium Pneumonitis
    8. Bariatosis
    9. Graphite Pneumoconiosis
   10. Byssinosis
F. Atelectasis
    1. Congenital
    2. Obstructive
        Massive—entire lung
        Lobar—single lobe
        Segmental—smaller segment
    3. Foreign body
    4. Bronchiogenic tumor
    5. Inspicated secretion—Massive Idiopathic Atelectasis
    6. Tuberculous granulations
    7. Disc-like Atelectases
    8. Anomalous fenestrated membrane
G. Emphysema and Cystic Disease
    1. Vesicular Emphysema
        a. Compensatory Expansion; (compensatory emphysema)
        b. Obstructive Expansion; (obstructive emphysema)
        c. Parenchymatous Vesicular Emphysema
        d. Bullous Emphysema
        e. Progressive Vesicular Pulmonary Emphysema
    2. Pulmonary Interstitial Emphysema
    3. Cystic Disease of the Lung
H. New Growth (Tumor) of Lung
    1. Primary Malignant
        a. Bronchiogenic Carcinoma
            Nodular type
            Diffuse (ulcerative) type
        b. Alveolar Cell (parenchymal) Carcinoma
        c. Sarcoma
    2. Metastatic
        a. Carcinoma
        b. Sarcoma
        c. Lymphoblastoma; Hodgkin's Disease; Lymphosarcoma, Leukemia
        d. Extramedullary Plasmocytoma
    3. Benign
        a. Bronchial Adenoma
        b. Cavernous Angioma
        c. Fibroma
        d. Tuberculoma
        e. Hamartoma
        f. Parasitic cysts
        g. Fluid Cysts
        h. Primary Amyloid Tumor
    4. Traumatic Pneumonia
    5. Traumatic Rupture Bronchus
    6. Explosive or "Blast" Effect on the Lung

        i. Paraffinoma
        j. Other rare forms; myoma, lipoma
        k. Infectious and vascular lesions resembling tumor
- I. Injuries to Lung
  - 1. Fractured ribs
    - a. Subcutaneous emphysema
  - 2. Hemorrhage into lung tissue
    - a. Gunshot and stab wounds
  - 3. Traumatic Pneumothorax
  - 4. Traumatic Pneumonia
- IV. Pleura
  - A. Thickening of pleura
    - 1. Dry pleurisy from infection
    - 2. Traumatic pleurisy
  - B. Generalized pleural effusion
    - 1. With pneumothorax
  - C. Localized pleural effusion
    - 1. Parietal
    - 2. Diaphragmatic
    - 3. Mediastinal (paravertebral)
    - 4. Interlobar
  - D. Pneumothorax
    - 1. Bilateral
    - 2. Artificial
    - 3. Spontaneous
    - 4. Interstitial Pulmonary Emphysema
    - 5. Traumatic
  - E. Tumors of the Pleura and Chest Wall
    - 1. Primary
    - 2. Secondary
    - 3. Pancoast Tumor
- V. Diaphragm
  - A. Contour
    - 1. Diaphragmatic adhesions
    - 2. "Scalloped" Diaphragm
  - B. Mobility
    - 1. Immobilization from Infection
      - a. Pleurisy—empyema
      - b. Peritonitis—subdiaphragmatic abscess
    - 2. Paralysis—phrenicotomy
  - C. Anomalies
    - 1. Eventration
    - 2. Diaphragmatic Hernia
    - 3. Congenital absence of diaphragm
    - 4. Diaphragmatic "Flutter"
- VI. Mediastinum—(Anatomy)
  - A. Mediastinitis
    - 1. Pyogenic
    - 2. Tuberculous
  - B. Adenopathy
    - 1. Hodgkin's Disease
    - 2. Tuberculosis
    - 3. Lymphosarcoma
    - 4. Metastatic malignancy
    - 5. Syphilis
    - 6. Boeck's Sarcoid
    - 7. Erythema Nodosum
    - 8. Periarteritis Nodosa
    - 9. Primary Amyloidosis
    - 10. Tularemia
    - 11. Mediastinal Hematoma
  - C. Primary Mediastinal Neoplasms
  - D. Thymus Gland
  - E. Substernal Thyroid
  - F. Pathology arising from the esophagus
  - G. Pathology arising from the spine
  - H. Mediastinal Emphysema

Chapter **XV**

NORMAL RESPIRATORY SYSTEM

The chest lends itself very readily to roentgenological examination; the air content of the lungs provides a medium of lesser density than the soft part structures which throws them into bold relief.

The position universally used for the primary examination of the chest is the erect anterior view; other accessory positions for demonstration of pathology in specific locations are posterior, right and left lateral; in upright, prone and lateral decubitus, (for technique see Manual of Roentgenological Technique). For unobscured examination of the upper lobe, the lordosis position is of value, (Zinn and Monroe). Much may be accomplished by the roentgenologic evaluation of pulmonary function through the correlation with clinical and other laboratory findings, (Barden and Comroe).

ROENTGEN ANATOMY

The lungs may be considered as two elastic bodies filling the pleural cavities on both sides, attached at the hilum regions only, and free to glide back and forth along the chest wall during respiration. They are divided by deep interlobar septa, on the left side into two and on the right into three lobes. These are covered by pleura which dips down to line the septa and is reflected back at the hilum to line the entire pleural cavity.

The "ligamentum pulmonale" is in reality not a ligament at all but is a vertical pleural fold running along the medial chest wall from the hilum to the diaphragm.

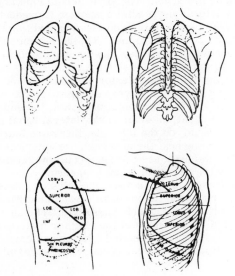

Fig. 146

TOPOGRAPHY OF THE LUNGS (Fig. 146). The location of the interlobar septa is very important in roentgen interpretation.

Anatomical descriptions based solely on autopsy material give all of the relationships too high; roentgenological and surgical observations on living individuals made during normal respiratory movements show these structures to be much lower.

On the right side the long, (oblique) interlobar fissure extends from a point posteriorly at the costovertebral articulation of the fifth thoracic vertebra downward and forward following the fifth rib or interspace to the mid-axillary line, where it dips down to a somewhat lower level following the sixth rib to its lower termination a short distance from the midline. A second, short fissure extends horizontally forward from the hilum region to the anterior chest wall at about the level of the fourth costochondral junction. These fissures divide the right lung into upper, middle and lower lobes.

On the left side a single, long (oblique) fissure leaves the vertebral column at a slightly higher level, (third to fifth rib) descending more obliquely along the fifth interspace or sixth rib. For all practical purposes the long (oblique) fissures on both sides may be considered as having similar locations. This divides the left lung into two lobes, an upper and a lower. A tongue-like prolongation of the lower portion of the upper lobe, or lingula, corresponds roughly to the middle lobe on the right. It is supplied by a separate bronchus.

Slight variations occur in the position of these fissures but the relationship described is the one most frequently encountered. The highly developed state of lung surgery makes accurate localization of surgical lesions of the lung imperative, (Brock), (Piersol's Anatomy).

Examination of autopsy specimens discloses that the lung fissures are often incomplete in their development. The major fissure of the left lung is complete in about 80% of all instances; the right major fissure about 70%. The middle lobe fissure on the right side is not complete in more than 1/3 of the instances, (Medlar).

The lung is further divided into smaller segments depending upon the bronchial subdivisions. Injection of the vascular supply of these segments with various colored gelatin solutions, clearly shows their extent and outline on the lung surface, (Brock). These are very important in recognition of areas of segmental involvement from infection, pneumonia or atelectasis.

THE BRONCHIAL TREE. (Figs. 147A, 147B and 147C.) The bronchial classification of Jackson and Huber is well suited to the needs of bronchoscopist,

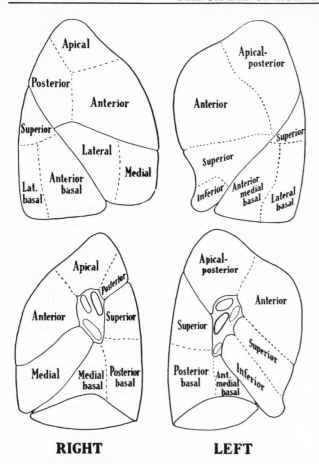

RIGHT   LEFT

Fig. 147A. The bronchopulmonary segments, shown in both anterolateral (above) and medial (below) aspects. The terminology used in this illustration as well as in Figs. 147B and 147C is that suggested by C. Jackson and J. F. Huber 9:319-1943 (Courtesy, Jackson and Jackson, Diseases of Nose, Throat and Ear. W. B. Saunders Co., 1945).

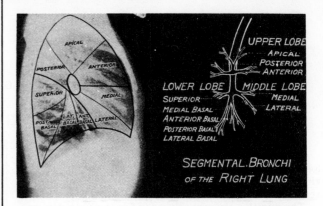

Fig. 147B. Segmental bronchi of right lung, showing relation to bronchopulmonary segments in right lateral bronchogram. (Courtesy, Jackson and Jackson, Diseases of Nose, Throat and Ear, W. B. Saunders Co., 1945).

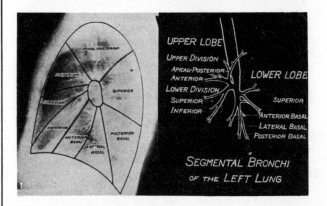

Fig. 147C. Segmental bronchi of _left_ lung, showing relation of bronchopulmonary segments in left lateral bronchogram. (Courtesy, Jackson and Jackson, Diseases of Nose, Throat and Ear, W. B. Saunders Co., 1945).

radiologist and surgeon. It has been adopted by the National Tuberculosis Association upon recommendation of the American Association of Thoracic Surgeons.

The trachea divides at the corina, into the right and left main stem bronchi. This is about the level of the fourth or fifth thoracic vertebra.

The right bronchus extends almost straight downward deviating only by a slight angle from the direction of the trachea, affording easier access for aspiration of material into this portion of the lung. A short distance from its origin, the right bronchus gives off an upper lobe branch which extends almost horizontally outward to supply the right upper lobe. It subdivides into an apical branch, which goes almost vertically upward, and posterior and anterior branches, which supply these portions of the upper lobe.

On the left side the bronchial branches to the upper lobe have substantially the same arrangement except that owing to the lower apical branches it is longer and also supplies the posterior portions.

The right bronchus, (the intermediate branch), continues downward where it divides into middle and lower lobe branches. The right middle lobe is supplied by lateral and medial branches; it presents itself to the chest wall only on these aspects so that there is no posterior branch. On the left side the lower portion of the upper lobe or lingula corresponds closely to the middle lobe on the right; it has branches to its superior and inferior portions. In the lower lobes the distribution is very similar: on the right side there are five bronchial branches, the superior, the medial basal, anterior basal, lateral basal and posterior basal; on the left side, there are four bronchial branches, the superior, the anterior-medial basal (combining these two segments) the lateral basal and the posterior basal branches.

The present highly developed status of lung surgery has rendered the recognition and identification of segmental involvement imperative. The surgical exterpation of segments of the lung for malignant disease and even for isolated tuberculous cavities, and infections is a matter of universal accomplishment.

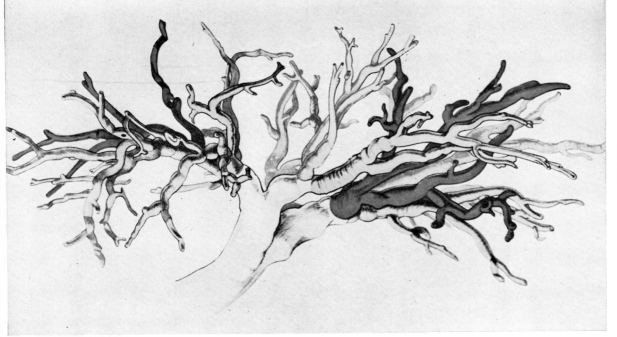

LEFT

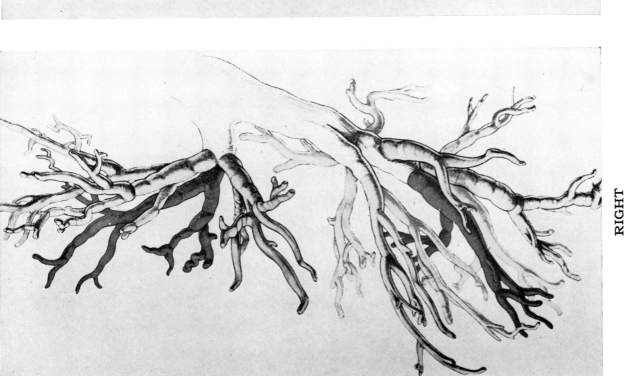

RIGHT

Legend—Drawing of a metal cast of the lungs showing bronchial branches for the various lobes, as viewed from in front—From R. C. Brock, Anatomy of the Bronchial Tree, Oxford University Press.

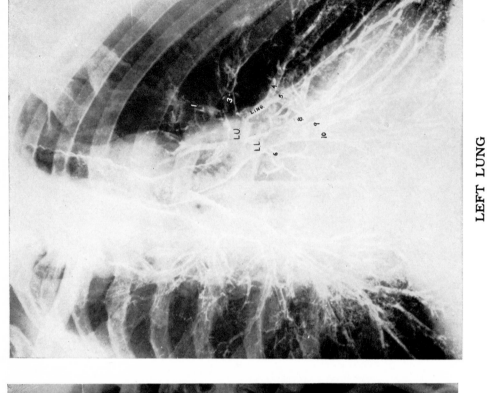

RIGHT LUNG

LOBES	SEGMENTS
Upper {	Apical (1) Posterior (2) Anterior (3)
Middle {	Lateral (4) Medial (5)
Lower {	Superior (6) Medial Basal (7) Anterior Basal (8) Lateral Basal (9) Posterior Basal (10)

LEFT LUNG

LOBES		SEGMENTS
Upper {	Upper Division	Apical-Posterior (1) Anterior (3)
	Lower (Lingular) Division	Superior (4) Inferior (5)
Lower		Superior (6) Anterior-Medial Basal (8) Lateral Basal (9) Posterior Basal (10)

Nomenclature of the bronchial tree and corresponding bronchopulmonary segments, from JACKSON and HUBER

For the identification of pathological involvement of the various lobes and their segments, roentgen examination is the most important means at our disposal. Bronchoscopic injection of the various bronchial subdivisions with radiopaque material followed by roentgen examination gives a clear, accurate indication of the distribution of the various bronchial subdivisions. For greatest accuracy, examination of segmental consolidation due to lobar pneumonia should be the best method of investigation. Lobar pneumonia consolidation neither reduces nor enlarges the size of the segment; it merely replaces the air-content with inflammatory exudate. The problem comes in being able to collect over a long period of time, sufficient cases of segmental consolidation from this cause.

Various injection methods utilized for this purpose, require removal of the lung from the chest in the cadaver, insertion of a catheter into the proper segment and injection of radiopaque solution.

Overdistension can usually be guarded against by mixing the radiopaque material with colored gelatin and carefully restricting the pressure so as to avoid distension.

The accompanying diagrams were redrawn from Kane I. J., Radiol. 59:229, 1952, by courtesy of author and publishers.

Bronchography*. Intratracheal injection of lipiodol renders the bronchial tree radio-opaque thus facilitating its roentgen examination.

The air content normally present in the trachea renders that structure readily examined by ordinary methods for displacement, constriction or other evidence of gross defect. For smaller lesions more detailed examination may be made by tracheography after filling the trachea with opaque oil. The technique of this procedure varies from that of bronchography; tracheography consists in filling the entire trachea momentarily for radiographic examination under general anaesthesia while bronchography consists in outlining the tracheal mucosa with opaqe oil under local anaesthesia, (for more detailed technique see Manual of Roentgenological Technique).

For bronchography the opaque oil, descending to the most dependent

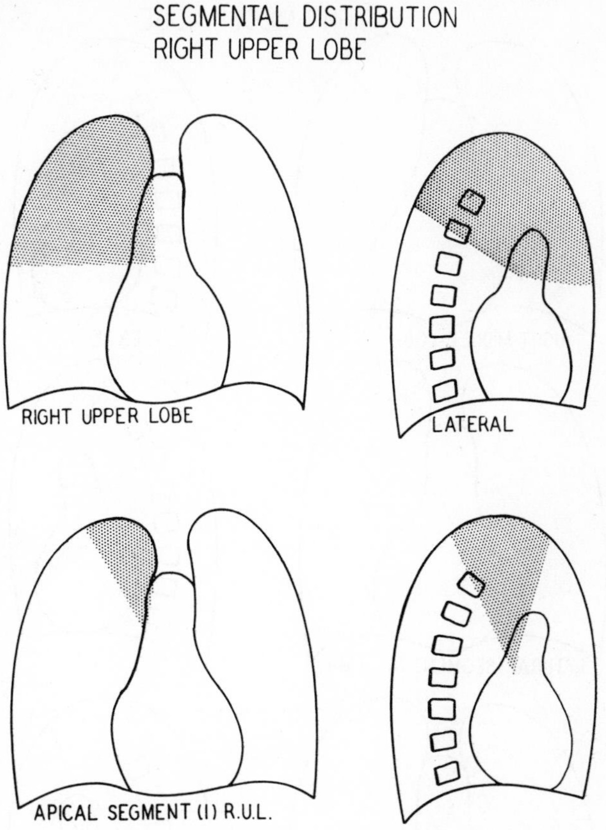

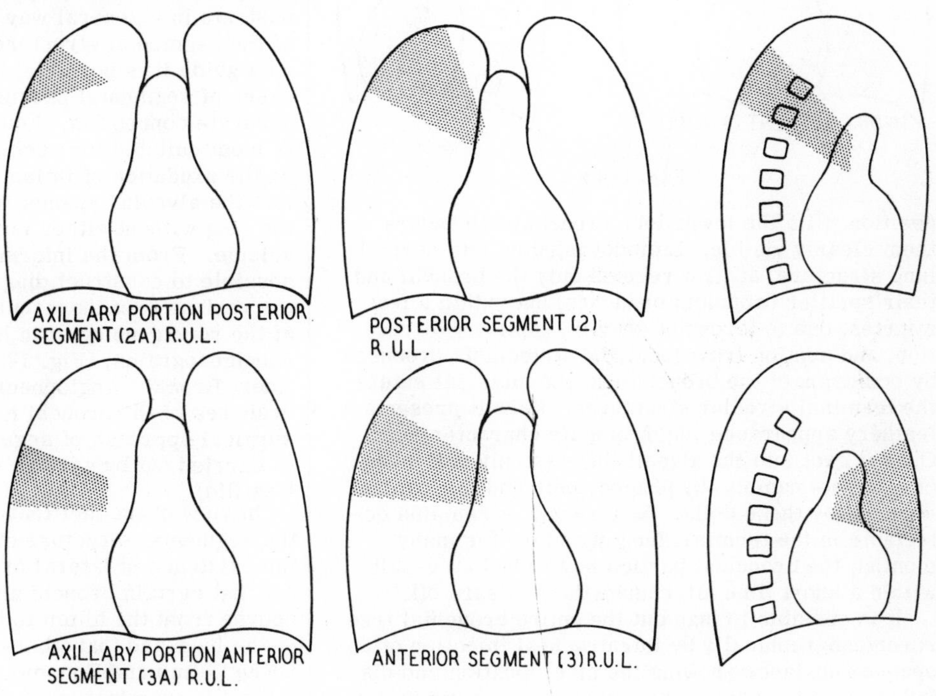

SEGMENTAL DISTRIBUTION
RIGHT UPPER LOBE

RIGHT UPPER LOBE — LATERAL

APICAL SEGMENT (I) R.U.L.

AXILLARY PORTION POSTERIOR SEGMENT (2A) R.U.L.

POSTERIOR SEGMENT (2) R.U.L.

AXILLARY PORTION ANTERIOR SEGMENT (3A) R.U.L.

ANTERIOR SEGMENT (3) R.U.L.

Fig. 148A

*An asterisk following any title indicates that roentgenographic reproductions illustrating this condition will be found in the pictorial supplement at the end of the chapter.

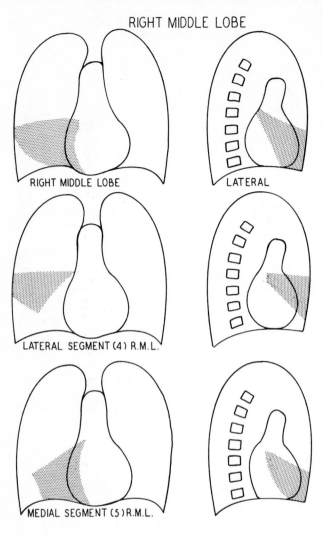

RIGHT MIDDLE LOBE

RIGHT MIDDLE LOBE   LATERAL

LATERAL SEGMENT (4) R.M.L.

MEDIAL SEGMENT (5) R.M.L.

Fig. 148B

position, fills the lower lobe bronchi and renders them clearly visible. Lipiodol injected into normal lung structure, at first reveals only the bronchi and their smaller bronchial branches, but within a few minutes, due to forces of gravity, capillary attraction, and suction from localized atelectasis produced by occlusion of the bronchioles, the material enters the terminal alveolar structures. Here it presents a feathery appearance which is quite characteristic. Once it gets into the alveoli there is only one means of escape—namely, by phagocytosis and mechanical removal by these cells. As a result, it remains detectable in the terminal lung structure for many months; the bronchial portion is coughed up usually within a short time after anaesthesia wears off.

It is possible to map out the entire bronchial tree roentgenographically by intratracheal injection of an opaque substance showing the size, location and distribution of the various branches (see accompanying plate). This means of examination finds its greatest usefulness in the detection and localization of bronchiectatic dilatation, and in bronchial obstruction from tumor or foreign body (q.v.). Numerous reports

are in the literature calling attention to the advisability of taking a "delayed" roentgenogram (1/2 to 1 hour) after injection of opaque media. It evidently requires time for viscid media to find its way into small pouch-like cavities. (Kane and Heiser; Abrams et al.) (For the technique of bronchographic examination see Manual of Roentgenological Technique.)

A new, water-soluble opaque medium, IODURON-B, has the advantage of rapid absorption so that the lung field becomes clear again in a very short time. In 45 minutes it is secreted in the urine producing very satisfactory pyelograms. It is 3.5 diiodpyridon-4-N acetic acid dissolved in the sodium salt of cellulose glycol acid ether. It is somewhat more irritating than lipiodol and requires more meticulous anaesthesia. It was reported by Fischer and Muelly. A similar water-soluble substance advocated by Cummins and Silver; and Holden and Crones, has definite advantages in bronchography.

Broncho-pulmonary Segments. The segmental structures have become very important because of the extension of surgery to these finer divisions of the lung. The combined efforts of the bronchoscopist, anatomist and surgeon have served to identify the bronchial branches and their corresponding lung segments (Jackson and Huber; Kramer and Glass; Niel, et al.; Brock; Boyden). Now it becomes the problem of the radiologist to identify and recognize pathology in these segments from the roentgenogram before surgical exploration. Making roentgen examinations of excised lungs after injection of the smaller branches of pulmonary arteries or terminal bronchial branches with radiopaque material will serve to demonstrate in a general way the size, form and location of the segmental structures. Using this information as a guide it is possible, by comparison with clinical cases of segmental pneumonia, to attain a much more accurate conception. Lobar pneumonic consolidation is most suitable for such a study since it is produced by the exudation of inflammatory cells and serum into the alveolar spaces, replacing the air content of the lung without either increase or decrease in lung volume. From the information thus obtained it is possible to construct diagramatic representations of the various bronchovascular segment for the guidance of the roentgenologist in his interpretation of chest roentgenograms, (Fig. 148), (Kane; Temple and Evans; Ader; Brock). Angiopneumography of special vascular branches of the bronchi has aided in the diagnosis of surgical approach of segmental lung pathology. This is carried out by cardiac catheterization, (Cicero and Castillo).

In view of the fact that "many authors in studying the segmental structure of the lung have recognized the existence of lateral or axillary regions, and point out that certain bronchi and arteries run a true lateral course from the hilum to the lateral or axillary parts of the lung, and that others deny their existence at all," DiGuglielmo and Bonomo of Stockholm have undertaken the examination of 500 cases of segmental lesions with an involvement of lateral subsegments of the lung, their constancy and radiological appearance. Correlation of roentgenological with other findings would indicate that the accompanying figures (148 E to L) represent most constant findings.

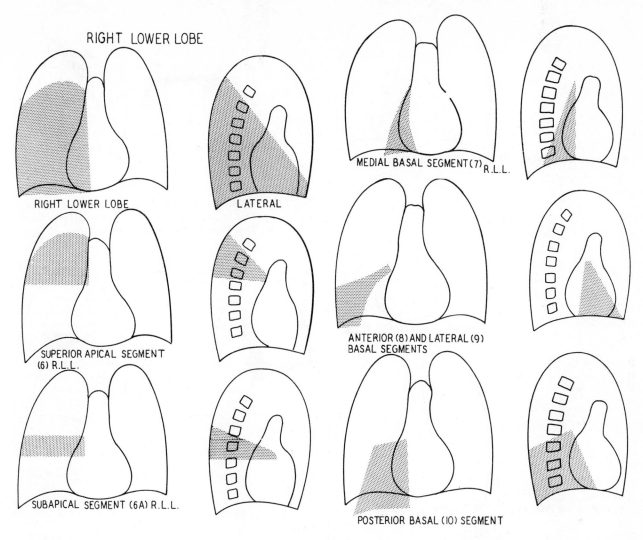

RIGHT LOWER LOBE

RIGHT LOWER LOBE

LATERAL

MEDIAL BASAL SEGMENT (7) R.L.L.

SUPERIOR APICAL SEGMENT (6) R.L.L.

ANTERIOR (8) AND LATERAL (9) BASAL SEGMENTS

SUBAPICAL SEGMENT (6A) R.L.L.

POSTERIOR BASAL (10) SEGMENT

Fig. 148C

ROENTGEN EXAMINATION OF LUNG FIELDS (Fig. 149). On roentgenographic examination the thoracic cavity is divided in the midline by the mediastinum. The mediastinal shadow is produced by the superimposed shadows of the thoracic spine behind, the sternum in front, and all intervening mediastinal structures, such as the heart and aorta, the trachea, the esophagus, and all associated lymphatics. The lung fields appear as two large radiolucent areas on either side of the mediastinal shadow. The bronchi, with their surrounding structures, produce branching linear markings in the lung fields, as they progress toward the periphery.

For purpose of study and description the lung field may be divided into three vertical zones, (Dunham); the inner one-third containing the hilum shadow, the middle one-third containing the larger bronchial branches, and the peripheral one-third containing the smaller bronchioles and parenchymal structure of the lung (Fig. 149).

The bronchial branches are maintained in a widely open condition by their cartilaginous rings.

Owing to their air content they produce linear markings of decreased density on the roentgenogram. They are accompanied in their course by blood vessels and lymphatics which divide and subdivide, becoming smaller and smaller as they progress from the hilum to the periphery. These structures, by reason of their blood and lymph content, produce shadows of greater density than that of the air-containing lung. They are supported by a surrounding peribronchial connective tissue framework which also adds its density to the formation of the linear markings of the lung. Since all of these structures are peribronchial in location, they are referred to as peribronchial markings. Or, since the chief structures concerned are the bronchi and the vascular structures, they are likewise frequently referred to as, "bronchovascular" markings. They all go to make up the lung markings seen in the roentgenogram.

Since the blood vessels are the densest structures, they contribute most to the lung markings seen on the roentgenogram. The anatomical arrangement

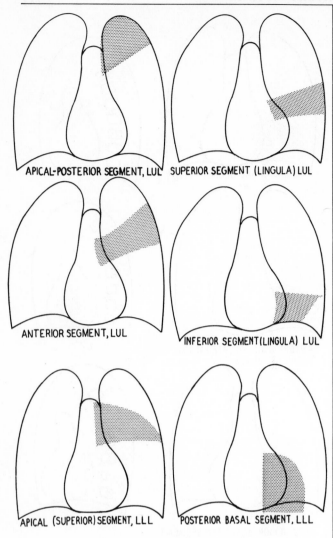

APICAL-POSTERIOR SEGMENT, LUL   SUPERIOR SEGMENT (LINGULA) LUL

ANTERIOR SEGMENT, LUL   INFERIOR SEGMENT (LINGULA) LUL

APICAL (SUPERIOR) SEGMENT, LLL   POSTERIOR BASAL SEGMENT, LLL

Fig. 148D

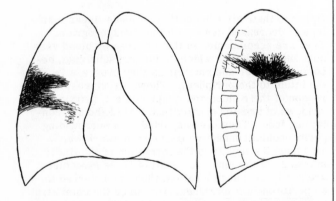

Fig. 148E. Consolidation of the lateral subsegment
of right upper lobe.
    a) PA. Band-shape density with clear cut
lower margin corresponding to horizontal fissure.
(RUL) b) Lateral. The opacity has a median location
and superimposes the point where two fissures meet.

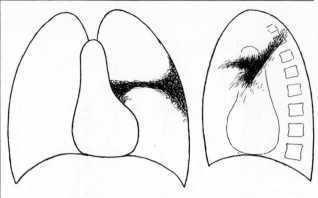

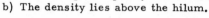

Fig. 148F. Consolidation of later subsegment of LUL.
(LUL) a) The triangular opacity is laterally located.
       b) The density lies above the hilum.

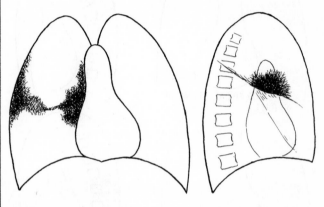

Fig. 148G. Consolidation of lateral subsegment of
R.U.L.
(RUL) PA and Lateral. Density is situated anteriorly above the horizontal fissure and corresponds to the
lateral branch of the anterior segment.

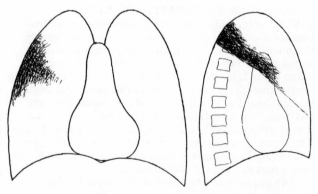

Fig. 148H. Consolidation of lateral subsegment of
R.U.L. PA, Lateral. The opacity is in contact only
with the oblique fissure and does not reach horizontal
fissure anteriorly. It corresponds to lateral branch
of the posterior segment.

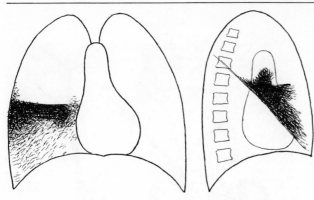

Fig. 148I. Consolidation of lateral segment of middle lobe. (R.M.L.) PA and Lateral.

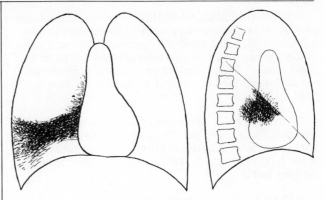

Fig. 148K

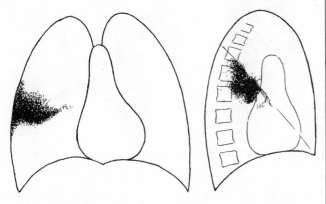

Fig. 148J. Consolidation of lateral subsegment of apical part of R.L.L.

(RLL) a) PA. Irregular opacity laterally situated and independent from horizontal fissure.

b) Lateral. The opacity is triangular and situated behind hilum. Directed superior from horizontal fissure and separated from thoracic wall posteriorly.

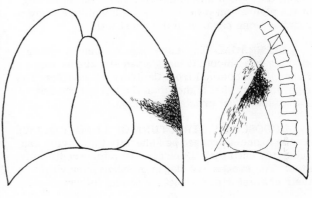

Fig. 148L

of the lung structures has been the subject of extensive, pains-taking research (Lodge). It has been found that the arteries accompanying the bronchi may vary in number, size, and distribution, but that as a general rule they are surprisingly consistent in their development, so much so that they can often be identified on the roentgenogram. "Pulmonary veins do not accompany arteries, possess no valves are fewer than arteries, have a lower total capacity than arteries and convey arterial blood. Near the heart they undergo the same rhythmical contraction as the heart itself. There are no anastamoses (with each other) in the pulmonary arterial tree."

HILUM. In the hilum region all of these structures are large, consequently their shadows are heavier. The hilum shadows present themselves as dense radiating structures on either side of the mediastinum near the center of the thoracic cavity. Normally, they occupy the zone in the inner one-third of the chest. Ordinarily the hilum glands play a very inconspicuous part in the production of this shadow.

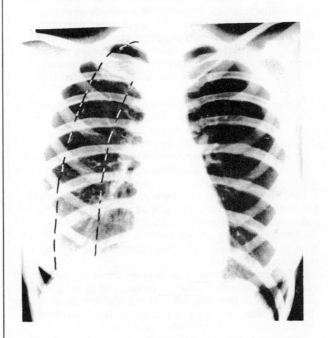

Fig. 149

PERIBRONCHIAL MARKINGS. As the bronchi and peribronchial structures proceed toward the periphery they divide and subdivide, producing in the roentgenogram markings which become finer and finer in appearance. These smaller peribronchial markings should be confined to the middle zone of the lung field.

PARENCHYMA. As the peribronchial markings progress to the very periphery of the lung, they feather out into imperceptibility as the parenchyma of the lung is reached. This forms the outer zone of the lung fields.

PLEURA. Ordinarily the pleural covering of the normal lung cannot be visualized in the roentgenogram; only when inflammation results in thickening of the pleura can it be seen as a ribbonlike shadow running along parallel to the chest wall.

DIAPHRAGM. The diaphragm is seen on either side, as two smooth dome-shaped structures separating the abdominal from the thoracic cavities. The right is somewhat higher than the left but the left shows somewhat greater excursion.

MICROSCOPIC STRUCTURE OF LUNG (Fig. 150). As the bronchi proceed peripherally they divide and subdivide until their branches are microscopic in size. The successive stages of subdivision with their characteristic structure are as follows:

Bronchi— larger air passages having cartilaginous rings which divide into
Bronchioles— smaller air passages having cartilaginous rings which divide further into,
Br— Respiratory Bronchioles— minute bronchial subdivisions, having a muscular coat but no cartilaginous rings. They are called respiratory bronchioles because of the atria or air sacs which spring directly from them. These in turn terminate in,
d.a.— Ductus Alveolaris—small ducts which lead to the atria; and,
a— Atria— vestibules of air sacs,
s.al.— Sacculi Alveolares— air sacs,
c—Alveoli Pulmonum— terminal alveoli of the lung or air cells.

As these bronchi and their subdivisions progress toward the periphery they are accompanied by the pulmonary and bronchial vessels and lymphatics.

The pulmonary artery carries venous blood to the lung parenchyma for aeration, constituting the main pulmonary circulation.

The bronchial artery is derived from the systemic circulation, carries arterial blood, and is embedded in the bronchial walls, providing nourishment to these structures. This is one of the few locations in the body provided with two circulations.

At each bronchial division there is a corresponding division of the vessels and lymphatic channels. Progressing outward from the hilum the bronchial

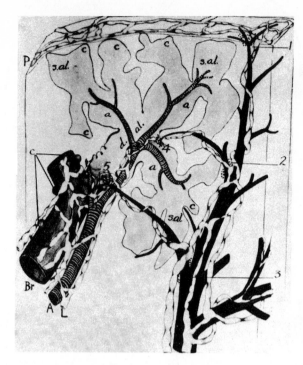

Diagrammatic representation of Primary Lobule

—From William Snow Miller

Fig. 150

artery supplies the bronchial tree with nourishment out as far as the respiratory bronchiole; from this point peripherally the pulmonary artery supplies by far the greatest portion of nourishment to the lung tissue. The two circulations mix in a plexus of capillaries which completely surround the terminal respiratory structures.

The lymph flow in the lung is in two directions; from the region of the respiratory bronchioles there is one system of lymphatic drainage inward through the lymphatic channels which accompany the bronchi inward to the hilum glands, the other outward from the region of the respiratory bronchioles toward the periphery, over the pleural surface of the lung and thence back to end at the hilum region of the lung also. Lymphoid deposits are present in the crotches of the subdividing bronchioles; lymphatic vessels, however, do not extend to the alveolar wall.

Such a terminal bronchiole with its final subdivisions, and terminal air sacs, together with its accompanying blood vessels, lymphatics, and surrounding peribronchial connective tissue is called a "primary lobule," (Wm. Snow Miller, The Lung, Chas. C. Thomas, Pub.).

ANOMALIES OF DEVELOPMENT. Anomalous development may occur in any of the lung structures. There may be agenesis of the lung, with a) complete aplasia, b) a tiny pocketing of the trachea but no lung tissue, or, c) extreme hypoplasia with the bronchi fully developed but small, ending in a fleshy mass without lobe formation lying in the mediastinum (Deweese and Howard). Or there may be atresia of the trachea or bronchi with development of congenital bronchiectasis or lung cysts; there may be defects in the diaphragm or complete absence of one side. Anomalous development of the lobes and interlobar septa may occur in any location in the lungs. Two such variations are commonly seen (Fig. 150A): the Azygos Lobe (A) (Bendick and Wessler), being a subdivision of the right upper lobe along its medial side by persistence of a cordlike remnant of the azygos vein; the other common anomalous development is the Accessory Inferior Lobe (I) indicated as a triangular shadow in the medial side of the base of the lung. An anomalous middle lobe has been reported on the left side (Hardman). Instances have been reported of simultaneous occurrence of an area of congenital cystic disease of the lung with failure of communication with the normal bronchi with associated blood supply by aberrant arteries from the aorta directly to the lung parenchyma, (Lalli, et al.). This gives rise to severe pulmonary sequestration with signs and symptoms which are relieved only by operation. Similar instances have been reported by Bruwer, et al., and Jensen and Wolff.

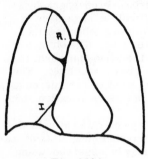

Fig. 150A

Pectus excavatum, a funnel-shaped deformity of the chest with the lower end of the sternum markedly depressed, and pectus carinatum, the so-called "keeled breast" or "chicken breast" are two relatively common deformities of the chest. The former may be so great as to interfere with proper function, it is amenable to corrective surgery; the latter rarely needs correction. Neither deformity is well visualized roentgenographically without application of barium-impregnated gauze over the chest wall to outline the deformity.

PHYSIOLOGY OF RESPIRATION

The lungs may be considered as elastic inflatable bags, fixed at the hilum, free to move elsewhere and to expand within closed thoracic cavities. The trachea and bronchi communicate directly with the inside of the bag permitting air to enter. The lungs are in close contact with the thoracic wall at all points; the "pleural cavity" is only a potential space, it does not exist unless it is filled with something such as air (pneumothorax) or fluid (hydrothorax). During normal respiration the thoracic cavity is enlarged by muscular contraction; the lungs, being closely adherent (cohesion) to the chest wall, are pulled outward with it. Being elastic they expand to fill the enlarged

thoracic cavity. During expiration the air is forced out by the "milking" action of the lungs and the elastic recoil of the lungs and thoracic wall. Forces which tend to aid in expansion of the lungs during inspiration are: the muscular contraction causing enlargement of the thoracic cavity, negative pressure in the thoracic cavity, and cohesion of the parietal and visceral pleurae. Factors which tend to hinder inflation of the lungs and which must be overcome are: friction of air as it passes into the constantly diminishing air passages, and the natural elasticity of the lung. Factors favoring expulsion of air in expiration are: elastic recoil of lung and chest wall, together with muscular action. The factor which has to be overcome during expiration is, the friction of air in being pressed out of smaller structures of the lung.

RESPIRATORY FUNCTION. The principle function of the lung is the aeration of the blood; the two structures concerned in this, the alveolar air and the capillary network, come into close relationship in the terminal air cells. There is still some controversy as to just how this is accomplished. The alveolus is lined by a continuous ring of flat epithelial cells as demonstrated in the microscopic sections shown by Wm. Snow Miller, from a case of acute pneumonia in which a zone of edema had completely lifted off the epithelial ring.

In viewing the microscopic structures of the alveoli it seems hardly possible that the thin delicate wall between two air cells could be composed of two layers of flat epithelium for the lining membranes of the alveoli, with intervening interstitial tissue in which the blood capillaries are located. Yet that this is the case has been amply demonstrated by cases in which this space has been attacked by inflammation such as virus pneumonia, or edema.

The blood capillaries form a sheath covering the alveoli on either side, presenting their epithelial lining in close contact with that of the respiratory lining of the alveolus. Gaseous exchange between the blood stream and alveolar air takes place readily by atomic diffusion through these two membranes.

Heavy strands of elastic tissue stretch like guy wires over the alveoli limiting their distention during inspiration and assisting in their elastic recoil, during expiration. The capillary network lying over the alveoli is in turn protected from squeezing by two adjacent over-distended alveoli by this regulatory mechanism. The best indication of what might happen without the protection afforded by the elastic tissue to the alveoli is the observation of the results of their over-distention as seen in diseases such as emphysema in which the capillary network is so completely squeezed by the enlarged alveoli that they are almost obliterated.

The capillaries are directly exposed to the changes in pressure in the pleural cavity however; that these changes during respiration, aid the circulation of the blood through the capillaries there can be no doubt. The decrease in intra-thoracic pressure during inspiration, applied directly to the capillary network, increases their engorgement, and causes temporary stasis, thus favoring aeration of the blood.

By this means the blood volume of the lung can be increased 50%. The air volume is increased by even a greater percent so that the roentgenogram of the chest during full inspiration shows greater illumination and brilliancy; during expiration the ratio of air volume to blood volume decreases so that the roentgenogram taken in this phase of respiration loses its brilliancy.

If anything should interfere with the normal circulation of the blood through the lung, such as an embolus, infarction of the involved segment of the lung may take place. The circulation of the lung is peculiar in that it is one of the few places provided with two circulatory systems: the bronchial from the systemic circulation and the pulmonary confined to the lungs. These two circulations mix in a capillary network surrounding the terminal bronchioli and air cells. If the bronchial circulation remains intact it may be sufficient to maintain the nutrition of the lung structure and necrosis may not take place; if on the other hand, infarction involves the circulation from both bronchial (systemic) and pulmonary vessels, necrosis will result.

The alveoli communicate with adjacent air cells by small openings or pores of the same lobule; these form a means of colateral ventilation which probably prevents collapse of small segments of the lung in the case of minor blockages of the smaller air passages.

In the face of edema or inflammation, these pores are soon clogged and this mechanism is of no avail. Atelectasis of small segments of the lungs which follows occlusion of small bronchial branches is evidence of the fallibility of these openings to prevent segmental collapse.

Occlusion of the larger air passages is followed by atelectasis of the involved portion of the lung, by simple process of absorption of the entrapped air by the circulating blood.

The lymphatic vessels lie in the interstitial spaces but do not form a capillary sheath about the alveoli; at the level of the ductuli alveolares they anastomose with the perivascular lymphatics and accompany them to the pleural surface. They all empty into the right thoracic duct which, because of its small calibre constitutes a "bottle neck" in the absorption of any great amount of exudate in the lungs or pleura.

The water and electrolyte balance is maintained between the circulating blood and interstitial tissue of the lung, as elsewhere in the body by the simple expedient of thirst. Excessive amounts of water are rapidly removed from the lung by direct absorption into the circulation with little if any change in the lymph flow.

The lymphatics maintain the proteid balance by returning proteid lost through edema or inflammation back into the blood stream. Any edema in the lungs leads at once to pronounced increase in lymph flow. Anoxia is one of the main conditions which favors edema, and since edema itself results in anoxia by filling the alveoli and obstructing the access of air to the respiratory epithelium it is obvious that a vicious circle is soon established. The rapidity with which edema of the lungs once started progresses to almost complete obscuring of the lung, is very evident in the roentgenogram.

The question of peristalsis in the bronchi and trachea is one which has never been definitely settled. Fluoroscopic observation of peristaltic contractions has never been made (Fleischer). A series of tracheal contractions during cough have been demonstrated roentgenographically, but these give more the impression of spasmodic contractions to expel mucus (DiRienzo). (See editorial by R. P. Barden.)

RESTORATION OF FUNCTION AFTER OPERATIVE PROCEDURES. In recent years advance in technical operative methods has made possible operative resection of the involved area of the lung (Graham). It devolves upon the roentgenologist, however, to localize closely the areas of lung involvement. This localization must be done by lobes since the operative procedure consists in removal of the affected lobes entirely. For this purpose bronchography is essential. It is no more difficult or hazardous to remove the right middle and lower lobes together than to remove only the lower lobe. The oblique views serve well to outline the various bronchi thus enabling localization to the lobes they supply. The lingula of the left upper lobe must be considered as a separate lobe for purposes of this localization since it is frequently involved.

Ware and Strauss have demonstrated a method by which reexpansion of the remaining lung after operative removal of a segment may be observed, using metal clips fastened to the lung margins.

Bronchography is especially valuable for determination of the reexpansion of the remainder of the lung after surgical removal of a lobe or segment (q.v.).

A study of compensatory reexpansion of this type by Boyer would indicate that the remaining bronchi with their associated parenchymal structures fan out and expand to fill up the space produced by removal of a segment of the lung from whatever cause. As a general rule following loss of the upper lobe, the remaining lower lobe bronchi fan out into the upper lobe space, whereas in lower lobe deficiency the remaining upper lobe branches swing down into the space left vacant by loss of the lower lobe. The greatest suction force is exerted on the structures immediately adjacent to the defect. The structures at the periphery are less restrained and freer to move, whereas those at the hilum are more restricted; as a result the suction force is greatest on most pendulous portions of the lung and the bronchi are displaced accordingly. Even the main stem bronchi may be displaced upward or downward depending upon the degree and character of the force exerted. Lung biopsy of diffuse pulmonary disease processes of the pleura or lung tumors is no longer the formidable surgical problem which it formerly was. Theodos, et al. have pointed out the relatively simple procedure which can be carried out through a small incision under local anaesthesia. The benefit derived therefrom may be decisive in the diagnosis and subsequent procedure.

DIFFERENTIAL DIAGNOSIS OF PULMONARY LESIONS. The differential diagnosis of lung pathology depends upon an analysis of the roentgenogram and correlation with the clinical history even more so than that of the bony structure (q.v.); so much so that it is hazardous in any instance to make a diagnosis in any condition without correlation of the pathological findings with the history and clinical manifestations.

Similar elements in analysis are essential to those considered under the diagnosis of bone lesions.

Roentgen diagnosis of pulmonary lesions required: 1) detection of pathology in the roentgenogram which presupposes a thorough acquaintance with the normal, 2) its proper evaluation, requiring a profound knowledge of the various lung changes resulting from various diseases, 3) correlation of roentgen manifestations with various elements of the history and clinical findings and, 4) an exercise of judgment as to the greatest degree of probability under the circumstances.

The lung is made up of so many varying tissues, of both the conventional variety, found elsewhere in the body, and of special varieties peculiar to the lung structures itself; subject to so many types of reaction, from infection, injury and malignant disease; requiring such varied periods for the course of the diseases, and exciting such varying types of reaction for the healing of the disease processes that only a profound knowledge of the mechanism of diseases can a differential diagnosis be reached with any degree of accuracy, (for a comprehensive study of the mechanism of disease the reader is referred to "Pathologic Physiology: Mechanisms of Disease," by W. A. Sodeman and his collaborators).

Fibrous tissue is the universal reparative structure of the lung. It responds to toxicity of infections, to the destruction of trauma; it seeks to limit detrimental processes and sometimes by excessive deposits defeats its own purpose. A critical analysis of the various conditions presents various methods of fibrous tissue response. Mitchum and Brady have analysed their roentgenographic appearance.

Chapter XVI

PATHOLOGY OF THE RESPIRATORY ORGANS

LARYNX

The laryngeal cartilages and other soft tissue structures are well outlined by the surrounding air (Fig. 151A & B). Ordinary roentgenographic examination of the larynx gives the greatest information in the lateral position, whereas, examination by the body section method is best suited to the postero-anterior position.

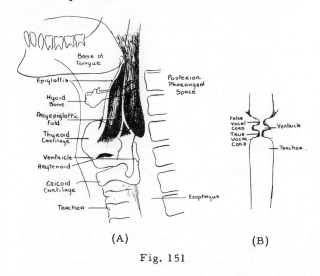

(A)   (B)

Fig. 151

In the lateral position (A) two examinations are made, one during phonation, pronouncing the letter a, a, ----, the other during forced expiration (valsalva exercise). Structures to be identified are:

Larger cartilages forming the framework of the larynx, thyroid and cricoid cartilage and the other smaller cartilages if calcified.

Ventricle, the air-filled space between the true and false cords.

Arytenoid cartilages, the small pyramidal cartilage giving attachment to the cords.

Epiglottis, the large spoon-shaped cartilaginous structure projecting upward over the glottis and protecting it during deglutition.

Aryepiglottic fold, or fold of mucous membrane between the aryetenoid cartilages and epiglottis.

Vestibule, the space just above the epiglottis.

Pyriform sinuses, the pouchlike structures which extend downward on either side of the larynx.

Vellecula, the two small crescentic pouches higher up.

Trachea, the air passage below the larynx extending to the lung.

Triticeous cartilages, small round or oval cartilages in the lateral hypothyroid ligament, (Grossman).

Other adjacent structures, posterior pharyngeal wall, base of tongue, hyoid bone.

In the postero-anterior position, (B) body section roentgenography gives most information. The entire air passage way is well outlined in "cross section." Two constrictions are produced by the false and true cords with intervening rounded area for the ventricle. On either side the pyriform sinuses may be clearly visible. Lower down the air passage again widens as it passes into the trachea.

Conditions in which laryngeal examination is helpful in diagnosis are:

1. Tumors of pharynx--projecting out into pharyngeal space.
   a. Papilloma--visualization of actual outline of growth.
   b. Carcinoma; Lymphoblastoma--infiltration laryngeal wall.
2. Paralysis of vocal cords--failure to visualize ventricle.
3. Laryngocele--large air-filled pouch on either side of the larynx.
4. Retropharyngeal infiltration; abscess or tumor bulging of the retropharyngeal structures into pharynx.
5. Infections--failure to visualize ventricles.
   a. Tuberculosis
   b. Syphilis
   c. Diphtheria.

For a more detailed consideration of the technique of laryngeal and hypopharyngeal examination and demonstration of lesions in these regions see articles by Welin.

TRACHEA

FOREIGN BODIES IN TRACHEA (Fig. 151C). Disclike foreign bodies, such as coins, lodging in the trachea, tend to assume an "on edge" position in the sagittal plane. This is due to the fact that the cartilaginous tracheal rings are complete with the exception of the posterior portions where the defect is bridged across with elastic tissue; therefore the only position in which the tracheal diameter can be increased is in the anteroposterior direction. Gianturco and Miller have described a new instrument for insertion of a catheter into the upper trachea to facilitate the rapid injection of contrast medium into the lung. They used Dionosil - oily which was absorbed within one week. Disclike foreign bodies, lodging in the esophagus, on the other hand, assume a "flat" position in the frontal plane; only very rarely have disc-

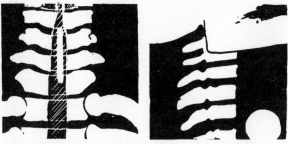

Fig. 151C

like intratracheal foreign bodies been reported as lodged in a frontal plane. This is due to the fact that the esophagus is flattened from before backward, making the transverse diameter the widest dimension. Open safety pins and other foreign bodies of this type may also take on similar positions but sharp-pointed objects may be retained in any position.

TRACHEAL DISPLACEMENT.   The trachea, because of its air content and the surrounding soft tissues, shows in the anteroposterior roentgenogram as a dark streak superimposing the cervical spine. In newborn infants it measures 3.5 to 4.5 mm., (Donaldson and Tompsett), whereas in the adult it measures about 1.5 cm. wide in the midline contained within the upper mediastinal shadow. Ordinarily the tracheal cartilages are not visible, in later life they may become visible due to calcification.

The trachea may be displaced from its normal midline position either by scar tissue retraction resulting from some adjacent inflammatory process, pressure from a tumor or growth, or by variation in intrathoracic pressure on the two sides from atelectasis. It may be pushed over by a new growth or hyperplasia of an otherwise normal structure.   Enlargement of the thyroid gland may cause considerable degree of tracheal displacement; it is always advisable therefore to determine by roentgenographic examination any deviation of the trachea from its midline position before goitre operation.

Retropharyngeal abscess may cause marked forward displacement of the pharynx and trachea.

TRACHEAL COMPRESSION (Fig. 152).   Compression of the trachea from hyperplasia of adja-

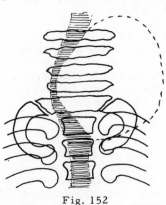

Fig. 152

cent organs or from new growths is usually readily demonstrable. Tracheal compression from thymic enlargement in infants may be very difficult to demonstrate; it can best be shown in the lateral chest roentgenogram. Tumors of the thyroid and especially substernal lobulations of the gland may cause pressure on the trachea easily demonstrated roentgenographically. Such enlargements of the gland or exten-

sion into the substernal region can be readily seen at roentgen examination. Acute hemorrhage into the thyroid gland in adenomatous goitre may cause rapid enlargement of the shadow of the thyroid with dangerous or fatal tracheal compression. Occasionally, pressure on the trachea from goitre, maintained for a long period of time, may result in permanent collapse of the trachea from pressure atrophy of the cartilaginous structures requiring tracheotomy and the permanent wearing of a tracheotomy tube.

CONGENITAL ANOMALIES.   Congenital absence, deformity, maldevelopment, or fusion of the tracheal rings may result in difficult respiration. Deficiency of the cartilaginous rings posteriorly in the newborn may result in tracheal collapse with each inspiration without the presence of any other constricting factor.

Buckling of the trachea in young infants may be due to soft cartilaginous rings. This gives rise to alarming inspiratory dyspnea. Atresia is more common in the bronchial region (Evans). Fenestrated membranes covering the tracheal orifice is another anomaly which has been noted.

Cutaneous sinuses in the lateral cervical region caused by bronchial cleft cysts occur above the hyoid bone; the thymopharyngeal duct is the origin of such sinuses if they occur below the hyoid bone, (Parsons).

Injection of the small duct in the neck will show the sinus to be either complete, communicating with the esophagus internally, forming a fistula to the outside or incomplete showing either internal or external orifice. Tracheography, (pp. 225 and 321) may be most helpful in detection of pressure defects from adjacent abnormal structures; since these are most diagnostic of aortic anomalies and pressure defects from abberant vessels such as right aortic arch, left ligamentum arteriosum anomalous innominate or left common carotid and abberant right subclavian, this particular method of examination is confined largely to vascular lesions, (q.v.).

Thickening of the tracheal wall with deposit of bony plaques have been demonstrated by Carr and Olsen by use of tomography. This rare but important condition produces cough, expectoration, hemoptysis, fever and attacks of obstructive pneumonitis.

TUMORS OF TRACHEA AND LARYNX. Papillary growths and other tumors springing from the tracheal wall may project not only forward into the lumen of the trachea but posteriorly, encroaching upon the esophagus as well.   Esophageal examination with barium mixture, in the oblique position, will disclose the impression of the tumor mass on the esophagus. Such tumors are rare in the trachea but more common in the larynx. Laryngoceles have been reported bulging outward from the larynx.

Small tracheal diverticula have been reported, (Drymalski, et al; Addington, et al).

BRONCHI

BRONCHIAL PATHOLOGY

BRONCHIAL IRRITATION. Bronchial irritation from inhalation of irritating and corrosive gases, such as nitrogen pentoxide, sulphur dioxide, etc., gives a most striking example of increase in the number and size of the lung markings. This is due, in the acute stage, to blood vessel dilatation from active congestion and edema from the irritation; in the later stages, after ulceration has been replaced with fibrosis, the increase in lung markings persist from the fibrosis. There may be no apparent parenchymatous changes and yet the disability may be very real and permanent. Inhalation of flames in a fire produces a similar picture with even greater indication of edema. (See lung involvement.)

The caustic action of zinc chloride contained in the smoke which is used to produce a smoke screen, when inhaled is evident roentgenographically as an intense congestion and edema of the bronchi and lungs. This may be severe enough to cause death by liberation of corrosive acid substances, (Whitaker).

BERYLLIUM used as an alloy in manufacturing processes has lead to many instances of poisoning. Inhalation of fine particles of this metal during the fusing process causes intense irritation of the skin, eyes, nose, throat and bronchial mucous membrane. Roentgenographically the hilum shadows are accentuated and a sunburst of heavy markings radiates outward into both lung fields producing a more intense reaction than any other condition. Recovery leaves evidence of pulmonary fibrosis; (q. v.).

ACUTE RESPIRATORY INFECTION* (Fig. 153). Perhaps the most common type of bronchial pathology with which we have to deal is bronchitis associated with acute respiratory infection. Since the peribronchial markings are formed by the bronchi, blood vessels, lymphatics, and peribronchial connective tissue, it is obvious that any pathological condition which would increase the density of any of these structures would cause an accentuation of their appearance in the roentgenogram. The exact nature of the causative agent cannot always be determined, but it is usually possible to differentiate conclusively between such conditions as bronchial inflammation and passive pulmonary congestion. In acute bronchitis there is an accentuation of the peribronchial lung markings of both lungs, usually most pronounced in

the hilum regions and lower lobes; the hilum shadows become enlarged extending into the middle zone of the lung field; the smaller bronchial markings, by reason of their accentuation from inflammation may extend well to the periphery of the lung into the third or outer zone.

Acute respiratory infection may be caused by either bacterial or viral infection; these cannot be differentiated when they involve the bronchial structures only.

If confined more or less to the larger bronchial branches, the main manifestation is seen as an enlargement of the hilum shadows. The appearance produced in bronchitis is an accentuation of the larger trunk markings, especially those supplying the lower lobes, radiating downward and outward as linear shadows. Adenopathy of the hilum glands can also cause enlargement of the hilum shadow but in this instance the appearance is that of more rounded nodular structures than one of radiating character.

BRONCHIOLITIS. At times infection seems to have a predilection for the terminal bronchioles causing widespread roles, without distinctive roentgen findings. After prolonged observation of such cases one is forced to the conclusion that this is primarily a clinical diagnosis in which roentgen examination plays little if any part. On healing there is a tendency to formation of minute fibrous tissue nodules or even multiple pin-point calcifications. They may be confused with the minute infiltrations of miliary tuberculosis. Usually the two conditions may be differentiated clinically by the relative mildness of the symptoms in bronchiolitis. In recent years it has been thought that these cases may be due to mycotic infection such as Histoplasmosis.

"INFLUENZA" or VIRUS BRONCHITIS, (Fig. 154). Different types of acute respiratory infection, when confined to the bronchial and peribronchial regions, often may not have any roentgen characteristics by which they can be distinguished from ordinary bacterial infection. Virus infection may be confined entirely to these regions leaving the parenchymal structures entirely free from infection. If the parenchyma is involved, a pneumonic process is indicated;

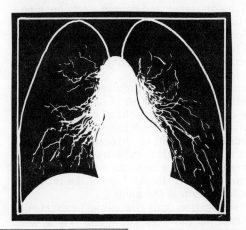

Fig. 153

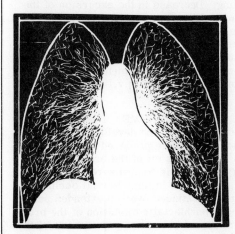

Fig. 154

*An asterisk following any title indicates that roentgenographic reproductions illustrating this condition will be found in the pictorial supplement at the end of the chapter.

virus pneumonia has other distinguishing characteristics (see virus pneumonia).

ASTHMA. Asthma itself produces no characteristic roentgen picture; there is some increase in lung markings but no evidence of other abnormality. Only when, as a result of long-standing chronic involvement, emphysema results, is there any recognizable variation from the normal appearance.

BRONCHOSTENOSIS

ETIOLOGY AND RESULTS OF BRONCHOSTENOSIS. Bronchostenosis may be caused either by internal occlusion of its lumen or by external pressure on the wall of the bronchus.

The principal causes of bronchostenosis are due to internal occlusion.

If there is complete occlusion of a bronchus from any cause, so that no air can enter or leave the obstructed portion of the lung, then within a very short time, often only a few hours, the entrapped air remaining is absorbed by the circulating blood and that portion of the lung becomes atelectatic. This presents such a characteristic roentgen picture that it can be readily recognized--see section on Atelectasis.

Complete stenosis of a bronchus by external pressure is very rare. The lung is elastic and the bronchi are readily displaced; only very firm pressure by a large mass would be expected to cause bronchial occlusion from external pressure. When this does occur, it is usually due to pressure on the smaller bronchioles.

Large tumors of the lung or mediastinum, or large masses of mediastinal lymphnodes may, by their pressure, produce bronchial stenosis. Large aneurysms of the aorta or enormous dilatation of the left auricle of the heart may, under exceptional circumstances, cause sufficient pressure to result in complete bronchostenosis and atelectasis. These are all very rare, however. Instances have been encountered where bronchostenosis has been caused by dense external adhesions following inflammation.

Partial occlusion of a bronchus from external pressure results in deficient expansion of this portion of the lung which is compensated for by the adjacent normal lung. Decrease in the excursion of the involved segment of the lung removes one of the most important aids to pulmonary blood flow, favoring stagnation of the circulation and edema of the parenchymal structure. This, in turn favors infection and if this should occur all of the elements necessary for development of bronchiectasis (q.v.) are present.

MIDDLE LOBE SYNDROME. The middle lobe lends itself very readily to the development of such a condition. The abrupt angle produced by the middle lobe bronchus as it comes off of the bronchial tree renders it very susceptible to pressure from an enlarged lymph gland at the hilum. Partial occlusion of the bronchus, if continued over an extended period of time, causes bronchiectatic dilatation of the bronchus with infection and indurative pneumonitis of the surrounding lung structure.

Roentgenologically the middle lobe becomes densely consolidated; although airless it is not contracted to the same extent as atelectasis. On bronchographic examination the bronchial structures may not fill readily, but on delayed examination after a short interval the opaque material will be found pooled in the dilated bronchial structures.

Microscopically the lung shows chronic indurative pneumonitis from infection surrounding the dilated bronchi with varying degrees of airlessness. Lobectomy is the only alternative for cure, (Graham).

BRONCHIAL DILATATION

BRONCHIECTASIS* (Fig. 155). Bronchiectasis is a dilatation of the bronchi due to pathological changes in the bronchial walls and adjacent structures.

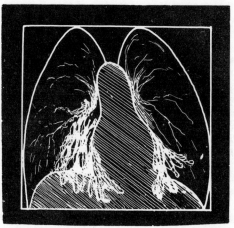

Fig. 155

It may be congenital or acquired. The congenital form is due to some congenital fault in development of the bronchial structure. The bronchi develop by a budding process which starts in the hilum region and progresses outward as the lung develops. Any fault in the natural progression of the process leaves immature bronchial pouches which are often devoid of elastic or muscular tissue and consequently have no means of resisting abnormal dilatation. Such air-filled dilatations of the bronchi in the strict sense may be considered as bronchiectasis but in the absence of infection we choose to designate them as air cysts, or pneumatoceles.

By common consent, the acquired type represents the condition which we think of as bronchiectasis. In this condition the bronchi of a portion of the lung become dilated with induration and thickening of their walls as a result of chronic infection. The dilatation may be tubular (cylindrical), saccular or cystic in type, depending upon the extent and character of the involvement. Regardless of the type, the underlying pathogenesis is the same.

Much investigation both clinical and experimental would indicate the following facts concerning the development of bronchiectasis:

1. The primary site of involvement is in the bronchiole just beyond those showing cartilaginous rings in which the main support of the bronchial wall is from musculature and elastic tissue.

2. Infection plays an important if not an essential part in the development of bronchiectasis. Such infection may be supplied by bronchopneumonia, whooping cough, lung abscess, tuberculosis or by infection from bronchial occlusion by bronchogenic tumor, foreign body, etc.

3. The bronchial epithelium is stripped up and destroyed and the entire bronchial wall is invaded with varying degrees of inflammatory involvement.

4. Destruction of the bronchial musculature results in abolition of normal rhythmic movements of the bronchial wall and loss of muscular tone whereby the bronchus is maintained as a narrow tubular structure changing in calibre with each phase of normal respiration.

5. Elastic tissue of the bronchiole is intimately connected with its musculature and is probably also destroyed or badly damaged as a functioning structure because of infiltration of the bronchiolar wall.

6. Bronchiolar dilatation occurs because the bronchiolar wall loses its support and becomes a structure incapable of resisting increase in intrabronchiolar pressure during inspiration and incapable of elastic recoil during expiration.

7. Atelectasis of the portion of the lung parenchyma supplied by the involved bronchiole occurs early in the process as a result of complete continuous occlusion from infected secretions. The entire parenchymal area becomes "drowned" in infectious secretion.

8. Fibrosis finally results not only within the infected parenchymal tissue but in the areas of peribronchial involvement as well. Contraction of the fibrous tissue serves to constrict the tissues and shorten the bronchiole.

9. Compensatory emphysema fills in any space defect caused by fibrous contraction.

10. Re-epithelization of the granulating surface of the bronchial lining with squamous cells completes the picture.

A complete discussion of the subject will be found in the monograph, "Bronchiectasis" by Lisa and Rosenblatt.

The multiple saclike dilatations of the bronchi form large reservoirs for the accumulation of mucous secretion and products of infection. This gives rise to the characteristic clinical symptoms: expectoration, frequently of large amounts of mucopurulent sputum especially in the morning; afternoon fever and the other indications of infection, and occasional hemorrhage.

Examination by military personnel has disclosed that bronchiectasis may very frequently be present with a minimum of classical signs (Evans and Galinsky). Recurrent basal bronchopneumonia, persistent peribronchial infiltration or a contracted segment of the lung should lead to investigation by bronchographic methods (intratracheal injection of iodized oil) in an effort to detect bronchial dilatation.

Roentgenologically, the chronic bronchial inflammation causes increase in size and number of the peribronchial lung markings in the involved area; if the inflammation is very great the surrounding tissue may become consolidated due to chronic indurative pneumonitis. Such areas of pneumonitis occur very commonly in the cardiophrenic regions giving the appearance of triangular areas of consolidation, (Richards). The lower lobes in the regions of the cardiophrenic sinuses are most frequently involved; these areas may be so completely overshadowed by the breasts and domes of the diaphragm that the pathology may go undetected in the ordinary roentgenogram. They are very frequently retrocardiac in the left lower lobe and are completely overshadowed by the heart (Block), and without lipiodol injection may be completely missed. Any portion of the lung may be involved. Pontius and Jacobs have reported a case in which there was apparent reversal of the bronchietatic process with restoration to normal. For surgical procedures for the extirpation of the disease see p. 231.

BRONCHOGRAPHY IN BRONCHIECTASIS*. Intratracheal injection of lipiodol finds its field of greatest usefulness in detection of this condition. In bronchiectasis, since there is only chronically infected mucous membrane remaining, no absorption can take place and the individual has no other means of ridding himself of infection other than by cough. Within a few hours, most of the opaque material is coughed up leaving the bronchiectatic bronchioles with only a scant amount of opaque oil; there is no evidence of alveolar filling distal to the dilated branches. DeRienzo has pointed out that expulsion of lipiodol from bronchiectatic (dilated) bronchi by coughing requires contraction of musculature; therefore, this is a good criterion upon which to base the estimation of the contractile muscle tissue still present; this may be used as an index of the severity of the disease.

Use of serial examinations may be found especially valuable when bronchiectasis occurs distal to a chronic bronchial constriction as in partial segmental obstruction from pressure of a calcified lymphnode, (Abrams, et al.).

As larger and larger broncho-pulmonary segments of lung are rendered functionally inert as a result of bronchiectatic involvement, the remaining aerated lung undergoes compensatory expansion to fill up the lost space; this causes rearrangement of the bronchial structures which supply the lung structure. Boyer has made a study of the arrangement of the various bronchial structures which occurs during this compensating process.

Water-soluble opaque media has the advantage of rapid absorption so that the lung field becomes clear again in a very short time. IODURON-B, reported by Fischer and Muelly, is absorbed from the lung and excreted in the urine within 45 minutes; incidentally making very satisfactory pyelograms. It is 3.5 diiodpyridon-4-N acetic acid dissolved in the sodium salt of cellulose glycol acid ether. It is somewhat more irritating than Lipiodol requiring more meticulous anaesthesia.

Dionosil, a 50% suspension of N-propyl, 3:5 di-iodo-4-pyridone-N-acetic acid; with added sodium caboxymethyl cellulose for a suspension agent; besides absorption in three or four days it has an additional advantage, Don has found it a safe material for bronchography in active but stable tuberculosis patients. Dionosil has also been investigated by Nice and Azad. Niknejad, et al. have recently undertaken a comprehensive analysis of bronchographic media, including "XUMBRADIL," a new agent.

BRONCHOLITHIASIS. Broncholithiasis is a condition in which numerous calcified deposits throughout the lungs, by reason of their position in close proximity to bronchi, erode through the bronchial walls and are expectorated. During the process of erosion hemorrhage may occur. Such concretions if large may remain impacted in the bronchus resulting in segmental atelectasis. The original cause of the calcifications is usually old healed tuberculous or fungus infection. If they cause only partial occlusion they may cause bronchiectatic dilation.

ANOMALIES
CONGENITAL BRONCHIECTASIS. This is an anomalous condition in the development of the bronchial buds of the lung. For some unknown reason, during the process of the development of the lung the budding process of the bronchi becomes arrested leaving rudimentary bronchial pouches in the central zone and the development of the peripheral lung structures is stopped. These are held open by cartilaginous rings and fill readily with lipiodol on tracheal injection. If a major portion of the lung fails to develop in this way it is called agenesis of the lung, (q.v.). If the parenchymal portion of the lung shows abnormal development it may result in dilatation of alveolar structures when it is called cystic disease of the lung, (q.v.).

DEVELOPMENTAL ANOMALIES have been reported such as partial obstruction of a bronchus by a fenestrated membrane,--local constriction of the lumen with or without congenital bronchiectasis and cyst formation.

BRONCHO-ESOPHAGEAL FISTULA. Broncho-esophageal fistula may be congenital; in congenital atresia of the esophagus (see esophageal strictures), there is usually a nonpatent portion of the esophagus which is represented only by a fibrous cord. Frequently the distal portion of the esophagus communicates through a fistulous opening with the trachea or a large bronchus. The atresia of the esophagus can be readily demonstrated by administration of lipiodol, but the fistulous tract, being connected only with the lower esophageal pouch, does not show. The presence of gas in the stomach and intestines is evidence of existence of such a fistula even though it cannot be seen, since otherwise air could not get into the gastrointestinal tract in a newborn infant.

Acquired broncho-esophageal fistula is usually the result of carcinoma of the esophagus which has eroded through into a bronchus. Very rarely it may

be due to bronchial tuberculosis. The fistulous tract is usually quite clearly demonstrable on administration of opaque material (iodized oil). Such a condition is, in itself, incompatible with life for any great length of time.

PATHOLOGY OF THE LUNGS

CIRCULATORY DISTURBANCES

PASSIVE PULMONARY CONGESTION (Fig. 156). Since the density of the blood vessels is especially responsible for the lung markings seen in the roentgenogram, any pathological process which causes engorgement of the vessels will therefore produce an apparent increase in the size and number of the lung markings. In passive pulmonary congestion from cardiac failure, this increase in markings has a distinctive appearance; it is most evident in

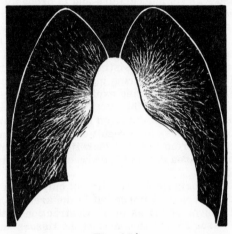

Fig. 156

the inner zones of the lung field. The hilum shadow is enlarged and encroaches upon the middle zone of the lung field, showing broad heavy markings radiating outward from the hilum into the middle zone; here they stop rather abruptly with relatively little extension into the peripheral zone. This gives a bilateral "sunburst" effect which is quite characteristic in its appearance. There is associated enlargement of the cardiac shadow, from cardiac decompensation. A similar appearance may be produced by passive congestion from pressure of a mediastinal mass, without cardiac enlargement.

PULMONARY HYPERTENSION. Certain cardiac anomalies give rise to pulmonary hypertension; through recognition of these signs of pulmonary hypertension it may be possible to obtain some indication of their cause. Carmichael, et al., "using these signs were able not only to detect the presence of pulmonary hypertension but also to correlate the magnitude of the changes with the degree of hypertension."

The criteria employed were: enlargement of the heart, enlargement of the right ventricle, prominence of the main pulmonary artery, prominence of the perihilar vessels, disproportion between the size of the enlarged central pulmonary arteries and narrowed peripheral pulmonary arteries, tortuosity of peripheral arteries, and the presence of fine horizontal lines at the periphery of the lungs near the costophrenic angle, ("Kerley's lines").

By the use of these criteria it was possible not only to recognize pulmonary hypertension but to predict its degree with some accuracy.

Keats, et al., applying these criteria for the detection of hypertension in congenital heart disease found that, "the only one of these criteria which proved applicable was disproportionate narrowing of the peripheral pulmonary arteries as compared to the proximal arteries."

CHRONIC MASSIVE THROMBOSIS OF THE PULMONARY ARTERIES, (Fig. 157). Westermark first described this condition as a wedge of translucency in the lung field due to contraction of the peripheral branches of the pulmonary artery. Even massive thrombosis of the pulmonary arteries is apparently not incompatible with life at least for periods of a few months to a year. Aitchison and McKay have added the use of angiography in the demonstration of this condition. Keating, et al. have described this condition pointing out the roentgen findings whereby it may be recognized and the syndrome which accompanies the condition. They consider it as 1) chronic congestive heart failure without congestion of the lung, 2) the strain put upon the right heart results in right ventricular hypertrophy and if observed over sufficient time during its development, the electrocardiographic findings should show change by serial records from left to right axis deviation, 3) roentgenologically the pulmonary vessels may become enormous in size with a tendency to be comma-shaped, trailing out to a point below, due to gradual thrombosis of the vessel. The lungs show abnormally

radiolucent fields as a result of pulmonary ischemia from cutting down of the blood supply. 4) The condition is characterized by a subacute course with relatively mild symptoms leading to sudden death. It remains to be seen whether early recognition and surgical intervention may possibly alter this course.

PULMONARY EDEMA*(Fig. 158A).

If edema of the lung supervenes, then there is added to the picture of congestion, small blotchy areas of exudation seen throughout the periphery of the lung. Some pleural effusion usually develops very soon after the onset of edema of lungs. The bases are most affected.

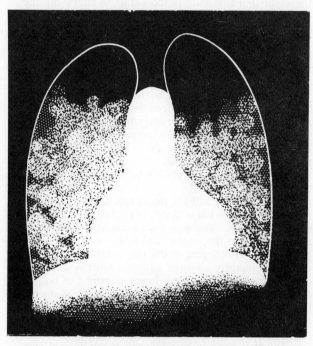

Fig. 158A. Edema Lungs

The mechanism by which edema of the lungs occurs is closely associated with the minute anatomical construction of the lung. The alveolus is lined by a single layer of flat epithelial cells forming a delicate membrane which offers little resistance to permeation of fluid. The alveoli are covered by a capillary sheath in close contact with the epithelial lining. This capillary network is subject to the influence of changes in intrathoracic pressure without the usual form of vaso-motor control. Lymphatic vessels also run in the interstitial space up to the alveoli but do not cover them; they empty into the right thoracic duct but are inadequate in carrying off any large amounts of fluid. The negative pressure in the pleural cavity is a constantly acting force tending to draw water out of the lung.

The balance in pressures between the blood stream and surrounding tissues which is concerned in production of edema elsewhere in the body, is not the only force concerned in production of edema in the lungs. Retardation of flow in the blood vessels results in passage of water from the capillaries into

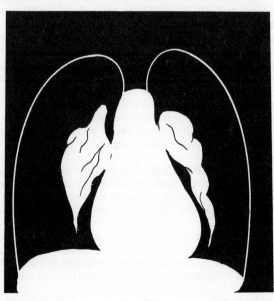

Fig. 157

the surrounding tissues and through the alveolar walls into the alveoli themselves. As fluid collects it backs up into the smaller bronchioles resulting in their obstruction and thereby preventing any air from entering that segment of the lung.

A potent factor in the production of edema is anoxia. The alveolar membrane does not receive its oxygen from the circulating blood but depends upon the inspired air with which it comes in contact; the cutting off of the air supply gives rise to anoxia. This in turn favors edema.

The lymphatics, whose function it is to restore the balance of blood proteins from the interstitial tissue, are extremely inadequate in the lungs since the right thoracic duct is too small to carry off any excessive amount of fluid. The process, therefore, has a tendency to become worse and worse (Drinker).

The water and electrolyte balance is regulated by thirst; this serves the normal individual as a means of maintenance of a relatively constant internal equilibrium between intracellular and extracellular regions (Muether). It has been shown that water or 0.9 % salt solution introduced into the trachea passed rapidly from the lungs directly into the blood stream with very little increase in lymph flow, so that this represents another means by which absorption of fluid occurs from the lung. Serum, on the other hand, absorbs very slowly probably only by the lymphatics (Courtice and Phipps).

Acute edema of the lungs can be produced by over-administration of fluid, especially during post-operative care. The super-abundance of fluid merely flows over into the interstitial tissue and lung spaces, causing water-logging of the lung. Roentgenographically this usually appears as large blotchy areas of increased density over the lower portions of both lung fields; if it persists long enough small amounts of fluid may occur in the costophrenic sinuses. The most dependent portions of the lung show the most pronounced involvement. Strangely enough the condition does not have to be bilateral; if the patient lies on one side, the water-logging has a tendency to occur in the dependent lung. Discontinuing the administration of fluid results in prompt restoration of the lung to normal.

Azotemic edema, (Fig. 158B) or edema caused by retention of nitrogenous waste products in the blood, associated with acute glomerulonephritis and other conditions causing anaphylactic reaction, produces a more or less characteristic picture roentgenographically. The hilar regions and inner zones of the lungs present blotchy areas of increased density similar to that seen in ordinary pulmonary edema, radiating outward toward the periphery of the lungs but stopping short of the outer edges, leaving a clear (aerated) peripheral zone throughout the lung (Rendict, et al.). The picture is in no way similar to edema of the lung from cardiac failure: in this case the blood is dammed back on the capillary circulation, and there is an accumulation of edematous fluid within the alveoli. In the case of azotemic edema some other mechanism must be at work since the zone of parenchymal tissue over 3 centimeters in width remains, not only perfectly clear and well

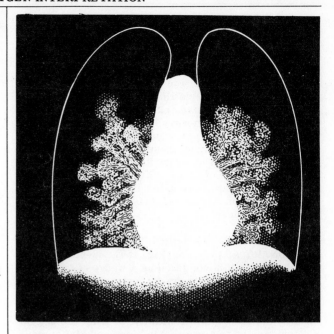

Fig. 158B. Azotemic edema

aerated, but shows normal respiratory change under auscultation; the edema, therefore must be in the perivascular regions. In azotemic involvement, then, the edema must be for the most part in the interstitial spaces about the bronchi and vascular structures as they radiate outward from the hilus regions and the vascular stasis must be mostly in these vessels and not in the capillaries.

Azotemic edema is commonly associated with the initial acute manifestation of many of the collagen diseases (q.v.) especially those with allergic manifestations. Perhaps it represents the profound collagen disturbance associated with sensitization reactions of many varying types.

It has been shown by Trueta et al that a bypass mechanism probably exists in the kidney circulation under such circumstances, permitting the blood to pass through the kidney by a shunt in the circulation before the parenchymal portion is reached, resulting in anuria. Perhaps this is manifestation of a similar mechanism in the lung; blood may be shunted through the proximal vascular branches, with a very limited amount reaching the capillary structures for aeration. This would explain the extreme dyspnea and cyanosis of such patients with maintenance of respiratory function and absence of physical signs.

HAEMOSIDEROSIS. Haemosiderin may be deposited in the lungs in any disorder causing pulmonary hemorrhage but so far as is known, in only two diseases can the deposits be shown roentgenographically.

1. Pulmonary siderosis in children; a rare condition characterized by anemia and occasional hemoptysis. The roentgen manifestations are miliary shadows in the lung due to focal accumulations of iron pigment.

2. In mitral stenosis after repeated attacks of

pulmonary congestion where it also manifests itself by miliary deposits, which look like the picture produced by passive pulmonary congestion but the radiating lines take on a finely beaded appearance even after all symptoms of congestion have disappeared. The involvement may be unilateral. Special staining methods have shown this to be due to iron pigment, (Pendergras, et al.). Cliff has called attention to an idiopathic form of the disease in which the picture is very similar but the cause unexplained.

Fine parallel linear striations have been reported in the cardiophrenic regions of patients with hemosiderosis from chronic pulmonary congestion. Microscopic evidence indicates that these are hemosiderin deposits in the interlobular septa. They may resemble areas of discoid atelectasis and like this condition may be transient. The coexistence of both indications of passive pulmonary congestion and hemosiderosis may occur, (Fleischer and Reiner).

Somewhat similar fine linear markings have been reported by Kerley which may be due to engorged lymphatics or other edematous channels.

Haubrich has determined, as a result of microscopic examination of the nodules, that they frequently show partial calcification.

EOSINOPHILIC INFILTRATION (LOEFFLER'S SYNDROME). A peculiar type of transient recurrent eosinophilic infiltration in the lung structure has been described, (Loeffler). The lack of fever and the eosinophilia of 30 to 40% suggest an allergic basis for the reaction.

Roentgenographically the lesions vary widely in their extent and character, from fine infiltrations to large coalescing areas of blotchy consolidation often resembling edema. Rapid absorption of exudate readily rules out tuberculosis.

Autopsy findings (Bayler, et al. and Bergstrand) show pneumonic exudate predominating in eosinophiles, focal granulomatous lesions, and necrosis. Perivascular lesions were noted similar to those seen in periarteritis nodosa. This would indicate an allergic basis of the condition, (Henderson and Peirce) (Heiken and Weise). One distinctive roentgen finding is the tendency for development of wide elongated streaks of infiltration in the lung field often obliquely or vertically placed (Hennell and Sussman).

A tropical form of disseminated bronchopneumonia associated with eosinophilia has been described (Hodes and Wood).

EMBOLISM; THROMBOSIS; INFARCT OF LUNG* (Fig. 159). It has been our impression that pulmonary infarction varies greatly both in severity of clinical symptoms and in roentgen manifestations, depending upon the source of the emboli.

The clinical picture of pulmonary embolism is often quite alarming. The origin of such emboli may be from clots in the femoral vessels or mural thrombi in the chambers of the heart. It occurs as a postoperative complication or develops following trauma, such as fracture. The patient experiences a sudden sharp, agonizing pain in the chest, with a sense of oppression and extreme dyspnea, often spitting up frothy blood-tinged sputum.

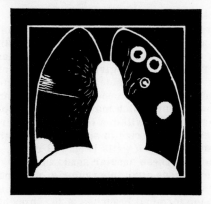

Fig. 159

Roentgenographically, often nothing distinctive can be seen in the chest film at this time.

If the area is small and sufficient blood supply reaches the area from the bronchial artery, pulmonary infarction will not develop, (Shapiro and Rigler). Two or three days later, if the portion of lung involvement is large, a triangular shadow or oval base at the periphery of the lung may develop, (Kirklin and Faust). If infection and necrosis supervene, lung abscess results. If the patient survives and the area of infarction is small resolution and absorption may ultimately take place; if large, it may undergo organization.

Infarcts of the pulmonary artery from this source tend to occur in the periphery of the lungs where the planes of the pleura come together. When well established they form small dense areas of consolidation, with their sides perpendicular to the pleural surface back into the lung. The costophrenic sinus is a frequent place of occurrence, (Fig. 159 right side).

Or the areas of infarction may take on unusual appearances, giving rise to large irregular, rounded areas of consolidation in the lung which may be very confusing. This is especially true when they occur as a result of endocarditis (Levy). Here also, if infection supervenes, exudation and abscess formation may develop after a few days. Organized infarcts show a dense rounded well defined border occurring frequently at the intersection of pleural planes, as for example in the costophrenic sinus. At autopsy they are found to be due to dense fibrous masses.

Pulmonary infarcts which develop as a result of vascular thrombosis from a failing pulmonary circulation are apt to be more insidious in their clinical manifestations and yet more definite in their roentgen findings.

Such patients often do not have the acute severe symptoms experienced by emboli which originate from some remote location. Usually however, their roentgen manifestation is immediate showing much larger areas of infarction. Such emboli seem to recur frequently.

Hanbury et al. have reported the occurrence of such silent infarcts in association with carcinoma of the lung.

Linear planes of fibrosis may result from small organized infarcts which look very much like disc atelectasis.

Thrombosis of the terminal branches of the bronchial artery as well as the terminal division of the pulmonary artery may occur from infection with certain strains of bacteria which seem to have an affinity for the vascular system, giving rise to infarcts of unusual type (Fig. 159, left side). These may appear as rounded nodules from one-half to two or three centimeters in diameter, which may retain their solid structure or may rapidly, within a few hours, undergo central liquefaction giving rise to spherical cavities with smooth uniformly thick walls (Fig. 159 right), (Sante and Hufford). These annular shadows may arise from other causes also; tuberculosis, malignant occlusion of vessels, polycythemia, etc., any process which occludes the terminal branches of the bronchial artery. A case has been reported in which similar nodules were produced by Friedlander Bacillus infection associated with septicemia, (Bulgrin).

Pulmonary Ischemia (Fig. 157). Ischemia of the lung occurs from chronic thrombosis of the pulmonary artery (q.v.) or any other condition which cuts down or obliterates the flow of blood through the pulmonary vessels (Keating, et al.; Woesner, et al.). Necrosis of lung tissue does not take place since the bronchial artery still furnishes nutrition to the lung structure.

POLYCYTHEMIA. Polycythemia is of two varieties; true polycythemia (vera), which is of unknown etiology, and secondary polycythemia which occurs as a physiological compensation to a variety of other conditions which interfere with the proper aeration of the blood. Polycythemia vera produces an extreme increase in the lung markings of the lower lobes similar to that seen in pulmonary congestion but without cardiac enlargement. Soft rounded nodules one centimeter or more in diameter may appear and disappear within three weeks, or they may remain permanently.

Polycythemia may occur secondary to sclerosis of the pulmonary artery (Ayerza's Disease), because of insufficient blood flow through the lungs. It may occur also as a result of a shunt between the arterial and venous circulations from arterio-venous aneurysm or angioma of the lung.

Primary Sclerosis of the Pulmonary Artery, (Pulmonary Arteriolar Sclerosis; Atheroma of the Pulmonary Artery; Ayerza's Disease).

This is a rare condition characterized by hyperplastic sclerosis of the pulmonary artery, causing progressive diminution of blood flow through the lungs. There is some indication that syphilis may be the underlying cause in these cases.

Clinically the patient shows intense cyanosis, dyspnea, clubbing of the fingers and cough without valvular lesions or cardiac enlargement. The pulse is regular. There is dilatation of the pulmonary curve and of the right chambers of the heart with ultimate cardiac enlargement, and associated signs of a failing circulation such as edema of the extremities, etc. Polycythemia occurs secondary to the reduction of blood volume pushed through the lungs;

the hemoglobin may be as high as 126% and the red count 7.5 million.

Pathologically the pulmonary vessels show hyperplastic sclerosis of the media layer with narrowing of the lumen to a small fraction of its normal size. Atheromatous degeneration often occurs. There may be thrombosis of the branches of the pulmonary artery. Toward the periphery the pulmonary arterioles show typical histological changes of thromboangitis obliterans. Sclerosis of the smaller vessels appears as small round and sharply defined opacities uniform in size toward the periphery, giving an appearance which closely resembles pneumoconiosis but distinguishable from it by absence of emphysema (Kerley).

Roentgenologically there is a generalized increase in lung markings throughout both lungs, especially pronounced in the hilum regions. Numerous small rounded nodules, larger than miliary tubercules and not so numerous or symmetrically placed as in miliary tuberculosis, are present throughout the lungs. The appearance is very similar to that sometimes produced by silicosis or sarcoidosis. There is usually no indication of emphysema.

The cardiac shadow is not enlarged (until the terminal stage) but there is definite accentuation of the pulmonary and right auricular curves. These findings correlated with the clinical symptoms usually serve to make the diagnosis.

BACTERIAL INFECTIONS OF THE LUNG

PNEUMONIA

We used to think of pneumonia as being of two or three distinct types: lobar, broncho or lobular, and possibly septic. All other forms were considered as atypical manifestations of these three types of involvement. Now, we are convinced that this large group of so-called, "atypical pneumonias" is comprised of many kinds of infections; virus and rickettsial pneumonias of many kinds.

These atypical forms may produce very similar symptoms to ordinary bacterial pneumonic involvement with widely varying physical signs. It therefore devolves upon the roentgenologist to at least point out the possibility of an atypical form of pneumonia even though the exact type of infection cannot always be determined from the roentgenographic examination. As a guide for the evaluation of these various forms of pneumonic involvement the following roentgenological analysis may be found helpful:

1. Lobar pneumonia*--massive homogeneous areas of involvement starting at the periphery in the alveolar structure and rapidly spreading to lobar distribution representing the response to infection with a definite bacterium, the pneumococcus.

2. Bronchopneumonia--clusters of peribronchial infiltrations representing extension of bacterial infection through the bronchial mucosa into the adjacent lung structure as a response to many types of

bacterial organism.

3. Septic lobular pneumonia--blotchy areas of pneumonitis irregularly scattered throughout the lung fields as a result of blood-borne infection from some distant septic infection, often the streptococcus.

4. "Glandular type" of pneumonic involvement where the first manifestation seems to be an adenopathy of the hilum nodes, followed by infiltrative processes throughout the periphery of the lung possibly arising in the parenchymal lymphoid deposits, such as tularemia, measles and possibly whooping cough.

5. Interstitial (virus) pneumonias; atypical pneumonias of unknown etiology, characterized at the onset by accentuation of the hilum shadows and lung markings of the lower lobes probably due to an acute active pulmonary congestion, rapidly followed by haziness of a definite area of the lung from interstitial edema and clusters of infiltrations in the periphery.

By careful analysis of the roentgen findings it may be possible to at least group the types of pneumonic involvement into these general classes.

LOBAR PNEUMONIA* (Fig. 160). In lobar pneumonia the alveolar spaces are completely filled with serofibrinous exudate, containing many polynuclear cells completely replacing the air in the portion of the lung involved but not affecting the interstitial tissue. This extensive pouring out of serofibrinous exudate into the alveoli results in a homogeneous consolidation. The disease usually affects an entire lobe so that certain definite characteristics are produced in the roentgenogram. With extension to the pleura, the diaphragm

becomes immobilized in a high position, due to resulting pleural pain.

To completely understand the characteristic appearance produced by consolidation of the various lobes it is necessary to know the position occupied by the interlobar septa, as they appear in the roentgenogram. The main pleural fissure runs from the region of the fifth or sixth dorsal vertebra posteriorly, downward and forward to the anterior shadow of the diaphragm. On the right side a second pleural fissure starts at the hilum and runs horizontally forward producing an upper and middle lobe (see Topography of the Lung).

If the x-ray tube is centered about the fifth or sixth dorsal vertebra posteriorly, at a target-film distance of about four to six feet, the divergent beam of x-rays falls almost exactly along the plane of the interlobar pleura between the upper and middle lobes on the right side (Fig. 160A). In upper lobe consolidation this produces a uniformly dense shadow in the roentgenogram occupying the upper portion of the lung, having an abrupt, straight line lower border running from the hilum to the periphery.

Middle lobe consolidation (Fig. 160B), by reason of the fact that its upper border is on the same plane as the adjacent lower border of the upper lobe, assumes a straight line upper border running outward from the hilum to the periphery. The shadow is much smaller in extent than upper lobe involvement since the size of the lobe is smaller. The consolidated lobe presents a wedge-shaped structure to the rays, thickest portions above and thinnest portion below;

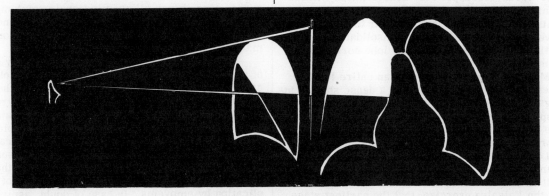

Fig. 160A

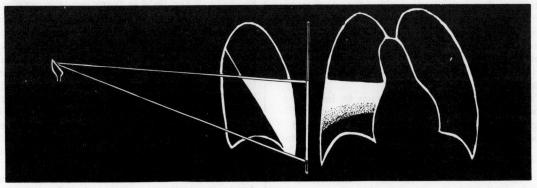

Fig. 160B

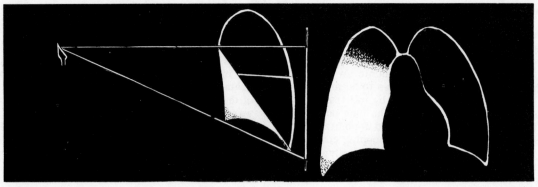

Fig. 160C

this results in the shadow being densest above, and feathering out into normal lung density below.

Lower lobe consolidation (Fig. 160C) is much more extensive and presents a much larger shadow, overlapping the middle lobe. The x-rays must traverse the greatest thickness in the midportion, therefore the shadow is densest in this region; both upper and lower portions are wedge-shaped in outline so that both upper and lower borders feather out into normal lung density.

On the left side there are but two lobes, the upper lobe on this side corresponding to the combined upper and middle lobes on the right side. As a result the shadows produced by left upper lobe pneumonia should correspond to the combined shadows of upper and middle lobe consolidation on the right side. In other words, left upper lobe consolidation extends down farther than right upper lobe involvement and presents a hazy lower border, similar to that seen at the lower border of middle lobe consolidation. The projecting lingula of the left upper lobe corresponds to the middle lobe on the right.

Massive lobar pneumonia of an entire lung is evidenced in the roentgenogram as a dense shadow involving one entire side of the chest without mediastinal displacement since there is no actual change in volume of the lung, merely replacement of air with serifibrinous exudate.

Lobar pneumonic consolidation has been reported in an anomalous azygos lobe, (Turnbull).

It may be shown by radiographic examination during the Valsalva exercise, that the earliest stage of the "consolidation" as seen in the roentgenogram is due to vascular engorgement since the shadow seen in the roentgenogram is completely dispelled by this maneuver (Westermark). Exudation which follows must be rapid and must be directly through the alveolar walls since the bronchial structures remain free and there is no roentgenological manifestations of atelectasis.

The initial site of consolidation in lobar pneumonia must be considered as the periphery of the lung in the alveolar spaces. Where only a part of a lobe is involved it may form a triangular shadow, base at the periphery of the lung and apex inward. This is frequently the case in children. In certain instances the consolidation appears roentgenographically to be in the hilum region; in view of more re-

cent developments it is most likely that hilum pneumonias of this sort are due to interstitial pneumonia of the virus type. The area of involvement spreads rapidly in lobar pneumonia, so that the full extent of the consolidation is usually present within twenty-four to forty-eight hours after the initial onset.

At the time of crisis, there is no apparent change in the area of consolidation but within a few days after crisis resolution begins and progresses rapidly, the density of the consolidation becoming less and less and the lung markings again reappearing as resolution progresses; complete resolution and restoration to normal should occur within two to three weeks. Other lobes of the lung, often remotely situated, may be successively involved. In this event, each lobe goes on to consolidation, resolution and restoration to normal following the usual sequence even though all constitutional symptoms continue. This leads one to assume that lobar pneumonia is a local disease of the lungs with constitutional manifestations.

If a shadow remains and there is not evidence of progressive favorable resolution three weeks after crisis, this is indication of complication; if the remaining shadow is central within the lung there is possibility of a lung abscess; if the shadow remaining is peripheral, the condition is probably due to pleural effusion, localized or in the general pleural cavity. A small amount of "protective serous fluid" usually accompanies lobar pneumonia; it is important that such protective fluid be not adjudged as evidence of complication by empyema. In case of doubt, aspiration and cell count on a small portion of the fluid should be made; if the fluid is frank pus, the conclusion is obvious; if it is clear or turbid fluid with many polynuclear leukocytes even with some pneumococci present it may be due entirely to "protective fluid" and may absorb completely within a short time without pus formation; if the cell count shows predominance of lymphocytes, beware of a tuberculous complication. Transitory atelectasis has been observed very rarely at the end of resolution as indicated by displacement of the mediastinal structures. It results from resolution of the pneumonic process with some occlusion of the bronchus still remaining. It may recur more frequently in children.

Lobar distribution of pneumonic process may be due to many other organisms besides the pneumococcus. The staphylococcus occasionally produces lobar involvement; Friedlander bacillus has been encountered; caseous tuberculous pneumonia is a very common cause. Tularemia under conditions which involve inhalation of the organisms has been shown to produce massive alveolar lesions (Bihss and Berlin).

In the various stages of acute rheumatic fever, large homogeneous areas of increased density have been noted giving the appearance of pneumonic consolidation.

Chemotherapy has done much to lower the mortality of this disease and to control complications. Even though the temperature may fall to normal within twenty-four hours after sulpha drug or penicillin therapy the roentgen picture remains the same.

In recent years classical lobar pneumonia has shown great reduction in morbidity and severity of symptoms. Complications have almost disappeared. This may be due to the fact that early treatment with chemotherapy promptly stamps out infection and prevents spread.

BRONCHOPNEUMONIA* (Fig. 161). In bronchopneumonia, on the other hand, infection spreads from the bronchi to the surrounding peribronchial structures. Isolated groups of infiltrations cluster about the bronchi, especially in their lower portions, like bunches of grapes clinging to the vine. Roentgenologically this results in blotchy areas of infiltration in

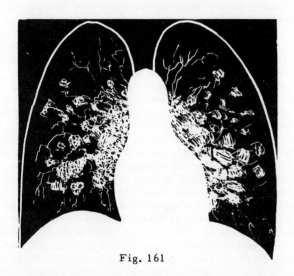

Fig. 161

the lower lobes--usually bilateral. There may be much greater involvement on one side than another, giving the impression of unilateral involvement. The lower lobes are the site of predominant involvement, a fact which distinguishes this condition from tuberculosis.

Bronchopneumonia may be associated with multiple small abscesses; under this condition it is referred to as necrotizing pneumonia. These are usually of bacterial origin.

SEPTIC PNEUMONIA* (Fig. 162). Septic lobular pneumonia is usually encountered in association with streptococcus septicemia following septic infection of some sort affecting all structures of the lung

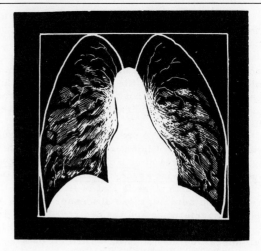

Fig. 162

alike, alveolar as well as interstitial. Staphylococcus septicemia may also result in this type of pneumonic involvement. The infection is blood-borne, so that it may lodge in any portion of the lung.

Roentgenologically it produces poorly defined blotchy areas of infiltration throughout the lungs. This was a very serious condition since it was only part of a general septic infection. If the patient survived, small abscesses developed or resolution occurred with scar formation resulting in small discreet shadows in the lung, depending in size and location upon the degree of original involvement. The advent of chemotherapy with sulpha drug and penicillin therapy has done much to reduce the mortality in this condition.

FRIEDLANDER BACILLUS PNEUMONIA (Fig. 163A, B, C). Friedlander Bacillus pneumonia is an unusual type of pneumonia encountered from time to time. At autopsy it presents no distinctive feature and cannot be differentiated from lobar pneumonia except by isolation of the Friedlander Bacillus. It presents four more-or-less defined phases in its development, giving rise to distinctive roentgen findings (Kornblum).

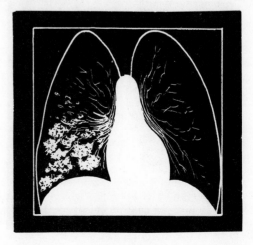

Fig. 163A

1. The stage of bronchopneumonic involvement with clusters of infiltrations about the bronchi, especially of the lower lobes (Fig. 163A).

2. These bronchopneumonic areas rapidly coalesce to form the second stage--that of pseudolobar involvement. If seen for the first time during this stage the condition may not be distinguishable roentgenographically from ordinary lobar pneumonia (Fig. 163B).

3. The third stage presents the most unusual feature of this type of infection. With incredible rapidity, the entire area of consolidation breaks down resulting in extensive abscess formation (Fig. 163C).

4. The fourth stage is that of fibrosis. If the patient should survive, these abscesses may be evacuated by expectoration and the destroyed areas in the lung may heal by scar tissue formation, or multiple small abscesses may remain, walled off by heavy deposits of fibrous tissue which become organized scar tissue and result in chronic diffuse interstitial fibrosis.

In certain instances, where the pseudolobar involvement is massive, the involved lung actually in-

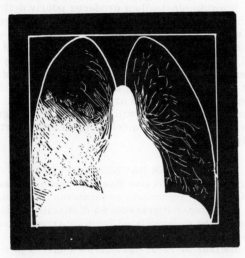

Fig. 163B

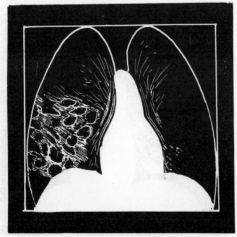

Fig. 163C

creases in size to the point of displacement of the mediastinal structures to the opposite side giving rise to an appearance of fluid under pressure or new growth. This probably represents the period when streptomycin has controlled the infection (with subsidence of fever), but products of inflammation have not yet been removed.

An unusual case of Friedlander Bacillus pneumonia has been reported, (Bulgrin) in which the only lung lesions were nodular masses similar in some respects to those seen in bronchial artery thrombosis. There was no evidence of annular shadow development in this case, however.

Until recently Friedlander Bacillus infection has always been thought of as an acute, very serious pneumonic involvement. Recently, however, a chronic form has been reported associated with chronic nasal sinus infection and lung involvement (Peirce and Li-Liang). The roentgen findings may show only as increased bronchovascular markings throughout both lung fields resembling the picture sometimes seen with fungus infection. Friedlander's bacillus has also been encountered as the case of acute osteomyelitis (q.v.).

Streptomycin has proved to be almost specific for this infection. Without chemotherapy very few patients survive the acute pneumonic form. This drug has been equally effective in the chronic form associated with nasal sinus infection.

Other unusual types of pneumonia have been reported from Paratyphoid infection and from Brucillosis. Both are dependent upon laboratory tests for establishment of the diagnosis. Holmes has recently pointed out that while streptomycin is the drug of choice in treatment of the disease, both aureomycin and chloramphenicol have been successfully used. Lung surgery for drainage or resection of tension cavities, etc., has a place in the healing of the fibrotic stage after medication has completely controlled the infectious stage.

Melioidosis is a very rare infection resembling glanders, caused by a similar organism, malleomyces pseudomallei, a gram negative bacillus transmitted by rats and other animals from foreign countries. On roentgen examination the chest shows mottled or slightly nodular densities resembling pneumonitislike virus infection or tuberculosis with degeneration into cavities. Streptomycin is of no perceptible value. For 6 months there is gradual increase in infiltration like tuberculosis. The condition is chronically progressive for years. Chloromycetin seems to have some temporary restraining action. Intestinal involvement and extension to all of the viscera may occur before death.

"GLANDULAR TYPE" OF PNEUMONIC INVOLVEMENT

Tularemic pneumonia is an example of this type of pneumonic involvement. The initial site of inoculation is in some remote location, usually through a wound sustained as a result of handling rabbits or other game which are infected with tularemia. Formation of an intractable wound is followed by regional and later by general glandular infection. Hilar adenopathy is the first indication of pulmonary involvement with subsequent retrograde spread along the bronchial lymphatics outward toward the periphery of the lung. Confluence of infiltrative exudate at the periphery of the lung soon results in parenchymal consolidation of varying degrees. This may result in abscess formation.

This type of pneumonic involvement as a result of tularemic infection is dependent upon this type of lymphatic inoculation. As previously mentioned, tularemic infection, if inoculated directly into the lung structure by inhalation, may produce a massive homogeneous pneumonic exudate of lobar pneumonic type (q.v.). This is an example of two different types of pneumonic response to infection with the same organism depending upon the method of inoculation.

The specific agglutination reaction may be necessary to determine tularemic infection. Dennis and Boudreau have reported on the x-ray manifestations in 14 cases of the pleuropulmonary type emphasizing early recognition and institution of proper therapy.

MEASLES PNEUMONIA may well be of the same character. In measles enlargement of the hilum nodes is a well-known entity, followed by a lobular type of pneumonia in the periphery. It may well be that this is due to direct infection with the measles organism.

Both sarcoid and erythema nodosum may produce bulky hilar enlargement. Both may spread to the periphery of the lung and may show miliary infiltrations like miliary tuberculosis ultimately clearing.

WHOOPING COUGH is associated with adenopathy but the roentgenogram would indicate more the picture of aspiration than any other type of pneumonic involvement.

VIRUS (INTERSTITIAL) PNEUMONIAS*--ATYPICAL PNEUMONIAS "PNEUMONIAS OF UNKNOWN ETIOLOGY--VARIETY X"

In this classification are included many types of unusual pneumonic involvement of uncertain or unknown etiology. Among these are virus pneumonias of many types, such as Epidemic "Influenzal" Pneumonia A and B, Psiticosis (Parrot Fever), and other types of virus pneumonia having special growth and cultural characteristics. A psiticosis-like, ornithotic (bird-borne) disease and lymphogranuloma venereum, two recently recognized viruses are apparently widespread among birds and domestic animals such as pigeons, chickens and mice. These spread to man and give rise to the syndrome called virus pneumonia (Reimann).

All of these atypical pneumonic processes have similarities pathologically and roentgenologically. In contradistinction to lobar pneumonia, these atypical infections attack the interstitial tissues of the lung affecting all structures of the lung alike, producing a profound disturbance in this structure. The alveolar walls are thickened and edematous and the lining alveolar cells lose their flat appearance becoming cuboidal in character showing numerous mitotic figures, evidence of profound inflammation. The alveoli are filled with gelatinous exudate, almost devoid of cells (only a few lymphocytes, mononuclear and red cells), which forms a hyaline membrane about the alveolar margin hampering exchange of air which accounts for the intense cyanosis of the patients. Inclusion bodies may be found in cells in some of these diseases.

A similar basic reaction in lung tissue from practically all of these widely varying types of interstitial infections suggests a similar fundamental type of involvement. Attention is called by Ackerman, et al. to the similarity in appearance of areas of organizing virus pneumonia to that of carcinoma of the lung. The similarity in appearance may be due to subsequent infection of the unresolved pneumonia by other bacteria.

DIFFUSE (HAMMON-RICH) FIBROSIS. Aside from the ordinary types of massive fibrosis associated with healing of lung destruction from injury or infection and fibrosis associated with emphysema and cystic disease Hamman and Rich have reported an idiopathic diffuse type of fibrosis which may be rapidly fatal, usually lasting from 4 to 24 weeks. Gough has pointed out that this type consists of a "diffuse progressive interstitial proliferation of fibrous tissue with hyaline membranes lining the alveoli and with esosinophilic leucocytes in the interstitial tissue in most cases. Cyanosis and cor pulmonale developed." "Heppleston . . . showed that even in this advanced stage the fibrosis was mainly due to increased reticulin rather than collagen formation. By staining with silver the difference could be clearly shown between this interstitial type of fibrosis and the intra-alveolar type such as occurs in unresolved lobar pneumonia."

The cause of Hammon-Rich fibrosis is not known and no bacteria or other organisms have been found in the lesions. Some authors such as Rubin, Kahn and Pecker (1952) consider the condition to be of virus origin. The prognosis is hopeless and death is due to cardiac or respiratory failure. At autopsy the lesions are found to be very extensive throughout both lungs. There is only slight dilatation of the air spaces in contrast to the honeycomb appearances of certain other forms of diffuse interstitial fibrosis.

VARICELLAR PNEUMONITIS. In recent years isolated cases have been reported where virulent chicken-pox infection has been attendant with extremely severe pneumonitis causing death of the individual. The roentgen picture is in no way distinctive from any other type of viral pneumonia. At autopsy the chicken-pox vesicles can be seen on the surface of the lung.

Roentgenologically these may also produce appearances similar in many respects to each other. The onset may be acute with: 1) accentuation of the hilum shadows and lung markings radiating outward into the lung substance like a "sunburst" (without any manifestation of adenopathy), followed by; 2) clusters

of fine infiltrations near the periphery which may coalesce to form blotchy areas of dense consolidation.
These areas may be single or multiple; unilateral or
bilateral, usually taking on a segmental appearance,
but they are never homogeneous or lobar in distribution. 3) Resolution and absorption usually requires
about two to three weeks but may be delayed for six
to eight weeks; 4) often leaving evidence of fine infiltration in the periphery of the lungs (near the costophrenic sinuses) long after the febrile reaction has
subsided. If the site of involvement is in the upper
lobes, and resolution is prolonged, the residual infiltration may very readily be mistaken for pulmonary
tuberculosis. A number of such instances have been
observed where organizing virus pneumonitis, persisting for months, gave an erroneous appearance
suggestive of neoplasm. These types of infection in
themselves are not usually fatal but they may pave
the way for secondary invaders. A well-known example of the dual type of infection was seen in the
epidemics of "Influenzal" Pneumonia, which occurred
in 1918-19. These produced such bizarre roentgenological findings as to make classification practically
impossible.

Chicken pox pneumonia has been reported by
Tan et al. in which the lungs were studded with multiple chickenpox lesions. Similar vesicolon lesions
were present throughout the abdomen studding all of
the viscera. These cases were only rarely fatal.
Endress and Schnell have made a comprehensive
study of this condition collected from publications and
of their own, with infiltration and areas of consolidation throughout the lungs and areas of necrosis. They
report as high as 42% mortality in some epidemics.
It is evident therefore that the extent of the lesions is
not an indication of the severity of the disease.

RICKETTSIAL PNEUMONIA. Rickettsial pneumonias, or those conveyed by the bite of small in-
sects such as lice or ticks, are probably similar to
others of virus type, giving similar roentgenological
and pathological pictures. Some of those which have
been most completely investigated are Q Fever,
Toxoplasmosis and Alveolar Adenomatosis. Rosen
has reported 15 cases of virus pneumonia in poultry
workers following handling of turkeys.

Q FEVER, caused by Rickettsia Burneti which
is transmitted by a tick bite, is a known causative
agent of one of the atypical pneumonias. A number of
different strains of Q fever have been isolated: Bal-
kan, Mediterranean, Italian, American and Pan-
American.

It has been pointed out (Denlinger and Carter)
that cattle and unpasteurized milk are reservoirs of
this infection and that many cases have originated
from these sources. Irons and Hooper have described
an outbreak which occurred among stock handlers and
slaughter house workers in Texas in 1947. Clinically,
there are chilly sensations, fever, anorexia, headache and hacking cough. Roentgenologically the condition resembles atypical pneumonia of other cause,
showing lobular and segmental consolidation with confluence of mottled infiltrations and possibly minimal
pleural effusion. Aureomycin seems to be the only

antibiotic of value. Positive diagnosis is made only
after isolation of the organism or by demonstration
of specific antibodies during convalescence.

TOXOPLASMOSIS is a disease characterized by
intense pneumonic involvement caused by Toxoplasma,
a plasmoidal-like organism, possibly also rickettsial
in origin through the bite of a tick. The discovery by
Pinkerton and Henderson of the pathogenicity of Toxoplasma for adults has opened a new phase in the possibilities of plasmodial infection.

JAAGSIECKTE ALVEOLAR ADENOMATOSIS.
Within the last few years a peculiar type of virus infection (Jaagsieckte) epidemic among sheep has been
found to be infectious for man. It is of especial importance since the proliferation of alveolar cells
which it produces is not unlike the appearance seen
in primary alveolar carcinomatosis, suggesting a possible close relationship between virus infection and
the production of tumors,--adenomatosis (Hildebrand).
The microscopic picture shows the alveolar epithelial
cells piled up on each other often still leaving an
aerated space in the alveolus.

The roentgen picture shows peculiar fine mottled areas throughout the lung fields which would be
excepted from the microscopic picture but this is not
characteristic since alveolar carcinomatosis gives a
similar picture.

SPIROCHETAL INFECTION

SYPHILIS, although common elsewhere in the
body, rarely involves the lung. Three types have been
described: 1) gummatous, 2) interstitial and, 3) lobar
pneumonic. Cases have been reported where large
consolidated areas in the lung ascribed to gumma have
disappeared after salvarsan administration, but this
is not sufficient proof to establish them as syphilitic
in nature. A few have been proved at autopsy. A
chronic interstitial fibrosing type has been described
as showing a shadow in the hilum region extending
outward into the lung; it is by no means distinctive.
The lobar pneumonic type (white pneumonia) occurs
only in the stillborn (McIntyre).

LEPTOSPIROSIS—(Weils disease) (Silverstein).
This is a disease produced by any of a group of Lepto-
spiral spirochetes. The disease is still rare in this
country; hogs and cattle are the chief animal hosts.
The condition is characterized by symptoms of acute
infection, chills, high fever, cerebral and urinary
symptoms, jaundice, hemorrhagic diathesis and an enlarged spleen. Roentgenologically, there are diffuse
blotchy areas of infiltration throughout the lungs due
in most part to edematous and hemorrhagic areas.
The appearance is not distinctive of the disease.

COLLAGEN DISEASES

We have, in the past, thought of connective tissue,
merely as a construction framework of the body to
support the cellular elements; it is difficult for us
therefore to think of interstitial tissue as the primary
site of any specific pathological process. Recent ob-

servations would indicate however, that certain diseases may be intimately connected with derangement of the collagenous tissues of the body.

Connective tissue maintains itself by proliferation of fibroblasts, the same as any other cellular tissue. It is the great reparative structure of the body which repairs the destruction wrought by disease. Beyond this little is known of its function in combating disease.

Steinberg has summarized briefly some of the pertinent facts concerning our knowledge of connective tissue:

Connective tissue is composed of two essential elements: (a) fibrillar material, and (b) interfibrillar substance.

(a) These fibrils under electron microscopic examination show cross-striations of regular periodicity (646 Å); they divide like the branches of a tree. These fibrous elements are composed of collagen reticulin and elastic fibers; they are proteins of high molecular weight. Collagen, when heated in aqueous solution, becomes amorphous gelatin. "Embryonic collagen fibers are soluble in salt-free dilute acid and when these solutions are treated with salt or neutralized, the proteins precipitate as fibers which possess the same fine structure as the native fibers."

(b) The interfibrillar substance in turn is composed of at least two components: (1) an amorphous ground substance, and (2) a cement substance. Little is known of the chemistry of the amorphous ground substance.

The cement substance proper serves as a bed for the fibrous elements. It contains protein and mucopolysaccharides. There are four known mucopolysaccharides. Of these, hyaluronic acid is best known. This acid is hydrolyzed by a specific enzyme, hyaluronidase, known as the "spreading factor" in streptococcus and other infections which contain this enzyme. It has been suggested that this action is produced by effect on the cement substance. Observations by clinicians would seem to indicate the possible involvement of this collagenous material as the basis of the pathological process in a number of conditions known as "collagen diseases."

The conditions most commonly identified with this group are as follows:

Hypersensitive states resulting in sensitization reactions to foreign protein; serum reaction.

Drug sensitization, possibly by combination of sensitizing agent with albumin inside (or outside) the body.

Blood incompatibility in transfusions.

Acute glomerulonephritis (with azotemic edema).

Periarteritis (polyarteritis) nodosa, resulting in reaction, centered more particularly about blood vessels. Gradual occlusion of the smaller blood vessels of the extremities leading to periosteal proliferation of the long bones demonstrable by radiographic examination giving rise to localized symptoms of pain and clinical manifestations of hypertension.

Rheumatic pneumonitis, in which transitory joint involvement is a prominent feature.

Rheumatoid arthritis, proliferation of synovial membrane of joints.

Disseminated lupus erythematosus, associated especially with butterfly skin lesions on nose, cheeks, and involvement of serous membranes, pericardial, endocardial, pleural, and abdominal.

Dermatomyositis.

Scleroderma.

These widely differing groups of diseases would seem, on first consideration, to have little to identify them with a common etiology. They have been observed on so many occasions to develop similar signs and symptoms during the course of the disease, however, that the possibility of a common etiological factor must be considered (Kampmeier). Each has some predominant clinical or pathological characteristic by which it can be identified, such as manifestations of foreign protein reaction; in hypersensitive states, in drug sensitization and in blood transfusions with incompatible blood; anuria and azotemic edema in glomerulonephritis; periarterial proliferation with resulting high blood pressure in periarteritis nodosa; multiple joint manifestations and certain characteristic pathological cell formations in rheumatic pneumonitis; butterfly skin reaction on nose and face in lupus, together with occurrence of certain characteristic cells known as lupus erythematosus cells.

Yet, in all, there is an associated common fundamental pathological lung reaction which seems to establish a common denominator for all of these diseases. The widely divergent clinical manifestations of these diseases would indicate that any such common etiological factor might lie in the involvement of a common structure such as the connective tissue (Banks).

Correlation of roentgenological and pathological findings should throw some light on the nature and character of these diseases.

The collagenous connective tissue is an all pervading substance present in all tissues throughout the body. It would be reasonable to suppose that any disease process affecting this structure would manifest itself in the lung as well as in the other organs and structures of the body, and that possibly these changes might be observed by roentgen examination of the lungs. By utilizing the lungs as a roentgen window we may be able to observe any pathological process which is taking place elsewhere in the body.

One of the most common types of anaphylactic reaction is that due to sensitization to drugs. Such cases are usually mild, being accompanied by urticarial reaction, eosinophilia, constitutional reaction, etc., rarely causing death. Few autopsies, therefore, are available. Such mild cases show little, if any, demonstrable roentgen manifestations in the lung since the dose is so small and the reaction so mild.

Occasionally, however, the reaction to such agents is prompt and severe, coming on immediately and causing death within a few days. Similar anaphylactic reaction occurs from foreign protein injection and from blood transfusions with incompatible blood. These amount to essentially the same circumstances; the injected material constitutes a foreign protein to which the body is sensitive (Rich, and Longcope and Winkenwerder).

In such cases the lung fields may rapidly assume a characteristic picture; the hilar regions and inner zones of the lungs present dense, blotchy areas of increased density similar to that seen in pulmonary edema, radiating outward toward the periphery of the lungs, but stopping short of the outer edges, leaving clear peripheral zones. The picture differs from that produced by acute pulmonary edema from cardiac failure in that it stops abruptly before it reaches the outer margins of the lung, and it is not associated with enlargement of the cardiac shadow which would be expected in such cases. Furthermore, the shadow may vary from the blotchy appearance of edema described above to one of heavy linear markings radiating outward from the hilus like a sunburst, but in no case extending into the peripheral zones, the exact location in which one would expect the greatest amount of edema. This, then, is the form of antigenic lung reaction which previous experience has indicated is associated with anaphylactic states. Garland and Sisson, after extensive investigation have likewise concluded that collagen diseases are a group of disorders characterized anatomically by generalized alterations of the connective tissue, especially of its extracellular components. The etiology is not known; several workers have produced fibrinoid changes of the connective tissues experimentally, by mechanical and by chemical means.

AZOTEMIC EDEMA. Since such reactions are invariably associated with acute glomerulonephritis resulting in suppression of urine with accumulation of excessive nitrogenous waste products in the blood, this specific type of reaction has been designated as, "azotemic edema", (q.v.). If the condition progresses it may encroach more and more on the peripheral lung tissue, narrowing down the outer clear zone of uninvolved lung.

Microscopically there is marked thickening of the interstitial space with edema of the alveolar wall; the alveolar spaces are filled with clear gelatinous material with few cellular elements usually mononuclears, plasma cells or lymphocytes. A homogeneous hyalin membrane forms along the alveolar walls. In short, the picture is basically similar to that found in pneumonitis from the various types of virus infection. It is possible therefore that the toxins produced by these diseases may be similar in character to those associated with urinary suppression from glomerulonephritis or may be attendant with such kidney damage. At any rate they are not specific for virus infections.

Similar microscopic findings in the lungs of newborn infants dying shortly after birth has given rise to an assumption that this is a specific disease which has been labeled "hyalin disease of the lungs" (Meschen, et al).

When azotemic edema occurs as a result of anaphylactic shock, it is of grave significance; it may, however, develop from impairment of kidney function from other causes for example, exposure to cold in which case it may not be of such grave prognostic significance.

All of the collagen diseases as listed, down to and including periarteritis (polyarteritis) nodosa are associated with acute anaphylactic reaction; the others are more chronic having periods of activity which may be associated with disturbances in kidney function and transitory edema.

POLYARTERITIS (Periarteritis) NODOSA. Polyarteritis nodosa is pretty well established as a sensitization reaction to foreign proteid probably horse serum. It is characterized by small subcutaneous nodules. Microscopically these represent small herniations of the vessel walls. When the lesions occur in the lungs the tiny perivascular nodules, when widely disseminated throughout the lungs, may give an appearance of miliary lesions similar to sarcoidosis or tuberculosis. In acute, often fatal, cases the extreme reaction of the perivascular structures of the hilum results in a dramatic roentgenological picture; heavy vascular markings radiate outward from both hilum regions like sun-bursts fading out toward the periphery of the lungs.

Such cases are very rare however; they were observed in the armed forces in a very small percentage of individuals immediately following serum inoculations. Lung involvement of any sort is very rare; only 4 cases out of 108 collected by Swanberg.

Doub, et al., recognize the acute oedematous reaction of polyarteritis but have found that it may not resolve directly but pass through a destructive inflammatory necrotizing reaction, invading one or all of the vascular coats as well as the surrounding tissue. They recognize four stages; the degenerative, characterized by oedema and a fibrinous exudate about the inner elastic membrane, the muscular walls being separated by the exudate. The acute inflammatory stage where there is infiltration of the media and adventitia by polymorphonuclear leukocytes and eosinophiles followed by necrosis of the wall. Secondary thrombosis is first seen in this stage and infarction of organs may result.

The stage of granulation or repair is characterized by a change of polymorphonuclears and eosinophils, to a round cell infiltration with fibroblastic proliferation.

The healed stage is seen as scar formation in the areas of involvement aneurysms, stenosis of vessels and irregular nodules of scar result.

Rogers and Roberto have called attention to the similarity of the lesions of Wegener's granulomatosis and periarteritis nodosa.

ASPIRATION PNEUMONITIS

ASPIRATION PNEUMONITIS. Aspiration of ordinary food material into the lungs as a result of laryngeal paralysis or from any other cause, aside from the immediate danger of asphyxiation, is not ordinarily attended with grave symptoms. Aspiration of vomitus, however, is dangerous in direct proportion to the amount and quantity of digestive juices and hydrochloric acid which it contains. This may result, after a short space of time, in edema of the lungs, dyspnoea and death. Roentgenographically the picture is that of profound edema of the lungs.

LIPOID PNEUMONITIS.* Lipoid pneumonia is

a condition in which the lung structures become inflamed from introduction of irritating oils. The use of oil as a vehicle for other medication, for nose drops and sprays of the upper respiratory passages, must be viewed with concern.

Various oils act differently when introduced into the lung.

Vegetable oils such as those used as vehicles with lipiodol (poppy seed oil) and lipiodine (oil of sesame), when highly refined and freed from all traces of fatty acids, cause no evidence of inflammation even after long sojourn in the lung; only if they become rancid do they cause any irritation.

Animal oils, especially cod liver oil, contain a large amount of fatty acids even when fresh; when rancid the fatty acid content is increased. Such oil remaining for a long time in the alveolar spaces is constantly subjected to the air, a condition which favors further rancid development of the oil. The inflammatory cellular reaction produced by this oil is extreme and may even cause death.

Microscopically, the oil droplet can be seen in the alveoli having a stringy appearance with an extreme degree of inflammatory infiltration involving all of the surrounding structures of the lung.

Mineral oil is also harmful, but in another way. Unlike animal and vegetable oils, mineral oil is chemically inert, acting as a foreign body in the lung parenchyma. The oil, aspirated into the lungs, enters the finer bronchi which become occluded. Air absorbed by the blood from the alveoli causes the oil to be sucked into the terminal structures. Here it remains for a long period of time because it cannot be removed except by phagocytosis. The oil cannot be saponified and therefore cannot be ingested by the phagocytes. In the long continued contact it produces a proliferative bronchopneumonia with involvement of all lung structures. Accumulation of oil in the lymphatics in the interstitial tissue may form paraffinomas of considerable size. Pinkerton has demonstrated the formation of paraffinomas (as large as 1.0 by 1.5 cm.) from aspiration of oil over a long period of time.

Microscopically these appear as rounded globular deposits of oil enmeshed in heavy almost acellular lar fibrous tissue. At the edge of the involved area where the oil is in close contact with the tissues, a violent cellular reaction is seen. We have observed the development of bronchiogenic carcinoma along the margins of paraffinomas of this type. Aspiration biopsy may be of value in establishing the diagnosis in cases of doubt. (Nathanson, Frenkel and Jacobi.)

Roentgenographically the lung picture presents an appearance of shaggy consolidation extending outward from the hilum regions into lower lobes, especially on the right side. The picture is one of massive irregular consolidation with interstitial inflammation and fibrosis. Paraffinomas produced in this way are not distinguishable roentgenographically from other types of inflammatory process without the history of oil aspiration.

Davis, et al., have reported 6 cases of lipoid pneumonia in which the roentgen findings could easily have been mistaken for tumor. Steinberg and Finby

have also pointed out large masses resembling tumors which may readily be overlooked.

Where large amounts of oil have been aspirated, the development of a paraffinoma may be observed over a period of years as the oil droplets are removed from the periphery and concentrated as large rounded masses in the central hilar zone.

KEROSENE (INTOXICATION) CHEMICAL PNEUMONITIS--The ingestion and aspiration of kerosene by children is not an uncommon occurrence. Kerosene may be detected in the lungs within thirty minutes after ingestion, by process of absorption into the blood stream and excretion by the respiratory tract. Aspiration of vomitus may also facilitate lung involvement. Its harmful effects have been ascribed to irritation of the mucous membrane; depression of the central nervous system and vascular damage to the lungs (Gershon-Cohen, et al). It is accompanied by pronounced dyspnea and intense cyanosis, which is sometimes alarming. This usually subsides within five to fourteen days, but may be fatal (approximately 2%).

Roentgenologically, the lung fields show blotchy areas of edema, especially in the lower lobes, which gradually disappear as the symptoms subside, leaving no indication of permanent damage to the lung structure (Reed, E. S., et al).

LUNG ABSCESS*

Abscess of the lung (Fig. 164A) implies the actual destruction of the parenchymal structure of the lung by invasion of pathogenic organisms, usually pyogenic. Roentgenographically, this results in a more-or-less circumscribed radiolucent area in the lung field in which the lung markings have disappeared, surrounded by an area of consolidation due to cells and serum thrown out as a defense mechanism to combat the infection. There may be a stage before actual lung destruction is evident in which the appearance is merely that of consolidation. Such consolidations, however, rarely take on the appearance of lobar consolidation, appearing, usually even in the early stages, as circumscribed areas of consolidation. The central area of destruction may be visible even before rupture of the abscess cavity.

Lung abscess may develop as a result of primary infection of the lung by many types of pathogenic organisms, from aspiration or embolism or it may follow ordinary pneumonia. In general, abscess formation presents a similar appearance regardless of the type of infection; certain types of bacteria, however, have characteristics which may betray their type. For instance, fusospirochetal organisms (of Vincent's Angina) have a tendency to produce large ragged cavities which spread with extreme rapidity and are attended with foul-smelling sputum (gangrene of the lung). Friedlander Bacillus abscesses are usually extremely extensive following rapidly upon pneumonic involvement. Abscesses of lung following streptococcus septic pneumonia are usually multiple,

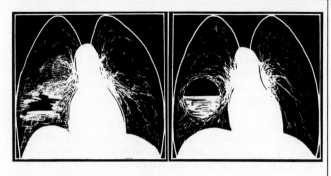

Fig. 164A   Fig. 164B

isolated areas of destruction occurring within areas of parenchymal infiltration.

Certain facts about the severity of the infection may be inferred from the roentgen appearance, produced by the infection; a wide zone of consolidation about an abscess cavity usually indicates its acute nature (Fig. 164A) and suggests a satisfactory constitutional reaction; if the zone of consolidation is very thin or absent in a patient who is obviously toxic and very sick, this indicates a poor constitutional reaction, having much the same significance as a low leukocyte count in the presence of overwhelming infection. Chronic lung abscess also may have a thin wall of reaction (Fig. 164B).

If the abscess becomes chronic, healing may take place by heavy deposits, layer upon layer of fibrous tissue, giving rise to a single rounded nodule two or three centimeters in diameter resembling a metastatic tumor nodule. This may be the source of solitary fibromatous tumors occasionally seen in the lung (q.v.). Its solitary character and its failure to change over months of observation serve to establish its benign character. Occasionally a tiny central area of necrosis may still be demonstrated by an overexposed film or by body section roentgenography. Such nodules may be identical in appearance with those produced by fibroma, hamartoma, tuberculoma or cyst.

A lung abscess may be evacuated spontaneously by rupture into a bronchus or into the general pleural cavity; or it may be removed surgically. In either event it is remarkable with what rapidity the consolidation surrounding an abscess disappears after complete evacuation of the abscess cavity. In our experience about one-third of such patients recover spontaneously; the remainder require chemotherapy or operative procedure. It is remarkable with what success chemotherapy is sometimes attended. Only after failure of chemotherapy should surgery be resorted to. Many surgeons feel that the operative risk is no greater on acute than chronic abscesses and that only a short time should be devoted to conservative treatment.

Accurate localization of lung abscesses with reference to their relationship to the lobes and fissures of the lung is essential for effective surgical approach.

Multiple small abscesses may develop in as-

sociation with bronchopneumonia but these are usually readily controlled with chemotherapy.

CHRONIC DIFFUSE INTERSTITIAL FIBROSIS * (FROM PYOGENIC AND PNEUMONIC INFECTION) (Fig. 165). Multiple small lung abscesses throughout the lung if untreated may stimulate so much fibrous-tissue formation that they become virtually encapsulated. Such fibrous tissue becomes organized and scar tissue results, thus effectually sealing up the infection in many foci. Scar tissue, wherever it occurs, contracts. Contraction of such a large amount of scar tissue in this location results in a decrease in size of the lung and pleural cavity on the affected side, a

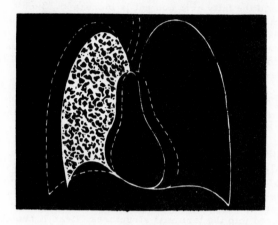

Fig. 165

condition which shows quite plainly in the roentgenogram; there is narrowing of the side of the chest affected, the ribs are more closely approximated and the intercostal spaces are narrower than normal, the diaphragm is elevated. In addition to this, the lung, from which all of the air has been squeezed by scar-tissue contraction, becomes solid in appearance showing irregular cavities due not so much to the tiny abscesses as to bronchiectatic cavities which result from the effect of scar-tissue traction on the bronchial walls. Massive atelectasis of the lung produces a similar appearance with the exception that the consolidation in this instance is homogeneous, never presenting evidence of cavity formation from the atelectatic involvement.

PULMONARY TUBERCULOSIS

FIRST INFECTION WITH PULMONARY TUBERCULOSIS IN CHILDHOOD* (Fig. 166). First infection with pulmonary tuberculosis usually occurs in childhood, although it may, in certain unusual circumstances, be deferred until adult life. Tubercule bacilli are inspired into the lung and lodge in alveolar structure. The initial infection may occur in any location of the lung. The lesion is small and usually cannot be detected during its active stage; not until calcium salts are deposited in the healed lesion can its presence be detected. The principal reaction to the infection is in the hilum lymph nodes; these

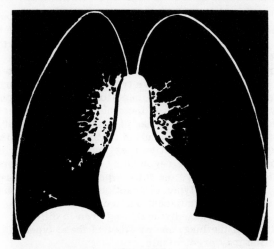

Fig. 166

become large and caseous as a result of the tuberculous infection which they drain. This is known as Ghon's phenomena. In a large majority of instances healing takes place with fibrosis and calcification and the individual recovers carrying with him throughout life these calcifications from old childhood infection. The original calcifications within the lung are usually few in number but occasionally an instance is encountered where multiple calcareous deposits are disseminated throughout both lungs. These may be due to healed disseminated tuberculosis but there is some indication that these may be due to healed mycotic infection, notably histoplasmosis. There is more convincing proof that histoplasmosis heals by calcifications of this type.

That there may be some tendency for calcareous tuberculous deposits to disappear is indicated from two cases observed by Wallgreen over a period of ten years in which he witnessed disappearance of small calcareous lesions and reduction in size of others from 2-1/2 mm. to pin-head size. Obviously a large percentage of childhood tuberculous infections get well since such a large percentage of adults bear the evidence of old healed childhood infection.

Roentgenographically, then, childhood infection with tuberculosis is recognized primarily by enlargement of the hilum glands rather than by detection of the initial lesion of parenchymatous infection; any calcification present should be suggestive evidence of a healed tuberculous process.

Such caseous glands usually retain the infection within their capsules, but occasionally rupture of the capsule occurs and the infection may be disseminated. If dissemination occurs into the surrounding lung structure, a diffuse zone of infiltration radiating out into the lung may be seen in the roentgenogram; if rupture occurs into a blood vessel, miliary tuberculosis results. In such cases tubercle bacilli usually cannot be found in the sputum in children, but examination of stomach washings may confirm the diagnosis in a doubtful case.

With the establishment of the diagnosis of childhood tuberculous infection, the physician's responsi-

bility is not over; it must be remembered that all pulmonary tuberculosis originates from contact with another person having the disease, so that examination of those in immediate and constant contact with the child is essential in order to ascertain the source of infection. A large factor in the recovery of the child is removal from the source of infection. Streptomycin and other antibiotics are of extreme value in prevention and cure of spread in childhood infections.

ADULT REINFECTION WITH PULMONARY TUBERCULOSIS* gives quite a different picture (Fig. 167). Here the site of initial reinfection is at the periphery of the lung, usually in the apex or first interspace of the upper lobes. The organisms, lodging in the parenchyma of the lung in this region grow and form colonies. There is a latent period of 10 to 20 weeks before development of the disease after exposure. The body, in its attempt to remove the infection, throws out a defense of endothelial cells and lymphocytes and microscopic tubercles are formed. These, as they enlarge, coalesce and finally become of sufficient size so that they become macroscopically visible and roentgenologically demonstrable. They appear as tiny infiltrations two to three millimeters in size in the apices or at the periphery of the upper lobes. Just why the initial tuberculous lesions should be in the apex of the lung is not definitely known; certain factors in the anatomic structure and function of the lung, however, may be contributory to the cause as suggested by Wm. Snow Miller; as the bronchi extend towards the periphery of the lung they divide and subdivide becoming smaller and smaller; after a time they reach the stage of division in which the bronchiole loses its cartilaginous rings and has budlike projections of air sacs from its walls; since it aids in respiration it is called a respiratory bronchiole. Up to this point the bronchi are supplied with blood from the bronchial artery; from this point peripheralward the pulmonary artery supplies the lung structure. In the region of the respiratory bronchiole, the two circulations mix and it may be that some retardation of flow results; this may be a

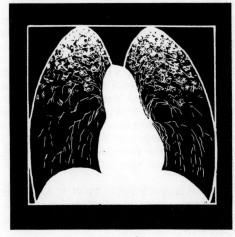

Fig. 167

factor in the lodgment and favorable growth of tubercle bacilli in this location.

Lymphatic drainage from such an area of infection is likewise in two directions; from the respiratory bronchiole drainage in inward by way of the lymphatic channels which accompany the bronchi, and also peripherally over the surface of the pleura and back to the hilum by this accessory route. This also may in some way favor growth of tubercle bacilli in this region. The fact that the upper portion of the lungs is subject to least expansion also may play a part.

The defense of the body against tuberculous infection is conducted principally by lymphocytes, mononuclears, epithelioid and giant cells. Polymorphonuclear cells play only a minor role. As the site of initial involvement in adult reinfection is drained toward the hilum, the lymphatic channels become engorged producing the appearance of a "fanlike" arrangement of the lung markings (Dunham's Fan). If the channels in this direction become blocked or overwhelmed, the infected area is drained peripherally toward the edge of the lung, over the surface of the lung to the hilum; the engorgement of the pleural lymphatics results in pleural thickening which can be detected roentgenographically as a narrow line running along parallel to the outer margin of the pleural cavity. Thickening of the interlobar pleura on the right side is sometimes seen under these conditions but it is of course not distinctive of the disease. In adult reinfection with tuberculosis the regional hilum glands do not show the same degree of enlargement and reaction as seen in the childhood type of first infection.

The disease may spread:

1. By continuity of tissue; as the disease progresses the individual infiltrations enlarge and coalesce, forming areas of consolidation.
2. By the respiratory system; sputum containing tubercle bacilli may be coughed up into the trachea and be aspirated into some other adjacent bronchus, thus inoculating some new remote region of the lung, even on the opposite side.
3. By the lymphatics; should the infection be too severe and extensive to cope with, tubercle bacilli, drained to the regional nodes, may again become active and produce new foci of infection.
4. By the blood stream; a caseous tuberculous lesion, eroding into a blood vessel may dump its infectious contents into the blood stream to be carried to the tissues supplied by the vessel involved. If this is some small vessel of the pulmonary circulation, disseminated pulmonary tuberculosis will result; if a larger vessel of the systemic circulation, miliary tuberculosis follows.

TYPES OF BODILY REACTION.* As a general rule there are three types of bodily reaction excited by tuberculous infection:
1. Exudative
2. Destructive
3. Fibrotic

When infection first becomes established mononuclear cells, lymphocytes and other body tissue cells and serum exude about the infection in an attempt to destroy it. Epithelioid and giant cells appear as a characteristic part of the reaction. This constitutes the infiltrative or exudative type of reaction; it may succeed in conquering the infection and the reaction may go no further. If, on the other hand, the bacterial infection is too great, areas of destruction or cavity formation occur as a result of toxins produced; this constitutes the destructive reaction. Finally, any destroyed area may be replaced by fibrous-tissue formation, and we have the third type of reaction, fibrosis. All of these types of reaction may be going on at the same time in adjacent portions of the lung.

In different individuals and even in different portions of the lung, one or other of these types of reaction may predominate.

Reinfection type of adult tuberculosis has its initial onset in the basal portions of the lungs in 1.5% of all instances. This is of special concern since in this location it has a tendency to abrupt onset passing quickly to a moderately advanced or far advanced stage with cavity formation often within 30 days. Prompt action with pneumothorax and chemotherapy is essential, (Cherry).

Favis after examination of a large number of tuberculous patients by planigraphic method has determined that while this method is helpful in detection of pulmonary cavities, it is by no means an absolute diagnostic method.

ACUTE CASEOUS TUBERCULOUS PNEUMONIA* (Fig. 168). In acute caseous tuberculous pneumonia we have an extreme example of the eduative type of reaction. This condition is characterized by an acute pneumonic consolidation usually involving an entire lobe, similar in appearance to lobar

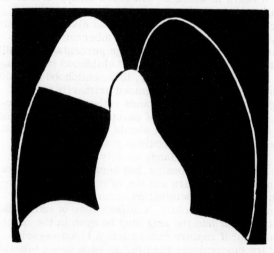

Fig. 168

pneumonia of pneumococcic origin and indistinguishable from it. Tubercle bacilli are usually absent from the sputum at this time. As the disease progresses long beyond the time for crisis, suspicion is aroused as to its tuberculous nature. The right upper lobe is the most frequent site of involvement although any portion of the lung may be involved. It often requires three months before cavity formation occurs in the consolidated area; not until this time are tubercle bacilli demonstrable in the sputum. From then on dissemination of the infection to the remainder of the lungs usually occurs; formerly few patients survived this disease; today, with the advent of antibiotic therapy the outlook is less gloomy. Just why tuberculous infection should exhibit such a marked pneumonic reaction such as this in some individuals is not entirely clear. Some feel that it is the reaction in a previously sensitized individual; it is a matter of clinical observation that in persons showing this type of reaction there is rarely any manifestation of previous tuberculous infection.

EPITUBERCULOSIS. An unusual type of sensitization reaction is seen in epituberculosis; in this case a gelatinous consolidation devoid of bacteria fills the lobe of the lung; (inoculation of a guinea pig with this material fails to show tuberculosis). Recovery with complete resolution results. This type cannot be distinguished roentgenologically from true caseous tuberculous pneumonia; the lack of severe clinical symptoms may be a clue to the true nature of the condition. It is a rare manifestation and almost always occurs in children.

EXCAVATING TUBERCULOSIS.* In certain instances, a tuberculous infection may show a great tendency to produce destruction; large irregular cavities develop sometimes completely excavating an entire lobe or lung. Such instances are extreme examples of the destructive action of the infection. Tuberculous cavities may be classified under three types, the acute cavity with ragged irregular walls which develops rapidly in the center of an area of caseation; the rounded cavity with a smooth thin fibrous wall which develops more slowly within a small area of tuberculous infiltration and the cavity with healing fibrotic walls which is due to its chronicity.

Rounded, smooth, thin-walled "tension cavities" may develop as a result of check valve action of granulations at the bronchial communication.

FIBROSIS AND HEALING.* Tuberculous lesions tend to heal by fibrosis whether they be small foci of infiltration within the lung or large areas of parenchymal involvement. As fibrous tissue organizes it contracts displacing adjacent movable structures to which it is attached; the hila of the lungs are displaced upward from apical scarring, the pleural septa are displaced by fibrous processes in the adjacent lobes; an entire lung may be involved causing narrowing of the entire side of the chest resulting in chronic interstitial fibrosis. Fibrosis may even result in healing of more extensive areas of caseation necrosis and cavity formation. Even large cavities may undergo gradual reduction in size and final obliteration by fibrosis. Some "heal" by conversion into a solid nodule (Pagel and Simmonds), such lesions presenting the appearance of rounded well-defined nodules in the lung,

are found on pathological examination to be due to layer upon layer of fibrous tissue with varying degrees of caseation necrosis in the center. These probably represent the "healing" of "closed cavities." Similar fibrotic nodules may occur as a "healing" stage in pyogenic lung abscesses; under these conditions however they are usually solitary and there are no manifestations of tuberculous infection in the chest. Calcification may or may not occur. Increased homogeneous density of such a nodule usually indicates heavy calcium deposit within an encapsulated caseous nodule. Ultimate obliteration of the infection may occur leaving only a fibrous nodule.

Radiologists have always hesitated to declare the degree of activity of tuberculous lesions from a single roentgen examination—and rightly so. Extensive surveys have shown, however, that he can probably conjecture an opinion with greater accuracy than he had formerly supposed. The conclusions of Birkelo and Rague indicate that: "activity can be determined accurately by roentgen examination and more rapidly and economically than by bacteriological methods."

"699 cases of minimal tuberculosis followed from 2 to 5 years show that their activity was correctly determined from the first roentgen examination in 86% of the cases (using large films and a roentgenologist's interpretation)."

CHRONIC DIFFUSE INTERSTITIAL FIBROSIS

TUBERCULOUS* (Fig. 169). Some individuals respond with an extreme degree of fibrous tissue reaction giving rise to such large quantities of fibrous tissue that it in itself becomes a menace. Chronic interstitial pneumonia is similar in every respect, whether the condition is produced by pyogenic infection or tuberculosis. There is one feature by which the tuberculous nature of such a condition may be suspected, namely by the appearance of manifestations of tuberculous infection in the opposite lung. It would be inconceivable that such an extensive tuberculous involvement of one side would not show some extension of the tuberculous infection to the opposite lung.

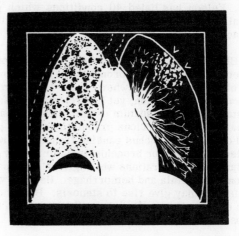

Fig. 169

MILIARY TUBERCULOSIS.* If a focus of tuberculous infection, such as a caseous gland, breaks through into a blood vessel, tubercle bacilli are disseminated by the blood stream throughout the distribution of the vessel involved. If that be the pulmonary circulation, dissemination of the disease to all or a part of the lungs occurs; if it is the abdominal circulation, peritoneal involvement results; if it is the blood supply of the central nervous system, tuberculous meningitis results. If the tuberculous material is inoculated into the systemic circulation, general miliary tuberculosis will result.

Roentgenographically, miliary tuberculosis of the lungs manifests itself as uniformly distributed tiny infiltrations, all of similar size since they were all disseminated at the same time and therefore have all had the same time for growth. Correlation of the roentgen findings with the patient's clinical symptoms, however, is essential since there are a number of other conditions with which it may be confused. With miliary tuberculosis there is usually high fever, great prostration and evidence of toxicity; in most of the other conditions with which it might be confused such constitutional symptoms are lacking.

Bronchiolitis occurs predominantly in infants and young children. It is a respiratory infection affecting mainly the terminal bronchiolar structures, with all attendant symptoms of infection. There are crepitant and subcrepitant roles throughout the chest, but no other evidence of disease. Pathologically, these small foci of infection may be the site of minute fibrous lesions on healing. Roentgenologically, however, there is little if any diagnostic evidence of the disease.

The nodular type of silicosis also may under certain circumstances resemble miliary tuberculosis; here also there are no confirming constitutional symptoms.

Other rarer conditions which may produce similar pictures are: miliary carcinomatosis, miliary deposits in lymphatic leukemia, mycotic infection such as aspergillus, histoplasmosis; miliary lesions associated with sarcoidosis and erythema nodosum. Inhalation of irritant dust particles such as silica and beryllium produce miliary nodules which may be confusing. Felson has listed 40 conditions which produce miliary lesions of the lung with notes on different reaction.

BRONCHIAL TUBERCULOSIS. Tuberculous involvement confined to a bronchus may not show evidence of involvement elsewhere in the lung on roentgenographic examination; yet tubercle bacilli may be a constant finding on sputum examination. It may be associated with tuberculous granulations which pile up and occlude a bronchus causing transitory areas of atelectasis (q.v.) or bronchiectasis or it may be associated with ulcerations which give rise to perforation with fistula and hemorrhage. Healing with scar tissues may give rise to stenosis. Bronchoscopic examination is the only method by which the diagnosis can be made.

NATIONAL TUBERCULOSIS ASSOCIATION AND AMERICAN TRUDEAU SOCIETY CLASSIFICATION (Diagnostic Standards, 1950). In order to come to some common ground of understanding, the National Tuberculosis Association has decided upon a classification to denote the extent and degree of pulmonary involvement. From the roentgenological standpoint the essential features of this classification are as follows:

Extent of Pulmonary Lesions

Minimal
Slight lesions without demonstrable excavation confined to a small part of one or both lungs. The total extent of the lesions, regardless of distribution, shall not exceed the equivalent of the volume of lung tissue which lies above the second chondrosternal junction and the spine of the fourth or body of the fifth thoracic vertebra on one side.

Moderately Advanced
One or both lungs may be involved but the total extent of the lesions shall not exceed the following limits:
Slight disseminated lesions which may extend through not more than the volume of one lung, or the equivalent in both lungs.
Dense and confluent lesions which may extend through not more than the equivalent of one-third the volume of one lung.
Total diameter of cavities less than 4 cm.

Far Advanced
Lesions more extensive than moderately advanced.

SURGICAL METHODS IN TREATMENT OF TUBERCULOSIS. The last decade has seen the development of the surgical treatment of tuberculosis to a high degree. Artificial pneumothorax is considered by most experts on tuberculosis as the greatest single advancement in the treatment of tuberculosis in the last twenty years; today antibiotic therapy has largely replaced pneumothorax as a therapeutic measure.

ARTIFICIAL PNEUMOTHORAX.* To be best suited for pneumothorax therapy, the involvement should be unilateral. By inducing pneumothorax on the affected side, the lung is freed from the chest wall and is partially collapsed. In this state it does not engage in the full degree of respiratory excursion and is, therefore, put somewhat at rest, favoring healing of the disease. Therapeutic pneumothorax to be effective must frequently be maintained over long periods. Re-expansion of the lung after such a long period of inactivity causes considerable decrease in its function.

There is some interchange of air as indicated by the fact that in recent years bilateral pneumothorax has been used as a therapeutic measure, without danger to the patient. Pneumothorax is frequently performed to cause collapse of cavities. This it may accomplish but not necessarily from compression. It may, by changing the relationship of its bronchial communication, abolish the check valve action which permits air to enter but not leave the cavity, and thus obliterate the cavity. Or it may even in certain instances intensify this action causing the cavity to blow up larger. By reducing the elastic recoil of the rest of the lung the process of natural healing by fibrosis is enhanced.

PNEUMOLYSIS.* Pleural adhesions between the parietal and visceral pleurae adjacent to a cavity motivate against its obliteration. Often such adhesions are strandlike and are confined to this location in the lung. Pneumolysis by severing of such adhesions with an electrocautery is possible by using a thoracoscope introduced into the chest cavity (Jacobeus). This operative procedure is very readily carried out and may effectively promote ultimate healing of a cavity.

PHRENICOTOMY* (Fig. 170). The same principle of rest for the involved lung is carried out in paralyzing the diaphragm from section of the phrenic nerve. If the nerve is completely severed, the diaphragm becomes paralyzed, flapping paradoxically, upward on inspiration, downward on expiration. If any nerve fibers remain by cross innervation from the opposite side, the diaphragm is merely immobilized in a high position, and paradoxical action may not develop.

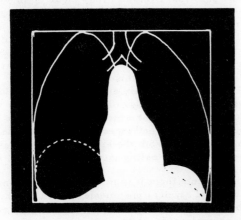

Fig. 170

PNEUMOPERITONEUM* in association with phrenicotomy may aid in still further displacement upward of the diaphragm on the affected side. It would not seem to be of much value for any other condition in the treatment of pulmonary tuberculosis.

THORACOPLASTY* (Fig. 171). Where large chronic cavities are present which cannot be collapsed by pneumothorax, in suitable cases, thoracoplasty can be utilized to collapse the involved side of the chest. The operation consists in removal of several inches of bone from part or all of the ribs on one side of the chest, causing collapse of the entire side of the thorax and compression of any cavities present. Even such compression may not result in obliteration of the cavity.

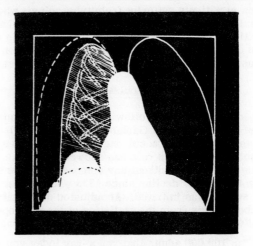

Fig. 171.

EXTRAPERIOSTEAL IVALON PACK. This is a procedure used by thoracic surgeons in collapse treatment of pulmonary tuberculosis. The peristeum is stripped from the ribs allowing the parietal and visceral pleura to fall inward thus creating an extrapleural space, which is then packed with Ivalon. The Ivalon is usually removed in three to five months and a small thoracoplasty is performed. In some cases the material is left in situ indefinitely.

Cohen has demonstrated the development of milkman's pseudofractures following the extraperiosteal Ivalon pack and concludes that this phenomenon is the result of trophic disturbance from loss of periosteal nerve and blood supply.

LOBECTOMY.* In recent years actual surgical removal of an entire disease-infected lobe has been practiced where conditions warrant. The development of atelectasis in a lobe of a patient under pneumothorax therapy is viewed with grave alarm by some clinicians (since it favors rapid spread of the disease), so much so that they feel that it is better to run the risk of lobectomy than to retain the diseased atelectatic lobe.

ASPIRATION OF CAVITIES. Direct aspiration of cavities through the chest wall and lung, for purposes of relief of tension produced by partial obstruction, and for medication, has not met with any great degree of success.

ANTIBIOTIC AND OTHER MEDICATION. Chief of the antibiotics to find favor in the treatment of tuberculosis was streptomycin. There can be no doubt of its efficacy in this field; the hopes at first entertained, however, that it would eliminate the disease have been dispelled and this type of therapy has assumed a more conservative form, utilizing various forms of the drug in an effort to find one which will be safe and at the same time beneficial.

At the same time it is necessary to urge precaution in the use of certain agents, even though used for the treatment of other diseases, in the presence of pulmonary tuberculosis. Numerous reports have been made of the rapid progression of pulmonary lesions in patients suffering from tuberculosis where A.C.T.H. or Cortisone was given for the treatment of arthritis. This is what would be suspected since the action of these agents is to inhibit bodily reaction and fibrous tissue development (King, et al.; Popp, et al.).

Surveys in Tuberculosis Prevention

In the discussion following a symposium on "Chest Surveys" Henry Garland (San Francisco) stressed the fact that according to the U. S. Statistics the tuberculosis death rate has showed a continuous decline since 1900, without any demonstrable variation in the rate of decline since 1933 when miniature chest survey was initiated. An adjusted death rate for tuberculosis from the statistics of the Metropolitan Life Insurance Co. corroborated these findings.

"In 100,000 adults that you x-ray today you will pick up about 50 new cases of active pulmonary tuberculosis. You will also detect about 8 unsuspected primary bronchogenic cancers and 57 cases of heart disease. Enlarged or arteriosclerotic hearts, for which little can be done make up a large proportion of the latter group. It seems to me that we should bear in mind the low potential yield in most routine admission survey programs."

George Jacobson (Los Angeles) in further discussion concluded:

"1) Mass survey with it has served a purpose but it is an uneconomical tuberculosis case-finding method and it is doubtful that future community-wide surveys should be conducted. 2) The admission chest x-ray program, particularly in large general hospitals is the most efficient tuberculosis case-finding method which is available today.

"One other feature of this is the prevention of tuberculosis among hospital personnel. Prior to 1951 we averaged approximately 15 cases of tuberculosis among our interns, residents and nurses. Since 1951 we haven't had a single case. The cost per examination, as closely as we can estimate it has been seventy-six cents per film."

MYCOTIC INFECTIONS

There are over 100,000 species of fungi; with few exceptions they are not pathognomonic for man. Fungi are commonly encountered on bread or grain, cheese and other organic materials.

The types which have been found causing pulmonary infection are: actinomycosis, blastomycosis, coccidioidomycosis, moniliasis, aspergillosis, cryptococcosis (torula) and histoplasmosis.

Fungus infections of the lung are relatively rare. In their acute form they resemble any other type of acute infection and cannot be differentiated except by finding the specific organism in the sputum. When such infection becomes chronic it may resemble tuberculosis very closely, both clinically and roentgenographically. Being granulomas they react in lung tissue like the granuloma of tuberculosis.

Actinomycosis and blastomycosis in their acute form resemble any other type of respiratory infection. In their chronic forms they may be indistinguishable from tuberculosis. Even miliary lesions may occur. There is a tendency to produce subcutaneous abscesses. The diagnosis can only be made with certainty by finding the organism. A special strain of actinomyces found in French West Indies, named Nocardosis, after its discoverer presenting much the same picture as our type of actinomycosis infection is described by Gundersen and Nice. For a recent review of roentgen pulmonary findings, see Hawley and Felson.

PRIMARY COCCIDIOIDOMYCOSIS. Infection occurs by inhalation of dusty soil containing the spores of the fungus in its vegetative phase. Transmission does not occur from person to person. The infection is prevalent in the San Joaquin Valley in California; by now it is found in many southwestern states, especially Arizona and Texas. Only two to five percent of the cases show associated skin eruption or bone involvement.

During the acute stage there are symptoms of a respiratory infection with fever. This lasts for 3 or 4 days and then subsides but the lung lesions persist. Areas of infiltration and consolidation may be present and cavities may develop. Annular ringlike shadows have been reported. Acute dissemination may occur throughout the lungs (Huntel, et al.).

The pulmonary findings may clear up in 2 weeks or it may become chronic and last for many years. There may be an associated adenopathy; this is almost always present in fatal cases. Patients with mediastinal involvement are usually very sick. Some lesions calcify. In its chronic stage it closely resembles tuberculosis (Jamison and Carter).

Roentgenographically enlarged nodular hilum shadows are almost always encountered with or without lobular or sublobular areas of infiltration in the periphery of the lung and increased peribronchial markings radiating from the hilum to these areas. Cavities are rare. Healing is slow, requiring 2 to 4 months.

In its acute form it is mistaken for influenza or other forms of atypical pneumonia, and in its chronic form the roentgen findings may resemble tuberculosis, lymphomatous deposits, sacroidosis or fungus infection. The final diagnosis depends greatly upon the geographical location in which the patient lives, the complement fixation test, and identification of the organism (Rakofsky and Knickerbocker).

Persistence of residual pulmonary lesions of various forms has been observed in war veterans, showing little, if any, change over two to five years (Bass, et al.).

MONILIASIS. Monilia infections also resemble acute inflammatory processes similar to pyogenic bacterial infection. The diagnosis can only be made by finding the organism in the pus or sputum. It seems to thrive on carcinomatous tissue and is therefore often encountered in association with carcinomatous growths.

ASPERGILLOSIS (Fig. 172). Aspergillus infection produces a somewhat different picture. In its most common form there are countless numbers of small soft rounded infiltrations uniformly scattered throughout both lung fields. It does not resemble disseminated infiltrative tuberculosis since the lesions are so widespread and uniform in distribution and symptoms are so mild; it does not resemble miliary tuberculosis since the individual lesions are much larger and the patient does not present the appearance of profound illness. The only condition which it resembles is second-stage silicosis where myriads of silicotic nodules are seen throughout the lung fields; the history, of course, will exclude this. It is usually seen in farmers or men who handle grain, since the fungus is usually derived from wheat. Pigeon-feeders, who fill their mouths with wheat and blow the granules forcibly into the mouths of pigeons to force-feed them, frequently acquire the disease. It is also frequently associated, as a secondary invader, with carcinoma of the lung.

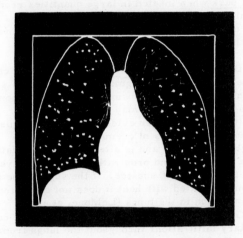

Fig. 172

Chortis in Greece reports the clinical and radiological similarity of acute aspergillosis and tuberculosis. Both infect the bronchial mucosa and peribronchial lymphatics and glands; necrosis and cavity formation may occur in either, and fibrosis and even calcification occur as a terminal reaction. Penicillin and sulfonamides will cure aspergillosis if infection is early.

It heals with multiple calcified lesions of unequal size, resembling healed lesions of tuberculosis. It is quite probable that other types of fungus infection such as coccidioides and histoplasma also heal in a similar manner by multiple calcifications; recently confirmation has been found for calcification of histoplasma nodules in a few reported instances. Microscopic concretions seen within the alveolar structures showing in the roentgenogram give a similar appearance to miliary calcifications wide spread throughout the lungs, (Petranyi and Zsebok). The exact cause is not known, but it is thought to be due to some episode of pneumonia or such infection which occur in childhood.

Pulmonary Intracavity Fungus Ball. Levin has described an unusual condition associated with fungus infection of the lungs, known as a pulmonary intracavity fungus ball. This is a rare but very spectacular pathological development which may occur especially in association with moniliasis or aspergillosis in which a ball of myelia develops free in a pulmonary cavity which communicates with the bronchial tree. Roentgenographically a dense, feathery bordered mass, roughly round or oval in shape, with a feathery border may be detected within a large pulmonary cavity which communicates with a bronchus.

CRYPTOCOCCOSIS (Torulosis). Cryptococcus infection of the lung is extremely rare, only 250 cases have been reported up to 1956; the great majority of these within the last 3 years. Improved cultural methods will probably account for an increasing number in the future.

Bonmati, et al. investigating the roentgen findings find that they fall into three groups: 1) Pseudotumorous lesions of varying size and number with rounded well defined margins and similar to indistinguishable other granulomatous lesions such as tuberculoma, 2) Disseminated small miliary nodular lesions distributed throughout both lungs such as monilia infection, 3) Infiltrative lesions of varied types. This group consists of small irregular areas of infiltration, patchy or linear, which resemble some other fungus disease or tuberculosis; such lesions although small may be associated with well defined ro rounded areas of cyst-like cavity formation. Healing may take place by fibrosis; calcium deposit is rarely encountered. Pleural effusion rarely accompanies the infection.

Spread to involvement of the meningeal structures develops in the large percentage of cases, ultimately causing death. In the past no medicinal remedy had been found of curative value; recently certain newly found drugs give promise of some success. Total surgical extirpation is occasionally successful. Of 14 cases resected by Bonmati, et al. 6 were found to later have infection of the central nervous system; this is often the case. Berk and Gerstl have reported a case in which surgical removal of the pulmonary focus resulted in eradication of the disease without recurrence over a four-year period.

HISTOPLASMOSIS. Histoplasma has long been known as a rare but potent cause of acute lung infection. Microscopically the large oval cells with multiple inclusion bodies can be demonstrated and identity can be established by cultural methods.

Clinically they produce evidence of pneumonic involvement which, in acute form, almost always results fatally within a short time.

Michael, et al., and Riley have made a very interesting investigation of the disease with special reference to birthplace and have found it to predominate in the Mississippi Valley and the South.

Roentgenographically the irregular areas of infiltration and consolidation bear nothing distinguishing them from other types of atypical pneumonic involvement. Fissel has recently reported acute fulminating cases of this type in which Cortisone therapy was beneficial and even curative after all other types of antibiotic agents had been futile.

It is believed that there may be a milder, more chronic form which ultimately results in recovery with calcification of the lesions.

In recent years an attempt has been made to connect histoplasma infection with patients showing multiple small calcified areas in the lung, because of the fact that individuals having such findings have a positive skin reaction with histoplasma antigen, and often are negative to tuberculin test. Serviansky and Schwarz, skin testing large groups of patients having such multiple calcifications, feel that they can differentiate those due to histoplasmosis from those of tuberculous origin.

Many instances of soft nodular infiltrations widely disseminated throughout the lung fields have been encountered in patients showing little if any symptoms of infection. While many of these are recognized as mycotic infection, the specific organism often cannot be identified even by most careful cultural methods. A report of the United States Public Health Service (Bunnell and Furcolow) indicates that mycotic organisms may be recovered for culture from stomach washings in a similar manner to that used for recovering tubercle bacilli. Utilizing this method, they were able to recover histoplasma capsulatum in a patient having soft nodular lesions widely disseminated throughout the lungs. The patient has been under observation for 3 years and has never had acute symptoms; "the lung lesions appear to be calcifying."

Since then other apparently authentic cases have been reported which would indicate a benign form of the disease which ultimately heals with calcification, thus bearing out the possibility that multiple calcifications throughout the lungs may indeed be due to healed histoplasmosis. It is probable, therefore, that a large percentage of such patients may not have been suffering from tuberculosis infection at all.

As a result of skin testing individuals having large numbers of calcium deposits in the spleen with Histoplasmin and Tuberculin Serviansky and Schwarz have found a positive histoplasmin and negative tuberculin reaction.

Jacobson and Zucherman have found less dense but definite splenic deposits in sickle cell anemia.

There is a recent report of a negro boy, aged twelve, who had a febrile reaction, with a roentgenogram of the chest which showed a large infiltrative lesion in the left lung. It required four months for resolution of the lesion and clearing of the roentgenogram. Tuberculosis and histoplasma were positive; other fungi negative. Complement fixation for histoplasma was positive in the yeast phase (Kunstadter, et al.). "In this patient the precursor phase of pulmonary calcification due to histoplasmosis was established for the first time. It was possible to demonstrate the progress of the primary phase of histoplasmosis from onset of the first symptoms through the stage of pulmonary infiltration, to final clearing of the lesion and beginning calcification. There was roentgen evidence that consolidation occurred eighty-five to ninety days or more before the histoplasma test became positive."

Chronic cavities removed surgically have been found to harbor histoplasma in their walls (Hodgson, et al.).

PULMONARY ALVEOLAR MICROLITHIASIS. In this condition millions of minute, sand-like granules of calcific density are spread uniformly throughout the lungs. They pack the alveoli even obscuring the heart shadow except on somewhat over exposed film. The etiology is unknown.

The condition is asymptomatic for years but ultimately leads to death. Microscopically the calcific deposits are within the alveoli with little if any other involvement or inflammatory cell reaction other than fibrosis.

MAPLE BARK SPORES. Certain spores of maple bark when inhaled in large quantities produce a peculiar infiltration in the bases of both lungs which usually clears up spontaneously on removal from the source of infection.

BAGASSE DISEASE. This is a condition caused by inhalation of small fragments of sugar cane stalk. After about 2 months exposure an acute pneumonic process develops which may cause death.

It causes roentgen evidence of acute lobular pneumonia with areas of edema and congestion throughout the lungs and is attendant at the outstart by fever, dyspnea and prostration. In a few days or weeks the symptoms subside. If the sugar cane is previously treated with heat it does not cause irritating reaction in the lungs (LeMone, et al.).

Greenspan and Fineberg have reported a case of miliary infiltrations throughout the lungs from Salmonella Bacteremia with associated spinal involvement. There was partial clearing after three months.

PNEUMOCONIOSIS

The continuous inhalation of certain types of dust particles over long periods may result in peribronchial fibrosis, resulting in great disability, and even death. The picture is entirely different from that produced by inhalation of irritating chemical materials (see Bronchial Irritation).

SILICOSIS*(Fig. 173). The special commissions of many governments and the efforts of individual physicians have combined to throw considerable light on this unusual malady, (Pancoast and Pendergrass; Pendergrass and Robert). These researches have indicated rather clearly that the offending substance in dust which causes it to become harmful is silica and that any dust is harmful in direct proportion to the silica which it contains. Organic dust causes irritation; chemical dust may cause toxicity but neither causes the same degree of fibrosis and lasting

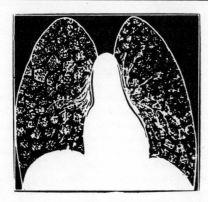

Fig. 173

damage as silica. Only the smallest particles of silica, 10 microns or less in size, are harmful since these are the only ones which can be breathed well down into the alveolar structure; larger particles are removed by the natural forces of elimination, ciliary motion, mucous secretion, and expectoration. Once these dust particles become deposited in the alveoli they cannot escape except by phagocytosis and elimination through the lymphatics. Ordinarily phagocytic cells become autolyzed and disintegrate but the silica acts in some manner as a preservative and the lymphatics may become clogged with cells.

In cases of massive silica inhalation, the lymphatics may become so loaded that this material fills the lymph nodes of the chest and flows over by way of the thoracic duct into the abdominal lymphatics where it is deposited in the lymph glands. Here it is deposited at the periphery as an "egg-shell" deposit.

Small rounded nodules or whorls of collagen develop along the lymphatic channels. Strangely enough, when examined microscopically, these whorls of collagen show a minimum deposit of silica on dark field illumination (Cole). When this occurs it gives rise to an appearance of beading along the lung markings throughout the lungs. As the disease progresses, this beaded appearance gives place to large blotchy areas of fibrosis or collagen deposits throughout the lungs. These large collagen deposits are frequently in the apices of the lower lobes. They often are bilateral giving the appearance in the anterior roentgenogram of a pair of "angel wings." At this stage of the disease diaphragmatic adhesions and pleural thickening are likely to occur and tuberculous infection of the lung usually supervenes, involving, not the apices as in ordinary tuberculosis, but occurring within the area of fibrosis.

The condition does not always pass through these definite stages but may manifest itself at once as large massive areas of fibrosis or collagenous deposit.

Not all individuals exposed to hazardous dust inhalation contract the disease. Ordinarily 5 to 10 years are required to develop the disease; rarely does it develop under two years of heavy dust exposure although some cases of acute silicosis have been recorded.

Silica is soluble to a certain extent in alkali; the solubility rate determines the rapidity of pathological changes which develop. For this reason the mixture of alkali with silica in certain types of abrasive soaps accentuates its harmful effect. Under these conditions silicosis may develop within 14 months. This also explains the continuous development of the disease after removal from exposure.

Apparently the smaller the particles, the more severe the symptoms; in industries in which there is fusion of quartz or silica, very severe symptoms appear very quickly and the disease is more apt to be fatal. On rare occasions there may be associated pneumothorax (Shaver).

Disability in silicotics is due to the inadequate oxygen supply resulting from the thickening and rigidity of the alveolar walls due to collagen deposits (Cole), and associated emphysematous changes. Capillary engorgement and edema of the air sacs and terminal bronchioles result causing inadequate aeration of the blood. The degree of disability cannot be estimated from the roentgen appearance, but is most reliably determined by respiratory function tests (Hammon).

In recent years many efforts have been made to alleviate the harmful effects of silica. The inhibitory effects of inhalation of aluminum dust and aluminum hydrate upon the action of silica has been demonstrated in animal experiments (Denny, et al) (Gardner, et al). The possibilities of such methods for the control of the disease are evident.

Roentgenologically, "a useful classification of the appearance of the silicotic process, which does not imply that there is progression of development or that there is a parallel degree of disability, has been developed.

In first degree silicosis, the nodules are barely visible and are associated with preservation or exaggeration of linear markings.

In second degree silicosis, the nodules are 2 to 3 mm. in diameter and largely obscure the linear markings.

In third degree silicosis, the nodules are larger than 3 mm. in diameter and there may be multiple, scattered, small areas of coalescence " (Pendergrass and Robert).

In the chronic stages there is coalescence and development of large blotchy areas of fibrosis throughout the lung; diaphragmatic restriction and adhesions; occasionally small collections of pleural effusion. Cavity formation without associated tuberculosis is so rare that from a practical standpoint any evidence of lung destruction may be taken as indication of tuberculous disease. A few instances have been reported of cavity formation without tuberculosis. There are evident differences in the roentgen picture in patients in whom tuberculosis develops in association with silicosis and in those in which silicosis develops on a previous tuberculous infection.

Any complication such as tuberculosis, emphysema, spontaneous pneumothorax, or cardiac enlargement gives a very unfavorable prognosis.

Once silicosis has become established it does not resolve but may become progressively worse even for a time after the individual is taken away from the sources of dust inhalation. Cases have been recorded in which, even after years away from harmful dust, fibrosis from exposure of previous years had developed into extreme disability. In the nodular stage it must be differentiated from sacroid, erythema nodosum, various forms of mycotic infection, leukemia and the lung lesions seen in tuberous sclerosis.

ASBESTOSIS. Certain silicates also produce similar changes in the lungs. Most prominent among these is asbestos. The individual lesions are softer in appearance; otherwise there is no distinctive difference between this and other types of silica involvement. The asbestos fibers can be detected microscopically in the lung so that the disease differs from that of silicosis.

ANTHRACOSIS. Anthracosis occurs from inhalation of coal dust over a long period of time. Hard coal is most injurious but even this usually requires twenty years or more exposure. The harmful effect is from the silica inhaled and not from the carbon; the greater the silica content the more likely the dust is to be harmful.

TREMOLITE TALC. This is also a silicate mineral (calcium magnesium silicate changes to talc) which produces fibrotic changes in the lung after prolonged inhalation (ten years or more) of fine particles

Clinically symptoms are more pronounced than in asbestos workers or silicosis patients: a) limited chest expansion, b) fatigue, c) curving or clubbing of nails and d) cardiac hypertrophy.

They seem distinctly sicker than silicosis patients.

Roentgenologically there is fine diffuse mottling of lung field similar to the appearance in asbestosis. Soft conglomerate fibrosis may occur causing emphysema and pleuritis. Like other forms of silica inhalation it predisposes to tuberculosis.

One unusual feature is "talc plaques." These are simply aggregations of actual talc dust which has remained in the periphery of the lung unable to be disposed of in any manner. These deposits are seen on the visceral pleura including the region of the diaphragm and occasionally the pericardium. They vary in size from single linear deposits a few centimeters long near the diaphragm to massive deposits of bizarre shapes extending over large parts of the pleural surface (Siegal, et al.).

CALCICOSIS. Calcicosis also is due in reality to the silica content of the dust not to the calcium salts; calcium being a natural constituent of the body causes little, if any, disturbance.

SIDEROSIS (ARC-WELDER'S LUNG). Siderosis or fibrosis from inhalation of iron particles from grinding has never been definitely established as a definite entity.

In recent years, however, it has been demonstrated (Groh) that the lungs of arc-welders present a uniform mottled appearance indistinguishable from silicosis due to inhalation of fine iron particles (hematite, Fe_2O_3). These do not excite fibrosis, however, and do not result in lasting disability (Sander). Microscopically they merely represent aggregates of iron oxide in the lymphatics of the lung.

BERYLLIUM PNEUMONITIS (Pascucci). The inhalation of fine particles of dust containing beryllium (used in the manufacture of fluorescent electric lamps and beryllium copper alloys) results in a delayed chemical pneumonitis. It produces an intense irritative reaction on the mucous membranes of the nose, throat, and respiratory system, extending well down into the finer lung structures. This requires an average exposure of 16 months.

Clinically there is dyspnoea, cough, fatigue, lassitude, and loss of weight. Anorexia and cyanosis develop and there is a low-grade fever. All have polycythemic blood counts.

Pathological examination shows that the "predominant finding is a granulomatous reaction infiltrating or completely obliterating the interstitial tissue." The granulomata consist of conglomerate masses and, in some cases, of foci of dense hyaline material and cellular infiltration of lymphocytes, plasma cells, and macrophages. Many multinucleated giant cells, with or without inclusion bodies, may be present. Mediastinal nodes in some cases may be infiltrated by a similar granulomatous process.

Roentgenographically, there is in the acute form widespread, diffuse involvement of both lungs, most intense in the mid-portion; radiating outward into both lungs from the hilum regions; the apices and costophrenic sinuses remaining free. There are two types of lesions, fine granulations and nodular infiltrations, depending upon the size. In the granular type the infiltrations may be so small and diffuse as to present a stippled "sand paper" appearance and there may be an associated reticular pattern. In the nodular type (which may well be a later development due to coalescence of the finer lesions) the lesions may be 4 to 5 mm. in size; they are more discrete and less numerous.

Sufficient time has not elapsed to warrant conclusions as to prognosis. The lesions may be slowly progressive finally causing death by respiratory and cardiac failure. Or, more commonly, there is a notable clearing of the lung fields but with a persistence of very fine nodulation. This may be followed by diffuse fibrosis six to nine months later with progression to very extensive involvement. Bruce has noted restricted air volume, hypoxemia and a tendency to develop emphysema of the lower lobes as a late manifestation resulting from fibrosis.

The roentgen pattern of the chronic form may be considered as a gradual transition from: 1) a diffuse granularity in all parts of the lung with gradual development of 2) a diffuse reticular pattern on the granular background and slightly enlarged indistinct hilar shadows with final development of 3) distinct nodules appearing uniformly throughout the lungs.

DeNardi, et al., have indicated the ultimate prognosis as very poor; 35% die, 50% remain static with chronic invalidism and only 15% show progressive recovery.

Not all cases go through these stages; there are many examples of remissions and exacerbations. There may be coalescence of lesions in some instances, basal emphysema, occasional slight pneumothorax. There may be some increase in cardiac size and enlargement of the pulmonary curve due to impairment of the pulmonary circulation; cor pulmonale is usually the ultimate cause of death.

BARIATOSIS is a condition which follows the inhalation of barium sulphate. It does not produce fibrosis or disability. Dense nodulation occurs throughout the lungs from collections of the opaque barium dust. These are large and more dense than silicotic nodules.

GRAPHITE PNEUMOCONIOSIS. Pneumoconiosis due to graphite mixed with a small amount of silica is of especial interest because of the massive consolidated areas with extensive necrosis. This is evidently due to lack of blood supply, not to associated tuberculous infection with cavity formation. There is no associated fever nor can tubercle bacilli be found. There is no true pneumoconiosis from graphite alone (Dunner and Bagnoll).

BYSSINOSIS, or pneumoconiosis, due to cotton fibers, gives the appearance in the roentgenogram of numerous soft rounded nodules throughout the lung fields. It does not result in fibrosis or permanently damage the lung structure (McCarthy and Akenhead).

ATELECTASIS

CONGENITAL ATELECTASIS, (Fig. 174). Congenital atelectasis may be present even in well-developed newborn children usually without evident cause. When it does occur it presents various degrees of consolidation within the lung field; it may impart a granular appearance to an entire lung field or may be confined to lobular areas, — patchy atelectasis. In still-born babies both entire lungs present the solid appearance of completely atelectatic lungs.

The chest is cone-shaped because expansion has never taken place; there is no deviation of the trachea or other mediastinal structures to either side because there is no variation in pressure within the chest cavity on either side.

HYALINE MEMBRANE DISEASE, A FORM OF ATELECTASIS. Little is definitely known about the basic cause of this disease. "The condition is seen most frequently in premature or debilitated infants shortly (even within 24 hours) after birth; they may be born by section or of diabetic mothers. It is never found in still born infants. Almost immediately breathing may become labored with sternal and costal retraction. It may progress rapidly to death. At autopsy the lungs appear dark red to purple from excessive engorgement with few or no gross air-filled spaces. Microscopically the capillaries are engorged and the alveoli and alveolar ducts may be collapsed. The few remaining air spaces are lined with a hyaline-like material," (Feinberg and Goldberg).

OBSTRUCTIVE ATELECTASIS.* Bronchial occlusion is the most frequent cause of atelectasis.

If complete obstruction of a bronchus occurs from any cause, so that no air can enter or leave the obstructed portion of the lung, then the entrapped air remaining is absorbed by the circulating blood and the involved portion of the lung becomes atelectatic. If the occlusion is in the main stem bronchus on either side, the entire lung becomes atelectatic (Fig. 175A). In its atelectatic state the lung becomes quite as dense as consolidation from pneumonia or tumor. This pronounced increase in density is due to engorgement of the vascular structure due to the pull on the vessel walls from collapse of the air cells. The collapsed lung, being devoid of air content, is smaller in volume than the normal air-containing lung; insofar as there is no associated pneumothorax and the surface of the lung remains closely applied to the chest wall, it is obvious that the side of the chest involved must become narrower from the suction effect produced by the shrinking lung volume. This suction effect is also manifested in retraction of the trachea, heart, and other

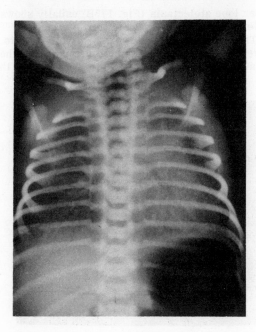

Fig. 174

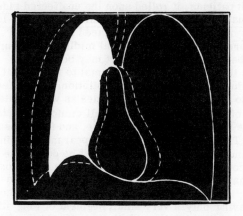

Fig. 175A - Massive atelectasis, entire lung

mediastinal structures toward the involved side, pulling up of the diaphragm and narrowing of the interspaces of the ribs on the involved side. This picture could hardly be confused with massive pneumonia of an entire lung since pneumonia does not cause any change in volume of the lung and consequently these phenomena do not appear.

Roentgenologically, then the signs of massive atelectasis of an entire lung from whatever cause, are:

1. A dense homogeneous shadow over one entire lung;
2. Narrowing of the affected side of the chest;
3. Contraction of the intercostal spaces;
4. Retraction of the trachea, heart, and other mediastinal structures toward the involved side;
5. Elevation of the diaphragm.

The picture resembles that of diffuse chronic interstitial pneumonia except that in this instance no bronchiectatic cavities are produced since there is no scar-tissue traction on the bronchial walls.

MASSIVE (ATELECTATIC) COLLAPSE OF LUNG* (Fig. 175A).

Another condition in which spontaneous atelectasis of an entire lung occurs under rather peculiar circumstances is known as Massive (Atelectatic) Collapse of the lung. This has been defined, (Bradford) as "a condition in which the lung, previously well aerated, suddenly without apparent cause, such as pleural effusion or bronchial occlusion, loses its air content and collapses." It is encountered most frequently at the present time as a postoperative complication, although it occurs not uncommonly after severe injury to the pelvis, abdomen, or chest. It seems to be independent of the type of anesthetic used at operation or may develop without previous anesthesia of any sort. There are no pathological findings to explain the cause of the condition. Atelectasis follows plugging of the bronchus by mucus, either a small inspissated plug of thick tenacious secretion or large amounts of watery mucus ("drowned lung"). The mystery which still surrounds the condition is: just what happens to abolish the cough reflex and allow mucus to accumulate in a bronchus in sufficient quantity to produce atelectatic collapse?

Such patients, if rolled upon the unaffected side and caused to cough may show reinflation of the lung almost immediately. The displaced mediastinal structures resume their normal midline position; often the apex beat of the heart may be followed across the chest from its abnormal to its normal position during the process of reinflation. The affected side of the chest again becomes as wide as its fellow of the opposite side, and all clinical symptoms such as pain, dyspnea, rapid pulse, and fever disappear. The lung loses its dense appearance within a few minutes, indicating that it must be due to the profound congestion which accompanies the condition.

It may be possible to have associated pneumothorax, if a major portion of an entire lung is occluded, leaving only a very small segment of lung still in free communication with the outside air; overdistention of the small remaining aerated portion, as the full pressure of the collapsing lung may be exerted upon this single small volume of remaining tissue (attempting compensatory emphysema), causes it to burst. Atelectasis of the various lobes produces characteristic pictures (Figs. 175A to F).

Position of the patient must play some part in the development of atelectasis since it tends to redevelop if the patient again lies on his back. Likewise, spontaneous massive atelectasis has been repeatedly encountered in debilitated infants who are allowed to remain for long periods lying on their backs. Lubert and Krause have analyzed the forces involved in the complete atelectic collapse of the lung and emphysematous expansion in the opposite lung with special reference to its appearance in the lateral view.

LOBAR ATELECTASIS* (Figs. 175A to F).

If atelectasis occurs in a single lobe, then the retraction of the chest wall is not so evident and the mediastinal displacement is not so pronounced. This is because the remaining inflated portion of the lung undergoes compensatory expansion to make up for the loss of volume of the collapsed portion.

During the process of compensatory expansion, the bronchial structures rearrange themselves to conform to the newly acquired shape of the remaining aerated lung. The lung being freely movable at the periphery and more confined in the hilum region causes the bronchi to fan out upward to fill defects in the upper lobe and downward to fill in lower lobe defects. The greatest pull is exerted upon the closest structures with less and less force exerted on the more remote lung structures. This is most strikingly demonstrated in right middle lobe atelectasis where normally aerated lung structures are intimately associated with the collapsed middle lobe on either side.

Upper lobe atelectasis (Fig. 175B) usually shows some deviation of the trachea toward the involved side. There is usually an upward arch imparted to the lower border of the lobe due to retraction of the atelectatic upper lobe. The peripheral margin at the

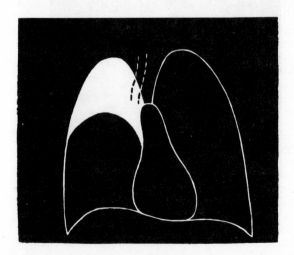

Fig. 175B - Right Upper lobe

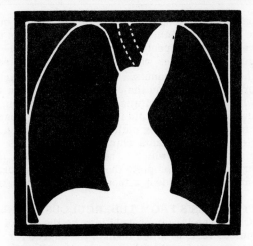

Fig. 175C - Left Upper lobe

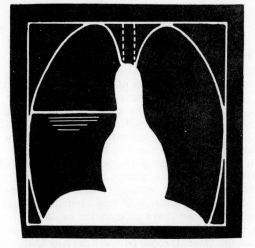

Fig. 175D - Middle lobe, anterior view

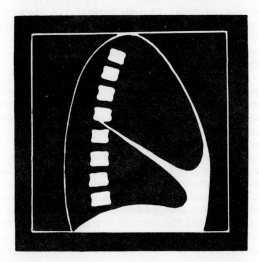

Fig. 175E - Middle lobe, Right lateral view

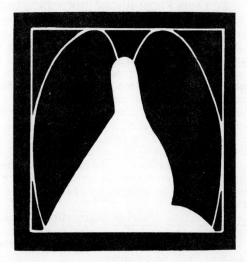

Fig. 175F - Lower lobe

lateral chest wall retains its normal position since the intact pleura will not permit elevation of this outer portion of the lobe. On the left side, (Fig. 175C), collapse of the upper lobe permits the lateral margins of the lobe to elevate somewhat higher since it is not confined by the extra middle lobe septum.

Atelectasis of the middle lobe (Fig. 175D) may be very difficult to detect in the anterior chest roentgenogram; the wedge-shaped shadow of the collapsed middle lobe presents only slight obstruction to the passage of the x-ray beam in this position and the slight haze produced may be entirely overlooked. The lordotic position and right lateral view are of value in its proper visualization. In the lordotic position the rays are projected horizontally across the upper margin of the middle lobe, visualizing more clearly its consolidation. Lateral view projection (Fig. 175E) discloses the location of all of the interlobar septa and shows the atelectatic middle lobe as a pancakelike structure between the upper and lower lobes.

Lower lobe atelectasis (Fig. 175F) results in an extreme degree of collapse of the lobe, forming a dense triangular structure obscuring the cardiophrenic sinus. It is sometimes amazing to see how small a structure the lower lobe can shrink to.

The most commonly encountered conditions causing occlusion are:
1. Foreign bodies
2. Bronchiogenic tumors
3. Inspicated bronchial secretions - "Idiopathic massive collapse"
4. Tuberculous granulations
5. Developmental anomalies of the bronchus

SEGMENTAL ATELECTASIS. If only a small segment is collapsed there may be some displacement of the adjacent lung septa but there is usually no manifestation of mediastinal displacement.

Reference to the diagram showing segments of the lungs supplied by small bronchial branches will aid in identification of the bronchial branches involved. When atelectasis occurs these segments become much smaller. They contract in the line of least resistance.

Microscopic and clinical evidence of porelike openings between the walls of adjacent alveoli of the same lobule would seem to indicate an accessory means for ventilation of the alveolar structures in case of bronchiolar obstruction (Van Allen and Lindskog). Van Allen found in healthy lungs that if the first branch of a bronchus was left unobstructed neither emphysema nor atelectasis would follow obstruction of the other branches due to collateral respiration. It would seem from this that atelectasis of smaller segments of lung structure would be impossible and yet there is abundant evidence that this does occur. Any inflammation or oedema quickly seals the interalveolar pores depriving that section of lung of its collateral respiratory mechanism.

ATELECTASIS FROM BRONCHIOGENIC TUMOR* (Fig 176). Whatever the cause of obstruction, the results are similar. One of the most frequent causes is bronchiogenic tumor. Such tumors, springing from the mucosal or submucosal layers of a bronchus grow out into its lumen, gradually increasing in size until it causes complete occlusion. The tumor itself may present only a small rounded shadow for a considerable period of time until complete occlusion occurs; then, suddenly, atelectasis develops in the occluded portion of the lung. If this happens to be in the right upper lobe bronchus, the rounded, lower margin of the tumor on the inner side, plus the concave lower border of the atelectatic upper lobe on the outer side, produces a characteristic "S"-shaped curve.

In left upper lobe bronchus obstruction, the atelectatic upper lobe contracts fan-shaped upward, sometimes to a very small size since there is no horizontal fissure to limit its collapse.

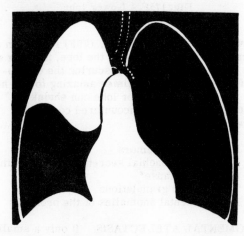

Fig. 176

FOREIGN-BODY ATELECTASIS. If occlusion of a bronchus is due to an opaque foreign body its presence can be readily recognized roentgenographically. If, on the other hand, the foreign body is of nonopaque consistency, it cannot be visualized; only by the secondary manifestations which it causes can its presence be suspected. Rather common nonopaque foreign bodies which are frequently aspirated into the lungs are peanuts. These are particularly dangerous inasmuch as the peanut contains essential oils which are very irritating to the lung tissues, causing infection and rapid formation of lung abscess, especially in very young children. If obstruction is complete, the atelectasis which develops causes dense consolidation which is readily detectable; if obstruction is not complete the presence of a foreign body may not be evident without special examination.

ATELECTASIS FROM TUBERCULOUS GRANULATIONS. The larger bronchi may be the site of tuberculous lesions which furnish the source for tubercle bacilli found in the sputum when the parenchymal lung structure shows no evidence of the involvement. Acute lesions may be ulcerative or hyperplastic, or both. Chronic lesions are fibrosclerotic producing varying degrees of stenosis. In the acute stage the lumen of the air passage may be narrowed by edema; in the chronic stage it may be stenosed by scar tissue contraction.

The air passage can be interfered with in still another manner; ulceration from infection caused by pressure of a bronchiolith may destroy a portion of the supporting cartilaginous ring of a bronchus permitting it to collapse and impede expiration (Chamberlain and Gordon).

These bronchial lesions cannot be visualized roentgenographically but their presence may be suspected from other manifestations which they produce. Transient atelectasis, balloon or check-valve cavities, sudden disappearance of a cavity and unexplained spread of the disease are all presumptive evidence of their existence. Bronchoscopy may be necessary to determine their presence.

COMPRESSION ATELECTASIS may occur due to long standing pressure on the lung structure from large tumors, aneurysms, etc. Under such conditions the expansion of the mass makes up for the loss of volume of the lung and there is no change in actual size.

DISC or PLATELIKE ATELECTASES (Fig. 177) are flat areas of atelectasis which occur in the bases of the lungs usually associated with restricted dia-

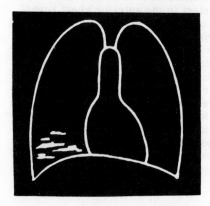

Fig. 177

phragmatic movement. These appear in the roentgenogram as dense bands extending horizontally across the lower lung fields. They usually disappear within a few days after resuming normal function.

ANOMALOUS FENESTRATED MEMBRANES have been reported causing local constriction of the lumen with or without atelectatic development. The fenestrations may be sufficiently large to permit satisfactory passage of air under normal conditions, whereas slight edema or infection may cause complete obstruction.

EMPHYSEMA and CYSTIC DISEASE

Emphysema may be defined as the presence of an excessive amount of air in the lungs; it may be vesicular if contained within overdistended alveoli or interstitial if it has escaped into the interstitial tissue of the lung.

COMPENSATORY EXPANSION; (COMPENSATORY EMPHYSEMA). Vesicular emphysema may be due merely to overexpansion of the otherwise normal lung. If any portion of the lung loses volume from any cause, such as atelectasis or operative removal, the remainder of the aerated lung, being still in free communication with the outside, undergoes compensatory expansion to fill up the lost space. The alveolar structures merely undergo inflation and increase in size; no pathological change is created within the parenchymal structures. Such a condition is known as compensatory expansion or emphysema.

OBSTRUCTIVE EXPANSION*; (OBSTRUCTIVE EMPHYSEMA), (Fig. 178A and 178B). If a nonopaque foreign body, lodged in a main stem bronchus on either side, does not completely obstruct, atelectasis will not develop. During inspiration (Fig. 178A), the bronchus becomes slightly larger in diameter permitting a small amount of air to enter the distal segment of the partially obstructed lung; on the expiration (Fig. 178B) the bronchus becomes smaller in calibre clamping down tightly upon the foreign body and preventing expulsion of air from that portion of

the lung. As a result, since any air absorbed by the circulating blood is continually replenished, atelectasis does not develop, but rather an increase in radiolucency appears on the involved side as a result of the overdistention with air. This condition is known as obstructive emphysema or obstructive expansion. This series of phenomena are readily seen on fluoroscopic examination. The diaphragm is immobile and depressed and does not move with respiration; the affected side of the chest retains its full volume during expiration while the unaffected side becomes narrower and denser in appearance as the air is expressed from the lung in normal respiratory movement; as a result of the varying pressure on the two sides of the chest during the various phases of respiration, the mediastinum swings back and forth like a pendulum across the chest with each respiratory movement (Manges).

Lobar or segmental emphysema of this type may be caused by buckling of the bronchus due to flail cartilaginous ring which may be so severe as to require lobectomy for relief (Fischer, et al).

This form of emphysema is merely a physiological response of the normal lung to a decrease in function elsewhere; there is no variation in the elastic tissue, the lung merely expands more because of an increase in the size of the pleural cavity. Ross Golden has demonstrated emphysema of small lung segments due to foreign body in smaller air passages. Small emphysematous segments of the lung may not produce demonstrable change in the adjacent lung structures but may result in displacement of the interlobar septa and hilum shadows.

PARENCHYMATOUS VESICULAR EMPHYSEMA. Parenchymatous vesicular emphysema, on the other hand, results from definite structural changes in the lung tissue. Loss in elasticity of the elastic tissue permits over-distension of the vesicular structures; air enters freely causing unrestricted distension of the air sacs to their maximum size, but air cannot leave the distended vesicles because of their loss of elastic recoil.

The terminal air sacs become dilated and in many cases their walls become destroyed, leaving the air spaces separated only by the alveolar septa. As a result, there appears on the roentgenogram, first, increased radiolucency of the lungs, and second, the

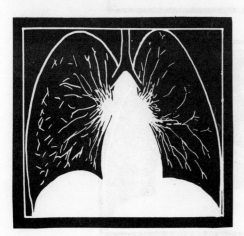

Fig. 178A

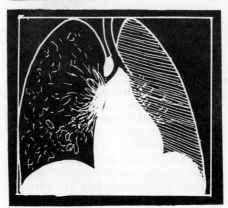

Fig. 178B

formation of a terminal network of finer lung markings which extend well to the very periphery of the lungs. This appearance has been referred to as "arborization or reticulation." Emphysema, when well established, affects the contour of the chest; the posterior ribs become horizontal and the anterior portions angulate abruptly downward, resulting in an increase in the anteroposterior diameter. Most cases do not progress to serious disability.

BULLOUS EMPHYSEMA*. Ordinary parenchymal emphysema may progress to the formation of large blebs and bullae throughout the lung; the septa between alveolar structures continue to rupture forming larger and larger air sacs until they constitute thin-walled blebs on the pleural surface and bullae throughout the lung. Spontaneous rupture of pleural blebs (q.v.) constitutes one of the most frequent causes of pneumothorax.

PROGRESSIVE VESICULAR PULMONARY EMPHYSEMA (Fig. 179A). This is a condition in which pleural bleds and bullae form at the periphery of the lung. The etiology is unknown. In its simplest form it manifests itself by spontaneous rupture of one of these distended vesicles resulting in pneumothorax. In its most grave form it results in progressive unrelenting vesicle formation which may over a period of months or years result in almost complete replacement of the lung. This condition has been referred to as "vanishing lung." A number of cases have been reported in which death ensued (Price and Teplick). Fortunately it is very rare.

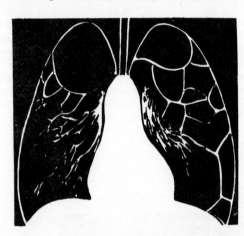

Fig. 179A

PULMONARY INTERSTITIAL EMPHYSEMA* (Hamman's Disease). Rupture of distended emphysematous bullae into the interstitial tissue of the lung results in interstitial emphysema. Air thus introduced into the interstitial tissue travels by way of the interstitial spaces toward the periphery of the lung and into the mediastinum, (q.v.) producing a characteristic appearance of halo about the heart often accompanied by spontaneous pneumothorax from rupture of pleural blebs and finally by complete atelectasis from avascularization by pressure on the vascular structures from within their fibrous

interstitial sheaths. Herrnheiser and Whitehead have pointed out the existence of air-filled pseudocysts within the lung which may be associated with this condition, but caution against too readily diagnosing the condition from these signs alone.

CYSTIC DISEASE OF LUNG (Fig. 179B, C and D). Cystic formation in the lung is being encountered with greater and greater frequency, (Peirce and Dirkse), (Kirklin). This may be congenital or acquired. The origin of congenital cysts of the lung is not fully understood; they probably represent accidental enclosures of bronchial or lung structure occurring during fetal development. They may show tracheal attachment or esophageal involvement and

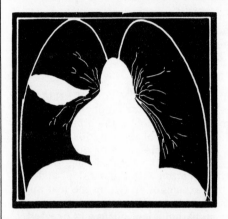

Fig. 179B

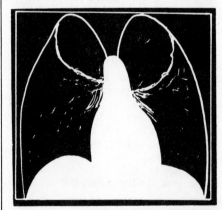

Fig. 179C

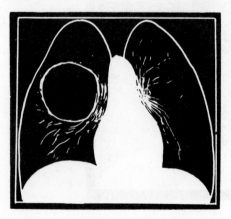

Fig. 179D

have been demonstrated in new-born infants. They are of two types, those containing fluid and those containing air—pneumatoceles. The fluid cyst may be the initial state of the cyst formation; that this may rupture, allowing egress of the fluid and collapse of the cyst resulting either in subsequent healing and obliteration of the defect, or in formation of a check-valve of mucous membrane allowing the cyst to be filled with air on each inspiratory movement but preventing expulsion of air on expiration by its valve-like action, thus causing it to become fully inflated with air. The extreme pressure maintained within the cyst may account for inhibition of further secretion by its secretory membrane.

Air cysts (pneumatoceles) vary in character depending upon the place of origin in the bronchial tree. If they originate in association with the larger bronchi which have cartilaginous rings they spring from the bronchial walls like herniations of multiple diverticula always maintaining a patent connection with the bronchus from which they originate. Roentgenographically they may appear as multiple rounded, thin-walled air spaces often spoken of as "honey-combed." The term is not well chosen as descriptive of the condition since the air spaces are much too large to resemble a honey comb. Lipiodol injected into the trachea will run out readily into the cystic structures of the larger bronchi. The "honey-combed" appearance of the lung may very readily be mistaken for tuberculous cavities. These air-filled vesicles do not change in size with respiration but maintain their constant pressure. This may become so great that it exerts sufficient pressure on the weak portion of the mediastinum to cause herniation to the opposite side. The farther out in the bronchial tree the air cysts originate, the thinner their walls and the more completely closed their communicating openings will be until those which occur at the periphery of the lung become pleural blebs and bullae; lipiodol injected into the lung will not extend out into them.

That lung cysts are not always congenital but may be acquired has been amply proven. Numerous instances have been observed where, in a previously healthy lung, cysts, both fluid and air-containing, have developed during the course of an inflammatory process in the chest such as lung suppuration, pneumonia or pleurisy.

Roentgenologically such cysts may be recognized in perfectly healthy individuals having no history or symptoms of disease. Only after prolonged observation is the diagnosis justifiable. The fluid cysts (Fig. 179B) may appear in the mediastinum or in the pleural cavity itself; they present smooth well-defined rounded shadows of uniform density; if rupture occurs a fluid level may be visualized.

Isolated "balloon" cysts (pneumatoceles) (Figs. 179C and 179D) are rounded well-defined radiolucent areas, devoid of lung markings, showing thin defining membranes; they occur most frequently in the upper lobes and may be bilateral.

While we have observed such cysts without change over many years in adults, we have also seen rapid expansion and death in infants, due to acute pressure on the great vessels. They are, therefore, a poten-tial danger in children. Under such circumstances, surgical removal may be justifiable (Warring).

Pulmonary tension disorders may take on many variable forms especially in children (Campbell and Silver). It is difficult to understand how pressure high above that of atmospheric can be built up in tension cysts when their filling occurs primarily as a passive process to equalize air pressure from respiratory movements. There must be some other intermediate space which being filled with air during ordinary respiration, is pressed upon by the musculature during the expiratory phase.

Pulmonary cysts of this type show a natural tendency to spontaneous regression during early infancy (Coffey), but should be watched carefully for any tendency to undue enlargement.

Air cysts of this type may be confused with annular shadows which result from septic thrombosis of the terminal bronchial vessels (q.v.). Annular shadows of this type have much thicker and more uniform walls. When multiple they do not cluster in a honey comb arrangement but each retains its own characteristic appearance. They may show some remnant of solid structure in their centers.

Fibrotic and cystlike changes have been noted in the lungs in association with cystic pancreatitis in infants and young children (q.v.). Recent observations would indicate that this peculiar disease owes its pathological symptoms to the thick glarry mucous secretion with which it is attended wherever it may be found in the body. It has therefore been designated as mucoviscidosis (Farber).

Congenital cystic-adenomatoid malformations of the lung are also described by Craig, et al. in which numerous air cysts much smaller in size are present associated with large masses of adenomatous tissue. The clinical symptoms are cyanosis, rapid respiration and an absence of respiratory distress or fever in newly born infants. Surgical resection is the treatment recommended.

NEW GROWTHS OF THE LUNG
(Jackson and Jackson)

Primary new growths of the lung may be either malignant or benign. Malignant growths are much more numerous than the benign and predominate in the male sex; benign growths are less common and occur most often in women.

MALIGNANT TUMORS*. Within the last few decades, primary carcinoma of the lung has risen to incidence from a rare disease to one second only to carcinoma of the stomach. The alarming increase in this disease has lead to a diligent search for the cause. The pronounced increase in cigarette smoking has directed suspicion to this as a possible cause; breathing of atmosphere visciated by large quantities of carbon monoxide and other gases contained in the exhaust fumes from so many automobiles may also be another possible source of bronchial irritation; many other conditions likewise present themselves as possible etiological factors. A summary of the classification of malignant tumors of the lung almost universally accepted (Rubin) is as follows:

Bronchiogenic carcinoma
    (1) Epidermoid; (squamous cell) carcinoma
    (2) Adenocarcinoma; may contain mucous cells
    (3) Undifferentiated carcinoma; small spindle or round cells; "oat-cell"; Pancoast tumor

Parenchymatous tumors
    (4) Alveolar cell carcinoma
Connective tissue tumors
    (5) Sarcoma of the lung, very rarely

Pleural tumors
    (6) Endothelioma (mesothelioma)

The site of origin and characteristics of their growth are largely responsible for the roentgenologic manifestations which they produce. From the roentgenologic viewpoint, bronchiogenic carcinoma may be considered as of two types; one a nodular type in which the growth springs from the bronchial epithelium, tends to remain local, and finally, by its growth, produces atelectasis of the segment of the lung in which it is located.

BRONCHIOGENIC CARCINOMA, NODULAR (POLYPOID) TYPE* (Fig. 180A). This type of malignant neoplasm produces a nodular growth originating from the bronchial epithelium, having a tendency to remain local, enlarging gradually until the bronchus is occluded, resulting in atelectasis of the portion of the lung which it supplies (Fig. 180B). When it involves the upper lobe, the combined appearance of the under convex margin of the bronchial carcinoma medially and upward concave margin of the lower edge of the upper lobe peripherally, produces an S-shaped curve which is quite characteristic of the condition in this location. Obviously, there is a much earlier period during its development when the small nodular growth just partially occludes the bronchus, causing obstructive emphysema. Detection in this early stage is most desirable. Only closest observation, using inspiration and expiration films, will

make possible the detection of this phenomenon.

Bronchography is of special value in the detection of early carcinomatous lesions of this type. By careful, repeated examinations it is possible to detect and prove the constancy of minute filling defects even in the smaller bronchioles; this requires precise painstaking examination which can only be perfected after extensive practice (Farinas). Such bronchiogenic carcinomatous lesions may occur at any location in the lung. In their early development they may present the appearance of a solitary rounded nodule very similar to benign tumors (q.v.), from which a differential diagnosis may be very difficult. Small amounts of calcium occurring in the lesion do not definitely rule out its malignant character, (O'Keefe). Rather extensive deposits of the laminated type favor healed granuloma; of the "popcorn" variety, indicate hamartoma.

Rigler has observed that notching of such a solitary nodule is always indication of malignancy, but does not hazard an opinion as to its cause. Such malignant solitary lesions may occur any place in the lung.

Present day thoracic surgery is no greater risk than the chance of retaining a potentially malignant lesion.

BRONCHIOGENIC CARCINOMA, DIFFUSE INFILTRATIVE (ULCERATING) TYPE* (Fig. 180C). Bronchiogenic carcinoma of this type springs from the deeper layers, forms a more bulky mass and tends to break down and ulcerate so early that the condition cannot be differentiated from a lung abscess. Even at autopsy the lesion is thought to be a pyogenic abscess, and indeed it is, except that it is within a carcinoma of the lung. Not until microscopic examination of the abscess wall is made, is its true malignant nature recognized. Only rarely does atelectasis occur in this type of bronchiogenic carcinoma. The destruction seen in these tumors is primarily due to the vulnerability of this specific type of growth, pyogenic infection is a secondary complication.

When carcinoma of the lung presents itself in the typical nodular form, the diagnosis is usually quite evident; unfortunately, however, there are so many other bizarre forms which it may present that often not until microscopic examination of the tumor tissue is made, is malignancy suspected.   A malignant

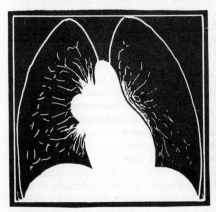

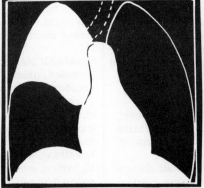

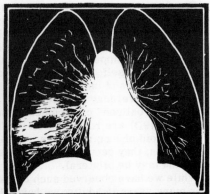

Fig. 180A   Fig. 180B   Fig. 180C

abscess wall may be so uniform and smooth that it may resemble a pneumatocele or air cyst of the lung. Only by correlation with the clinical history can a correct diagnosis be made with any appreciable consistency.

Investigation of the clinical symptoms accompanying carcinoma of the lung has convinced us of the importance of the following symptoms:

1) In an individual 50 years of age or older,
2) Having a duration of illness of 3 months or longer,
3) With progressive weakness and loss of weight without demonstrable cause,
4) Without fever or other signs of infection,
5) With possibly a cough,
6) Or possibly blood streaked sputum or hemoptysis at any time during the disease.

These symptoms coupled with a persistent area of infiltration or consolidation give the best criterion for the diagnosis of carcinoma of the lung.

Many additional aids are available for confirmation of the diagnosis of malignant neoplasm.

Body section radiography or bronchography will demonstrate a block of the bronchus in 90% of instances. Bronchoscopy will show a tumor in 85%; it has a rather characteristic bronchoscopic picture and the microscopic appearance is usually quite characteristic (Howe). Cytological examination of bronchial secretion will also be of aid in detection of malignant cells in a high percentage of instances (Rigler).

In smaller bronchial branches bronchiogenic carcinoma may be suspected if inspiration-expiration films show small areas of obstructive emphysema (Rigler and Kelby).

PRIMARY ALVEOLAR CARCINOMA* (Davis and Simon). Primary carcinoma of the lung may arise from the alveolar structure of the lung. Simultaneous development of such tumors from multiple areas throughout the lung has been amply proved. Microscopically there is overgrowth of alveolar cells over a wide area causing encroachment upon but not at first filling the alveolus; remaining air in the alveoli give the roentgen appearance of small granules throughout the affected portions of the lung. Starting simultaneously in multiple foci (a condition unique in the realm of malignant tumor genesis), it gradually extends to involve more and more of the lung substance; when fully established it appears as a diffuse homogeneous area of consolidation. Because of lack of metastases it is considered by some to be a benign overgrowth of cells which causes death by obliteration of all air spaces.

Microscopically it resembles closely the adenomatosis resulting from jaagsiekte virus disease occurring in sheep.

Here again the clinical history is essential for the diagnosis. 1) the lack of fever, 2) the chronic character of the disease, 3) the progressive weakness and loss of weight, all serve to aid in establishing the diagnosis. It may be difficult to differentiate from the benign insidious types of adenomatosis of the lung, or from some cases of atypical pneumonia or mycotic infection. Monilia infection is a frequent complicating condition.

Primary Carcinoma of Lung with Associated Mycotic Infection. Not infrequently, malignant growths of the lung become associated with mycotic infection; Monilia, Aspergillus, Saccharomyces, etc. It would seem that they furnish especially favorable soil for growth of yeast organisms. Such combined involvement may present a troublesome picture for the radiologist. If the fungous infection is identified in pure culture, it may be assumed that the pathology present is due entirely to this infection. It has been our experience, however, that wherever such mycotic infection is identified, the possibility of carcinoma must always be considered. There does not seem to be a similar tendency for metastatic carcinomatous lesions to develop mycotic infection. Possibly because the growth is more rapid and the lesions less closely associated with the bronchi.

Pancoast Tumor. Pancoast tumor ("superior sulcus" tumor) is not due to any specific cell; many types of cell structure have been found in such tumors. By "superior sulcus" is meant the superior rounded apical portion of the chest. This tumor has one characteristic by which it can usually be recognized: associated erosion and destruction of the adjacent ribs (by which the character of the tumor is recognized), and pressure on the adjacent nerve structures. This would suggest the invasion or origin within the chest wall.

While such tumors may not have a common cellular structure, certain features which characterize tumors of this region bind them together as a special entity. These are: extensive destruction of the adjacent ribs (by which the character of the tumor is recognized) and pressure on the adjacent nerve structures.

Primary Sarcoma of the Lung. This is a very rare tumor, producing a roentgen picture often indistinguishable from other types of neoplasm. There are a few characterizations of its growth however which may offer a clue as to its true nature. Carcinomatous tumors arise from bronchial epithelium and tend to be confined to bronchial structures; they enlarge by multiplication of cells in all directions, hence have a tendency to rounded nodule formation; any degree of variation from spherical formation must be attributed to variability in the factors influencing growth of the cellular structures as they divide and subdivide.

Sarcomatous tumors on the other hand spring from the connective tissue which is all pervading and while they grow and enlarge by multiplication of cells they do not tend to be confined by any limiting structure. This is shown by a tendency of such tumors to spread along the planes of the interlobar septa.

METASTATIC LUNG TUMORS*. Secondary metastatic tumors of the lung may be either of carcinomatous or sarcomatous variety, or of the type seen

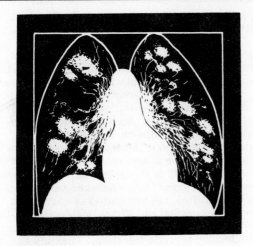

Fig. 180D

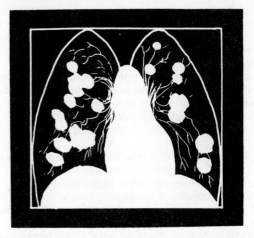

Fig. 180E

in lymphoblastomatous conditions. Metastatic malignancy in the lungs usually appears as multiple rounded nodular growths from a few millimeters to a few centimeters in diameter widely scattered throughout the lungs. Carcinomatous nodules (Fig. 180D) are usually less numerous and less well defined than sarcomatous metastases. Sarcomatous nodules (Fig. 180E) may be as clearly outlined as if a number of coins were actually placed upon the film. They are, therefore, sometimes referred to as coin lesions of the lung. Widespread miliary metastases throughout the lungs may occur with carcinoma, sarcoma or lymphoid deposits of Hodgkin's, or leukemia. The lacework type of infiltration seen in tuberous sclerosis may be difficult to differentiate.

Massive metastatic involvement is a frequent development from hypernephroma, although this may be of the distinctly nodular variety.

Occasionally, a peculiar type of metastatic spread is seen in carcinoma of the breast directly through the chest wall into the mediastinum and peribronchial lymphatic structures. Roentgenographically this appears as an accentuation of the bronchial branches radiating outward abruptly from the hilum regions giving a sunburst effect. Celis, et al. have pointed out the importance of the thoracic duct in the spread of malignant disease.

Lymphoblastomata; Hodgkins Disease; Lymphosarcoma. These diseases affect the lymphatic structures manifesting themselves primarily as bulky adenopathy of the hilum glands, spreading, retrograde, along the pulmonary lymphatics outward like a sunburst giving rise to a roentgen picture which is distinctive of this type of spread of malignant disease. As the disease progresses coelescence and enlargement of the lymphoid deposits may produce massive areas of consolidation indistinguishable from other types of malignant involvement.

Another kindred type of malignant tumor which sometimes starts as a pulmonary lesion is extramedullary plasmocytoma of the lung (Rozsa and Frieman). The picture is not characteristic; it may

present itself only as an area of diffuse infiltration or as a large massive, well-defined consolidation involving an entire lobe. The bone may be secondarily involved or may be free. Diagnosis is made by biopsy and surgical resection offers hope of cure.

Kruckenburg tumors can, under unusual circumstances, spread from their original location in the stomach directly upward by way of the lymphatics into the lungs, without ovarian involvement. Roentgenologically they may produce a picture very similar to the lymphatic spread of Hodgkin's disease.

Hepatomas often cause widespread microscopic metastases in the lungs which cannot be detected roentgenologically but are quite evident on microscopic examination.

When there is no evidence of primary lesion, metastatic involvement may be difficult or impossible to diagnose (Russo and Cavanaugh).

GRANULOMAS OF LUNG

Granulomas are collections of granulation tissue which have developed in response to tissue reaction in an effort to rid the body of infection. Such infection may be pyogenic, tuberculous, mycotic or possibly viral. The occurrence of such granulomas in the lung renders them very amenable to roentgen examination; due to the surrounding air-filled lung it is possible to effectively examine them as to their location, size, shape, form and outline, and the consistency of their structure.

Pyogenic granuloma, from the walling off of small areas of pyogenic abscess in the lung, may present the appearance of a small discrete, well-rounded nodule, which on section presents the appearance of a central focus of remaining pyogenic infection, surrounded by layer upon layer of dense fibrous tissue like the skins of an onion. Roentgenologically the density may appear uniform throughout or there may be a slightly rarified central zone, best observed on body section examination; rarely is there any calcification. There is ordinarily little if any change over long periods of time.

Tuberculoma. In a similar manner old tuberculous lesions may become encapsulated with formation of well-defined rounded nodules. They are usually limited by a dense fibrous capsule with a greater amount of central destruction and calcium deposit. As time goes on, liquifaction of the granuloma may result in complete caseation necrosis within the fibrous capsule and excessive calcium deposit. They have a tendency to multiple occurrence.

Mycotic Granuloma. Similar solitary, rounded nodular lesions may occur as a result of mycotic infection. They may bear no distinctive roentgen difference from tuberculous granulomatous lesions and cannot be differentiated.

Kerley has endeavored by arterial injection to determine the role played by vascularity in the site of occurrence and character of these solitary nodular tumors. By an analysis of the sites of tuberculomas he has found that these granulomatous masses never occur anteriorly and are likewise very rare in the posterior middle and anterior basillor segments. Fully 80% of tuberculous granulomas occur in the apical segments; this seems parallel to the predominating site of such infection. Carcinoma may occur in any location.

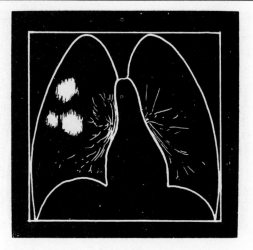

Fig. 181

BENIGN TUMORS

Benign tumors of the lung occur most frequently in young individuals; they are more apt to contain calcium deposits, but their benign character cannot be depended upon from the detection of a small amount of calcification alone; only if the calcium deposit is of the laminated concentric type as in old healed infection or of the "pop corn" variety as occurs in hamartoma can it be relied upon as a definite sign of benign character, (O'Keefe, et al.).

Bronchial adenomas, when they occur in the peripheral segments of the lung take on a similar rounded nodular appearance, without calcification and may not be differentiated from other nodular lesions, (Bluth).

BRONCHIAL ADENOMA. This is a tumor of bronchial origin very similar in all respects to bronchiogenic carcinoma with the exception that it is slow and insidious in its growth, often lasting for years. Many observers feel that it is also potentially malignant. We have followed such a patient for four years, only to have the growth take on malignant characteristics after that period. About 12% undergo such malignant changes.

CAVERNOUS HEMANGIOMA* (Fig. 181). Benign tumors of the blood vessels of the lung, although quite rare, present a striking clinical and roentgenological picture. Cavernous hemangioma (Goldman) occurring in the lung have the effect of producing an arteriovenous fistula. If the shunting of the circulation is sufficient, cyanosis, dyspnea, clubbing of the fingers, cardiac enlargement and polycythemia may occur. A bruit may be heard over the lesion in the chest. Roentgenographically there is one or more rounded, well-defined, dense area in the lung which remains with little change over a long period of time (Sloan and Cooley). Fluoroscopic examination while the Valsalva Exercise is carried out will show a diminution in size of the angioma. These lesions are prone to bleed into the surrounding lung structure giving an appearance of irregular lung consolidation. Fever produced by foreign protein reaction of the extravasated blood completes the picture of inflammatory process. If first seen during such a period the diagnosis of pneumonia is very apt to be made. A similar condition may arise from an arteriovenous aneurysm of the pulmonary circulation from gunshot wound or similar trauma. Lobectomy removes the vascular fistula and all the symptoms disappear. The size of the heart is not affected by a pulmonary fistula as it is with a fistula of the systemic circulation. Angiocardiographic examination will definitely confirm the diagnosis of blood vessel tumor.

Other rare forms of benign tumor are: fibroma, myoma, lipoma, tuberculoma, hamartoma and various forms of cysts.

Tumors having their origin in the mediastinal region, lymphoblastomata, dermoids and neurofibromata, often invade the lung. (See mediastinal tumors).

FIBROMA* (Fig. 182). Benign fibroma is a relatively rare tumor of the lung. They are 1 to 6 centimeters in size and present no unusual features from a tumor nodule of malignant type except that they remain stationary in size over a long period of time. They are usually solitary and probably most frequently have their origin in chronic infection from healing of a lung abscess by layer upon layer of fibrous tissue walling off the infection. On cut section this gives an onion skin appearance. A small area of remaining infection can sometimes still be detected in the center. At this final stage they may resemble malignant nodules.

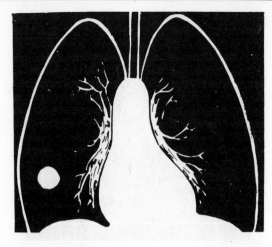

Fig. 182

TUBERCULOMA.* In a similar manner old tuberculous lesions may become encapsulated with formation of well-defined rounded nodules. Old encapsulated caseous nodules are usually denser due to excess of calcium salts, and have a greater tendency to multiple occurrence. An ever increasing number of instances are being reported of solitary granulomatous lesions believed to be tuberculous granulomas turning out on section of the resected specimen to be granulomas of other type especially histoplama and coccidiodal with only occasionally one of tuberculous origin (Zimmerman).

PARASITIC CYSTS—ECHINOCOCCUS CYSTS of the lung show at the outstart only very blurred images; these later on develop into large well-defined rounded masses. The disease is very chronic lasting over a period of months or years. During this time cysts may disappear and others develop. High eosinophilia and other tests help to confirm the diagnosis.

HAMARTOMA produces a well-defined, rounded tumor in the lung field much the same as that seen with fibroma, except that there is usually irregular calcium deposited throughout the mass. Such tumors are not true neoplasms; they are merely collections of all histologic elements which make up mature bronchi or lung tissue; cartilage usually predominates with irregular calcification or ossification throughout the mass often spoken of as "pop corn" variety, (Stein, et al.). This is characteristic of the tumor.

FLUID CYSTS.* Cystic tumors containing fluid are not uncommonly found in the lung. They are usually rounded and smooth in outline, and vary in size from a few centimeters to lesions almost filling an entire side of the chest cavity. They may rupture, discharging their fluid, and disappear within a short time leaving a normal lung picture; or they may remain following rupture as large air cysts or pneumatoceles. Peabody, et al. have reported

carcinomatous development in such innocent-appearing cysts.

PARAFFINOMA OF THE LUNG. Introduction of paraffin-base oils, such as mineral oil, as a vehicle for medication into the lungs, sets up an irritating reaction in the lung when the oil reaches the alveolar spaces (Pinkerton). Macrophages which take up the oil particles cannot digest them because they are inert and cannot be saponified. They are removed by way of the lymphatics and collect in the lymphatic structures near the hilum, where the phagocytes are destroyed and the oil coalesces into large inert masses. Heavy fibrous tissue reaction about the oily particles results in so-called paraffinoma formation. Davis, et al. have reported cases of lipoid pneumonia in which a solitary deposit of lipoid reaction in the lung has occurred resembling tumor. There is evidence to suspect that such collections may stimulate carcinomatous degeneration.

PRIMARY AMYLOID TUMOR.* This is a very unusual type of tumor (Weismann, et al.); it is not a neoplasm in the true sense of the word since it does not result from multiplication of cell structures. It is a primary deposit of amyloid material, not the involvement commonly developing secondary to chronic suppuration in tuberculosis. The amyloid material is of grayish-yellow color and rubbery in consistency. Its etiology is not understood. There is no manifestation of infection; it occurs as a homogeneous material surrounding the bronchial and vascular structures of the lung and may invade and occlude the bronchial or arterial lumen. When this occurs they bleed spontaneously and profusely.

Reimann's classification of amyloid disease is as follows:

(1) Primary (atypical or systematized without any other associated disease).

(2) Secondary (typical of the ordinary form which follows prolonged suppuration).

(3) Tumor-forming (single or multiple localized).

(4) Amyloidosis in association with multiple myeloma.

Other rare forms of benign tumor are myoma and lipoma. Tumors having their origin in the mediastinal region, lymphoblastoma, neurofibromata, dermoids and other cyst-like structures such as meningocele may encroach upon the lung. (See mediastinal tumors.)

A number of other conditions may simulate tumors during some stage of their development but usually there are other symptoms which aid in differentiation. Lobar pneumonia, for instance, may start with consolidation of smaller segments of the lung, which, when viewed "on end," give the impression of rounded nodules. Of course the high temperature and elevated white count indicate the inflammatory nature of the disease.

Mycotic infection, especially torula, may show as its initial lesion a large solitary more or less rounded area of consolidation in the lung showing little change over a period of months, without fever or other signs of inflammation. Detection of the organism in the sputum or spread to meningeal involvement will clinch the diagnosis.

Aneurysm of the aorta or other large vessels may produce a rounded well-defined mass without signs of inflammation which remains unchanged over a long period of time and may simulate tumor. Angiocardiography should establish the diagnosis.

Differential Diagnosis of Solitary Nodular Lesions in the Lung

The problem of differentiation of solitary circumscribed nodules in the lung presents itself. No physical characteristic of location, size, shape, form or outline, or density is specifically diagnostic. A small rounded nodule of soft tissue density, which, if multiple, would be diagnosed as a metastatic lesion, at once becomes a diagnostic problem if it occurs as a solitary lesion.

Good, et al., in a study of 156 such cases found that only 10% were really metastatic having a primary lesion elsewhere in the body; that, exclusive of these, only 25% of the remainder were primarily malignant. Of the remaining 68% over 40% were due to granulomatous lesions, representing the healed stages of pyogenic infection, tuberculosis or fungus lesion (especially coccidioidal mycosis).

Calcium deposits within the tumor of the laminated type or of the "pop corn" variety were found to be the only reliable sign of its benign character. This occurred principally in tuberculomas, hamartomas or coccidioidal granulomas and was best detected in certain instances by body section radiography, (O'Keefe, et al.). Rigler and Heitzman have demonstrated by planigraphic examination of solitary spherical nodules of the lung a notching or umbillication of the border which is highly indicative of its malignant nature. The absence of this sign is of no significance.

INJURIES TO THE LUNG

FRACTURED RIBS*. Fractures of the ribs, in themselves, are not usually very dangerous; they may, however, by protrusion of a sharp fragment, cause injury to the pleura or underlying lung, or if the fragments are widely separated, the intercostal artery may be ruptured and serious hemorrhage result.

An unusual cause of fractures of the ribs may occur from coughing as a result of the shearing stress which occurs between the origin of the external oblique and costal slips of the latissimus dorsi. Herniation of the lung has been reported following such fractures (Mann).

SUBCUTANEOUS EMPHYSEMA* (Fig. 183). Rupture of the lung in this way results in pneumothorax and collapse of the lung. If a flaplike wound is made in the pleura, each respiratory movement may pump air out into the subcutaneous tissues, causing subcu-

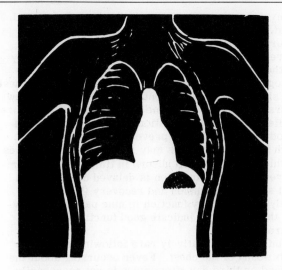

Fig. 183

taneous emphysema. This is indicated in the roentgenogram by dark streaks of air beneath the skin, stripping up the fascia planes and working in between the muscles. Clinically, the condition produces a crackling sensation on palpation of the soft parts. If air should extend inward into the mediastinum it becomes quite dangerous. It produces a distinctive picture (see mediastinal emphysema).

HEMORRHAGE INTO LUNG* (Fig. 184). Injury to the lung, by penetrating wound, such as gunshot or stab wound of the chest, is usually responsible for hemorrhage into the lung. It is possible for a bullet to go completely through the lung without causing any detectable change in the roentgenogram; likewise a sharp object may penetrate the lung without leaving roentgenographic evidence. Usually, however, such mishaps result in hemorrhage into the lung substance; roentgenologically, this appears as an irregular blotchy area of increased density in the lung field about the site of the injury. This may not be present immediately after injury; blood does not clot as readily in the chest cavity as it does when exposed to the outside air, consequently slight hemorrhage may continue for considerable period after injury. Bleeding into the general pleural cavity may continue for

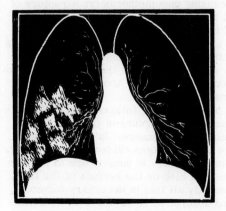

Fig. 184

many days, even weeks, producing hemothorax and fluid. Fluid blood can even be aspirated from the pleural cavity many months later. One should not therefore lull oneself into a sense of false security on the basis of negative findings in a single roentgenogram taken immediately after injury to the chest, but should make subsequent examination after a few hours or days to determine any change in the picture.

Repeated early aspiration, if large quantities of blood are present, will prevent fibrinous pleuritis. Such fibrinous exudates may reach 1/4 to 1/2 inches in thickness; they will absorb in time if left to themselves, but if reexpansion is delayed decortication will speed reexpansion and recovery (Barden). A study of pulmonary function in nine patients receiving this treatment indicate good functional results (Caroll, et al).

Infection is relatively rare following gunshot or stab wound of the chest. Fever occurring about the second or third day after injury is not necessarily indicative of pneumonia or other infection; it may be the result of foreign protein reaction from absorption of the byproducts of blood disintegration. This is especially true in patients showing massive hemothorax. Lung abscess rarely occurs from trauma to the chest (approximately 1%) unless there has been actual penetration of the chest wall and introduction of infection from the outside. Hemorrhage into the lung substance from injury to the lung usually absorbs without mishap; occasionally however an arteriovenous aneurysm of the lung may develop; this appears as a persistent clearly outlined, well-rounded shadow well out in the lung field. Its pulsation cannot usually be seen, but it may be detectable by kymographic study. Roentgen examination during valsalva exercise may show some decrease in size of the vascular shadow from expression of blood due to increased pulmonary pressure.

If the fistulous opening between the vessels is large and the exchange of blood is sufficiently great, secondary circulatory changes may result similar to those which occur with cavernous angioma of the lung; cyanosis, dyspnea, clubbing of the fingers and ultimately polycythemia. Hypertrophic pulmonary osteoarthropathy may develop.

TRAUMATIC PNEUMOTHORAX*. Pneumothorax may occur after trauma to the chest without a mark being left on the chest wall. An automobile may pass over the chest causing pneumothorax from rupture of the lung without fracturing the ribs or leaving any visible trace of injury upon the chest wall.

Mention has already been made of pneumothorax as a result of puncture of the lung from fractured ribs.

Examination with the patient in the lateral decubitus position has been emphasized by Abo, as a means of detecting minimal pneumothorax.

Spontaneous pneumothorax, following even slight exertion, may occur from rupture of the lung by increased intrapulmonary pressure. In such instances, the lung may not show roentgen evidence of pathology. Pneumothorax in such cases is usually due to rupture of an emphysematous bleb on the surface of the lung. Rest in bed is usually all that is necessary for complete healing and absorption of the air with re-expansion of the lung. Occasionally instances are noted where a pleural fistula results and reinflation does not occur, even over a long period of time. Intratracheal injection of lipiodol may result in closure of the fistula and reexpansion of the lung. Where this is not successful, dusting of the pleural cavity with talcum powder at open operation may produce pleural adhesions and reexpansion. (See mediastinal emphysema).

TRAUMATIC PNEUMONIA. Pneumonia sometimes follows trauma to the chest even where there is no fracture, contusion or laceration. There is usually a latent period of three or four days before the pneumonic consolidation develops; pain may be an outstanding symptom during this period. It is of the lobar type and runs a typical course of lobar pneumonia. This is a very rare occurrence, however. Contrary to observations of some other publications it is our experience that actual pneumonia rarely occurs as a result of trauma to the chest (Phillips).

TRAUMATIC RUPTURE OF A BRONCHUS near the tracheal bifurcation has been reported from accidental injury, (Hodes, et al.). This resulted in permanent occlusion of the bronchus forming a blind pouch with permanent atelectasis of the lung.

Injury of the lung structure from explosion from flash of the flame into the lung results in an immediate picture of oedema and hemorrhage into the lung structure; dilatation of the heart with pulse rate as high as 140 per minute, and extreme shock. This may gradually clear within a few days or may cause death.

EXPLOSIVE OR "BLAST" EFFECT ON THE LUNG (Savage). The subjection of the thorax to intense explosion results in production of more or less characteristic pathological lesions in the lung. Multiple capillary hemorrhages in the periphery of the lung coalesce to form areas of alveolar and interstitial consolidation over the surface of the lung, often most pronounced in the costophrenic regions.

Roentgenologically this condition gives rise to a diffuse "fluffy" mottling somewhat similar to that seen in silicosis.

At autopsy the lungs were large, but in most instances did not show significant changes on the surface. Only on section was the "spatter" of hemorrhages evident.

Traumatic Torsion of the Lung

This extremely rare injury presents on x-ray examination, "a curved striated pattern extending from the hilus upward to the apex, with a partial pneumothorax". In the case reported by Parks, death followed six hours after an automobile wheel passed over the chest.

"At autopsy, the left lung was found to be rotated anteriorly with its base assuming a superior position and its apex in an inferior position. The inversion was 180° above a transverse (coronal) axis through the left hilus. The curved striated pattern represented the inverted vascular trunks supplying the left lower lobe then in the apex of the left thoracic cavity. The torsion was believed to have been brought about by the sudden compression of the left lower chest by the weight of the vehicle causing displacement of the lower lobe cephalad. The sudden release of the pressure allowed the expanded upper lobe to move more caudad and occupy the space normally filled by the lower lobe." A similar case has been previously reported by Stratemeier and Barry.

THE PLEURA

THICKENING OF THE PLEURA* (Fig. 185). Dry pleurisy occurs as a result of infection, inflammation, or trauma applied to the chest wall. Whatever the cause, it appears roentgenographically as a fine ribbon-like shadow running along parallel to the chest wall at the outer margin of the lung. Ordinarily, the normal pleural covering of the lung does not show on x-ray examination, only when it becomes thickened from infection or inflammation does it become evident. In the early stages of dry pleurisy, especially when localized to a small area, pleurisy may not be evident at x-ray examination; a pleural friction rub may be clearly demonstrable and yet no thickening of the pleura may be demonstrable roentgenographically.

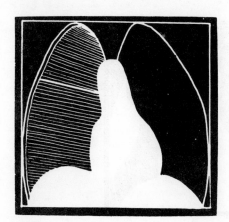

Fig. 185

TRAUMATIC PLEURISY*. Dry pleurisy following injury to the chest is not an uncommon occurrence. It follows about three or four days after trauma to the chest wall and is represented roentgenographically by a thickened pleura over the site of former trauma; it usually subsides and heals spontaneously without lasting disability with strapping of the chest.

PLEURAL EFFUSION

FREE IN PLEURAL CAVITY* (Fig. 186). Large effusions free in the pleural cavity frequently occur from inflammation or injury. As fluid collects in the pleural cavity it gravitates to the most dependent position, the costophernic sinus; this is

the first portion of the lung field to be obscured. As the fluid continues to increase in quantity it fills the lower portion of the thorax pressing against the elastic air-filled lung. Being attached at the hilum region only, the lung is free to float upward on the surface of the fluid at the periphery, but is restrained at its central attachment. This imparts a curved upper border to the fluid line extending from the midline upward toward the axilla, roentgenological evidence of the "S" curve of Ellis demonstrable on physical examination (Fig. 186A). As still further accumulation of fluid occurs in the chest, the lung is floated upward and becomes compressed along the mediastinal border; since it is almost impossible to express all of the air from the lung in such a manner this gives rise to an important differential roentgen sign in diagnosis of pleural effusion, namely, the presence of a remnant of aerated lung along the medial side of the apex (Fig. 186B). Pneumonic consolidation, on the other hand, produces a uniform shadow. Very large pleural effusions, by their weight, cause shifting of the mediastinum to the opposite side; under such circumstances the remaining aerated portion of the lung on the medial side of the apex may be displaced behind the mediastinal shadow and not be visible, but the mediastinal shift in itself is enough to establish the diagnosis (Fig. 186C). Any condition which causes a loss of resiliency of the lung such as bronchial obstruction, emphysema, infiltrative exudate, either infectious or malignant, will cause a variation in the

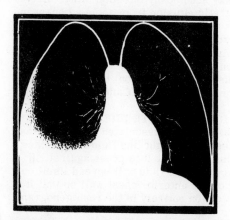

Fig. 186A

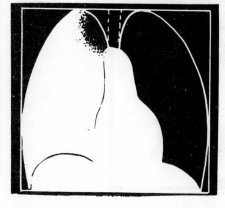

Fig. 186B

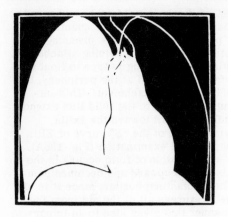

Fig. 186C

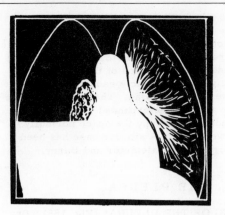

Fig. 187

curved upper border usually assumed by effusion free in the pleural cavity, causing it to take on the appearance of a ribbonlike density along the peripheral margin of the lung field. Very small collections of pleural effusion hidden in the posterior cul-de-sac beneath the dome of the diaphragm may be detected by examining the patient while lying on the affected side (in the lateral decubitus); this position permits the fluid to flow readily up along the side of the chest between the free margin of the lung and the chest wall (Fig. 186D) (Rigler).

    Pleural effusion occurs most commonly as a result of irritation, exposure to cold, trauma, pulmonary congestion from failure of circulation or oedema of lungs. It may accompany infection either direct or as a sympathetic effusion from some adjacent infection such as pneumonia, lung abscess, or subdiaphragmatic abscess. It may be due to metastatic malignant involvement. Under unusual circumstances pleural effusion may be caused by rupture of a subphrenic abscess (amebic infection) through the diaphragm into the pleural cavity (Campbell).

PLEURAL EFFUSION WITH PNEUMOTHORAX*

(Fig. 187). When there is associated pneumothorax, pleural fluid seeks a straight line fluid level, since there is no elastic body for it to press against. If the patient lies prone the fluid will spread itself out in a thin layer on the anterior chest wall so that it may escape detection entirely in the roentgenogram.

LOCALIZED PLEURAL EFFUSION*.

Pleural effusion may become entrapped by adhesions between the pleural layers wherever they come in contact with each other. This may be at the periphery of the lung between the parietal and visceral pleura (Fig. 188), or in the interlobar spaces (Fig. 189). Localized pleural effusion, no matter where it occurs, presents certain characteristics, namely, a dense shadow at the periphery of the lung with a rounded convex border directed in toward the compressible lung. If the localized pocket is on the anterior or posterior aspect of the chest it may be necessary to examine the patient fluoroscopically, turned in many positions in

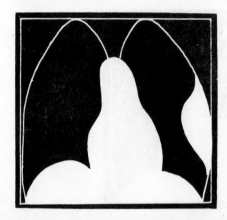

Fig. 188

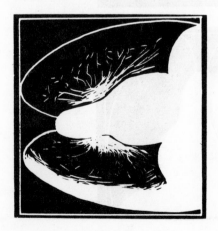

Fig. 186D

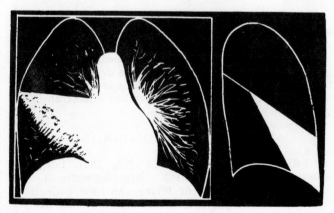

Fig. 189A   Fig. 189B

order to view the collection in profile. Such localized collections may be diaphragmatic—infrapulmonary, (Rothstein and Landis), (Fig. 190), between the diaphragm and the lower portion of the lung or along the mediastinal border (Fig. 191). Such paramediastinal collections of localized effusion may extend entirely along the mediastinal margin or they may be confined to the upper or lower portions. The location of the short fissure on the right side often is the site of the boundary of the localized effusions. In the bases they assume a triangular form. Examinations made in the upright position with inspiration and expiration will avoid many pitfalls in diagnosis.

Localized effusion on the anterior or posterior chest wall may produce such a slight shadow in the

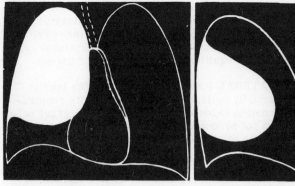

Fig. 192A   Fig. 192B

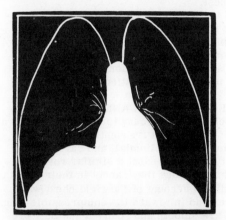

Fig. 190

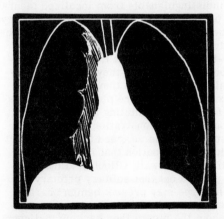

Fig. 191

anterior view of the chest that it may be entirely overlooked in the roentgenogram. The vague indication of a fluid level or a slight increase in density of the lung in any position should be investigated in all positions.

When the interlobar space is the site of localized pleural effusion, a lateral view of the chest may be the essential factor in determining the diagnosis (Figs. 192A and B); at such examination a shadow running along the interlobar septum indicates interlobar effusion. The lordosis position may be of aid in detecting this condition (see Manual of Roentgenological Technique), (Levitin). Juxta or extra pleural effusion, or collections of fluid between the parietal pleura and the chest wall, are occasionally encoun-

tered especially in patients who are undergoing pneumothorax treatment for tuberculosis (Levine and Hurst).

PNEUMOTHORAX* (Fig. 193). Normally the pleural cavity is only a potential space. The visceral pleura covering the lung is in intimate contact with the parietal pleura lining the chest cavity. Not until the pleural space becomes filled with something, such as fluid or air, does it become an actual cavity. Since there is a negative pressure within the pleural cavity any connection with the outside atmospheric pressure will permit air to enter, allowing collapse of the lung from its natural elastic recoil. A flap-valve action of the pleura may permit building up of sufficient pressure within the pleural cavity to cause pressure on the mediastinum (q.v.); pressure pneumothorax. With pressure pneumothorax a weak spot in the anterior mediastinum may cause bulging into the opposite lung field.

Roentgen Manifestations. Collapse of the lung results in removal of the lung markings from the outer portion of the lung field. The outer zone of the lung field assumes a darker, more homogeneous appearance; the margin of the collapsed lung can be readily traced.

The degree of collapse of the lung is dependent upon the size of the opening into the pleural cavity; the larger the opening, the greater the amount of air which can enter with each inspiration. With a small

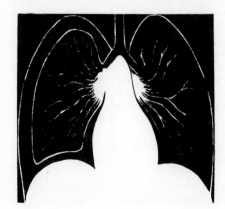

Fig. 193

opening, the lung will not continue to collapse to its smallest size, since with the next expiratory phase part of the air will be expelled through the opening in the chest wall as well as through the natural channels; an equilibrium is rapidly established.

BILATERAL PNEUMOTHORAX*. The lung in this partially collapsed state continues its respiratory function to some extent so that if too great collapse is not produced it is possible for an individual to live with bilateral partial pneumothorax.

ARTIFICIAL PNEUMOTHORAX*. Artificial pneumothorax is used very extensively in treatment of pulmonary tuberculosis, sometimes bilaterally.

SPONTANEOUS PNEUMOTHORAX*. Spontaneous pneumothorax occurs most frequently as a result of disease process in the lung. Many instances are encountered, however, where no disease process is demonstrable roentgenologically. Lung collapse with pneumothorax occurs suddenly after exertion, often of a very trivial character. Such instances are probably due to rupture of an emphysematous bleb on the surface of the pleura. Rest in bed usually results in healing of the rent and absorption of the air within a few weeks. Subsequent recurrence may develop, however. The writer has encountered a case in which five attacks occurred within a period of six months; one full month of bed-rest resulted in complete healing, no subsequent attack having occurred for more than ten years. Occasionally cases are encountered where a pleural fistula is established and reexpansion does not occur. Intratracheal injection of lipiodol may occlude the fistula permitting reexpansion of the lung. If this fails, dusting of the pleural cavity with talcum powder may cause pleural adhesions and reexpansion of the lung.

SPONTANEOUS INTERSTITIAL PULMONARY EMPHYSEMA—MEDIASTINAL EMPHYSEMA. Rupture of a pleural bleb or bulla usually results in spontaneous pneumothorax because they are usually so superficially located. Very rarely rupture may be into the interstitial tissues of the lung. Herrnheiser and Whitehead have been able to show the resultant air cysts in the interstitial tissue of the lung. Traversing the interstitial tissue and vascular sheaths to the hilum, the air finds its way to the mediastinum (q.v.); from here it passes upward extending into the subcutaneous tissues of the neck. The symptoms may be very severe simulating coronary occlusion. Clinically a loud clattering sound may be heard almost across the room with each heart beat. This is due to the heart beating against the air-filled mediastinum. Death may result from pressure of the air bubbles within the vascular sheaths. Mediastinal emphysema is a dreaded complication of tracheotomy; operations of this type should not be undertaken unless there is certainty that the operation will relieve the tracheal obstruction and eliminate the dyspnoea.

Roentgenographically there is a uniform linear zone of decreased density outlining the heart due to air in the mediastinum giving the impression of a "halo" about the heart (Fig. 207B). In addition air can be seen in the cellular tissues of the neck. Lateral-view examination of the chest shows a large collection of air in the anterior mediastinum in front of the heart. A needle thrust into the anterior mediastinal space may be a life-saving measure.

TRAUMATIC PNEUMOTHORAX*. Pneumothorax may result from trauma applied to the chest wall without fracture of the ribs or in fact without even a mark on the chest. The passage of an automobile tire across the chest of a young child may produce such a result. Several instances of pneumothorax have been encountered in divers, striking the surface of water flat upon the chest.

Puncture of the lung from the sharp end of a fractured rib or as a result of stab wound of the chest may result in pneumothorax. If fluid is associated with pneumothorax it takes on a straight-line fluid level in the most dependent portion, which changes with change of position of the patient.

TUMORS OF THE PLEURA AND CHEST WALL (Fig. 194), (Hochberg). Primary tumors of the pleura are very rare. Those most frequently encountered are endothelioma (mesotheliomia), and sarcoma. Regardless of type they present a similar roentgenological appearance. Since they cannot in their growth expand outwardly on account of the rigid chest wall, they naturally extend in toward the compressible lung. Their margins are smooth and rounded and they present a picture indistinguishable from localized pleural effusion at the periphery of the lung. Sometimes they may protrude between the ribs to the outside, producing rounded notches of pressure atrophy on the ribs as the dumbell-type tumor passes through the interspace. Later on in their course they may cause associated pleural effusion. Often they form multiple small nodules studding the entire pleural cavity. Aspiration of the fluid and substituting air will permit their roentgenographic demonstration. If the tumor moves with respiration it is attached to the lung; if it remains fixed it is an indication that it probably is still confined to the chest wall, (Blount). Finby and Steinberg have pointed out that solitary primary pleural tumors of this type may present benign characteristics for years; but when they show rapid multiplication throughout the pleura they become malignant

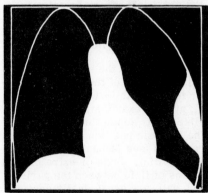

Fig. 194

SECONDARY TUMORS OF PLEURA. Secondary tumors of the pleura produce a very similar appearance; they are usually multiple, however. Many types of malignant growths may cause metastatic involvement of the pleura but the one in which such involvement seems, in our experience, to be the most frequent, is hypernephroma. Such secondary nodules may be mistaken for primary tumors, since hypernephroma, in its original site, may remain dormant for a long time and may not incite symptoms indicative of its presence.

PANCOAST TUMOR (Stein). These represent a peculiar group of tumors described by Pancoast occurring in the region between the root of the neck and apex of lung. They give rise to a peculiar clinical syndrome resulting from involvement of the brachial plexus and cervical sympathetic chain. This consists of pain around the shoulder and down the inner side of the forearm on the affected side, atrophy of muscles of the hand and Horner's Syndrome, namely, unilateral miosis, ptosis of the upper eyelid, exophthalmos and anhidrosis of face and neck.

Roentgenologically the Pancoast's "Superior Pulmonary Sulcus Tumor" shows a sharply defined shadow in the apex of the lung, destruction of one or more of the upper three ribs posteriorly, erosion of the transverse processes and bodies of the corresponding vertebrae. There may be slight indentation and displacement of the trachea to the opposite side.

Microscopically they are produced by a variety of different cell tumors. Some feel that they may be bronchiogenic in origin.

Few are operable. X-ray therapy may be used for palliation; the average survival is about 13 months.

DIAPHRAGM

The two leaves of the diaphragm form fibromuscular partitions between the abdomen and the chest on either side. Their excursion during respiration can be clearly visualized fluoroscopically. Their contour is normally rounded and smooth, with dome-shaped upper borders. This dome-shaped character produces a deep sulcus where the diaphragm attaches to the chest wall. Laterally, this sulcus is known as the costophrenic angle or sulcus; medially, as the cardiophrenic angle or sulcus; posteriorly and anteriorly, it is referred to as the posterior and anterior costophrenic sulcus respectively.

DIAPHRAGMATIC ADHESIONS (Fig. 195). The smooth rounded contour of the diaphragm may be disturbed by diaphragmatic adhesions. Any inflammatory process in the chest, whether by pyogenic or tuberculous infection, or by new growth, if it involves the diaphragmatic pleura, may result in diaphragmatic adhesions. Roentgenologically this condition is recognized by sharp upward projections in the diaphragmatic contour known as "tenting of the diaphragm." Fluoroscopic examination shows restriction of the diaphragmatic movement in these

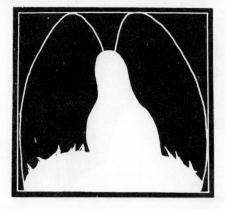

Fig. 195

regions on deep inspiration. Accentuation of the costal attachments gives a somewhat similar appearance except that they are uniform in spacing and location.

"SCALLOPING" DEFORMITY OF THE DIAPHRAGM (Fig. 196). In contradistinction to the tenting type of deformity, the diaphragm may show a "scalloped" appearance, with points downward producing smooth rounded portions projecting upward toward the chest. Simultaneous induction of pneumothorax and pneumoperitoneum indicates that this is due to accentuation of the costal attachments of the muscular segments of the diaphragm. It is of no significance as an indication of active disease.

Bulging of a flail segment (usually inner) with a rounded relaxed portion may be the result of trauma or may be congenital. It probably represents a localized partial herniation. In our experience it is seldom of any special importance. Such cases have been reported by Rossetti, and Hollander and Dugan.

Adhesions are apt to occur where the septa come in contact with the diaphragm.

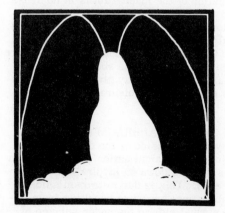

Fig. 196

IMMOBILIZATION OF THE DIAPHRAGM (Fig. 197). Any inflammation or infection of the parietal pleura above, or the parietal peritoneum beneath, results in immobilization of the diaphragm in a high position, Nature's effort to splint the diseased area.

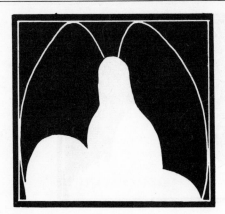

Fig. 197

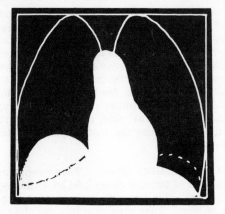

Fig. 198

Pleurisy causing extreme pain, even though it does not involve the diaphragmatic pleura itself, will result in immobilization of the diaphragm. A good example of this is seen in lobar pneumonia; although the involvement may be confined to the upper lobe, the pain incident to the associated parietal pleural involvement will reflexly cause immobilization of the diaphragm in a high position. If inflammation or infection is confined to the lung or interlobar space, pain is not an accompaniment and diaphragmatic movement is not restricted; as soon as the infection spreads to involve the parietal pleura, pain results and diaphragmatic immobilization develops.

Inflammation and infection of the peritoneum below the diaphragm may likewise result in immobilization in a high position. This is frequently seen as a postoperative observation where there is pain from insult to the parietal peritoneum. Subdiaphragmatic abscess results in immobilization also; infection in this location cannot usually be demonstrated except by aid of pneumoperitoneum (q.v.). This defense immobilization of the idaphragm is in no sense due to spasm of the diaphragm, spastic contraction should be in a low position; nor is it due to paralysis, since with paralysis the diaphragm should be a flail membrane free to respond to any changes in pressure between the pleural cavity and the abdomen.

Subdiaphragmatic abscess may give rise to a sympathetic serous effusion in the pleural cavity above the diaphragm, (Beye).

PARALYSIS OF THE DIAPHRAGM (Fig. 198). Complete paralysis of one side of the diaphragm results in so-called "paradoxical action"; that is, when the uninvolved side goes down on inspiration, the paralyzed side ascends. This is due to transmission of the increased abdominal pressure resulting from depression of the normal side to the under surface of the paralyzed side causing it to ascend. Complete paralysis of the diaphragm, however, is rarely encountered; even after section of the phrenic nerve as a therapeutic measure in tuberculosis, the phenomenon may not develop. This is probably due to cross innervation of the diaphragm from the opposite side.

ANOMALIES OF THE DIAPHRAGM. Several types of anomalous development of the diaphragm are encountered.

EVENTRATION (Fig. 199). Eventration is a condition in which the diaphragm persists in an unusually high position, usually on the left side. It may move with respiration, a condition which will distinguish it from immobilization of the diaphragm in a high position due to inflammation. However, it may be restricted in its excursion or even show some paradoxical action depending upon the degree of muscular development. Instances have been encountered where the elevation was so great (extending to the third rib) that the stomach, spleen, most of the small

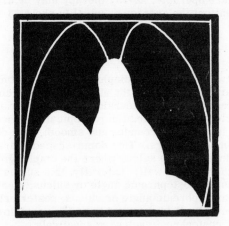

Fig. 199

intestines and a portion of the colon were displaced high up into the thoracic cage; distension of the stomach and intestines resulted in mediastinal displacement and pressure on the recurrent laryngeal nerve!

DIAPHRAGMATIC HERNIA (Fig. 200). Diaphragmatic hernia may be congenital or may be acquired by severe trauma to the abdomen. It usually occurs on the left side, where the diaphragmatic structure is not so well protected. A flail hernial

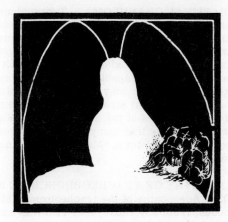

Fig. 200

sac protruding into the chest cavity may contain large portions of the stomach, small and large intestines, and other abdominal organs. The occurrence of peculiar shadows above the diaphragm especially on the left side should always be investigated. The administration of a barium meal should show clearly the presence of these structures in the chest. The herniation of these organs may be reduced at times with the return of all abdominal structures to their normal position beneath the diaphragm, so that the appearance will vary at different examinations. Hiatus herniation of the stomach back through the esophageal orifice is probably the most common defect. In such diaphragmatic hernias ulcerating erosion from trauma caused by constant irritation at the margin of the hernial orifice may cause hemorrhage and anemia; the ulcers usually cannot be detected on roentgen examination. Herniation through the right diaphragm is a very rare condition but it does occur at times; it may contain intestine or only a lobule of the liver. Intestinal coils between the right diaphragm and the liver are encountered without actual hernia.

CONGENITAL ABSENCE OF ONE SIDE OF THE DIAPHRAGM. A number of cases have been reported in which there was congenital absence of one side of the diaphragm. Oritt and Hyde have reported cases of pneumothorax associated with spontaneous pneumoperitoneum from rupture of an ulcer due to a hole in the diaphragm forming a communication with the chest.

DIAPHRAGMATIC "FLUTTER." A rare but interesting disturbance which may affect the diaphragm is diaphragmatic "flutter." This is a condition in which numerous secondary contraction waves become superimposed upon the ordinary diaphragmatic contraction. These are rapid, fully 240 to 300 per minute; they can be observed fluoroscopically, occurring simultaneously on both sides. A peculiar shuffling sound over the anterior portion of the chest, which accompanies the phenomenon, gives the impression of a rapid heart beat. Tracing of the dia-

phragmatic contractions, likewise, reveals the secondary waves; the electrocardiographic tracing is essentially normal. The radial pulse is normal and slow, 60 to 88 per minute. It may be accompanied by severe precordial pain, giving the impression of an anginal attack.

Phrenic nerve crush (both sides) sometimes relieves the condition and all symptoms and signs disappear. In other instances, the condition still appears at intervals. The cause of this unusual phenomenon is not known (Porter).

MEDIASTINUM

The mediastinum is a very important space. It is bounded by the sternum in front, the spine behind, the diaphragm below, and on either side, by the reflection of the visceral pleurae at the hilum regions. The mediastinum is divided into inferior and superior portions. The inferior part is further divided into the anterior, middle and posterior portions; the superior portion (or the part above the level of the 3rd or 4th thoracic vertebra), is not so satisfactorily subdivided.

The middle mediastinum is occupied by the heart, the great vessels; the anterior portion is in front of the heart between it and the sternum while the posterior mediastinum is behind it extending to the spine. It is occupied by some of the most vital structures in the body.

Roentgenologically, the mediastinum, when seen in the anterior or posterior chest views presents a composite impression of the sternum in front, the dorsal spine behind, and all intervening structures contained in the mediastinal space. The anterior mediastinum constitutes a weak partition between the two sides of the chest. In case of pressure pneumothorax on one side, the deviation of this weak portion can be seen bulging into the opposite chest cavity. The oblique projections are best adapted for less obstructed views of these various organs, such as the esophagus and aorta. Examination in the upright position in full inspiration and expiration will avoid many pit-falls in diagnosis. Pathological involvement of these various structures which it contains will be considered in greater detail under the system of which they are a part. Roentgen examination of the mediastinum is never complete without esophageal examination with a barium swallow.

MEDIASTINITIS; PERI-ESOPHAGEAL ABSCESS (Fig. 201). The mediastinal space itself is subject to infection from disease of the structures which it contains. Perforation of the esophagus by a foreign body or as a result of instrumentation may inoculate pyogenic infection into the mediastinal space with production of peri-esophageal abscess. Retropharyngeal abscess and infections of the neck may spread by continuity of tissue directly into the mediastinum. A very rare instance of mediastinitis has been reported from extension of a pyogenic osteomyelitis of the thoracic vertebrae to the mediastinal space (Solomon and Brockman). The loose cellular character of the alveolar tissue within this space renders such extension very easy and rapid. The

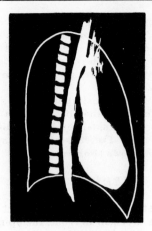

Fig. 201

relative inaccessibility of the space for surgical drainage makes it important to recognize threatened mediastinal invasion as promptly as possible. In recent years, mediastinal infections have been attacked surgically with greater success. Administration of a small amount of opaque mixture will often disclose the perforation of the esophagus whereby infection has gained entrance into the peri-esophageal tissues, this extruded opaque medium presenting a dense irregular shadow on the surrounding esophageal. tissues. The advent of chemotherapy aids greatly in treatment and prognosis.

TUBERCULOUS MEDIASTINITIS (Hawes).

Tuberculous mediastinitis is perhaps the most frequently encountered type of mediastinal infection. Breaking down of caseous tuberculous tracheobronchial lymph nodes results in spread of the infection to the mediastinal space. Irregular fibrosis of the mediastinum may result from Nature's effort to limit the infection, showing roentgenographically as a hazy fibrotic appearance of the mediastinal space. Tuberculous abscess may even result with formation of fistulous tracts discharging to the surface, usually posteriorly in the lumbar region. Such tracts have been demonstrated by opaque oil injection to have their origin in the mediastinal space. Suppuration may not occur however; the only manifestation may be from fibrosis. Obstruction to the vena cava from mediastinal fibrosis may be the only lesion present.

Tuberculous adhesions to the esophagus may cause traction on the esophageal wall very clearly demonstrable roentgenographically. This may result in traction diverticula. Enlarged mediastinal nodes may, from pressure displace the esophagus, or the tuberculous process may even involve the esophageal wall forming a tuberculoma which projects into the lumen.

The pericardium may become involved with tuberculous pericarditis resulting in tugging of the diaphragm and adjacent pleural structures with each heart beat corresponding to the clinical manifestations of Broadbent's sign.

MEDIASTINAL GRANULOMA.

Tuberculous granuloma may result from coelsence of caseous nodes to form a rounded, well-defined mass projecting outward into the lung field from the mediastinum. There is usually associated calcareous deposit often at the periphery of the capsule. It may progress to complete caseation and may even rupture into the surrounding mediastinal structures from pressure. Study of 16 such cases at the Mayo clinic by Kunkel, et al., would indicate that many different stages may be present so that the term "Mediastinal Granuloma" is suggested.

ADENOPATHY OF TRACHEOBRONCHIAL NODES (Fig. 202).

Adenopathy of the tracheobronchial lymph nodes, from any cause, may result in an irregular widening of the mediastinal shadow. Such adenopathy is usually due to tuberculous infection, Hodgkin's disease, lymphosarcoma, secondary malignant involvement of the glands, or syphilis. While the specific nature of the involvement cannot under all circumstances be definitely determined, still these processes have certain characteristics which frequently betray the nature of their etiology. Tuberculous adenitis, for instance, almost always exhibits some calcareous deposits; Hodgkin's disease and lymphosarcoma show large groups of glands, nodular in outline, extending well out beyond the hilum regions into the mid-zone of the lung field; carcinomatous metastases, on the other hand, are smaller, and tend to cluster about the bronchi, producing peribronchial radiations into lung fields; syphilitic adenopathy of the tracheobronchial glands is a possibility, but, in our experience, it has been exceedingly rare.

In addition to hilum or mediastinal adenopathy, Hodgkin's disease may involve the parenchymal structures producing infiltrations in the lung resembling tuberculosis, metastatic carcinoma, bronchopneumonia, Boeck's Sarcoid, or erythema nodosum.

A nodular appearance simulating adenopathy may be produced by saccular dilatation of the esophagus from cardiospasm but this can be readily recognized by demonstration of a fluid level after the administration of a barium meal.

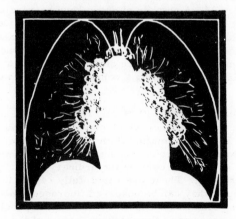

Fig. 202

Thrombosis of the pulmonary artery produces accentuation of the hilum shadow which may resemble adenopathy, but this can usually be recognized by the trailing off of the lower end of the vascular shadow into a point, and by the appearance of hyperaeration of the lungs which accompanies the condition without the other evidences of emphysema.

BOECK'S SARCOID. The etiology is unknown. The roentgen findings may be very bizarre in their appearance, having at the outstart only pronounced adenopathy of the hilar nodes usually with a zone of aerated lung between the mass of nodes and the mediastinum. Symmetry of hilar node involvement and their enormous size, "potato nodes," is emphasized as of great diagnostic importance (Garland). Months later linear markings radiate outward into the lungs and miliary infiltrations may appear throughout both lung fields, possibly representing involvement of the minute lymphoid deposits in the lungs. This is the most distinctive picture of sarcoidosis. At this stage it may resemble silicosis but there is no history of exposure to silica dust. Larger areas of consolidation may occur or in other instances the entire picture may fade with complete recovery and restoration to normal; this requires months or years, and regression is in reverse order to that of acquiring the lesions. Often the diagnosis is clinched by biopsy of associated subcutaneous lymph gland involvement or of concurrent skin nodules. The small joints may show characteristic punched-out areas of bone involvement with disintegration of the trabecular structure, (Fig. 145) or there may be thickened pigmented areas of skin involvement.

In recent years the favorable response of this disease to treatment with cortisone has been noted.

ERYTHEMA NODOSUM. This condition, thought to be related in some way to allergy, is characterized by glandular enlargement often massive in size in the hilum regions, transitory nodular infiltrations throughout the lungs, acute erythematous skin lesions occurring usually in sites subject to trauma. There may be little if any constitutional manifestations other than fatigue. Kerley, based upon his observation of 37 cases (all adults), feels that there is a distinct similarity between the findings in this condition and sarcoidosis.

Roentgenologically the outstanding characteristic is the enormous lymph node enlargement in the hilum regions, with associated skin lesions and without pronounced constitutional reaction.

PRIMARY AMYLOIDOSIS of the lungs. The following classification of amyloidosis has been proposed (Reimann, et al.).
1. Primary
    Systemic type—a generalized disease of the mesoderm
    Localized type—in which one or two organs in particular are involved
2. Secondary—following chronic lung suppuration
3. Amyloidosis associated with multiple myeloma

4. Tumor forming amyloidosis
Secondary amyloid degeneration of organs such as the liver, spleen, and kidneys in association with long standing infections such as tuberculosis of the spine is well known. A primary form which occurs without such antecedent infection is not so well understood, (Dirkse).

The characteristics ascribed to the primary form by Lubarsch are as follows:
1. Almost complete absence of amyloid in organs most involved in typical amyloidosis such as spleen, liver, and kidneys.
2. Presence of amyloid in organs and parts not usually involved, such as heart, lungs, and skin.
3. The occasional occurrence of tumor-like nodules of amyloidosis.
4. The frequent failure of deposits to react to the specific strains for amyloidosis.
5. The absence of a preceding or concomitant disease to which the presence of amyloidosis may be ascribed.

The disease is insidious in its onset, often being ushered in by a respiratory infection. There are no distinctive physical signs or symptoms. Some cough, dyspnea, cardiac enlargement and swelling of the extremities are noted. An alarming symptom which we have noted in association with amyloid tumors is repeated profuse pulmonary hemorrhages which almost cause exsanguination.

Roentgenologically, in a recent report after examination of 21 cases Wang and Robbins concluded, "that the roentgen changes described in various organs are not pathognomonic of amyloid disease." " . . . clinical data and laboratory tests may lead to a correct diagnosis. The recognition of primary amyloidosis is difficult but the diagnosis may be suggested roentgenologically and confirmed by tissue biopsy."

TULAREMIA. The hilar adenopathy of tularemia is often indistinguishable from sarcoidosis erythema nodosum or Hodgkin's disease. The disease may spread out along the lymphatics like sarcoid or Hodgkin's disease also. Specific agglutination for tularemia reaction will clinch the diagnosis. The disease is usually very acute with high fever and great prostration.

MEDIASTINAL HEMATOMA. Traumatic mediastinal hematoma has been described by Endress showing local mediastinal enlargement, usually of the superior mediastinum, following trauma. This is readily recognizable in the anterior view but less demonstrable in the lateral position. It undergoes absorption and disappearance after bed rest.

MEDIASTINAL TUMORS (Fig. 203). Mediastinal tumor is not an uncommon occurrence. Tumors in this region usually present themselves as large rounded well-defined masses, extending outward on both sides into the lung fields. They are often in very close relationship to the aorta and frequently resemble aneurysm of this structure. Roentgenologically they may show transmitted pulsation from the aorta,

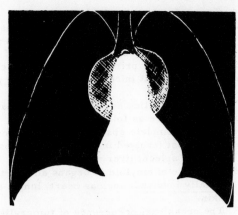

Fig. 203

but their pulsation is never of the expansile type seen in aneurysm, however. Even with kymographic examination it may be difficult to demonstrate expansile pulsation. If both sides of the shadow can be obtained on the kymogram, expansile pulsation can be determined.

Obstruction to the superior vena cava by pressure from a mediastinal mass, whether primary or metastatic may give rise to massive engorgement of the superfiscial veins over the chest and neck; this is a confirmatory sign of great clinical value (Roswit, et al.).

According to Harrington in most instances the type of tumor may be adjudged from its location:
1. Anterior mediastinum - teratoid tumors (these include teratomas and dermoid cysts).
2. Middle mediastinum - Lymphoblastomata (including Hodgkin's disease, lymphosarcoma and leukemia).
3. Posterior mediastinum - Neurogenic tumors.

The lymphoblastomata are often amenable to deep x-ray therapy, showing immediate regression or disappearance, but rarely are they cured by such methods. A rather peculiar tumor of this type, known as a leukosarcoma seen in children, regresses promptly with very small doses of radiation; after an interval of two to three months the child suddenly develops a high leucocyte count, 300,000 to 400,000, with the blood picture of leukemia, even though at first the blood picture had been normal. Deep x-ray therapy has little effect on teratoid tumors or neurogenic tumors, so that theraputic exposure to the roentgen-ray can be used as a diagnostic sign. They may be successfully removed by modern surgical methods. Calcium deposits occur in dermoids and aneurysms; this is always indication of the benign nature of a lesion. In dermoid cysts the fatty contents may rise to the top giving an appearance in the roentgenogram similar to a fluid level or the light zone may surround the cyst. Tooth structures may be demonstrated.

Neurogenic tumors are benign neoplasms which frequently arise from the nerve tissue posteriorly;

they may extend into the spinal canal forming dumbbell tumors or may by pressure erode the vertebral bodies or other surrounding bony structures. They can be successfully removed by operation. They are usually benign but may take on sarcomatous degeneration. On the other hand, intrathoracic meningocele may very readily be mistaken for neurofibroma of the lung. Their extra pleural nature can be demonstrated by pneumothorax and by pantopaque in the spinal canal (Byron, et al), (Sengpiel, et al).

Other rarer types of mediastinal tumor are: bronchiogenic cysts, pericardial celomic cyst (located anteriorly in close relationship to the pericardium), fibroma, chondroma, and lipoma. Recent reports of the mediastinal tumors operated in the army would indicate that bronchiogenic cysts are not as uncommon as formerly supposed - at least in younger individuals (B. Blades). Some rare types of cyst formation found in the mediastinum are congenital in origin: bronchial, esophogeal, gastroenteric, and cystic lymphangioma. Parasitic cysts such as Echinococcus cysts are very unusual in this country (Laipply). Extension of meningoceles or dumbell tumors of the spinal cord may extend into the mediastinum or thorax simulating the appearance of lung tumor, (Baker and Curtis). Davis and Simonton have recently reported bronchogenic mediastinal cysts occurring just below the carina or bifurcation of the trachea. Scheff, et al., have reported dense rounded shadows extending into the lung field from hematomas resulting after sympathectomy. For a comprehensive review of mediastinal tumor the reader is referred to Hever and Andrus.

THYMUS GLAND (Fig. 204). The thymus gland occupies the anterior portion of the superior mediastinum. It is normal structure in infants up to two years of age, and is almost always visible in the roentgenogram. It increases in size from birth to about eighteen months, decreasing from this period until about two years of age, when it should no longer be demonstrable roentgenographically as a definite structure. It may form a keystonelike shadow, base downward, above and overlapping the aorta, or it may present a well-defined triangular shadow along

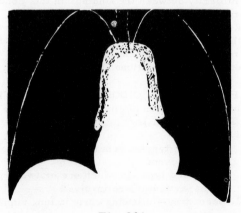

Fig. 204

the right hilum region. The mere visualization of
the thymus does not indicate pathological enlargement. Only if, by its pressure on the trachea, it
causes clinical symptoms of respiratory obstruction
can it be designated as pathological. Lateral-view
examination has been recommended to detect such
compression of the trachea (Pancoast and Pendergrass). Examination in upright position in inspiration and expiration and lateral view examination
should be made to avoid pitfalls in diagnosis.

SUBSTERNAL THYROID (Fig. 205). Tumors
of the thyroid gland not only cause displacement of
the trachea but usually cause some stenosis also. An
accessory lobe of thyroid gland may extend down into
the thorax behind the upper portion of the sternum,
forming a shadow in the upper portion of the mediastinum. Such shadows can usually be identified by
tracing their borders up into the neck. Sudden enlargement of substernal thyroid causing alarming
dyspnea with evident increase in size on roentgenographic examination may erroneously suggest growth
of a tumor; such sudden enlargements are occasionally encountered as a result of spontaneous intracapsular hemorrhage. Occasionally intrathoracic
goiter may occur in the posterior mediastinum resembling new growth (Pancoast and Pendergrass).

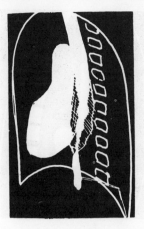

Fig. 206A

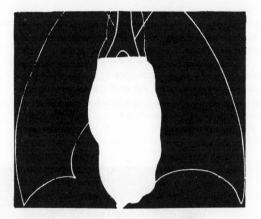

Fig. 206B

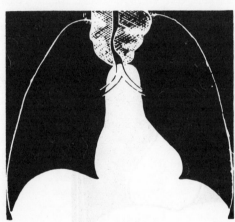

Fig. 205

Diverticula may be so large as to cast confusing
shadows (Fig. 206C).

Short esophagus, with thoracic stomach, can
often be detected from the appearance of the gas bubble in the stomach seen through the cardiac shadow.
Once suspected the diagnosis is easily confirmed by
the administration of a barium meal (Fig. 206D).

Intrathoracic gastric cysts or cysts composed

MEDIASTINAL INVOLVEMENT BY ESOPHA-
GEAL PATHOLOGY. Carcinoma of the esophagus
(Fig. 206A) rarely produces sufficient shadow to be
detectable in the ordinary roentgenogram; it rarely,
if ever, resembles tumor arising primarily from the
mediastinal structures. Cardiospasm (Fig. 206B),
however, is occasionally accompanied by such marked
dilatation of the esophagus that it bulges over beyond
the mediastinal margins on the right side, giving the
impression of a bulky nodular growth—often a fluid
level can be seen which betrays the true character
of the condition. In any event administration of a
barium mixture will definitely disclose the esophageal dilatation. There may be associated infiltration in the lung from aspiration of food material.

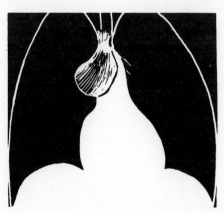

Fig. 206C

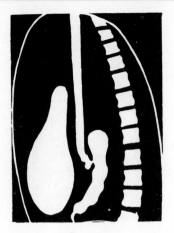

Fig. 206D

of gastric mucosa are occasionally found in the mediastinal space. These are congenital in origin, benign, and of no pathological significance.

Cold abscess from tuberculosis of the spine, confined by the spinal muscles (Fig. 207A), may produce a fusiform shadow resembling mediastinal pathology; lateral-view examination will localize the disease to the spinal column.

MEDIASTINAL EMPHYSEMA (Fig. 207B). Emphysema of the mediastinal space manifests itself as a "halo" of air about the heart. This is due to collection of the air in the anterior mediastinal space, shown beautifully in the lateral roentgenogram.

It may be due to spontaneous rupture of an emphysematous bleb into the interstitial tissue of the lung. Or it may develop after traumatic laceration of the neck or chest wall by air being sucked into the tissues during respiration. Forbes and Salmon have demonstrated that mediastinal emphysema and pneumothorax are frequent complications of tracheotomy especially where the operative procedure does not relieve the dyspnea. Air sucked in through the wound passes into the mediastinum by way of the interstitial tissue of the lung causing spontaneous pneumothorax and death. It has been shown that the air spreads along the vascular sheaths and that the entrapped air presses on the vascular walls and causes circulatory embarrassment (Macklin). A needle inserted through the chest wall into the anterior mediastinal space may be a life-saving measure. (See Spontaneous Interstitial Pulmonary Emphysema.)

For a review covering "Fifty Years of Progress in Roentgenology of the Chest," the reader is referred to an article by that title published by Wm. J. Tuddenham, Am. J. Roentgenol., 75:659, 1956.

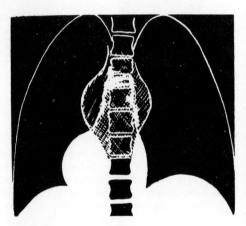

Fig. 207A

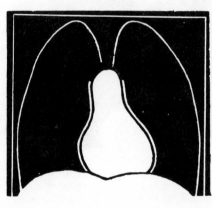

Fig. 207B

QUESTIONS ON THE CHEST

Questions marked with a dagger deal with rare and less-important conditions.

1. Why does the chest lend itself so readily to roentgenographic examination?

2. Describe briefly the appearance of the lung field and indicate the anatomical structures producing the various densities seen in the roentgenogram.

3. Describe briefly the minute anatomy of the lung as outlined by Wm. Snow Miller.

4. Show by diagram the position of the interlobar septa of the lungs.

5. Name and indicate the position of three arbitrary zones of the lung described by Dunham, and indicate their importance in determining the pathological accentuation of the lung markings.

6. What causes the linear markings of the lung? How may they be accentuated? What is the roentgen manifestation of bronchitis? Of irritant gas inhalation?

7. What are the x-ray characteristics of massive atelectasis and upon what physiological process do these findings depend? Under what conditions does it develop?

8. What is the appearance of atelectasis when a single lobe alone is involved? What is meant by disc atelectasis?

†9. Why is an atelectatic lung as dense as pneumonic consolidation while a lung shrunken to even smaller size from pneumothorax still remains relatively radiolucent?

†10. What are the radiological findings in opaque and nonopaque foreign bodies in the lung: (a) With complete obstruction? (b) With partial obstruction?

†11. Describe the succession of events when a bronchiogenic tumor enlarges and obstructs a bronchus. What are the characteristics of atelectasis from bronchiogenic tumor of an upper lobe bronchus?

12. How may bronchiectasis be demonstrated roentgenographically? What are its roentgenological manifestations?

13. Describe the appearance of the lung fields, in passive pulmonary congestion following pulmonary embolus; in edema of the lungs. What is meant by postoperative edema?

14. What types of pneumonic involvement may be recognized roentgenographically? What may be the first manifestation of lobar pneumonia as seen in the roentgenogram? Show by diagrams the characteristic x-ray appearance of consolidation of the various lobes.

15. What x-ray evidence have we that lobar pneumonia is a local disease of the lung (with constitutional manifestation) running a limited course?

16. In children what other condition is frequently confused with lobar pneumonia clinically?

17. What changes are seen in the roentgenographic appearance of lobar pneumonia immediately after crisis? How long before resolution is complete?

18. What is meant by "protective" fluid and how may it be detected?

19. What complications are commonly encountered with lobar pneumonia, and how are they manifested in the roentgenogram?

20. Describe the roentgen picture in bronchopneumonia; in septic pneumonia. What four stages are recognized in Friedlander Bacillus Pneumonia?

21. What are the manifestations of atypical pneumonia? Of glandular type?

22. What is the roentgenographic appearance of lung abscess, and how does it differ in appearance from pneumonic consolidation? To what causes may it be due and what is the outlook for recovery?

23. What are the x-ray characteristics of chronic diffuse interstitial fibrosis of the lung and to what process is it due? How may it be differentiated from massive atelectasis?

24. What are the x-ray manifestations of childhood type of first infection with pulmonary tuberculosis? What conditions must be differentiated in making the diagnosis? What is the greatest factor in treatment of the disease?

25. What are the x-ray manifestations of reinfection with adult-type pulmonary tuberculosis?

26. By what methods does pulmonary tuberculosis spread and how may this be indicated in the roentgenogram?

27. How may the minute anatomy of the lung favor lodgement and growth of tubercle bacilli?

28. Give American Tuberculosis Association classification of stages of pulmonary tuberculosis.

29. How does pulmonary tuberculosis heal and what manifestation of healing can be seen in the x-ray? Can activity of a lesion always be determined roentgenologically?

30. What is meant by caseous tuberculous pneumonia and how is it manifested in the roentgenogram? Differentiate from lobar pneumonia.

†31. What is epituberculosis? How may it be differentiated from caseous tuberculous pneumonia?

32. How does miliary tuberculosis develop and what is the roentgenographic picture of the disease? How does it differ in appearance from mycotic infections; sarcoid; erythema nodosum?

33. What surgical procedures are of value in the treatment of pulmonary tuberculosis?

†34. In general do mycotic infections of the lung have any characteristic manifestations? What is the picture of aspergillus infection in the acute stage? After healing?

35. Describe briefly the picture of established silicosis.

36. What primary tumors of the bronchi are recognized? Of the lung? Describe the development of fluid and air cysts of the lung.

†37. What effect does trauma have on production of acute inflammatory diseases of the chest, pneumonia, pleurisy, etc.? How can subcutaneous emphysema be detected roentgenographically? To what is spontaneous pneumothorax due? What is progressive vesicular pulmonary emphysema?

38. What are the roentgenographic findings in interstitial hemorrhage from stab wound or gunshot wound of the lung? What difference in appearance is there between ordinary effusion and hemothorax? Does blood show the same tendency to clot in the pleural cavity as it does elsewhere?

39. What is the characteristic appearance of fluid free in the pleural cavity? Pleural effusion associated with pneumothorax? Localized pleural effusion?

40. What is the characteristic appearance of pneumothorax? Under what conditions does spontaneous pneumothorax occur?

†41. What is the characteristic appearance of tumors of the pleura? Can they be differentiated roentgenographically from localized pleural effusion?

42. To what are the following conditions of the diaphragm due?
         tenting
         scalloping
         immobilization
         paradoxical action
         eventration
         hernia

43. Name the common conditions which give rise to mediastinitis.

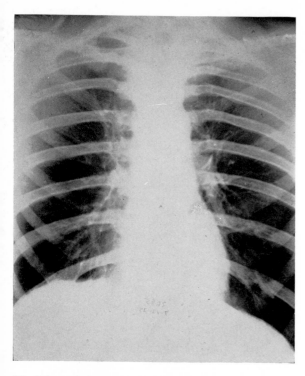

Healthy adult chest showing the hilum shadows and lung markings extending outward into the lungs. These shadows are produced by the combined densities of the blood vessels, lymphatics and bronchial structures.

Pulmonary Emphysema following chronic bronchitis and asthma. Lipiodol injection shows filling of bronchial branches but not of alveolar structures.   →

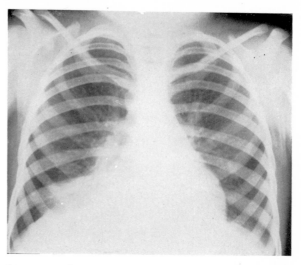

Acute respiratory infection produces an increase in the bronchovascular markings of the hilum regions and lower lobes. In this case the infection was due to aspiration of material from accessory nasal sinus infection causing induration in the cardiophrenic sinus so called "Sinus Lung."

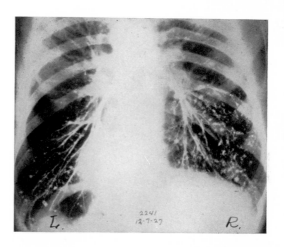

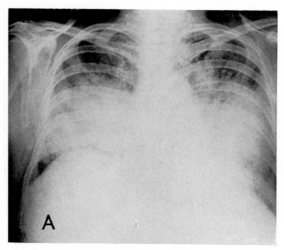

Azotemic oedema of the lungs a form of antigenic pneumonitis associated with acute glomerulonephritis. Note peripheral clear zone of lung tissue.

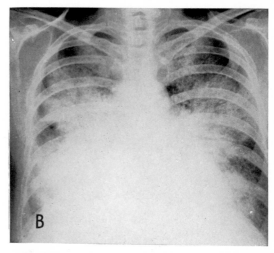

Antigenic pneumonitis (azotemic oedema) associated with periarteritis nodosa.

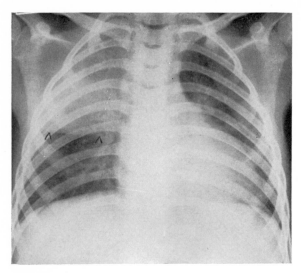

Right upper lobe lobar pneumonia, showing dense homogeneous consolidation of the right upper lobe with a sharply outlined lower border. Characteristic of consolidation of the right upper lobe.

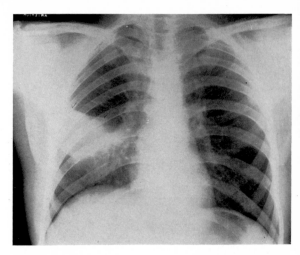

Right middle lobar pneumonia, showing homogeneous consolidation extending from hilium region to periphery with sharply outlined lung density. Characteristic of middle lobe consolidation.

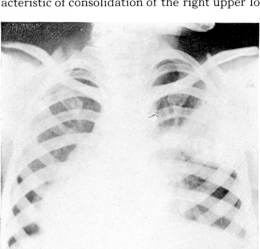

← Segmental lobar pneumonia showing triangular consolidation of lower segment of right upper lobe.

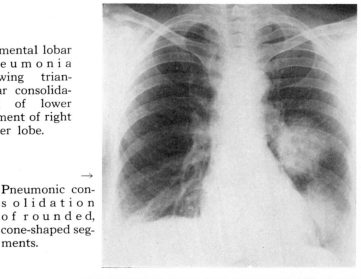

→ Pneumonic consolidation of rounded, cone-shaped segments.

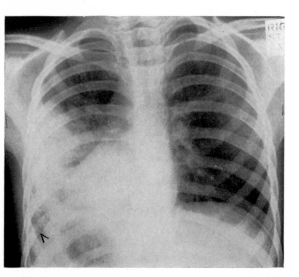

Left lower lobar pneumonia, showing a dense homogeneous shadow involving the lower two-thirds of the lung field, fading out into the normal lung density above and below; the costophrenic angle is the last location to lose its aeration. Characteristic of lower lobe consolidation.

Bronchopneumonia, showing multiple peribronchial infiltrations in the right lower lobe. The lower lobes are the site of predilection and the lesions originate as extensions from the bronchi.

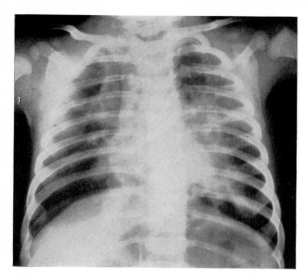

Lipoid pneumonia, showing the shaggy irregular peribronchial infiltration extending outward from the hilum regions into both lower lobes. This may result from repeated aspiration of oils.

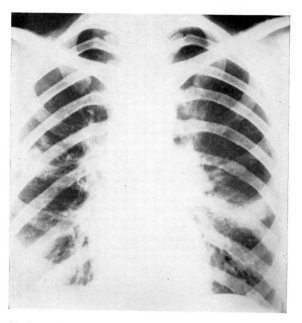

Tularemic pneumonia. A primary lymphatic type of tularemic pneumonia starts with hilar adenopathy and increase in lung markings radiating outward into both lungs.

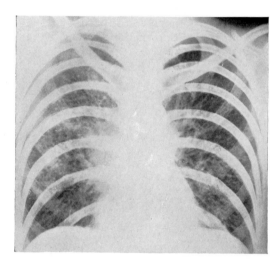

Atypical pneumonia of virus type ultimately causes irregular areas of lobular consolidation throughout the lung.

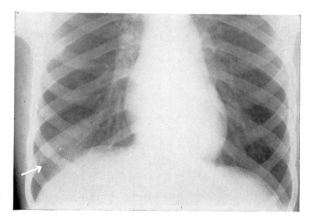

Attenuated lobular pneumonia, showing patch of infiltration in costophrenic sinus; lasts for six weeks with little if any fever or other symptoms—disappears spontaneously.

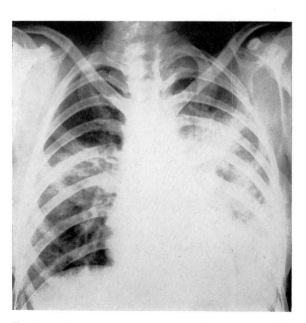

Septic lobular pneumonia, showing small areas of infiltration caused from blood-borne septic infection. This causes an appearance of blotchy infiltration throughout the lungs.

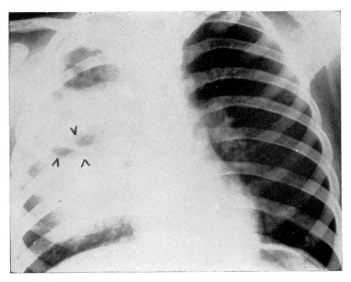

Lung abscess following tonsillectomy. Note the area of destruction shown within a large area of consolidation in the lung.

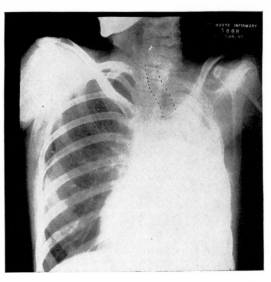

Chronic diffuse interstitial fibrosis of the lung resulting from multiple abscesses in the lung or pleura with overstimulation of fibrous tissue. The organized scar tissue results in narrowing of the involved side of the chest and approximation of the ribs and elevation of the diaphragm.

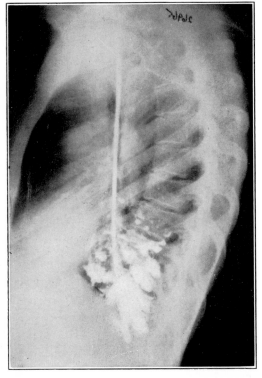

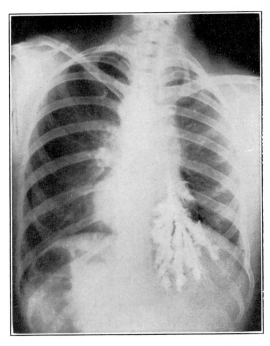

Bronchiectasis, showing the dilated lower lobe bronchi on the left side filled with Lipiodol. In the lateral view a small catheter is seen extending into the lower lobe bronchus for the purpose of injecting a small portion of the lung. Bronchiectatic dilatations may extend far down below the dome of the diaphragm and be invisible in the ordinary postero-anterior view.

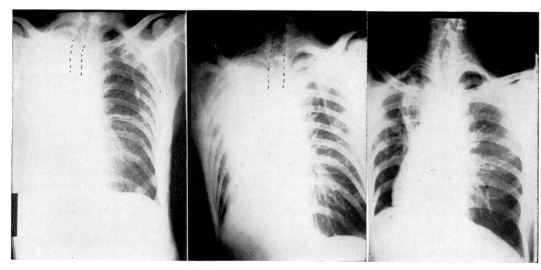

Massive atelectatic collapse of the lung following a kidney operation. Occlusion of a bronchus by mucus results in absorption of the air in the portion of the lung supplied by the bronchus. As a result the lung is reduced in volume and atelectasis results. Since there is no pneumothorax and the lung is closely applied to the chest wall the entire side of the chest is reduced in size; there is narrowing of the side of the thorax and approximation of the ribs, displacement of the heart and mediastinal structures toward the involved side and elevation of the diaphragm. If the patient is caused to lie upon the unaffected side and cough to dislodge the mucus, the lung will re-expand within a few minutes under direct fluoroscopic examination.

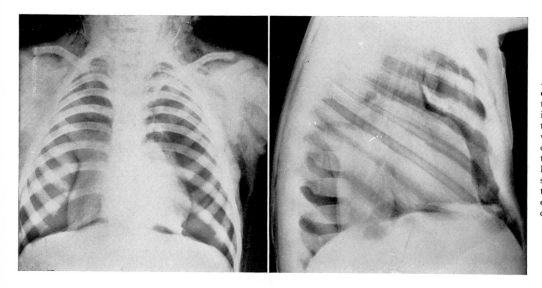

Anteroposterior and lateral roentgenograms of the chest. Air introduced into the mediastinum through a tracheotomy wound may be forced outward through the interstitial tissues of the lung to the finest lung structures, causing rupture of the alveoli, bilateral pneumothorax and death.

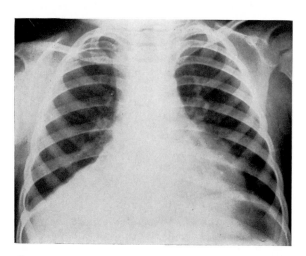

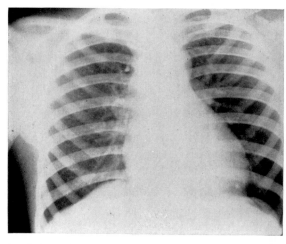

Complete atelectasis of the right lower lobe from occlusion by a foreign body. When a single lobe of the lung becomes atelectatic and reduces in size, the remaining portion of the lung expands, equalizing the pressure, and the signs of contraction of the chest wall and mediastinum are much less evident. Same patient after re-expansion.

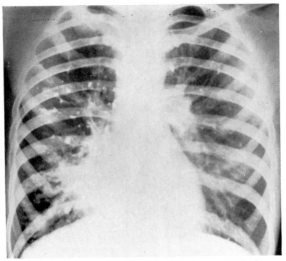

First infection with tuberculosis in a child showing a pronounced glandular reaction and extension of the disease beyond the nodes.

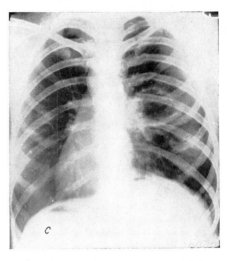

Activation of a previously quiescent tuberculous lymph node remaining from childhood tuberculous infection. Note the large cavity in the hilum region. Patient succumbed in a short while from disseminated tuberculosis.

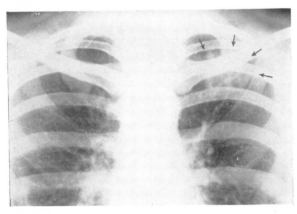

Minimal pulmonary tuberculosis, showing definite tuberculous infiltration in the right apex and infra-clavicular region. Compare with the opposite healthy side.

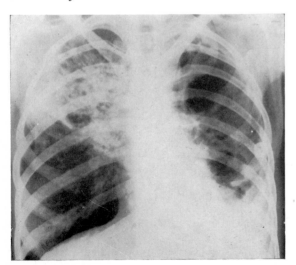

Far advanced pulmonary tuberculosis, showing a dense area of consolidation throughout the upper half of the right lung and involvement of the entire left lung by consolidation and cavity formation.

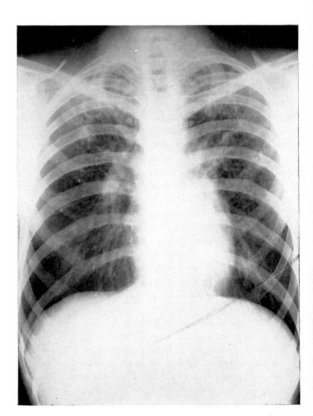

Moderately advanced pulmonary tuberculosis, showing areas of infiltration throughout the right upper lobe with extension into the infra-clavicular region on the left. There is no evidence of cavity formation.

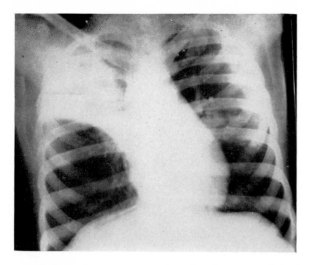 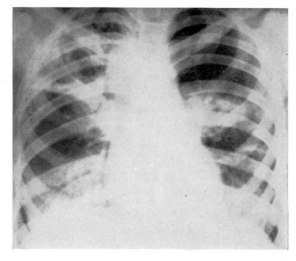

Caseous tuberculous pneumonia, showing consolidation of the right upper lobe resembling lobar pneumonia. Three months later showing cavity formation.

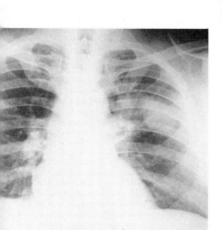 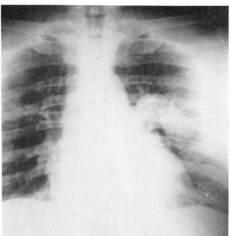 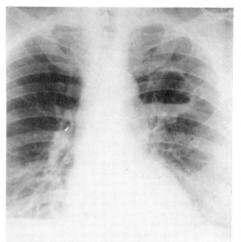

Left: Nodular tuberculous lesion in left lung with some hilar adenopathy, mistaken for bronchiogenic tumor. Middle: After treatment with 200 K.V. x-ray therapy, lesion assumes S-shaped appearance probably from caseation. Right: One year later, development of cavity.

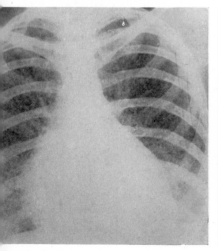 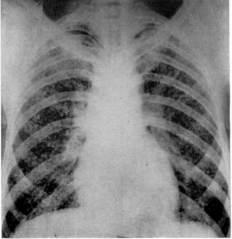 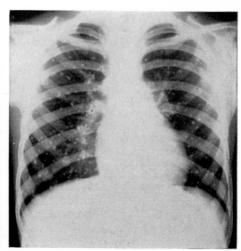

ary tuberculosis, showing wide-
ad involvement by uniform, small
rculous lesions due to blood stream
mination.

Silicosis, showing widespread involvement of both lungs by small fibrous
nodules resembling miliary tuberculosis
but without clinical evidence of the disease.

Numerous tiny calcareous deposits
throughout the lungs. These represent
healed disseminated lesions, due possibly to tuberculosis or histoplasmosis.

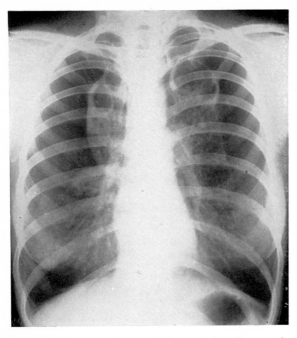

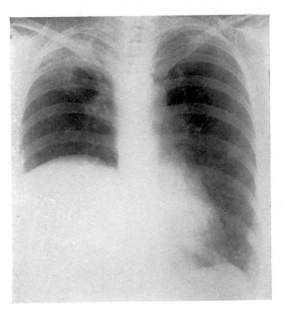

Phrenicotomy or section of the phrenic nerve causes diaphragm to assume a high position; used to help rest the lung in tuberculosis.

Bilateral pneumothorax with partial collapse of both lungs; used to decrease excursion of the lungs in pulmonary tuberculosis.

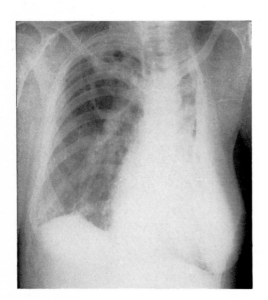

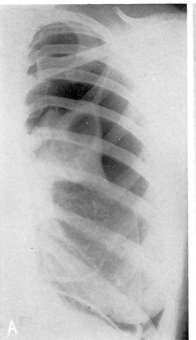

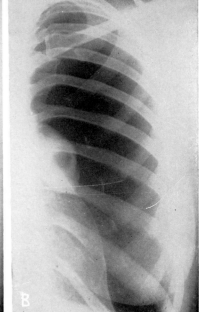

Thoracoplasty or surgical removal of rib structure permits collapse of a section of the chest wall in an effort to compress cavities.

Pneumolysis or severance of a pleural adhesion allowing the lung collapse more effectively.

A. Before operation showing strand-like adhesion.

B. After operation showing severing of adhesion and collapse of lung.

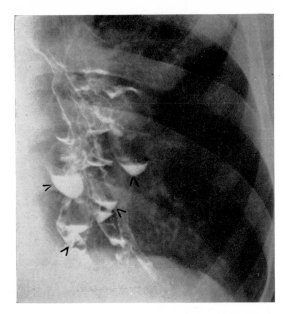

Congenital Bronchiectasis; Note pouches filled with Lipiodol projecting out from large bronchi. These cyst-like structures in the lung appear as multiple, thin-walled rings showing no sputum or other evidence of infection.

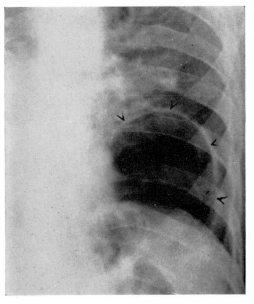

Large rounded thin-walled pneumatocele about 10 cm. in diameter in the left pleural cavity just above the diaphragm behind the heart. The history indicated that this was present for over ten years.

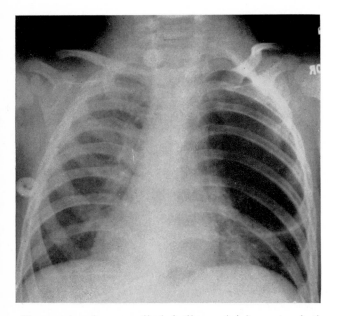

Pneumatocele; so-called balloon (air) cyst of the lung. *A.* Large solitary pneumatocele indicated by the dark well-circumscribed area in the right lung field which is devoid of lung markings. This examination was made at full *inspiration.*

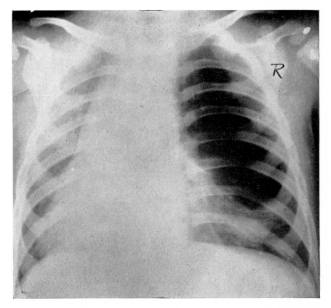

B. Same patient; examination in full *expiration* shows no reduction in size of pneumatocele but definite displacement of the heart and mediastinal structures to the opposite side due to increased pressure in the right chest.

LUNG TUMORS

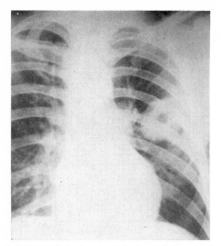

A large nodule in the left lung field with a central rarefied area, due to layer upon layer of fibrous tissue, walling off a pyogenic lung abscess.

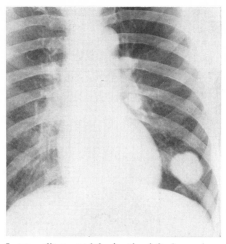

Large solitary nodule in the left lower lung field having the density of calcium. Tubercu'oma filled with calcium-containing caseous materials.

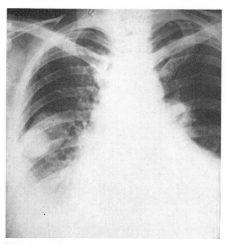

Nodular lesion due to interlobar effusion encapsulated in the interlobar region on the right side which might be mistaken for tumor.

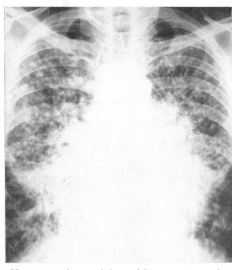

Numerous tiny nodules arising spontaneously at many points throughout both lungs simultaneously due to alveolar carcinoma. This is an unusual type of carcinomatous involvement which resembles the lesions seen in the lungs of virus disease (jaagsiekte) in sheep.

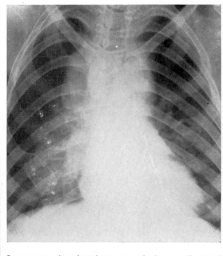

Large massive involvement of the mediastinal glands in Hodgkin's Disease. Note the bulky mediastinal shadow extending out on either side into the lung fields.

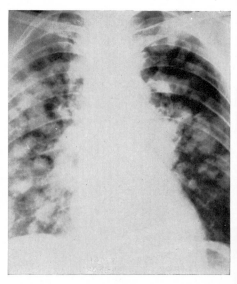

Metastatic involvement, secondary to carcinoma of the breast.

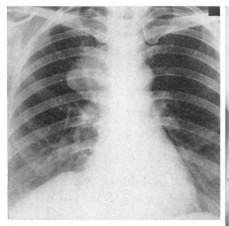

The commonest type of nodular growth due to bronchiogenic carcinoma. It has well defined borders, usually springs from larger bronchial branches and does not tend to break down and ulcerate.

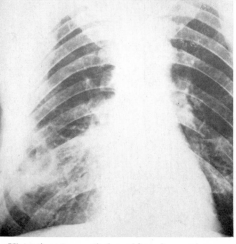

Ulcerative type of bronchiogenic carcinoma showing early breaking down of the tumor with secondary infection and abscess formation. This cannot be differentiated from pyogenic abscess, without microscopic examination.

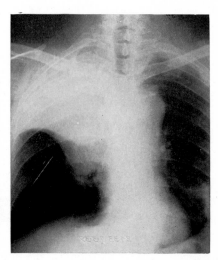

Bronchiogenic tumor occluding the bronchus of the right upper lobe resulting in right upper lobe atelectasis. This "S" shaped curve is characteristic of the condition (Ross Golden).

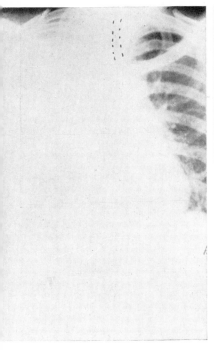

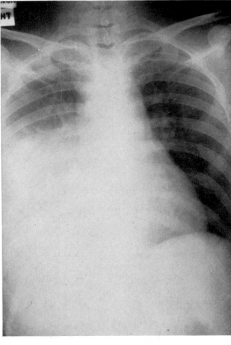

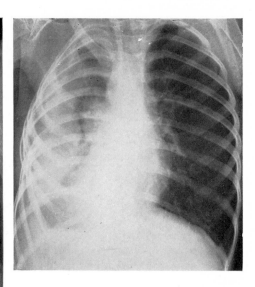

Pocketed pleural effusion localized to the lateral chest wall showing the characteristic rounded margin bulging in toward the compressible lung.

ge pleural effusion in a child causing lacement of the heart and medias- structure to the opposite side from weight of the fluid.

Large pleural effusion in an adult. Note the hazy concave upper border with remaining aeration of the upper mediastinal portion of the lung. This is always seen where the heart and mediastinal structures are fixed in position.

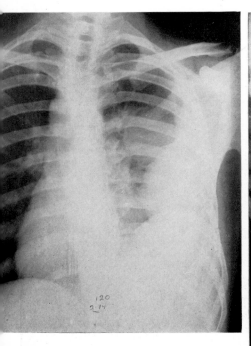

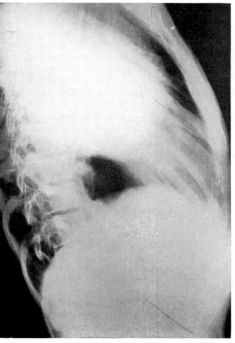

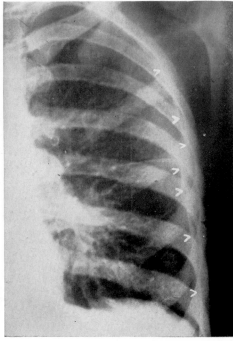

localized pleural effusion in the left al cavity. The sharply outlined inner r indicates that the effusion must be zed.

Lateral view showing the sac-like collection of localized pleural effusion.

Marked thickening of the parietal pleura shows as a ribbon-like shadow extending along the parietal chest wall.

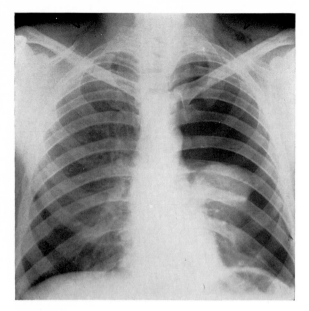

Pneumothorax from fracture of a rib showing complete collapse of the lung with removal of the lung markings from the outer lung field. Arrows indicate the fracture of the rib and air in the subcutaneous tissues of the neck.

Pneumothorax with associated pleural effusion in the recumbent position. In this position the fluid spreads itself out in a thin layer on the anterior chest wall and is not demonstrable in the radiograph.

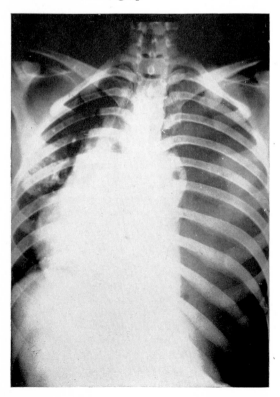

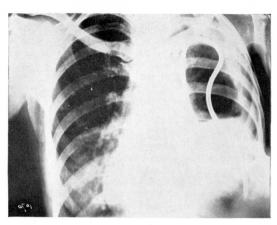

Empyema cavity showing a drainage tube in place.

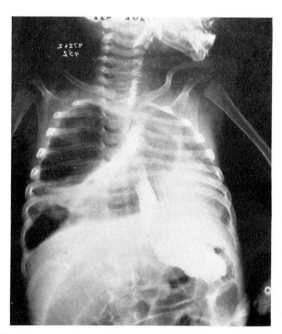

Pressure pneumothorax right chest, with displacement and herniation of mediastinum to left.

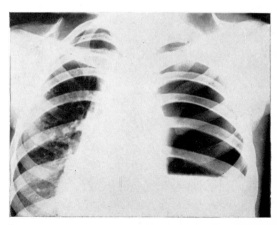

Same case in the upright position showing a fluid level.

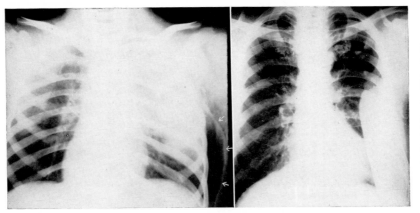

Subcutaneous emphysema with interstitial pulmonary hemorrhage due to fracture of the ribs from an automobile accident. Note large pocket of air in subcutaneous tissues.

Subpleural hematoma caused by injury from a batted ball received at twelve years of age. The organized hematoma has persisted into adult life.

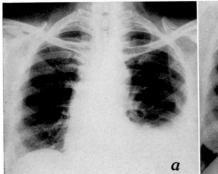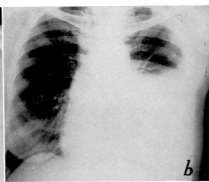

A. Hemothorax from rupture of intercostal artery due to fractured ribs. The blood, free in the pleural cavity, takes on the characteristic appearance of ordinary pleural effusion.

B. Same patient a month and a half later showing considerable increase in amount of fluid. Blood does not clot as readily in the pleural cavity and bleeding may continue for long periods.

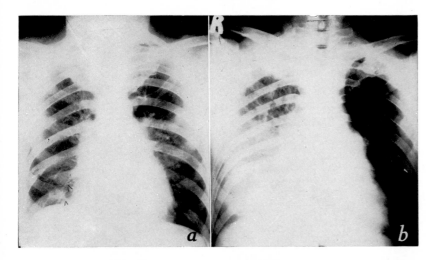

A. Delayed interstitial pulmonary hemorrhage from fracture of the ribs as the result of a fall. Examination after injury showed some separation of the fragments but little evidence of injury to the underlying lung.

B. Further examination a short time later revealed hemorrhage into the lung structures.

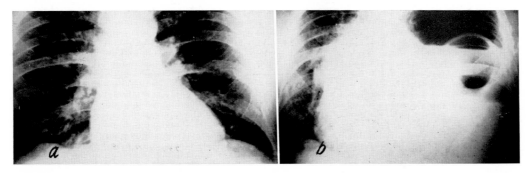

A. Stabwound of chest without apparent injury.
B. Sudden complete spontaneous rupture of partially healed lacerated wound of diaphragm several months later, on exertion, with herniation of abdominal viscera into chest and exsanguination.

Bilateral pneumothorax from fractured ribs as a result of an automobile passing over the body. Complete collapse of the left lung and partial collapse of the right. About one week later he coughed up a blood clot and from then on the left lung rapidly expanded.

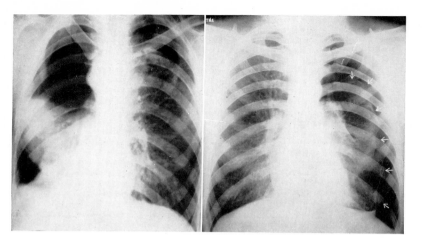

Traumatic pneumothorax from penetrating wound of the chest. Note collapse of the lung without evidence of hemorrhage into lung structures or pleural cavity.

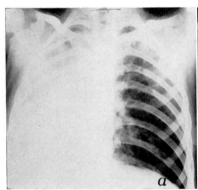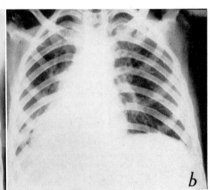

A. Massive (atelectatic) collapse of the lung following seven days after injury to spleen from an automobile accident.

B. Complete reinflation after rolling patient upon the uninvolved side and causing him to cough. This dislodges the plug of inspissated mucus and permits free entrance of air resulting in immediate reinflation of the lung under direct fluoroscopic vision.

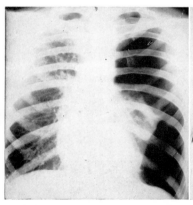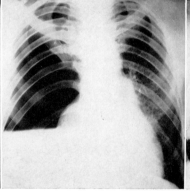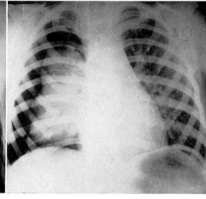

Progressive spontaneous pneumothorax following exertion showing almost complete collapse of the lung. Process of collapse was slow but continuous requiring more than an hour to become complete. Spontaneous pneumothorax is usually due to rupture of an emphysematous bleb.

Spontaneous hemopneumothorax with complete collapse of the lung. Hemorrhage is a very unusual complication of spontaneous pneumothorax. Three days after this examination he suddenly died. Death was due to acute pressure on the great vessels from **pressure** pneumothorax.

Pneumothorax and atelectasis following injury to the lung from removal of a cylindrical glass bead from the right main stem bronchus. A sharp broken corner of the bead caused laceration of the lung during bronchoscopic removal. Note the consolidated collapsed lung from atelectasis and the free air in the pleural cavity.

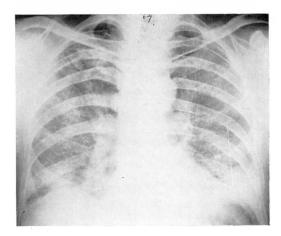

Infarcts of the pulmonary circulation have a tendency to occur at the periphery of the lung where the planes of the pleura form an angle with each other. These become consolidated, showing in the roentgenogram as areas of increased density, margins perpendicular to the pleural plane, inner edge may be rounded and smooth.

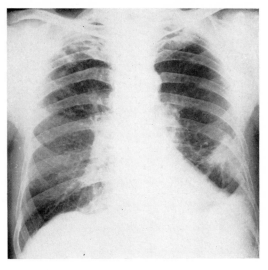

Organization of infarcts commences almost immediately. Even within a few days microscopic evidence of beginning organization is present; complete organization requires several weeks.

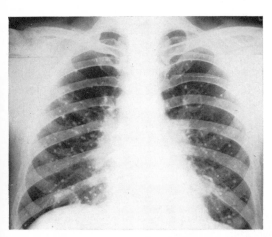

At times annular shadows originating in a similar way persist for more than a year.

Sometimes ordinary infarcts, if infected, develop central necrosis.

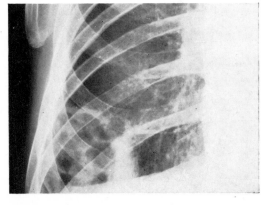

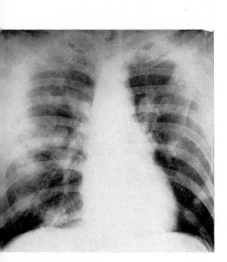

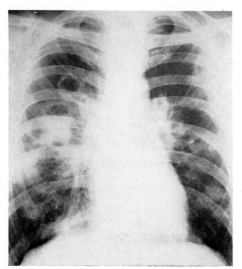

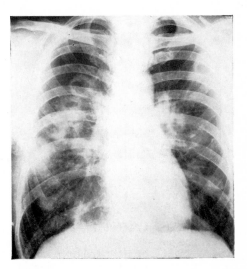

Numerous rounded nodular areas appearing throughout the lungs during the course of an acute systemic streptococcus infection. Second film made later the same day shows that some of the nodules have broken down in their centers leaving annular shadows. Third examination several days later showed still further involvement. Probably due to thrombosus of bronchial as well as pulmonary artery.

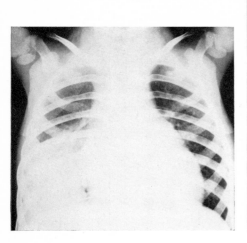 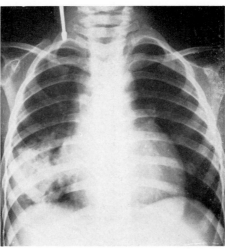 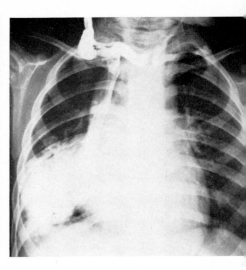

Appearance of lobular consolidation in right lower lung resembling pneumonia due to arterio-venous fistula from angioma of lung.

Same patient, showing persistence of rounded area of mottled density three months later. Canula in jugular vein for opaque injection.

Same patient, showing direct vascular connection with angioma of lung. Operated by Dr. J. L. Mudd with complete pneumonectomy and cure.

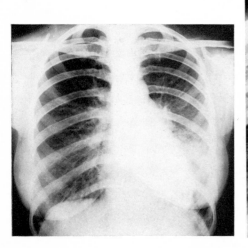 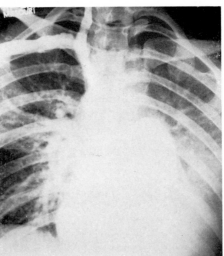 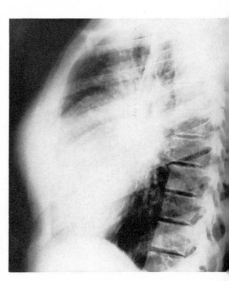

Diffuse increase in lung markings, left lung, young woman, chief complaint spontaneous pulmonary hemorrhage.

Angiogram of same patient after injection of Diodrast into right decubital vein, showing normal vascular structure in right lung, but no opaque material entering left lung. Operated by Dr. J. L. Mudd, primary amyloid tumor was found growing into and occluding pulmonary vessels.

Same patient. Lateral view showing dense hilum shadow due to tumor ramifying into hilar vessels.

Roentgen Anatomy and Physiology

Zinn, B., and Monroe, L., "The Lordotic Position in Fluoroscopy and Roentgenography of the Chest," Am. J. Roentgenol., 75:682, 1956.

Barden, R. P., and Comroe, J. H., "Roentgenologic Evaluation of Pulmonary Function," Am. J. Roentgenol., 75:668, 1956.

Brock, R. C., The Anatomy of the Bronchial Tree, Oxford Press, London, 1946.

Chynn, K. R., and Sante, L. R., "Roentgenologic Method for Demonstration of Bronchopulmonary Segments in Fully Expanded Cadaver Lungs in Situ," Am. J. Roentgenol., 75:779, 1956.

Medler, E. M., "Variations in Interlobar Fissures," Am. J. Roentgenol., 57:723, 1947.

Jackson, C., and Huber, J. F., Diseases of the Nose, Throat and Ear, W. B. Saunders, 1945.

Kane, J., and Heiser, S., "Indications for Delayed Roentgenogram in Bronchography," J. Thoracic Surg., 24:70, 1952.

Abrams, H. L., Hencky, G., and Kaplan, H. S., "Delayed Films in Bronchography," Calif. Med., 78:104, 1953.

Fischer, F. K., and Muelly, K., "Water-Soluble Opaque Medium for Bronchography IODURON-B," Schweiz med. Wchnuschr., 78:1025, 1027, 1948.

Cummins, C., and Silver, C. P., "Bronchography with Rapidly Eliminated Compound 'Dionosil,'" Brit. J. Radiol., 26:435, 1953.

Holden, W. S., and Crone, R. S., "Bronchography using DIONOSIL Only," Brit. J. Radiol., 26:317, 1953.

Jackson, C., and Huber, J. F., "Correlated Applied Anatomy of Bronchial Tree and Lungs with System of Nomenclature," Dis. Chest, 9:319, 1943.

Kramer, R., and Glass, A., "Bronchoscopic Localization of Lung Abscess," Ann. Otol., Rhin., and Laryng., 41:1210, 1932.

Neil, J. H., Gilmoor, W., and Gwynne, F. J., "Broncho-Pulmonary Segments," M. J. Australia, 2:165, 1937.

Boyden, E. A., "Intrahilar and Related Segmental Anatomy of Lung," Surg., 18:706, 1945.

Kane, I. J., "Segmental Localization of Pulmonary Disease on the Postero-anterior Roentgenogram," Radiol., 59:229, 1952.

Temple, H. L., and Evans, J. A., "Bronchopulmonary Segments," Am. J. Roentgenol., 63:26, 1950.

Cicero, R., and Del Castillo, H., "Lobar and Segmental Angiopneumonography in Pulmonary Disease," Acta Radiol., 54:42, 1956.

DiGuglielmo, L., and Bonomo, B., "The Significance of the Lateral Subsegments of the Lung in Pulmonary Disease," Acta Radiol., 44:217, 1955.

Lodge, T., "The Anatomy of the Blood Vessels of the Human Lung as Applied to Chest Radiology," Brit. J. Radiol., 1:77, 1946.

Miller, William Snow, The Lung, Chas. C. Thomas, 1937.

Deweese, E. R., and Howard, J. C., "Congenital Absence of a Lung," Radiol., 42:389, 1944.

Bendick, A. J., and Wessler, H., "The Azygos Lobe of the Lung," Am. J. Roentgenol., 20:1, 1928.

Hardman, G. I., "The Anomalous Middle Lobe of the Left Lung," Brit. J. Radiol., 21:70, 1948

Lalli, A., Carlson, R. F., and Adams, W. E., "Intralobar Pulmonary Sequestration," Arch. Surg., 69:797, 1954.

Bruwer, A. J., Clagett, T., and McDonald, J. R., "Interlobar Pulmonary Sequestration," Am. J. Roentgenol., 71:751, 1956.

Jensen, V., and Wolff, A., "Congenital Intralobar Pulmonary Sequestration with Anomalous Artery from the Aorta," Acta Radiol., 45:357, 1956.

Boyer, R. C., "Bronchography in Chronic Lobar Collapse," Am. J. Roentgenol., 69:28, 1953.

Fleischer, F. G., "Bronchial Peristalsis," Am. J. Roentgenol., 62:65, 1949.

DiRienzo, S., "Radiologic Exploration of the Bronchus," Chas. C. Thomas, 1949; Radiol., 53:168, 1949.

Barden, R. P., "Clinical Radiology and Studies of Pulmonary Function," Editorial, Am. J. Roentgenol., 77:1084, 1957.

Ware, P. F., and Strauss, H. K., "Lung Expansion Patterns Following Upper Lobe Segmental Resection," Radiol., 67:516, 1956.

Theodos, P. A., Albbritten, F. F., Jr., and Breckenridge, L., "Lung Biopsy in Diffuse Pulmonary Disease," Dis. Chest, 27:637, 1955.

Mitchum, W. R., and Brady, B. M., "Differential Diagnosis of Fibrosing Lung Lesions," Radiol., 68:36, 1957.

Pathology of the Respiratory Organs, Larynx and Trachea:

Grossman, J. W., "The Triticeous Cartilages," Am. J. Roentgenol., 53:166, 1945.

Weilin, S., "Diagnostic Radiological Aspects of Hypopharyngeal Cancer," Brit. J. Radiol., 26:218, 1953; Am. J. Roentgenol., 69:796, 1953.

Weilin, S., "The Roentgenologic Diagnosis and Follow Up of Hypopharyngeal Cancer," Am. J. Roentgenol., 69:796, 1953.

Gianturco, C., and Miller, G. A., "Bilateral Bronchography," Radiol., 65:57, 1955.

Donaldson, S. W., and Thompsett, A. C., "Tracheal Diameter in the Normal New Born Infant," Am. J. Roentgenol., 67:785, 1952.

Evans, W. A., Jr., "Congenital Obstructions of the Respiratory Tract," Am. J. Roentgenol., 62:167, 1949.

Parsons, P. B., "Lateral Cervical Sinus," Am. J. Roentgenol., 67:757, May 1952.

Ferguson, C. F., and Flake, C. G., "Tracheographic and Bronchographic Studies as Aids in Diagnosis of Congenital Malformations of Tracheobronchial Tree and Aortic Arch in Infants and Children," Ann. Otol., Rhin., and Laryng., 63:1056, 1954.

Carr, D. T., and Olsen, A. M., "Tracheopathia Osteoplastica," J.A.M.A., 155:1563, Aug. 28, 1954.

Drymalski, G. W., Thompson, J. R., and Sweany, H. C., "Tracheal Diverticula," Am. J. Roentgenol., 60:403, 1948.

Bronchial Pathology:

Whitaker, P. H., "Radiological Appearances of the Chest Following Partial Asphyxiation by a Smoke Screen," Brit. J. Radiol., 18:396, 1945.

Graham, E. A., Burtord, T. H., and Mayer, J. H., "Middle Lobe Syndrome," Postgrad. Med., 4:29, 1948.

Lisa, J. R., and Rosenblatt, M. B., Bronchiectasis, Oxford Press, 1943.

Evans, W. A., and Galinsky, L. J., "Diagnosis of Bronchiectasis in Young Adults; Prebronchographic Roentgen Manifestations Observed among Military Personnel," Am. J. Roentgenol., 51:537, 1944.

Richards, G. E., "The Interpretation of the Triangular Basal Shadows in Roentgenograms of the Chest," Am. J. Roentgenol., 30:289, 1933.

Block, E. G., Sandock, L. F., and Mitchell, E. B., "Retrocardiac Bronchiectasis," Am. J. Roentgenol., 60:219, 1948.

Pontius, J. R., and Jacobs, L. G., "The Reversal of Advanced Bronchiectasis," Radiol., 68:204, 1957.

Don, C., "Bronchography with Dionosil in Pulmonary Tuberculosis," J. Faculty Radiol., 6:189, 1955.

Nice, C. M., and Azad, M., "The Use of Dionisil in Bronchography," Radiol., 66:1, 1956.

Niknejad, I., Aurelius, J. R., Peterson, D. H., and Rigler, L. G., "The Current Status of Bronchography with Water-Soluble Media," Am. J. Roentgenol., 75:701, 1956.

Abrams, H. L., Hencky, G., and Kaplan, H. S., "The Use of Delayed Films in Bronchography," Radiol., 61:317, 1953.

Boyer, R. C., "Bronchography in Chronic Lobar Collapse," Am. J. Roentgenol., 69:28, 1953.

Pathology of the Lungs—Circulatory Disturbances:

Carmichael, J. H. E., Julian, D. G., Jones, G. P., and Wren, E. M., "Radiological Signs in Pulmonary Hypertension - Significance of Line B of Kerley," Brit. J. Radiol., 27:393, 1954.

Keats, T. E., Kreis, Van A., and Simpson, E., "Roentgen Manifestations of Pulmonary Hypertension in Congenital Heart Disease," Radiol., 66:693, 1956.

Westermark, N., "On the Roentgen Diagnosis of Lung Embolism," Acta Radiol., 19:357, 1938.

Aitchison, J. D., McKay, J. M., "Pulmonary Artery Occlusion Demonstrated by Angiography," Brit. J. Radiol., 29:398, 1956.

Keating, D. R., Burkey, J. N., Hellerstein, H. K., and Feil, H., "Chronic Massive Thrombosis of Pulmonary Arteries," Am. J. Roentgenol., 69:208, 1953.

Drinker, C. K., Pulmonary Edema and Inflammation, Harvard University Press, 1945.

Muether, R. O., "Water Balance," J. Missouri State M. A., 43:599, 1946.

Courtice, F. C., and Phipps, P. J., "The Absorption of Fluids from the Lungs," J. Physiol., 105:186, 1946.

Rendicht, R. A., Levy, A. W., and Cove, A. M., "Pulmonary Manifestations of Azotemia," Am. J. Roentgenol., 46:802, 1941.

Truetta, J., Barclay, A. E., Franklin, K. J., Daniel, P. M., and Prichard, M. M. L., Studies of the Renal Circulation, Chas. C. Thomas, Springfield, Illinois.

Loeffler, W., "Differential Diagnosis of Infiltrations in Relation to Other Manifestations; Time of Retrogression of Early Infiltrates," Beitr. Klin. Tuberk., 79:338, 1932.

Loeffler, W., "Die flüchtigen lungeninfiltrate mit eosinophilie," Schweiz. Med. Wschr., 66:1069, 1936.

Loeffler, W., and Maier, C., "Zur frage der pathogenese des eosinophilen infiltrates," Praxis, 33:529, 1944.

Bayley, E. C., Lindberg, D. O. N., and Baggenostoss, A. H., "Loeffler's Syndrome," Arch. Path., 40:376, 1945.

Bergstrand, H., "Morphological Equivalents in Polyarthritis, Rheumatica, Periarteritis, Nodosa Transient Eosinophilic Infiltration of the Lung and Other Allergic Syndromes," J. Path. and Bact., 58:399, 1946.

Henderson, A. T., and Pierce, C. B., "Transitory Focal Pulmonary Edema and Eosinophilia," Am. J. Roentgenol., 58:391, 1947.

Heiken, C. A., and Weise, E. R., "Loeffler's Syndrome," Am. Rev. Tuberc., 63:480, 1951.

Hennell, H., and Sussman, M. L., "The Roentgen Features of Eosinophilic Infiltrations in the Lungs," Radiol., 44:328, 1945.

Hodes, P. J., and Wood, F. C., "Eosinophilic Lung (Tropical Eosinophilia)," Am. J. Med. Sc., 210:288, Sept. 1945.

Pendergras, E. P., Lame, E. L., and Ostrum, H. W., "Hemosiderosis of the Lung due to Mitral Disease," Am. J. Roentgenol., 61:443, 1949.

Wyllie, W. G., Sheldon, W., Bodian, M., and Barlow, A., "Idiopathic Pulmonary Haemosiderosis (Essential Brown Induration of Lungs)," Quart. J. Med., 17:25, 1948.

Cliff, J. M., "Idiopathic Pulmonary Hemosiderosis," Brit. J. Radiol., 26:102, 1953.

Fleischner, F. G., and Reiner, L., "Linear X-ray Shadows in Acquired Pulmonary Hemosiderosis and Congestion," New England J. Med., 250:900, 1954.

Haubrich, R., "Miliary Hemosiderosis of Lungs with Partial Ossification," Fortschr. Geb. Rontgenstrahlen, 81:440, 1954.

Hanbury, W. J., Cureton, R. J. R., Simon, G., "Pulmonary Infarcts Associated with Bronchogenic Carcinoma," Thorax, 9:304, 1954.

Shapiro, R., and Rigler, L. G., "Pulmonary Embolism without Infarction," Am. J. Roentgenol., 60:460, 1948.

Kirklin, B. R., and Faust, L., "A Clinical and Roentgenological Consideration of Pulmonary Infarction," Am. J. Roentgenol., 23:265, 1930.

Levy, H., "Atypical Roentgen Appearance of Pulmonary Infarction in Patients with Heart Failure," Am. J. Roentgenol., 35:635, 1936.

Sante, L. R., and Hufford, C. E., "Annular Shadows of Unusual Type Associated with Acute Pulmonary Infection," Am. J. Roentgenol., 50:719, 1943.

Bulgrin, J. G., "Unusual Friedlander's Bacillus Pneumonia Associated with Septicemia," Radiol., 50:526, 1948.

Kerley, P., "The Inferior Accessory Lobe of the Lung," Brit. J. Radiol., 5:234, 1936.

Lung Infections—Bacterial and Viral Pneumonias:

Sante, L. R., "Correlation of Roentgenological and Pathological Findings in the Pneumonias," New England R. R. Soc., 4:1, 1947.

Sante, L. R., "Roentgen-ray Classification of the Pneumonias with Special Reference to the Tissues Involved," J. Missouri State M. A., 43:93, 1946.

Sante, L. R., "A Study of Lobar Pneumonia and Its Pulmonary Complications," Am. J. Roentgenol., 10:351, 1923.

Studdert, T. C., and Turnbull, A. K., "Pneumonia of Lobe of Azygos Vein," Brit. J. Radiol., 20:119, 1947.

Westermark, N., "On Influence of Intra-alveolar Pressure on Normal and Pathological Structure of Lungs," Acta Radiol., 25:874, 1944.

Bihss, F., and Berland, H. I., "Roentgenological Manifestations of Pleuropulmonary Involvement in Tularemia," Radiol., 41:431, 1943.

Kornblum, Karl, "The Roentgen-ray Diagnosis of Pulmonary Infections with Friedlander's Bacillus," Am. J. Roentgenol., 19:513, 1928.

Holmes, R. B., "Friedlander's Pneumonia," Am. J. Roentgenol., 75:728, 1956.

Oderr, C. P., and Shaw, J. F., "Roentgen Findings in a Case of Chronic Melioidosis," Am. J. Roentgenol., 76:94, 1956.

Dennis, J. M., and Boudreau, R. P., "Pleuropulmonary Tularemia: Its Roentgen Manifestations," Radiol., 68:25, 1957.

Ackerman, L. V., Elliott, G. V., and Alanis, M., "Localized Organizing Pneumonia: Its Resemblance to Carcinoma," Am. J. Roentgenol., 71:988, 1954.

Sante, L. R., "Pulmonary Infection in Tularemia," Am. J. Roentgenol., 25:241, 1931.

Sante, L. R., "A Study of Influenzal Pneumonia by Serial Roentgen-ray Examinations," J. Missouri State M.A., 18:43, 1921.

Reimann, H. A., The Pneumonias, W. B. Saunders, 1938.

Hamman, L., and Rich, A. R., "Acute Diffuse Interstitial Fibrosis of the Lung," Bull. Johns Hopkins Hosp., 74:177, 1944.

Gough, J., "Generalized and Primary Fibrosis of the Lungs," Brit. J. Radiol., 29:641, 1956.

Tan, D. Y. M., Kaufman, S. A., and Levene, G., "Primary Chickenpox Pneumonia," Am. J. Roentgenol., 76:527, 1956.

Endress, Z. F., and Schnell, F. R., "Varicella Pneumonitis," Radiol., 66:723, 1956.

Rosen, B., "Ornithosis as an Occupational Hazard," Radiol., 65:373, 1955.

Pinkerton, H., and Henderson, R. G., "Adult Toxoplasmosis," J.A.M.A., 11:807, 1941.

Jacobson, G., Delinger, R. B., and Carter, R. A., "Roentgen Manifestations of Q Fever," Radiol., 53:739, 1949.

Irons, J. V., and Hooper, J. M., "Q Fever in the United States," J.A.M.A., 133:815, 1947.

Pinkerton, H., and Henderson, R. G., "Adult Toxoplasmosis, Previously Unrecognized Disease Entity Simulating Typhus-Spotted Fever Groups," J.A.M.A., 116:807, 1941.

Sante, L. R., "Roentgen Manifestations of Adult Toxoplasmosis," Am. J. Roentgenol., 47:825, 1942.

McIntyre, M. C., "Pulmonary Syphilis; Its Frequency, Pathology and Roentgenological Appearance," Arch. Path., 11:258, 1931.

Silverstein, C. M., "Pulmonary Manifestations of Leptospirosis," Radiol., 61:327, 1953.

Hildebrand, E., "Pulmonary Adenomatosis," Am. Rev. Tuberc., 57:281, 1948.

Steinberg, C., "Vitamin E in Collagen in the Rheumatic Diseases," Ann. New York Acad. Sc., 52:380, 1949.

Collagen Diseases:

Kampmeier, R. H., "Vascular Diseases due to Hyper-sensitivity; So-called Diffuse Collagen Disease," Am. Pract. and Digest Treat., 1:113, 1950.

Banks, B. M., "Is There A Common Denominator in Scleroderma, Dermatomyositis, Disseminated Lupus Erythematosus, Libman-Sacks Syndrome and Polyarteritis Nodosa?," New England J. Med., 225:433, 1941.

Rich, A. R., "Hypersensitivity to Iodine as a Cause of Periarteritis Nodosa," Bull. Johns Hopkins Hosp., 77:43, 1945.

Longcope, W. T., and Winkenwerder, W. L., "Anaphylaxis Serum Disease, Urticaria, and Angioneurotic Edema," Nelson's Loose Leaf Medicine, N. Y., 2:631, 648.

Meschan, I., Marvin, H. N., Gordon, V. H., and Regnier, G., "The Radiographic Appearances of Hyalin Disease of the Lung in the New Born," Radiol., 60:383, 1953.

Garland, L. H., and Sisson, M. A., "Roentgen Findings in the 'Collagen' Diseases," Am. J. Roentgenol., 71:581, 1954.

Doub, H. P., Goodrich, B. E., and Gish, J. R., "The Pulmonary Aspects of Polyarteritis (Periarteritis) Nodosa," Am. J. Roentgenol., 71:785, 1954.

Rogers, J. V., and Roberto, A. E., "Circumscribed Pulmonary Lesions in Periarteritis Nodosa and Wegener's Granulomatosis," Am. J. Roentgenol., 76:88, 1956.

Saville, P., "Polyarteritis Nodosa with New Bone Formation," J. Bone and Joint Surg., 36B:327, 1956.

Aspiration Pneumonitis:

Pinkerton, H., "Reaction to Oils and Fats in Lung," Arch. Path., 5:380, 1928.

Nathanson, L., Frenkel, D., and Jacobi, M., "Diagnosis of Lipoid Pneumonia by Aspiration Biopsy," Arch. Int. Med., 72:627, 1934.

Davis, E. W., Hampton, A. O., Bickham, C., and Winship, T., "Lipoid Pneumonia Simulating Tumor," J. Thoracic Surg., 28:212, 1954.

Steinberg, I., and Finby, N., "Lipoid (Mineral Oil) Pneumonia and Cor Pulmonale Due to Cardiospasm," Am. J. Roentgenol., 76:108, 1956.

Sante, L. R., "The Fate of Oil Particles in the Lung and Their Possible Relationship to the Development of Bronchiogenic Carcinoma," Am. J. Roentgenol., 62:788, 1949.

Sante, L. R., "Lung Abscess," Radiol., 4:183, 1922.

Gershon-Cohen, J., Bringhurst, L. S., and Byrne, R. N., "Roentgenography of Kerosene Poisoning," Am. J. Roentgenol., 69:557, 1953.

Reed, E. S., "Kerosene Intoxication," Am. J. Dis. Childhood, 79:623, 1950.

Sante, L. R., "Pulmonary Tuberculosis," Radiol., 6:504, 1926.

Miller, William Snow, "Tuberculous Lung in which Large Emphysematous Bulla was Mistaken for Cavity," Am. Rev. Tuber., 28:359, 1933.

Cherry, H. H., "Basal Onset of Reinfection Tuberculosis," Am. J. Roentgenol., 59:82, 1948.

Favis, E. A., "Planigraphy (Body Section Radiography) in Detecting Tuberculous Pulmonary Cavitation," Dis. Chest, 26:255, 1954.

Sante, L. R., "Tuberculous Lobar Pneumonia," Am. J. Roentgenol., 11:55, 1924.

Pagel, W., and Simmonds, F. A. H., "The Healing of Cavities," Am. J. Med. Sc., 197:281, 1939.

Birkelo, C. C., and Rague, P. O., "Accuracy of Roentgen Determination of Activity of Minimal Pulmonary Tuberculosis," Am. J. Roentgenol., 60:303, 1948.

Sante, L. R., "Cirrhosis of Lung," Radiol., 3:128, 1924.

Sante, L. R., "Study of Miliary Tuberculosis," Radiol., 3:467, 1924.

Felson, B., "Acute Miliary Disease of the Lung," Radiol., 59:32, 1952.

Jacobeus, H. C., "The Cauterization of Adhesions in Pneumothorax Treatment of Tuberculosis," Surg., Gynec., Obst., 32:493, 1921.

Cohen, S. L., "Milkman's Pseudofractures of the Ribs Following Extraperiosteal Ivalon Pack," Radiol., 65:587, 1955.

King, E. Q., Johnson, J. B., Batten, G. S., and Henry, W. L., "Tuberculosis Following Cortisone Therapy," J.A.M.A., 147:238, 1951.

Popp, C. G., Ottosen, P., and Brasher, C. A., "Cortisone and Pulmonary Tuberculosis," J.A.M.A., 147:241, 1951.

Garland, L., Moderator, "Chest Surveys," Radiol., 65:19, 1955.

Gunderson, G. A., and Nice, C. M., "Nocardiosis," Radiol., 68, 31, 1957.

Hawley, C., and Felson, B., "Roentgen Aspects of Intrathoracic Blastomycosis," Am. J. Roentgenol., 75:751, 1956.

Mycotic Infections:

Huntel, W., Jr., and Horsman, R. K., "Acute Disseminated Coccidioidal Granuloma," Am. Rev. Tuberc., 63:476, 1951.

Jamison, H. W., and Carter, R. A., "Roentgen Findings in Early Coccidioidomycosis," Radiol., 48:323, 1947.

Rakofsky, M., and Knickerbocker, T. W., "Roentgenological Manifestations of Primary Pulmonary Coccidioidomycosis," Am. J. Roentgenol., 56:141, 1946.

Bass, H. E., Schamer, A., and Berke, R., "Coccidioidomycosis," Arch. Int. Med., 82:519, 1948.

Chortis, P., "Pulmonary Aspergillosis in Greece," Dis. Chest, 22:206, 1952.

Petranyi, G., and Zsebok, Z., "Micolithiasis Alveolaris Miliaris Pulmonum," Radiol. Clin., 23:202, 1954.

Levin, E. J., "Pulmonary Intracavity Fungus Ball," Radiol., 66:9, 1956.

Bonmati, J., Rogers, J. V., and Hopkins, W. A., "Pulmonary Cryptococcosis," Radiol., 66:188, 1956.

Berk, M., and Gerst, B., "Torulosis Producing Solitary Pulmonary Lesion," J.A.M.A., 149:1310, 1952.

Fissel, G., "Acute Fulminating Histoplasmosis," Am. J. Roentgenol., 76:60, 1956.

Serviansky, B., and Schwarz, J., "Calcified Intrathoracic Lesions Caused by Histoplasmosis and Tuberculosis," Am. J. Roentgenol., 77:1034, 1957.

Bunnell, I. L., and Furcolow, M. L., "A Report on Ten Proved Cases of Histoplasmosis," Public Health Reports, 63:299, March 5, 1948.

Kunstadter, R. H., "Primary Histoplasmosis with Recovery of Histoplasma Capsulatum from the Blood and Bronchial Secretions," J. Lab. and Clin. Med., 34:1290, 1949.

Serviansky, B., and Schwarz, J., "The Incidence of Splenic Calcifications in Positive Reactors to Histoplasmin and Tuberculin," Am. J. Roentgenol., 76:53, 1956.

Jacobson, G., and Zuckerman, S. D., "Roentgenologically Demonstrable Splenic Deposits in Sickle Cell Anemia," Am. J. Roentgenol., 76:47, 1956.

Hodgson, C. H., Weed, L. A., and Clagett, O. T., "Pulmonary Histoplasmosis," J.A.M.A., 145:807, 1951.

Sossman, M. C., Dodd, G. D., Jones, W. D. and Pillmore, G. U., "The Familial Occurrence of Pulmonary Alveolar Microlithiasis," Am. J. Roentgenol., 77:947, 1957.

LeMone, D. V., Scott, W. G., Moore, S., and Koven, A. L., "Bagasse Disease of the Lungs," Radiol., 49:556, 1947.

Greenspan, R. H., and Fineberg, S. B., "Salmonella Bacteremia," Radiol., 67:860, 1957.

Jacobs, L. G., Gerstl, B., Hollander, A. G., and Berk, M., "Intraabdominal Egg-Shell Calcifications Due to Silicosis," Radiol., 67:527, 1956.

Pneumoconiosis:

Pancoast, H. K., and Pendergrass, E. P., Pneumoconiosis, Paul Hoeber, 1926.

Pendergrass, E. P., and Robert, A. G., "Some Considerations of the Roentgen Diagnosis of Silicosis and Conditions that May Simulate It," Radiol., 50:725, 1948.

Cole, L. C., Lung Dust Lesions, Am. Med. Films Inc., White Plains, N.Y., 1948.

Shaver, C. G., "Further Observations of Lung Changes Associated with the Manufacture of Alumina Abrasives," Radiol., 50:760, 1948.

Cole, L. G., and Cole, W. G., Pneumoconiosis, J. B. Pierce Foundations, N.Y., 1940.

Denny, J. J., Robson, W. D., and Irwin, D. A., "The Prevention of Silicosis by Metallic Aluminum," Canadian M. A. J., 40:213, 1939.

Gardner, L. U., Dworski, M., and Delahant, A. B., "Aluminum Therapy in Silicosis," J. Indust. Hyg. and Toxicol., 26:211, 1944.

Siegal, W., Smith, A. R., Greenburg, L., "The Dust Hazard in Tremalite Talc Mining, Including Roentgenological Findings in Talc Workers," Am. J. Roentgenol., 49:11.

Groh, J. A., "Benign Pulmonary Changes in Arc-Welders: Arch-Welders' Siderosis," Ohio State Med. J., 40:732, 1944.

Sander, O. A., "Further Observations in Lung Changes in Electric Arc Welders," J. Indust. Hyg. and Toxicol., 26:79, 1944.

Pascucci, L. M., "Pulmonary Disease in Workers Exposed to Beryllium Compounds," Radiol., 50:23, 1948.

Bruce, R. A., et al., "Further Observations on the Pathological Physiology of Chronic Pulmonary Granulomatosis Associated with Beryllium Workers," Am. Rev. Tuberc., 62:29, 1950.

DeNardi, J. M., Van Ordstrand, H. S., and Curtis, G. H., "Beryllosis," Cleveland Clin. Quart., 19:171, 1952.

Dunner, L., and Bagnoll, J. R., "Graphite Pneumoconiosis Complicated by Cavitation due to Necrosis," Brit. J. Radiol., 19:165, 1946.

McCarthy, P. V., and Akenhead, W. R., "Pneumoconiosis due to Cotton Dust (Byssinosis)," Radiol., 46:46, Jan. 1946.

Feinberg, S. B., and Goldberg, M. E., "Hyaline Membrane Disease," Radiol., 68:185, 1957.

Atelectasis:

Bradford, J. R., "Massive Collapse of the Lung," Oxford Lose Leaf Med., 2:127, 1920.

Sante, L. R., "Massive (Atelectic) Collapse of the Lung," Ann. Surg., 88:161, 1928.

Sante, L. R., "Massive (Atelectic) Collapse of the Lung," Acta Radiol., 9:434, 1928.

Sante, L. R., "Massive (Atelectic) Collapse of the Lung, with Especial Reference to Treatment," J.A.M.A., 88:1539, 1927.

Lubert, M., and Krause, R., "Total Unilateral Pulmonary Collapse," Radiol., 67:175, 1956.

Chamberlain, J. M., and Gordon, J., "Bronchial Adenoma Treated by Pulmonary Resection," J. Thor. Surg., 14:144, 1945.

Van Allen, C. M., and Lindskog, G. E., "Collateral Respiration in Lung; Role in Bronchial Obstruction to Prevent Atelectasis and to Restore Patency," Surg. Gynec. and Obst., 53:16, 1931.

Loosli, C. G., "Intralveolar Communications in Normal and in Pathologic Mammalian Lungs," Arch. Path., 24:743, 1937.

Keating, D. R., Burkey, J. N., Hellerstein, H. K., and Feil, H., "Chronic Massive Thrombosis of Pulmonary Arteries," Am. J. Roentgenol., 69:208, 1953.

Woesner, M. E., Gardiner, G. A., and Stilson, W. L., "Pulmonary Embolism does not Necessarily Mean Pulmonary Infarction," Am. J. Roentgenol., 69:380, 1953.

Emphysema:

Herrnheiser, G., and Whitehead, J. P., "Pulmonary Interstitial Emphysema," Brit. J. Radiol., 26:519, 1953.

Manges, W. F., "The Roentgen-Ray Diagnosis on Non-Opaque Foreign Bodies in the Air Passages," Am. J. Roentgenol., 79:288, 1922.

Fischer, H. W., Potts, W. J., and Holinger, H., "Lobar Emphysema in Infants and Children," J. Pediat., 41:403, 1952.

Golden, R., "Abnormally Wide Respiratory Movement of Lower Lung Structures," Am. J. Roentgenol., 44:325, 1940.

Sante, L. R., "Cystic Disease of the Lung," Radiol., 33:152, 1939.

Peirce, C. B., and Dirkse, P. R., "Pulmonary Pneumatosele (Localized Alveolar or Lobular Ectasia)," Radiol., 28:651, 1937.

Kirklin, B. R., "Congenital Cysts of the Lung from the Roentgenologic Viewpoint," Am. J. Roentgenol., 36:19, 1936.

Warring, F. C., Jr., and Lindskog, G. E., "Surgical Management of Giant Air Cysts of the Lungs," Am. Rev. Tuberc., 63:579, 1951.

Campbell, J. A., and Silver, R. A., "Roentgen Differentiation of Pulmonary Tension Disorders in Infants and Children," Radiol., 61:161, 1953.

Coffey, J., "Natural Regression of Pulmonary Cysts During Early Infancy," J. Pediat., 11:48, 1953.

Farber, S., "Some Organic Digestive Disturbances in Early Life," J. Michigan Med. Soc., 44:587, 1945.

Craig, J. M., Kirkpatrick, J., and Neuhauser, E. B. D., "Congenital Cystic Adenomatoid Malformation of the Lung in Infants," Am. J. Roentgenol., 76:516, 1956.

Price, A. H., and Teplick, G., "Progressive Bilateral Bullous Emphysema," Arch. Int. Med., 77:132, 1946.

New Growths of the Lung:

Jackson, C., and Jackson, C. L., Disease of Nose, Throat, and Ear, W. B. Saunders, Philadelphia, 1946.

Rubin, E. H., Diseases of Chest, p. 460, W. B. Saunders Co., Philadelphia, 1947.

Farinas, P. L., "Recent Progress in the Bronchoscopic Examination of Bronchogenic Carcinoma," Am. J. Roentgenol., 44:370, 1940.

O'Keefe, M. E., Good, C. A., and McDonald, J. R., "Calcification in Solitary Nodules of the Lung," Am. J. Roentgenol., 77:1023, 1957.

Rigler, L. G., and Heitzman, E. R., "Panigraphy in the Differential Diagnosis of the Pulmonary Nodule," Radiol., 65:692, 1955.

Rigler, L., "A New Roentgen Sign of Malignancy in Solitary Pulmonary Nodule," J.A.M.A., 157:907, 1955.

Celis, A., Kuthy, J., and del Castillo, E., "The Importance of the Thoracic Duct in the Spread of Malignant Disease," Acta Radiol., 45:169, 1956.

Rigler, L. G., "Planigraphy in the Diagnosis of Bronchiogenic Carcinoma," Am. J. Roentgenol., 58:267, 1947.

Rigler, L. G., and Kelby, G. M., "Emphysema: An Early Roentgen Sign of Bronchiogenic Carcinoma," Radiol., 49:578, 1947.

Davis, M. W., and Simon, T. P., "Alveolar Cell Tumor of the Lung," Am. Rev. Tuberc., 62:594, 1950.

Rozsa, P. E., and Cavanaugh, C. J., "Diagnosis of Pulmonary Metastases," Radiol., 60:198, 1953.

Kerley, P., "Nature of Round Intrapulmonary Tumors," Acta Radiol., Supp. 116, p. 256, 1954.

Zimmerman, L, E., "Demonstration of Histoplasma and Coccidioides in So-Called Tuberculomas of the Lung," Arch. Int. Med., 94:690, 1954.

Davis, E. W., Hampton, A. O., Bickham, C. E., and Winship, T., "Lipoid Pneumonia Simulating Tumor," J. Thoracic Surg., 28:212, 1954.

Goldman, A., "Cavernous Hemangioma of the Lung," Dis. Chest, 9:479, 1943.

Sante, L. R., "Cystic Disease of the Lung," Radiol., 33:152, 1939.

Sante, L. R., "Fate of Oil Particles in the Lung," Am. J. Roentgenol., 62:788, 1949.

Weismann, R. E., Clagett, O. T., and Macdonald, J. R., "Amyloid Disease of the Lung Treated by Pneumonectomy," J. Thoracic Surg., 16:269, 1947.

Good, A., Hood, R. T., and Macdonald, J. R., "Significance of a Solitary Mass in the Lung," Am. J. Roentgenol., 70:543, 1953.

Bluth, I., "A Note on the Roentgen Features of Bronchial Adenoma of the Peripheral Type," Radiol., 68:193, 1957.

Hood, R. T., Jr., Good, C. A., Clagett, O. T., and McDonald, "Solitary Circumscribed Lesions of the Lung," J.A.M.A., 152:1185, 1953.

Thornton, T. F., Jr., Adams, W. E., and Bloch, R. G., "Solitary Circumscribed Tumors of the Lung," Surg. Gyn. and Obst., 78:364.

Sloan, R. D., and Cooley, R. N., "Congenital Pulmonary Arteriovenus Aneurysm," Am. J. Roentgenol., 70:183, 1953.

Stein, J., Jacobson, H. G., Poppel, M. H., and Lawrence, L. R., "Pulmonary Hamartoma," Am. J. Roentgenol., 70:971, 1953.

Injuries to the Lung:

Mann, L. S., Olson, K. C., Walls, W. S., "Lung Hernia," Surg., 25:127, 1949.

Barden, S. P., "Important Sequelae and Complications of Hemothorax Resulting from Penetrating Wounds of the Pleural Cavity," Am. J. Roentgenol., 59:525, 1948.

Carroll, D., McClemeny, J., Himmelstein, A., and Cournaud, A., "Pulmonary Function Following Decortication of the Lung," Am. Rev. Tuberc., 63:231, 1951.

Abo, S., "Roentgenographic Detection of Minimal Pneumothorax in the Lateral Decubitus Position," Am. J. Roentgenol., 77:1066, 1957.

Sante, L. R., "Roentgenological Manifestations of Injuries to the Chest," Minnesota Med., 24:819, Oct. 1941.

Phillips, E., "Pneumonia Following Nonpenetrating Pulmonary Injuries," J.A.M.A., 133:161, Jan. 18, 1947.

Hodes, P. J., Atkins, J. P., and Johnson, J., "Traumatic Bronchial Rupture with Occlusion," Am. J. Roentgenol., 60:448, 1948.

Savage, O., "Pulmonary Concussion ("Blast") in Non-Thoracic Battle Wounds," Lancet, 1:424, 1945.

Parks, R. E., "Traumatic Torsion of the Lung," Radiol., 67:582, 1956.

Stratemeier, E. H., and Barry, J. W., "Torision of the Lung Following Thoracic Trauma," Radiol., 62:726, 1954.

Pleura:

Sante, L. R., "Roentgen-ray Diagnosis of Pleural Effusions, General and Local," J.A.M.A., 88:215, 1927.

Campbell, W., "A Case of Secondary Amoebiasis of the Lung," Brit. J. Radiol., 19:120, 1946.

Rothstein, E., and Landis, F. B., "Infrapulmonary Pleura Effusion," Brit. J. Radiol., 23:490, 1950.

Levitin, J., "Interlobar Empyema," Am. J. Roentgenol., 56:156, 1946.

Levine, M. H., and Hurst, A., "Tomographic Exploration of Juxta Pulmonary Pathology in Extrapleural Plombage," Brit. J. Radiol., 23:493, 1950.

Sante, L. R., "Pneumothorax," Radiol., 11:126, 1928.

Hochberg, L. A., "Endothelioma (Mesothelioma) of the Pleura," Am. Rev. Tuberc., 63:150, 1951.

Blount, H. C., Jr., "Localized Mesothelioma of the Pleura," Radiol., 67:822, 1956.

Finby, N., and Steinberg, I., Roentgen Aspects of Pleural Mesothelioma," Radiol., 65:169, 1955.

Stein, J. J., "Primary Cancer of the Lung with Special Reference to Apical Lung Tumors," Am. J. Roentgenol., 60:58, 1948.

Diaphragm:

Sante, L. R., "Basal Exudates of Subphrenic Origin," Am. J. Roentgenol., 44:350, 1940.

Rossetti, M., "Partial Relaxation of Right Hemidiaphragm," Radiol. Clin., 23:212, 1954.

Hollander, A. G., and Dugan, D. J., "Hernia of Liver," J. Thoracic Surg., 29:357, 1955.

Beye, H., "The Thoracic Complications of Subdiaphragmatic Infections," J. Thoracic Surg., 1:655, 1932.

Oritt, J. E., and Hyde, L., "Transdiaphragmatic Eventration of Peritoneum Secondary to Pneumoperitoneum," Am. Rev. Tuberc., 69:1045, 1954.

Porter, W. B., "Diaphragmatic Flutter with Symptoms of Angina Pectoris," J.A.M.A., 106:992, 1936.

Mediastinum:

Herrnheiser, G., and Whitehead, J. P., "Pulmonary Interstitial Emphysema," Brit. J. Radiol., 26:519, 1953.

Solomon, H. A., and Brackman, A. L., "Pyogenic Osteomyelitis of the Thoracic Spine Presenting as Primary Pulmonary Disease," Am. J. Roentgenol., 49:219, 1943.

Hawes, L. E., "The Roentgenological Changes in the Esophagus in Tuberculous Mediastinitis," Am. J. Roentgenol., 51:575, 1944.

Kunkel, W. M., Jr., Clagget, O. T., and MacDonald, J. R., "Mediastinal Granuloma," J. Thoracic Surg., 27:565, 1954.

Garland, L. H., "Pulmonary Sarcoidosis: The Early Roentgen Findings," Radiol., 48:333, 1947.

Kerley, P., "The Etiology of Erythema Nodosum," Brit. J. Radiol., 16:199, 1943.

Svanberg, Tore, "Roentgenological Pulmonary Changes in Periarteritis Nodosa," Acta Radiol., 26:307, 1945.

Reimann, H. A., Koucky, R. F., and Eklung, C. M., "Primary Amyloidosis Limited to Tissue of Mesodermal Origin," Am. J. Path., 11:977, 1935.

Dirkse, P. R., "Primary Amyloidosis of the Lung," Am. J. Roentgenol., 56:577, 1946.

Wang, C. C., and Robbins, L. L., "Amyloid Disease," Radiol., 66:489, 1956.

Endress, Z. F., "Traumatic Mediastinal Hematoma," Am. J. Roentgenol., 70:576, 1953.

Roswit, B. R., Kaplan, G., and Jocobson, H. G., "The Superior Vena Cava Obstruction Syndrome in Bronchiogenic Carcinoma," Radiol., 61:722, 1953.

Byron, F. X., Alling, E. E., and Samson, P. C., "Intrathoracic Meningocele," J. Thoracic Surg., 18:294, 1949.

Sengpiel, G. W., Rucizka, F., and Lodmell, E. A., "Lateral Intrathoracic Meningocele," Radiol., 50:505, 1948.

Blades, B., "Mediastinal Tumors," Ann. Surg., 123:749, May 1946.

Laipply, T. C., "Cysts and Cystic Tumors of the Mediastinum," Arch. Path., 39:153, 1945.

Baker. J. M., and Curtis, G. M., "Intrathoracic Meningocele," West. J. Surg., 61:209, 1953.

Davis, J. G., and Simonton, J. H., "Mediastinal Carinal Bronchogenic Cysts," Radiol., 67:391, 1956.

Scheff, S., Bednarz, W. W., and Levene, G., "Roentgenologic Aspects of Retropleural Hematomas Following Sympathectomy," Radiol., 68:224, 1957.

Heuer, G. J., Andrus, De W., "The Surgery of Mediastinal Tumors," Am. J. Surg., 50:146, 1940.

Pancoast, H., and Pendergrass, E., "Roentgenologic Aspect of Pneumonoconiosis and Its Differential Diagnosis," J.A.M.A., 101:587, 1933.

Sweet, R. H., "Intrathoracic Goiter Located in the Posterior Mediastinum," Surg., Gynec. and Obst., 89:57, 1949.

Macklin, C. C., "Transport of Air Along Sheaths of Pulmonic Blood Vessels from Alveoli to Mediastinum," Arch. Int. Med., 64:913, 1939.

NORMAL HEART AND GREAT VESSELS

I. Roentgen Anatomy
   A. TOPOGRAPHY of HEART and AORTA
   B. Methods of Examination
      1. Fluoroscopy
      2. Roentgenography
         a. Anterior Position
         b. Right Anterior Oblique
         c. Left Anterior Oblique
         d. Lateral
      3. Teleroentgenography
      4. Orthodiography
      5. Plastic Reconstruction
      6. Kymography
      7. Scanography

PATHOLOGY of HEART and ASSOCIATED STRUCTURES - ACQUIRED

I. HEART
   A. Position
      1. Retraction from Pleuropulmonary Adhesions
      2. Displacement from Intrathoracic Pressure Changes
      3. Pressure of Adjacent Structures
      4. Congenital Anomalies
   B. Size and Shape
      1. Conditions Influencing Size
      2. Cardiac Measurements
         a. UNGERLEIDER and CLARK'S METHOD
         b. CLAYTOR and MERRIL'S TABLES
         c. HODGES and EYSTER'S PREDICTION TABLES
   C. Form and Outline
      1. Enlargement of Various Chambers
         a. Left Ventricle
         b. Left Auricle
         c. Right Ventricle
         d. Right Auricle
      2. Valvular Disease
         a. Mitral
         b. Aortic
         c. Tricuspid
         d. Pulmonary

      3. Cardiac Aneurysm (infarct)
      4. Other Conditions Showing Change in Cardiac Outline
   D. Contractibility
      1. Contraction of Various Chambers
      2. Amplitude or Force of Contractions
      3. Rate
      4. Rhythm — Sequence
      5. Reversal Point of Pulsation on Left Border (where character of pulsations change)
   E. Mobility — influenced by mediastinal fibrosis, as seen on fluoroscopic examination with,
      1. Patient in Right and Left Lateral Decubitus Positions
         a. In Children
         b. In Adults
      2. Patient in Anterior Position on Deep Inspiration and Expiration
         a. Fixed Mediastinum
         b. Pendulum Movement of Heart and Mediastinum with Relative Changes in Intrapulmonary
            Pressure on the Two Sides During Respiration
   F. Abnormal Calcification
      1. Valves
      2. Arteries
      3. Pericardium
   G. Relationship of Heart to Surrounding Structures
      1. Bony structures (spinal deformity)
      2. Pathology of Adjacent Soft Tissue Structures
         a. Mediastinal Tumors—cysts
         b. Esophageal Pathology—cardiospasm
         c. Diaphragmatic Hernia
         d. Thoracic Stomach

293

II. Aorta and Great Vessels
   A. Aortitis
      1. Arteriosclerotic
      2. Syphilitic
   B. Elongation and Tortuosity

   C. Aneurysm
      1. Ascending Arch
      2. Transverse Arch
      3. Descending Arch
      4. Dissecting
   D. Arterio-Venous Fistula

III. Pericardium, Pericardial Outline
   A. Acute Pericarditis
   B. Pericardial Effusion
      1. Differentiation from Cardiac Dilatation
   C. Chronic Constrictive Pericarditis
   D. Pleuropericardial Adhesions

IV. Congenital Anomalies of Heart and Associated Structures
   ANGIOCARDIOGRAPHY
   CATHETERIZATION OF THE HEART
   A. Anomalies of Structural Development of the Great Vessels
      1. Persistent Patent Ductus Arteriosus
      2. Coarctation of the Aorta
      3. Right Aortic Arch
         a. With Left Descending Aorta
         b. With Right Descending Aorta
      4. Vascular Rings
         a. Double Aortic Arch
         b. Right Aortic Arch and Left Ligamentum Arteriosus
         c. Other Anomalies of the Aortic Arch
      5. Anomalous Right Subclavian Artery
      6. Aortic Septal Defect
      7. Anomalies of the Pulmonary Veins
      8. Idiopathic Dilatation of Pulmonary Artery
      9. Arterio-Venous Fistula of the Lung
    10. Abnormal Pulmonary Artery Associated with Intralobar Broncho-Pulmonary Sequestration
   B. Anomalies of Cardiac Position
         a. Dextra Cardia
         b. Situs Inversus
   C. Anomalies of Structural Development of the Heart
      1. Tetralogy of Fallot
      2. Tricuspid Atresia
      3. Complete Transposition of the Great Vessels—Associated with Pulmonary Stenosis
      4. Pulmonary Stenosis with Intact Ventricular Septum but with Auricular Septal Defect or
         Patent Foramen Ovale
      5. Ebstein's Anomaly
      6. Truncus Arteriosus and Pseudotruncus
      7. Eisenmenger's Complex
      8. Auricular Septal Defect
         a. Isolated Defect
         b. Lutembacher's Syndrome
      9. Ventricular Septal Defect —Maladie de Roger
    10. Pure Pulmonic Stenosis
    11. Other Types of Congenital Heart Disease
         a. Aortic and Subaortic Stenosis
         b. Congenital Idiopathic Hypertrophy
         c. Origin of coronary Arteries from Pulmonary Artery
         d. Idiopathic Dilatation of Pulmonary Artery
         e. Cor Triloculare bi-ventricularis
         f. Cor Triloculare bi-atriatum
         g. Cor Bi-loculare
         h. Aortic Atresia
         i. Congenital Mitral Stenosis or Atresia

D. Diagnostic Approach - Roentgen Survey
E. Heart Muscle Defects
    a. Idiopathic Hypertrophic Enlargement (Glycogen Heart)
F. Pericardial Defects—Celomic Cysts

Chapter XVII

CIRCULATORY SYSTEM

NORMAL HEART AND GREAT VESSELS

A. Topography

Being dense structures, the heart and great vessels are thrown into bold relief by the surrounding air-filled lungs.

The heart and aorta lie in the midline and occupy the mid-portion of the mediastinal space. Roughly pyramidal in shape, the heart lies in the chest with the apex below and slightly to the left and the base upward in the region of the attachment of the large vessels (Fig. 210A). The right auricle and auricular appendage make up almost the entire right side of the heart; whereas, the right ventricle forms the anterior portion of the heart from its broad base in contact with the diaphragm below to its upper termination in the conus arteriosus and pulmonary artery. The left auricle on the other hand makes up in greater part the upper posterior portion of the heart and the left ventricle extends along the left side and posteriorly extending upward and terminating in the aorta.

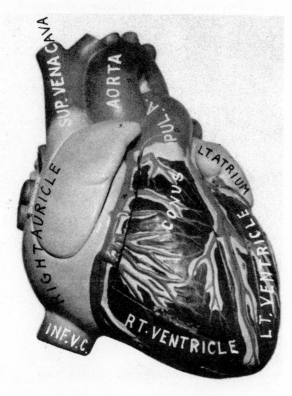

Fig. 210A. Anterior View.

The blood, flowing into the right auricle from the superior and inferior vena cava, is ejected by contraction of this chamber through the tricuspid valve into the right ventricle. Passing into the right ventricle the blood is projected in a stream between the posterior wall and interventricular septum to the apex, known as the "inflow tract"; in passing out of the ventricle, the blood stream is projected between the anterior wall and adjacent portion of the interventricular septum or "outflow tract." Similarly in passing through the left ventricle the blood is projected through the mitral valve, between the posterior wall and the interventricular septum, to the apex constituting the "inflow tract" and outward between the anterior wall and interventricular septum from the apex to the aortic valve, representing the "outflow tract."

Thus in passing through the various chambers of the heart, the blood undergoes a swirling motion. These inflow and outflow tracts are of importance since ventricular enlargement begins with accentuation of the structures going to make up these tracts.

Since roentgenography is concerned chiefly with the silhouetted outline of the cardiac shadow, let us consider the various chambers of the heart which go to make up its outline (Fig. 210B). Only where these cardiac chambers present themselves in profile can their outlines be recognized, therefore, roentgenographic examination is essential in several positions. The optimum positions for examination are: 1) the anterior view, 2) the right anterior oblique and 3) the left anterior oblique views, (see Manual of Roentgenological Technique).

In the ANTERIOR VIEW; the right auricle (RA) produces the large sweeping curve on the right side of the cardiac shadow. Below, just before the right auricular curve meets the diaphragmatic shadow, the right ventricle (RV) contributes very slightly to the outline. Above, the aorta (A) extends upward forming a prominent curve; the superior vena cava (SVC) may produce a linear shadow above and lateral to this. A.A. represents the aortic arch, and A.K. the aortic knob.

The right ventricle (RV) presents itself anteriorly. It extends downward to form the inferior border of the heart but in this location the cardiac shadow fuses with that of the abdominal structures; in no position does it form or contribute to the cardiac silhouette except perhaps at the extreme lower portion of the right border.

On the left side, the left ventricle (LV) forms the predominating lower curve. Immediately above this is a smaller curve or depression produced by the

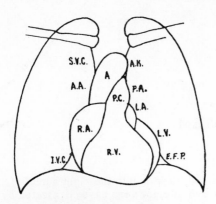

Fig. 210B. Anterior View.

left auricular appendage (LA), often indistinguishable in normal individuals. On fluoroscopic examination however, the extent of the left ventricular curve can be readily detected by observation of the point of reversal in the pulsation of the left border. During systole the left ventricle pulls upward, forward and inward while the auricle and pulmonary portions expand outward and upward. The point of reversal pulsation serves to identify the left ventricular portion. Another small curve above the auricular curve is produced by the pulmonary artery (PA) as it arches upward from the left ventricle. The inferior vena cava (IVC) may show as an oblique line at the lower right margin of the cardiac silhouette as it extends into the right auricle and the superior vena cava (SVC) runs along parallel to the aortic shadow above on the right side. The triangular shadow (EFP) in

the left cardiophrenic region is due to an epicardial fat pad.

The arch and descending portions of the aorta form a prominent knob at the highest point in the cardiac outline. The aorta ascends on the right, arches over and descends on the left side.

The pericardium is attached below and on either side to the upper portion of the diaphragm; from this position it extends upward, enclosing the heart, and is attached to the great vessels. It is a thin, elastic membrane which does not interfere in any way with the cardiac movements. The small curved shadow at the cardio-phrenic sinus (where the heart margin meets the diaphragm) is due to a triangular epicardial fat pad.

The RIGHT ANTERIOR OBLIQUE VIEW (Figs. 210C and D), (with patient turned about 45°; right breast to the film), presents another aspect of the heart in its relationship to the adjacent structures. The optimum position for examination must be secured in each individual instance by fluoroscopic examination. In this view, the anterior cardiac outline presents a large sweeping curve which may be due entirely to the right ventricle (RV) or may show the margin of the left ventricle in its lowest portion depending upon the degree of rotation of the patient and the configuration of the heart. The pulmonary conus (PC) above produces a sharper curve in the cardiac outline. The posterior border shows the right auricle (RA) below and the left auricle (LA) above. The pulmonary artery (PA) is viewed, "on end," as an oval shadow at the root of the aortic arch.

The upper end of the cardiac shadow merges into the aorta as it ascends, arches posteriorly and descends, overlapping the spinal column. The margin of the inferior vena cava (IVC) forms a triangular shadow at the posterior inferior margin as it enters

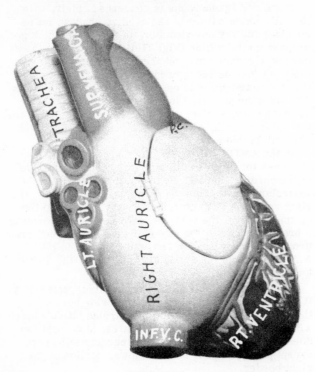

Fig. 210C

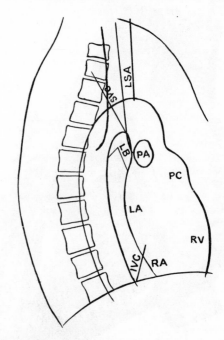

Fig. 210D. Right Anterior Oblique View.

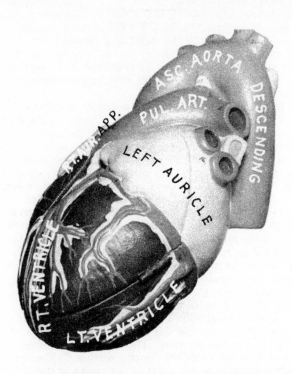

Fig. 210E. Left Anterior Oblique View.

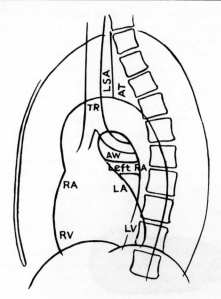

Fig. 210F. Left Anterior Oblique View.

the heart and the shadow of the superior vena cava may be recognized above as it crosses the mid-portion of the aortic arch. The trachea and its bifurcation is evident near the aortic arch and the left main stem bronchus (LB) can usually be seen within the arch of the aorta. The esophagus passes downward posterior to the aorta coming into close relationship with the left auricle in its descent.

The LEFT ANTERIOR OBLIQUE VIEW (Fig. 210E and F) (with the patient turned 45°; left breast to the film), presents the left ventricular curve (LV) posterior and the right ventricle anteriorly (RV). In this view the auricular curves are above the ventricular curves in each instance.

The aortic arch sweeps around in a full arch and the descending aorta is plainly seen throughout its entire descent. The tracheal (TR) bifurcation is clearly seen; the clear space enclosed by the sweep of the aortic arch is known as the aortic clear space or window (AW); it is traversed by the left main branch of the pulmonary artery (LPA). Above the arch is a triangular space, formed below by the upper border of the aortic arch, posteriorly by the upper thoracic spine and anteriorly by the left subclavian artery (LSA), representing the aortic triangle (AT).

The esophagus, as it passes through the mediastinum, comes into close relationship with the various vascular structures, and may serve as a guide in the detection of any displacement or enlargement of these structures (Fig. 224).

In the RIGHT ANTERIOR OBLIQUE VIEW as the esophagus passes downward through the mediastinal space the adjacent organs leave their impression on its anterior aspect. Above, the impression made by the aortic arch is most prominent; just below the arch, is the "bronchial impression" a shallower less pronounced depression usually caused by the left main stem bronchus (or occasionally by the right bronchus or the trachea) depending upon any slight deviation of these structures. Lower down where it passes behind the heart it is in close contact with the left auricle serving to demonstrate by its displacement the degree of enlargement of this chamber (this is the only means by which left auricular enlargement can be demonstrated). At the lower end, just before it pierces the diaphragm, the esophagus crossed over in front of the descending aorta which leaves a slight impression on its contour. Under certain pathological conditions, an enlargement of the pulmonary artery may produce an impression on the esophagus.

In the left anterior oblique and postero-anterior positions, the esophagus is not deviated from its straight course in the normal individual.

Deformity of the spine and thorax from kyphoscoliosis may result in rotation or other faulty position of the heart and great vessels which may give an impression of cardiac enlargement and may influence its function.

B. Methods of Examination

Fluoroscopy is a particularly valuable method for examination of the heart because it permits observation of the cardiac movements during its entire cycle. Observe the valvular area for possible calcareous deposits—calcified valves can best be detected fluoroscopically by their dancing movement with the cardiac beat. Not only the vigor of contraction, but rhythm and sequence of the beat can be closely observed. The relationship of the apex beat to the cardiac shadow can usually be clearly made out by palpation during fluoroscopy. The relative size of the cardiac shadow can be estimated, and careful observation by this method can often differentiate cardiac enlargement from pericardial effusion. Proceed with the fluoroscopic examination of the various contours of the cardiac shadow with the patient first in the anterior, then in the right anterior oblique, and finally in the left anterior oblique positions.

In the anterior position, the left border of the heart forms a prominent outward curve over the lower one-third to one-half of the cardiac border; this is produced by the lateral wall of the left ventricle and represents the outflow tract of that chamber. Above this, two less prominent curves are produced by the pulmonary artery and aortic knob with occasionally an intervening bulge between the pulmonary and left ventricular curves produced by the left auricle or auricular appendage. The movement of the left ventricle with each contraction is inward, whereas, that of the structures above is outward and upward, so that a point of "adjacent opposite pulsation" is created which is readily detectable with each heart beat, marking the location of the left auriculo-ventricular septum. In this manner it is possible to determine enlargement of the outflow tract of the left ventricle, dilatation of the outflow tract of the pulmonary artery or conus, and prominence of the aorta as it arches across. Normally the right border of the heart presents the rounded prominent contour of the right auricle; below, an angular shadow is cast by the inferior vena cava, and above, the ascending aorta extending upward to the arch; a shadow paralleling the aorta sometimes seen extending upward into the thorax is produced by the superior vena cava and innominate vein. The right ventricle forming the base of the cardiac shadow cannot be visualized.

A barium swallow should show the esophagus descending to the right in close contact with the aortic arch as it proceeds downward. The intimate contact of the esophagus with the aorta permits an accurate measurement of the width of the aorta in teleroentgenographic examination.

In the right anterior oblique position the anterior border is formed by the right ventricle and pulmonary artery (representing the outflow tract of this chamber). There should be considerable space intervening between this border of the heart and the anterior chest wall; obliteration of this space is indication of dilatation of the outflow tract of the right ventricle. The contour above the conus is due to the ascending branch of the aorta as it proceeds upward to form the arch. The posterior margin of the cardiac outline is produced by the confluent margins of the right auricle below and left auricle above, with a small angular shadow produced by the inferior vena cava below the lower margin of the right auricle. Unless one or the other is enlarged, the auricular contours cannot be distinguished from each other. The esophagus extends downward between the anterior surface of the aorta and the posterior surface of the heart so that it can be used as an indicator of any change in the cardiac outline of the portions with which it comes in contact. Normally, when filled with barium, the esophagus shows two impressions on its anterior aspect, the aortic arch above, and the right bronchus just below. As the esophagus reaches its lower end, it passes anterior to the aorta to traverse the diaphragm. Normally the esophagus should pass downward in a gentle curve; any enlargement of the left auricle is manifested by pressure of its contour on the anterior margin of the esophagus at the auricular level.

In the left anterior oblique position, the lower portion of the cardiac outline is produced by the right ventricle which extends upward along the anterior margin to form the lower curve. On the anterior aspect the right auricular appendage and ascending aorta extend above this to complete the anterior margin. Posteriorly the lower curve is produced by the left ventricle; its junction with the right ventricle is marked by an indentation, the interventricular groove, which is seen best by fluoroscopic examination with deep inspiration. This groove may be very difficult to detect by roentgenographic examination and may fall below the diaphragmatic shadow; the left auricle forms the remainder of the posterior curve; a shallow indentation, the auriculoventricular groove, marks their point of union.

In this view the arch of the aorta is opened, disclosing all portions of the structure as it arches over to its descending portion. This clear space beneath the arch is known as the "aortic window." The trachea bifurcates at the level of the arch and the left bronchus angulates downward through the aortic window; the right bronchus seems foreshortened. The left pulmonary artery traverses the aortic window in an almost horizontal position. The brachiocephalic vessels ascend anterior to the trachea above the ascending portion of the aorta.

Roentgenographic examination of the chest made in the anterior position will give a rough estimate as to the position and size of the heart and will direct attention to any obvious pathology. Supplemented by the right and left anterior oblique views it serves to give a good indication of the outline of the various chambers of the heart. For a more accurate estimation of the cardiac size and outline however, other methods must also be utilized.

TELEROENTGENOGRAPHIC EXAMINATION

For a more accurate estimation of the size of the cardiac shadow teleroentgenographic examination may be resorted to. This consists in examination of the chest at six-foot target-to-film distance, to produce more nearly parallel rays and to insure therefore less distortion in size and shape. It is advisable to give one full second exposure so as to secure the maximum size of the cardiac outline during diastole. Under these conditions the resulting cardiac silhouette is within less than one centimeter of the size which would result if the rays were parallel. By means of a barium swallow the relationship of the esophagus to the heart and other structures can be noted.

ORTHODIOGRAPHY. Orthodiographic examination accomplishes a similar purpose. Under fluoroscopic examination, with the diaphragm shut down to about a one-inch square so as to project the central ray tangentially across every point on the cardiac outline, an outline drawing of the true size of the cardiac shadow is made with a wax pencil on the glass of the fluoroscopic screen or on a superimposed sheet of celluloid. To carry out this procedure, provision must be made for fixation of the screen, and independent movement of the tube. By this method the central x-ray beam is used to map the heart size eliminating the magnification produced by a diverging x-ray beam. It gives most accurate results if done carefully. It is time consuming, however, and holds no advantages over teleroentgenographic examination and has been largely displaced by the radiographic method.

PLASTIC RECONSTRUCTION. Methods have been devised whereby outlines of the cardiac shadow made in numerous positions of rotation have been utilized for the construction of plastic models of the heart.

KYMOGRAPHIC EXAMINATION. For accurately recording the depth of the contraction of various portions of the different chambers, and for their correlation in the cardiac cycle, the kymograph may be used. This consists of a sheet of lead in which multiple parallel slits about 1 mm. wide have been cut about 1 cm. apart. This is interposed between the chest wall and the cassette, remaining stationary in place during the exposure. The cassette itself is moved for a distance equivalent to the interval between slits on the lead shield. As the cassette descends a graphic outline of the pulsations of each portion of the cardiac outline intersected by the slits in the lead shield will be recorded on the roentgenogram for the period of time necessary for the cassette to traverse the distance between two slits. By careful measurement of the time and depth of contraction of the various chambers, the rhythm of the cardiac cycle and force can be investigated. The peaks of the curve represent diastole; the valleys systole. By this method noncontractile scars from infarcts in the cardiac muscle can be demonstrated, and the expansile pulsation of aneurysm may be differentiated from the transmitted pulsation seen in mediastinal tumor.

The kymograph has found its greatest usefulness in the following conditions.

1. Constrictive pericarditis; here the restricted movement is clearly shown.
2. Ventricular hernia (cardiac aneurysm) may be well shown, due to the paradoxical action of the herniated portion of the ventricle with each heart beat, due to its thin, flaccid wall.
3. Advanced mitral disease; the periods of contracture in the cardiac cycle establish the identity of the chamber. Only in advanced mitral disease does the conus show.
4. Cardiac infarcts; only after a prolonged period however. It may take weeks before they show as noncontractile plateaus on the ventricular surface.

5. Pericardial effusion; there is restricted movement or it may be entirely absent.

The faults of kymography as a precise instrument for diagnosis are as follows:

1. It does not record the full contraction of the heart chambers due to the divergence of the beam.
2. It does not demonstrate the movement of the same point throughout the cycle.
3. The rotation of the heart during contraction also presents different effects on the wave produced.
4. The cephalo-caudal movement as the heart contracts is another source of errors.
5. The effect of respiration on the heart is a source of error; inspiration causes diminution of waves at base of the heart.
6. The photographic record is a summation of the densities presented at various times during the exposure in which superimposed shadows of various contracting chambers may modify or nullify each other.

As a result we are forced to the conclusion that this method of examination is of limited usefulness. Measurement of the exact size of the cardiac shadow in one direction may be accomplished by the scanograph.

SCANOGRAPH. This apparatus devised by Millwee is of value in measuring the true size of objects by means of the roentgen rays. It consists of a narrow slit-like ray field 2 mm. wide projected by movement of the x-ray tube over the part to be examined from one end to the other. Employing only the central ray it measures accurately the dimension of all structures in one direction, along the line of movement; in the direction perpendicular to the line of movement the image is still subject to the same distortion caused by the divergence of the x-ray beam. (See Manual of Roentgenological Technique).

PATHOLOGY OF THE HEART AND ASSOCIATED STRUCTURES

1. HEART. Pathology of the heart and associated structures may well be considered under the following headings:

A. Position
B. Size and Shape
C. Form and Outline
D. Contractibility
E. Mobility
F. Abnormal Calcification
G. Relation to Adjacent Structures

A. Position of Heart—Normal in midline in middle mediastinum.
   Displacement to either side, rotation or elevation, caused by:
1. Retraction from Pleuropulmonary Adhesions from:
   a. Tuberculosis—lungs and pleura
   b. Pyogenic infections of lungs and pleura

2. Intrathoracic Pressure Changes
   a. Pleural effusions (large) causing mediastinal pressure on both inspiration and expiration.
   b. Massive tumors of lung or pleura causing pressure on both inspiration and expiration
   c. Obstructive emphysema— due to partial bronchial occlusion; by foreign bodies, tumors or bronchial secretions—causing pressure during expiration
   d. Bullous emphysema causing pressure during expiration—vanishing lung, solitary cyst (air or fluid) of lung
   e. Atelectasis; massive or lobar, causing retraction
3. Deformity from Pressure of Adjacent Structures
   a. Bony structures (deformity of spine)
   b. Pathology of adjacent soft structures—mediastinal tumor, esophageal pathology, cardiospasm (massive), diverticulum (large), tumor (large)
4. Congenital Anomalies
   a. Dextrocardia
   b. Situs Inversus
   c. Other developmental Anomalies

B. Size and Shape of Heart

Roughly, the size and shape of the normal heart compare very closely with the right fist—it is surprising how closely this relationship is maintained. In the ordinary anterior chest roentgenogram a rough estimate of the size of the heart may be made by comparison of the transverse diameter of the thorax at its widest point. This ratio is called the cardiothoracic index and it should not exceed 1:2.

Cardiac hypoplasia, is frequently encountered in individuals who from some intercurrent disease disease such as pulmonary tuberculosis have had to spend long periods of time at rest in bed; this can readily be understood. Occasionally however, for some reason which is not clear, the heart may become progressively smaller in an otherwise healthy individual even without bed rest.

In tuberculosis of the adrenal gland, Addison's disease, the heart may be reduced materially in size, returning to normal within a short time after administration of sodium chloride.

Reduction in size of the heart does not seem to be the determining factor in cardiac pathology; enlargement of the heart beyond normal limits is the most striking evidence of disease. Under certain circumstances the heart may show physiological enlargement.

ARTERIO-VENOUS FISTULA. A fistula of this character may be due to anomalous development or may be due to trauma. A fistulous opening between the arterial and venous system shunts a portion of the arterial blood back through the veins without performing its function in supplying some distal part or organ. Owing to the loss of peripheral resistance the arterial pressure drops and less arterial blood gets to the part. The larger the opening and the nearer the fistula is to the heart the greater the effect. Since the blood reaching the part is reduced, the heart beats faster and becomes larger in order to deliver sufficient blood to the part for normal function.

On operative closure of the fistula, normal circulation is soon established, the burden is taken off of the heart and it reduces to normal size. This change in size of the cardiac shadow is readily observed roentgenographically.

GENERALIZED CARDIAC ENLARGEMENT. The healthy heart does not undergo much enlargement under any condition. It has been demonstrated (Roesler) that even under vigorous exercise the heart does not undergo much enlargement; it beats faster and stronger and thus causes acceleration of the circulation but any change in size is extremely slight. Likewise, hypertrophy of the heart from prolonged exertion as seen in athletes does not result in much actual cardiac enlargement; the heart muscle may become thicker but any actual increase in the size of the heart is very slight. The detection of enlargement of the heart therefore is a very important indication of pathology.

Under certain conditions the heart may show generalized enlargement. Severe, prolonged anemia, myxedema, and residence at high altitude have been known to cause cardiac enlargement. In myxedema, the pulsations are weak, with radiologic findings similar to pericardiac effusions.

Myocarditis, either inflammatory or toxic, can cause generalized cardiac enlargement. Large, globular hearts have been noted in vitamin B deficiency, beriberi. Severe, prolonged thyrotoxicosis causes some, but not great heart enlargement, unless failure or auricular fibrillation develops. The heart, as are other internal organs, is increased in size by acromegaly.

The heart appears large in pregnancy and with obesity. In both of these conditions, elevation of the diaphragm and a more transverse position of the heart makes the heart appear larger than actual size. With obesity, deposition of epicardial fat increases size of the cardiac contour.

CARDIAC MEASUREMENTS. Authorities are agreed that cardiac enlargement is the most consistent indication of cardiac disease. For ascertaining an estimate of the normal cardiac outline, Bardeen made numerous examinations of healthy adult men and women. He devised a method for measurement of the transverse diameter of the cardiac shadow, and for estimating the area. These were correlated with height, weight, and age of the individual (Fig. 211A). The distance from a line running down the midline to the extreme extent of the right border of the heart (MR), plus the measurement from the same vertical line to the extreme left border (ML) determines the maximum transverse (TD) diameter. The area of the cardiac shadow can be secured by outlining with a planimeter or by superimposing a sheet of celluloid on which centimeter squares have been ruled. The information necessary for proper carry-

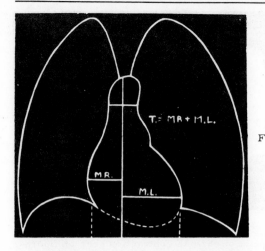

Fig. 211A

ing out of the examination includes: sex, age, height and weight. (See U.S. Army X-ray Manual, 1st Edition). The measurements secured from the teleroentgenogram are compared with the normal found in Bardeen's. To be normal the values should fall between those estimates for a person of this age and sex, for same height and for the same weight. Ten percent variation above or below these values must be considered abnormal.

Using teleroentgenographic measurements with the tube at six foot distance, Ungerleider and Clark have tabulated reference prediction tables for transverse diameter of the heart (see tables) for use in life insurance-examinations (Assn. of Life Ins. Med. Directors of America). These values are slightly higher than those made by orthodiographic method; they are probably the most widely used today.

Another method of measurement gives a more accurate idea of the true length and breadth of the heart (Fig. 211B). A line is drawn from the junction of the great vessels and right auricle obliquely downward to the apex; this is the oblique diameter and indicates the length of the heart (LD). Lines perpendicular to this diameter are drawn on the left to the junction of the left auricular and left ventricular curves (BL); on the right to the junction of the right auricular curve, with the diaphragm (BR). The sum of these two diameters represents the breadth of the heart (BD).

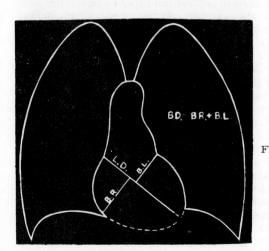

Fig. 211B

This is a more accurate measurement of the heart in the regions of the various septa. For an estimation of the area of the cardiac shadow the curved line of the cardiac outline is merely projected to bridge across between the left ventricle and right auricle.

A method has been recommended for estimation of cardiac size using a ratio of area of the cardiac outline to the area of the chest (Newcomer and Newcomer). These areas are estimated in the following manner: from a teleroentgenogram obtain the transverse diameter, TD, and the long diameter of the heart, LD. The product of these two equals the area of the "cardiac rectangle." Now obtain the area of the "thoracic rectangle" by multiplying the transverse diameter of the thorax measured at the upper level of the leaf of the diaphragm, by the height measured from a horizontal line drawn through the upper margins of both apices.

$$\frac{\text{Rectangle of heart (long x transverse diameter)}}{\text{Rectangle of lung (transverse diameter x height)}} = \%$$

Any heart above 28% is abnormal.

Eyster and Hodges have deducted a very intricate mathematical formula for the prediction of the size of the cardiac shadow.

$$\text{Est.T.D.} = +0.1094 \times \text{Age} - 0.1941 \times \text{Height} + 0.8179 \times \text{Weight} + 95.8625$$

If the heart is 5 mm. wider in transverse diameter than the Predicted Diameter obtained by this formula, the chances are 3 to 1 that the widening is pathologic. A slide rule is available for rapid calculation of this formula; their table of calculated values (see accompanying charts), will be found more simple to use, (Hodges and Eyster). These values are for orthodiographic measurements for males; 0.8 should be subtracted for female patients. They are slightly smaller than the figures obtained by Teleroentgenographic measurements.

More recently, it has been stressed that the normal ranges of cardiac dimensions are quite large and overlap the pathological ranges to a great degree. Study of the frontal plane area, (obtained by multiplying together the long diameter, the broad diameter, and the factor 0.735) correlated with the transverse thoracic diameter is recommended by Hilbish and Morgan. They feel this is simple and practical and gives one of the highest degrees of accuracy in estimating true cardiac size. If the heart size from this formula is above the normal range, the heart is certainly enlarged, but if the size is within the stated normal range, the heart may still be considerably enlarged. The greatest use of cardiac measurement is in comparing the patient's own heart size at intervals to note whether there has been change from previous films or change on subsequent films.

Claytor and Merril have compiled a table for average measurement of cardiac values for the rapid practical use; perhaps the cardio-thoracic ratio is the most reliable for rapid rough estimation of cardiac size.

Heart Measurement in Children. Cardiac measurement in children has also been worked out, and nomograms have been provided for this purpose in children above three or four years of age, (Meyer). No fully reliable method has been devised for the prediction of normal cardiac size in children under three years due largely to the wide variations in chest size and shape, general body size, and the great changes which may take place in heart size and chest volume during different phases of respiration, both in health and disease. See nomogram and chart on pp. 307-309.

Within recent years it has been found possible to activate x-ray apparatus by light projected on to a selenium cell, causing an x-ray exposure to be made. If the apparatus is delicately adjusted exposures can be made by the deflection of an electrocardiograph, in complete systole or diastole. With suitable apparatus for rapid changing of films, two successive exposures can be taken of these two phases in the cardiac cycle. From the variation in the sizes of the cardiac outlines during these two phases the difference in heart volume can be calculated, and thus the amount of blood expelled per beat can be determined. Up to the present time this is too delicate a procedure to be used as a practical method.

All of these methods give strikingly similar results — one which most nearly satisfies the needs of the individual radiologist should be selected and adhered to.

C. Form and Outline

By and large, hearts fit individuals; the tall slender hyposthenic individual has a slender vertical heart, whereas the short, stocky hypersthenic person normally possesses a horizontal heart. Any variation would at once suggest an abnormal condition. The first manifestion of failure of any chamber of the heart, to perform its function is indicated by enlargement; (Taussig). Under certain circumstances the enlargement of various chambers imparts "characteristic" shapes to the cardiac outline such as the "Coeur en Sabot" or "Wooden Shoe" heart, etc. Such shapes are not always characteristic however, and give no indication as to the structures involved. Analysis of the appearance of the cardiac outline with reference to enlargement of the various chambers furnishes a much better conception of the underlying pathology.

The contours of the various chambers of the heart are further modified by lesions affecting the blood stream as it flows into or out of the chamber.

The accompanying diagrams indicating the cardiac contours in various heart lesions have been reproduced with the permission of the New York Heart Association.

Left ventricular enlargement is manifested by elongation and bulging of the left ventricular curve (Fig. 212). Location of the point of reversal pulsation along the left border by fluoroscopic examination will show the upper extent of the left ventricle and indicate the degree of elongation of the left ventricular chamber. This represents the outflow tract or heavy muscular portion along the lateral wall con-

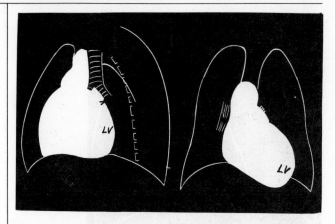

Fig. 212. Left Ventricular Enlargement. The reversal point of cardiac contraction seen on fluoroscopic examination in the anterior view (right figure) along the left border of the heart marks the upper extent of the left ventricular shadow and indicates its size. Enlargement of outflow tract is shown by extension to left and downward below diaphragm.

In the left anterior oblique view (left figure), the inflow tract causes posterior upward enlargement without elevation of the left bronchus. The interventricular groove can frequently be seen on fluoroscopic examination on the inferior border of the heart through the stomach bubble.

cerned in expressing the blood from the heart into the systemic circulation.

As the musculature becomes less and less efficient, blood remaining in the chamber prevents adequate function of the inflow tract during diastole causing ultimate enlargement of this portion of the chamber also. This portion of the left ventricle presents itself in profile along the posterior portion of the heart and is best seen in the left anterior oblique view. The enlarged chamber bulges posteriorly without causing any encroachment upon, or displacement of the left bronchus.

The left auricle occupies the left upper posterior portion of the heart; with its appendage it forms a small portion of the left cardiac outline just above the left ventricular curve (Fig. 213). Enlargement of the left auricle is first indicated by posterior bulging of this chamber into the retrocardiac region. As it does so it displaces the esophagus, with which it is in close relationship. This can be best observed in the right anterior oblique view; the barium-filled esophagus which normally courses almost straight downward through the mediastinum will be seen to bulge backward in a sweeping curve as it passes over the posterior portion of the heart. This is the only absolute means for diagnosis of left auricular enlargement. There is only one condition in which it may not be valid; elongation of the transverse portion of the aortic arch pulls the esophagus away from the left auricle; when this occurs the esophagus can no longer be used as a means of detecting left auricular enlargement. Enlargement of the left auricle may assume massive proportions; in one instance it formed a mass which almost filled the right pleural cavity, which at autopsy was found to contain more

HODGES AND EYSTER'S PREDICTION TABLE FOR ORTHODIOGRAPHIC MEASUREMENTS*

Predicted T–D = + 0.1094 × A − 0.1941 × H + 0.8170 × W + 95.8625

I				II			
Stature Cm.	In.	Area, Sq. Cm.	Transverse Diameter, Mm.	Weight Kg.	Pounds	Area, Sq. Cm.	Transverse Diameter, Mm.
150	59	66.7	66.74	50	110	17.00	40.90
151		67.57	66.55	51	112.2	17.34	41.71
152		68.44	66.36	52	114.4	17.68	42.53
153	60	69.31	66.16	53	116.6	18.02	43.35
154		70.18	65.97	54	118.8	18.36	44.17
155	61	71.05	65.77	55	121	18.70	44.98
156		71.92	65.58	56	123.2	19.04	45.80
157		72.79	65.39	57	125.4	19.38	46.62
158	62	73.66	65.19	58	127.6	19.72	47.44
159		74.53	65.00	59	129.8	20.06	48.26
160	63	75.40	64.80	60	132	20.40	49.07
161		76.27	64.61	61	134.2	20.74	49.89
162		77.14	64.42	62	136.4	21.08	50.71
163	64	78.01	64.22	63	138.6	21.42	51.53
164		78.88	64.03	64	140.8	21.76	52.35
165	65	79.75	63.83	65	143	22.10	53.16
166		80.62	63.64	66	145.2	22.44	53.98
167		81.49	63.45	67	147.4	22.78	54.80
168	66	82.36	63.25	68	149.6	23.12	55.62
169		83.23	63.06	69	151.8	23.46	56.44
170	67	84.10	62.86	70	154	23.80	57.25
171		84.97	62.67	71	156.2	24.14	58.07
172		85.84	62.47	72	158.4	24.48	58.89
173	68	86.71	62.28	73	160.6	24.82	59.71
174		87.58	62.09	74	162.8	25.16	60.52
175	69	88.45	61.89	75	165	25.50	61.34
176		89.32	61.70	76	167.2	25.84	62.16
177		90.19	61.50	77	169.4	26.18	62.98
178	70	91.06	61.31	78	171.6	26.52	63.80
179		91.93	61.12	79	173.8	26.86	64.61
180	71	92.80	60.92	80	176	27.20	65.43
181		93.67	60.73	81	178.2	27.54	66.25
182		94.54	60.53	82	180.4	27.88	67.07
183	72	95.41	60.34	83	182.6	28.22	67.89
184		96.28	60.15	84	184.8	28.56	68.70
185	73	97.15	59.95	85	187	28.90	69.52
186		98.02	59.76	86	189.2	29.24	70.34
187		98.89	59.56	87	191.4	29.58	71.16
188	74	99.76	59.37	88	193.6	29.92	71.98
189		100.63	59.18	89	195.8	30.26	72.79
190	75	101.50	58.98	90	198	30.60	73.61
191		102.37	58.79	91	200.2	30.94	74.43
192		103.24	58.59	92	202.4	31.28	75.25
193	76	104.11	58.40	93	204.6	31.62	76.06
194		104.98	58.21	94	206.8	31.96	76.88
195		105.85	58.01	95	209	32.30	77.70
196	77	106.72	57.82	96	211.2	32.64	78.52
197		107.59	57.62	97	213.4	32.98	79.34
198	78	108.46	57.43	98	215.6	33.32	80.15
199		109.39	57.23	99	217.8	33.66	80.97
200	79	110.22	57.04	100	220	34.00	81.79

To find normal transverse diameter for a given individual, add T–D figure for stature to T–D figure for weight and to this total add 1 mm. for every decade of age; e.g., height, 6 feet; weight, 187 pounds; age, 50 = 134.86 mm. T–D or 60.34 + 69.52 + 5. The figures of this table are valid for orthodiagrams and for male subjects. The hearts of female subjects of same stature, weight and age are slightly smaller in size. Bainton has suggested to subtract .8 cm. for T–D of female.

From F. Y. Hodges and J. A. E. Eyster. Arch. of Int. Med. 1926, 37; 706.

HEART MEASUREMENTS

From CLAYTOR and MERRIL'S Table

Wt. in lbs.	MEN	Transverse diameter in cm. M.R. + M.L.	Longitudinal diameter in cm.
109–117	Min.	10.7	11.8
	Ave.	10.9	12.6
	Max.	11.3	13.5
118–126	Min.	11.0	12.0
	Ave.	11.8	13.2
	Max.	12.5	14.0
127–135	Min.	11.0	12.0
	Ave.	11.9	13.4
	Max.	13.1	14.5
136–144	Min.	11.5	12.5
	Ave.	12.3	13.5
	Max.	13.0	15.0
145–162	Min.	12.0	14.0
	Ave.	12.4	14.6
	Max.	13.8	15.3
163–181	Min.	11.0	14.0
	Ave.	12.9	14.7
	Max.	13.4	15.8

Wt. in lbs.	WOMEN	Transverse diameter in cm. M.R. + M.L.	Longitudinal diameter in cm.
91–99	Min.	9.9	12.0
	Ave.	10.2	12.1
	Max.	10.5	12.3
100–108	Min.	10.0	11.5
	Ave.	10.7	11.9
	Max.	11.1	12.4
109–117	Min.	10.2	10.5
	Ave.	11.0	12.2
	Max.	12.2	13.8
118–126	Min.	9.6	11.2
	Ave.	11.2	12.4
	Max.	12.6	13.3
127–135	Min.	10.0	12.2
	Ave.	11.1	12.7
	Max.	11.8	13.2
136–144	Min.	10.9	12.3
	Ave.	11.6	12.9
	Max.	12.8	14.2
145–159	Min.	10.6	11.8
	Ave.	11.7	12.6
	Max.	12.6	13.2

**Theoretical Transverse Diameters of Heart Silhouette
for Various Heights and Weights**

T.D. of Heart	HEIGHT																		
	5'0"	1"	2"	3"	4"	5"	6"	7"	8"	9"	10"	11"	6'0"	1"	2"	3"	4"	5"	6"
100 mm	83	85	86	87	89	90	92												
101 "	85	86	88	89	91	92	93	95											
102 "	87	88	90	91	92	94	95	97											
103 "	88	90	92	93	94	96	97	99	100										
104 "	90	92	93	95	96	98	99	101	102										
105 "	92	93	95	96	98	99	101	103	104	106									
106 "	94	95	97	98	100	101	103	104	106	108									
107 "	95	97	99	100	102	103	105	106	108	110	111								
108 "	97	99	100	102	104	105	107	108	110	112	113								
109 "	99	101	102	104	106	107	109	110	112	114	115	117							
110 "	101	102	104	106	108	109	111	113	114	116	118	119	121						
111 "	103	104	106	108	109	111	113	115	116	118	120	121	123	125					
112 "	105	106	108	110	111	113	115	117	118	120	122	124	125	127	129				
113 "	106	108	110	112	113	115	117	119	121	123	124	126	128	129	131	133			
114 "	108	110	112	114	115	117	119	121	123	125	126	128	130	132	133	135	137		
115 "	110	112	114	116	117	119	121	123	125	127	129	130	132	134	136	138	140	141	
116 "	112	114	116	118	120	121	123	125	127	129	131	133	134	136	138	140	142	144	146
117 "	114	116	118	120	122	124	125	127	129	131	133	135	137	139	141	143	144	146	148
118 "	116	118	120	122	124	126	128	129	131	133	135	137	139	141	143	145	147	149	151
119 "	118	120	122	124	126	128	130	132	134	136	138	140	142	143	145	147	149	151	153
120 "	120	122	124	126	128	130	132	134	136	138	140	142	144	146	148	150	152	154	156
121 "	122	124	126	128	130	132	134	136	138	140	142	144	146	148	150	152	154	156	159
122 "	124	126	128	130	132	134	136	138	140	143	145	147	149	151	153	155	157	159	161
123 "	126	128	130	132	134	136	139	141	143	145	147	149	152	153	155	157	160	162	164
124 "	128	130	132	134	137	139	141	143	145	147	149	152	154	156	158	160	162	164	166
125 "	130	132	134	137	139	141	143	145	147	150	152	154	156	158	160	163	165	167	169
126 "	132	134	137	139	141	143	145	148	150	152	154	156	159	161	163	165	167	170	172
127 "	134	137	139	141	143	146	148	150	152	154	157	159	161	163	166	168	170	172	175
128 "	136	139	141	143	146	148	150	152	155	157	159	161	164	166	168	171	173	175	177
129 "	139	141	143	146	148	150	152	155	157	159	162	164	166	169	171	173	176	178	180
130 "	141	143	145	148	150	152	155	157	160	162	164	167	169	171	174	176	178	181	183
131 "	143	145	148	150	152	155	157	160	162	164	167	169	172	174	176	179	181	183	186
132 "	145	148	150	152	155	157	160	162	164	167	169	172	174	177	179	181	184	186	189
133 "	147	150	152	155	157	160	162	165	167	169	172	174	177	179	182	184	187	189	192
134 "	150	152	155	157	160	162	164	167	169	172	174	177	179	182	184	187	189	192	194
135 "	152	154	157	159	162	164	167	169	172	175	177	180	182	185	187	190	192	195	197
136 "	154	157	159	162	164	167	169	172	175	177	180	182	185	187	190	193	195	198	200
137 "	156	159	162	164	167	169	172	175	177	180	182	185	188	190	193	195	198	201	203
138 "	159	161	164	167	169	172	174	177	180	182	185	188	190	193	196	198	201	204	206
139 "	161	164	166	169	172	174	177	180	182	185	188	190	193	196	198	201	204	206	209
140 "	163	166	169	171	174	177	180	182	185	188	190	193	196	199	201	204	207	209	212
141 "	166	168	171	174	177	179	182	185	188	190	193	196	199	201	204	207	210	212	215
142 "	168	171	174	176	179	182	185	188	190	193	196	199	202	204	207	210	213	216	218
143 "	170	173	176	179	182	184	187	190	193	196	199	202	204	207	210	213	216	219	221
144 "	173	176	178	181	184	187	190	193	196	199	201	204	207	210	213	216	219	222	224
145 "	175	178	181	184	187	190	193	196	198	201	204	207	210	213	216	219	222	225	228
146 "	178	180	183	186	189	192	195	198	201	204	207	210	213	216	219	222	225	228	231
147 "	180	183	186	189	192	195	198	201	204	207	210	213	216	219	222	225	228	231	234
148 "	182	185	188	192	195	198	201	204	207	210	213	216	219	222	225	228	231	234	237
149 "	185	188	191	194	197	200	203	206	210	213	216	219	222	225	228	231	234	237	240
150 "	187	191	194	197	200	203	206	209	212	215	219	222	225	228	231	234	237	240	243
151 "	190	193	196	199	203	206	209	212	215	218	222	225	228	231	234	237	241	244	247
152 "	192	196	199	202	205	208	212	215	218	221	224	228	231	234	237	241	244	247	250
153 "	195	198	201	205	208	211	214	218	221	224	227	231	234	237	240	244	247	250	253
154 "	198	201	204	207	211	214	217	221	224	227	230	234	237	240	244	247	250	253	257
155 "	200	203	207	210	213	217	220	224	227	230	233	237	240	243	247	250	253	257	260
156 "		206	210	213	216	220	223	227	230	233	236	240	243	247	250	254	257	260	264
157 "				216	219	222	226	229	233	236	239	243	246	250	253	257	260	263	267
158 "						225	229	232	236	239	243	246	249	253	256	260	263	267	270
159 "								235	239	242	246	249	253	256	260	263	267	270	274
160 "										245	249	252		259	263	266	270	274	277
161 "												255	259	263	266	270	273	277	281
162 "												259	262	266	270	273	277	280	284
163 "														269	273	277	280	284	288
164 "														273	276	280	284	287	291

Refer to paper entitled "A Study of the Transverse Diameter of the Heart Silhouette with Prediction Table Based on the Teleroentgenogram" presented to the Association of Life Insurance Medical Directors of America by Dr. Harry E. Ungerleider of the Equitable Life Assurance Society, and Dr. Charles P. Clark, of the Mutual Benefit Life Insurance Company. (1938)

UNGERLEIDER and CLARK'S PREDICTION TABLE, based on Teleroengenographic Measurements of the Heart. (Am. Heart J., 17:92, 1939).

PREDICTED AREA FROM WEIGHT AND HEIGHT, AND ACTUAL AREA FROM LONG AND BROAD DIAMETERS

$[A = \pi/4\ L \times B]$ FOR ORTHODIAGRAM AND TELEOROENTGENOGRAM

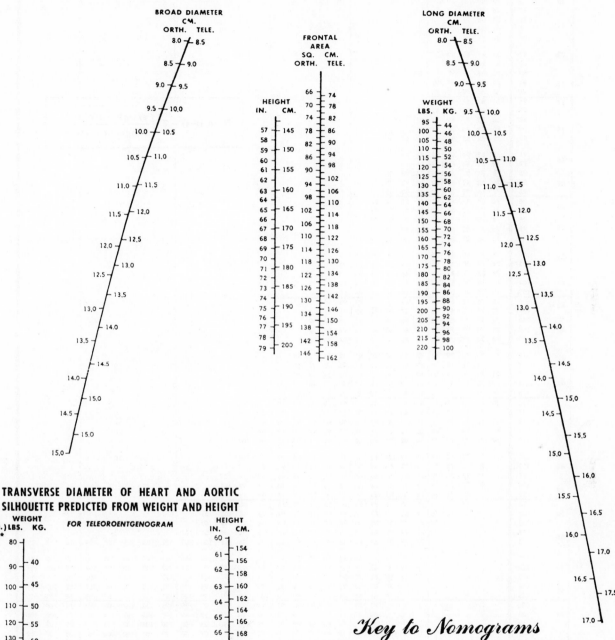

BROAD DIAMETER CM.
ORTH. TELE.

FRONTAL AREA SQ. CM.
ORTH. TELE.

HEIGHT IN. CM.

LONG DIAMETER CM.
ORTH. TELE.

WEIGHT LBS. KG.

TRANSVERSE DIAMETER OF HEART AND AORTIC SILHOUETTE PREDICTED FROM WEIGHT AND HEIGHT

TRANSVERSE DIAMETER (MM.) HEART AORTA* **WEIGHT LBS. KG.**

FOR TELEOROENTGENOGRAM

HEIGHT IN. CM.

*FOR AORTIC DIAMETER ADD 1 MM. FOR EACH 3 YRS. OVER AGE 43 AND SUBTRACT 1 MM. FOR EACH 3 YRS. UNDER 43

Key to Nomograms

The values for actual (or predicted) area are read at the point at which a straight line extending from the long and broad diameters (or weight and height) intersects the cardiac area scale. Orthodiagram values are on the left, teleoroentgenogram values on the right. In the lower nomogram the predicted transverse diameter of the heart (left side of scale) or aortic arch (right side of scale) is obtained as an extension of a straight line connecting height and weight. A correction for age, as indicated, is necessary for the aortic diameter. Values exceeding 10% above the predicted are abnormal.

Adult Nomograms—Courtesy Picker X-Ray Corp.

TABLE FOR PREDICTION OF TRANSERVSE CARDIAC DIAMETER IN CHILDREN

WEIGHT LBS. (top scale): 35 40 45 50 55 60 65 70 75 80 85 99

$$D \text{ (in cms)} = 2\sqrt{\frac{\text{Weight (in kilos)}}{\text{Height (in meters)}}}$$

HEIGHT IN.	CM.	14	15	16	17	18	19	20	21	22	23	24	25	26	27	28	29	30	31	32	33	34	35	36	37	38	39	40	41
30	76	86	89																										
	77	86	89																										
31	78	85	88	91																									
	79	85	88	91																									
	80	84	87	90																									
32	81	84	87	90	92																								
	82	83	86	89	92																								
	83	83	86	89	91																								
33	84	82	85	88	91	93																							
	85	82	85	88	90	93																							
34	86	81	84	87	90	92																							
	87	81	84	86	89	92	94																						
	88	80	83	86	89	91	93																						
35	89	80	83	85	88	91	93																						
	90	79	82	85	88	90	92	95																					
	91	79	82	84	87	90	92	94																					
36	92	79	81	84	87	89	91	94																					
	93	78	81	83	86	89	91	93	96																				
	94	78	80	83	86	88	90	93	95																				
37	95	77	80	82	85	88	90	92	95																				
	96	77	80	82	85	87	89	92	94	96																			
	97	76	79	82	84	87	89	91	94	96																			
38	98	76	79	81	84	86	88	91	93	95																			
	99	76	78	81	83	86	88	90	93	95	97																		
	100	75	78	81	83	85	88	90	92	94	96																		
39	99	76	78	81	83	86	88	90	93	95	97																		
40	101	75	77	80	82	85	87	89	92	94	96																		
	102	74	77	80	82	84	87	89	91	93	95	98																	
	103	74	77	79	82	84	86	88	91	93	95	97																	
41	104	74	76	79	81	84	86	88	90	92	94	97																	
	105	73	76	78	81	83	86	88	90	92	94	96	98																
42	106	73	76	78	80	83	85	87	89	91	93	96	98																
	107	73	75	78	80	82	85	87	89	91	93	95	97																
	108	72	75	77	80	82	84	86	88	91	92	95	97	99															
43	109	73	75	77	79	82	84	86	88	90	92	94	96	98															
	110	72	74	77	79	81	83	86	88	90	92	94	96	98															
44	111	71	74	76	79	81	83	85	87	89	91	93	95	97	99														
	112	71	74	76	78	80	83	85	87	89	91	93	95	97	99														
	113	71	73	76	78	80	82	84	86	89	91	92	94	96	98														
45	114	70	73	75	78	80	82	84	86	88	90	92	94	96	98	99													
	115	70	73	75	77	79	82	84	86	88	89	92	94	96	97	99													
46	116	70	72	75	77	79	81	83	85	87	89	91	93	95	97	99													
	117	70	72	74	77	79	81	83	85	87	89	91	93	95	96	98	100												
	118	69	72	74	76	78	81	83	85	87	88	90	92	94	96	98	99												
47	119	69	71	74	76	78	80	82	84	86	88	90	92	94	96	97	99												
	120	69	71	73	76	78	80	82	84	86	88	90	92	94	95	97	99	100											
48	121		71	73	75	77	79	82	84	86	87	89	91	93	95	97	98	100											
	122		70	73	75	77	79	81	83	85	87	89	91	93	95	96	98	100											
	123		70	72	75	77	79	81	83	85	87	89	91	92	94	96	98	99	101										
49	124		70	72	74	76	79	81	82	84	86	88	90	92	94	95	97	99	101										
	125			72	74	76	78	80	82	84	86	88	90	92	93	95	97	98	100										
50	126			72	74	76	78	80	82	84	86	87	89	91	93	95	96	98	100	102									
	127				73	76	78	80	82	83	85	87	89	91	93	94	96	98	100	101									
	128					75	77	79	81	83	85	87	89	90	92	94	96	97	99	101									
51	129					75	77	79	81	83	85	86	88	90	92	94	95	97	99	101	102								
	130						77	79	81	82	84	86	88	90	92	93	95	96	98	100	102	102	104	105	107	108	110	111	112
52	131						76	78	80	82	84	86	88	89	91	93	94	96	98	100	101	102	104	105	106	108	109	110	112
	132						76	78	80	82	84	85	87	89	91	93	94	96	98	99	101	102	103	105	106	107	109	110	111
53	133						76	78	80	82	83	85	87	89	90	92	94	95	97	99	101	102	103	104	106	107	108	110	111
	134								79	81	83	85	87	88	90	92	93	95	97	98	100	101	103	104	105	107	108	109	111
	135								79	81	83	84	86	88	90	91	93	95	97	98	100	101	102	104	105	106	108	109	110
54	136									81	82	84	86	88	89	91	93	94	96	98	99	101	102	103	105	106	107	108	110
	137									80	82	84	86	87	89	91	92	94	96	97	99	100	102	103	104	106	107	108	109
	138										82	84	85	87	89	90	92	94	96	97	98	100	101	103	104	105	107	108	109
55	139										82	83	85	87	88	90	92	94	95	97	98	99	101	102	104	105	106	107	109
	140											83	85	86	88	90	91	93	95	96	98	99	101	102	103	105	106	107	108
56	141												84	86	88	89	91	92	95	96	97	99	100	102	103	104	106	107	108
	142												84	86	87	89	91	92	94	96	97	98	100	101	103	104	105	106	108
	143														87	88	90	92	94	95	97	98	100	101	102	104	105	106	107
57	144														87	88	90	92	93	95	96	98	99	101	102	103	105	105	107
	145															88	90	91	93	95	96	97	99	100	102	103	104	105	107
58	146															88	89	91	93	94	96	97	99	100	101	103	104	105	106
	147																	89	91	92	94	97	98	100	101	102	104	105	106
	148																89	90	92	94	95	96	98	99	101	102	103	104	106
59	149																88	90	92	93	95	96	98	99	100	102	103	104	105
	150																88	90	92	93	94	96	97	99	100	101	103		
	151																		91	93	94	95	97	98	100	101	102		
60	152																		91	92	94	95	97	98	99	101	102		

Refer to papers entitled "The Anthropometric Index and the Transverse Diameter of the Heart (prediction table for children)— *Boletín Clínica de Marly*—Vol. XI—#5-6-7-8 (May to December) 1949

NOTE: Predictions for subjects over 60" (152 cm.) may be found in a parallel chart "HEART SIZE MEASUREMENTS" prepared by the Medical Department of the Equitable Life Assurance Society of the United States. Copies are available from Picker X-Ray Corp.

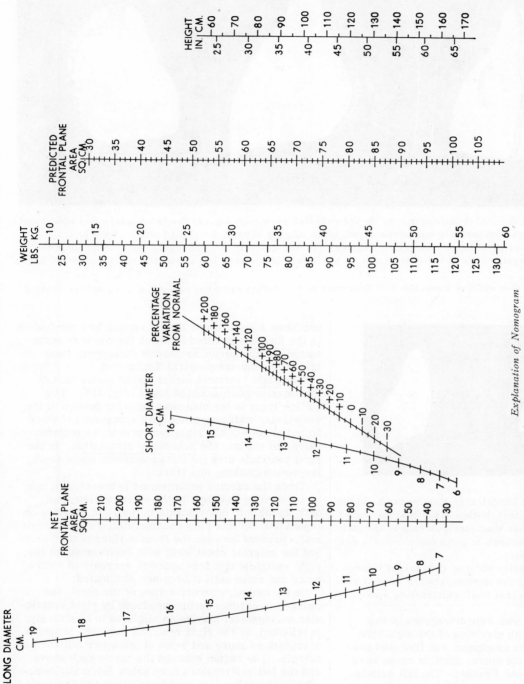

Explanation of Nomogram

The nomogram is applicable only to children between the ages of three and sixteen years, inclusive. If the stature is greater than 170 cm., use the adult nomogram (1). The chest film must be taken with the anterior chest surface next to the film at a target-film distance of 72 inches.

The long and short diameters are measured directly on the chest film with a transparent centimeter ruler. The values are transferred to the nomogram, the ruler is placed across the scales for *long* and *short diameters*, the *net frontal plane area* being read where the ruler intersects that scale. Next, the ruler is placed across the scales for *body weight* and *height* and the *predicted frontal plane area* is read where the ruler intersects that scale. Finally, the ruler is placed so that it connects the values for *net* and *predicted frontal plane area*, the *percentage variation from normal* being read on the sloping center scale at the point intersected by the ruler.—Meyer, **R. R. Radiol. 53:363, 1949.**

Photostatic copies of this nomogram, 14 × 17 inches, may be obtained from the University of Chicago Bookstore, 5802 Ellis Ave., Chicago 37, Ill., at $1.50 each.

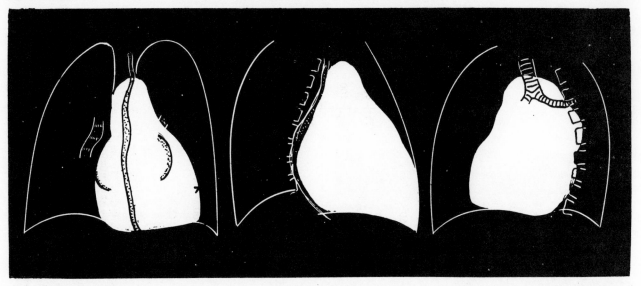

Fig. 213. Left Auricular Enlargement. In the anterior view (left figure) the left auricle lies above and posteriorly; it enlarges posteriorly and to the right, often bulging beyond the right border of the heart.

In the right anterior oblique view (center figure), the auricular mass impresses its contour upon the barium-filled esophagus. This is the only means of positively identifying left auricular enlargement.(Schorr, et al.).

In the left anterior oblique view, the left bronchus is carried upward because of upward enlargement of the left auricle.

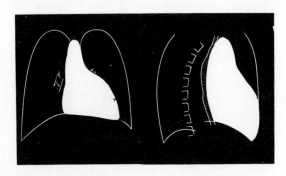

Fig. 214. Right Ventricular Enlargement. In the anterior view (left figure), little change may be seen in cardiac contour other than straightening of the left border of the heart and loss of pulmonary curve since enlargement is anterior.

In the right anterior oblique view (right figure), the anterior margin of the cardiac shadow almost extends to the anterior chest wall, obliterating space.

than 2,000 cc. There was wide divergence of the main stem bronchi, with elevation of the right side from pressure, and the esophagus was flattened posteriorly and followed the aorta. Similar cases have been reported (Daley and Franks). The left auricle enlarges upward also carrying with it the left bronchus which it not only displaces but even constricts from pressure; this can best be observed in the left anterior oblique view. There may be some accentuation of the left auricular curve as seen in the anterior view but this is relatively slight compared to the posterior bulging of the chamber. It can be differentiated from the pulmonary conus which sometimes

produces a prominence in this region, by examination in the lordosis position in which the conus is accentuated and the auricular shadow disappears (see Manual of Roentgenological Technique).

The right ventricle makes up the major part of the anterior portion of the heart (Fig. 214). The outflow tract is the muscular anterior portion of the ventricular wall concerned with expression of blood from the apex of the right ventricle to the pulmonary valve and out into the pulmonary circulation. In the right ventricle also the first manifestation of enlargement is along this tract.

Since the cardiac enlargement is anterior, it may be impossible to detect in the anterior view, and only possible to demonstrate in the right anterior oblique view. In this view considerable distance is normally present between the front surface of the heart and the anterior chest wall; with enlargement of the right ventricle this free space is encroached upon more and more until it becomes eliminated.

In the ordinary anterior view of the chest, the changes in cardiac outline produced by right ventricular enlargement may be so slight as to be entirely overlooked, as the right ventricle becomes larger it overshadows more and more of the upper left cardiac margin. The region between the aortic knob above and the left ventricular curve below (normally occupied by the pulmonary artery or conus and the auricular depression or prominence), is filled in by the overshadowing enlarged right ventricle, giving the appearance of straightening of the contour.

As enlargement progresses, the inflow tract also becomes involved. This is the tract between the tricuspid valve and the apex through which blood is injected into the ventricle. This causes a deepening of

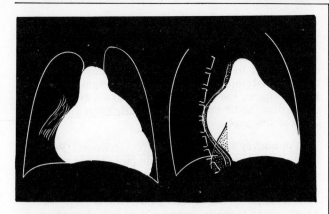

Fig. 215. Enlargement of Right Auricular Appendage and Auricle. Enlargement of the right auricular appendage is first manifestation; the enlargement of the body of auricle follows later. Best seen in right anterior oblique view as an elongation of the horizontal segment of the auricular curve. Enlargement of the body of the right auricle shows as a downward and backward projection of the cardiac shadow through which the barium-filled esophagus seems to run.

the ventricle which can be observed in the left anterior oblique view.

The right auricle lies posteriorly; it receives blood from the inferior vena cava below and the superior vena cava above; the portion between these vessels is called the body of the auricle (Fig. 215). The auricular appendage extends anteriorly. The smooth rounded curve on the right side of the heart is produced by the right auricle. The first manifestation of enlargement is in the appendage, the body of the auricle follows later.

Enlargement of the appendage is best seen in the right anterior oblique view as an elongation of the horizontal segment of the right auricular curve. Enlargement of the body of the right auricle is best observed in the right anterior oblique view as a downward and backward projection of the cardiac shadow through which the barium filled esophagus seems to run.

VALVULAR DISEASE. Valvular disease is most commonly encountered in the left side of the heart; right sided valvular lesions, although they do occur, are most frequently in conjunction with other left sided valvular deficiencies. The mitral valve is undoubtedly the most frequent site of involvement. Rheumatic fever and chorea rank high as etiological factors.

Mitral Valvular Disease. Rheumatic lesions of the mitral valve result in stenosis or insufficiency or both stenosis and insufficiency.

Mitral Stenosis. Stenosis of the mitral valve prevents delivery of the normal quantity of blood to the left ventricle. An excessive accumulation of blood in the left atrium results in dilatation of that chamber. The left ventricle remains unchanged. The aorta, too, is unaffected or may even be small when the amount of blood reaching this vessel is greatly diminished.

As the condition progresses the blood stream is dammed back through the pulmonary circulation to the right ventricle, causing enlargement of this chamber also. With severe and long standing stenosis pulmonary hypertension and its concomitant changes in the lung vasculature pattern become apparent.

Four radiologic features of left atrial enlargement are the appearance of the left auricular appendage in the P-A view, a double density in the right cardiac shadow in P-A view, the posterior displacement of the esophagus in the right anterior oblique view, and the backward and upward displacement of the posterior heart contour in left anterior oblique view. Any one of these four features may be present in normal individuals, but when any two or more are present, the significance is greater (Kaye), and left atrial enlargement is more likely to be actually present. Most radiologists feel that esophageal displacement is the most reliable sign of left atrial enlargement.

As the right ventricle enlarges, it extends to the left, since the unaffected or undersized left ventricle offers no resistance; this causes a counter-clockwise rotation of the heart to the left, the distended right ventricle assuming more and more of the left cardiac contour.

Since, generally speaking, the best surgical results in mitral valvular disease are obtained in mitral stenosis, it is important to determine if the left ventricle is enlarged, as it is with mitral insufficiency. In pure mitral stenosis, the left ventricle is small, and the aorta is not prominent.

The changes in the roentgenographic appearance of the pulmonary vasculature in mitral stenosis are not specific for mitral stenosis, but are characteristic of pulmonary hypertension. They consist of enlargement of the main pulmonary artery and main branches, with abrupt diminution in the caliber of the vessels more peripherally. In early or less severe mitral stenosis, such lung changes are not usually present. The more long-lasting or more severe the stenosis, the more likely are lung vessels patterns of this type to be observed. Correlated with pulmonary hypertension and the gross enlargement of the hilar vessels and clearing of the peripheral vasculature, is the presence of small horizontal lines about one inch long seen near the costophrenic angles, the "B" lines of Kerley, (Carmichael).

The rate or the degree of disappearance of the cardiac and lung signs of mitral stenosis and pulmonary hypertension in the post surgical period is variable, and not necessarily correlated with the symptomatic improvement.

Mitral Insufficiency. Mitral regurgitation without associated stenosis is rarely encountered. In this condition left ventricular enlargement occurs as well as left atrial and rgiht ventricular enlargement, and two lesions must be differentiated with the help of clinical studies. The presence of a distended left ventricle prevents expansion of the right ventricle to the left so that this chamber is forced to expand upward causing less rotation of the heart and a greater prominence of the pulmonary artery. The systolic expansion of the left atrium, described as characteristic of a mitral regurgitation, is thought not to be reliable since it is seen often with mitral stenosis alone.

Combined Mitral Stenosis and Insufficiency. Radiologic findings consist of those already described.

Angiocardiography. This procedure is not needed for the routine diagnosis of mitral valvular disease. In pure mitral stenosis, prolonged, dense opacification of the left atrium is observed. In mitral insufficiency or combined stenosis and insufficiency, mixing of the opaque material between the left atrium and ventricle with uniform density is seen, (Zinsser).

Aortic Valvular Disease. Most aortic lesions are luetic or arteriosclerotic in origin, although some undoubtedly do follow rheumatic fever. Both stenotic and insufficiency lesions produce some enlargement of the left ventricle but with regurgitation dilatation may be extreme. The left cardiac border is characterized by marked convexity in these lesions, and the aortic knob is prominent. Depending in part on syphilytic or arteriosclerotic involvement of the aortic wall itself, either with or without associated hypertension, the aorta becomes dilated and has increased pulsatile qualities. In aortic insufficiency, prominence of the aortic knob is noted. The left atrium shows no enlargement unless cardiac decompensation supervenes. The right cardiac chambers are normal, and the pulmonary vessels are not unusual.

Tricuspid Valvular Disease. Tricuspid valvular lesions are very rare. They may become part of the picture of other valvular lesions as a result of rheumatic fever however. Both cause marked right auricular enlargement however. With stenosis, as on the left sided insufficiency, blood is delivered to the right ventricle in smaller amounts and this structure remains small; the damming back of the blood in the auricle however, extends to the superior and inferior venae cavae (upper engorged vessel is visualized but lower is obscured by auricular enlargement).

Pulmonary Valvular Disease. Lesions of the pulmonary valves are often associated with other congenital cardiac defects such as interauricular septal defects. The effects on the cardiac outline vary widely with the extent, character and location of the lesion so that it often is impossible to determine with any degree of certainty the character of the lesion present from roentgen examination. In pulmonary valve stenosis the pulmonary artery may show marked reduction in size depending on the degree of the stenosis. Or, the pulmonary artery may be thin-walled and dilated. If the stenosis is great, marked enlargement of the conus and right ventricle may be present.

Pulmonary valve insufficiency permits regurgitation of blood resulting in expansile pulsations in the pulmonary arterial branches seen in the hilar regions. On fluoroscopy this collapsing pulsation can be noted in the pulmonary vessels, giving the appearance of a "hilar dance."

showing material change in the heart shadow. Follow-up examination however usually discloses gradual increase in the size of the heart, most marked in the left ventricle, later involving the right side also. Broadening of the aortic shadow may be evident early in the disease or there may be elongation and tortuosity of the aorta.

Pulmonary Emphysema—Effect on Heart. Pulmonary emphysema presents an obstacle to the passage of blood through the lungs which results in right ventricular hypertrophy and dilatation which may not be recognizable in the ordinary anterior view of the chest (since there is ordinarily no actual cardiac malalignment). Angiocardiography with present technic not reliable for differentiation between mitral stenosis and insufficiency.

Poorer than clinical methods, (McAfee, et al.). Only in the right anterior oblique view is the prominence of the conus and pulmonary artery and enlargement of right ventricle noted. Right heart failure ultimately results in death with the systemic circulation all but unimpaired.

Cardiac Decompensation. As long as the heart performs its function, regardless of the pathological lesion present, the circulation is maintained and there is no ill effect. As soon as the left heart fails to maintain the systemic circulation, there is a burden thrown upon the right heart through the engorged pulmonary circulation. This is indicated roentgenographically by accentuation of the lung markings of the hilum regions radiating outward into the lung fields, but fading out before they reached the periphery. Accentuation of the right auricular and pulmonary artery curves with enlargement of the heart to the right soon becomes evident in the roentgenogram.

COR PULMONALE. Any disease which seriously affects the pulmonary circulation may produce an effect upon the heart, by pulmonary hypertension. Such diseases as emphysema, asthma, advanced stages of silicosis and other conditions causing fibrosis of the lung, and sclerosis of the pulmonary vessels themselves (Ayerza's disease) may cause this condition. Rigler and Hallock describe the condition as a right heart enlargement and failure. Hypertrophy and dilation of the right side of the heart, especially the right ventricle, occurs; this may easily escape detection in the ordinary anterior view of the heart because of the location of the right ventricular chamber. In the right anterior view, however, the enlarged right ventricle can be seen approaching the anterior chest wall.

ACUTE CORONARY DISEASE. Angina pectoris may accompany any type of disease of the heart or great vessels. In a great number of cases in adults, however, the disease is primarily due to arteriosclerosis or spasm of the coronary artery. This causes no change in the appearance of the cardiac outline. Occasionally, even small scars in the cardiac muscle from infarcts may be demonstrable on kymographic examination. By painstaking examination these small portions of the cardiac musculature can be shown to be without motion during normal contraction of the adjacent parts.

Although roentgenographic examination shows no demonstrable change in cardiac outline in this disease, it sometimes is associated with acute pulmonary edema which is quite striking. This may be due to shock and impairment of the circulation, since the edema is most pronounced at the most dependent portion. It clears rapidly with recovery. Calcareous deposits may at times be demonstrable in the coronary arteries.

CARDIAC ANEURYSM.* Cardiac aneurysm is found very rarely at autopsy; rarer still is it diagnosed in vivo. They occur most frequently as dilated pouches from the left ventricle, due to atrophy of isolated areas of the ventricular wall from gradual thrombosis of the coronary arteries. In cardiac aneurysm, the narrowing of the coronary artery, is from arteriosclerosis and the final occlusion is from thrombosis. For a cardiac aneurysm to develop, the rate at which occlusion occurs must be too slow to produce sudden death and too rapid to permit capillary compensation.

Roentgenologically cardiac aneurysm may show abnormal bulging of the ventricular wall with pulsation which is abnormal in the cardiac cycle. Pulsation may be absent or even be paradoxical if the aneurysmal sac is small compared to the size of the chamber itself. Aneurysms near the apex are usually readily visualized; those near the base are most frequently confused with other cardiac curves.

In differentiation of this curve from that produced by other rounded structures such as tumor of adjacent organs, etc., recourse must be had to observation of the changes in cardiac cycle during heart beat. Sayman has called attention to the changes in cardiac contour in cardiac aneurysm during forced inspiration and expiration.

In cardiac aneurysm, the accessory bulge over the left ventricular region becomes accentuated during forced inspiration and disappears resuming a normal contour during forced expiration.

Similar changes occur in cardiac infarct during its immediate occurrence; the flattened area over the left ventricle is accentuated during forced inspiration, and the heart assumes its normal contour during forced expiration. Kymographic studies show decrease in amplitude of the heart beat over the infarcted area and increase in cardiac contraction after exertion.

In "total cardiac aneurysm of the heart" there is paradoxical respiratory expansion of the heart.

Unusual curves near the base of the heart are most frequently due to dilatation of the pulmonary conus or the sinus of valsalva or more rarely to sclerosis of the pulmonary artery in Ayerza's disease or coronary aneurysm.

D. Contractibility: On fluoroscopic examination of the heart, observation of the rate, rhythm and forcefulness of the beat are of importance and sometimes are of decisive diagnostic value. The heart beat of course can be accurately determined by the pulse rate, but correlation of the systolic contractions of the heart with the pulse beat under fluoroscopic observation will often detect extra systoles which do not come through into the systemic circulation. The rhythm with which the ventricular beat follows auricular contraction can be observed and any arhythmia noted. Observation of the nodal point of reversed contraction on the left cardiac border is of prime diagnostic importance; this point should be transferred to the teleroentgenogram for further diagnostic consideration.

The forcefulness of the beat may lead to the diagnosis. A small or normally sized heart with feeble ventricular contractions in a person suffering from dyspnoea on slight exertion at once suggests constrictive pericarditis. Whereas, a feeble or absent beat of an enormous cardiac shadow suggests the possibility of pericardial effusion. If, under such conditions, the apex beat can be palpated well within such an enlarged cardiac shadow, it is definite confirmatory evidence of pericardial effusion. If in addition vigorous pulsation is seen above, without pulsation of the lower portion of the cardiac shadow, this is additional evidence of pericardial effusion.

Vigorous ventricular contractions which seem out of all proportion to the symptoms especially in children (in whom emotional reaction incident to the examination can be ruled out) are very frequently encountered in patent ductus arteriosus.

E. Mobility: Ordinarily the normal heart, remains unchanged in its position during respiration since any change in thoracic pressure is bilateral and equal. Any chest pathology which results in an inequality of pressure on the two sides will result in deviation of the elastic mediastinal structures to one side or the other. This elasticity of the mediastinal structures can be demonstrated by examining the patient while lying on his side on a stretcher before the vertical fluoroscope, first on one side and then on the other. In certain pathological conditions, the mediastinal fibrosis may limit the lateral movement of the mediastinum under such conditions. In chronic mediastinitis, study of the esophagus may show deviation in its course from scar tissue reaction, (see mediastinitis).

Unusual tugging of the adjacent portion of the diaphragm with each heart beat may be due to pleuropericardial adhesions, corresponding to the clinical manifestations of Broadbent's Sign.

F. Abnormal Calcifications
INTRACARDIAC AND INTRAPERICARDIAL CALCIFICATIONS. Calcification of the heart valves and other intracardiac and intrapericardial calcifications have been demonstrated roentgenologically by Sosman and Wosika. (Fig. 216). These are usually

---

*An asterisk following any title indicates that roentgenographic reproductions illustrating this condition will be found in the pictorial supplement at the end of the chapter.

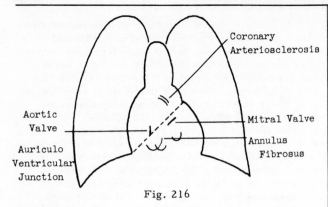

Fig. 216

more readily demonstrated by fluoroscopic than roentgenographic examination. This is because of the fact that their constant dancing motion blurs their roentgenographic image whereas it aids their detection by fluoroscopy. Sosman lists the following conditions necessary for successful fluoroscopic detection:

1. Preparation of the eyes
*2. Type B fluoroscopic screen and fine focus tube
3. For calcified valves look along the auriculoventricular junction
4. Valves will show as dancing shadows
5. Valves are seen best with deep held inspiration
6. Valves are found best in slight R.A.O. position
7. Valves are identified best in the marked L.A.O. position; the mitral being in the posterior third of the heart shadow; aortic valve in the middle third
8. Other calcified areas which can be found and identified are:
   a. Calcified coronary arteries
   b. Calcified pericarditis
   c. Calcified infarcts
   d. Calcified endocarditis
   e. Calcified tumor

*A fluoroscopic screen of even greater brilliance has been developed.

Calcified valves are most readily detected on inspiration with the patient in the posterior-anterior or slight R.A.O. position in the region of the auriculoventricular plane.

This plane is readily located by determining the auriculo-ventricular junction (point of reversal pulsation) on the left border of the heart and connecting it to the lowest point of the right auricular curve where it meets the diaphragm. This plane should lie at about 45° from the horizontal. Searching fluoro-

scopically in the region of this line, rotating the patient 15 to 20° into a modified right anterior oblique position, dancing shadows of calcified valves should be most readily detectible. The patient should hold his breath to eliminate confusion from movement of calcified bodies in the lung. Since the aortic and mitral valves are located so closely together they usually cannot be differentiated in this view. Calcified valves can best be identified with the patient in the extreme left anterior oblique position.

In the left anterior oblique view the aortic valve still remains almost in the center of the cardiac shadow while the mitral valve is displaced well into the posterior third of the cardiac shadow.

The dancing movement of the shadows caused by calcified valves is far in excess of any other calcium deposits in the lung or hilum region with which they may be confused. Their amplitude of movement is similar to that of the ventricular contraction. Once detected their movement may be confirmed by kymographic examination, (Rigler). For radiographic demonstration of valves rapid exposure (1/20 second or less) is essential. The target film distance may be reduced to 4 feet or less in order to gain speed of exposure with considerable advantage. It is even possible to demonstrate calcified valves by body section examination.

Care must be taken not to mistake calcified rings at the base of the valves as in the valves themselves. Calcified and even ossified areas in the heart muscle from old infarcts are usually larger and are easily identified (Brean, et al.). Pericardial calcification appears as a shell about the heart. (Davies and Steiner.)

G. Relation of Heart to Surrounding Structures

Spinal curvature may cause definite displacement and rotation of the heart and great vessels, so that it falsely appears the heart is enlarged from intrinsic disease. Pectus excavatum results similarly in displacement of the heart to the left, giving the appearance of enlargement erroneously. Mediastinal tumors may by their size and location affect the heart. Esophageal tumors are not so likely to be of sufficient bulk to encroach upon the heart but the enormous esophageal dilatation associated with cardiospasm may often displace the heart.

Herniation of a portion of the stomach through the diaphragm, as a true hernia through the diaphragm either congenital or acquired, or hiatus hernia may so encroach upon and displace the heart as to interfere with its normal action and cause pain.

"Duplication of Cardiac Shadow," by the gas bubble of the stomach herniated through the diaphragm to a position in the mediastinum behind the heart, may often lead to diagnosis of this condition, otherwise unsuspected (Nemec), (Fig. 217).

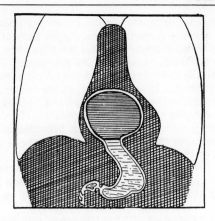

Fig. 217

II. AORTA AND GREAT VESSELS

ARTERIOSCLEROTIC AORTITIS*(Fig. 218). The aortic shadow, consisting of the superimposed shadows of the ascending and descending portions, should not exceed 6 cm. in width; any diffuse enlargement of the aorta beyond this measurement is indication of aortitis. This does not represent the true width of the aorta. The close apposition of the esophagus to the left side of the aorta makes it possible to more accurately determine this measurement. Actually the true width of the aorta, measured from the barium-filled esophagus to the left border of the aortic knob should not exceed 3 cm. (H. Roesler). This may be due either to arteriosclerosis or syphilis. The aorta ascends on the right, arches across and descends on the left side. In the young adult individual the ascending and descending portions are superimposed in the anterior chest roentgenogram. As the individual advances in years, the vessel walls become less elastic, and the vascular loop tends to untwist itself. In old age, the vessel walls may become very rigid and inelastic and atheromatous degeneration may occur. The aortic shadow may become broadened far exceeding normal limits,

indicating aortitis. This is attended by calcareous deposits in the aortic walls which are clearly visible roentgenographically. The process may be so pronounced that the entire aorta appears to be calcified. Any appearance of calcareous plaques in the aortic wall is evidence then of arteriosclerotic aortitis.

SYPHILITIC AORTITIS. If progressive broadening of the aortic shadow develops in a relatively young individual, this is suspicious of syphilitic aortitis. Wolkin has pointed out that syphilitic aortitis is often associated with calcareous deposits in the wall of the ascending aorta either with or without aneurysmal dilatation. This is in contradistinction to arteriosclerotic aortitis in which calcareous deposits are in the arch and descending portions.

With angiocardiography injection of opaque media, (Diodrast or Urokon) into the circulation permits direct measurement of the width of the aorta, (See Manual of Roentgenolic Technique).

ELONGATION AND TORTUOSITY OF THE AORTA. Elongation of the aorta usually occurs in conditions in which excessive amounts of blood are rapidly pumped into the vessel and then suddenly released as in aortic insufficiency; or in increased blood pressure where the increase in pressure within the vessel produces a tendency to uncoil and elongate the loop produced by the aorta between its cardiac origin and its diaphragmatic attachment. Where this condition is maintained for a considerable period of time, the aorta finally becomes so elongated that tortuosity results. Dilatation of the aortic structures soon supervenes, depending upon the degree of elasticity of the vessel wall.

Elongation of the aorta is seen best in the left anterior oblique view. Just as a loop of rubber hose tends to uncoil and elongate when subjected to the stress of fluid under increasing pressure, so the aortic loop tends to uncoil. The ascending limb of the aorta in place of going vertically upward, forms a broad circular sweep toward the anterior chest wall; the transverse portion circles upward even above the sternal notch, and, the descending portion sweeps far backward to lie in the trough to the left and posterior to the thoracic spine.

The displaced aorta produces pronounced changes in the esophagus due to pressure in this abnormal position. In the anterior view of the chest the esophagus shows a marked deviation to the left in its course through the upper portion of the mediastinum. This deviation of the esophagus is usually associated with the appearance of an additional curve along the left upper border of the heart due to the left border of the descending aorta. In the left anterior oblique position the esophagus deviates backward drawn by adhesions from the backward displaced descending portion of the aorta.

PULMONARY VEINS IN HEART DISEASE. Attention is called by Steinbach, et al. to examination of the pulmonary vessels, especially the pulmonary veins with body-section roentgenography for evaluation of the degree of pulmonary congestion in heart disease.

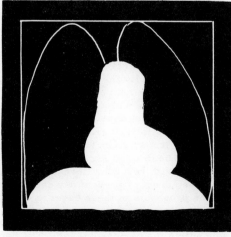

Fig. 218

The size of the pulmonary veins correlates well with the amount of pulmonary blood flow. Large veins occurred in cases of intracardiac shunts with left to right flow, patent ductus arteriosus, and pulmonary window. Small pulmonary veins have been found in pulmonic volvular stenosis, tetrology of Fallot and pulmonary thrombosis. In mitral stenosis and in mitral insufficiency the pulmonary veins are usually of normal size rather than enlarged. Occasionally they may be smaller than normal, even though the right ventricle, pulmonary artery and left atrium are definitely enlarged, due probably to constriction of the peripheral vessels.

AORTIC ANEURYSM*(Fig. 219). Syphilitic aortitis is the forerunner of aneurysm. With the fewer number of cases being seen due to improved primary treatment; aneurysm of arteriosclerotic nature are now becoming more common. When the effects of syphilitic involvement become too great on the aortic wall, the wall gives way and a bulging aneurysmal sac develops. Roentgenologically this appears as a rounded sacculation springing from the aorta. They may be recognized fluoroscopically by their expansile pulsation, that is, with the inrush of blood at each heart beat, the aneurysmal sac becomes suddenly distended simultaneously in all directions. The larger the sac, the greater difficulty is experienced in detecting the expansile character of the pulsation. This is only natural since the same amount of blood injected by the heart at each contraction into the aneurysmal sac will cause greater expansion in a sac of small size than in one of larger dimension. Likewise, mediastinal tumors often present a similar well-defined, rounded appearance; owing to their close association with the great vessels, pulsation of a transmitted character is often observed. Under such conditions only angiocardiographic examination by injection of opaque material into the blood stream may aid in differentiating the conditions (See Manual of Roentgenological Technique).

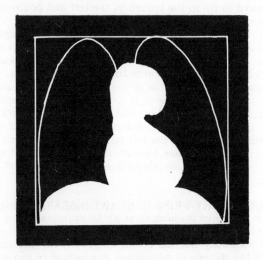

Fig. 219

Aneurysmal dilatation of the ascending aorta bulges out to the right from the region above the cardiac origin of the vessel; in this location expansile pulsation must be relied upon for diagnosis. Aneurysms arising from the transverse arch because of their relationship to the trachea, cause pressure of this structure to the right and forward as seen in the anterior and left anterior oblique views. The transverse arch passes beneath the left bronchus so that any dilatation of this portion of the aorta will cause elevation of the left bronchus, characteristic seen very clearly in the anterior and left lateral views of the chest. Aneurysms of the descending arch bulge to the left at any location in the descending aorta.

DISSECTING ANEURYSM.* Rupture into the walls of the aorta with slow but steady dissection of its coats results in obliteration of the normal curves shown on both sides of the aorta, constituting a dissecting aneurysm. Such aneurysms may dissect between the vascular coats far down into the abdomen presenting painful palpable masses.

The roentgenological diagnosis depends upon the roentgen observation of a rapid succession of changes in the aorta over a relatively short period of time, and to do this serial films are needed. Expansile pulsation is rarely of value in the diagnosis since in such aneurysms the sac frequently becomes filled with clotted blood. At times the aneurysmal pathway will again rupture back into the aorta lower down and the patient may survive and live for a long time with this condition. Only by close correlation of the physical signs and symptoms with the radiological findings can the diagnosis be made.

One would think that angiocardiography, or injection of opaque material (70% Diodrast, NeoIopax, or Urokon) would serve to outline the vascular structures and prove with certainty the presence of such a dissecting aneurysm but this is often not the case since the blood is frequently clotted in its extravasated sac.

III PERICARDIUM

ACUTE PERICARDITIS. Purulent inflammation of the pericardial sac can result especially in children from septic infection. Starting with no other manifestation than a sore throat it is possible for infection of the pericardial sac to take place with very few signs to lead to its detection.

Roentgenographically the heart shadow may show little if any enlargement and the heart beat may be within the range of normal as indicated fluoroscopically. The diagnosis depends upon physical signs. The prognosis is very grave but some patients do recover. It may go on to frank pericardial effusion which can be drained successfully or the patient may recover with resulting fibrosis of the pericardial sac. The advent of present day chemotherapy may change the prognosis in these cases.

PERICARDIAL EFFUSION. Normally the heart moves freely within the pericardial sac. The pericardium is attached below to the diaphragm and above to the hilum of lung and great vessels. Any accumulation of fluid within this sac will influence the contour of the cardiac shadow. When the amount of fluid is small, it gravitates to the lower portion of the sac, filling the cardiophrenic sinuses and straightening out the normal cardiac curves. With small pericardial effusions, then, the roentgen appearance of the cardiac outline may be one of a "triangle suspended from the neck" (Fig. 220A).

As the effusion increases in size, the sac bulges outward beyond its diaphragmatic attachment on either side at the bottom due to the weight of the fluid. This again imparts curves to the lower portion of the cardiac outline not unlike the appearance of ordinary cardiac dilatation (Fig. 220B). Differentiation between these two conditions sometimes taxes the greatest resourcefulness of the roentgenologist. Since the pericardial fluid is practically of the same density as the heart it is impossible to distinguish the cardiac outline within the pericardial fluid. Several methods are at our command, however. First fluoroscope the patient in an upright position and note the force of the heart beat. If definite contractions occur, ventricular following auricular contraction in normal sequence, then we can eliminate pericardial effusion of more than very small size. But, as only too often happens,

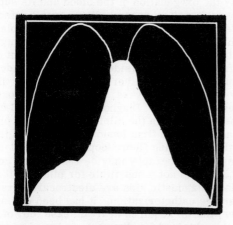

Fig. 220A

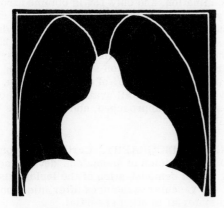

Fig. 220B

the detection of contraction by this means is impossible. If, by palpation under fluoroscopic observation, a definite apex beat can be located, well inside the region of the apical shadow, and, if at the same time there is evidence of only shallow contraction of the cardiac outline, this is definite evidence of existence of pericardial effusion.

Several confirmatory tests can be made which are based upon the shift of the pericardial fluid. If the patient is observed under the fluoroscope, lying first on one side and then on the other, it will be found that the most dependent portion of the cardiac shadow loses its beat, and the uppermost portion develops a more vigorous contraction. When this evidence is obtained it is absolute indication of pericardial effusion.

Or the following method may be resorted to: Two anterior roentgenograms of the chest taken under precisely similar conditions of exposure, distance, and position, one in upright position and the other recumbent, may show bulging of the lower portion of the cardiac shadow in the upright position from the weight of the fluid. If the fluid is under great tension, the variation in appearance may be so slight that a decisive opinion cannot be rendered.

If there is associated pneumopericardium a definite level is imparted to the fluid which changes the level on change of position of the patient. Clinically there is a splashing sound on oscultation. Dassel and Kirsh report two such cases from spontaneous rupture of a gastric ulcer into the pericardium. A linear shadow along the left side of the cardiac shadow has been demonstrated by Kremens which is probably due to an excessive distribution of pericardial fibrosis or fat.

CHRONIC CONSTRICTIVE PERICARDITIS* (Calcification of Pericardium). As a result of previous pericardial infection the pericardial sac may become obliterated and the resulting fibrous tissue may become organized causing constriction of the heart by its contraction. If the original infection was of tuberculous character, calcium deposit in the pericardium may be demonstrable in the roentgenogram; it may require overexposure of the roentgenogram or a due lateral view for its demonstration. It is in itself evidence of constrictive pericarditis. Stewart, et. al. have outlined the following findings as most conclusive roentgen signs of chronic constrictive pericarditis:

1. Small heart, when the patient has signs of heart failure (fluid in the chest, ascites, liver enlargement, etc.) and small aorta.
2. Calcification of pericardium.
3. Decrease in pulsation in ordinary anterior fluoroscopic examination of chest; the heart appears to be "standing still."
4. Limitation of motion of the heart with change in position of patient.
5. Decreased pulsation of the aorta and of the lateral margin of the heart in roentgenkymograms.

Of these, calcification of the pericardium, if present, is the most reliable sign. It must be associated with signs of obstruction to be of significance since the area of constriction may be localized to a position in which it causes little functional impairment.

In talc workers, deposits of this opaque dust may accumulate in the pericardium and pleura giving rise to the appearance of calcium deposits.

In absence of calcification the most commonly observed sign is a small flattened aortic knob or complete absence of the knob formation.

Small size of cardiac shadow is of most importance but large heart does not rule out constrictive pericarditis.

On fluoroscopic examination, decrease in excursion of the cardiac border may be detected over the area constricted by pericardial thickening; there may be limitation of lateral shift of the heart on changing position of the patient and limitation of elongation of the heart with descent of the diaphragm or evidence of pleuropericardial adhesions. Operative removal of the constricting pericardial band may result in complete relief and cure of the disease. In other cases only slight relief may be experienced. Some patients may not suffer too much disability from the condition.

PLEUROPERICARDIAL ADHESIONS (Fig. 221). Adhesive pericarditis may develop to such a degree that the entire pericardial space becomes obliterated. Although there may be some hint of cardiac embarrassment in the electrocardiograph, still roentgenographic examination may give little if any indication of its presence. Teleroentgenographic examination shows no cardiac enlargement, nor does fluoroscopic examination disclose any distinctive variation in cardiac impulse. If, however, pleuropericardial adhesions develop, then with each beat the heart can be seen tugging at the diaphragm and adjacent lung structures. Clinically this is known as Broadbent's sign. Kymographic examination may aid in diagnosis.

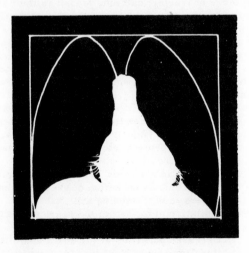

Fig. 221

Such a condition materially embarrasses the circulation; it can be relieved in some instances by relaxing the adhesions to the chest wall by a cardiolysis operation. Clinically, this tugging of the diaphragm and pleura is manifested by traction seen with each heart beat on the posterior aspect of the thorax low down near its spinal attachment.

IV. CONGENITAL ANOMALIES OF HEART AND ASSOCIATED STRUCTURES

Congenital anomalies of circulatory development show wide variation from normal, (Fig. 222). To bring order to the great body of descriptive material on this subject, an arbitrary classification must be introduced to separate anomalies of development of the great vessels from anomalies of development of the heart itself. This separation cannot be absolute, since some conditions are composed of defects in both the heart and great vessels, like transposition of the great vessels. In general, cardiac lesions resolve themselves into septal defects, valvular malformations, and variations in the chambers of the heart and great vessels. The response of the heart to these various defects is proportional to their severity in disrupting the cardiac function. If this disorganization of function be minimal and not affect materially the oxygenation of the blood and its supply to the tissues, such an anomaly like a small defect in the interventricular septum may be compatible with long life and may not even be detectable roentgenologically. If the cardiac lesion allows a shunt of blood from right to left side of the heart, inadequately oxygenated blood is delivered to the tissues. Disability may then be severe, and the roentgenographic changes pronounced. Diagnosis of congenital cardiac diseases begins with the clinical history and physical examination as the firm foundation. Radiological examination, including fluoroscopic study is all-important; Angiocardiography may be essential in certain cases, but it is not a substitute for other methods. Auxiliary diagnostic aids are electrocardiography and cardiac catheterization. It has been estimated (Dexter) that in acquired heart disease, 60% of all information obtained for diagnosis is based on the history. 25% of the information is derived from the physical examination, and only 15% is obtained from laboratory procedures like EKG and x-ray. In congenital heart disease, however, only 15% of the diagnostic information comes from the history and 25% is furnished by the physical findings, with x-ray, EKG and cardiac catheterization studies supplying an overwhelmingly important 60% of the information. It is only by correlation of all available information that a diagnosis can be approached, and sometimes even this fails.

ANGIOCARDIOGRAPHY.* Certain symptoms may lead to the suspicion of anomalous development but for the actual demonstration of the lesion, visualization of the vascular structures after injection of opaque material is often essential.

Angiocardiography is a method introduced by Robb

NORMAL CIRCULATION

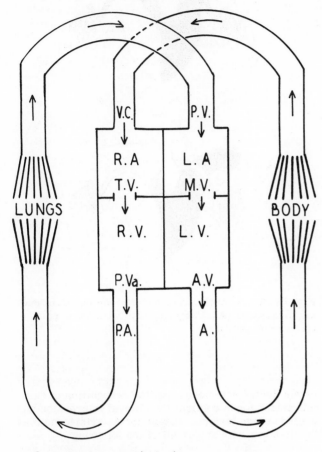

V.C. Superior and inferior vena cava

R.A. Right atrium

T.V. Tricuspid valve

R.V. Right ventricle

P.Va. Pulmonary valve

P.A. Pulmonary artery

P.V. Pulmonary veins

L.A. Left atrium

M.V. Mitral valve

L.V. Left ventricle

A.V. Aortic valve

A. Aorta

Fig. 222

and Steinberg for the visualization of the vascular structures of the heart and lungs. Opaque material, usually 70% Diodrast or Urokon, rapidly injected into a vein, renders the blood opaque to x-rays permitting the visulization of the heart and vascular structures

as it passes through. This method has been found to be of great aid in the detection of cardiovascular defects in congenital heart lesions. Apparatus has been devised for making x-ray exposures in rapid succession so as to visualize the various chambers and vessels of the heart as the opaque material is propelled through the circulation, (See Manual of Roentgenological Technique). The right posterior oblique position of the chest seems best suited to this examination.

The risk of angiocardiography to the patient is low but appreciable. Death has occured in 26 instances in 6824 angiocardiographies, most of the fatalities occurring in children with congenital heart lesions (Dotter and Steinberg). Morgan estimated a higher mortality rate, 1%. Angiocardiography is of little value in diagnosis of non-cyanotic congenital heart disease. Shunts are either not present or when they are present are left to right shunts which are not well visualized. In cyanotic disease, angiocardiography is of great value, demonstrating right to left shunts, septal defects, and malpositions of the great vessels. It should be remembered that little of the present angiocardiographic information has been confirmed by anatomic studies.

CATHETERIZATION OF THE HEART (Schnitker). Catheterization of the heart by passing a long opaque ureteral-like catheter through the vein of the arm and superior vena cava into the right auricle, ventricle and pulmonary artery and its branches, permits the taking of blood pressure readings and samples of blood for oxygen determination, (cc. per liter O_2) from locations in the various chambers of the heart; this may be the only effective means of making a diagnosis in certain conditions since the roentgen picture may not be characteristic. Multiple blood samples for oxygen saturation values are withdrawn and pressure recordings are made from the chambers and vessels. As the tip is guided by fluoroscopic control further knowledge of position of chambers and communications between chambers is obtained. An associated determination is the blood oxygen saturation of a peripheral artery (femoral). Cardiac catheterization is valuable in studying the pulmonary artery in both cyanotic and non-cyanotic disease. Stenosis is indicated by a pressure drop as the catheter enters the pulmonary artery from the right ventricle. Valuable assistance is given in the diagnosis of left to right shunts on the basis of abnormally high oxygen contents of right heart blood. The passage of the catheter tip into an over-riding aorta or through a septal defect is positive evidence of these anomalies. Failure to do so does not exclude their presence. Lowered oxygen content of peripheral arterial blood indicates a right to left shunt.

A. ANOMALIES OF STRUCTURAL DEVELOPMENT OF THE GREAT VESSELS. Two of the best understood anomalies of development of the vascular structures are patent ductus arteriosus and coarctation of the aorta.

1. PERSISTENT PATENT DUCTUS ARTERIOSUS,* (Fig. 223 A-1, A-2 and A-3). The ductus arteriosus

PATENT DUCTUS ARTERIOSUS

Fig. 223 A-1

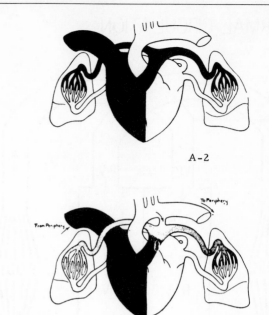

A-2

A-3

Fig. 223 A-2 & A-3. The flow of blood in patent ductus arteriosus (A-3) as compared with the normal
circulation (A-2).

functions during intrauterine life and normally closes
at birth or shortly thereafter with establishment of the
pulmonary circulation. Under certain circumstances,
the exact nature of which is not clearly understood,
it may remain as a persistent communication between
the pulmonary and systemic circulations. The shunting of arterial blood into the pulmonary artery may
result in the pulmonary blood flow reaching two to
four times that of the systemic flow. Due to the increased strain on the left ventricle, persistent disability eventually develops, and life expectancy of untreated cases is about 35 years. Congestive failure
and subacute bacterial endocarditis and endarteritis
are the ultimate causes of death in three fourths of
the untreated cases. There may be dyspnea on exertion, palpitation and increased fatigability but
symptoms may be completely lacking. Cyanosis is
practically never seen with the isolated lesion, and
then only with cardiac failure or sclerosis or obstruction of the pulmonary vascular bed. (When patent ductus is accompanied by other abnormalities of
the heart and great vessels, cyanosis may be present due to the associated lesions). A continuous ma-
chinery-like murmur is almost always present above
and to the left of the pulmonary area on auscultation.
A systolic thrill in the second left intercostal space,
a rapid heart beat, and an increased pulse pressure
are usually present.

ROENTGEN EXAMINATION. The roentgen examination cannot be relied upon solely to diagnose

patent ductus arteriosus, but the recognition of certain findings can confirm the clinical impression and
exclude other lesions. Patent ductus arteriosus may
be attendant with any or all of the following:

a. Enlargement of the left ventricle,
b. Accentuation of the pulmonary artery segment,
   (convexity of the pulmonic curve) and increased pulsation of the pulmonary artery and
   its main branches, which in some instances
   may be so great as to constitute "hilar dance,"
c. Increased vascularity of the lung fields,
d. Dilatation of the left auricle,
e. Vigorous beat of heart on fluoroscopic examination out of all proportion to physical demand.
f. Dilatation of the proximal aorta.
g. Moderate increase in overall heart size.

If apprehension can be excluded as a cause of the
forceful, rapid beating, then this, in our experience,
is of greatest diagnostic value. The diagnosis can
almost always be made on the basis of the characteristic murmur, a situation unique in congenital heart
disease. In the infant and very young child, the typical murmur may be absent and other diagnostic
methods must be used. When pulmonary hypertension
develops, the right ventricle enlarges.

ANGIOCARDIOGRAPHY.* Almost all cases of
patent ductus can be diagnosed by the clinical history
and physical findings, mainly the characteristic ma-

chinery murmur. Only in the very young and in the rare questionable case, and when other defects are suspected, cardiac catheterization and angiocardiography are indicated. When the catheter can be passed into the pulmonary artery, arterialized blood and a pulmonary artery hypertension may be recorded. Occasionally the catheter can be passed through the ductus into the aorta.

Angiocardiography may be used to visualize the pulmonary vessels and aortic arch. Dilatation and elevation of the main pulmonary artery and its left branch can be seen, as well as re-opacification of the left pulmonary artery at time of aortic opacification in the cardiac cycle. More important, a bulge of the aortic wall can be demonstrated in the region where the ductus leaves the aorta. This bulging described as the infundibulum of the ductus, is usually visible best in the left anterior oblique position, but is also seen in the A-P and left lateral views. Visualization of the ductus itself by angiocardiography is exceptional. Thoracic aortography by retrograde injection into carotid or brachial artery (see Manual of Roentgenographic Technique for procedure) will demonstrate more constantly the presence of a ductus. Opacification of the pulmonary artery is more frequently seen by this injection than the ductus itself. When the acutal ductus is not visualized, observing of the infundibulum provides the only means of establishing the exact position of the ductus. A very slight bulge in this region of the aorta should be interpreted with caution for it is seen sometimes when no patent ductus is present. The value of this finding is still in dispute since this infundibulum sign occurs at the site of a normal increase in aortic-caliber. In normal individuals, the bulge has never been seen to project more than one millimeter.

Many cardiac anomalies are associated with one or more of the roentgenographic findings of patent ductus arteriosus: Inter-atrial septal defect, mitral stenosis, Eisenmenger's complex, idiopathic dilatation of the pulmonary artery, interventricular septal defect and pulmonic stenosis. Differentiation is made by other criteria.

SURGICAL OPERATION. In 1939 a patent ductus arteriosus was first successfully ligated (Gross and Hubbard); this has been followed by a rapid advance of surgical procedures for the alleviation of anomalous development in congenital heart disease.

Operative ligation of the ductus re-establishes the normal flow of blood. The procedure now routinely performed with a low mortality rate drastically changes the prognosis for the better. Individuals with a patent ductus are susceptible to the development of bacterial endarteritis and endocarditis. If the patient is suffering from streptococcus viridans infection of this nature, operative ligation of the ductus will result in sterilization of the blood stream and complete recovery of the patient in a high percentage of cases, althrough the operative mortality is somewhat higher under such circumstances. Postoperatively after a sufficient time interval, the roentgenographic findings revert to normal.

2. COARCTATION OF THE AORTA,* (Fig. 223 B-1, B-2, B-3 and B-4). Another anomaly now of great practical importance is coarctation. Since 1945 this has been a surgically correctible form of hypertension. In more than 90% of the cases, the site of constriction of the aortic lumen is between the origin of the left subclavian artery and the region of the ligamentum arteriosum. Hypertension is present in the vessels proximal to the constriction, with a lower pressure and a diminished or absent pulse in the vessels below the lesion. Physical examination alone can make the diagnosis in most cases, by the discrepancy of blood pressure readings in the upper and lower extremities. Blood is conveyed beyond the region of constriction by collateral circulation through the intercostal, subscapular, and internal mammary arteries; in this way the circulation is maintained. The arteries partaking in the collateral circulation become enlarged and tortuous. Individuals with coarctation have a lowered life expectancy due to the hypertension and its complications, namely cerebrovascular accidents and cardiac failure.

COARCTATION OF THE AORTA

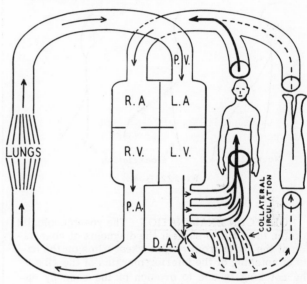

Fig. 223 B-1

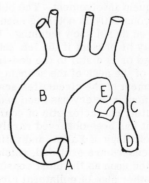

Fig. 223 B-2

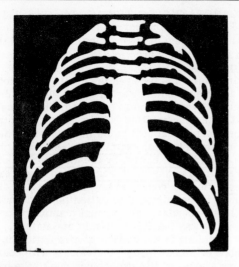

Fig.223B-3. Coarctation of aorta. Note notching of posterior ribs from dilated intercostal vessels resulting from collateral circulation.

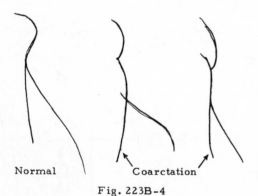

Normal   Coarctation

Fig. 223B-4

ROENTGEN EXAMINATION. The roentgenologist is often the first to suggest the diagnosis of coarctation of the aorta from routine chest films on the basis of notching of the inferior margins of the ribs. The notching is due to erosion of the bone by enlarged, tortuous, pulsatile intercostal arteries, part of the collateral circulation. Ribs four through eight are most commonly involved; ribs three and nine show infrequent involvement. The older the patient, the more constantly is notching seen. Infants and young children do not show notching. Unilateral notching only may be present if the left subclavian artery is involved or is distal to the constricted segment. Notching of the neck of the scapula assumed to be from enlargement of the circumflex scapular branch of the scapular artery has been seen. Notching is not absolutely characteristic of coarctation, however, since it has been observed rarely in neurofibromatosis, Tetralogy of Fallot, and without known cause. If these causes are excluded, notching of the ribs may be relied upon as the most constant sign of coarctation. Another sign of collateral circulation is dilatation of the internal mammary arteries seen as an increased soft tissue shadow on true lateral view of the chest.

A defect or break in the continuity of the distal aortic arch or a double aortic curve along the left border of the upper mediastinum is seen in about one third of the cases of coarctation, (Fig. 223B-3). This indentation usually indicates the site of the coarctation. The segment of curve proximal to the indentation, represents either the left subclavian or the proximal aorta. The distal segment of the curve delineates the post-stenotic segment. Other signs of coarctation such as absence or insignificance of the aortic knob on P-A view, tortuosity or dilatation of the ascending aorta, and left ventricular enlargement are either inconstant or not specific. They are helpful in evaluating each case, but are not diagnostic. Left atrial enlargement has been noted in small children evidently before collateral circulation develops, (Kjellberg).

SURGICAL OPERATION. Knowledge of the actual site and extent of the constricted segment before operation is helpful to the surgeon in preparing for the type of procedure and predicting the need for an aortic graft. The constricted or obliterated area is usually short so that resection of the area can be performed and continuity re-established by end to end anastomosis or by a short aortic graft. Rarely the area of constriction is long or located other than in the typical place, and longer grafts are needed to re-establish continuity of the aorta.

ANGIOCARDIOGRAPHY. Intravenous angiocardiography is not of much value. Thoracic aortography, in which the contrast medium is injected via a catheter introduced into the carotid or radial artery is much more accurate for giving the surgeon the anatomical information needed.

Cardiac Catheterization is not helpful or indicated in this or other lesions of the left side of the heart and aorta except to exclude any other suspected accompanying lesion.

3. RIGHT AORTIC ARCH*(Fig. 223C) is probably the most common anomaly of the great vessels. Normally the aorta ascends on the right, arches over to the left and descends on the left side. In the anterior view the aortic arch lies to the left of the esophagus, indenting that barium-filled structure as it courses downward through the mediastinum. In fact, the esophagus is in such close apposition to the aortic arch, that this method is used for the accurate measurement of the width of the aorta at this point. In the right anterior oblique position a shallow pressure defect is produced on the anterior margin of the esophagus by the aortic arch. In the left anterior oblique position the esophagus descends without significant indentation by other structures. In the anterior position the trachea may appear somewhat deviated to the right due to the normal position of the aorta on the left but there is no indentation of the tracheal wall as visualized either by lateral chest films or after lipiodol injection.

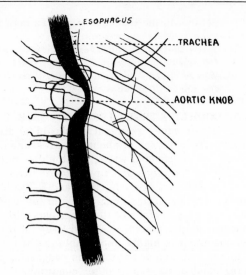

Fig. 223C. Right aortic arch with left descending aorta. R.A.O. View. The right aortic arch passes to the right of the esophagus and trachea, then passes posterior (dorsal) to the esophagus as it crosses the midline to descend on the left.

ROENTGEN EXAMINATION. In right aortic arch these relationships are changed. The aortic arch lies to the right of the esophagus. The roentgenologic sign of right aortic arch is displacement of the esophagus to the left on P-A view. Indentation of the esophagus on the right is the sign of right arch, regardless of the position of the descending aorta. The aorta may then descend either on the left or the right, the left descending course being far the more common. When the aorta descends on the right, there is no encroachment upon either the posterior or anterior surface of the esophagus in either oblique view. The aorta after coursing to the right of the esophagus and trachea and over the right main stem bronchus, descends to the right of the esophagus and trachea until about the level of the ninth thoracic vertebra where it swings to the left to go through the aortic hiatus of the diaphragm. When the aorta descends on the left from a right arch, the radiologic findings are the same in P-A view; the esophagus is indented on its right border. In the right anterior oblique view, however, the esophagus shows an indentation on its posterior aspect (instead of its anterior surface) below the level of the aortic arch where the descending aorta crosses the midline, swinging back to the left side. Neither of these anomalies, right arch with right descending aorta or right arch with left descending aorta is associated with symptoms due to encroachment upon the trachea or esophagus. They should be recognized as one of the anomalies of the great vessels occurring with either normal or congenitally abnormal heart.

Right aortic arch is present in about one-fourth of all Tetralogy of Fallot hearts, and is very frequent in other congenital heart lesions such as tricuspid

atresia. It is also seen in dextrocardia without transposition of other viscera.

SURGICAL SIGNIFICANCE. The recognition of the side of the arch is of importance to the surgeon who must determine which side of the chest should be explored to perform an anastomosis of the subclavian artery or the aorta to the pulmonary artery for congenital cyanotic heart disease. For the Potts-Smith aortic-pulmonary anastomosis, the side of the arch must be known for the aorta is the systemic vessels used, and the procedure on the left arch is technically easier than on the right arch. The Blalock-Taussig Procedure makes use of the subclavian artery preferably, and knowledge of the side of the arch and the probable position of the subclavian artery is desirable.

4. VASCULAR RINGS.* Many other variations occur in the development of the great vessels. Modern roentgenology now contributes much to the detection and diagnosis of these conditions. Anomalous placement of great vessels gives rise to symptoms secondary to encroachment upon the trachea and esophagus. In the infant and young child, wheezing and stridor, bouts of cyanosis, repeated respiratory infections, difficult breathing with retractions, dysphagia and regurgitation may be seen, or symptoms may not begin until late in life when dilatation and loss of elasticity of vessels cause changes in the relationships between the vessels and the trachea and esophagus.

Such symptoms in the young should call for an investigation of the esophagus and trachea by fluoroscopic examination aided by opaque contrast material. Diagnosis can be made from routine roentgenograms by these methods in the majority of cases. In a few instances, visualization of the trachea by the use of Lipiodol is necessary for complete diagnosis. Angiocardiography or retrograde aortography is rarely necessary. Many cases of respiratory difficulty which in previous years would have been blamed on an enlarged thymus are now known to be due to encroachment upon the esophagus and trachea by anomalous vessels.

Many other variations occur in the development of the great vessels. The evanescent character of the six pairs of embryonic arches, which replace each other in rapid transition as the heart ascends in the thorax, supplies the basis for a well recognized series of anomalies in which arrest has occurred at a point that is commonly mirrored in the hearts of the lower orders of vertebrates. The third pair of embryonic arches becomes the carotid arteries. The only embryonic arch that persists in its entirety in the normal human heart is the fourth left, which becomes the definitive aorta; the right fourth arch is normally suppressed in part, the cephalic portion only persisting as the innominate artery. Persistence of both fourth arches in their entire length results in a double aortic arch (Fig. 223 D-1). A right aortic arch may persist with total suppression of the left arch, or the caudal or distal portion of the latter may and usually does, coexist, giving rise to a right aortic arch with persistent left root, or left descending aorta. If suppression of the right or left fourth arch has occurred before the ascent of the subclavian, one of the latter will arise from the descending aorta or thoracic aorta, the right subclavian from a persistent right root, or the left subclavian from a left root, with a resulting aberrant subclavian artery. The sixth arches become the adult pulmonary artery.

Such pressure on the esophagus and trachea is not manifested in the ordinary roentgenogram but it may give clinical manifestations which should cause investigation to be made. Pressure defects on the esophagus and trachea should be looked for under the following conditions:

a. When there is dysphagia.
b. When there is wheezing or stridor. Inherent

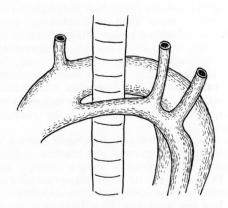

Fig. 223 D-1. Double Aortic Arch.

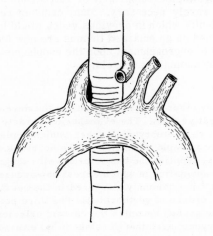

Fig. 223 D-2. Pressure defects on the anterior surface of the trachea may be produced either by a right subclavian artery or by an anomalous position of the innominate passing to the right of the trachea circling around it.

defects in the tracheal structure may produce similar symptoms.

c. When there are recurrent attacks of lung infection or pneumonia.
d. Where there is dyspnoea and retraction of the chest is present.

4 A. DOUBLE AORTIC ARCH*(Fig. 223 E-1, E-2, E-3, E-4). Roentgen examination should be directed at visualizing evidence of abnormal pressure on the tracheal and esophageal walls, and the determination of the side of the more prominent aortic arch and the side of the descending aorta, (E-1 and E-2). The most important finding in this regard is a pressure defect on the posterior surface of the esophagus with anterior esophageal displacement, (E-3 and E-4). If this finding is absent, it is highly improbable that a vascular ring is present, and any symptoms suggesting a vascular ring must be caused by other conditions.

An aberrant subclavian artery, which is not a "vascular ring" can cause symptoms when it passes anterior to the esophagus or anterior to the esophagus and trachea, as well as when it passes posterior to the esophagus. This is the exception to the above statement. An excellent all-inclusive classification of anomalies of the aortic arch has been made by Edwards with the functioning double aortic arch as the basic pattern and with division into two groups depending on the origin of the ductus arteriosus from the right or left pulmonary artery. Kirklin and Clagett and Stones and Effler have devised classification systems based on the finding of the position, either right or left, of the upper portion of the descending aorta. Since the position of the upper descending aorta can be determined roentgenologically, whereas the origin of the ductus can only be inferred, this is a more practical classification. The position of the descending aorta may be detected by observing the position of the esophagus adjacent to the upper portion of the descending aorta. The left descending aorta displaces the esophagus slightly to the right of the midline in its upper half so that the esophagus appears to be close to the right border of the spine in P-A view than the left. The right sided upper descending aorta gives a mirror image of this. Although the ductus arteriosus or the ligamentum arteriosus

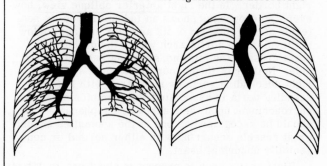

Figs. 223 E-1 and E-2. Pressure defects on trachea and esophagus from vascular ring caused by double aortic arch.

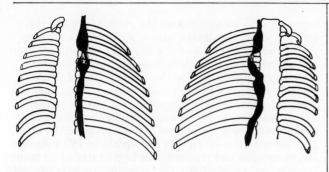

Figs. 223 E-3 and E-4. Compression deformity with forward displacement of esophagus due to double aortic arch.

lies on the same side as the upper descending aorta this is not always true.

In a double aortic arch with upper descending aorta on the left, the right aortic arch is usually the larger and is usually the functioning arch. The left aortic arch may be atretic in whole or in part. If the left arch is completely patent, a true double arch is present. If the vascular ring is sufficiently tight, both esophagus and trachea will be compressed. The right arch runs first to the right of the esophagus producing an indentation on the right side of the esophagus on P-A view. It then runs behind (dorsal to) the esophagus, producing a filling defect on the posterior aspect of the esophagus, seen best in the right anterior oblique position. The left arch may produce an indentation in the left side of the esophagus as seen in P-A view, so that bilateral pressure defects on the esophagus are seen. Filling of the trachea with opaque oil will disclose associated pressure defects on the trachea, usually on the right in P-A view. In the lateral view, there is narrowing and anterior displacement of the trachea at the level of the aortic arch. It may be possible from the appearance of the defects to determine which of the arches is smaller, anterior or posterior, but this is risky, since a small vessel has been known to produce a large defect. Almost always a vascular ring of the double aortic arch has encompassed both esophagus and trachea, but on one occasion the trachea alone was said to be enclosed. Relief of symptoms is obtained by ligation and division of the appropriate portion of the vascular ring.

When the aorta descends on the right, a mirror image to the left descending aorta is present in double aortic arch. The left aortic arch ascends on the left, crosses over the left main stem bronchus, and runs behind (dorsal to) the esophagus. The right arch ascends on the right anterior to the trachea and esophagus and joins the descending aorta after passing over the right main stem bronchus. This anomaly has been observed much less often than double arch with left descending aorta. At fluoroscopy with barium swallow, bilateral indentations are seen on the esophagus in the P-A view. Oblique views show the left arch coursing posterior to the esophagus displacing it anteriorly.

4B. RIGHT AORTIC ARCH and LEFT LIGA-MENTUM ARTERIOSUM, (Fig. 223F) (Neuhauser). Right aortic arch and left ligamentum arteriosum has been observed to produce tracheo-esophageal constriction. The ring in this type is due to a right aortic arch with right descending aorta and a ligamentum arteriosum passing from the right pulmonary artery to the left of the trachea and esophagus and then behind the esophagus to join the thoracic aorta on the right side just below the level of the aortic arch. The aortic arch produces a shallow but definite indentation on the right side of the esophagus in P-A view and LAO view. The findings are very similar to a double aortic arch, but the defect on the posterior margin of the esophagus is described as sufficiently different to indicate that the ligamentum is present, rather than an aortic arch. Relief of symptoms was obtained by division of the ligament.

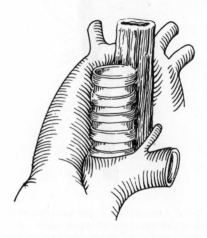

LA.-OBI.

Fig. 223F. Vascular ring produced by right aortic arch and left ligamentum arteriosum—after Neuhauser, Am. J. Roentgenol., 62:493, 1949.

4C. OTHER ANOMALIES OF THE AORTIC ARCH have been observed rarely. The complete and detailed classification of all the possible combinations of the vessels has been amply covered by Edwards. Single cases of unusual double arches, and unusual courses of one or more vessels have been reported: left ascending aorta with right arch and right descending aorta, left aortic arch with right descending aorta and associated with right or left ductus, right arch with left descending aorta associated with a persistent left aortic diverticulum giving origin to the left subclavian and ductus arteriosus. Right descending aorta may be arteriosclerotic; may give impression of mediastinal tumor, (Snider, et al.). Observations of encroachment on esophagus and trachea with a logical consideration of the possibilities in each individual case will be necessary.

5. ANOMALOUS RIGHT SUBCLAVIAN ARTERY*
(Fig. 223 G) may cause compression of the esophagus,
although the great majority are asymptomatic. This
anomaly, one of the most common, is believed to be
the result of abnormal disappearance of the right
fourth arch, the artery developing from a persistent
right dorsal aorta. This aberrant subclavian no
longer communicates with the ascending aorta, but
arises as the last branch from the aortic arch. It
arises usually about 1.5 cm. distal to the origin of the
left subclavian artery, and always courses upward to
the right, causing an imprint on the right posterior-
lateral wall of the esophagus at the level of the third
or fourth thoracic vertebra. The oblique esophageal
defect is above the level of the aortic knob, and is
best seen in P-A and L.A.O. views. The passage of a

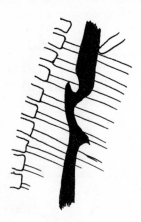

Fig. 223 G-1. Anomalous right subclavian artery as
seen in the right anterior oblique view. An oblique
pressure defect is seen on the posterior and lateral
aspect of the esophagus.

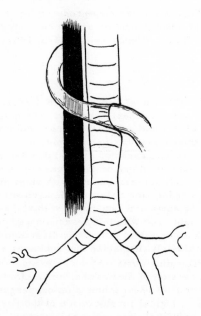

Fig. 223 G-2

ureteral type catheter down the right brachial artery
into the right subclavian artery and aortic arch has
given undoubted proof of the aberrant vessels position
in the living patient. Occasionally, severe lusoria
dysphagia is produced by the vessels; relief is obtained by division of the vessel. Usually this anomaly
does not produce symptoms and is noted as an incidental finding. In 80% of cases studies on anatomical
specimens, the aberrant subclavian crossed the midline between the esophagus and spine, in 15% between
the esophagus and trachea, and in 5% anterior to both
trachea and esophagus. The anterior position has not
yet been described radiographically.

6. AORTIC SEPTAL DEFECT, a very rare
anomaly, presents a picture very similar if not indistinguishable from patent ductus arteriosus (Gasul,
et al.). The abnormal opening in the aorta above the
valves is a communication between the aorta and
either the pulmonary conus or pulmonary artery.
The shunt of blood is from left to right, and cyanosis
is therefore not present. The hemodynamics are
practically the same as those of patent ductus, as
are the clinical, fluoroscopic and roentgenographic
and EKG criteria. Undependable points are a larger
heart than in patent ductus, and a murmur heard beneath the manubrium sterni, rather than the pulmonic
area.

Angiocardiography shows reopacification of the
pulmonary artery after filling of the aorta, but without visualization of the location of the communication
between aorta and pulmonary artery; these findings
are also compatible with patent ductus. Recently,
diagnosis by retrograde aortography has been reported. The contrast material from retrograde
aortography could be seen to enter the pulmonary
artery just above the semilunar valves.

7. ANOMALIES OF THE PULMONARY VEINS.

Return of Pulmonary Vein into Vena Cava or
Right Auricle (Fig. 223 H-1). Rarely anomalous
drainage of the pulmonary veins occurs. That is, one
or more and sometimes all of the pulmonary veins
drain into the right sided structures, the right atrium
or the great systemic veins, rather than into the left
atrium. The clinical and radiologic findings are dependent on whether this drainage is complete or incomplete.

Incomplete or Partial Anomalous Drainage of
the Pulmonary Veins, (Fig. 223 H-2) has clinical and
hemodynamic findings very similar, and often undis-
tinguishable, from atrial septal defect. The right
heart receives an increased blood flow, as does the
pulmonary circulation. The right atrial and ventricle
are enlarged. The pulmonary vessels, both central
and peripheral are large. A shunt of less than 50%
of the blood flow from the lungs into the right heart
is compatible with a normal life.

Cardiac catheterization is diagnositic if a
stream of arterialized blood is found in the vena cava.
A stream of arterialized blood in the right atrium indicates anomalous pulmonary vein return or an atrial
septal defect. Direct evidence is the passage of a
catheter into the anomalous vessel itself from the

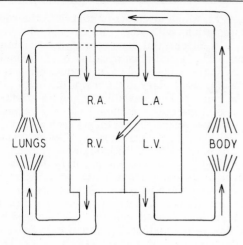

Fig. 223 H-1a.

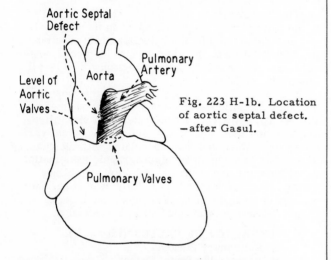

Fig. 223 H-1b. Location of aortic septal defect. —after Gasul.

to be enlarged, the right heart inconspicuous. Cyanosis is present, and a septal defect is necessarily present. Recognition of this anomaly should be a contraindication to surgical removal or collapse of the normal lung which would be disastrous.

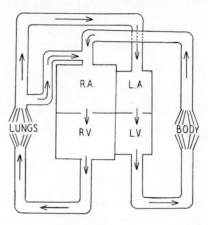

Fig. 223 H-2. Anomalous venous return of pulmonary vein into vena cava.

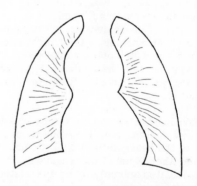

Fig. 223 H-3. "Figure of eight" configuration of complete anomalous pulmonary vein drainage into persistent left superior vena cava.

vena cava. Atrial septal defects may be present as an additional lesion, but are not necessary for survival.

Complete Anomalous Drainage of the Pulmonary Veins is incompatible with life unless there is a communication between right and left hearts. Right atrial and ventricular enlargement and prominence of pulmonary vessels, characteristic of left to right shunts, are present here, too. The aorta is relatively inconspicuous, and the left atrium is not enlarged.

A "figure of eight" appearance of a P-A chest film has been described (Fig. 223 H-3) as characteristic of complete pulmonary vein drainage into a persistent left superior vena cava, which in turn drains into the right superior vena cava via a left innominate vein. The anomalous venous channels form the upper half of the "eight", the cardiac contour, the lower. Confirmation may be obtained by intravenous angiocardiography, but the appearance is so typical it is seldom necessary.

Another anomaly is the entrance of one or both vena cavae into the left auricle. Little is known of this rare malformation. The left heart is reported

8. IDIOPATHIC DILATATION OF THE PULMONARY ARTERY is characterized by a large pulmonary artery without other signs of cardiac abnormality. Heart chamber enlargement is not present. The abnormally large main pulmonary trunk has no increased pulsations. The peripheral pulmonary vasculature is normal. This condition is of clinical importance, because it may be confused with more serious causes of pulmonary artery enlargement, such as pulmonary stenosis or left to right shunts. Angiocardiography and cardiac catheterization may be necessary to completely exclude these possibilities. A rare vascular anomaly of great vessels is an anomalous course of the pulmonary artery producing respiratory symptoms. Roentgenographically this appears as a pressure defect or indenture running across the esophagus similar to an aberrant subclavian attery, (Wittenborg, et al.).

9. ARTERIO-VENOUS FISTULA OF THE LUNG.
This subject is discussed under Chapter on Lung Diseases.

10. ABNORMAL PULMONARY ARTERY ASSOCIATED WITH INTRALOBAR PULMONARY SEQUESTRATION. Intralobar pulmonary sequestration is a partial or complete developmental separation of a portion of a lobe of a lung from its continuity with the normal bronchial tree. In this segment of the lung congenital cystic disease of the lung occurs.

The etiologic factor in intralobar sequestration is an anomalous artery that arises from the lower part of the thoracic or upper portion of the abdominal aorta or from one of the branches of the celiac axis, (Pryce, et al.).

B. ANOMALIES OF CARDIAC POSITION. Dextrocardia or a right-sided heart in which the apex points to the right may occur alone or it may be associated with total transposition of all of the viscera, (Situs Inversus). The heart is anatomically normal except for its being a mirror image. This anomaly is itself of no pathological significance and gives rise to no characteristic symptoms with one very rare exception; a high incidence of nasal sinus disease and bronchiectasis has been observed associated with situs inversus, (Kartagener's triad), suggesting possible congenital origin of bronchiectasis. Diagnosis is no problem if correct marking of the film is assured.

Dextrocardia in which other viscera are not transposed, however, may be associated with other heart defects; its recognition should stimulate search for other cardiac lesions.

DEXTROVERSION, as pointed out by Welsh, is an unusual type of dextrocardia resulting from congenital nonrotation of the heart, differing in its embryologic aspects from other types of dextrocardia. It may occur as an isolated anomaly or be associated with other congenital defects.

The diagnosis may be made on the basis of a normally functioning heart with normal chamber development (as detected by electrocardiogram) and roentgen indication of right-sided heart.

Location of the heart outside of the thorax is extremely rare. Radiological diagnosis is obvious if it should escape physical examination. Associated defects and cyanosis are said to be common.

C. ANOMALIES OF STRUCTURAL DEVELOPMENT OF THE HEART. Great credit must be accorded Maud Abbott whose early investigation and classification of congenital heart lesions is the groundwork upon which our present conceptions have been built. The meticulous work of Helen B. Taussig in analysis of the ordinary heart roentgenogram of the various anomalous congenital heart lesion has done much to advance our knowledge in this intricate diagnostic field. Countless others have approached the subject from various viewpoints in an effort to bring some sort of order out of diagnostic chaos. A "rational guide to the stepwise diagnosis of congenital malformations of the heart" has been recommended by Bing, et al, which attempts to correlate the roentgen manifestations with other clinical and laboratory findings, in a differential diagnosis of various cardiac anomalies. The initial classification is physiological; like most others it is based on an obvious clinical finding, cyanosis. Secondary divisions of the main groups are on the basis of lung vascularity and its effects on the size and shape of the pulmonary artery segment.

With but few exceptions, cyanosis indicates a right to left shunt of the circulation. The secondary differentiation is made on the basis of observable radiologic findings, seen on the ordinary anterior chest roentgenograms, and at fluoroscopic examination in optimum standard positions, indicative of the hemodynamic status. In certain specific conditions the diagnosis may depend upon findings obtained by other methods—for instance, physical examination will disclose a patent ductus arteriosus by a characteristic murmur; cardiac catheterization will be necessary for detection of varying pressure relationship for the diagnosis of pulmonic stenosis; the EKG is the determining diagnostic agent in the diagnosis of tricuspid atresia by the detection of left ventricular preponderance. In other special instances, angiocardiography or retrograde aortography may be all-important methods.

In an effort to simplify the subject, the most important congenital cardiac conditions as outlined by Bing et al., will first be illustrated by a simplified diagram and their anatomical and physiological variations described, and then correlated with the changes which they produce on roentgenographic examination in the anterior and right and left anterior oblique views. After each condition is fully described, a discussion of their differentiation along the lines of Bing's "stepwise diagnosis" will be undertaken.

1. TETRALOGY OF FALLOT*(Fig. 223I).
   a) Pulmonary Stenosis
   b) Ventricular Septal Defect
   c) Right Ventricular Enlargement
   d) Dextroposition of the Aorta

TETRALOGY OF FALLOT

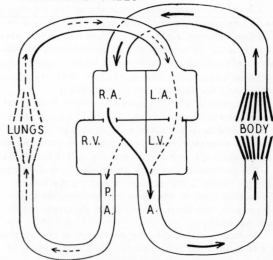

Fig. 223 I-1. Diagram of Circulation.

Table I. CLASSIFICATION OF CONGENITAL HEART DISEASE: CYANOTIC GROUP
(Reproduced with permission of authors and publisher, BING, et al, Correlation of Physiologic,
Radiologic and Electrocardiographic Findings, Ann. Int. Med., 37:664, 1952)

Pulmonary Flow less than Systemic Flow - Pulmonary Artery pressure Usually Decreased

Diagnosis	Fluoroscopic Findings				Electrical preponderance
	Lungs	Size and Shape Heart	Pulm. Window	Pulm. Seg.	
Tetralogy	clear	Elevated Apex, not enlarged, "Coeur en sabot"	clear	concave	right
Pseudotruncus	clear	Enlarged and Boot Shaped	clear	concave	right
Tricuspid Atresia	clear	Concavity of lower right border in PA Projection "Coeur en sabot"	clear	concave	left
Transposition of Great Vessels with Pulmonary Stenosis	clear	Enlarged. Narrow Mediastinal shadow in AP and Lateral positions	hazy	concave	combined heart strain
Ebstein's Disease with Patent Foramen Ovale	clear	Enlarged	hazy	convex	right
Pulm. arterio-venous fistula	round opacities	Enlarged or normal	hazy	convex	right or left with bundle branch block
Patent foramen ovale or auricular septal defect with pulm. stenosis	clear	Slightly enlarged	hazy	convex	right

Pulmonary Flow Greater than Systemic Flow and/or Pulmonary Artery Pressure Normal or Increased

Eisenmengers	vascular	Enlarged	hazy	convex	right
Complete transposition	vascular	Enlarged, Narrow mediastinal shadow in AP, widening in Lateral, absence of aortic knob	hazy		right
Patent ductus with reversed flow	vascular	Enlarged	hazy	convex	right
Truncus Arteriosis	vascular	Enlarged and boot shaped	clear	concave	left or right

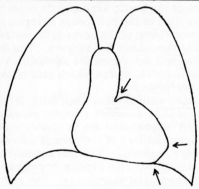

Fig. 2231-2. Tetralogy of Fallot showing "coeur en sabot," enlarged cardiac shadow to left of median line, prominent aorta, blunting and elevation of apex on left border (arrow). Second arrow indicates loss of pulmonary curve.

Table II. CLASSIFICATION OF CONGENITAL HEART DISEASE: NON CYANOTIC GROUP
(Reproduced with permission of authors and publisher, BING, et al, Correlation of Physiologic,
Radiologic and Electrocardiographic Findings, Ann. Int. Med., 37:664, 1952)

Pulmonary Flow Greater than Systemic Flow and/or Pulmonary Artery Pressure Normal or Increased

Diagnosis	Fluoroscopic Findings				Electrical preponderance
	Lungs	Size and Shape Heart	Pulm. Window	Pulm. Seg.	
Isolated Septal defect, auricular, uncomplicated	vascular	Enlarged	hazy	convex	right
Lutembacher's	vascular	Enlarged	hazy	very prominent	right
Ventricular septal defect	vascular	Enlarged, usually	hazy	convex	left or right
Patent ductus	vascular	Enlarged	hazy	convex	normal or left
Aortic septal defect	vascular	Enlarged	hazy		normal or left
Anomalous venous return with pulm. vein emptying into vena cava or right auricle	vascular	Enlarged	hazy	convex	right

Pulmonary Flow Equals Systemic Flow at Rest and After Exercise

Pure pulmonic stenosis	clear	Enlarged	hazy	prominent	right

The pulmonary stenosis dams back the blood into the right ventricle increasing the pressure in this chamber. The ventricular septal defect, usually in the upper portion, serves as an outlet for the blood in the right ventricle, which is under higher pressure, to pass through into the left ventricle. The aorta taking origin from the right ventricle, (dextroposition of the aorta), just above the defect, conveys deficiently oxygenated blood to the body tissues explaining the deep cyanosis.

This is the most common type of cyanotic congenital cardiac disease: It is seen most frequently in children but patients may reach adult life. A prominent feature of the disease is clubbing of the fingers and toes from the anoxemia which accompanies the defect. Polycythemia results as a compensatory feature and the red blood count may go as high as 12,000,000. The pulmonary artery is very hypoplastic.

Angiocardiography by injection of opaque material may give real information in this anomaly.

Pulmonary stenosis with marked reduction of blood to the lungs is usually very evident.

The interventricular septal defect and straddling position of the aorta serve as an easy pathway for opaque material in the right ventricle to escape simultaneously into both the pulmonary artery and the aorta, so that simultaneous appearance of opaque substance in the aorta and pulmonary circulation is evidence of this anomaly.

Tetralogy of Fallot is one of the few cardiac anomalies in which surgical intervention may be of value; accurate diagnosis is therefore essential.

The surgical production of an artificial ductus arteriosus has greatly improved the prognosis in this condition. This is accomplished either by anastomosis of the subclavian and pulmonary arteries (Blalock and Taussig) or of the aorta and pulmonary arteries (Potts, Smith and Gibson). Right-sided aortic arch is present in 20% of cases. Knowledge of the position of the aortic arch and its branches, the size and position of the pulmonary arteries, and the degree of overriding of the aorta is important in evaluation of the patient for surgery. The information obtained will determine the advisability and the type of anastomosis, and on which side of the chest it is to be performed.

On roentgen examination, when fully developed, the cardiac outline assumes a "coeur en sabot" or "boot-shaped" appearance due to elevation and blunting of the apex and loss of the normal convexity of the pulmonary segment. Pulmonary stenosis accompanying the condition also results in clearer lung fields from decreased vascularity. The right ventricle is enlarged, the aorta often dilated.

Angiocardiography demonstration of ventricular septal defect with overriding dextroposed aorta is shown by simultaneous filling of aorta and pulmonary artery with opaque material before left auricle or lung circulation is visualized. The anatomic details of the type of pulmonary stenosis is seen usually this being of the infundibular type or combined infundibular and valvular.

Cardiac Catheterization. Passage of a cardiac catheter from the right ventricle through the ventricular septal defect into the dextroposed aorta is observed. Pulmonary Stenosis is confirmed by the drop from a high pressure in the right ventricle to a low pressure in the pulmonary artery. Dextroposition of the aorta may be recognized by identical systolic pressures in the right ventricle and aorta or brachial artery.

Diagnostic Criteria. Cor en sabot. Loss of normal (concave) pulmonic curve on cardiac silhouette.

Diminution of hilum shadows and scarcity of bronchovascular markings in lung producing abnormally clear lung fields.

2. TRICUSPID ATRESIA (Fig. 223J).
   a) Atresia of Tricuspid Valve
   b) Right Ventricular Hypoplasia
   c) Pulmonary Artery Hypoplasia, and decrease in vascularity of lungs
   d) Left Ventricular Enlargement
   e) Patent Foramen Ovale or Atrial Septal Defect
   f) Patent Ductus Arteriosus or Interventricular Septal Defect or both

In tricuspid stenosis (Fig. 223 J-1) there is little if any blood going to the right ventricle through the tricuspid valve; the blood passes directly through an atrial septal defect or foramen ovale to the left auricle, thence to the left ventricle, and out by way of the aorta. Blood finds its way to the lungs through a ventricular septal defect into the pulmonary artery or via a patent ductus. The vascularity of the lungs decreased and the left ventricle is enormously enlarged.

In clinical course and physical findings, tricuspid atresia is very similar to Tetralogy of Fallot.

Roentgenologically, many of the cases have an appearance identical to Tetralogy of Fallot (Fig. 223 J-2). Other cases have a roentgen appearance of dextrocardia (without situs inversus) with a cardiac configuration similar or identical with that of the mirror image of Tetralogy of Fallot (Fig. 223 J-3). The so-called characteristic appearance of tricuspid atresia has been actually observed only in a minority of cases (Fig. 223 J-4). It consists of diminished convexity or actual concavity of the lower right border of the cardiac silhouette in the anterior view, which is the direct result of the insignificance of the right ventricle. In the left anterior oblique view, the cardiac shadow does not project toward the anterior chest wall beyond the shadow cast by the aorta. The left ventricle fails to clear the spine in the right anterior oblique view. All cases show absent pulmonary segment and clear lung fields and a clear aortic

TRICUSPID ATRESIA

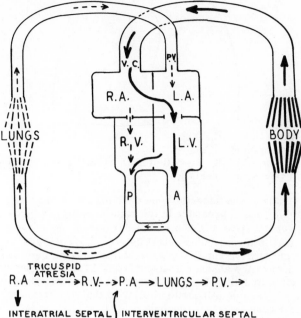

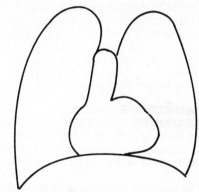

Fig. 223 J-1. Diagram of Circulation.

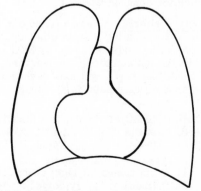

Fig. 223 J-2. Tricuspid atresia having an appearance identical with tetralogy, apex on left.

Fig. 223 J-3. Tricuspid atresia; mirror image to tetralogy, apex on right.

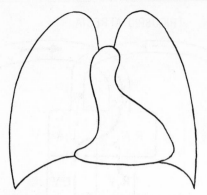

Fig. 223 J-4. So-called characteristic appearance of tricuspid atresia.

window. The superior vena cava may be visible due to increased pressure in the right auricle. Dispro-proportionate right atrial enlargement indicates a small interauricular septal defect. The enlarged right auricle rotates antero-laterally on the right to obscure the absence or hypoplasia of the right ventricle by filling the right border of the heart, produc-ing a cardiac silhouette similar to that of Tetralogy of Fallot.

Astley has described the shape of the left ventricle as characteristic for tricuspidatresia. The apex is rounded and blunt. Angulation and local prominence of the left superior cardiac border in its lateral and dorso-lateral aspects is considered due to the over-lapping of the enlarged left auricular appendage.

Angiocardiography should easily demonstrate the enlarged right atrium and failure of the right ventri-cle to fill with contrast medium. The presence of an interauricular septal defect may be directly demon-strated and its size estimated. The aorta and pul-monary artery both fill from the enlarged left ven-tricle.

Cardiac Catheterization. The Cardiac catheter may be seen passing directly from the right auricle into the left auricle, and it is unlikely that the cathe-ter could be made to enter the underdeveloped right ventricle.

Unless the contrast material is injected into the left ventricle by catheter (Kjellberg) anatomical de-tails of the pulmonary outflow tract will not have much chance for demonstration.

Diagnostic Criteria. A unique feature of tricus-pid atresia differentiating it from other cyanotic heart lesions is left axis deviation on EKG examina-tion, due to the left ventricular hypertrophy. Almost all other conditions have right axis deviation so that this becomes a reliable point in diagnosis.

3. TRANSPOSITION OF GREAT VESSELS, COM-PLETE AND ASSOCIATED WITH PULMONARY STENOSIS (Fig. 223K).
    a) Reversal of great vessels
      1) Aorta comes off right ventricle
      2) Pulmonary Artery comes off left ven-tricle

    b) Communication between right and left sides of heart is either by:
      1) Interventricular septal defect, or
      2) Patent foramen ovale or atrial septal defect
      3) Patent ductus
      4) Combinations of the above.

In this condition the great trunks are completely reversed (K-1 and 2); the aorta comes off of the right ventricle, the pulmonary artery is connected with the left ventricle. It will be seen that the venous blood returning to the right auricle passes into the right ventricle and is then pumped out unaerated again into the systemic circulation. The pulmonary circulation continues to pump aerated blood around and around through the lung. The only aeration which can be ac-complished is through a patent foramen ovale and persistent ductus arteriosus or any septal defect.

This arrangement results in the most profound cyanosis, present from birth, which is ever encoun-tered.

Roentgenological Manifestations, (K-3). The typical roentgenological findings are a narrow shadow of the great vessels in the P-A view, and a large globular heart. When the patient is turned into the left an-terior oblique position, there is a widening of the great vessel shadow, (K-4). The usual convex contour of the pulmonary artery is absent. Both ventricles are increased in size, contributing to the large globular heart. In contrast to most cyanotic lesions, the pulmonary vascular markings are prominent and hilar pulsations may be seen. When pulmonary sten-osis co-exists, however, the vascular lung markings are inconspicuous and differentiation from other con-ditions may be more difficult.

Angiocardiography. The most reliable sign of transposition of the great vessels demonstrated by angiocardiography is an anteriorly placed aorta with a high concentration of the radiopaque agent, at the same time the right ventricle has a high concentra-tion, best seen in the lateral view. The more com-plete the transposition, the more anterior is the ori-gin of the aorta. Associated ventricular or atrial septal defects may be demonstrated.

Diagnostic Criteria
1. Large globular heart (P-A view); enlargement of both ventricles.
2. Narrow shadow great vessels, becoming wider on rotation into left anterior oblique position.
3. Pulmonary artery segment concave.
4. Contrary to most cyanotic lesions, pulmonary vascular markings are prominent and hilar pulsation may be seen (unless pulmonary stenosis coexists).
5. On angiocardiography in lateral view; anterior-ly placed aorta with high concentration of radiopaque agent concurrently with filling of right ventricle.

TRANSPOSITION OF GREAT VESSELS
WITH HIGH INTERVENTRICULAR SEPTAL DEFECT

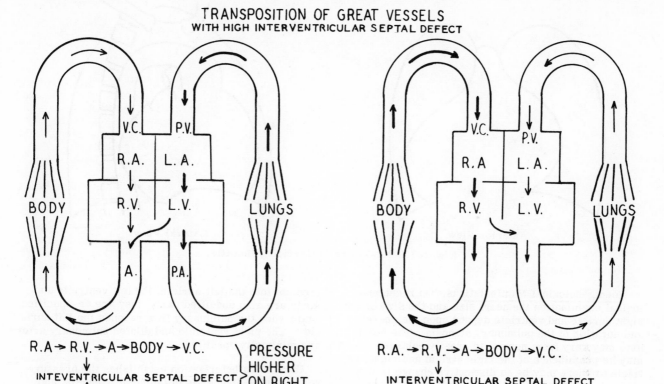

R.A → R.V. → A → BODY → V.C. \
↓ \
INTEVENTRICULAR SEPTAL DEFECT \
↑ \
L.A → L.V. → P.A. → LUNGS → P.V.

PRESSURE HIGHER ON RIGHT SIDE THAN LEFT THEN:

R.A. → R.V. → A → BODY → V.C. \
↓ \
INTERVENTRICULAR SEPTAL DEFECT \
↓ \
L.A. → L.V. → P.A. → LUNGS → P.V.

Fig. 223 K-1. Diagrams of Circulation.

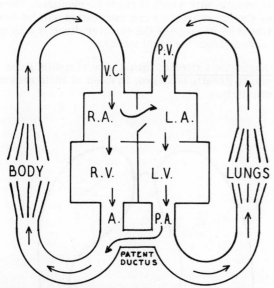

FORAMEN OVALE INTERMITTENTLY OPENS AND CLOSES DEPENDING ON THE RELATIVE PRESSURES IN THE RIGHT AND LEFT ATRIA WITH PATENT DUCTUS AND PATENT FORAMEN OVALE

Fig. 223 K-2. Diagram of Circulation.

Surgical treatment. Survival is short, and surgical creation of additional extracardiac and intracardiac shunts has not been very promising.

4. PULMONIC STENOSIS WITH AURICULAR SEPTAL DEFECTS, (Fig. 223L).
   a) Patentforamen ovale or auricular septal defect.
   b) Post Stenotic Dilatation of Pulmonary artery and its main branches.
   c) Normal or diminished lung circulation.
   d) Right Heart Enlargement.

When pulmonic stenosis is severe, increase in the right heart effort leads to right ventricular and auricular enlargement. The pressure in the right ventricle is high and the chamber wall hypertrophies. After a period of time, the right auricular pressure increases and the chamber dilates. If a septal defect is already present, a right to left shunt occurs. If no defect is originally present, stretching of the right auricle will cause the foramen ovale to become patent, allowing a similar right to left shunt.

Clinically the resulting cyanosis which may have been mild at birth becomes progressively worse. Dyspnea, physical incapacity and attacks of loss of consciousness are observed.

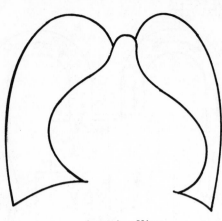

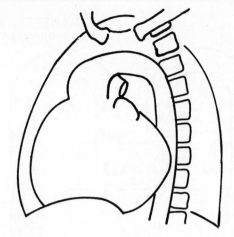

Anterior View   Lateral View

Fig. 223 K-3. Outline of Cardiac Silhouette.

<u>Roentgenological Manifestations</u>. On roentgenological examination the heart size and the size of the right auricle and ventricle depend upon the degree and duration of the pulmonary stenosis. The heart size may vary from normal to greatly enlarged; there may be prominence of the right atrium and right ventricle or there may be no distinctive change in their size. A prominence of the main pulmonary artery known as post stenotic dilatation with decreased or normal lung vascularity is characteristic. Decreased amplitude of pulsations in the right and left pulmonary arteries and increased amplitude of pulsations in the dilated main pulmonary artery is a cardinal feature, whether or not there is a right to left shunt.

<u>Angiocardiography</u> reveals a simultaneous filling of both auricles, evidence of the auricular defect and right to left shunt. With the early flow of contrast medium into the left auricle, the left ventricle and aorta are also opacified early; they are re-opacified again when the pulmonary flow reaches the left auricle. The right ventricle and dilated pulmonary artery are minimally opacified.

<u>Cardiac catheterization</u> establishes the pressure relationships diagnostic of pulmonic stenosis, and excludes a left to right shunt. Pressure changes indicative of pulmonary stenosis are recorded as the catheter is passed from right ventricle to pulmonary artery. The exclusion of left to right shunts is important in differentiating this lesion from other heart lesions with which it might be confused. Sometimes the interauricular communication will be demonstrated by passage of the catheter directly into the left auricle from the right auricle.

<u>Diagnostic Criteria</u>: Heart size variable, from normal to greatly enlarged; in itself of little help in differentiation.

PULMONARY STENOSIS WITH PATENT FORAMEN
OVALE OR AURICULAR SEPTAL DEFECT

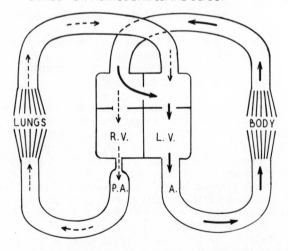

Fig. 223 L-1. Diagram of Circulation.

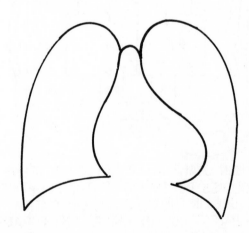

Fig. 223 L-2. Outline of Cardiac Silhouette.

Prominence of main pulmonary artery.
Decrease or normal lung vascularity.
Angiocardiography may be determining factor.

Surgical Consideration. The importance of differentiating pulmonic stenosis with intact ventricular septum from pulmonic stenosis with ventricular septal defect and dextroposed aorta is brought out when inappropriate surgery is performed under an incorrect diagnosis. Brock introduced the direct treatment of pulmonic stenosis (with intact ventricular septum) of pulmonary valvulotomy, obtaining excellent results. A Blalock or Potts-Smith procedure appropriate in pulmonary stenosis with ventricular septal defect and overriding aorta or with associated tricuspid atresia, when performed on "pure pulmonics" increases the strain on the right heart by elevating left auricular pressure and tending to close the valve of the foramen ovale. Rather than benefit, congestive cardiac failure supervenes.

5. Ebsteins anomaly consists of downward displacement of the tricuspid valve. It is a rare anomaly, but has a typical appearance (Fig. 223 L-3). The right atrium is greatly dilated and thin-walled. With the proximal portion of the right ventricle it forms a huge chamber which has weak pulsations, and empties poorly. The right ventricle receives a reduced blood flow. A right to left shunt may occur through a foramen ovale or interauricular septal defect. The heart is enlarged and globular with an appearance resembling pericardial effusion. The pulmonary segment is concave and pulsations in the pulmonary artery are absent due to the low pulmonary blood flow. The lung fields are abnormally clear.

Angiocardiography, although not needed for diagnosis reveals the enormous size and slow emptying of the right atrium. Some radiopaque material may be seen to go through the auricular septal defect.

Cardiac Catheterization: The catheter may be passed directly from the right to left auricles, when a septal defect exists. The catheter will indicate the large atrium from its coiling in this huge chamber.

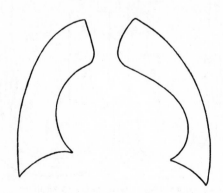

Fig. 223 L-3. Ebsteins disease with huge dilated right atrium.

6. TRUNCUS ARTERIOSUS (Fig. 223M).
   a) Aorta and pulmonary artery form single large arterial trunk.
   b) Overrides ventricular septal defect.
   c) Branches to send blood to both pulmonary and systemic circulations.
   d) Enlargement of both ventricles.

TRUNCUS ARTERIOSUS features a single great vessel combining the function of both aorta and pulmonary artery, receiving blood from both ventricles and carrying it to both systemic and pulmonary circulations. The associated incidence of a three cham-

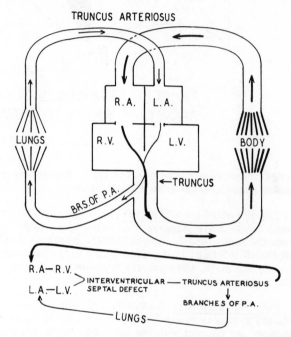

Fig. 223 M-1. Diagram of Circulation.

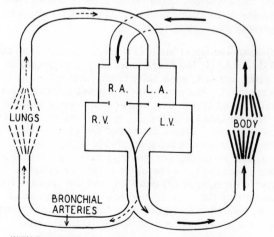

WITH THE BRONCHIAL ARTERIES AS ONLY SOURCE OF BLOOD SUPPLYING LUNGS CYANOSIS EVEN MORE MARKED

Fig. 223 M-2. Diagram of Circulation.

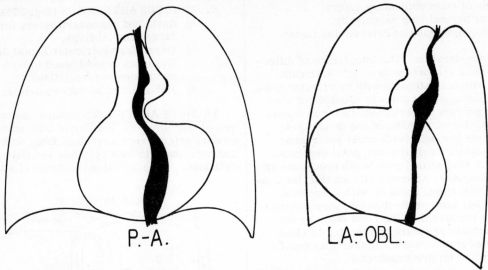

P.-A.   LA.-OBL.

TRUNCUS ARTERIOSUS WITH CIRCULATION TO LUNGS BY BRONCHIAL ARTERIES. INFANT. (AFTER TAUSSIG)

Figs. 223 M-3 and M-4.   X-ray Drawing.

bered or two chambered heart is high. The single vessel overrides the ventricular septum.

TRUE TRUNCUS ARTERIOSUS. When circulation to the lungs is via pulmonary arteries which arise from the main vessel, the condition is known as TRUE TRUNCUS ARTERIOSUS. Circulation to the lungs is usually adequate, and cyanosis is minimal. Roentgenologically the lung fields are vascular.

PSEUDO-TRUNCUS ARTERIOSUS. When a pulmonary artery is present and proceeds to the lungs but does not connect with the heart and aorta, the condition is known as PSEUDO-TRUNCUS ARTERIOSUS. The atretic pulmonary artery can carry no blood to the lungs, so pulmonary circulation is maintained by bronchial arteries. Such circulation is inadequate, resulting in intense cyanosis. The lung fields are relatively avascular, (Taussig).

Roentgenological manifestations: In both true and pseudo-truncus, the heart in infancy is enlarged to the right and left, especially from right ventricular enlargement. The single large vessel is prominent, usually found on the left, and conspicuously indents the barium-filled esophagus. In the Left Anterior Oblique position, Taussig describes the greatly enlarged right ventricle as making an abrupt angle with the aorta, and extending horizontally outward to the anterior chest wall. In the older child, the heart assumes a more vertical position, and the appearance is more like the boot-shaped heart of Tetralogy of Fallot, but tends to a greater enlargement. The pulmonary segment and pulmonary window are clear.

Angiocardiography may show the single trunk.

Surgical Treatment: An anastomosing operation such as the Blalock-Taussig is strongly indicated.

7. EISENMENGER COMPLEX (Fig. 223N).
   a) Same as Tetralogy of Fallot without pulmonary stenosis.
      1) High interventricular septal defect.
      2) Overriding dextroposed aorta.
      3) Minimal right ventricular enlargement except that there is no pulmonary stenosis.
   b) The pulmonary artery is normal or dilated and the lung fields vascular.

This is an uncommon but distinct entity; (A) consists of high interventricular septal defect, a dextroposed aorta, minimal right ventricular hypertrophy,

EISENMENGER'S SYNDROME

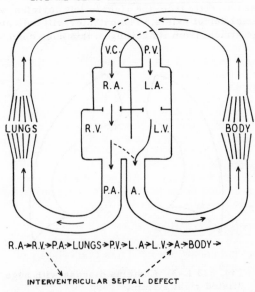

R.A→R.V.→P.A.→LUNGS→P.V.→L.A.→L.V.→A.→BODY→

INTERVENTRICULAR SEPTAL DEFECT

Fig. 223N-1. Diagram of Circulation.

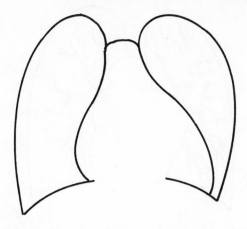

Fig. 223 N-2. Outline of Cardiac Silhouette.

and a normal or dilated pulmonary artery. It differs from the Tetralogy of Fallot in that the pulmonary artery is not stenotic, and the lung fields show normal or increased vascularity.

Cyanosis is frequently delayed. Cyanosis is not completely explained by a right to left shunt through the interventricular septal defect and the overriding aorta and secondary changes in the lungs have been suggested as a cause (Taussig).

Roentgenological Manifestations: (B) The roentgenographic appearance is related to the size of the pulmonary artery. When the pulmonary artery is normal the heart is of normal configuration or is boot-shaped, and may be enlarged. When the pulmonary artery is enlarged, the heart configuration resembles that of the Lutembacher syndrome or a mitral stenosis with pronounced fullness of the pulmonary conus, pulmonary artery, and right ventricle. The hilar vessels are prominent and are seen to pulsate differentiating this complex from Tetralogy, and isolated pulmonary stenosis.

Angiocardiography will show simultaneous visualization of the overriding aorta and the pulmonary arteries which are enlarged and engorged peripherally as well as centrally. The absence of pulmonary stenosis is confirmed by cardiac catheterization pressure studies.

Cardiac Catheterization: Cardiac catheterization is most important in differentiating Eisenmenger's complex from other cyanotic lesions. Absence of pulmonary stenosis is diagnostic when other radiographic and angiocardiographic findings are very similar to Tetralogy of Fallot. Identical pressures are recorded in the pulmonary artery, aorta, and right ventricle.

Diagnostic Criteria:
1. All elements of Tetralogy of Fallot are present except pulmonary stenosis and avascularity of the lung fields.
2. Instead, pulmonary artery is normal or dilated and the lung fields are vascular.

Surgical Consideration:
The necessity of differentiation of Eisenmenger's complex is clear if it is recalled that, with no diminution of pulmonary blood blow, the surgical creation of an artificial ductus arteriosus is not indicated but contraindicated.

8. AURICULAR SEPTAL DEFECT*(Fig. 223 O-1 and O-2) and LUTEMBACHER SYNDROME (Fig. 223 O-3 and O-4).
 a) Auricular septal defect.
 b) Marked right heart enlargement, both auricle and ventricle.

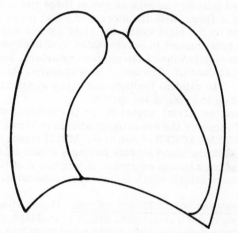

Fig. 223 O-1. Outline of Cardiac Silhouette.

AURICULAR SEPTAL DEFECT

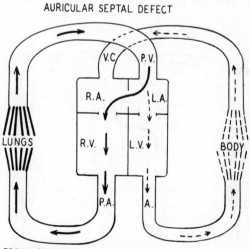

PRESSURE HIGHER L.A. THAN R.A
BLOOD FLOW:
R.A.→R.V.→P.A.→LUNGS→P.V.→L.A.→L.V.→A.→BODY→V.C.→R.A.
THROUGH AURICULAR SEPTAL DEFECT

Fig. 223 O-2. Circulation Diagram.

c) Pulmonary artery enlargement and increased activity - hilar dance. When associated with mitral stenosis (Lutembacher Syndrome) the pulmonary artery becomes enormous.
d) Lung fields vascular.
e) Small aortic knob.

The shunt of blood through the interauricular defect is predominantly from left to right since pressure in the left auricle is greater than in the right.
When the right auricle has an increased pressure due
to other anomalies, the flow is from right to left.
With the flow of blood from left to right, cyanosis is
not present. There results an increased work load
on the right heart with the pulmonary blood flow increased possibly as high as two to three times the
systemic flow. With the increased blood volume
pumped by the right heart, the right auricle and ventricle enlargement is accompanied by dilatation and
increased pulsation of the pulmonary artery, known
as "hilar dance." The aortic now appears relatively
small. The clinical findings and x-ray appearance
depend on the size of the defect.

When an atrial septal defect is combined with
mitral stenosis the resulting condition is known as
the LUTEMBACHER Syndrome. Mitral stenosis
dams back the blood stream putting a strain on the
right heart, causing enormous enlargement of the
pulmonary artery which is quite characteristic.

Roentgenological Manifestations: Outstanding
features of auricular septal defect are: 1) the marked
enlargement of both right auricle and ventricle as
seen in the anterior and right anterior oblique views,
2) in pure septal defect, the increase in size of pulmonary arteries and hilar shadows may not be re-

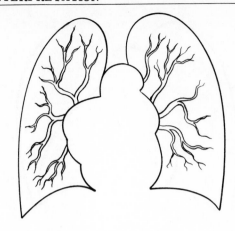

Lutembacher's Syndrome showing pronounced
fullness of pulmonary conus, prominent
hilar vessels and vascular lung fluid.

Fig. 2230-4

markable.

The roentgenographic picture is not pathognomic,
since any other circulatory abnormality which results in an increased resting blood flow or pressure
in the pulmonary circulation without an accompanying
disturbance in the systemic circuit will produce an
x-ray picture indistinguishable from that of interauricular septal defect. These are: Eisenmenger's
complex, cor pulmonale, patent ductus arteriosus and
large interventricular septal defect and anomalous
drainage of pulmonary veins. If a left heart lesion is
not present, the left auricle and ventricle are of normal size.

Angiocardiography shows the enlarged right atrium
and right ventricle and the large pulmonary artery,
while the left sided structures are of normal size.
Antero-posterior view is the best position for angiocardiography in the adult. The auricular defect is
seldom visualized since the shunt is from left to right,
except in children where the right sided temporary increase in pressure from the rapid injection of contrast medium may reverse the flow.

Cardiac Catheterization. Detection of arterialized
blood in the right atrium is diagnostic for a left to
right interauricular shunt. The interauricular communication is sometimes demonstrated by direct passage of the catheter from right to left atrium.

Diagnostic Criteria: The outstanding feature of
this condition is the pronounced enlargement of the
pulmonary artery with transmitted hyperactive pulsations - "hilar dance." Associated right heart enlargement.

LUTEMBACHER'S SYNDROME

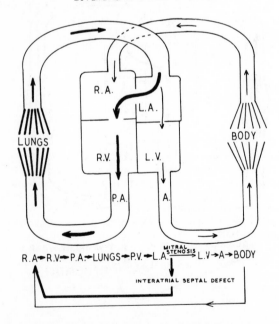

Fig. 2230-3. Diagram of Circulation.

VENTRICULAR SEPTAL DEFECT (MALADIE DE ROGER):
SMALL DEFECT, USUALLY NEAR BASE OF SEPTUM

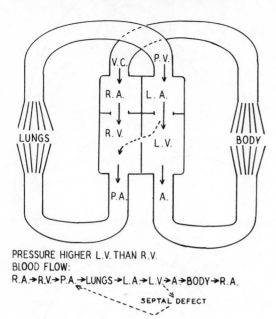

PRESSURE HIGHER L.V. THAN R.V.
BLOOD FLOW:
R.A.→R.V.→P.A.→LUNGS→L.A.→L.V.→A→BODY→R.A.
                              SEPTAL DEFECT

Fig. 223 P-1. Circulation Diagram.

HIGH VENTRICULAR SEPTAL DEFECT: AT BASE OF AORTA IN
THE MEMBRANOUS PORTION OF THE SEPTUM

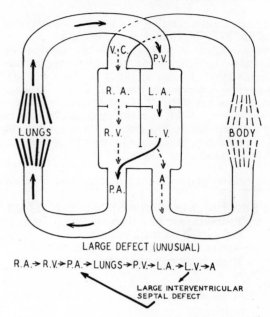

LARGE DEFECT (UNUSUAL)
R.A.→ R.V.→P.A.→ LUNGS→P.V.→L.A.→L.V.→A
                              LARGE INTERVENTRICULAR
                              SEPTAL DEFECT

Fig. 223 P-3. Circulation Diagram.

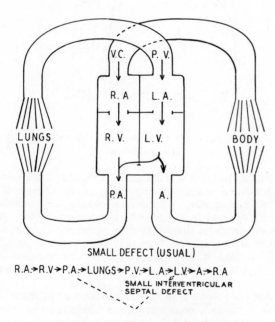

SMALL DEFECT (USUAL)
R.A.→R.V→P.A.→LUNGS→P.V.→L.A.→L.V.→A.→R.A
                              SMALL INTERVENTRICULAR
                              SEPTAL DEFECT

Fig. 223 P-2. Circulation Diagram.

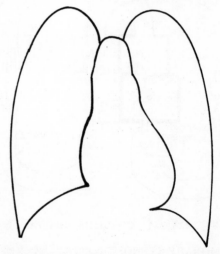

Fig. 223 P-4. Outline of Cardiac Silhouette.

9. VENTRICULAR SEPTAL DEFECTS (MALADIE DE ROGER) (Fig. 223P).

    a) Of small size, usually at base of septum.
    b) High ventricular septal defect; at base of the aorta, in the membranous portion of the septum.

VENTRICULAR SEPTAL DEFECTS of small size (Maladie de Roger) are seldom associated with char-acteristic x-ray findings (P-1). Only a small volume of blood is shunted from left to right hearts. The cardiac size and shape are normal. Cardiac catheterization is the best diagnostic means for interventricular septal defects.

When a high ventricular septal defect is present, the aortic septum fails to meet the ventricular septum, the left ventricle may pump a large volume of blood directly into the pulmonary artery. The pulmonary artery then becomes greatly dilated and the pulsations conspicuous. Both ventricles hypertrophy, (Taussig).

Roentgenological Consideration: Small septal defects rarely show any roentgenological evidence. In larger defects the fluoroscopic and roentgenographic findings closely resemble an auricular septal defect as previously described.

Cardiac catheterization is the best diagnostic means for interventricular septal defects.

The possibility of diagnosing an interventricular septal defect by detecting an increased oxygen content in the right ventricular blood as compared to the right auricle depends on the size of the opening. Small defects are difficult to detect and the procedure is unnecessary. A left to right shunt can be observed along with pulmonary hypertension in large defects, and the procedure is indicated when this lesion must be differentiated from others.

Angiocardiography is usually of no diagnostic value.

10. PURE PULMONARY STENOSIS (Fig. 223 Q).
   a) Post-stenotic dilatation of main pulmonary artery and its main branches.
   b) Normal or diminished lung vascularity.
   c) Right ventricular and atrial enlargement.

PURE PULMONARY STENOSIS

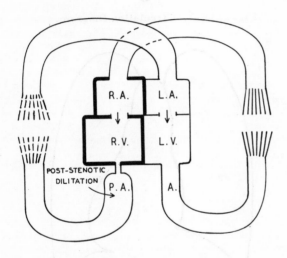

Fig. 223 Q-1. Circulation Diagram.

PULMONARY STENOSIS occurs most often in association with other defects, which have already been discussed, but it also occurs in a pure state, with overriding aorta and with intact ventricular septum. (Pulmonary stenosis with atrial septal defect is discussed on page 331.)

Pulmonary stenosis is valvular or infundibular in type. Infundibular stenosis may be circumscribed with the formation of a chamber, known as the third ventricle, or the entire length of the infundibulum may be narrowed and constricted. The right ventricle becomes hypertrophied in an effort to maintain cardiac output through the stenotic area. Secondarily the right atrium becomes enlarged and hypertrophied.

Clinical Symptoms: The clinical picture of PUL-

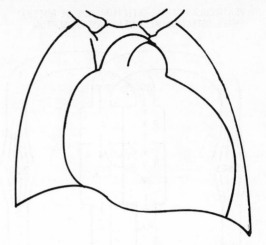

Fig. 223 Q-2. Pure Pulmonary Stenosis, Anterior View.

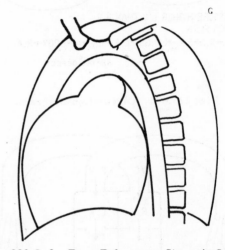

Fig. 223 Q-3. Pure Pulmonary Stenosis Severe, Lateral View.

MONIC STENOSIS WITH CLOSED SEPTA varies from no to severe symptoms depending on the degree of pulmonic stenosis. With mild stenosis, the individual may be normal in his activity and non-cyanotic. With severe stenosis, disability may be marked and cyanosis of the peripheral type may be observed. Associated septal defects account for severe cyanosis or late development of cyanosis from right to left shunts.

Roentgenologic: In valvular stenosis the main trunk of the pulmonary artery is dilated and has increased pulsations, but the peripheral lung vessels are narrowed. The right ventricle and atrium are enlarged, and hypertrophied depending on the severity of the stenosis. Infundibular stenosis may show these findings too, but they are not often characteristic and vary much more.

Angiocardiography confirms the enlargement of the main trunk of the pulmonary artery. The anatomy of the stenosis, whether valvular or infundibular, can be demonstrated, best in the lateral view and with six exposures per second, (Kjellberg).

Cardiac catheterization is the most reliable method of diagnosing pulmonic stenosis. An increased right ventricular pressure is recorded with a low or normal pulmonary arterial pressure. Fluoroscopic examination of the exact location of pressure change as the catheter is introduced or withdrawn will help in determining the presence of a valvular or infundibular stenosis. Study of oxygen content of blood samples from the right heart demonstrates the absence of septal defects.

Diagnostic Criteria: Prominence of the main pulmonary trunk; clear lung fields; right ventricular and atrial enlargement are confirmatory help in diagnosis. Diagnosis made by catheterization, but anatomic details can be supplied by angiography.

PRIMARY PULMONARY HYPERTENSION is not a cardiac lesion, but the primary defect in the lung vasculature results in cardiac changes which may be confused with other heart lesions. This condition is rare. Its importance is its resemblance to other forms of pulmonary hypertension, occurring secondarily to congenital cardiac lesions, such as PDA and VSD which are amenable to surgery. Radiologically, an enlarged right ventricle and a dilated, pulsatile main pulmonary artery are seen. The peripheral lung vessels are narrowed. The radiologist's diagnosis is made on the basis of exclusion of other heart lesions which are capable of producing pulmonary hypertension. Complete accuracy in the making of this diagnosis, requires catheterization to exclude a left to right shunt, or the pressure relationships of pulmonic stenosis. Angiocardiography offers aid in exclusion of a shunt.

11. OTHER TYPES OF CONGENITAL HEART DISEASE. Roentgenological examination plays a relatively minor role in the diagnosis of other types of congenital heart disease. AORTIC and SUBAORTIC STENOSIS produce left ventricular hypertrophy, and an ascending aorta which shows dilatation and increased pulsations.

ANEURYSM OF SINUS OF VALSAVA. Aneurysm of the left Sinus of Valsalva extends through the ventricular septum, finally rupturing into the right ventricle producing a left to right shunt.

The presence of the aneurysm causes little if any demonstrable effect upon the heart up to the time of rupture. There is no cyanosis. Rupture establishes a left-to-right shunt causing rapid enlargement of the heart and death.

Clinical Manifestations may be practically absent up to the time of rupture of the aneurysm which is attended with sudden pain. The clinical course is progressively downward after rupture has taken place.

Roentgenologically there is rapid, progressive general dilatation of the heart without other distinctive features.

CONGENITAL IDIOPATHIC HYPERTROPHY produces an enlarged heart. ORIGIN OF THE CORONARY ARTERIES FROM THE PULMONARY ARTERY is characterized by an increase in cardiac size, mainly left ventricle enlargement. IDIOPATHIC DILATATION OF THE PULMONARY ARTERIES occurs showing only large pulmonary vessels. The pulmonary conus is enlarged, the right ventricle less obviously so. The shadows of the pulmonary arteries may even simulate a mediastinal tumor. Angiocardiography demonstrates the dilated pulmonary vessels and with the help of cardiac catheterization excludes other lesions which are also characterized by right heart, pulmonary conus, and pulmonary artery enlargement and increased hilar pulsations.

Three chambered hearts are of two types: 1) COR TRILOCULARE BI-VENTRICULARIS (Fig. 223S) (having a common auricle and two ventricular chambers), has radiographic findings very similar to hearts with large interauricular septal defects. Cyanosis depends on the amount of mixture of blood. 2) COR TRILOCULARE BI-ATRIATUM, (having two auricles but a single ventricle), is characterized by dyspnea and cyanosis. The amount of oxygenated blood and the pulmonary findings vary, depending on the position of the great vessels. When the pulmonary artery arises from a rudimentary outflow chamber, little blood will be pumped into it. The hilar shadows will be insignificant and cyanosis intense. When the pulmonary artery is filled from the main ventricle, cyanosis is less and the hilar shadows are prominent. In either case, the heart is enlarged. Angiocardiography may demonstrate the single ventricle. Most of the patients succumb early, the ones with more adequate pulmonary blood flow surviving longer.

COR BI-LOCULARE (two chambers only) also shows an enlarged heart. Although the heart may be huge, the appearance is not distinctive. If the communications between the chambers are small, as in persistent ostium atrioventricularis communis, there may be little cyanosis and the heart is not unusual in size or shape.

AORTIC ATRESIA seldom presents a diagnostic problem because the patients live only a few days.

In CONGENITAL MITRAL STENOSIS OR ATRESIA, the left ventricle is non-functional. The right heart and the pulmonary conus are enlarged,

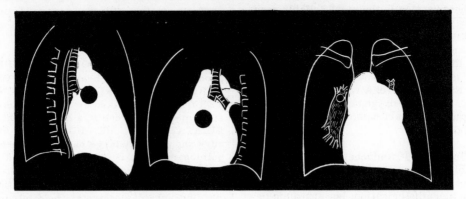

Fig. 223S. Interauricular septal defect and cor triloculare biventriculare give similar pictures depending upon the size of the defect.

but the roentgenographic appearance is not diagnostic (Taussig; Schnitker).

D. Diagnostic Approach; Roentgen Survey and Analysis of Congenital Cardiac Defects:

A cursory survey of the vast amount of clinical, radiological and laboratory data which is involved in the diagnosis of congenital heart disease is convincing evidence of the need for some means of correlation of the data if any consistency in diagnosis is to be accomplished.

More detailed analysis of certain elements in the roentgenological findings as outlined in Bing's tables may further assist in determining the ultimate diagnosis: vascularity of the lung fields, indicating the degree and character of pulmonary engorgement, may be a valuable aid in the primary division of cardiac anomalies into various groups; the shape and size of the cardiac shadow due to various chamber enlargements and the character of the pulmonic curve indicating the size of the pulmonary artery may be valuable in the final analysis.

In order to carry out this step-wise method of roentgen diagnosis, the roentgenogram must be examined for the presence of the various elements utilized for analysis in the tables; they must be evaluated and actually noted upon separate pieces of paper for each category examined. Further correlation of roentgen findings as shown in the various tables should then be made as an aid in establishing the ultimate diagnosis. This compilation of the same data in different groups for more ready comparison and analysis will naturally result in considerable repetition, but that is unavoidable.

Other special methods of examination such as electrocardiographic findings, angiocardiography and cardiac catheterization may have to be resorted to at times in an effort to make a final diagnosis.

Correlation of cardiac conditions with the degree of vascularity of the lung fields will indicate at once that they fall into several more or less distinct categories. It will be noted that, as a rule, clear lung fields (indicating a reduction in blood supply) usually go with a concave, (depleted) pulmonary artery seg-

ment and a relatively small heart, where as, vascular lung fields are usually associated with a convex pulmonary artery segment and an enlarged heart. This serves at once to partially divide the conditions under consideration. Of the convex pulmonary segment-vascular lung group, only one (complete transposition of the great vessels) is cyanotic; of the concave pulmonary segment-clear lung group, all are cyanotic.

It will be noted that in only three conditions, Ebstein's Disease, Pulmonary Stenosis with auricular septal defect, and Pure pulmonary stenosis, there are clear lung fields associated with a convex (dilated) pulmonary artery segment; this is explained by post-stenotic dilatation of the pulmonary artery not by increased blood flow. Of these only one, (pure pulmonary stenosis), is non-cyanotic.

Vascularity of the lung fields and concavity (depletion) of the pulmonary segment is present in two conditions,— Eisenmenger's and Truncus Arteriosus, — in neither case is it associated with any undue cardiac enlargement; in both instances the heart appears boot-shaped and both show cyanosis.

Convexity of the pulmonary artery segment is usually associated with cardiac enlargement. Enlargement of the pulmonary artery likewise is usually accompanied by increase in lung vascularity with the following exceptions:

Ebstein's Disease
Pulmonary Stenosis
    with auricular septal defect
Pure Pulmonary Stenosis

In these conditions, although the pulmonary artery is large (convex), the lung fields appear clear (avascular). This is due to post-stenotic dilatation of the pulmonary artery—"the Venturi principle, which states that if a stream bed gradually widens after a constriction the lateral pressure in the distal, wider tube is higher than in the constricted portion " (Wiggers). Of these Ebstein's disease and Pulmonary Stenosis with auricular septal defect or patent foramen ovale are cyanotic; pure pulmonary stenosis is noncyanotic. In Ebstein's disease cyanosis is delayed and symptoms may be mild; it is rarely diagnosed during life. Angiocardiographic studies may

TABLE III
VASCULARITY OF LUNG FIELDS

	DIAGNOSIS	HEART SIZE	PUL. ARTERY SEGMENT	LUNG FIELD	PULMONIC WINDOW	ANGIOCARDIOGRAPHY-CATHETERIZATION**	EKG PREPONDERANCE
CYANOTIC	Tetralogy of Fallot	Small Boot-Shaped	*Concave	Clear	Clear	Simultaneous filling aorta and pulmonary artery. Catheterization: Pressure changes indication of pulmonary stenosis. Catheter may pass from right ventricle into aorta	Right
	Pseudo-Truncus	Slight enlargement, both ventricles boot-shaped	Concave	Clear; post. mediastinal veins may be engorged	Clear	Right ventricle enlarged; may show single trunk	Right
	Tricuspid Atresia	May be boot-shaped, show typical concave right border	Concave	Clear	Clear	Failure right ventricle to fill. Right to left auricular shunt. Difficulty passing catheter into right ventricle	Left
	Transposition with Pulmonary Stenosis	When heart is not enlarged resembles Tetralogy of Fallot	Concave	Clear	Hazy	Pulmonary Artery extremely small	Right
	Ebstein's Disease	Enlarged	Convex (due to post stenotic dilatation)	Clear	Hazy	Very large slowly emptying auricle. Patent foramen ovale. Catheter may pass from right into left auricle	Right or Left Bundle Branch Block
	Pul. Stenosis with Auricular Septal Defect	Slight Enlargement	Convex (due to post stenotic dilatation)	Clear	Hazy	Early opacity left auricle; ventricle and aorta showing right to left auricle shunt. Catheterization establishes relationships diagnostic of pulmonary stenosis; excludes left to right shunt	Right
NON	Pure Pulmonic Stenosis	Enlarged	Convex-Prominent (due to post stenotic dilatation)	Clear	Hazy	Useful only to exclude septal defects and overriding aorta. Increased right ventricular pressure with low or normal pulmonary artery pressure	Right
CYANOTIC	Eisenmenger's	Both ventricles slightly enlarged. Appearance resembles boot-shape	Concave	Vascular	Clear	Angiocardiogram: Simultaneous visualization of overriding aorta and pulmonary arteries which are enlarged both centrally and peripherally. Absence of pulmonary stenosis based on pressure relationships	----
	Truncus Arteriosus	Slightly enlarged, boot-shaped	Concave	Vascular	Clear	Right ventricle enlarged; may show single trunk. Oxygen sat. of value in diagnosis	----
	Complete Transposition Great Vessels	Enlarged; Narrow Mediastinum; absent. Aortic Knob	Convex	Vascular	Hazy	Lateral view; aorta arises right ventricle anteriorly in PA view: aorta forms left cardiac border	Right
NON-CYANOTIC	Auricular Septal Defect	Enlarged	Convex	Vascular	Hazy	Right heart enlargement. Pulmonary artery enlarged. Left to right shunt determined by O_2 concentration in right auricle. Catheter may go thru auricular defect	Right
	Lutembacher's	Enlarged	Convex	Vascular	Hazy	Usually not necessary; pulmonary artery enormous	Right
	Ventricular Septal Defect (Large)	Unusually enlarged	Convex	Vascular	Hazy	Usually not useful or indicated. Catheterization best diagnostic means for ventricular septal defect	Left or Right
	Patent Ductus Arteriosus	Enlarged	Convex	Vascular	Hazy	Angiocardiography for demonstration of connection between aorta and pulmonary circulation	Normal or Left
	Aortic Septal Defect	Enlarged	Convex	Vascular	Hazy	Not useful. Findings indistinguishable from patent ductus	Normal or Left
	Anomalous venous return with pulmonary vein emptying into right heart	Enlarged	Convex	Vascular	Hazy	Usually not necessary. Anomalous vessels sometimes demonstrable. Catheterization: Entrance of arterialized blood into right auricle or vena cava catheter may be passed into right auricle	Right

* Boxes indicate distinctive diagnostic characteristics of each condition.
** An essential part of the cardiac catheterization technic is analysis of peripheral arterial blood by femoral puncture. Minor degrees of oxygen unsaturation not sufficient to give visible cyanosis may be thus detected. For further details on the findings in cardiac catheterization, see section following the tables.

TABLE IV
PULMONARY ARTERY SEGMENT

CONVEX SEGMENT — LARGE HEART*

	DIAGNOSIS	HEART SIZE AND SHAPE	PUL. ARTERY SEGMENT	LUNG FIELD	PULMONIC WINDOW	ANGIOCARDIOGRAPHY-CATHETERIZATION	EKG PREPONDERANCE
CYANOTIC	Ebstein's Disease	Enlarged	Convex	Clear	Hazy	Very large, slowly emptying right auricle. Patent foramen ovale. Catheter may pass from right into left auricle	Right or Left with Bundle Branch Block
CYANOTIC	Eisenmenger's (with large pulmonary artery): (when pul. artery is normal cyanosis may be delayed	Enlarged (when pulmonary artery is of normal size, heart may be boot-shaped).	Convex When pulmonary artery is of normal size, pulmonary artery segment may be concave	Vascular	Hazy	Angiocardiogram: Simultaneous visualization of overriding aorta and pulmonary arteries which are enlarged peripherally. Oxygen saturation necessary for diagnosis	Right
CYANOTIC	Pulmonary Stenosis with auricular septal defect or Patent Foramen Ovale	Only slight enlargement	Convex - due to post stenotic dilatation	Clear - (Avascular)	Hazy	Early opacity left auricle, ventricle and aorta showing right to left auricular shunt. Catheterization: Pressure changes in right ventricle and pulmonary artery indicative of stenosis. Excludes left to right shunt by O_2 determination	Right
NON-CYANOTIC	Auricular Septal Defect (with pul. art. normal size and small aorta)	Enlarged Right Auricle and Right Ventricle	Convex	Vascular	Hazy	Angiocardiography shows simultaneous filling both auricles indicating defect; actual defect seldom seen. Left to right shunt determined by O_2 concentration in right auricle. Catheter may pass from right to left auricle.	Right
NON-CYANOTIC	Lutembachers (cyanosis may occur later)	Enlarged	Convex Usually prominent	Unusually Vascular	Hazy	Usually not necessary; pulmonary artery enormous.	Right
NON-CYANOTIC	Large Ventricular Septal Defects	Unusually Enlarged	Convex (may be much enlarged)	Vascular	Hazy	Cardiac catheterization is the best method of detection	Left to Right
NON-CYANOTIC	Patent Ductus Arteriosus	Enlarged	Convex	Vascular	Hazy	Retrograde cardioangiographic injection into the carotid artery causes immediate appearance in the pulmonary artery. The ductus itself is rarely visualized.	Normal or Left
NON-CYANOTIC	Anomalous Pulmonary Venous Return to the right heart	Enlarged	Convex	Vascular	Hazy	Usually not necessary	Right
NON-CYANOTIC	Pure Pulmonary Stenosis	Enlarged	Convex, Prominent due to post stenotic dilatation	Clear Avascular	Hazy	Useful only to exclude septal defects and overriding aorta. Increased right ventricle pressure with low or normal pulmonary artery pressure	Right

* Boxes indicate distinctive diagnostic characteristics of each condition.

be necessary to demonstrate the enormous size of the right auricle and its slow emptying.

All of the remaining conditions show convex pulmonary artery segments and vascularity of the lung fields. Of these Eisenmenger's complex is the only one associated with cyanosis.

Auricular septal defect with normal sized pulmonary artery and small aorta can best be confirmed by angiocardiographic methods showing simultaneous filling of both auricles; and by cardiac catheterization. When Lutembacher's is present the enormous dilatation of the pulmonary artery segment with the general configuration of the heart is sufficient for a diagnosis.

Large Ventricular septal defects may cause an extreme vascularity of the pulmonary artery and lung structures. Cardiac catheterization is the best method for detection of this anomaly.

Patent ductus arteriosus is best demonstrated if physical signs are not conclusive by retrograde angiocardiographic injection of contrast medium into the cartoid. Immediate appearance in the pulmonary artery or lung circulation is indication of a patent ductus; the ductus itself is rarely visualized.

Boot-Shaped Heart:

This is a form of cardiac outline commonly encountered; it may or may not be accompanied by enlargement. It is most frequently associated with the Tetralogy of Fallot but occurs in several other conditions. It is due primarily to a combination of right ventricular enlargement from pulmonary stenosis and concave pulmonary artery segment.

This combination results in an indenture (concavity) at the site of the pulmonary artery segment with an elevation of the apex; there may be little if any recognizable enlargement of the heart, or moderate dilatation may be present. Rarely, if ever, is this a prominent feature.

Boot-Shaped Heart

Under proper circumstances, all may show a boot-shaped appearance of the heart.

It will be noted that all show concavity of the pulmonary segment (pulmonary stenosis) and all but two show the lung fields clear; in Truncus Arteriosus and Eisenmenger's only are the lung fields vascular—this serves to differentiate these two conditions from the rest. Further differentiation may be effected by the fact that Truncus Arteriosus patients always show cyanosis whereas in Eisenmenger's cyanosis may or may not be present. In Pseudo-Truncus the lung fields may be essentially clear but the posterior mediastinal veins may be tortuous and engorged. For definite differentiation angiocardiography may be of value.

Consideration of the conditions in which the lung fields are clear:
Tetralogy of Fallot

Pseudo Truncus
Tricuspid Atresia
Transposition of Great Vessels
    with pulmonary stenosis
Tricuspid atresia may be eliminated:
    1)   the typical concave right lower border of the heart if present caused by the hypoplastic right ventricle,
    2)   or in any event, by the left ventricular preponderance shown on EKG examination; in no other condition is it so consistently found in infants.

For the differentiation of:
    Tetralogy of Fallot
    Pseudo Truncus and
    Transposition of the Great Vessels,
        with pulmonary stenosis

Haziness of the pulmonic window in transposition of the great vessels with pulmonary stenosis, may be helpful but not dependable. Angiocardiography may be necessary for differentiation.

Angiocardiographic findings in:
Tetralogy may be quite decisive; simultaneous filling of the pulmonary artery and aorta before vascularization of the lung, in a patient showing a boot-shaped heart is almost certainly due to Tetralogy of Fallot. Pseudotruncus the right ventricular curve is enlarged; the pulmonary artery is small and does not connect with the heart or aorta; the lungs are supplied by the bronchial arteries. The single arterial trunk may be visualized. Transposition of the great vessels with pulmonary stenosis before extreme dilatation has occurred may show distinctive angiocardiographic findings in the lateral view; anteriorly placed aorta with high concentration of the radiopaque agent concurrently with filling of right ventricle.

Size and Shape of the Cardiac Silhouette
Enlargement of individual chambers of the heart can usually be recognized without difficulty and the cause detected by methods of roentgen examination previously described. Enlargement of more than one chamber, with complications such as septal defects, vascular atresia and other anomalies, may result in a picture so bizarre that it baffles all understanding of the underlying cause. Certain conditions, however, result in more or less constant pictures of cardiac enlargement such as large globular heart, boot-shaped heart, etc. The picture in globular enlargement of the heart is one of narrowing of the great vessels above, with gradual smooth symmetrical enlargement of the cardiac silhouette below. Comparison of the conditions in which it occurs may be helpful in differentiation.

Examination of the above table indicates that a globular type of cardiac enlargement most frequently results from enlargement of the right auricle and ventricle although it may result from bilateral enlargement of the ventricles, or even from enormous enlargement of the right auricle alone.

The non-cyanotic character of the condition when associated with auricular septal defects as seen in

TABLE V

BOOT-SHAPED HEART — DUE TO CONCAVE PULMONARY SEGMENT WITH ELEVATION OF APEX AND OTHER DISTINGUISHING FEATURES*

	DIAGNOSIS	HEART SIZE	PUL. ARTERY SEGMENT	LUNG FIELD	PUL-MONIC WINDOW	ANGIOCARDIOGRAPHY-CATHETERIZATION	EKG PREPONDERANCE
CYANOTIC	Tetralogy of Fallot	Tends to be small with elevation of apex Most truly boot-shaped; Right ventricle enlarged	Concave	Clear	Clear	Simultaneous filling of the pulmonary artery and aorta before vascularization of the lungs. Catheter may pass into aorta from right ventricle. Pressure changes indicative of pulmonary stenosis	Right
	Pseudo Truncus	Both ventricles slightly enlarged; Boot-Shaped	Concave	Clear; post-mediastinal veins may be engorged	Clear	Right ventricle enlarged; may show single trunk	Right
	Tricuspid Atresia	May be boot-shaped or have typical concave right border	Concave	Clear	Clear	Left ventricle enormously enlarged; right ventricle not visualized. Right to left auricle shunt. Difficulty passing catheter into right ventricle	Left
	Truncus Arteriosus	Slightly enlarged; Boot-Shaped	Concave	Vascular	Clear	Right ventricle enlarged, may show single trunk. Oxygen content of blood taken from common ventricle will be identical with that from femoral artery	Right
	Transposition of the Great Vessels with Pulmonary Stenosis	When heart is enlarged, resembles Tetralogy of Fallot	Concave	Clear	Hazy in LAO view	Angiocardiography may show pulmonary artery extremely small	Right
MAY OR MAY NOT BE CYANOTIC	Eisenmenger's with normal sized pul. artery	Both ventricles slightly enlarged. Gives appearance resembling Boot-Shaped Heart	Concave	Vascular	Clear	Angiocardiography; simultaneous opacification of both pulmonary artery and aorta. Oxygen Saturation arterial blood necessary for diagnosis	No value

* Boxes indicate distinctive diagnostic characteristics of each condition.

auricular septal defect with normal pulmonary artery and small aorta, and with Ebstein's Disease indicates inadequate right auricular pressure to establish a right to left shunt and serves to differentiate this condition from the others, all of which are associated with cyanosis.

Transposition of the great vessels, either with associated vascular shunts or with pulmonary stenosis can be differentiated by the convex pulmonary segment and vascular lung fields on the one hand, or by the concave pulmonary segment and clear, avascular lung fields on the other. Both show unusual narrowing of the mediastinal shadow.

Pulmonary stenosis with auricular septal defect shows in addition to the cardiac enlargement, a convex pulmonary artery segment associated with clear, avascular lung fields. This is due to post stenotic dilatation of the pulmonary artery.

TABLE VI

GLOBULAR ENLARGEMENT OF HEART;
Great vessels narrowed with gradual smooth bilateral widening
(does not include ordinary enlargement)*

	DIAGNOSIS	HEART SHAPE	PUL. ARTERY SEGMENT	LUNG FIELD	PUL-MONIC WINDOW	ANGIOCARDIOGRAPHY-CATHETERIZATION	EKG PRE-PONDER-ANCE
CYANOTIC	Transposition of Great Vessels with Shunts	Right auricle and ventricle enlargement. Aorta displaced anteriorly in Lat. and LOA views; narrow mediastinal shadow in AP view; widening, in lat. view; absence of aortic knob	Convex	Vascular	Hazy	Lateral view; aorta arises right ventricle, anteriorly. P-A view: aorta forms left cardiac border	Right
	Transposition of Great Vessels with Pulmonary Stenosis (when dilation is established)	Both Ventricles Enlarged Aorta small narrow mediast. shadow in P-A and LAT. positions	Concave	Clear	Hazy	Pulmonary artery extremely small. Catheterization of confirmatory valve	Combined heart strain
	Pul. Stenosis with Patent Foramen Ovale or Auricular Septal Defect	Enlarged right auricle and ventricle	Convex; Post-Stenotic dilatation	Clear	Hazy	Angiocardiography: simultaneous filling both auricles evidence of septal defect; right to left auricle. Catheterization: establishes pressure relationship diagnostic of pulmonary stenosis. Exclude left to right shunt by O_2 determinations	Right
	Ebstein's Disease	Right auricle tremendously enlarged	Concave	Clear (avascular)	Hazy	Angiocardiogram; enormously enlarged, slow emptying right auricle	Right or left with bundle branch block
NON-CYANOTIC	Auricular Septal Defect with pul. art. of normal size and small aorta	Enlarged right auricle and right ventricle	Convex	Vascular	Hazy	Simultaneous filling both auricles; evidence of septal defect and right to left shunt. Catheterization establishes pressure relationship of pul. stenosis. Left to right shunt determined by O_2 concentration in right auricle	Right

*Boxes indicate distinctive diagnostic characteristics of each condition.

E. Other causes of cardiomegaly in infants are often confused with the described congenital lesions. Enormous globular heart enlargement without apparent cause, occurring in infants or young children, can be due to abnormal, excessive glycogen storage in heart muscle, Von Gierke's Disease. Endocardial fibroelastosis and idiopathic myocarditis are two other causes of large hearts. Diagnosis is made mainly on clinical grounds.

F. PERICARDIAL DEFECTS. Celomic Cysts (Fig. 223T). During the developmental period defects may occur in the pericardial sac. A small segment of pericardial membrane may be completely pinched off giving rise to a pericardial celomic cyst or a small diverticulum or herniation of the pericardium may result. These usually occur on the right side near the cardiophrenic region and in the lateral view

are seen to be anteriorly at the anterior diaphragmatic attachment. Such anomalies are usually of no pathological significance.

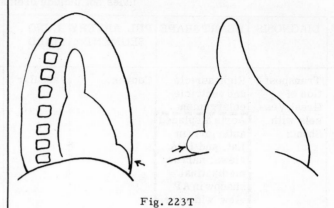

Fig. 223T

QUESTIONS ON THE CIRCULATORY SYSTEM

Questions marked with a dagger deal with rare and less-important conditions.

1. Describe briefly the topography of the heart and identify the curves produced by its various chambers on the cardiac silhouette.

2. Describe the methods of roentgen examination of the heart and indicate their advantages.

3. What is meant by teleroentgenographic examination? Orthodiography? What factors must be known to estimate the relationship of the cardiac silhouette with the normal?

†4. What is kymographic examination and how is it carried out? In what particular phase of cardiac function is this method of particular advantage? In what condition is it of value? What are its limitations?

5. What is the most consistent indication of cardiac disease?

6. How does valvular disease of the heart manifest itself in the roentgenogram? Show by drawings the characteristic appearance of the heart in: Mitral insufficiency,
    Mitral stenosis,
    Aortic insufficiency,
    Aortic stenosis.

7. What x-ray manifestations are there of cardiac decompensation? Coronary disease?

8. What are x-ray manifestations of acute pericarditis? Of chronic constrictive pericarditis?

9. How would you differentiate pericardial effusion from cardiac enlargement?

†10. What is the significance of intracardiac calcifications and how are they detected?

11. What are the common causes of aortitis and how may they be distinguished roentgenographically?

12. What are the roentgen characteristics of aneurysm of the aorta?

†13. What is meant by coarctation of the aorta and what are its roentgen manifestations?

†14. What are the roentgen manifestations of right-sided aorta? Indicate its clinical significance.

†15. Of what aid is roentgen examination in detection of patent ductus arteriosus and of what importance is it? When are angiocardiography or aortography and cardiac catheterization indicated?

†16. How does closure of an arterio-venous fistula affect the heart?

17. List causes for engorgement and enlargement of the pulmonary artery drawing from congenital and acquired lesions and lung diseases.

18. Outline roentgenologic investigation of a child with respiratory or swallowing difficulty.

19. Differentiate in so far as possible between the various lesions causing a boot-shaped heart and avascular lung fields.

20. Can all congenital cardiac lesions be diagnosed roentgenologically?

21. When is contrast visualization of coarctation indicated?

22. Which procedure provides better diagnostic information of pulmonary stenosis, cardiac catheterization or angiocardiography? Interauricular communication with left to right shunt? Interauricular communication with right to left shunt? Interventricular communication with left to right shunt? Interventricular communication with right to left shunt?

23. In what percentage of all congenital cardiac lesion do you think diagnosis can be made by history, physical examination, EKG, conventional roentgenologic procedures, that is, without resort to angiocardiography?

24. With what congenital lesions could rheumatic mitral disease be confused with roentgenologically?

25. How would a radiologist distinguish between Tetralogy of Fallot and pulmonic stenosis with inter-auricular communication? Of what significance would this be?

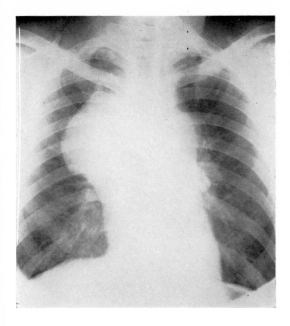

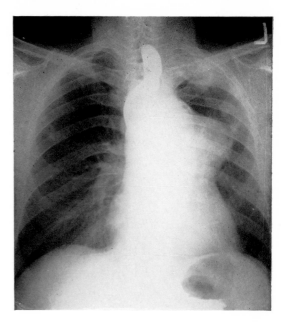

← Aneurysm of the ascending portion of the aorta bulging to the right.

➡ Aneurysm of the descending portion of the aorta bulging to the left.

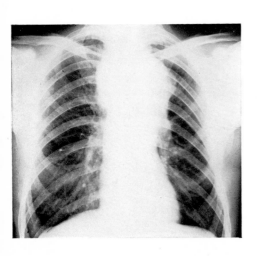

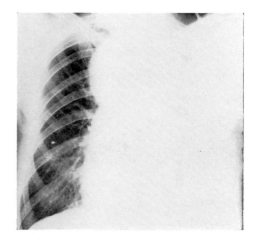

← Dissecting aneurysm. Aneurysm of the aortic arch dissecting its way along the vascular wall.

➡ Dissecting aneurysm; same patient 12 days later showing rupture with blood in the pleural cavity.

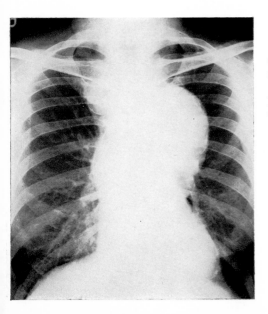

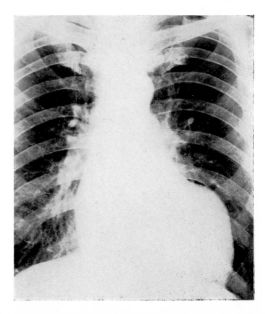

← Innominate aneurysm, associated with aneurysm of the aortic arch.

Note calcium deposit in vascular walls.

➡ Aneurysm of left ventricle; note unusual bulge.

CIRCULATORY SYSTEM

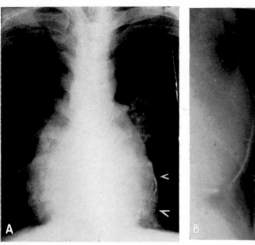

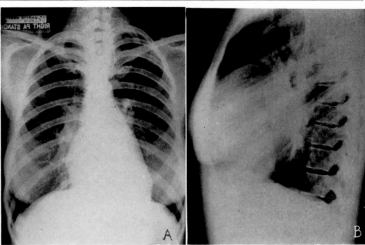

A. Constrictive pericarditis showing calcium deposits in pericardium. B. Detailed view.

A. Cor pulmonale showing; in A-P view straightening out of left border of heart and loss of aortic knob; in B. Lateral view, right ventricle enlargement to anterior chest wall.

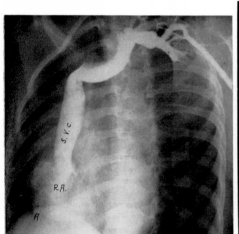

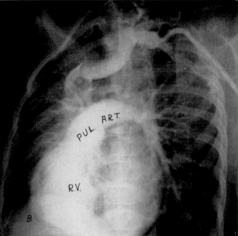

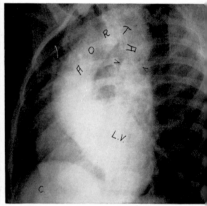

A. Coarctation of aorta demonstrated by intravenous injection thru left brachial, subclavian, innominate, and superior vena cava to right auricle. B. Extension from right ventricle thru pulmonary artery to lungs. C. Back to left ventricle, out thru ascending aorta to arch and descending portion showing coarctation (arrow).

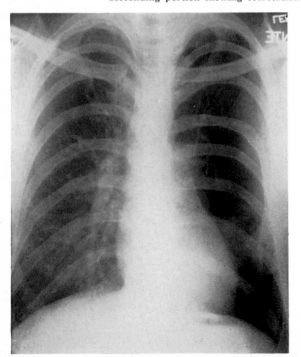

←
Coarctation of the aorta, a condition in which the aorta is constricted in a small section requiring collateral circulation to carry on systemic function. Note notching of ribs from dilated intercostal vessels.

→
Aortogram by retrograde injection into the carotid artery showing coarctation, (arrow), and post-stenotic dilatation of the aorta. Colateral circulation thru an enormously dilated internal mammary artery.

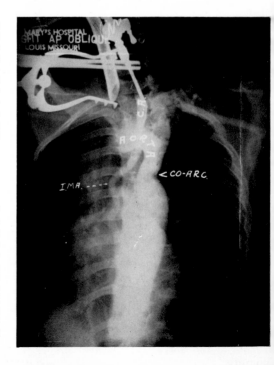

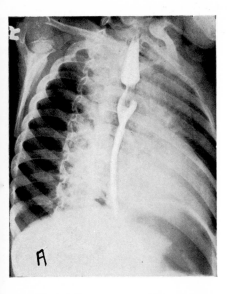

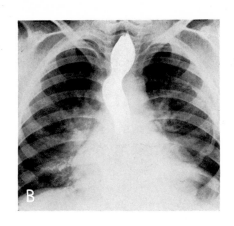

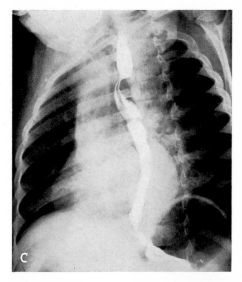

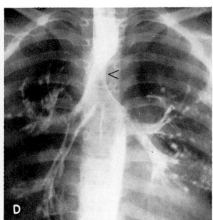

DOUBLE AORTIC ARCH showing characteristic pressure defects on esophagus and trachea.

A. Right Anterior oblique view.

B. Anterior view showing bilateral pressure defects on esophagus.

C. Left anterior oblique view.

D. Tracheal pressure defect seen after filling trachea with lipiodol.

E. Tomogram demonstrates not only tracheal defect but vascular arch as well.

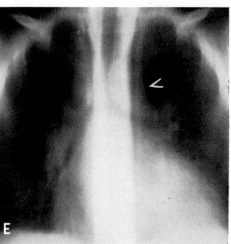

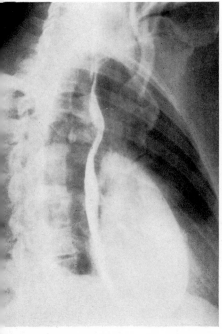

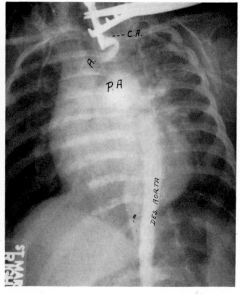

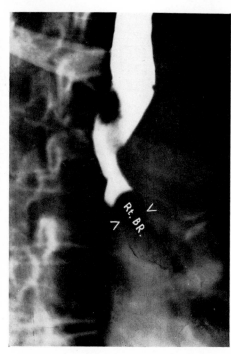

Right-sided aorta. Esophagus passes in front of the aorta. Developmental anomaly.

Opaque material injected retrograde thru the carotid into aorta, immediately appears in the pulmonary artery proving existance of patent ductus arteriosus even though it is not visualized.

Anomalous right subclavian artery causing pressure defect on barium-filled esophagus.

CIRCULATORY SYSTEM

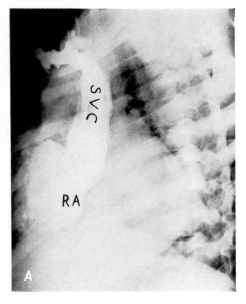

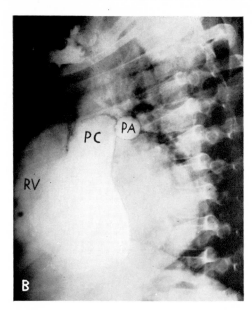

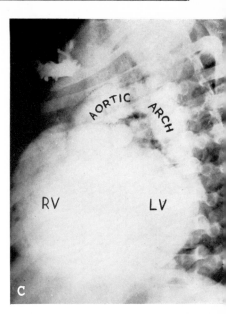

CARDIOANGIOGRAPHY. Injection of 80% Diodrast into circulation, Right Posterior Oblique position, for visualization of chambers of heart. A. Opaque injection entering thru superior vena cava into right auricle. B. Taken a few seconds later, right ventricle filled and pulmonary conus and artery visualized. C. Both right and left ventricles filled, aortic arch visualized.

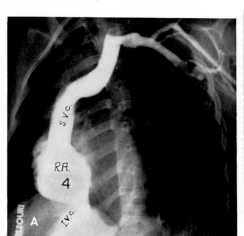

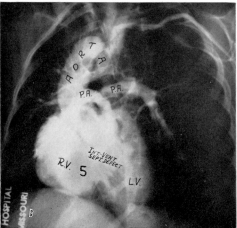

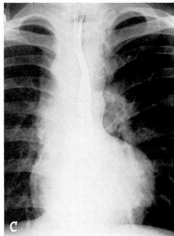

Tetralogy of Fallot showing, A. injection of opaque material into vein of right arm, filling of superior vena cava and right auricle. B. Passage into right ventricle and simultaneous discharge thru both pulmonary artery and aorta; scant lung vascularization from decrease in size of pulmonary artery. C. Characteristic boot-shaped heart in Tetralogy with deviation of barium column to left indicating right aortic arch; it is important to indicate aorta's position if operation is to be carried out.

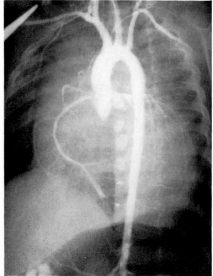

Retrograde injection of carotid artery into aorta. Aortic valve clearly shown. Coronary arteries well filled; descending aorta and its branches demonstrated.

Cardioangiographic examination showing rudimentary right ventricle, (from absence of tricuspid valve) and interventricular septal defect. Left ventricle reservoir for all ventricular blood. Reflux into inferior vena cava.

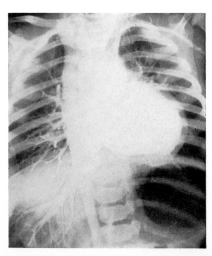

REFERENCES FOR CIRCULATORY SYSTEM

Pathology of the Heart and Associated Structures:

I. Heart

New York Heart Association, Nomenclature and Criteria for Diagnosis of Diseases of the Heart, New York, 1942.

Schwedel, J. B., "Clinical Roentgenology of the Heart," Annals of Roentgenology, Vol. 18, Paul Hoeber, Inc., New York, 1948.

Meyers, J. A., and McKinlay, C. A., The Chest and Heart, Vol. 2, Chas. C. Thomas, Pub., Springfield.

Ungerleider, H. E., and Gubner, R., "Roentgenology of the Heart and Great Vessels," Reprint, STROUD Diagnosis and Treatment of Cardiovascular Diseases, F. A. Davis Co., Philadelphia, 1950.

Roesler, H., Clinical Roentgenology of the Cardiovascular System, Chas. C. Thomas, 1943.

Bardeen, C. R., U.S. Army X-Ray Manual, 1st Ed., Paul Hoeber, 1918.

Millwee, R. H., "Spot Scanography," Radiol., 28:483, 1937.

Claytor, T. A., and Merril, W. H., "Orthodiagraphy in the Study of the Heart and Great Vessels," Am. J. Med. Sc., 138:549, 1909.

Hilbish, T. F., and Morgan, R. H., "Cardiac Mensuration by Roentgenologic Methods," Am. J. Med. Sc., 224:586, 1952.

Ungerleider, H. E., and Clark, C. P., "A Study of the Transverse Diameter of the Heart Silhouette with Prediction Table Based on the Teleroentgenogram," Am. Heart J., 17:92, 1939.

Ungerleider, H. E., and Gubner, R., Roentgenology of the Heart and Great Vessels, F. A. Davis Co., Phil., 1950.

Newcomer, E., and Newcomer, N. D., "Heart Measurements," Radiol., 27:52, 1936.

Hodges, F. Y., and Eyster, J. A. E., "Estimation of Transverse Cardiac Diameter in Man," Arch. Int. Med., 37:706, 1926.

Meyer, R. R., "A Method for Measuring Children's Hearts," Radiol., 53:363, 1949.

Equitable Life Insurance Company, Med. Dept., Heart Size Measurement Tables.

Schorr, S., Dreyfuss, F., and Frankel, M., "Evaluation of the Recumbent Esophagram in the Early Detection of Left Atrial Enlargement," Radiol., 67:186, 1956.

Kaye, J., "The Radiological Diagnosis of Mitral Valve Disease," Brit. J. Radiol., 26:242, 1953.

Carmichael, J. H. E., "Radiological Signs in Pulmonary Hypertension. The Significance of Lines B. of Kerley," Brit. J. Radiol., 27:393, 1954.

Doley, R., and Franks, R., "Massive Dilatation of the Left Auricle," Quart. J. Med., 18:81, 1949.

Rigler, L., and Hallock, P., "Azerza's Disease," Am. J. Roentgenol., 50:453, 1943.

Sosman, M. C., and Wosika, P. H., "Calcification in Aortic and Mitral Valves," Am. J. Roentgenol., 30:328, 1955.

McAfee, J. G., Hilbish, T. F., and Stewart, K. R., "Angiocardiography in the Preoperative Diagnosis of Mitral Stenosis and Insufficiency," Radiol., 67:321, 1956.

Rigler, L. G., "Roentgen Kymography in Demonstration of Calcified Valves of the Heart," Am. J. Roentgenol., 47:480, 1942.

Sayman, M. I., "A New Sign in the Diagnosis of Cardiac Aneurysm and Myocardial Infarction," Radiol., 67:242, 1956.

Brean, H. P., Marks, J. H., Sosman, M. C., and Schlesinger, M. J., "Massive Calcification in Infarcted Myocardium," Radiol., 54:33, 1950.

Finestone, A. J., and Geschickter, C. F., "Bone Formation in the Heart," Am. J. Clin. Path., 19:974, 1949.

Davies, C. E., and Steiner, R. E., "Calcified Aortic Valve," Brit. Heart J., 11:126, 1949.

Nemec, S. S., "Differential Diagnosis of Retrocardiac Shadows," Radiol., 50:174, 1948.

Steinbach, H. L., Keats, T. E. and Sheline, G. E., "The Roentgen Appearance of the Pulmonary Veins in Heart Disease," Radiol., 65:157, 1955.

Moragues, V., and Lynxweiler, C. P., Cardiac Anomalies; A Clinicopathologic Correlation, Wm. Wilkins Co., Baltimore, Maryland, 1954.

II. Aorta and Great Vessels:

Roesler, H., Clinical Roentgenology of the Cardiovascular System, Chas. C. Thomas, Springfield, Illinois, 1943.

Wolkin, A., The Significance of Calcification of the Ascending Portion of the Aortic Arch," Radiol., 62:101, 1954.

III. Pericardium:

Broadbent, W., "Adherent Pericardium," Brit. Med. J., 1:147, 1898.

Dassel, P. M., and Kirsch, I. E., "Nontraumatic Pneumopericardium and Pyopneumopericardium: Report of Two Cases," Radiol., 63:346, 1954.

Stewart, H. J., Carty, J. R., and Seal, J. R., "Contributions of Roentgenology to the Diagnosis of Chronic Constrictive Pericarditis," Am. J. Roentgenol., 49:349, 1943.

IV. Congenital Anomalies of Heart and Associated Structures:

Angiocardiography and Cardiac Catheterization

Robb, G. F., and Steinberg, I., "Visualization of the Chambers of the Heart, The Pulmonary Circulation, and the Great Vessels in Man," Am. J. Roentgenol., 41:1, 1939.

Dotter, C. T., and Steinberg, I., "Angiocardiography," Annals of Roentgenology, Vol. XX, Paul B. Hoeber, New York, 1953.

Schnitker, M. A., Congenital Anomalies of the Heart and Great Vessels, Oxford Univ. Press, New York, 1952.

_____, The Electrocardiogram in Congenital Cardiac Disease, Harvard Univ. Press, Cambridge, 1940.

Dotter, C. T., and Jackson, F. S., "Death Following Angiocardiography," Radiol., 54:527, 1950.

Dexter, L., "Cardiac Catheterization in the Diagnosis of Congenital Heart Disease," Bull. New York Acad. Med., 26:93, 1950.

Morgan, R. H., "Problems of Angiocardiography," Am. J. Roentgenol., 64:189, 1950.

Cournand, A., "New Methods in the Diagnosis of Congenital Cardiac Anomalies," Bull. New York Acad. Med., 27:277, 1951.

Cooley, R. N., "Angiocardiography in the Diagnosis of Congenital Cyanotic Heart Disease," J. Faculty Radiol., 2:249, 1951.

Dry, T. J., Edwards, J. E., Parker, R. L., Burchell, H. B., Rogers, H. M., and Bulbulian, A. H., (Mayo Clinic), Congenital Anomalies of the Heart and Great Vessels, Chas. C. Thomas, Pub., Springfield, Illinois.

Persistent Patent Ductus Arteriosus

Eppinger, E. C., and Burwell, C. "The Mechanical Effects of Patent Ductus Arteriosus on the Heart." J.A.M.A., 115:1263, 1940.

Gross, R. E., and Hubb, J. P., "Surgical Ligation of a Patent Ductus Arteriosus; Report of First Successful Case," J.A.M.A., 112:729, 1939.

Steinberg, M. F., Grishman, A., and Sussman, M. L., "Angiocardiography in Congenital Heart Disease," Am. J. Roentgenol., 50:306, 1943.

Kjellberg, S. R., Mannheimer, E., Ruhde, V., and Jonsson, B., Diagnosis of Congenital Heart Disease," Year Book Pub., Chicago, 1955.

Johnson, G., and Saltzman, G., "Infundibulum of the Patent Ductus Arteriosus Studies by Thoracic Aortography," Acta Radiol., 37:445, 1952.

Keith, J. D., and Forsyth, C., "Aortography in Infants," Circulation, 2:907, 1950.

Barclay, A. E., Franklin, J. K., and Prichard, M. M. L., The Fetal Circulation, Blackwell Scientific Pub., Ltd., London, 1944.

Coarctation of the Aorta

Sloan, R. D., and Cooley, R. N., "Coarctation of the Aorta," Radiol., 61:701, 1953.

Blackford, L. M., "Coarctation of the Aorta," Arch. Int. Med., 41:702, 1928.

Crafoord, C., and Nylin, G., "Congenital Coarctation of the Aorta and Its Surgical Treatment, J. Thoracic Surg., 14:347, 1945.

MacLaughlin, J. R., "Unilateral Costal and Scapular Notching Associated with Coarctation of the Aorta," Brit. J. Radiol., 24:688-690, December 1951.

Gross, R. E., "Coarctation of the Aorta; Surgical Treatment of One Hundred Cases," Circulation, 1:41, 1950.

Bruwer, A., and Pugh, D. W., "A Neglected Roentgenological Sign of Coarctation of the Aorta," Proceedings of Staff Meeting, Mayo Clinic, 27:377, 1952.

Anomalies of Aortic Arch

Edwards, Jesse E., "Anomalies of the Derivatives of the Aortic Arch System," Med. Clin. N. Am., 32:925-949, 1948.

Snider, G. L., Gildenhorn, H. L., and Rubenstein, L. H., "Dextraposition of the Descending Thoracic Aorta," Radiol., 67:333, 1956.

Kirklin, J. W., and Clagett, O. T., "Vascular Rings Producing Respiratory Obstruction in Infants," Proc. Staff Meet. Mayo Clin., 25:360-367, 1950.

Neuhauser, E. B., "Tracheo-Esophageal Constriction Produced by Right Aortic Arch and Left Ligementum Arteriosum," Am. J. Roentgenol., 62:493, 1949.

Abrams, H. L., "Left Ascending Aorta with Right Arch and Right Descending Aorta," Radiol., 57:58, July 1951.

Paul, R. N., "A New Anomaly of the Aorta; Left Aortic Arch with Right Descending Aorta," J. Pediat., 32:19, January 1948.

Lubert, M., Epstein, H. C., Mendelsohn, H., Freedlander, S. O., "An Unusual Variant of Double Aortic Arch," Am. J. Roentgenol., 67:763, 1952.

Neuhauser, E. B. D., "Roentgen Diagnosis of Double Aortic Arch and Other Anomalies of the Great Vessels," Am. J. Roentgenol., 55:1, 1946.

Aortic Septal Defect

Gasul, B. M., Fell, E. H., and Casas, R., "The Diagnosis of Aortic Septal Defect by Retrograde Aortography," Circulation, 4:251-254, August 1951.

Wittenborg, M. H., Tantiwongse, T., and Rosenberg, G. B. F., "Anomalous Course of Left Pulmonary Artery with Respiratory Obstruction," Radiol., 67:339, 1956.

Anomalous Right Subclavian Artery

Felson, B., Cohen, S., Courter, S. R., and McGuire, J., "Anomalous Right Subclavian Artery," Radiol., 54:340, March 1950.

Raphael, R. L., Schnabel, T. G., Jr., and Leopold, S. S., "A New Method for Demonstrating an Aberrant Right Subclavian Artery," Radiol., 58:89, 1952.

Gross, R. E., "Surgical Treatment for Dysphagia Lusoria," Ann. Surg., 124:532, September 1946.

Anomalies of the Pulmonary Vessels

Dotter, C. T., Hardesty, N. M., and Steinberg, I., "Anomalous Right Pulmonary Vein Entering the Inferior Vena Cava," Am. J. Med. Sc., 218:31-36, July 1949.

Snellen, H. A., and Albers, F. H., "The Clinical Diagnosis of Anomalous Pulmonary Venous Drainage," Circulation, 6:801-806, December, 1952.

Anomalies of Cardiac Position

Kartagener, M., "Zur pathogenese der bronchiektasien: Bronchiektasien bei Situs viscerum inversus," Beitr. Z. Klin. de Tuberk., 83:489, 1933.

Pryce, D. M., "Lower Accessory Pulmonary Artery with Intralobar Sequestration of the Lung," J. Path. and Bact., 58:457, 1946.

————, Sellors, T. H., and Blair, L. G., "Intralobar Sequestration of Lung Associated with an Abnormal Pulmonary Artery," Brit. J. Surg., 35:18, 1947.

Ebstein's Anomaly

Engle, M. A., and others, "Ebstein's Anomaly of the Tricuspid Valve," Circulation, 1:1246, 1950.

Truncus Arteriosus

Taussig, H. B., Congenital Malformations of the Heart, The Commonwealth Fund, New York, 1947.

Taussig, H. B., "Clinical and Pathological Findings in Cases of Truncus Arteriosus in Infancy," Am. J. Med., 2:26, 1947.

Auricular Septal Defect and Lutembacher's Syndrome

Healey, R. F., "The Roentgenographic Appearance of Interatrial Septal Defect," Am. J. Roentgenol., 63:646, 1950.

Pure Pulmonary Stenosis

Healey, R. F., Dexter, L., Elkin, M., and Sosman, M. C., "Roentgenographic Changes in Pulmonary Stenosis, Am. J. Roentgenol., 63:813, 1950.

Engle, M. A., and Taussig, H. B., "Valvular Pulmonic Stenosis with Intact Ventricular Septum and Patent Foramen Ovale," Circulation, 2:481, 1950.

Blount, S. G., McCord, M. C., Koniesu, S., and Lanier, R. R., "Roentgen Aspects of Isolated Volvular Pulmonic Stenosis," Radiol., 62:337, 1954.

Anomalies of Structural Development of Heart

Abbott, Maud, Atlas of Congenital Cardiac Disease, Am. Heart Assoc., New York, 1936.

Taussig, H. B., Congenital Malformations of the Heart, Commonwealth Fund, New York, 1947.

Bing, R. J., Lombardo, T. A., Bargeron, L. M., Taeschler, M., and Tulny, S., "Congenital Heart Disease; A Clinical and Physiological Correlation," Ann. Int. Med., 37:664, 1952.

Tetralogy of Fallot

Cooley, R. N., Bahnson, H. J., and Hanlon, C. R., "Angiocardiography in Congenital Heart Disease of Cyanotic Type with Pulmonic Stenosis or Atresia," Radiol., 52:329, 1949.

Tricuspid Atresia

Wittenborg, M. H., Neuhauser, E. B. D., and Sprunt, W. H., "Roentgenographic Findings in Congenital Tricuspid Atresia with Hypoplasia of the Right Ventricle," Am. J. Roentgenol., 66:712, 1951.

Cooley, R. N., Sloan, R. D., Hanlon, C. R., and Bahnson, H. T., "Angiocardiography in Congenital Heart Disease of Cyanotic Type," Radiol., 54:848, 1950.

Transposition of Great Vessels

Abrams, H. L., Kaplan, H. S., and Purdy, A., "Diagnosis of Complete Transposition of the Great Vessels," Radiol., 57:500, 1951.

Cooley, R. N., and Sloan, R. D., "Angiocardiography in Congenital Heart Disease of Cyanotic Type," Radiol., 58:481, 1952.

Astley, R., and Parsons, C., "Complete Transposition of the Great Vessels," Brit. Heart J., 14:13, 1952.

Pulmonary Stenosis with Auricular Septal Defect

Blalock, A., "Technique of Creation of an Artificial Ductus Arteriosus in the Treatment of Pulmonary Stenosis," J. Thoracic Surg., 16:244, 1947.

Blalock, A., and Taussig, H. B., "Surgical Treatment of Malformations of the Heart in which there is Pulmonary Stenosis or Pulmonary Atresia," J.A.M.A., 128:189, 1945.

Potts, W. J., Smith, S., Gibson, S., "Anastomosis of the Aorta to a Pulmonary Artery," J.A.M.A., 132:627, 1946.

Bing, R. J., Vandam, L. D., and Gray, F. D., Jr., "Physiological Studies in Congenital Heart Disease. II. Results of Preoperative Studies in Patients with Tetralogy of Fallot," Bull. Johns Hopkins Hospital, 80:121, 1947.

Eisenmenger's Complex

Bing, R. J., Vandam, L. D., and Gray, F. D., Jr., "Physiological Studies in Congenital Heart Disease. III. Results Obtained in Five Cases of Eisenmenger's Complex," Bull. Johns Hopkins Hospital, 80:323, 1947.

INDEX

TO

GASTROINTESTINAL

AND

BILIARY TRACT

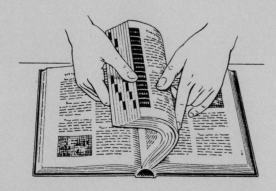

Esophagus

Stomach

Duodenum

Jejunum
and
Ileum

Appendix

Colon

Gall
Bladder

Bile
Ducts

PART III

GASTROINTESTINAL TRACT

ESOPHAGUS (Chapter XVIII)

  I. ANATOMY

  II. ROENTGEN EXAMINATION

  III. PATHOLOGY
     A. Foreign bodies
     B. Constriction or obstruction
     C. Diverticulum
     D. Miscellaneous lesions

STOMACH (Chapter XIX)

  I. ANATOMY

  II. RELATION OF GASTRIC TYPES TO HABITUS

  III. ROENTGEN EXAMINATION
     A. Normal stomach
     B. Organic pathology
     C. Functional lesions
     D. Corrective operative procedures

SMALL INTESTINE (Chapter XX)

DUODENUM

  I. ANATOMY

  II. ROENTGEN EXAMINATION

     A. Normal duodenum
     B. Organic pathology
       Intrinsic
       Extrinsic
     C. Other lesions from adjacent organs
     D. Functional

JEJUNUM AND ILEUM

  I. ANATOMY

  II. ROENTGENOLOGICAL EXAMINATION

  III. PATHOLOGICAL MANIFESTATIONS

APPENDIX

COLON (Chapter XXI)

  I. ANATOMY

  II. ROENTGENOLOGICAL EXAMINATION

  III. INDICATIONS OF PATHOLOGY

     A. Anomalies
     B. Colitis
     C. Obstruction
     D. Diverticula

GASTROINTESTINAL TRACT

The gastrointestinal tract is essentially a muscular tube having variations in thickness and calibre in different locations depending upon the functions it is called upon to perform. In its non-functioning state it is collapsed, presenting only a potential cavity, capable of expansion and enlargement, within certain normal limits to accommodate its contents. It traverses some of the most important regions of the body: the mediastinum in its course through the chest and the peritoneal cavity in its abdominal location. Being of soft-tissue structure, similar in density to the surrounding structures, it cannot be visualized in its natural state. To render it visible roentgenologically an opaque meal containing barium sulphate, 5 ozs. to a pint of buttermilk or other suitable medium, is used. Rugar, an extremely viscid opaque material, is especially valuable for demonstrating the mucosal relief; one-half teaspoonful is sufficient for examination of the esophagus, one teaspoonful for the stomach. This material, filling the gastrointestinal tract, produces a silhouette of the mucosal lining of the tract but does not disclose the thickness of the wall itself. Fortunately conditions of the gastrointestinal tract usually extend to involve the mucosal lining, giving evidence of their presence in the roentgenogram.

THE ESOPHAGUS Chapter XVIII

I. ANATOMY
II. ROENTGEN EXAMINATION
III. PATHOLOGY
    A. Foreign Bodies
        1. Opaque
        2. Nonopaque
    B. Constriction or Obstruction
        1. Benign
            Congenital atresia
            Stricture from caustic agents
            Esophagitis
            Syphilitic stricture
            Cardiospasm—achalasia
            Esophageal reflux
            Scleroderma
            Intramural tumors
        2. Malignant
            Carcinoma
    C. Diverticulum
        1. Pulsion
        2. Traction
    D. Miscellaneous Lesions
        1. Esophageal varices
        2. Post-cricoid web
        3. Congenital anomalies
            Atresia
            Short esophagus—thoracic stomach
            Diaphragmatic hernia
            Eventration of diaphragm
            Elongation of esophagus
        4. Peptic ulcer—reflux esophagitis
        5. Lower esophageal ring
        6. Nervous interference with esophageal contraction
            Bulbar palsy
            Curling or corkscrew (writhing) esophagus
        7. Injury to the esophagus
            Perforation
            Foreign body and other trauma
            Spontaneous

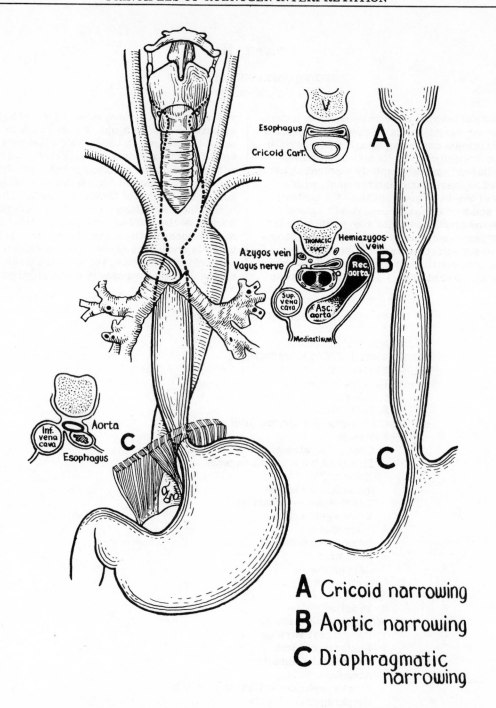

A Cricoid narrowing
B Aortic narrowing
C Diaphragmatic narrowing

Fig. 224. The esophagus as an indicator of pathology of the great vessels and heart. The esophagus in its course through the mediastinum is in close relationship to other structures. Anomalies or other variations of the great vessels or heart leave their impression upon the esophagus and give valuable aid in diagnosis. The normal relationship of the esophagus to the mediastinal structures is shown above. The three points of natural constriction are indicated, A, B, and C. Redrawn from Bockus, H.L., gastroenterology, W. B. Saunders Co.

Chapter XVIII

ESOPHAGUS

ANATOMY. The esophagus is the most muscular portion of the gastrointestinal tract; this is because its chief function is concerned with propulsion of food into the stomach.

Peristalsis throughout the gastro-intestinal tract, is produced by a gradient of nerve impulses which progresses from segment to segment of the muscular structure causing first a zone of relaxation of the muscular tone normally present, followed almost at once by a deep contraction. Normally waves progress in the esophagus at the rate of three to three-and one-half in two seconds. The mechanism of swallowing may be studied by high speed cineradiography (30 to 60 frames per second) showing the movements of the epiglottis and pharynx, (Saunders, et al.). This mechanism is regulated by Auerbach's plexus; any derangement of this nerve plexus may result in grave dysfunction. Esophageal contractions may be studied by Kymography (McLaren).

The nerve supply to the esophagus is from the sympathetic and vagus nerves, although the latter predominate. Their function is chiefly motor, with inhibition of the cardia. The sympathetic nerves exert a restraining influence but cannot be said to be antagonistic to the action of the vagi. The vagus nerves terminate in the myenteric plexuses; when they degenerate or their impulses are blocked, spastic contraction of the smooth muscle results. No actual sphincter muscle can be demonstrated at the cardia or elsewhere but the circular contraction of the smooth muscle fibers produces a function similar to a sphincter.

When there is obstruction, secondary more intense waves occur in the mid-portion. Localized segmental waves of the smooth musculature have been described as a result of faulty nerve stimulation.

The mucous membrane lining the esophagus is of squamous epithelium; it is arranged in longitudinal folds which does not have the structure of gastric rugae.

Roentgen Examination

Examination is made in both the upright and recumbent positions. Frequently a much better filling of the esophagus can be obtained in the lying position, utilizing thicker barium mixture, and its movements may be studied more leisurely.

As the esophagus passes downward (Fig. 224) it lies slightly to the right in its upper portion, inclines to the mid-line as it descends and passes slightly to the left in the lower portion; it is marked by indentations on its anterior margin from pressure of the aorta, left bronchus and diaphragm as it passes through. Just before the esophagus passes through the diaphragm an ovoid dilation is often seen between the diaphragm and a constriction ring in the lower esophagus; this is called the ampulla of the esophagus or "phrenic ampulla." Two small notches may be present due to insertion of the phreno-esophageal sheath.

Pathology

FOREIGN BODIES* (Figs. 225A and B). In its collapsed state the upper portion of the esophagus is flattened in its anteroposterior diameter; this causes flat or disclike foreign bodies, when they lodge in the esophagus, to assume a flat appearance in the anteroposterior view. Such foreign bodies, when lodged in the trachea, appear on end in the anteroposterior view, since the natural defect in the cartilaginous rings of the trachea in the mid-line posteriorly, is the only point permitting distention. The position which a disclike foreign body assumes in this region then determines its location in either esophagus or trachea. Instances have been reported in which disclike foreign bodies, lodged in the retrocardiac portion of the esophagus have assumed an on-end position.

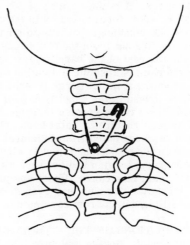

Fig. 225A

---

*An asterisk following any title indicates that roentgenographic reproductions illustrating this condition will be found in the pictorial supplement at the end of the chapter.

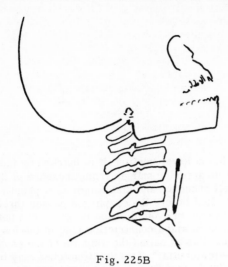

Fig. 225B

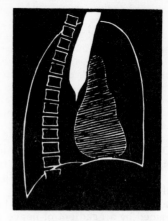

Fig. 226

At this level (Fig. 224) the esophagus assumes a more oblique position permitting this variation in position.

There are three major points of normal narrowing of the esophagus:

1. At the introitus, cricoid narrowing,

2. As it passes the aortic arch, aortic narrowing,

3. At the diaphragmatic hiatus, diaphragmatic narrowing.

Foreign bodies are most apt to lodge at one of these points of normal constriction. If the foreign body is composed of metal or some other radiopaque material it can, of course, be readily visualized; for the detection of non-opaque foreign bodies, such as fish bones, etc., other means must be resorted to. Close fluoroscopic observation, with ingestion of a barium sulphate mixture may disclose this opaque material clinging to the foreign body. A tiny pledget of cotton soaked in barium solution when swallowed will often stop at the site of the foreign body. Sharp foreign bodies are apt to perforate the esophageal wall and introduce infection into the surrounding mediastinal space. It is this chance of periesophageal abscess which makes foreign bodies in the esophagus so dangerous. Roentgenographically, a small stream of barium extending out from the esophagus and remaining after the rest of the barium meal has passed on into the stomach is absolute indication of perforation of the esophageal wall. Large irregular-shaped foreign bodies lodged in the esophagus over a long period of time may cause erosion through the wall into the adjacent structures. Fatal hemorrhage from such a cause has been noted from lodgment of a plate of false teeth in the esophagus for over eighteen months. Nonopaque foreign bodies, such as a large piece of beefsteak, may cause almost complete occlusion; their irregular margins may even give the impression of filling defect from carcinoma.

CONSTRICTIONS OF THE ESOPHAGUS may be benign or malignant. Benign stricture may be congenital or acquired, (q. v.).

BENIGN STRICTURE* (Fig. 226). Stricture of the esophagus is frequently seen after swallowing caustic agents—especially lye. In this instance the constriction is due to contraction of a ring of scar tissue which follows healing of ulcerations caused by the caustic agent. During the stage of acute esophagitis, examination will show irregular erosions which cause a stringy appearance of the barium mixture when it descends. After it has become chronic it is seen as a smooth conical constriction, apex downward, of varying length. Benign stricture may be produced anywhere along the esophageal length, but most are seen in the middle and upper thirds, except those secondary to reflux esophagitis which are in the lower third. See p. 363. Spasm of the esophagus may produce a somewhat similar picture but spasm is transitory, and organic stricture is permanently present. Such strictures can usually be dilated with continued passage of filiform bougies, although gastrostomy for feeding of the patient may be necessary in the meantime. At first, filiforms are introduced through an esophagoscope; later, by passing a thread through the opening into the stomach—larger and larger bougies can be successively passed through the opening.

SYPHILITIC STRICTURE. Syphilitic strictures are very rare. They present rounded smooth conical constrictions which may at first be relieved by antiluetic treatment, but later after a dense cicatrix has formed may require progressive dilatation similar to any other fibrous stricture. All other commoner causes must be eliminated before a diagnosis of syphilitic stricture is made. With the modern control of syphilis in its early stages, such strictures are becoming much less frequent.

CARDIOSPASM (ACHALASIA).* (Fig. 206B, 227). Cardiospasm is a condition in which extreme constriction of the esophagus at the cardiac orifice of the stomach may almost completely prevent the passage of food. The point of constriction seems to be very near the diaphragmatic orifice of the esophagus; the constricted region is smooth, conical and of short length, and beak-like. There is tremendous dilatation of the esophagus above the point of constriction.

In achalasia the esophago-gastric junction may be well above the diaphragm in cases of direct gastric herniation. In other instances the dilated esophageal junction extends down to the stomach by esophagoscopic examination and its position translated to fluoroscopy by placing a metallic brain clip at the mucosal junction and taking a biopsy of the mucosa.

A study using this transesophagoscopic biopsy and clip technic would indicate that the vestibule (part between the diaphragm and stomach) behaves quite differently than the body of the esophagus in this disease. The vestibule is capable of functioning normally but does not, probably because it receives no activating stimulus from the esophagus. It is concluded that in achalasia all of the esophagus as defined anatomically according to mucosal type, is diseased and that the potentially normal narrow segment below the area of dilatation is part of the stomach, (Palmer).

In no other condition is such extreme dilatation seen; the distended and lengthened esophagus, filled with retained food, may bulge to the right side of the mediastinum giving the appearance of a mediastinal new growth. An instance has been reported where it filled the entire right side of the chest (Kay). Rare cases have been reported where the bulging esophagus has herniated through the cardiac orifice down into the abdomen. This would indicate that the point of constriction is inherent in the esophageal muscle and independent of any spasmodic contraction of the diaphragm. On fluoroscopic examination, periodic ejection of a small stream of barium mixture is indication of its spasmodic nature. If small pieces of food material lodge in the apex of the obstruction the outline may appear irregular and the diagnosis may be in doubt for a time. The inconstancy of such irregularity at subsequent examination and the extreme dilation, eliminate the possibility of carcinomatous involvement. A case has been reported of volvulus of the enlarged esophagus, (D'Alessio).

The condition is thought to be due to a lesion of Auerbach's Plexus, causing the dysfunction; the vagus

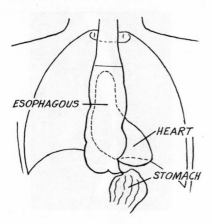

Fig. 227

acts on the smooth muscle of the esophagus through the plexus. Failure of dilator impulses leaves constrictor impulses unopposed; the extreme dilatation of the esophagus above is due to loss of tone, no waves are seen passing down the esophagus once this condition is established. When the myenteric plexus is degenerated or blocked experimentally the smooth muscle goes into spastic constriction.

The condition is not incompatible with life even over long periods; continuous eating finally crowds some food into the stomach. Long stasis of food in the esophagus may result in esophagitis. Attention has been called to the occasional association of cardiac achalasia with carcinoma of the esophagus. (Baer and Sicher). The degree of esophageal dilatation is never as great however, under these circumstances.

Ordinary antispasmodics such as Atropine and Benzedrine have no relaxing effect on the cardiospasm but the nitrites (amyl or nitroglycerine) relax the spasm within a few minutes causing ready flow of barium into the stomach. The effect is only transitory and cannot be used as a therapeutic procedure. A new drug, Octvlnitrite is said to be more effective (Grossmann), but in our experience it has not been very satisfactory. Injection of Mecholyl has been found to produce a lumen-obliterating contraction of the esophagus in cardiospasm which did not occur in other conditions suggesting that it might be used in doubtful cases as a confirmatory diagnostic measure, (Kramer and Ingelfinger). In the early stages, dilatation of the cardiac constriction by a hydrostatic pressure from a rubber bag inserted in the constriction may result in complete cure. Many operations have been advocated for this condition but none is wholly satisfactory. A transthoracic longitudinal splitting of the esophageal coats down to but not including the mucosa (Heller operation) seems to give good results with minimal complications in many cases.

ESOPHAGEAL REFLUX. In some infants relaxation or absence of sphincteric control at the cardia results in reflux of the stomach contents into the esophagus and spitting up of the ingested meal, on assuming the horizontal position. These symptoms may give rise to a mistaken impression of vomiting from pyloric stenosis. On roentgen examination the barium mixture flows back freely above the diaphragm moving in and out of the stomach synchronously with respiration. This has been attributed to a faulty mechanism at the cardia, (Astley and Carré). Normally: 1) the pinch cock action of the left diaphragm forms an oblique junction with the stomach; 2) gas pressure in the fundus of the stomach tends to prevent reflux, and 3) a certain degree of sphincter control is present at the lower end of the esophagus. Gastroesophageal incompetence occurs when there is loss of obliquity of the junction due to a wide hiatus produced by a tendency to formation of a thoracic stomach resulting in a poor pinch cock action; this likewise results in loss of the stomach bubble. Conway-Hughes after examination of a large series of adult patients having esophageal reflux, for other accompanying pathology has concluded that esophageal reflux is a relatively common condition, occurring in 20 per cent of all patients examined. It may be free, or may be forced, requiring abdominal pressure to produce. It is more frequent in women than in men.

It is a common finding in all age groups; pregnancy is not an important factor. It is most frequently found as an isolated lesion and does not occur commonly in those exhibiting poor tone or ptosis.

Symptoms may be referable to the throat; x-ray examination is readily conclusive after taking a pint of barium.

ESOPHAGEAL DISTURBANCES IN GENERALIZED SCLERODERMA.

In scleroderma certain very unusual changes are observed in the esophagus (Lindsay, et al.) These are characterized by: 1) atony and dilatation of lower esophagus with loss of peristaltic waves especially in the lower half; 2) dysphagia, especially while in the recumbent position with consequent delay in emptying the esophagus; 3) substernal pain about an hour after meals probably from regurgitation of the gastric contents into the lower esophagus; 4) chronic ulceration in lower esophagus near the ampulla, probably from the irritating effect of the gastric juice; 5) ultimately stricture formation just above the diaphragm from cicatrization. Considerable delay is also noted in emptying of the stomach and in passage of the barium through the intestines (Hale, and Schatzki) Pachyderma, or thickening and induration of the entire esophageal wall from inflammation may occur, giving rise to a roentgen picture of fine parallel longitudinal esophageal folds with irregular marginal indentations (Ludin). The constricted region is longer than that seen in cardiospasm, and not necessarily immediately at the cardia. Dilatation above the stricture is not as pronounced as in cardiospasm.

INTRAMURAL EXTRAMUCOSAL TUMORS OF THE ESOPHAGUS (Fig. 228A and B).

Intramural tumors of the esophagus cause rounded pressure defects on the esophagus which produce sharp, clearcut edges at the margins. They differ in appearance from pressure defects produced by adjacent extraesophageal structures such as the aorta or tumors of other types such as chordoma, or meningocele, in that structures of this type produce more gradual pressure without the sharp abrupt margin, (Sennett). The diagnosis is of great importance in that intramural tumors of this kind regardless of whether they occur in the esophagus, stomach or intestine are usually benign, (Schatzki, and Hawes). Benign tumors of the esophagus are very rare; those most commonly encountered are myoma, fibroma, lipoma and polypi. Cystic dysembryoma has been reported, (Truchot and Coutou).

MALIGNANT TUMORS OF ESOPHAGUS* (Fig. 228C).

Carcinoma is the most common type of involvement of the esophagus. It occurs most frequently in males (90%). The carcinomatous growth, springing from the inner mucosal lining of the esophagus, grows inward into the lumen, thus taking up part of the space ordinarily available for the passage of food. Such growths are relatively painless and may progress to large size before they give evidence of their presence by obstruction to swallowing. They may ultimately completely occlude the esophagus. On the administration of a barium mixture they show a silhouette of the inner margin of the growth giving the appearance of an irregular constriction—apex downward.

The defect and constriction from the tumor may be seen at any level of the esophagus, but the majority of malignant lesions are in the lower third, and next most frequent site on the middle third. Food particles impacted at the site of obstruction may conceal the true appearance of the lesion, or contrarily, may cause a benign lesion such as smooth stricture to have the irregular outline of a carcinoma.

Usually carcinomata can be distinguished from benign smoothly tapering or abruptly constricting lesions by their irregular contour, and also by the infrequency of appreciable dilatation of the esophagus above the lesion. Benign lesions are more compatible with longer life expectancy, and do not progress so often to complete obstruction, thus allowing dilatation above the lesion, sometimes of enormous degree.

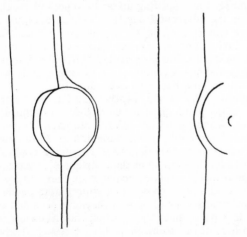

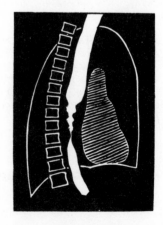

Fig. 228A   Fig. 228B   Fig. 228C

The short abdominal portion may be difficult to examine in detail in some cases. Retropneumoperitoneum may be of aid in visualizing lesions in this region (Antoine, et al.). Mediastinal tumors or bronchiogenic tumors and their lymph node metastases may cause pressure defects on the esophagus (Middleman). Later on they may extend into a bronchus with the establishment of a bronchoesophageal fistula. This is indicated at fluoroscopic examination by the escape of opaque mixture through the fistula into the bronchial tree. If complete occlusion has occurred, gastrostomy may be performed for prolongation of life. Freidenfelt has described a method of double contrast examination of the esophagus of use especially in cases of stricture for the differentiation of pathological lesions. This is accomplished by administration of a teaspoonful of effervescent powder (sodium bicarbonate and tartaric acid, equal parts) immediately washed down by a thin barium solution. A similar effect may sometimes be secured by merely swallowing air with the solution of barium, or by belching air and barium from the stomach.

Surgical resection is now feasible in a goodly number of cases although the five-year survival rate is disappointing. However, the ability to swallow normally for the remaining months or years of life makes justifiable an operation of this magnitude even when done purely for palliation.

Deep X-ray therapy given through a continuous port with complete rotation of the patient's body, using small repeated doses carried on over a protracted period has proved of some promise in the treatment of this disease.

The technic of intubation in obstructing carcinoma of the esophagus permitting the passage of a polyethylene tube past the stricture into the stomach, for palliative purposes, has been described by Leborne.

Using an ordinary intubation tube such as those used in anaesthesiology, inserted into the pharynx and upper esophagus, as a guide, a polyethylene tube with metal wire is passed down the esophagus to the point of stricture. By manipulation the tube is passed through the carcinomatous stricture into the stomach, where it remains permanently. False passage is encountered in less than 2 per cent of the cases.

DIVERTICULUM OF ESOPHAGUS.* A diverticulum is a pouchlike projection from the lumen of a hollow viscus. Diverticula of the esophagus may occur at any age; they may vary from a few millimeters to many, eight or ten, centimeters in size. Most diverticula give very few symptoms until by their size and location they interfere with the act of swallowing.

Diverticula of the esophagus are of essentially two types:

1. Traction and
2. Pulsion

Traction diverticula (Fig. 229A), as their name implies, are produced by scar tissue traction on the esophageal wall following mediastinal infections, such

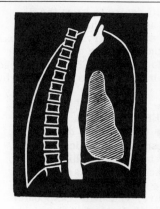
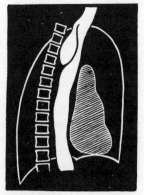

Fig. 229A   Fig. 229B

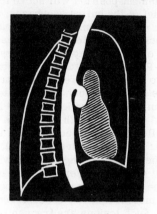

Fig. 229C

as tuberculous mediastinitis. They occur most commonly in the middle third on the lateral or anterior wall. They are usually small and solitary and are usually directed upwards. If examination with a barium meal is not made in the recumbent position they may be entirely missed. They are almost always of no clinical significance, not giving rise to symptoms and not requiring excision.

Pulsion diverticula (Fig. 229B) are more common; they usually occur high up in the neck near the junction of the pharynx and esophagus; although they may occur in any location in the esophagus (Fig. 229C). They are probably due to a deficiency in the musculature and a failure of the cricopharyngeus muscle to relax during swallowing; a pouch of the mucous membrane is formed by the natural process of swallowing. Once started, such diverticula may progress to enormous size causing obstruction by the pressure pouch on the esophagus.

They are best seen on flouroscopic examination; as the patient drinks, the thin barium sulphate mixture enters the diverticulum disclosing the saclike appendage. This retains the barium after the remainder of the solution continues on into the stomach. The neck of the sac is upward and the fundus or rounded end is downward, producing a form of shadow exactly opposite to that seen in any type of esophageal constriction. They arise from the posterior aspect of the esophagus, and usually protrude to the left side of the neck. The surgeon will desire to know the diverticulum's position, so as to plan his incision.

A dissecting (intramural) pharyngo-esophageal diverticulum separating the muscular coats of the esophagus as it extends downward has been described (Melamed, and Walker). Its contents is milked out by the act of swallowing.

ESOPHAGEAL VARICES (Fig. 230A). Another condition of the esophagus which can be detected by roentgen examination is esophageal varicosities. These are located mainly in the lower third of the esophagus near the cardiac orifice. Examination with barium mixture while lying down shows their elongated tortuous structure. One-half teaspoonful of Rugar administered with the patient in the right oblique recumbent position will serve to outline the mucosal relief of the entire esophagus; a number of radiographic examinations should be made from 5 seconds to one minute after the administration of Rugar. Use of a serial rapid film changer such as the Sanchez-Perez apparatus for cardioangiography making six to eight exposures at one-half to one second intervals has done much to facilitate this examination. Examination is made in forced inspiration and in forced expiration with the glottis closed; immediately following sustained Valsalva exercise is a good time for x-ray exposure, (Nelson). It has been shown that the varices change in size with change in intrathoracic pressure. Peristatsis may completely flatten out the folds causing their disappearance. The condition is most frequently encountered in cirrhosis of the liver. Such lesions are frequently accompanied by gastric varices of the fundus of the stomach. Varices often bleed, and the blood loss may be of massive proportions. Unfortunately varices are poorly demonstrated as a rule during the bleeding period, but barium swallow examination should be attempted because of the importance of localizing an upper alimentary tract bleeding lesion. Brick and Palmer, on examination of 172 patients with proved esophageal varices, with roentgen rays, found that 78.1% were detected where there was a history of hemorrhage and only 52.7% where there was no such history; only 22% of cases diagnosed by esophagoscopy were discovered by roentgen rays alone; indicating the need for improvement in roentgen methods.

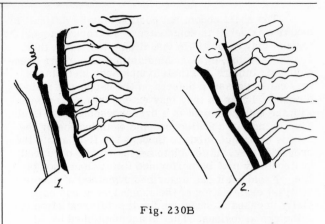

Fig. 230B

POST-CRICOID WEB (Fig. 230B$_1$ & B$_2$). The development of a weblike structure at the upper end of the esophagus in post-cricoid region, has been noted in association with dysphagia in patients suffering from sideropenia, an iron-deficiency state (Paterson-Brown Kelly; or Plummer-Vinson Syndrome). At the upper end of the esophagus the circular muscle fibres blend with the cricopharyngeus muscle; the longitudinal fibres are inserted into the cricoid cartilage itself. It is possible that the iron-deficiency state may have some effect on this muscular attachment, (Waldenstrom and Kjellberg).

Roentgenologically this web-like structure produces a small protrusion extending from the anterior wall, into the lumen like a thin shelf, as if a loop of thread were tied about the esophagus, (Fig. 230B$_2$). The lower portion of the pharyngeus muscle may form a smooth indentation of the posterior pharyngeal wall, (Fig. 230B$_1$), (Killian's Lip) as it passes this point in normal individuals; this is larger and should not be confused with the web structure. Such webs are associated with microcytic, hypochromic anaemia, glossitis, fissures at the corners of the mouth, achlorhydria and splenomegaly. Such strictures should be dilated under pharyngoscopic observation. They have been encountered with hypopharyngeal cancer, (Lindvall). Waldmann and Turnbull feel that they may be congenital in origin. Spiro has reported 12 cases.

CONGENITAL ATRESIA (Fig. 230D). Congenital atresia of the esophagus is seen in newborn infants. Obviously, if complete, it is not compatible with life. From the outset it is observed that the infant cannot eat properly but regurgitates its food almost immediately. X-ray examination with barium sulphate mixture or lipiodol discloses the atresia usually in the upper thoracic portion with formation of a blind pouch, (E). In congenital atresia a small segment of the esophagus is replaced by a fibrous cord, without lumen, the upper and lower segments being normal. Most often there is an associated esophagotracheal or bronchial fistula, (B), connecting with the lower segment, which permits air inspired through the trachea to be forced into the stomach and intestines, (I). A minority of cases do not have the associated tracheo-esophageal fistula, and these may diagnosed by absence of air in the stomach and intestines. Many of these infants develop a pneumonia

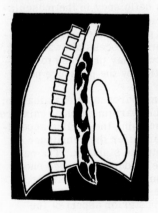   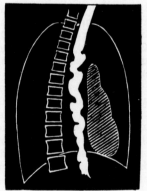

Fig. 230A   Fig. 230C

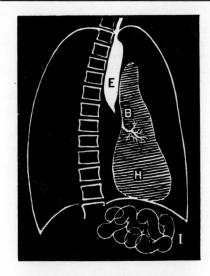

Fig. 230D

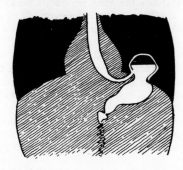

Fig. 231A

from aspiration, further adding to the morbidity. For this reason, early diagnosis is imperative. Hutton, in a study of 24 cases has found that the radiographic abnormality of web constriction found in the lower pharynx and upper esophagus are not the only ones encountered; but segmental webs or zones of constriction have been found in the lower esophagus also.

Slight congenital narrowing of the esophagus has been reported in infants near the level of the seventh thoracic vertebra which cause some difficulty in feeding. At about one year of age when the child partakes of solid food this difficulty becomes more pronounced. Roentgenologically the previous narrowing becomes a definite stricture in this location with dilatation of the proximal portion. Within a short time the fundus of the stomach may be pulled upward above the diaphragm finally developing into a partial thoracic stomach. Plain muscle may contract to one-fourth its ordinary length. Any irritating focus in the esophagus may cause retraction of the esophageal ampulla gradually dragging the stomach through the hiatus. An air bubble in the stomach may show through the cardiac shadow giving a clue to its presence even in the ordinary chest roentgenogram. A similar process may occur in adults from peptic ulcer of the esophagus. Thus it may be possible that short esophagus and thoracic stomach may not in all cases be congenital in origin, (Johnstone), and many observers think a true congenitally short esophagus to be a rarity.

Cysts lined by gastric mucosa have been reported in the mediastinum.

DIAPHRAGMATIC HERNIA.* (Fig. 231A) with protrusion of the stomach through a hernial sac into the thorax, carries with it the esophagus; in this case the esophagus is not shortened but is normal in length. (See Gastric Hernias.)

Eventration of the diaphragm may result in the stomach occupying an extremely high position with the esophagus following into the new location.

Elongation of the esophagus. The esophagus may become extremely elongated; an instance has been reported where almost the entire stomach was within the hernial sac of a scrotal hernia, (English; Lust).

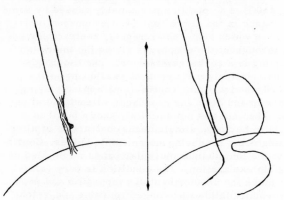

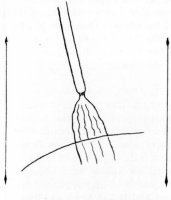

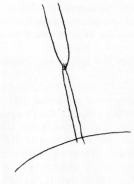

B. Peptic Esophagitis with ulcer.

C. Peptic Esophagitis with hiatal hernia.

D. Peptic Esophagitis with short constricted area, shortened esophagus, and small pouch-like gastric hernia. Ulcer may or may not be seen.

E. Peptic esophagitis and ulceration, possibly from aberrant gastric mucosa.

REFLUX ESOPHAGITIS AND PEPTIC ULCER of the lower esophagus are two related entities. Both are thought to be caused by reflux of acid gastric juice into the lower esophagus. There the mucosa cannot withstand the acidity and thus becomes inflamed, and eventually ulcerated. Early signs of esophagitis consist of spasm and slight narrowing of the inflamed region with distortion or loss of mucosal folds. Later the constriction may become more pronounced and more constant. Small erosions and ulcerations are seen, often extending over quite a length of the tube. Dilatation of the esophagus above the diseased area does not occur until later when permanent non-relaxing constriction is present. Whereas early changes may be reversible, continued disease leads to fibrosis and irreversible narrowing, (see Johnstone, Wolf). Robinson and Hennessy have reported two cases in which vomiting and collapse figured prominently.

Should localized ulceration persist, or undergo phases of healing and exacerbation resulting in additional fibrosis the constricted length may be quite limited. This type of finding is often seen at the esophagogastric junction, in association with a shortened esophagus and herniation of a pouch of stomach above the diaphragm. These cases have been referred to as congenitally short esophagus, but there is an increasing feeling that the shortening of the esophagus is acquired, that is, due to the fibrosis and spasm caused by reflux of peptic acid contents into the lower esophagus. The short constricted length in addition to showing distortion and loss of mucosa, may show a definite deep ulcer niche at the margin of the stomach and esophagus. The reflux of stomach contents into the esophagus can be demonstrated at fluoroscopy if the stenosis has not progressed too far.

Peptic esophagitis may result from severe, prolonged vomiting or from the trauma of indwelling gastric tube. Duodenal and gastric ulcers, and hiatus herniae, of several types, also predisposes to peptic esophagitis, and conversely peptic esophagitis may progress to herniation of the stomach supradiaphragmatically.

In addition to substernal and upper abdominal pain, hemorrhage either massive and acute or small and chronic is experienced by some. This should always be kept in mind when the "g. i. bleeder" is examined. Bleeding is from the discrete ulcer, or from the inflamed, fragile mucosa.

LOWER ESOPHAGEAL RING. Schatzki and Gary have reported a diaphragm-like localized narrowing in the lower esophagus just above the cardia sometimes associated with dysphasia and inability to swallow solid food of ordinary size. The cause is not known. Esophagoscopy often fails to disclose either an organic stricture or a definite sphincteric action. In one instance it has been observed by esophagoscopy to consist of a fibrosed band and it has been assumed that this may have resulted from healed peptic ulcer. Resection of this segment has given relief. A similar type of diaphragm-like lesion has been reported at the pyloric end of the stomach (q.v.). The same authors have recently presented their findings after

a study of 21 such cases, as follows:

1. A thin diaphragm-like constriction of the lower esophagus is not infrequently found if the esophagus is distended with barium mixture.

2. This narrowing represents a thin annual position of the wall of the esophagus which cannot be distended as well as the wall above and below this region.

3. The maximal diameter of the ring is usually constant for several years.

4. The ring occurs equally frequently in males and females. It is considerably more common in persons past the age of fifty.

5. The ring must be differentiated from simple muscular contraction of the esophagus and from hiatus hernia with or without esophagitis.

6. The cause of the ring is unknown. The ring is frequently associated with a hiatus hernia, and it appears likely that some upward displacement of the intestinal tube into the chest is present in all cases with rings.

7. In most instances the ring produces no clinical symptoms; in a smaller group of persons it results in dysphagia with characteristic sporadic episodes of difficulty in swallowing solid foods.

The authors have observed 21 patients with dysphagia. The question of whether or not dysphagia occurs depends primarily on the diameter of the maximally opened ring and to a lesser degree on the eating habits of the patient.

8. Satisfactory therapeutic results in the patients with dysphagia can usually be obtained by proper education of the patient. An occasional case will require surgery.

NERVOUS INTERFERENCE WITH ESOPHAGEAL CONTRACTION

Bulbar Paralysis. In bulbar palsy, myasthenia gravis and similar afflictions, the swallowing reflex is disturbed and barium mixture, in place of passing normally down the esophagus, is aspirated into the lungs.

"Curling" or Corkscrew-(Writhing) esophagus (Fig. 230C) is a condition presumably caused by some disturbance in the nerve control of esophageal peristalsis in which numerous irregular contractions appear throughout the esophagus giving the impression of curling in a corkscrew fashion. The esophagus may be relatively inactive until swallowing is attempted when writhing contractions appear playing rapidly up and down the esophagus without useful purpose. The cause is not definitely known but it is thought to be due to simultaneous contraction of alternate segments producing intermediate bulges. Contraction of the longitudinal muscular bands might also be a plausible explanation. The condition is very rare.

Since the development of esophagitis and peptic ulcer usually follows prolonged vomiting and retching causing irritating gastric juice to remain in long contact with the lower esophageal mucosa Dawson has also shown by a series of remarkable cases the development of ulceration in esophagitis, the contraction and shortening of the esophagus with herniation of stomach through the esophageal orifice.

Infection of esophagus with monilia albicans has become more prevalent in recent years since the widespread use of antibiotics and cortisone. With suitable technic the esophageal infection can be detected. Symptoms of the cases were a long history of leukopenia and splenomegaly, severe recurrent infection, long treatment with antibiotics and short treatment with cortisone.

Roentgen examination of the esophagus revealed essentially extensive mural changes without involvement of the esophagus itself. Aside from dysphagia there were not eeophageal symptoms. Roentgen examination of the esophagus showed the outline to be irregular and ragged, made up of small indentations and protrusions. Many of the cases are fatal, (Andren and Theander).

INJURY TO THE ESOPHAGUS

Esophageal Perforation. Perforation of the esophagus whether it be from foreign body or spontaneous rupture is a very serious condition which is frequently fatal unless promptly recognized and treated. Perforation from a foreign body is localized to a small area and usually gives ample indication of its presence. Increase in the retropharyngeal space or widening of the mediastinum with accompanying interstitial emphysema are the main diagnostic points. Administration of Lipiodol may demonstrate the fistulous tract into the surrounding tissues.

Spontaneous rupture of the esophagus is a less frequent but much more dramatic incident. The essential factor in its production according to GAY is, "a sudden increase in intra-abdominal pressure associated with spasm of the pylorus and cricopharyngeus muscles with resulting sudden increase in the intraluminal pressure of the lower esophagus." Under these conditions a spontaneous tear results in the distal end of the esophagus. This is its weakest part anatomically where the vessels and nerves enter. The tear extends longitudinally, involves all coats in the distal 3 inches of the esophagus. There is immediate dissection of the stomach contents into the mediastinum or pleural cavity. Emphysema extends into the mediastinum and subcutaneous spaces and there is frequently associated pleural effusion. In most cases this accident occurs during the act of swallowing in association with some other outside influence at the time such as hiccoughing, when the stomach is already distended. In a patient observed by us, the rupture occurred in the stomach and into the pleural cavity discharging a large amount of air and beer into the pleural cavity. Christoforidis and Nelson have reported a case in which the irregular rent formed a pouch which recovered spontaneously; usually the accident requires immediate operation. Migliaccio has reported a case which occurred five years after resection of the stomach. Bodi, et al., have also reported a case.

Dysphagia. In bulbar palsy (Madsen) x-ray examination reveals the cause of the dysphagia to be 1) passage of the barium mixture into the larynx and trachea, 2) its accumulation in the pharynx, 3) its retention in the valleculae, and pyriform fossae, and 4) its slow passage down the esophagus. Dysphagia has been encountered in association with the pressure of the sclerotic aorta upon the esophagus, (Keates and Magidson). Langton and Laws have reported 3 cases of carcinoma of the pancreas in which dysphagia was a prominent and early symptom; this seems to be very uncommon.

I. Anatomy
   Relation of gastric types to habitus
II. Roentgen examination
   Normal stomach
   1. Divisions of stomach
       Pars cardiaca
       Pars media
       Pars pylorica
   2. Normal landmarks
       Stomach bubble
       Lesser curvature
       Greater curvature
       Incisura cardiaca
       Incisura angularis
       Cardiac orifice
       Pyloric antrum
       Pyloric sphincter
       Duodenal bulb
   3. Peristalsis
       Hyper- and hypo-
       Reverse
   4. Gastric motility
       Motor barium sulphate meal
       Hyper- and hypo-motility
III. Organic pathology
   1. Gastric ulcer—roentgen characteristics
     a. Types
        Mucosal
        Submucosal
        Penetrating (through circular muscular layers)
        Perforating (through peritoneal layer
        Healed, hour-glass stomach
     b. Location of involvement
     c. Etiology of, influence of ischemia
     d. Roentgen observation during treatment of,
       Influence of bed-rest,
     e. Malignant degeneration of,
     f. Surgical intervention in,
   2. Gastric carcinoma—roentgen characteristics
     a. Types
        Polypoid fungating type
        Scirrhus type
     b. Location
        Fundus
        Pars media
        Pars pylorica
     c. Surgical treatment of,
   3. Linitis plastica—roentgen characteristics
     a. Carcinomatous
     b. Fibrotic
   4. Malignant lymphomata
     a. Hodgkin's disease
     b. Primary lymphosarcoma
   5. Gastric syphilis—roentgen characteristics
     a. Gumma of stomach
     b. Sclerosis
     c. Tabetic crisis
   6. Pyloric muscle hypertrophy
     a. In infants (congenital)
     b. In adults

7. Benign tumors of stomach—roentgen characteristics
    a. Myoma
    b. Fibroma
    c. Adenoma
    d. Angioma
    e. Neuroma—Schwannoma
8. Giant gastric rugae
9. Redundant gastric mucosa
10. Gastric polyps
11. Multiple polyposis
12. Gastritis
    a. Hypertrophic—alcoholic
    b. Atrophic
    c. Ulcerative
    d. Phlegmonous
    e. Emphysematous
    f. Post-irradiation gastritis
    g. Tuberculosis of stomach
13. Diapedetic hemorrhage from stomach without demonstrable lesion
In chronic abdominal infection;
    a. of gall bladder
    b. of appendix
    c. of diverticula
14. Foreign bodies
    a. Trichobezoar
    b. Phytobezoar
15. Diverticulum of stomach—roentgen characteristics
16. Gastric hernia and kindred lesions
    a. Esophageal orifice
    b. Diaphragmatic
    c. Eventration
    d. Ectopic stomach (scrotal femoral hernia)
    e. Thoracic stomach (congenital)
IV. Functional lesions—roentgen characteristics
    1. Gastric spasm
        Intrinsic origin
            Pylorospasm
        Extrinsic origin
            Reflex
    2. Gastroptosis
    3. Nervous indigestion
    4. Gastric neurosis
    5. Psychological effect on gastric function
    6. Cascade stomach
    7. Gastro-duodenal invagination, (intussusception)
V. Corrective operative procedures
    1. Gastroenterostomy—roentgen manifestations
        a. Marginal ulcer
    2. Vagotomy
    3. Gastric resection
    4. Perigastric hematoma from traumatic rupture of spleen

Chapter XIX

STOMACH

ANATOMY. The stomach is the most expanded portion of the gastrointestinal tract. It consists of four distinct coats:

1. The outer serous or peritoneal coat covering the stomach is similar in all respects to peritoneum elsewhere in the abdomen,

2. A muscular coat made up of an outer longitudinal and an inner circular layer of muscle fibers. At the cardiac or upper end, the stomach connects with the esophagus. A small ovoid dilation of the esophagus just above the diaphragm is known as the cardiac or diaphragmatic ampulla. There does not seem to be any definite muscular sphincter demonstrable at this orifice but the contraction of the smooth muscle fibers seems to function as if there were; Chevalier Jackson has demonstrated that the constriction demonstrable lower down is due to a pinch-cock action of the diaphragm. Occasionally a weak sphincteric action can be demonstrated but for the most part no actual change can be seen. Fluoroscopically, however, the lower esophagus behaves as if a sphincter were present especially if any of the acid contents of the stomach regurgitates into the esophagus. At the pyloric or lower end of the stomach there is, however, a very distinct thickening of the circular musculature forming the pyloric muscle or sphincter. Progressive contractions of segments of the muscular coat produce peristaltic waves by which the gastric content is propelled onward into the intestines. During the first few weeks of life the pyloric mechanism lacks proper coordination and an infant's stomach may not empty in eight or even, as much as twenty-four hours. Within the first seven to ten days of life any delay in gastric motility cannot be considered as pathological.

3. A coat of areolar tissue which furnishes a space for transmission of blood vessels. This loosely constructed layer permits passage of blood through the vessels without interference from peristaltic contractions. The blood supply to the stomach is from the gastric artery which passes to the lesser curvature just below the cardia and from the pyloric artery which passes along the lesser curvature from below upward. The greater curvature is supplied by the left gastroepiploic artery from above and the right gastroepiploic artery from below. Some observers believe that these vessels are of particular importance in the formation and healing of gastric ulcer. The nerves are from the right and left vagus and solar plexus of the sympathetic system. Auerbach's plexus is probably the site of the nerve control for peristaltic movement while Meissner's plexus influences gastric secretion by its distribution to the gastric glands.

4. An inner mucosal lining which furnishes the secretory portion of the organ. This is the most specialized layer of all; it is concerned with secretion of the gastric juice. It is thicker and less elastic than the other layers, being thrown into folds by contraction of the muscularis mucosa. As the stomach is filled these become ironed out but are never completely lost. These mucosal folds or rugae are continuous through the pyloric ring into the first portion or bulb of the duodenum which has led many observers to consider the first portion of the duodenum as a part of the stomach rather than the intestine.

The stomach usually occupies the position in the left upper quadrant of the abdomen, but occasionally it may be found on the right side. This may be due to a complete situs inversus, all of the organs being reversed, or it may be the only organ displaced, (Almy, et al.).

RELATION OF GASTRIC TYPES TO HABITUS.* In the cadaver the stomach is found high up under the ribs. Even at operation the stomach appears high up in the abdomen. This is because in each instance the subject is in the recumbent position. In active life, with the patient standing, the stomach extends much farther downward. Before this fact was appreciated a great deal of confusion resulted in the study of roentgenology by the various shapes and sizes in which the stomach was found. It remained for R. Walter Mills to definitely correlate habitus with stomach form (Fig. 232). If we represent diagrammatically the physical characteristics of a normal well-built individual by a square and designate this type of habitus as sthenic, the type of stomach normally possessed by such an individual should be tubular in shape—as wide above as it is below—with the pylorus to the right side and well above the umbilicus. A stomach having these characteristics is called an orthotonic stomach or one which exhibits normal tone.

Now if we progress toward more slender individuals, whom we may designate as of hyposthenic habitus, we find that their type of stomach is longer and more slender, narrower at the top and having a tendency to sag below, the greater curvature descending to or near the umbilicus and the pyloric end swinging over more to the left side. Such a stomach is known as the hypotonic type—it is normally found

---

*An asterisk following any title indicates that roentgenographic reproductions illustrating this condition will be found in the pictorial supplement at the end of the chapter.

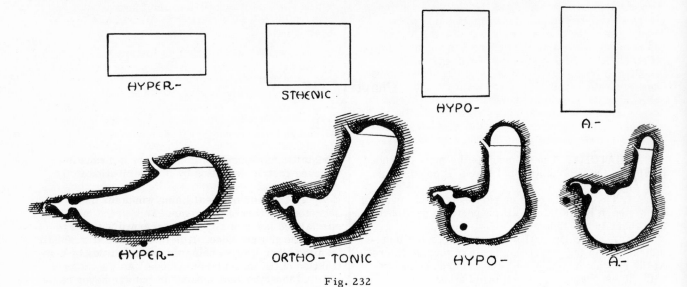

Fig. 232

in an individual of this type.

Still more slender individuals are designated as asthenic individuals and their stomachs sag far down below the umbilicus into the pelvis, being almost collapsed above, expanding into large sacs below. They frequently swing entirely over to the left of the umbilicus. Such stomachs are known as atonic stomachs.

Progressing in the opposite direction from the normal sthenic habitus to the short, fat stocky individual, designated as hypersthenic, we find their stomachs much higher in the abdomen, often well up under the rib margins, extremely wide above and narrow below; lying almost transversely across the upper abdomen with the pyloric end well to the right. Such stomachs are designated as of hypertonic type.

There can be no doubt that the intraabdominal pressure contributes greatly to the development of these various gastric types; indeed, it may be that it is the most important factor. As the intraabdominal pressure is raised by deposit of fat on the abdomen, the abdominal wall becomes less flabby and does not permit the sagging down of the abdominal contents. The influence of this support is seen mainly in the lower, more movable portion of the stomach, so that it is held up and not permitted to sag. Change in type of stomach to conform to habitus has been noted clinically when a patient by putting on weight changes his stature.

In its natural state the stomach, being of similar density to the surrounding structures cannot be visualized by roentgen-ray examination. Again it is necessary to resort to administration of radiopaque mixture—barium sulphate. Such a mixture filling the stomach does not render the stomach itself visible but merely provides a silhouette of the gastric lumen. Any defect in the mucosal lining can be readily visualized.

NORMAL LANDMARKS * (Fig. 233A and B). As the barium sulphate mixture enters the stomach

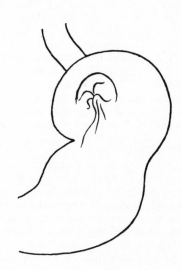

Fig. 233A

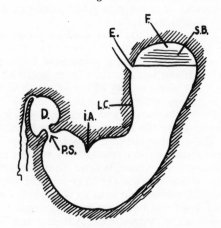

Fig. 233B

through the cardiac orifice of the esophagus it may leave a stellate and semilunar impression on the upper end of the stomach due to puckering of the esophageal mucosa as the orifice is seen "on end," (Fig. 233A). This must always be borne in mind as normal structure (Hodges, et al.). The barium descends along the lesser curvature to the lower portion of the stomach where it collects, gradually expanding the stomach from below as it fills. The portion of the stomach above the esophageal orifice is known as the pars cardiaca or fundus; that below the incisura angularis to the pyloric sphincter is known as the pars pylorica, and the intervening portion is designated as the pars media.

The esophageal opening (e) being below the highest point of the stomach permits the accumulation of any gas in the stomach above this point. This gives rise to the stomach bubble (s.b.) a gas collection always found in the fundus (f) of normal stomachs. As we proceed downward along the lesser curvature (l.c.) we come to an abrupt indentation at the point where the stomach assumes a more horizontal position; this is known as the incisura angularis (i.a.). At the lower end of the stomach there is a muscular ring known as the pyloric sphincter (p.s.) which relaxes periodically, permitting barium to be ejected into the duodenum, (d).

Contraction of the gastric musculature is concerned in maintaining its tone.

PERISTALSIS (Fig. 234). The stomach is emptied by peristaltic movement. Peristaltic contractions are successive ringlike contractions of the circular musculature produced by a gradient of nervous impulses which start at the fundus and progress downward toward the pyloric end, terminating at the pylorus by relaxation of the pyloric sphincter permitting small portions of the stomach contents to be ejected into the duodenum. They are diminished in carcinoma and increased in ulcer or pyloric stenosis. They may be increased in the normal stomach within a few minutes by administration of 1/25 grain of physostigmine sulphate by mouth. Muscular tone may be restored to an atonic stomach by the administration of 40 gm. syrup of ipecac which serves also to rid the stomach of any residue of food material (Seneque). A fine mucosal diaphragm has been reported as a rare occurrence in the prepyloric

Fig. 234

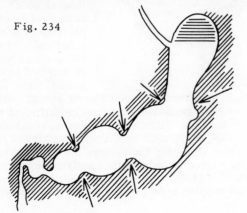

region of the stomach (Gross and Durham), but this does not seem to interfere with gastric motility or other functions.

GASTRIC MOTILITY. The emptying time of the stomach is influenced by the composition of the food material. Water begins to leave the stomach at once and is entirely ejected within an hour. A carbohydrate meal, in most individuals, requires four hours for complete ejection from the stomach. All normal individuals should show complete emptying in five hours. It is safe to say then, that retention in the stomach six hours after a carbohydrate barium meal is definite evidence of pathologic change. A purely protein meal requires longer— seven hours, whereas a fat meal requires the longest period for complete ejection—nine hours. It is obvious then that in testing gastric motility with a carbohydrate meal that no protein or fat be ingested during the test, or erroneous conclusions will be reached.

The first portion of the duodenum is triangular or "chocolate-drop" shaped and is smooth in outline. The second portion descends abruptly from the apex of the triangle for three or four inches to its most dependent position; this portion is not smooth like the first portion but assumes a feathery appearance similar to that seen in the small intestine. The horizontal portion of the third part is very short and the ascending portion of the third part again goes upward posterior to the pyloric portion of the stomach where it becomes the jejunum.

Hypomotility occurs, for instance, in generalized scleroderma where there is a peculiar atony of the stomach with some dilatation and lack of normal peristalsis resulting in prolonged retention. A similar lack of peristalsis is noted in the esophagus and intestines. Vagotomy or any drug or pathological process interfering with the vagus nerve will also cause retention. Certain drugs used in therapy may produce such side effects, such as Hexamethonium for high blood pressure as observed by Ettman, et al.; simple abdominal x-ray examination may serve to check upon the occurrence of such complications. Hypermotility occurs in association with linitis plastica, a condition in which carcinomatous infiltration of the pyloric sphincter prevents proper closure of this structure.

GASTROINTESTINAL EXAMINATION—ORGANIC LESIONS. Examination of the gastrointestinal tract is directed therefore, first to the detection of organic defects, and second to the detection of faults in its normal motility. Functional lesions of the gastrointestinal tract cannot be detected except insofar as they influence motility and tone. For this purpose the following procedure is carried out. A meal consisting of five to six ounces of barium sulphate in a pint of water, (skimmed milk or buttermilk), is administered on an empty stomach. (Be sure that barium sulphate—"pure for roentgen diagnosis," is used since many otherwise innocuous substances given in such large doses become actually harmful). Examine the esophagus and stomach during ingestion of the barium meal for any organic defects and for peristaltic action. After a five-hour interval re-examine the stomach and intestines; the barium mixture should have entirely left the stomach and progressed as far as the ascending portion of the colon, extending back into the terminal ileum. Twenty-four hours after ingestion, the barium mixture should have advanced beyond the ileocecal valve and should fill the large bowel. At forty-eight hour examination most of the barium mixture should be expelled from the colon, only a small residue remaining in the cecum and rectum. (For the technique of fluoroscopy and roentgenographic examination see Manual of Roentgenological Technique.)

GASTRIC ULCER* (Fig. 235A, B and C). The organic lesions of the stomach most frequently encountered are gastric ulcer and carcinoma. Gastric ulcer is a destructive process, producing a small rounded, punched-out area in the gastric mucosa which allows the escape of barium mixture beyond the natural contour thus producing a budlike projection, known as a niche. Since a large majority of gastric ulcers appear on the lesser curvature, they can usually be seen in profile without difficulty. When they occur on the anterior or posterior gastric wall, they may be hidden from view by the barium-filled stomach but manual pressure under fluoroscopic observation, approximating the anterior gastric wall to the posterior portion, presses out the opaque mixture from between them and leaves only the small rounded niche filled with barium mixture.

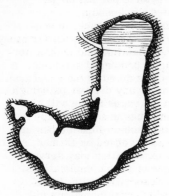

Fig. 235A

Gastric ulcers are so rarely encountered on the greater curvature that when they do occur in this location they must be considered as ulcerating carcinoma until proved otherwise. Occasionally, however, benign ulcers do occur in this location (Campbell). Attention has been called to the appearance of a so-called pseudo-niche on the greater curvature of the stomach which resembles the niche of true ulcer but cannot be substantiated on operative examination. The explanation of "localized spasm" about an area of superficial erosion does not seem tenable, (Moutier).

Much can be inferred as to the depth to which ulceration has occurred by the roentgen signs.

1. Mucosal ulcers confined to the mucous membrane retain tiny flecks of barium and on fluoroscopic examination, ride with the peristaltic wave.

2. Submucosal ulcers (Fig. 235A), which extend deeper into the submucosal layer, are slightly larger and remain more or less fixed in position during peristalsis; they do not ride with the wave.

3. Ulcers which have penetrated to involve the muscular coat result in persistent contraction of the circular muscular fibers of the stomach at this point (Fig. 235B). This gives rise to an incisura or indentation on the greater curvature opposite to the ulcer, resulting in a "B"-shaped deformity of the stomach.

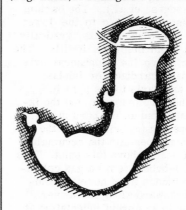

Fig. 235B

4. Perforating ulcers, which have perforated through the stomach wall to the peritoneal layer, show a small bubble of gas at the top of the perforated pouch (Fig. 235C). If complete rupture occurs, gas may be expelled into the peritoneal cavity giving rise to spontaneous pneumoperitoneum; this can be detected as a collection of gas under the diaphragm with the patient in the upright position. While the detection of free air in the abdominal cavity is indication of rupture of a hollow viscus, its absence cannot be construed as absolute indication that rupture of a hollow viscus has not occurred (Fig. 235D). If gas is not present in the viscus at the time of rupture, pneumoperitoneum does not occur. Pneumoperitoneum can be demonstrated in 80% of ruptured peptic ulcers; in rupture of typhoid ulcers the sign is absolutely diagnostic, since in typhoid fever the intestines always contain gas.

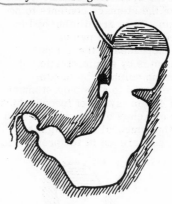

Fig. 235C

Gastric motility, or the emptying power of the stomach, depends primarily upon two things: the force exerted by the peristaltic waves to push food material through the pylorus, and the size of the opening through which it has to be expressed; if peristalsis is not sufficiently vigorous, the stomach will not be emptied in the normal time; if the orifice is narrowed by carcinoma or benign constriction, ordinary peristalsis may not be sufficient to force it through. Ulcer of the stomach, regardless of its location, may result in delayed emptying of the stomach; if it is near the pylorus it may delay emptying by reason of the spastic constriction which it causes; if it is higher up on the lesser curvature it may cause delay in emptying because of its inter-

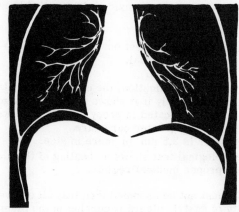

Fig. 235D

ference with normal peristalsis. Attention has been
called (Lilja) to the inhibitory effect on peristaltic
contraction of the pyloric portion of the stomach due
to gastric ulcer involving the incisura anguloris or
its immediate vicinity. The pyloric portion lies limp
like a bag and the pylorus remains widely open. This
is probably due to the involvement of the underlying
muscular coat by the ulcer. If obstruction of the
pylorus is complete, peristalsis may be reversed.
Reverse peristalsis always means that pathology is
present.

Roentgenological examination is also of value
in observing from time to time the state of healing
during treatment of an ulcer. As healing progresses,
the niche becomes smaller and smaller in size until
it can no longer be detected. If penetration of the
ulcer has been sufficiently deep to involve the circular muscle, the resulting scar formation may even
cause hour-glass contraction of the stomach. Scar
tissue formation retraction may cause shortening of
the lesser curvature resulting in elevation and displacement of the pyloric segment, (Hinds and Harper).
This is a condition which is rarely seen in recent
years, since examination by roentgen rays usually
results in earlier diagnosis.

Wilson and Wilson have pointed out the similarity of roentgen appearance of the outpouching of
pseudo-ulcerations of the stomach and duodenum
produced by traction diverticula. Persistence of the
appearance of the lesion is a sign favoring ulcer.
The traction type of diverticula are shallow and,
having a broad base empty readily; the usual type
occurring in the cardia have a narrow neck and retain barium for a long time.

For many years there has been much specula-
tion as to the cause of gastric ulcer, without arrival
at any definite conclusion.

Roentgenological observation of gastric ulcers
over a period of years has disclosed that the ulcers
heal with disappearance of their craters following
many varying forms of treatment. Advocates of the
theory of hyperacidity as a cause of gastric ulcer,
gave large doses of alkalies and under this treatment
roentgenological examination revealed healing of the
ulcers in many cases. Many drugs were used to control this hyperacidity. Others, feeling that excessive
alkalies merely stimulate further acid secretion, re-

lied upon diet alone, in the treatment of this condition;
in many instances there was healing of the ulcer, with
disappearance of the niche, at least temporarily.

The advent of surgical treatment of ulcer was
hailed with great enthusiasm and resection of the
ulcer and gastroenterostomy were practiced for a
time indiscriminately on large numbers of ulcer patients, on the theory that in the first instance this
eradicated the disease, and in the second the false
opening in the stomach permitted rapid egress of the
food, thereby relieving the stomach of its burden of
digestion. In many instances the patient was relieved
of symptoms, and niche formation disappeared and
the ulcer healed. It was only natural to assume that
the surgical procedure cured the patient.

The more or less successful results obtained by
these widely varying methods of treatment leads one
to seek some factor in the treatment common to all
methods. About the only thing common to all of these
methods of treatment is bed rest; how could rest,
even complete bed-rest influence the cause or healing
of gastric ulcer?

Every roentgenologist knows that by far the
greatest number of gastric ulcers occur on the lesser
curvature of large hypotonic stomachs which sag well
down in the abdomen; gastric ulcers rarely occur in
hypertonic stomachs.

What is there then about the hypertonic stomach
which protects it from ulcer formation, and what is
there about the hypotonic stomach which renders it
more susceptible to this condition? Could it be that
with the sagging down of the hypotonic stomach there
is a consequent pull on the omentum with a resulting
ischemia of the lesser curvature of the stomach?
This region is likewise rather poorly nourished under
normal circumstances. The more atonic the stomach
becomes, the more it pulls upon its omental attachment and the greater the amount of ischemia which
results. The hypertonic stomach, on the other hand,
is held high up by increased intra-abdominal pressure
caused by the abdominal fat, and the blood supply to
this portion of the stomach is not interfered with.
This is, of course, conjecture; no one really knows
what factors operate in the healing of ulcers. Theoretically then, on the basis of ischemia of the lesser
curvature of the stomach as the important factor in
the etiology of gastric ulcer, anything which would relieve the ischemia of the ulcer-bearing area, and
bring richer nourishment to the part, might be logically considered as a rational procedure for treatment.
Is it not possible, therefore, that rest--complete bed
rest--may be the important factor in all of these types
of treatment for gastric ulcer?

The influence of bed rest as a factor in the
treatment of gastric ulcer can be easily tested; simply
observe by roentgenological examination the changes
in the gastric ulcer over a period of a few weeks
while the patient, on a regular diet, without medication or other treatment of any sort, is maintained on
absolute bed rest. Under this treatment most ulcers
one centimeter or less in diameter heal within three
weeks; ulcers larger than this may require a longer
time, usually six to eight weeks.

If, after a few weeks of strict bed-rest regime,
there is no evidence of progressive healing of the

ulcer, then it may be assumed that you may be dealing with something other than a benign lesion. A superficial type of carcinomatous lesion has been reported which spreads in the submucosal tissues and is often associated with ulceration. On the other hand, the somewhat indurated margins of an ordinary benign ulcer can be mistaken for malignant involvement. At any rate, a trial period of a few weeks to observe the progress of the ulcer under bed-rest will not be amiss and will save operative removal of many benign ulcers.

What good does it do to put the patient to bed on his back to relieve the ischemia and cure the ulcer, if, by standing him on his feet again, the same conditions which gave rise to the ulcer in the first place are again produced? Won't he have recurrence at once? What can we do to avoid recurrence? Increase his intra-abdominal pressure by putting fat on his belly wall; correct any elements of anemia by blood transfusions if necessary and by administration of blood-building diet and medication. By such general measures, correcting conditions which theoretically gave rise to the ulcer in the first place you should be able to fortify the patient against a recurrence.

Little concern should be experienced for the two or three weeks' time utilized in carrying out the treatment of the patient in this manner, especially if roentgen examination indicates the benign character of the lesion; nor should the fear of benign ulcer undergoing malignant change deter such conservative action; this must certainly be a very rare occurrence. Many patients having large untreated ulcers observed off and on for years show no manifestations of malignant development.

On the basis of animal experimentation and clinical observations, Dragstedt, on the other hand presents the concept that peptic ulcers are usually due to an abnormal increase in the corrosive and digestive properties of the gastric content as a result of hypersecretion of gastric juice. Furthermore, that duodenal ulcers are usually due to a hypersecretion of gastric juice of nervous origin and gastric ulcers are usually due to hypersecretion of humoral or humoral origin.

Conditions Influencing the Benign or Malignant Character of Gastric Ulcers (Kirklin)

An ulcer may be considered as probably benign when:

1. The duration of the symptoms are 10 years or more.
2. The patient's age is 30 years or less.
3. There is a free hydrochloric acid determination of 40 or more.
4. At roentgenological examination the ulceration goes through the wall.
5. The lesion is found at roentgenographic examination on the lesser curvature.
6. The crater of the ulcer measures 2 cm. or less.
7. The stomach is of the B type.
8. The biological test shows reduction of size of the crater under medical treatment.

An ulcer may be considered as probably malignant when:

1. Symptoms are of recent onset.
2. In an elderly individual.
3. There is an achylia.
4. At roentgen examination, the ulcer is irregular in outline, especially if it shows a meniscus sign.
5. The lesion is located in prepyloric region, posterior wall or greater curvature.
6. The crater is 2.5 cm. or more in size.
7. The biological test shows no healing of the ulcer under proper medical regime.

It must not be assumed then that all or even a majority of gastric ulcers occurring in the older age group are malignant. Klein and Bradley found that the average age of occurrence of ulcer in this group was 55.3 years of age. In the group studies all of these were benign.

Preservation of the normal mucosal fold pattern in the stomach and in the vicinity of the ulcer is further evidence of benignicity. Sometimes the mucosal folds appear to converge at the site of the benign ulcer. Extreme large size of an ulcer should make the examiner suspicious of malignancy, but very large benign ulcers have also been observed. Elliott, et al., by careful statistical examination of 191 proved ulcer cases, have concluded that in determining the benign or malignant character of an ulcer, "the size or location of the ulcer was of no diagnostic significance". Rarely more than one ulcer may be present at the same time; yet Katz and Bierenbaum have reported that in from 2 to 12 per cent of cases, ulceration of the stomach shows multiple involvement. They have reported a case where there were 4 simulating gastric ulcers.

It would seem then that the treatment of gastric ulcer is largely medical. There are, however, three conditions under which surgical intervention is essential. These conditions are:

1. Uncontrollable hemorrhage.
2. Pyloric obstruction.
3. Perforation.
4. If there is any suggestion the lesion is neoplastic.

Vickers reports a case in which a large gastric ulcer developed under Cortisone therapy and disappeared on discontinuing the therapy only to recur on again resuming Cortisone treatment.

GASTRIC CARCINOMA* (Fig. 236A and B). In carcinoma of the stomach we have the reverse process, i.e., an overgrowth of tumor springing from the mucosa and extending out into the lumen of the stomach, taking up part of the available space. This does not permit complete filling-out of the stomach, the portion occupied by the new growth giving rise to a "filling defect." Such tumors are ragged and irregular, frequently extending completely around the stomach to the lesser curvature; if they do this they give rise to an "X"-shaped deformity. Subsequent

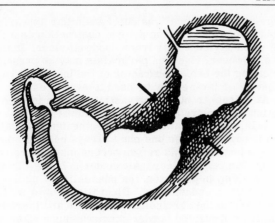

Fig. 236A

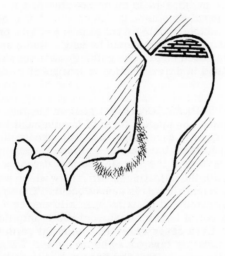

Fig. 236B

growth may completely occlude the pyloric orifice. They may occur at any location in the stomach. If on palpation a definite mass can be felt which corresponds to such a defect, then 95 times out of 100 (Carman), the diagnosis can be established as carcinoma. They frequently undergo destruction in the center of the growth giving rise to large indurated ulcerations. Pressure of the hand causes the barium-filled crater to remain while the indurated border describes a crescentic shape within the lumen of the stomach (Fig. 236B)—known as Carman's Meniscus sign, this is always indication of malignancy. Benign gastric ulcers, on the other hand, are sharply outlined and punched-out in appearance; they do not ordinarily have indurated borders nor do they infiltrate and obliterate the surrounding rugal markings.

Carcinoma of the stomach is commonly of two types: the polypoid, fungating type which is soft and bulky, growing into the lumen, and the scirrhous type which is hard and infiltrates the wall but does not ordinarily produce an isolated mass.

A superficial type of carcinoma of the stomach has been reported (Golden, and Stout), in which the growth occurs in the mucosal layers and spreads superficially without formation of a demonstrable tumor mass. These areas are always small and are frequently associated with an ulceration. They do not spread to involve the stomach in anything like the manner in which linitis plastica does.

Their close association with gastric ulcer again brings up the question of the possibility of malignant development in the walls of a primary benign ulcer. If this ever occurs it must be extremely rare.

Carcinoma of the stomach may progress to enormous size before pain and other secondary manifestations give evidence of its presence. By the time the symptoms have called attention to the disease, the local lesion has usually progressed to such size that it involves the surrounding organs and cannot be successfully removed.

Kendig, et al. have reported a case in which extensive stippled calcification was present throughout a large carcinomatous gastric cancer.

If the growth is so situated that it interferes with normal function then it may give symptoms much earlier in the course of the disease and thereby bring the patient for examination while the growth is still small. Therein lies the challenge to the roentgenologist to detect such lesions while they are yet small. Even during this stage, however, resection offers little hope for recovery of the patient. It is a very prevalent disease claiming almost three times as many deaths in the United States as active warfare and twice as many as auto accidents (Livingston and Pack). Photofluorographic surveys of the public have been proposed as a means for early detection of carcinomatous lesions of the stomach in an effort to improve the results of surgical resection. Up to 40 years of age the incidence of carcinoma of the stomach is very small; beyond that age period however it increases to 1 case in 900 population. The recent experimental work in increasing the brightness of the fluoroscopic image, using a Schmidt optical system or other methods, has brought some encouragement along this line.

Small carcinomatous lesions of the fundus near the cardiac orifice are among the most difficult to detect. Close observation of the first few swallows of barium mixture as it enters the stomach may disclose spattering of the mixture rather than the smooth descent along the lesser curvature seen in normal individuals. Examination in both erect and lying positions is essential. At times a small carcinomatous growth may be demonstrated by introducing air or gas into the stomach by a stomach tube or drinking a bottle of soda water; the gas bubble surrounds the tumor making it more readily visible. Artificial pneumoperitoneum has been advocated as an adjunct to x-ray examination for the more precise demonstration of tumors in the region of the fundus (Meneghini and de Marchi).

Kirklin and Gilbertson give the signs of carcinoma of the fundus as:

1. Distortion or partial stenosis of the lower portion of the esophagus with or without dilatation above,

2. Abnormally retarded outflow of barium into the stomach,

3. Continuous outflow of the barium instead of spurting,

4. Polypoid growths project as rounded prominences and cause deviation of path of barium; less frequently the column of barium splits as it hits the tumor.

Such lesions, however, have a very difficult surgical approach and are rarely curable. Care must be taken not to mistake the stellar and crescentic deformity of the end of the esophagus viewed on end as an actual organic lesion. Attention has been called to the occurrence of esophagogastric varices in the fundus near the esophageal orifice which may cause filling defect resembling new growth, (Evans and Delany). Some very helpful points in the diagnosis of lesions of the cardiac end of the stomach are discussed by Malenchini and Roca .

In the pars media, carcinamatous lesions are usually quite readily recognizable. When they involve the greater curvature they may be confused with the appearance produced by pressure of gas in the adjacent colon.

Carcinomatous lesions of the pyloric region are more apt to interfere with normal gastric motility, so that they may give symptomatic evidence of their presence while still small. This region is likewise more readily examined roentgenologically. In this region gastric resection can be more readily and more effectively carried out. Surgical statistics, however, indicate the rather hopeless status of surgical resection for carcinoma of the stomach as a whole; these show only a small number of patients (less than 5 per cent) living five years after operation for carcinoma of the stomach. Resection of pyloric carcinoma, however, when grouped alone shows as much as 18 per cent five-year recoveries in recent years   (Bell).

Scirrhus carcinoma (Fig. 237A) of the pylorus often presents such a small, smooth primary lesion that no filling defect can be visualized and the presence of the growth must be assumed from the obstruction which it produces. The gastric enlargement and atony which occurs with this type of growth is enormous. There often is complete obstruction, the stomach lying passively, showing little if any peris-

large "sickle-shaped" residue. A similar appearing residue may result from pyloric obstruction as a result of constricted scar from duodenal ulcer. In this case, however, vigorous peristalsis may be present, indicating the benign character of the lesion. Syrup of Ipecac or lavage may be used to evauuate the stomach from troublesome gastric residue in preparation for a more satisfactory examination.

In the differentiation between benign and malignant prepyloric ulcer one must always bear in mind that carcinoma in this region occurs much more commonly than benign ulcer, (Alexander). In any ulcer over 2.5 cm. in diameter, the possibility of malignancy must be considered. Ulceration, however, is secondary to the carcinomatous growth and there is usually an indurated border-meniscus sign; likewise the ulcer is rarely in the exact center of the indurated area. Carcinoma is attended with profound anemia; this is sometimes so pronounced that it stimulates pernicious anemia. In case of doubt, all methods available should be put to use; gastroscopy is a very helpful aid and should be used. Rubin and Nelson have added exfoliative cytology as a very effective method in differentiation of malignant gastric lesions.

LINITIS PLASTICA (Fig. 237B) or "leather bottle stomach" is another form of involvement which is most frequently carcinomatous. It presents no actual filling defect but usually a diffuse thickening of the entire wall of the stomach so that it can be rolled beneath the palpating hand. The walls are so thick that peristaltic waves cannot occur. The pyloric ring is infiltrated and remains open allowing immediate pouring out of barium mixture directly into the duodenum. Even cases where no malignant cells can be found ultimately turn out to be malignant; Ewing expresses the opinion that the fibrous tissue cells crowd out and kill the cancer cells.

Certain cases have been observed however, in which fibrous tissue, not malignant infiltration, produces the induration, similar in some respects to cirrhosis of the liver. Syphilis is said to be the cause of such fibrosis, however, we have never encountered a proven case of this type.

Linitis plastica, regardless of its etiology, is a fatal disease. This condition gives rise to a profound anemia and leads to starvation and death. The disease is most common between forty and sixty years

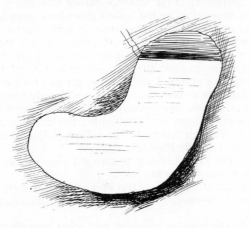

Fig. 237A

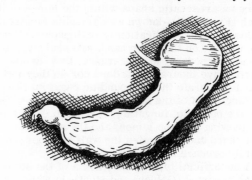

Fig. 237B

and occurs most frequently in males. The superficial infiltrating types of carcinoma of the stomach described by Golden in which the mucosal and submucosal layers are the locations of main involvement are not of the linitis plastica type. Boeck's sarcoid rarely involves the stomach. Sirak investigating the literature has found that these cases invariably have the clinical symptoms of ulcer and roentgen findings of linitis plastica.

MALIGNANT LYMPHOMATA

HODGKIN'S DISEASE OF THE STOMACH.

Hodgkin's involvement of the stomach is essentially of three types (Jungmann):
1) Ulcerative type with multiple flat ulcers
2) Tumorlike type involving the prepyloric region producing a filling defect with narrowing of the gastric lumen and five hour gastric retention
3) A type in which the entire stomach is involved like polyposis of the stomach.

Primary lymphosarcoma involves the wall of the stomach in a thick, bulky filling defect—much the same as Hodgkin's or even carcinoma. It may cause smooth infiltration of the stomach wall with little if any detectable filling defect. It is said to represent 1 to 2 % of malignant tumors of the stomach (Jenkinson, et al.).

Lymphosarcoma of the stomach may have the appearance of carcinoma. Irregularity, enlargement, and stiffening of the gastric folds are also signs of the lymphomatous involvement of the stomach, either localized or generalized. A bizarre mucosal pattern should make the examiner suspicious of neoplastic involvement. Since gastritis can also give very similar findings, a differentiation is often extremely difficult to make. Valuable aid can be obtained many times from the gastroscopist. Exploration and microscopic examination of the stomach biopsies are needed on occasion for accurate diagnosis. Wang and Petersen, after a study of 165 cases of malignant lymphoma have concluded that these tumors mimic so many other benign and malignant lesions of the gastrointestinal tract that they seldom can be diagnosed without biopsy.

SYPHILIS OF THE STOMACH. Syphilis of the stomach is an extremely rare disease. It occurs as a manifestation of the tertiary stage of the disease (gumma) and produces an infiltrative type of lesion similar in appearance to carcinoma. This gives rise to a visible filling defect on fluoroscopic examination but frequently no mass can be detected on palpation: this has been spoken of as the most characteristic finding. Then again, the lack of physical weakness, anemia, etc., which would be expected with carcinomatous involvement of this extent aids in establishing the diagnosis. The disappearance of the lesion after anti-luetic treatment is confirmatory but not conclusive evidence of its luetic nature.

Tabetic crises are of different origin and are not associated with any demonstrable type of organic pathology of the stomach.

Mendl, et al. have reported the roentgen findings in a case of congenital syphilis. They consider that a positive Wasserman reaction is not sufficient to establish the diagnosis of the gastric lesion. Isolation or identification of the Spirochaete pallida is essential.

PYLORIC MUSCLE HYPERTROPHY. (Fig. 238A). In infants this is termed congenital hypertrophic pyloric stenosis. Symptoms begin early, usually at about three weeks of age. It is characterized clinically by vomiting, (often of the projectile type); hyperperistalsis with visible peristaltic waves progressing from left to right across the upper abdomen, marked loss of weight from lack of retained food, constipation from the same cause, and often a palpable mass representing the hypertrophied pyloric muscle. A detailed study of the anatomical structure reveals the complicated muscular arrangement of the pyloric canal, (Thorgersen). In typical cases, the diagnosis can be made without radiological examination. The dehydration and fluid imbalance should be attended to before x-ray examination is begun.

Roentgenologically, the stomach is large and atonic, it may lie dormant or there may be showers of peristaltic waves which fade out at the pylorus without forcing any appreciable amount of stomach contents through the pylorus. A small threadlike channel of barium may be forced through the pylorus and the rounded impression of the hypertrophied pyloric muscle may leave its imprint on the adjacent stomach. A tumor mass produced by the hypertrophic pyloric muscle can often be palpated. Examination made at hourly intervals will fail to show any great amount of gastric emptying for three or four hours.

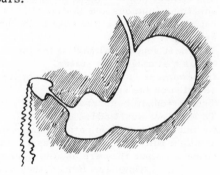

Fig. 238A

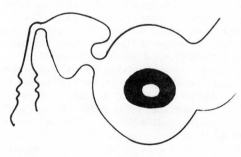

Fig. 238B

Many of these signs are not always present how-ever; greatest reliance must be placed upon the threadlike shadow produced by the barium as it passes through the pyloric sphincter. In very young infants, within the first four weeks, too much reliance must not be placed upon prolonged gastric retention even up to six hours.

Likewise, in a small percentage of new born in-fants a similar lack of nervous coordination may ef-fect the cardiac orifice and stomach contents may merely run back up into the esophagus on assuming the horizontal position and yet this may give rise to similar symptoms of regurgitation.

That spasm must be in some way associated with pyloric hypertrophy is indicated by the fact that atropine aids in relieving this condition.

Plastic operative procedure on the pylorus usually relieves the condition.

In adults hypertrophy of the pyloric muscle occurs much less frequently, and yet there are cases in which there are no other findings to explain the gastric distress and discomfort which the patient experiences. The roentgen findings which seem to be most constant in these cases are elongation of pre-pyloric area with " crescentic indentation of the bulbar base" (Kirklin), from pressure of the hypertrophic pyloric muscle.

BENIGN TUMORS OF THE STOMACH. Benign tumors of the stomach are relatively rare, compris-ing probably less than 5%.

Roberts, quoting Moore, Schindler, and Buck-stein gives the roentgen signs of benignancy as fol-lows:

1. The tumour has a smooth round appearance.
2. Junction of tumour and gastric wall is clear-cut and the angles at the edge of the growth are acute.
3. The most superficial part of the tumour often shows a simple ulcer crater.
4. If the tumour is considerable mobility may be noted on the screen.
5. The surrounding mucosa is intact.
   To these we would add:
6. On fluoroscopic examination, benign tumors are as a rule more readily pressed out on palpation since they are usually thinner and softer in consistency. In fact, they are some-times so readily obliterated by slight pres-sure that they may readily escape detection.

Tumors of this type are chiefly some form of myoma, fibroma, lipoma, adenoma and occasionally angioma or neurogenic tumor. They lack the infiltra-tive border of malignant disease. They are inter-mural and often do not disturb the mucosal folds. A solitary large lipoma involving the pyloric portion of the stomach occupying the greater curvature has been recorded by Rogers and Adams. They may spread out between the layers below the mucosal sur-face and are often called "iceberg tumors" because only one-tenth of the tumor shows above the surface.

Extraluminal growths of this sort produce a rather clear margin similar somewhat to that of foreign material in the stomach. Leiomyoma (smooth muscle), Schwannoma (nerve sheath) tumors and aberrant pancreatic deposits may produce rounded filling defects; there may be associated central ulcer-ation producing a doughnut-like appearance, (Evans and Weintraub; Littner and Kirsch). Such benign tu-mors may remain intact, but if they do ulcerate this is an indication that they may be undergoing malignant change. They are extramucosal tumors arising from the underlying muscular layer frequently with over-lying degenerative ulcerative changes. There may be calcium deposits in the tumor. Davis and Adams have reported nine cases.

There is no single radiographic appearance. If removed the outlook for leiomyoma is favorable; for lieomyocarcoma is more favorable than adenosar-coma. Neurofibromas have been reported in the stomach in neurofibromatosis, (Von Recklinghausen's Disease) in association with multiple neurofibromatous nodules all over the body, (Gillespie). Primary amy-loid tumors have been reported in the stomach. They produce a picture very similar to carcinoma, have areas of ulceration and are prone to massive hemor-rhage, (Cooley). Flannery and Caster have pointed out certain diagnostic criteria of hemangioma of the stomach; the tumor feels like a "mass of worms" and may disclose the presence of phleboliths.

Sarcoidosis of the gastrointestinal tract is very rare, but it may affect almost any part. Eso-phageal involvement in the only case reported (Kerley, 1950) takes on the form of a stricture.

When it involves the stomach it may take on the appearance of a granuloma but the definite di-agnosis can only be made by biopsy. Roentgeno-logically it may show narrowing of the stomach, or may take on other appearance as of a carcinoma-tous mass or may not show roentgen evidence at all.

In the small intestine it may be indistinguish-able from regional ileitis. The colon is very rarely if ever involved, (Allen, et al.).

IDIOPATHIC MULTIPLE HEMORRHAGE SAR-COMA, (KAPOSI'S DISEASE). This is, as its name implies, a condition of unknown origin in which mul-tiple spontaneous hemorrhagic sarcomatous lesions arise, especially in the skin of the extremities al-though there are usual associated visceral lesions. The most frequent occurrence is in the gastrointes-tinal tract where it may develop without associated skin lesions. It occurs most frequently in Italians and in Russian or Polish Jews.

Roentgenologically the lesions of Kaposi's dis-ease appear as multiple centimeter-sized tumors in the mucosa and submucosa which are readily shown by pressure with apparently healthy tissues between involved areas. Hemorrhage is a common accom-panying symptom which may direct attention to the condition, (Grove).

GIANT GASTRIC RUGAE (Fig. 239A). Some-times the rugae of the stomach become so enor-mously enlarged that they actually simulate gastric carcinoma. Only by careful fluoroscopic examina-tion tracing the rugal folds is this mistake avoided.

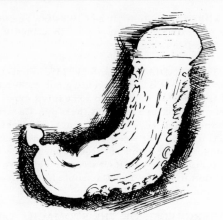

Fig. 239A

When this condition occurs it usually involves the entire stomach. The differentiation of the benign, large and distorted folds from carcinoma or lymphoma is often so difficult that surgery is necessary to exclude malignancy, and even then with the aid of frozen section tissue diagnosis errors are made.

REDUNDANT GASTRIC MUCOSA. Very rarely the gastric mucosa may become loose and redundant hanging in folds and even at times projecting through the pylorus, simulating tumor of the duodenum. Small polypoid growths of the pylorus having a similar appearance may likewise project through into the duodenal cap producing rounded defects. (Fig. 239B). It may be impossible to differentiate. Redundant gastric mucosa, however, is softer in texture usually producing a less clearly defined margin; it is usually a mushroom or umbrella-shaped defect near the pyloric orifice with lobulation due to antral folds. An elaborate investigation by Rappaport, et al, would indicate that it has no specific symptomatology and is found in association with a wide variety of other conditions. It usually was found in overweight individuals who indulged in excessive rapid eating. All other conditions must be ruled out before this is considered as a primary cause of gastric difficulty (New).

GASTRIC POLYP (Fig. 239B). Small polypoid growths occur most frequently in the pyloric region. If they are sufficiently close to the pyloric ring they may protrude through the pylorus into the duodenal bulb. Roentgenographically they may appear as smooth rounded filling defects alternately protruding through the pylorus into the bulb and retracting into the prepyloric region of the stomach. If the pedicle is thick and the bulb is large and well filled, the polyp may be overshadowed in the bulb but may be suspected from the elongated appearance of the gastric mucosal folds as they project through the pylorus. Review of the literature by Richards would indicate that these are primarily benign growths.

They may be formed from many various tissues; a complete classification has been developed.

Such polyps may be the source of prolonged bleeding eventually even simulating the clinical picture of pernicious anemia, (Rigler, et al.). Gall stones which have ulcerated through the gall bladder and become impacted in the duodenum or pyloric end of the stomach may produce a similar appearance, (deFeo and Meigher).

GASTRIC GRANULOMA. First recognized by Vanek, this condition was described as a "gastric submucosal granuloma with eosinophilic infiltration."

Recognized roentgenologically the lesion presents itself as a fairly well circumscirbed elevated lobular mass, several centimeters in size. Histologically it consists of loose fibrous tissue with a cellular infiltrate that is dominated by eosinophils, (Rigler, et al.). Smith has described similar lesions with illustration of relationship of granulomatous mass to the gastric rugae and microscopic sections showing the marked vascularity of the lesion.

MULTIPLE POLYPOSIS (Fig. 240). Under certain conditions the gastric mucosa may give rise to multiple polypi. These are soft pedunculated structures projecting into and partially filling the stomach. Roentgenologically they produce a mottled appearance of the stomach especially near the pyloric end where the stomach becomes narrower. Under fluroscopic examination pressure with the hand discloses even more clearly the mottled appearance characteristic of this condition. If the distribution is not too extensive operative resection may be carried out. The appearance produced by hypertrophied gastric rugae and redundancy of the mucosa may be so similar that differentiation is very difficult from this condition.

GASTRITIS. Gastritis may be 1) hypertrophic, 2) atrophic, 3) ulcerative, 4) phlegmonous or 5) emphysematous.

Hypertrophic and atrophic gastritis are not often accurately diagnosed roentgenographically. Mere hypertrophy or atrophy of gastric rugae is not a criterion of the condition of the mucosa. Gastroscopy offers a means by which the mucosa can be directly visualized, and should be made on the gastroscopic findings, not the roentgenographic. Large, irregular folds of the stomach which are not as pliable as normal suggest gastritis. Lymphomatous involvement of

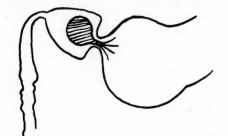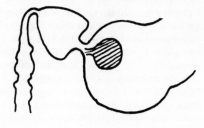

Fig. 239B

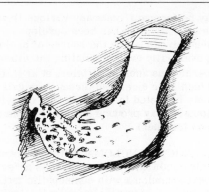

Fig. 240

the stomach simulates these findings; the stomach with a bizarre mucosal pattern should be viewed with suspicion. Much reliance rests on gastroscopy and the clinical pattern.

The ulcerative erosive form, with superficial mucosal ulcerations can occasionally be demonstrated roentgenographically by mucosal relief. This is frequently caused by chronic alcoholism and may be attended by massive gastric hemorrhage (Walk).

Phlegmonous Gastritis from low grade sub-mucosal pyogenic infection of the stomach wall may result in enormous thickening of the tissues resembling a carcinomatous mass. It is usually attendant with excessive alcoholic consumption and rupture of the gastric wall may occur with air free in the abdomen (Miller and Nushan). Antibiotics may have some influence on the condition.

Lumsden has reported a case in which the gastric wall was found at x-ray examination to have gas bubbles outlining its wall. This was discovered in an 83-year-old man. At autopsy the cause was ascertained as Bacillus Welchii infection. There was no history of gastroscopy or other indication of trauma. He points out two other causes of gas occurring in the gastric wall; cystic pneumatosis (or gas cysts of the stomach wall) which may be solitary or multiple of varying size, as large as 10 cm., either on the mesenteric or antimesenteric side. Unless these cysts cause obstruction they may be symptomless. They are often associated with gastric or duodenal ulcer. Interstitial gastric emphysema in which trauma seemed to play a part such as gastroscopic examination or tearing of an old ulcer site.

Emphysematous Gastritis is due to a phlegmonous inflammation of the stomach caused by gas-forming organisms. The condition has been reported (Weens) following drinking concentrated hydrochloric acid in a suicidal attempt. Roentgenologically the gastric wall filled with air bubbles is easily demonstrated by barium sulphate mixture within the stomach as a radiolucent zone. An instance has been reported in an infant caused by gastric infection with gas-forming organisms (Henry). This may be somewhat akin to cystitis emphysematosa, a condition occurring in diabetic patients where the bladder wall

is filled with air bubbles. It has likewise resulted following prickling of the mucosa with a needle during surgical operation.

POST-IRRADIATION GASTRITIS. Post-irradiation gastritis is not a disease entity but rather a reaction of the gastric mucosa to excessive exposure of the gastric mucosa to radiation therapy. Gastroscopic examination reveals the blanching effect with superficial ulcerations seen elsewhere on mucous membranes. There is no roentgen appearance which is characteristic nor can its extent or severity be adjudged by this method. The flat superficial ulcerations likewise cannot be visualized.

TUBERCULOSIS OF THE STOMACH. Tuberculosis of the stomach is very rare. Unless it is associated with extensive tuberculous lesions elsewhere in the body it is hazardous to make the diagnosis. It may take the form of a smooth niche on the lesser curvature of the stomach producing exactly similar roentgensigns as benign gastric ulcer. The most significant roentgen findings are simultaneous involvement of stomach and duodenum, presence of fistulae and sinuses, and signs of external pressure by enlarged lymph nodes. Microscopic examination is necessary for final diagnosis, (Ostrum and Serber).

HEMORRHAGE; DIAPOEDETIC. Massive hemorrhages from the gastro-intestinal tract are most frequently associated with ulcer or cancer. Smith, Good and Gray reported that 95% of cases with melena or hemorrhage of non colonic origin were found in the upper gastro-intestinal tract (duodenum or above).

MASSIVE HEMORRHAGE. Massive hemorrhage from the upper gastrointestinal tract is most often due to bleeding peptic ulcer of the duodenum or stomach. Gastric carcinoma is an uncommon source of heavy, fast bleeding. Benign tumors of the stomach have a high incidence of associated hemorrhage, but their occurrence is so low in general, that these lesions are not an important source of bleeding.

Massive hemorrhage from the stomach not infrequently is encountered without demonstrable organic lesion roentgenologically. Even at autopsy, for these hemorrhages without a demonstrated ulcer or tumor can be fatal too, the source of blood loss is not revealed. Gastric hemorrhage may be due to gastritis, and many appear to be related to excessive acute and chronic ingestion of alcohol in one of its many forms. Such hemorrhages are of diapedetic type with blood oozing from the mucosa.

It is felt that a diagnosis should be made in the bleeding patient as soon as possible. This opinion presupposes that surgery has much to offer the acutely, massively bleeding patient. For the internist to know that an operable lesion is present, for example an ulcer of the duodenum, is important. Or it is important to know that the definite source of bleeding cannot be demonstrated, causing nonoperative treatment to be considered more strongly. (Esophageal varices are to be considered in every case of upper alimentary tract bleeding. See page 361.)

A modified gastrointestinal examination is utilized for the bleeding patient, (Hampton). Since many of these patients are in precarious condition secondary to the blood loss, the patient remains recumbent. The esophagus is first examined for varices, tumors and hiatus hernia with thin barium in small amount. Attention is then turned to the stomach. By turning the patient on his right side and then back again, barium is made to coat the stomach wall and enter the duodenal bulb. This maneuver is repeated as needed with multiple films being obtained. A double contrast effect from the stomach gas bubble rising into the antral region and bulb is desired, this being facilitated by turning the patient to the left, making these structures uppermost. The entire examination is carried out without palpation of the abdomen, and with the least disturbance to the patient. After a sufficient number of films have been made of the air-barium contrast effect, the esophagus can be re-examined with thick barium. The patient is then placed in the prone position, and additional films made.

For the detection of the source of small, insidious hemorrhages from the gastrointestinal tract, Henry has proposed an ingenious modification of the gastrointestinal examination. Veriopake (ordinarily used for gall bladder examination) 6 ounces mixed with 2 or 3 teaspoonsful of hydrogen peroxide is administered by mouth as a medium for gastrointestinal examination. In the presence of blood the peroxide liberates gas bubbles which may be readily visualized on x-ray examination, disclosing the bleeding point. A serious drawback is the fact that sometimes in a normal individual bubbles form within the small intestine, so that the method has been restricted by its originator to those cases of insidious bleeding (tarry stools) where the source of the bleeding cannot otherwise be found.

FOREIGN BODIES IN THE STOMACH, (Bezoar). Foreign bodies are frequently swallowed, passing into the stomach. If they are composed of some opaque substance they can be readily visualized at ordinary roentgen examination; if not of radiopaque material they may be visualized by administration of a small amount of barium sulphate mixture. Ordinarily any foreign body which will pass the cardiac orifice of the stomach, will pass through the pylorus also; occasionally, however, one sees foreign bodies which may remain for a long time in the stomach. In one instance a pearl button from a lady's coat about one inch in diameter remained in the stomach of a four-year-old child for over three months before it was spontaneously passed; since there were no distressing symptoms it was thought best to refrain from any operative procedure, depending upon time to increase the size of the stomach to the point where the pyloric opening would be large enough to pass the foreign body. Sharp pointed foreign bodies are dangerous only insofar as they may cause perforation of the stomach or intestinal walls. In over twenty years' observation the writer has seen but one instance in which this occurred after the foreign body had reached the stomach. In one instance, a tie pin three inches in length re-

mained in the stomach eight days before it passed the pyloric orifice; it could be observed fluoroscopically, presenting first the blunt end and then the sharp end to the pylorus, but it finally passed without injury to the patient. A fever thermometer was seen to remain in the loop of the duodenum for eight days before passing. Insane individuals often have a mania for swallowing foreign objects. Sometimes these remain for a long time in stomach; in one such instance which we have observed, 856 metallic foreign bodies found in the stomach were later removed surgically. If there is any doubt about the lodgment of a foreign body in the stomach it may be localized to this location by administration of a carbonated drink,(Roberts). Brizzola has reported a method for the successful removal of metallic foreign bodies such as bobby pin, too long to pass the curve of the duodenum, by introduction of a Alnico-V magnet into the stomach.

Swallowing of hair over a long period of time results in formation of a hair ball in the stomach (Fig. 241) known as trichobezoar. A substance which frequently is the cause of phytobezoar formation is persimmons. The skins of this fruit, especially if not completely ripe, remain in the stomach to form large foreign bodies. Roentgenologically these appear as large irregular radiolucent areas in the midst of the barium-filled stomach. Their appearance is quite characteristic. It is said that trichobezoar float on top of the barium mixture while phytobezoar sink. These must be carefully differentiated from extra-luminal tumors arising in the stomach wall and projecting into the stomach beneath an intact mucosa. An unusual case of radiopaque phytobezoar has been described by Canlas and Fildes in which the bezoar was rendered radiopaque by long-standing medication with bismuth taken as an antacid.

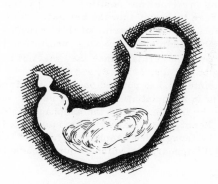

Fig. 241

DIVERTICULUM OF STOMACH (Fig. 242A). True diverticula of the stomach are uncommon. The gastric wall is so strong and muscular that the conditions which ordinarily give rise to them rarely develop. They are most frequently encountered in the cardiac portion and must be differentiated from hiatus hernias of the stomach back through the esophageal opening, and from ulcers high on the lesser curvature.

The fact that they have no rugal markings and are below the diaphragm serves to differentiate them

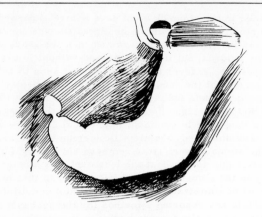

Fig. 242A

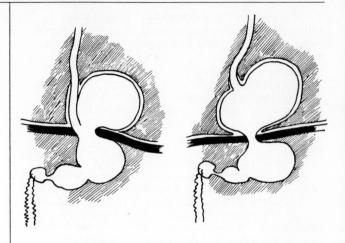

Fig. 243A   Fig. 243B

from hiatus or other diaphragmatic hernia. Likewise a diverticulum should be larger on inspiration than expiration; the opposite should be true of hernia (E. Pendergrass). The Mayos have found diverticula equally frequent in the pyloric region; 43 percent. Vascular interference predisposes to ulceration and hemorrhage. Diverticula have also been reported arising from the greater curvature of the stomach.

GASTRIC HERNIA: HIATUS HERNIA (Fig. 242B), Johnstone). Herniation of a portion of the stomach back through the esophageal hiatus is not an infrequent occurrence especially in extremely stout individuals, in the older age group. In the upright position herniation may not be observed but with the patient lying in the recumbent position the abdominal pressure causes a small pouch of the stomach to protrude back through the cardiac orifice, the esophagus remaining in its normal position. The gastric rugae may be seen following into the herniated portion. Paraesophageal hiatus hernia of this sort may more properly be considered as hiatus insufficiencies rather than true hernias since they may not have sacs, (Harrington), (Figs. 243A, B, and C).

Kleinfelter has pointed out that symptoms of dysphasia in association with hiatus hernia may be produced by invagination of the esophagus into the hernia. Roentgenologically the barium coated mucosa of the invaginated esophagus gives a "Jack-in-the-Pulpit" appearance which is quite characteristic.

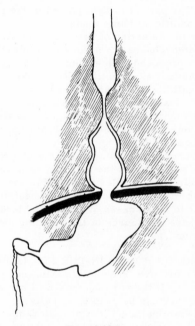

Fig. 243C

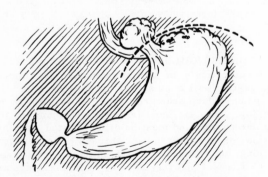

Fig. 242B

Hiatus hernia is demonstrated easier if the patient is examined with barium swallow in the recumbent or Trendelenburg (head down) position. To this is added a maneuver to increase the intraabdominal pressure, such as coughing, grunting, raising of the legs. Marchand recommends the use of an inflated football bladder for pressure upon the upper abdomen. Reducible hiatus hernia is frequently difficult to demonstrate. When the hernia is incarcerated, it is simple to demonstrate by barium swallow. The herniated stomach may cause considerable displacement of the distal esophagus. An upright chest film may give the first indication of an incarcerated hiatus hernia. The gas bubble of gas-fluid level within the herniated stomach superimposes the heart on P-A view, and is posterior to the heart on lateral view, (Fig. 206D, p. 284, and Fig. 217, p. 314). Whether the hernia has a sac or not cannot be determined by x-ray study is not important, but it is of value to know whether the hernia is incarcerated or not.

They may continue to enlarge becoming true pulsion hernias, however, due to continued increase in abdominal pressure, pushing the esophagus, fundus of the stomach and all structures upward through the weakened diaphragm into the chest. The stomach may become completely inverted, (Marks).

Herniation through the postero-lateral portion of the diaphragm, the foramen of Bochdalek, is less frequent than periesophageal herniation. This occurs most frequently on the left, but does occur on the right also.   Numerous cases of this type have been observed where the entire stomach and a large part of the small intestine and colon have protruded into the pleural cavity. Even the pancreas has been reported herniated into the chest, (Poppel et al.). There may even be congenital absence of one-half of the diaphragm with the abdominal viscera extending into the chest. Such hernias are most frequently congenital, although rare instances have been described in which "extensive crushing injuries or lacerations may have given rise to the condition." Whenever there is doubt about the nature of any pathological process existing in the left lower chest, always examine the gastro-intestinal tract to rule out diaphragmatic hernia.

In the newborn and young child, severe respiratory distress may be the first indication of diaphragmatic hernia. Plain film examination is often confusing, making barium studies necessary.

Eventration of the diaphragm is a congenital thinning of one side which permits a high position of this leaf of the diaphragm. The diaphragm may extend as high as the second or third rib permitting the entire stomach, a greater portion of the small intestine and a portion of the colon to protrude into the chest; gas-filled intestines in this location may cause mediastinal displacement to the opposite side and pressure on the recurrent laryngeal nerve.

Hernias through the foramen of Morgagni are rare. Stomach, colon or other abdominal contents herniate into the chest through the opening behind the sternum and anterior to the heart.

Inguinal hernias have been observed where the major portion of the stomach was in the scrotum; constant drag on the esophageal end has elongated that structure to such a degree that herniation through the ring was made possible, (English). Femoral hernias of a similar nature have also been encountered.

Thoracic stomach occurs in association with congenitally short esophagus with the stomach lying entirely or in part within the thorax. Under such circumstances the stomach is small in size and the esophagus is attached to the highest point of the fundus of the stomach. There is evidence to indicate that this condition is only rarely congenital and may develop by traction of the longitudinal muscle fibers of the esophagus in association with esophageal peptic ulcer or esophagitis, (Fig. 243C). It may give rise to unusual digestive disturbances. However, it may not cause any abnormal symptoms and is not incompatible with a long normal life.

Volvulus of the Stomach. This is a condition in which the stomach undergoes wide rotation with reference to its fixed points; either the esophageal and duodenal openings, (organoaxial) or rotation on the axis of mesenteric attachments of the stomach (mesenterio-axial). Rotation of a portion of the stomach with a spiral twisting between involved parts causing the stomach to be divided into pouches constitutes the only pathology of the condition. The roentgen diagnosis then should consist in detection of a definite spiral rugal pattern of gastric mucosa with displacement of the normal structures and consequent development of enormous gas-dilated segments of the stomach. The condition is made possible by the existence of a long mesentery or omentum. Correction is surgical. Jenkinson and Bate have reviewed the subject and reported an interesting case. de Lorimier and Penn have emphasized the differentiation of kindred lesions and have emphasized certain management hazards.

FUNCTIONAL LESIONS OF THE STOMACH

GASTRIC SPASM (Fig. 244). Spasm of the stomach may be due either to intrinsic gastric or duodenal lesions, or to extrinsic causes. Peptic ulcer is the most important cause of spasmodic contraction of the stomach.

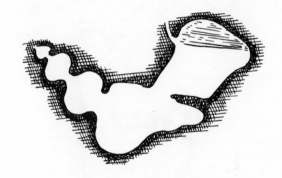

Fig. 244

A persistent deep incisura on the greater curvature opposite a niche, from spasm of the circular musculature, may give a classical picture of penetrating ulcer until spasm is relieved by administration of atropine and it disappears. Or the peristaltic waves may become deep and persistent and the pyloric sphincter may remain tightly closed from reflex spasm.

The pyloro spasm associated with hypertrophy of the pyloric muscle seen in young infants is probably also due to reflex causes.

Gastric spasm occurs from extrinsic causes as well. A deep incisura may develop in the mid-portion of the stomach which may remain almost like an organic stricture, from reflex irritation of acute inflammation of the appendix or gall bladder, or from a duodenal ulcer. Spasmodic constriction can be readily differentiated from organic stricture, however, by the administration of an antispasmodic.

Tincture of Belladonna to its full physiological activity will relax spasm in a few hours or amyl nitrite inhalation will cause relaxation of the spasm at once. Spasmodic contractures disappear under anesthesia.

GASTROPTOSIS * (Fig. 245). Gastroptosis is a condition in which the stomach hangs down much lower in the abdominal cavity than the habitus of the individual would indicate as normal. It usually is associated with ptosis of the other abdominal viscera. Relaxation of the abdominal wall probably is the chief etiological factor; the possibility of an endocrine basis is suggested by the frequent association of other manifestations of endocrine disorders in these individuals: chronic interstitial mastitis of breasts and dysmenorrhea. The condition may give rise to vague digestive disturbances, and, when the colon is affected, to symptoms simulating appendicitis. A large percentage of patients in whom appendectomy fails to relieve symptoms will be found to have this condition. An abdominal support will give temporary relief but permanent relief will only be attained by strengthening the belly wall by abdominal exercise and increasing the fatty layer on the abdomen.

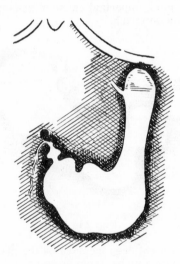

Fig. 245

NERVOUS INDIGESTION. That very evident digestive upsets can actually occur as the result of "nervous" interference with normal gastric function, there is no doubt. The individual, who in his business is keyed up to a high state of nervous strain, may develop inhibitions to normal gastric secretion and function which will result in extreme digestive distress.

Headache, nausea or an intense emotional upset may cause almost complete inhibition of peristalsis with large six-hour gastric residue.

Roentgenologically there may be no manifestations of such interference with normal function. Gastric peristalsis may progress in a normal manner or there may be manifestations of inhibition of function with absent peristalsis.

GASTRIC NEUROSIS. Certain individuals develop gastric distress and digestive disorders for which no organic basis can be found and which cannot be explained on the basis of high business pressure or worry. Such individuals may continually eliminate articles from their diet until they are subsisting on a few unusual articles of food, the nature of which would seem to belie the possibility of even a functional indigestion. It will usually be found that such individuals are suffering from some endocrine dysfunction. Careful search must always be made first for every other possible source of the disturbance before the condition is attributed to gastric neurosis.

Psychological Influence on Gastric Function. Attention has been called to the effects of the threat of a hypodermic injection and disturbance caused by a gun shot on the rate and character of peristaltic contractions of the stomach. Complete but temporary inhibition occurred in some patients, in others the effects were not so prompt nor so lasting. There is evidence, however, that distasteful experiences can interfere with gastric function, (Jungmann and Venning).

CASCADE STOMACH (Fig. 246). A condition known as "cascade stomach" in which the stomach

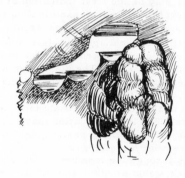

Fig. 246

is displaced to the right by gaseous distention of a highly placed splenic flexure of the colon which crowds it over, often gives rise to very distressing symptoms. By reason of this displacement, the stomach is converted by its natural curvature into a number of pouches which fill successively when in the upright position, giving the effect of a cascade. Having the patient lie on his face immediately relieves the pressure on the stomach and does away with the malformed appearance. Naturally, direction of treatment to the colon relieving the constipation and gas has a beneficial effect on the digestive disturbance.

In many instances such pressure of gas in the splenic flexure of the colon and stomach gives rise to symptoms attributable to cardiac pathology such as coronary attacks. Usually symptoms are functional only and on assuming the prone position they disappear, (Davies).

GASTRO-DUODENAL INVAGINATION, (INTUS-SUSCEPTION), (Jungmann; Poppel and Herstone). This is a very unusual condition in which there is marked enlargement of the antrum and pyloric end of the stomach engulfing the duodenum and adjacent structures. The duodenal cap seems to be drawn into the stomach. The invaginating process does not seem to produce acute symptoms and it may be tolerated for years without its true nature being discovered. It does not produce complete obstruction and may not interfere materially with emptying.

Roentgenologically the intussuscepted duodenum and stomach forms a large rounded mass in the region of the pyloric antrum. It is readily recognized since the normal longitudinal gastric folds end abruptly at the mass and are replaced by the rounded projections of barium which seem to encircle the mass. The findings are very similar to those of intussusception elsewhere in the intestines. Operative resection is the only curative measure.

CORRECTIVE OPERATIVE PROCEDURES

GASTROENTEROSTOMY*,--MARGINAL AND JEJUNAL ULCER (Fig. 247). After gastroenterostomy, the stomach usually empties rapidly through the artificial opening. Pernicious vomiting developing after operation may be due to formation of a vicious circle--food from the stomach passing into the proximal loop of the duodenum is emptied back into the stomach again through the gastroenterostomy opening thus going around and around. Atresia of the distal loop also may cause pernicious vomiting. To obtain a successfully functioning gastroenterostomy it is necessary that the pyloric end be either entirely closed or its function impeded. Even with a large gastroenterostomy opening the food material may continue to pass through the natural route. Pouch formation may occur at or near the stoma in which peristalsis is inhibited permitting retention of secretion for a long time. These may militate against satisfactory function of the gastroenterostomy and

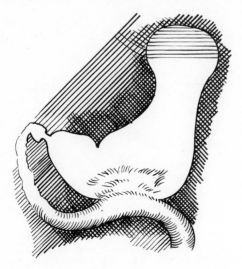

Fig. 247

should be searched for, (Lands). Position of the patient after ingestion of food may play an important part in the establishment of a successfully functioning gastroenterostomy; fluoroscopic examination may aid in finding the most satisfactory position. Retrograde intussusception of the jejunum into the stomach has been reported by Palmer, in patients having a gastroenterostomy opening; such instances are very rarely observed.

Marginal ulcerations may develop at the edges of the stoma; they may have an irregular orifice and may show a definite crater of the descending loop several centimeters from the orifice (jejunal ulcer). These are difficult and at times impossible to detect; development of pain and symptoms of indigestion after gastroenterostomy in an individual showing spasticity of the intestinal loop are suggestive of development of marginal ulcer even though actual ulcer may not be demonstrable. Vagotomy in such cases usually causes prompt relief of the symptoms of the marginal or jejunal ulcer, (Dragstedt, et al.). Banthine, a drug recently developed, acting upon the vagus nerve, has also been found most satisfactory in dealing with this condition. Surgical resection of the ulcer area and further resection of the stomach is sometimes necessary if more conservative means fail.

A rather rare but very spectacular complication is the spontaneous development of jejuno-gastric intussusception of the intestine through the gastroenterostomy opening into the stomach. Under such conditions the coiled up intestinal loop shows clearly within the stomach, (Wisoff).

Prolapse of the gastric mucosa may occur through the gastroenterostomy opening into the intestine resembling carcinoma (Maisel and Weintraub).

Vagotomy has been practiced to try to control the gastric hyperacidity in duodenal ulcer.

After vagotomy the patient usually experiences almost immediate symptomatic relief, and healing of the ulcer. Roentgen observation, however, reveals complete lack of peristalsis with dilatation and atony of the stomach usually for a period of eight to ten days. It may be weeks or even years before normal function is restored. Under such circumstances it may be necessary to do a gastroenterostomy. Organic obstruction from scar tissue or other cause is obviously a contraindication to vagotomy in the first place.

Sufficient time has not yet elapsed to evaluate properly the ultimate effects of the procedure. In properly selected cases, it is of definite value.

GASTRIC RESECTION. While it is true that most benign ulcers will heal with bed rest alone, without special diet or medication, still there are many in which the possibility of ulcerating carcinomatous lesions cannot be ruled out. Obviously such lesions require surgical resection. It may be said then that any patient in whom a trial period of bed rest does not show prompt healing of the lesion should be subjected to surgical exploration.

In duodenal ulcer however, with persistent hypersecretion, gastric resection has been advocated with the idea of removing the acid-secreting gland-bearing portion of the stomach. This procedure has met with the most clinical success; it does have the disadvantage of removal of a large part of an important organ   (requiring the patient to eat smaller amounts at more frequent intervals). Marginal ulcer may develop, or the patient may experience a variety of unpleasant symptoms and disturbances in alimentation. The procedure is not entirely an unmixed blessing.

Postoperative complications after partial resection of the stomach have been discussed by Hajdu, et al. He lists these as follows and illustrates the roentgen pictures produced:

Group A. Obstruction occurs as a result of small intestine herniating through the gap between the anastomosis and the transverse colon, either from right to left or from left to right.

Group B. A long afferent loop attached to the lesser curvature of the gastric stump is present. Obstruction results from volvulus, kinking or strangulation.

Group C. Obstruction results from constricting bands, local post-operative adhesions, or traction and misplacement of the greater omentum. This is the least well defined group.

Perigastric Hematoma from Traumatic Laceration of Spleen. Rupture of the spleen from injury may be attendant with certain roentgen signs which are diagnostic. Such injury is frequently attendant with considerable maceration of this organ and slow oozing of blood which plasters the injured organ to the adjacent wall of the stomach giving rise to perigastric hematoma in the following roentgen signs which may be diagnostic (Solis-Cohen and Levine).

Obliteration of splenic shadow.
Gaseous dilatation of stomach.
Serration of adjacent gastric wall (pars media and cardica) with increased density along greater curvature.

SPLENIC CALCIFICATIONS. Schwarz, et al., investigating a large number of spleens having calcium deposits, found that in the endemic areas they were most frequently due to Histoplasma Capsulatum. Aneurysms of the splenic artery are not uncommon. They are usually readily recognized by their larger amount of calcification in the vessel walls. They may attain six inches in diameter, enough to cause marked pressure on the adjacent stomach. Their cause is probably due to arteriosclerosis but trauma may play a part.

Hexamethonium is a widely used drug for the control of high blood pressure. Ettman, et al. have found that its prolonged use is apt to result in untoward gastrointestinal symptoms. It results in delay in gastric emptying from diminished peristalsis but in gastric secretion was only slightly altered. Constipation was most marked result, even progressing to a dynamic ileus.

THE SMALL INTESTINE (Chapter XX)

THE DUODENUM

I. ANATOMY

II. ROENTGEN EXAMINATION

A. Normal duodenum

   1. Anatomical divisions—roentgen characteristics

III. PATHOLOGY

A. Intrinsic organic lesions

   1. Duodenal ulcer

   2. Duodenitis

   3. Duodenal diverticulum

   4. Duodenal tumors— Ampulla of Vater

   5. Duodenal obstruction—atresia

   6. Megaduodenum

B. Extrensic lesion affecting duodenum

   1. Neoplasms of the periampullar region

   2. Tumor of head of pancreas

     a. Carcinoma

     b. Cyst

C. Other lesions from adjacent organs

   1. Aberrant pancreas

   2. Pressure defects from gall bladder and adjacent organs

   3. Periduodenal and pericholecystic adhesions

   4. Pancreatic lithiasis

   5. Acute hemorrhagic pancreatitis

   6. Gas abscess of pancreas

   7. Biliary fistula and duodenocolic fistula

D. Functional conditions

   Spasm of duodenum

Chapter XX

SMALL INTESTINE AND APPENDIX

THE DUODENUM

ANATOMY OF DUODENUM. The duodenum is the upper portion of the small intestine. It is located high up in the abdominal cavity and is closely fixed to the posterior abdominal wall; it is largely retroperitoneal and has no mesentery. It is divided into three portions; the first short (superior) portion forming an extension from the pyloric end of the stomach; the second descending portion which passes downward beneath the transverse colon to the level of the third or fourth lumbar vertebra; the transverse section, of the third portion, passes horizontally to the left; from here it turns upward to form the ascending section of the third portion joining the jejunum. The duodenojejunal flexure is usually the highest fixed point of the small intestine. The flexure is suspended by the fibromuscular ligament of Trietz which passes downward behind the pancreas from the lumbar portion of the diaphragm. Within the curve of the duodenum lies the head of the pancreas. The bile and pancreatic ducts empty into the second portion at the ampulla of Vater.

ROENTGEN EXAMINATION

Roentgenologically the first portion of the duodenum appears as a smooth triangular structure or "bulb," filling by ejection of food material from the stomach, and emptying at its upper apical end, by contraction, into the second portion. Many observers feel that the first portion of the duodenum might better be considered as a terminal division of the stomach since it has more of the characteristics of the gastric mucosa than of the intestinal lining; rugae similar to those seen in the stomach run out into the bulb. With the second position of the duodenum we have the commencement of the feathery appearance seen in the small bowel as a result of the plicae circularis (valvulae conniventes). The ampulla of Vater cannot usually be visualized unless, by some disease, the orifice is held open permitting ingress of a tiny quantity of barium.

PATHOLOGY
INTRINSIC ORGANIC LESIONS

DUODENAL ULCER* (Fig. 248). The most common intrinsic lesions of the duodenum are duodenal ulcers. These occur almost entirely in the first portion of the duodenum. They are more commonly encountered than gastric in a ratio of 15 or 20 to one. Contrary to previous impressions, duodenal ulcer is not uncommonly found in children (Aye). It is thought to be influenced by some emotional state.

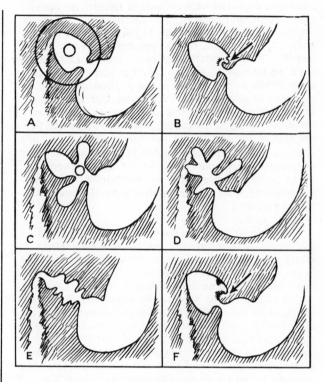

Fig. 248

Roentgenologically duodenal ulcer, if acute, may show a niche similar to that seen in the stomach from gastric ulcer. Since they frequently occur on the posterior or anterior duodenal wall, they may escape detection if pressure is not exerted on the bulb to approximate these two surfaces (A). At times they occur on the margin and can be seen in profile (B). In hypersthenic individuals, where compression is impossible, the use of Hampton's maneuver to introduce air into the bulb may facilitate demonstration of an ulcer crater, (Meyer).

Spasm may cause contracture of the bulb producing the characteristic cloverleaf deformity (C) or a similar modification (D). In more chronic cases the scar tissue contraction resulting from the ulcer produces an irregular deformity of the bulb (E and F). Such deformity, if constant at all examinations, is evidence of duodenal ulcer. Spasm of the duodenum may occur as a result of adjacent inflammation, such as cholecystitis, but this is not constant and is relieved by antispasmodics. Perforating duodenal ulcer may, on rare occasions, show a small

---

*An asterisk following any title indicates that roentgenographic reproductions illustrating this condition will be found in the pictorial supplement at the end of the chapter.

niche with a bubble of air similar to perforating gastric ulcers, but in the case of the duodenum the wall is thinner and complete rupture into the peritoneal cavity takes place more readily. Since many ulcers of the duodenum are on the posterior wall, the portion which is not covered with peritoneum, it is possible for walling off of the perforation to occur without infection of the peritoneal cavity. Usually, however, ruptured ulcer requires immediate operation to avoid peritonitis. The likelihood of recovery depends upon the speed with which operative procedure is instituted, so that prompt diagnosis is essential. It is, of course not permissible to administer anything by mouth, so that reliance must be placed upon detection of air free in the peritoneal cavity as evidence of perforation. Wherever this is found it is indication of rupture of a hollow viscus; free air is not found in all cases, however, since air is not always present in the duodenum at the time of rupture (80%). Duodenal ulcer is frequently a cause of intestinal hypermotility. Peptic ulcers rarely occur in the 2nd portion of the duodenum; when they do, however, they may resemble a small diverticulum, (Elkeles).

Perforation of the duodenum may occur in its uncovered portion into the retroperitoneal tissues. While this may result from erosion of a peptic ulcer in the cases recorded it has most frequently resulted from severe trauma applied to the abdomen, such as a kick of a horse or blow to the abdomen. Roentgenographically the distinguishing features are: air visualized in the retroperitoneal structures, fixed in the tissues without moving on changing position of the patient. The air most frequently extends along the interstitial space: under the left leaf of the diaphragm between it and its peritoneal covering; along the transverse mesocolon; the root of the mesentery of the small intestine; about the kidneys; down along the side of the cecum; along the psoas muscle or along the great vessels through the diaphragm into the mediastinum (Jacobs, et al.).

Mortality is high; prompt recognition and operative procedure is the only means of combating the infection. A few cases have been reported of spontaneous recovery.

Cases have been reported where rupture occurred during gastro-intestinal examination with escape of the barium into the adjacent tissues. This caused no special irritation and remained fixed in the tissues for many years, (Hayden).

DUODENITIS. This is a condition which resembles duodenal ulcer both clinically and roentgenologically. It is an inflammation of the duodenal mucosa showing hyperemia, stippling of the mucosal surface and even superficial ulcerations which bleed easily. There is irritability and tenderness on pressure. Microscopically there is cellular destruction, congestion, and oedema, with leukocytic infiltration.

The criteria for roentgen diagnosis are:

a) Irritability of the duodenal bulb with rapid emptying.

b) Pronounced but unstable deformity of the duodenal bulb and second portion of the duodenum,

c) Absence of a niche or crater,

d) Absence of gastric retention,

e) Coarse reticulated appearance of the mucosal pattern.

With subsidence of the inflammation the duodenum returns to normal; whereas, duodenal deformity from duodenal ulcer, once present always remains (Kirklin).

DIVERTICULUM OF DUODENUM (Fig. 249A and B). Duodenal diverticula may occur in any portion of the duodenum but they are more frequent in the second portion. Roentgenologically they appear as rounded pouches from a few millimeters to several centimeters in diameter, budding off from the duodenum, (Fig. 249A). They do not empty by peristaltic action and in the upright position may show a bubble of gas over a fluid level, (Fig. 249B). Such diverticula may extend posteriorly into the retroperitoneal tissues and be very difficult to detect at operation. They may become the site of inflammation and infection and giving rise to troublesome

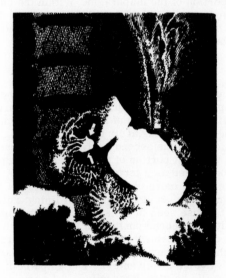

Fig. 249A

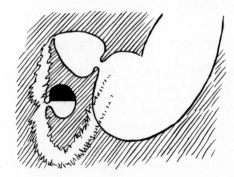

Fig. 249B

symptoms. They may ulcerate showing typical niche formation within the diverticulum, (Whitmore). They may be the source of hemorrhage. Usually, however, they are incidental findings in a gastrointestinal examination.

DUODENAL TUMORS. Benign polyps, either having their origin within the duodenum itself or originating in the prepyloric area of the stomach and protruding through into the duodenal bulb are most important because of their tendency to bleed periodically over extended periods giving rise to such grave anemic states as to suggest pernicious anemia (Fig. 239B), (Rigler). Other types of benign tumors occasionally encountered are: adenoma, angioma, fibroma, leiomyoma, neuroma, carcinoida, aberrant deposits of pancreatic tissue. These usually take on a small rounded form with smooth edges. Melamed and Pantone have reported a case of hematoma of the duodenum following abdominal trauma. The diagnosis was made on the basis of an intramural "tumor" of the bowel which spontaneously disappeared within the next few weeks.

Malignant lesions of the first portion of the duodenum are so rare that they can almost be discarded as a clinical entity. In the distal portion of the duodenum they are less uncommon (Mendl and Tanner). Such carcinomatous growths occurring in this region usually arise from the ampulla of Vater.

BRUNNER'S GLANDS. Hyperplasia of Brunner's glands may produce roentgenologically visible multiple nodules in the duodenum. The nodules give a "cobblestone" or "Swiss cheese" appearance when barium is partially displaced from the bulb by pressure. The nodularity is observed mainly in the bulb and in the upper duodenum, a distribution corresponding to the anatomic description of the normal glands. The hyperplasia is thought to be related to hyperacidity, since the glands help neutralize gastric acidity. Symptoms are vague and non-specific or similar to those of ulcer. Medical treatment is advised.

NEOPLASMS OF THE PERI-AMPULLAR REGION (Brunschwig and Templeton). Most carcinomatous lesions of the duodenum arise in the structures of the Ampulla of Vater or its immediate vicinity. They may be polypoid and project into the duodenum and may attain considerable size causing dilatation of the duodenum at this site with accompanying filling defect. They may be small with indurated rolled margins presenting only small defects or they may present the reverse "3" defect, (Frostberg).

Clinically, pain not usually of the colicky type, persistent jaundice and pronounced progressive loss of weight are the fundamental symptoms which are encountered in this condition.

Resection of the entire duodenum, head of pancreas and pylorus is feasible. Freedman, et al. have reported 5 cases of primary carcinoma and 3

cases of benign tumors of the duodenum with excellent informative comparison of the roentgen picture and the postoperative specimens.

Because of the difficulty often encountered in evaluation of the duodenal bulb, and the frequent accessibility of compression, Hinkel and Moller have perfected a technique for the barium-gas examination of this structure, with only minor modifications of Hampton's technique.

1. After the esophagus, stomach and duodenal bulb have been examined with barium in the usual manner (including pressure films of the stomach and duodenal bulb in the erect position), the patient is given one ounce of carbonated beverage and the table is brought to the horizontal position. This amount of beverage neither obliterates the mucosal pattern nor dilutes the barium appreciably. When there is a large gas bubble in the cardia the carbonated beverage is omitted.

2. The patient is rolled towards his left (right anterior oblique with respect to the fluoroscopic screen) until the gas rises into the antrum and bulb. Usually the bulb is seen projected through or just to the left of the spine.

3. Spot films are made in rapid succession. Photo-timing is a great convenience, and a rotating anode tube under the table provides excellent detail.

4. If the gas does not enter the bulb promptly the left lateral position may be utilized.

MEGADUODENUM. Uncapher and Holder have presented a comprehensive outline of the etiology of megaduodenum:

1. Congenital
    A. Intrinsic
        a. Diaphragms or valves.
    B. Extrinsic
        a. Duodenal bands or peristent cholesysto-duodenocolic membrane.
        b. Annular pancreas.
        c. Aberrant superior mesenteric vessel.
        d. Faulty rotation of the intestine.
        e. High fixation of the ligament of Treitz with acute angulation of the duodenum.
2. Acquired
    A. Intrinsic
        a. Tumor
        b. Ulcer in second or third portion of duodenum or in upper jejunum.
        c. Foreign bodies
    B. Extrinsic
        a. Tumor or enlarged lymph nodes
        b. Inflammatory or postoperative adhesions
        c. Arteriomesenteric occlusion
3. Idiopathic

They reported a case in which there was no apparent reason for the duodenal dilatation and McClenahan mentioned the possibility suggested by Sturtevant that such cases of enormous duodenal dilatation might be due to dissolution of the controlling nerve plexuses which regulate duodenal motion much the same as those of Auerbach and Meissner in the colon causing the development of megacolon; this however has not yet been proved, (Goin and Wilk).

DUODENAL ATRESIA AND OBSTRUCTION.

When there is a congenital atresia or complete stenosis of the duodenum, symptoms of high intestinal obstruction present in the new born period. Persistent vomiting in the first few days of life justifies radiographs in recumbent and upright positions. An extremely large gas-filled dilated stomach and duodenum without gas in other intestinal loops is typical. Examination with the infant in head down position will better outline the duodenum. Barium when given should be used cautiously and in as small amount as feasible, but most often the diagnosis is made with certainty on plain films.

When stenosis is not complete, symptoms may not be severe enough to require examination until later in infancy or childhood. The appearance on plain films may not be so pronounced or characteristic, but barium study will demonstrate the duodenal obstruction.

The descending duodenum is also obstructed by an extrinsic mechanism when bands of reflected peritoneum related to an incompletely rotated cecum compress it. Symptoms may be present in the immediate newborn period or not until much later. The findings on plain films and gastrointestinal barium study are very similar to other types of duodenal obstruction, already discussed, except that obstruction is far less likely to be complete, and gas is therefore to be seen in the lower small bowel. Barium enema will reveal the defect in colon rotation, with the cecum being seen not in the right lower abdominal quadrant, but in the right or left upper abdomen, in close relation to the stomach and duodenum.

EXTRINSIC LESIONS AFFECTING THE DUODENUM

TUMOR AND OTHER PATHOLOGY OF THE PANCREAS (Fig. 250A). The duodenum, by displacement from its normal position and pressure defects on its normal contour, gives clues as to the existence of other pathological conditions in adjacent organs. Carcinoma or cyst of the head of the pancreas may, owing to the enlargement of the head of the pancreas,

spread out the curve of the duodenum into a large circular structure, smooth and rounded on the inner margin, which when it occurs, is quite characteristic of the disease. Tumors in other portions of the pancreas may be detected by displacement of the stomach, colon, and other surrounding structures. Cysts and tumors of the body and tail can produce significant pressure defects on the left kidney, demonstrable on intravenous or retrograde pyelography in the recumbent position. The persistence of the defects when the patient is upright would suggest fixation to the kidney, (Chamberlin).

Before carcinoma of the head of the pancreas attains sufficient size to cause duodenal displacement it may be detected by its effect on the mucosal layers of the duodenum giving rise to a deformity described as an inverted figure three, (P. S. Friedman) on the outer duodenal border (Fig. 250B), or on the inner side of the loop, (Fig. 250C). Stiennon has concluded after extensive investigation that the Epsilon configuration is actually due to edema of the minor and major duodenal papillae.

INTERMURAL HEMATOMA OF DUODENUM.

Felson and Levin have reported a novel condition of the duodenum in which there appeared to be narrowing and almost complete obstruction in its second portion with the development of a coiled-spring appearance at its junction with the third portion as if there was a rotary volvulus, associated with a mass due to hematoma of the intramural layers. The etiology is not known. There was no history of trauma. Castigliano reports a large tumor mass in the region of the head of the pancreas, thought at first to be due to carcinoma, which disappeared completely under antisyphilitic treatment and has remained well for 14 years.

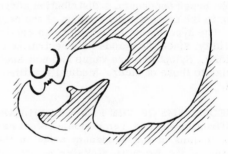

Fig. 250B

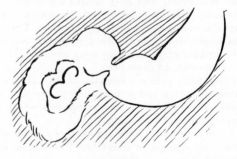

Fig. 250C

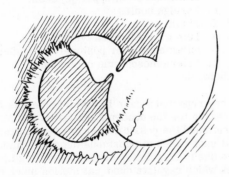

Fig. 250A

ANNULAR PANCREAS. Annular constriction of the duodenum from encirclement by the pancreas presenting a smooth constriction of the duodenum in its descending portion. The constriction retards the free flow of the duodenal contents and results in six-hour gastric retention, (Lehman; Feldman and Weinberg) (Fig. 250D).

Complete obstruction of the duodenum results in enormous gaseous distension of the stomach with gas. According to Hope and Gibbons it may be possible to observe an indenture on the duodenum in location of its portion which may give a clue as to its cause. Differentiation as to the causative lesion may be impossible.

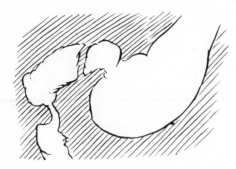

Fig. 250D

OTHER LESIONS OF THE PANCREAS, (Poppel). Aberrant deposits of pancreatic tissue may occur at any place in the duodenum or pyloric region of the stomach. They appear merely as small benign tumor masses of any other sort, arising extra-mucosally.

PANCREATIC CALCIFICATION

PANCREATIC CALCULI. Pancreatic calculi are rare. They may lie within the duodenal loop, but frequently form a series of multiple deposits extending throughout the pancreas across the upper abdomen, (Keats). Various observers have located these multiple small calcareous deposits in the smaller ducts, or in the parenchymal tissue itself. McGeorge, et al., have concluded that, "These areas of calcification may appear to be in the parenchyma because the lining epithelium of the radicals become denuded, most likely due to pressure, necrosis, infection and stassis." They may be associated with fibrocystic changes in the lungs.

"The characteristic microscopic appearance of our cases of diffuse calcification of the pancreas is the replacement of most of the parenchyma by dense, acellular fibrous tissue, with marked dilatation and deformity of the ducts, absence of most of the ancini, preservation of some of the Islands of Langerhans and chronic inflammatory round cell infiltration."

Both the lung and the pancreas are developed from the same embryological structure which probably explains their relationship in this disorder. The lungs show varying degrees of fibrocystic changes and bronchiectasis often with patches of bronchopneumonia which may serve to direct suspicion to the pancreatic disorder. Often a bronchogram may be necessary to show the cystic changes. A celiac type may have associated intestinal symptoms. It may have some connection with fat soluble vitamin A deficiency. The islands of LANGERHANS are usually not affected until late in the process. The small intestine may assume the appearance of a deficiency state (SAGE). The repeated attacks of upper respiratory infection, with cough wheezing respiration and dyspnoea, leading even to much more serious results and as lung abscess and empyema has served to emphysize the pulmonary aspect of the condition. The essential alteration of the mucus-secreting glands in all locations serves to emphasize these as the primary defect of the disease. This has led FARBER to suggest the name, "mucoviscidosis."

Poppel et al. have reported an instance in which the pancreas was herniated into the chest.

Small gall stones may occlude the Ampulla of Vater causing bile to enter the pancreatic duct resulting in acute hemorrhagic pancreatitis. In this condition there may be an accumulation of fluid in the lesser peritoneal cavity causing a mass between the stomach and transverse colon. The diaphragm is held in a high position (RIGLER).

Gas abscesses of the pancreas have been reported which are recognized by the changing fluid level within the abscess cavity.

GALL-BLADDER PRESSURE (Fig. 251). The pressure of an enlarged gall bladder or other adjacent organ on the duodenum, may be readily manifested.

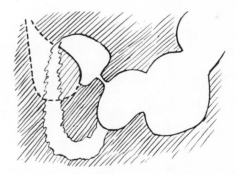

Fig. 251

PERIDUODENAL AND CHOLECYSTIC ADHESIONS. Periduodenal and pericholecystic adhesions following inflammatory conditions in this region may give rise to irregularity of the duodenal bulb which may simulate ulcer or duodenitis. It has been found, however, that deformity of the duodenal bulb from this cause represents such a small percentage of cases that they may be, for practical purposes, disregarded--

any constant deformity of the bulb being adjudged as evidence of duodenal ulcer.

Metastatic carcinomatous lymph nodes have been demonstrated causing a pressure defect on the 3rd portion of the duodenum, (McCort).

BILIARY FISTULA (See Biliary Tract, Figs. 273C & D, and p. 433). When erosion of a gall stone or of malignant growth causes a fistula between biliary tree and duodenum, deformity of the duodenum of varying degree may be seen with barium meal. The diagnosis is easily made by observation of gas in the arborizations of the bile ducts on plain films, or by the outlining of these ducts by ingested barium. Very rarely the biliary calculus responsible for this abnormal communication between biliary system and intestine is seen still in the duodenum.

Duodenocolic fistula is less often encountered. Carcinoma of the hepatic flexure, ruptured duodenal ulcer, ulcerative colitis, and tuberculous lymphadenitis have been known to produce this lesion, best detected by a barium enema, (Clayton and Thornton).

A plastic tube can be inserted into the pancreatic duct, (Doubilet), after transduodenal section of the sphincter of Oddi, and opaque material may be injected for visualization of the pancreatic duct system. The tube may be inserted into the duct for 4.5 centimeters and brought out through the duodenum and choledochus alongside a T-tube. In the event of postoperative oedema and inflammation the opaque material may pass through the epithelium, but as the inflammation subsides it assumes its normal form. Cysts and pseudocysts, abscesses, etc., may be visualized.

Gallstone Impaction in Duodenum. Erosion of gall stones into the duodenum and impaction into the bulb is a rare condition, which rarely is precisely diagnosed. Administration of a barium meal will demonstrate the filling defect produced by the stones, but often their nature cannot be recognized. Figiel and Figiel have pointed out that with cholecystography the fistulous tracts produced by the migrating stones become visualized and establish the correct diagnosis.

I. ANATOMY

II. ROENTGEN EXAMINATION

III. PATHOLOGICAL MANIFESTATIONS

1. Small intestinal obstruction—complete
2. Paralytic ileus
    Generalized
    Localized—associated with abscess
3. Localized spastic (sympathetic) ileus
4. Mesenteric thrombosis
    a. Arterial
    b. Venous
5. Vovulus of small bowel
    a. Twisting—acute
    b. Rotary—subacute, of terminal ileum
        WANGENSTEEN apparatus—for aspiration gastric contents
        MILLER-ABBOTT tube—for deflation of gas-distended intestine
6. Abdominal hernias
    a. Inguinal
    b. Femoral
    c. Ventral
    d. Umbilical
    e. Obturator
    f. Sacrosciatic
    g. Petite's triangle
    h. Pudendal
    i. Foramen of Winslow
    j. Mesenteric—Richter's
    k. Paraduodenal
    l. Intersigmoid
    m. Recto-genital pouch
7. Meconium ileus
8. Fetal meconium peritonitis
9. Intestinal emphysema—pneumatosis cystoides intestinalis
10. Incomplete intestinal obstruction
        Cold physiological salt solution—barium meal for small intestinal examination
        Rehfuss tube—for small intestinal enema
11. Regional enteritis; terminal ileitis; ileo-jejunitis
12. Tumors of small bowel
13. Multiple polypi
14. Diverticula; MECKEL'S
15. Nutritional disorders
        Avitaminosis
        Steatorrhea
        Sprue
        Celiac disease
        Amyloidosis
        Other deficiency states
16. Intestinal parasites—round worms
17. Peritoneal exudates

ANATOMY. The jejunum and ileum constitute the remainder of the small bowel. In these portions of the small bowel the valvulae conniventes produce a more "feathery" pattern than the picture produced by the stomach and duodenal bulb. These markings are most pronounced higher up in the intestines and become less evident as we progress downward,—a fact which is utilized in intestinal obstruction to determine the probable location of the obstructive lesion. Sloan has undertaken a most informative, painstaking study of the roentgen appearance of the small intestine. Barium meals composed of different food material produce different intestinal patterns; water mixture alone passes rapidly into the intestines and produces a more solid smooth pattern of the intestinal loops, whereas a carbohydrate meal produces a more feathery appearance in the intestine.

ROENTGEN EXAMINATION

Normally, a purely carbohydrate meal should leave the stomach and completely traverse the entire small bowel in five hours, only a small amount remaining in the terminal ileum. Greater advancement than this indicates hypermotility; delayed passage indicates hypomotility. If physiological saline solution is used as a vehicle, the barium mixture leaves the stomach at once and usually reaches the cecum within an hour or less. This is used for examination of the small intestines. If the stomach is not emptied after six hours it is evidence of pathology. A striking example of intestinal hypermotility is seen in diarrhea of infants associated with intestinal infection. This is usually associated with excessive intestinal gas but occasionally however the lack of intestinal gas is a striking feature of the condition; the cause of this apparent discrepancy is not known, (Margulis, et al.).

PATHOLOGY

SMALL INTESTINAL OBSTRUCTION. * (Fig. 252A, B, C.) A review of the physiology of intestinal obstruction may aid in understanding the clinical symptoms and roentgen signs which develop. With complete obstruction of the intestine a definite chain of roentgen signs and symptoms rapidly develop (Case).

At the outstart, there is an effort of the bowel to overcome the obstruction which results in vigorous peristalsis. In the upper portion of the bowel this is without purpose since it meets with the obstructing lesion, but in the portion of the bowel below the obstruction it succeeds in stripping the distal portion of its contents. This is a very important point since it explains two points in the diagnosis first, that it is possible to have a bowel movement after obstruction has taken place; and second, that the bowel distal to the obstruction becomes stripped of its contents both fecal and gaseous and remains empty lying limp and flaccid. A finger introduced into the rectum will indicate the rectum empty with the rectal wall relaxed and flaccid falling loosely in folds about the examining finger. This also explains the roentgen sign which

is of such great importance: the lack of gas in the distal loop and rectum in intestinal obstruction.

Then, the portion of the bowel proximal to the obstruction, unable to rid itself of its contents, rapidly fills with gas. The origin of the gas which rapidly collects to distend the proximal intestinal loops is

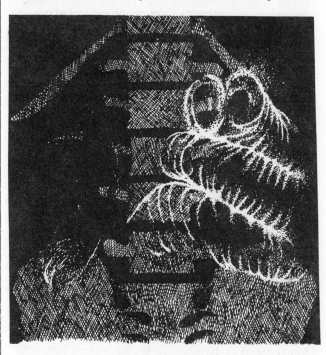

Fig. 252A

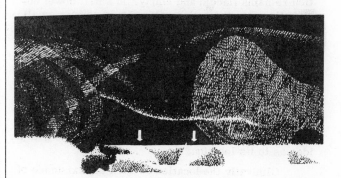

Fig. 252B

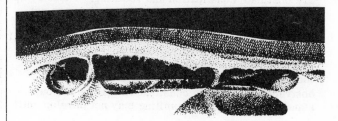

Fig. 252C

not fully understood but it probably results from many causes; the products of putrification, swallowing of air, fermentation, but probably the most important source is the gaseous interchange between the intestine and the blood stream which is probably disturbed by the uneven pressure produced on the venous return by the increasing distention of the intestine. Roentgenographically these gas-filled loops of bowel take on a characteristic appearance. Because of the extreme dilatation of the small bowel, the valvulae conniventes are stretched and accentuated giving the roentgen appearance of so-called, "herring bone" design, and the loops of gas-distended bowel arrange themselves back and forth across the abdomen in a "step-ladder" fashion. The abrupt looping of the gas-distended loops of bowel are often likened to "hair-pin" turns. These signs are best demonstrated in the anterior prone position of the abdomen. Within a few hours after obstruction fluid is excreted into the bowel giving rise to the roentgen appearance of multiple fluid levels. This is due to partial interference with the blood supply squeezing the blood vessels between the intestinal coats. These fluid levels are best demonstrated roentgenographically in the upright or lateral views (Figs. 252B and C). Large amounts of intestinal fluid are repelled back into the stomach by reverse peristalsis in an effort to rid the body of this toxic material and fecal vomiting occurs. The continued excretion of fluid into the bowel explains the source of such voluminous amounts of material which are sometimes vomited with intestinal obstruction, and the dehydrated state of the body tissues which develops.

At times it may be difficult to decide whether the small intestine or the colon is the portion of the bowel which is distended; a barium enema will soon decide this question. It will be recalled that the rectum and portion of the bowel distal to the obstruction remains flaccid and empty. In small bowel obstruction then the entire colon should remain small in calibre building up slowly even to its ordinary size as more and more of the barium enema is administered. There is no danger to be feared from a barium enema and frequently the information obtained is decisive.

The higher up in the small intestines the obstruction occurs, the more pronounced are the intestinal markings, so that it may be possible from the roentgen appearance of the distended bowel to gain an idea as to its location.

Clinically the location or even the existence of obstruction may be in doubt, so that obstructive lesions of both the small and large bowel must be considered. Among the most prominent symptoms are obstinate constipation and vomiting. These symptoms are invariably present, although they are not always sufficiently evident at the onset to justify a diagnosis of obstruction. In complete small intestinal obstruction vomiting may be the most prominent symptom, the constipation may be entirely overlooked; whereas, in complete large intestinal obstruction, obstinate constipation may be the outstanding symptom and vomiting may not develop until

much later. If the vomiting is fecal, this is, of course, a definite indication of obstruction. Intermittent colicky pains are usually a feature of acute small intestinal obstruction but they may not be very intense and later on, after the patient becomes extremely toxic, all manifestations of pain may cease and the patient may even experience a feeling of well being. Gaseous distension is present of course, but it remains for the roentgenological examination to determine its character and location. If peristalsis is visible through the abdominal wall, as it occasionally is in very thin individuals, it is additional evidence of existence of obstruction.

The most common cause of small bowel obstruction is postoperative abdominal adhesions. These are sometimes accompanied by exudation. Peritoneal veils and constricting membrane provide the obstructing medium in only a small percentage of cases. Primary malignancy is extremely rare, although secondary growths are responsible for obstruction in a greater percentage of instances. Strangulated hernias produce a goodly number of cases; under such circumstances the diagnosis is usually so self-evident that the patient is rarely sent for roentgenological examination. Complete obstruction has been described as a result of a number of other causes: volvulus occasionally associated with intussusception, impacted gallstones at the ileocecal valve, Ascaris worms, eating of grasshoppers in the Belgian Congo, fetal remnants following abortion, fibroids, (secondary), and very rarely, primary growth. When it occurs in association with congenital atresia of the bowel, the findings are the same but the symptoms are much milder.

Regardless of the cause, the roentgen findings of intestinal obstruction are the same.

The roentgen signs then upon which the diagnosis of intestinal obstruction is made are:

1. Gas distended loops of intestine, above the obstruction; flaccid empty bowel below the obstruction. The rectum must not contain gas or fecal material.
2. "Herring bone design" (produced by accentuation of valvulae conniventes with small bowel dilatation), "ladder pattern" due to arrangement of gas-distended loops on top of each other, and "hair-pin turns." The loss of valvulae conniventes is said to be evidence of gangrene of bowel.
3. Multiple fluid levels in the dilated intestinal loops.

These signs are best demonstrated by roentgenographic examination in the following positions:

1) a flat film examination of the entire abdomen in an effort to disclose any gas-filled intestinal loops. (Fig. 252A.)
2) examinations should also be made with the patient in the upright or lateral decubitus to disclose any fluid levels, or free air in the abdomen. (Fig. 252B.)
3) another examination in the transabdominal position (with patient lying on his back, x-ray beam directed horizontally across abdomen) should be made, not only to demonstrate fluid levels but to show exudate between the gas-filled intestinal loops. (Fig. 252C.)

These usually are sufficient to determine the diagnosis. It is always best to make the diagnosis without any injection or administration of barium sulphate if possible. If there is any doubt about the identity of the loops of the bowel, a barium enema may be given. If the evidence from these procedures is not conclusive a few swallows of barium sulphate mixture may be given by mouth and the course of the ingested material followed through the intestinal tract. We never hesitate to give small quantities of barium sulphate, two or three swallows of the mixture by mouth, even in patients where complete obstruction is suspected; larger quantities are inadvisable, since they may produce intestinal masses which interfere with subsequent operative procedure. Frimann-Dahl has had similar experience with the use of small quantities of barium by mouth in exceptional cases.

GENERALIZED PARALYTIC ILEUS.* In generalized paralytic ileus on the other hand (Fig. 253), there is no mechanical occlusion to the passage of material, merely a lack of propulsive force to push material through; the bowel lies distended with gas, unable to pass its contents along owing to paralysis. In such instances there is no definite localization of the lesion; gas is present throughout the bowel, and the rectum should be dilated equally as much as the remainder of the bowel.

Generalized paralytic ileus of this type may be due to general periotenal irritation such as peritonitis from infection, appendiceal or other abdominal abscess, subdiaphragmatic abscess, retroperitoneal abscess (q.v.), etc. Reflex inhibition from trauma either external or postoperative may cause ileus. There can be little doubt of the influence of the sympathetic nervous system on intestinal movement and gas formation.

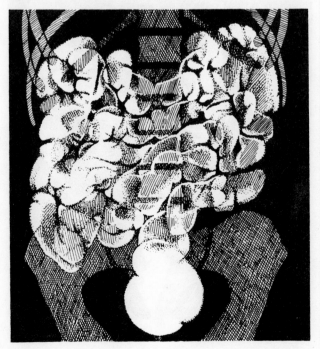

Fig. 253

The sudden appearance of gas-filled loops of small bowel in association with ureteral colic from passage of a stone or ureteral catheterization, which sometimes is observed, suggests the possible influence of the sympathetic nervous system, in gas formation by its influence on the circulation.

The acute development of gas in the intestines in shock is another manifestation of influence of the sympathetic nervous system, probably acting through the retarded circulation. A case of paralytic ileus complicating myocardial infarct has been described.

To the surgeon or clinician the points of prime importance are:

1. The establishment of the fact that an obstruction is present and that the meteorism is not due to paralytic ileus;
2. Its localization to a specific portion of the small or large bowel as nearly as possible;
3. The detection of any complicating conditions which may tend to throw light on the etiology or govern the method of treatment.

Usually the differentiation between small intestinal obstruction and paralytic ileus should be readily made from correlation of the history and symptoms with the X-ray findings. At times, however, the differentiation between the two conditions becomes quite difficult.

ABSCESS. Paralytic ileus frequently develops with abdominal and other localized abscesses, such as appendiceal, pelvis, subdiaphragmatic and retroperitoneal, (q.v.). Those infections which are associated with gas-forming bacteria may present numerous gas bubbles associated with the abscess. The extensive gas distention produced by paralytic ileus may obscure the smaller gas deposits unless they are especially borne in mind. The use of stereoscopic films of the abdomen is most effective in detecting such isolated gas deposits and separating them from the gas-filled loops of bowel. This is especially true in the diagnosis of retroperitoneal abscess, (Bird, et al.). If the abscess is not produced by gas-forming organisms, this sign is of no aid and other methods must be utilized for diagnosis (q.v.).

LOCALIZED PARALYTIC OR SPASTIC ILEUS* has been observed in which isolated sections of intestines become filled with gas as a result of extreme pain or local irritation from infection or other reflex cause—such as that seen when urethral catheterization is carried out for pyelography, and as seen in acute pancreatitis.

Localized paralytic or spastic ileus of this type may involve an isolated loop of bowel adjacent to or walling off a localized infection such as an appendiceal abscess, or it may be due to a reflex inhibition from pain. If these elements are borne in mind, it will be less difficult to come to a conclusion about this condition.

Another very important point of differentiation is the fact that the gas-filled loops of the bowel in spastic ileus are never as great as in true mechanical obstruction; they do not undergo extreme distention.

Young has been able by consideration of an abdominal survey film to suggest the cause of such reflex dilatation by its location and clinical signs.

MESENTERIC THROMBOSIS.* (Figs. 254A and B). Mesenteric arterial thrombosis, when fully established, causes similar gaseous dilatation of the bowel resembling intestinal obstruction roentgenologically. It is attended with excruciating abdominal pain and collapse, however, conditions which serve to differentiate it from simple obstruction. The clinical picture is one of acute abdominal emergency with symptoms out of all proportion to those of intestinal obstruction.

Occlusion of the superior mesenteric artery produces pronounced nervous stimulation resulting in intense contraction of all of the muscles of the gut.

Operative procedure at this stage discloses the entire gut drawn up into a knot from the severity of the reaction. Roentgen examination at this stage reveals only a bizarre pattern of gas distribution. After a few hours the contraction relaxes and gas distention of the bowel results. As the bowel relaxes, blood entrapped in the mesenteric veins drains back into the bowel, presenting the picture of multiple fluid levels similar in roentgen appearance to those from intestinal obstruction. Their cause in this case is due to blood, not transudate; a bloody stool, therefore, is a good clinical sign of mesenteric obstruction.

The superior mesenteric artery supplies all of the bowel, both small and large, up to the transverse colon near the splenic flexure. This is the artery most frequently involved. As a result, gaseous dilatation is confined to these regions of the gut, the colon beyond this point retaining its tone and normal appearance. It is difficult at times to clearly visualize the true extent and location of the gas distention, however, and for better evaluation it may be neces-

sary to perform a barium enema. As the barium enters the distal portion of the colon, it will fill normally, showing small caliber and tone; the barium will flow without obstruction through the zone of apparent obstruction near the splenic flexure of the colon into the gaseous dilated proximal portion of the colon, thus proving the presence of arterial mesenteric obstruction (Rendich and Harrington).

MESENTERIC VENOUS THROMBOSIS,* on the other hand, is not attended with such severe symptoms. Stasis from interference with return of the venous blood results in edema and waterlogging of all of the tissue, and transudation into the intestinal lumen and even the peritoneal cavity. The clinical picture is one of continuous severe hemorrhage although there is no actual bleeding. Roentgenologically, there is no evidence of gas-distended loops of bowel—a few tiny globules of gas may be present but for the most part the entire abdomen presents an homogeneous blank appearance.

Prompt surgical resection of the involved bowel is the only method which has met with success. Up to 1948 only 116 cases with successful resection have been reported (Benjamin).

Volvulus of Small Intestine
Volvulus or twisting of a loop of bowel 180° or more is usually associated with, if not instigated by, a long mesentery. Prompt diagnosis is essential if anything is to be accomplished for the patient. Yet it is in this very condition which our diagnostic acumen is least acute. One would think that twisting of the mesentery sufficient to produce complete occlusion of the intestine would result in the same roentgen

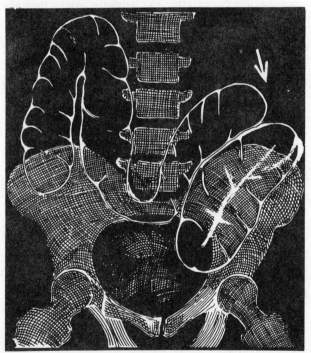

Fig. 254A. Arterial Mesenteric Thrombosis.

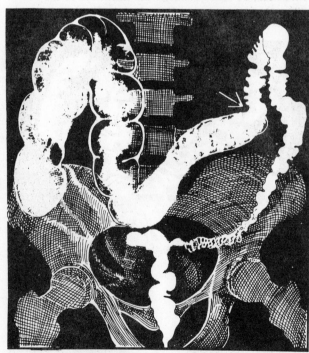

Fig. 254B. Arterial Mesenteric Thrombosis.

signs of intestinal obstruction produced by other causes, yet this does not seem to be the case. A few small gas-containing loops of bowel may be seen near the site of involvement, but these do not take on the appearance presented by other cases of intestinal obstruction but appear more like the isolated loops of gas-containing bowel seen in localized spastic ileus which develops in response to pain. Perhaps the simultaneous occlusion of the vascular supply and intestinal continuity might explain the lack of development of the signs associated with complete intestinal obstruction.

We have always looked upon gaseous distention of the bowels and their fluid content which develops in complete intestinal obstruction as manifestation of interference with normal gaseous interchange and fluid balance between the intestine and its blood supply.

Perhaps development of these signs is dependent upon the gradual interference with the blood supply, the venous return being first affected, followed by arterial occlusion only after sufficient gaseous pressure is built up in the distended intestine. In volvulus, the blood supply is reduced suddenly and in a different manner; both venous and arterial vessels are restricted at their sources simultaneously. This would explain the lack of gas distention and fluid levels in the twisted loop of bowel provided the process was sudden and complete, as it usually is in volvulus of the small intestine. Where the large bowel is involved the process is more gradual and gaseous distention may be enormous as it is in the cecum and sigmoid. This does not explain, however, why gas distention and fluid levels do not appear within the bowel proximal to the volvulus assuming that complete intestinal obstruction is produced. Perhaps we cannot assume that complete intestinal obstruction has occurred and that sufficient continuity of the intestine remains to prevent the development of these signs. Perhaps the primary fault is one of interference with the blood supply and that complete intestinal obstruction is a secondary development which occurs only as a late complication if at all. At any rate, this series of circumstances make volvulus of the small bowel the outstanding condition in which roentgen diagnosis may be of little value.

Mellnis and Rigler, attempting to throw some light on the subject by an analysis of the pathological and roentgenological findings, have suggested two signs, one a "coffee bean" sign consisting of a closed loop of gas-distended intestine, the other a so-called "pseudo-tumor" sign which represents fluid-filled intestinal loops. The one may be easily mistaken in any case of intestinal obstruction, the other may be difficult to detect.

Volvulus of the entire small bowel in the immediately postoperative period is a condition which also may occur. It is of unknown origin according to Gannon and Harrington. They suggest that it may be due to the paralytic ileus that usually follows operation, especially where extensive manipulation of the bowel is carried out during operation.

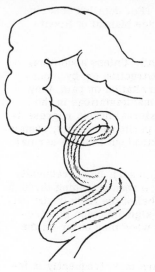

Fig. 254C

SUBACUTE ROTARY VOLVULUS OF THE TERMINAL ILEUM— (Fig. 254C). Subacute volvulus of the terminal ileum has been described (Tiscenco), in which the patient has symptoms of intermittent obstruction. Roentgenologically the terminal portion of the ileum can be seen turning in one or more loops with the mucosal folds drawn out into parallel lines, twisted upon themselves. The cecum may also be involved in a similar type of rotary ileus, q.v.

WANGENSTEEN APPARATUS. One of the most distressing and most harmful conditions associated with obstruction and other small bowel lesions is the uncontrolled vomiting. By this means the patient is dehydrated from excessive loss of fluid and becomes increasingly nauseated and toxic by loss of HCl. Wangensteen has developed an apparatus for constant drainage of the stomach contents through a stomach tube, which, with administration of salt solution subcutaneously serves to replace the body fluids and electrolytes and restore the body to a more normal physiologic state. This has in itself lowered the mortality of intestinal obstruction tremendously but from the x-ray standpoint it may serve to mask the x-ray findings. It is better to establish the diagnosis before any such methods are resorted to.

MILLER-ABBOTT TUBE. This ingenious device consists of a long double-barreled rubber tube, one tube within the other. The outer tube is connected to a small rubber balloon near its end and the inner tube bearing a small metal tip, opens freely on the end. This tube is passed downward through the esophagus and stomach into the duodenum where the small balloon is inflated to fill the lumen of the bowel; then by constant suction on the other tube the gas and intestinal contents of the distended small bowel are sucked out and the tube passes downward by peristalsis to the point of obstruction. When the gas distention is relieved, few obstructions are found to be absolute, and the normal passage of the bowel may be re-established. A small amount of barium solution may be injected into the intestine at the point of obstruction and it may be possible to determine its cause. The tube may be left in place to guide the surgeon at operation. Direct fluoroscopic examination is utilized to introduce and guide the tube through the stomach and intestines. A few cc. of mercury placed in the bag facilitates the passage of the tube into the duodenum. Multiple positionings of both tube and patient are often necessary before the tube enters the duodenum. (For detailed description of passage of the tube see Manual of Roentgenological Technique.)

ABDOMINAL HERNIAS. Unless abdominal hernias cause intestinal obstruction or, by incarceration cause peritoneal irritation or pain, they usually do not cause other manifestations in the bowel. They are merely external hernia representing out pouchings from the peritoneal cavity, containing loops of bowel which extend out into the hernial sac.

Inguinal hernias of this sort, most frequently encountered in the male, are seen extending through the inguinal ring far down below the floor of the pelvis into the scrotum. The sigmoid colon is a frequent site of such hernias, when they occur on the left side.

Femoral hernia occurs most frequently in female patients; it is not so readily demonstrated.

Ventral hernias of the anterior abdominal wall and umbilical hernias often become saclike and contain large quantities of intestinal structures; their extent and content can usually be readily demonstrated.

Hernias have been encountered passing through every conceivable weak spot in the peritoneum, such as the obturator foramen (obturator hernia), the sacrosciatic notch (sacrosciatic hernia), Petite's triangle (Petite's hernia), through the inguinal canal down into the vulva of a female patient (pudendal hernia). For the most part they do not produce any unusual picture different from any other type of hernia other than their position.

There are, however, a few internal hernias which are important because of the structures they involve. The most important internal hernias are; herniation through the Foramen of Winslow, paraduodenal hernias and mesenteric or other types of Richter's hernia.

Newman and Frische have reported a case of abscess of the lesser peritoneal cavity in which the entrapped infection caused pressure on the fundus and lesser curvature of the stomach giving the impression of an intraluminal defect. The abscess caused a distension of the lesser peritoneal sac but was homogeneous in appearance and could hardly have been mistaken for a hernia.

Hernia into the Lesser Peritoneal Sac Through the Foramen of Winslow. Herniation of the small intestines and even a portion of the ascending colon through the Foramen of Winslow into the lesser peritoneal sac is a type rarely seen. Roentgenographically the gas distended loops of bowel are seen above the lesser curvature and the stomach seems to "hug" the extraneous loops giving the appearance of a double contour to the lesser curvature. The barium column stops abruptly at the site of incarceration. The sac may contain small bowel entirely or the hepatic flexure and part of the transverse colon may enter the hernia, (Cimmino; St. John).

Paraduodenal Hernia (Fig. 254D). This unusual hernia originates in the paraduodenal fossa beneath the root of the jejunal mesentery. Parsons quotes Callander's explanation that this type of herniation is due not to incomplete or malrotation of the colon but to invagination of an area of the descending mesocolon medial to the ascending branch of the left colic artery and inferior mesenteric vein by the jejunum and ileum while the descending colon is mobile and is not yet fused with the primitive posterior parietal peritoneum. They felt that the name should be changed to "hernia into the descending colon." They also felt that the right paraduodenal hernia should be called, "hernia behind the ascending colon."

The roentgen findings in right- and left-sided hernias are described as follows: (Exner)

RIGHT	LEFT
1. The intestines appear in a bag.	1. Same
2. The coils cannot be displaced.	2. Same
3. The axis is to the right of midline.	3. The axis is to the left of midline.
4. With the patient upright, the corpus of the stomach hangs down and to the left. The pylorus and antrum are not displaced.	4. The stomach rides high over the mass.
5. Absence of small intestine in pelvis not always true.	5. Same
6. No clear space between stomach and the mass.	6. There is a clear space between stomach and mass.
7. Exit from the mass by change in the appearance of the intestine can be demonstrated.	7. Same
8. The ascending colon lies behind the mass.	8. The ascending colon always lies to right of the mass.
9. There is an abnormal degree of stasis.	9. Same

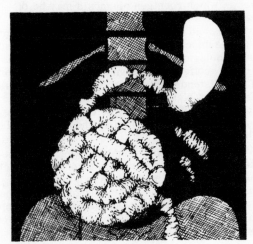

Fig. 254D

Similar displacement is caused by non-rotation of the colon; so this anomaly must always be ruled out by barium enema.

Mesenteric Hernia* ; Richter's Hernia (Fig. 254E). This is a condition in which a knuckle of bowel, herniated through a small opening in the mesentery, becomes incarcerated or strangulated. Even if complete obstruction does not occur, there is marked gaseous distention of the involved bowel from localized spastic ileus as a result of pain. Efforts of the intestine to free itself result in a circular pattern of gas-distended intestinal loops.

Roentgenologically these gas-distended loops arrange themselves in a concentric circular pattern about the point of incarceration giving rise to a picture which is quite characteristic.

Intersigmoid Hernia (Gotlieb). This is a very rare condition, only twenty cases have been previously reported.

"Close to the iliac artery near its bifurcation there is situated an orifice which leads into the sigmoid fossa behind the sigmoid mesocolon. The fossa extends upward varying in depth from a few millimeters to a few centimeters. The fossa results from the physiological adhesions between the posterior layer of the mesocolon and the parietal peritoneum at the disappearance of the descending mesocolon in the seventh month of intrauterine life with turning over of the descending colon to the left. The physiological adhesions starting at the splenic flexure leave a gap in the lower border, the so-called intersigmoid fossa. The catching of the duodenum or jejunum in the fossa produces an internal intersigmoid hernia or retroperitoneal hernia."

Roentgenological examination reveals the intermittent obstruction of the small intestine with gas distended loops of bowel stopping at the region of the sigmoid near the brim of the pelvis. Barium enema shows narrowing of the sigmoid with gas-distended small bowel originating at this point in left side.

Herniation of Rectogenital Pouch. In certain instances of relaxation of the pelvic floor, the recto-

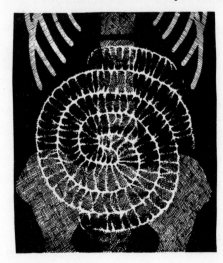

Fig. 254E

genital pouch may herniate downward between the anterior rectal wall and the pelvic structures. Lateral view examination in the upright position especially when bearing down will demonstrate the barium-filled colon or small bowel protruding well down into this pouchlike structure (Wallen). Wolf and Marshak have observed the characteristics of the bowel after infarction from segments due for instance to reduced incarcerated hernia. It is often important to know if the formerly strangulated segment of bowel is viable or if immediate operation is desirable. They found that if infarction had taken place the reduced segment of bowel would show tubular stenosis with effacement of of the mucosal pattern and conical transition to the proximal dilated bowel.

Since the various tissues of the small bowel may present different degrees of resistance to the necrotic process which follows, some of the structures may remain viable longer than others and it is proper to refer to partial infarction. It is possible therefore to relieve certain such cases by resection. The Miller-Abbott tube may be helpful in localizing such areas.

MECONIUM ILEUS. This is a congenital condition seen in new-born infants due to cystic fibrosis of the pancreas with occlusion of its ducts. The ducts and glands are filled with pancreatic secretion but it cannot escape into the intestine, (Baggenstoss, et al.).

Without the pancreatic secretions, failure of digestion of protein and fats occurs. The meconium becomes consequently thickened and inspissated, and readily blocks the intestinal lumen. Gaseous dilatation and other findings of intestinal obstruction supervene. A bubble appearance of areas in the abdomen may be noted on the plain films, due to the admixture of air and meconium. In uncomplicated meconium ileus, demonstration of dilated loops of small bowel with no fluid levels on the upright films of the abdomen warrants the diagnosis. When obstruction progresses to gangrene, perforation, and peritonitis fluid levels may be present, (White). Barium enema will show a very small caliber colon, for the obstruction is in the small bowel.

Seventeen cases of meconium ileus have been analyzed by Herson who found that intestinal obstruction with large bubbles of gas in a young infant was the most reliable sign of this condition.

Intestinal obstruction in newborn and very young children is indicated by essentially the same roentgen findings as in the adult. Agenesis of the myenteric plexus of the newborn, volvulus of the midgut, ileo-ileo intussusceptions and duplications of the small bowel, as well as the colon, cause small bowel obstruction.

Meconium (Fetal) Peritonitis. Newborn infants suffer from this disorder, a peritonitis due to the presence of meconium in the abdominal cavity during fetal life. It is usually associated with an obstructing lesion of the intestine of congenital origin. The meconium reaches the peritoneum through defects in the intestinal wall, but the site of perforation may never be satisfactorily demonstrated. The roentgen signs are those of intestinal obstruction plus calcific densities, often in multiple streaks throughout the abdomen. The calcifications result from deposition of lime in the meconial masses. Calcifications should be looked for in the scrotal region. Operative relief of the primary obstruction may result in recovery, (Neuhauser; Pratt).

Lester, quoting Boikan (1930) states that "the intestinal perforation in meconium peritonitis is due to obstruction caused by atresia, volvulus or string formations in about one-half of the cases. Meckel's diverticulum has been reported to be the exciting cause in two cases, (Mookherjee, 1955; Boikan, 1932)."

Obstetric or other traumata may occasionally give rise to perforation, (Zillner, 1884). In the remaining cases the disease will be associated with pancreatic fibrosis, leading to a putty-like consistency of the meconium and failure of its peristaltic propulsion through the intestine.

PNEUMATOSIS CYSTOIDES INTESTINALIS,
(Lerner and Gazin; Schorr, et al.). This is a condition in which cystic bubbles of gas collect in the mucosal wall of the small intestine or colon similar in every respect to gastric or bladder involvement by a similar process. A zone of lesser density produced by the air cysts is present outlining the mucosal layer of the intestine, intervening between the intestinal wall and any barium content which may be introduced. The etiology is unknown.

Roentgenologically care must be taken not to mistake the appearance of bowel partially filled with air before the barium enema, with this condition. It may interfere with motility but does not seem to be of any grave pathological significance and it subsides spontaneously. There may be air free in the peritoneal cavity from rupture of the cysts but this is associated with infection. The same lesions also involve the colon. Ramos and Powers have recently reported in detail the findings in such a case involving the colon. The operative specimen revealed thousands of gas-filled cysts occurring within the mucosal layer of the intestine resembling polyps. Rosenbaum has reported a fatal case following rupture of one of the cysts of the colon. Roentgenologically the diagnosis should not be difficult; gas-filled polypoid-appearing lesions projecting into the lumen of the intestine, usually the small intestine, although the large intestine may also be involved, (McGee, et al.).

INCOMPLETE INTESTINAL OBSTRUCTION.
The problem of partial intestinal obstruction still remains. It is partial obstruction of the small bowel which gives us the greatest difficulty in diagnosis. In partial obstruction there are no gaseous-dilated loops of bowel to direct our attention to the true pathology unless complete obstruction intermittently occurs. Occasionally gas may collect in the small intestines with partial obstruction, but there is never the extreme distention which gives rise to the characteristic picture of bowel obstruction.   The only

means by which we can detect the partial obstruction is by the retardation of flow of intestinal contents through this region of the gut. To accomplish this, it is desirable to follow the barium meal through the intestinal tract, making examinations at frequent intervals until the barium has passed completely through the small bowel. The detection of malformed small intestinal loops, constant at all examinations in any location, is the basis for the diagnosis of partial obstruction. By this method incarceration of intestinal loops in hernias, partial obstruction from postoperative adhesions or peritoneal folds, tuberculous peritonitis, localized exudate, tumors, etc., can be shown. Regional enteritis, especially when it involves the terminal ileum (terminal ileitis) may be detected by this method. The roentgen findings may not be characteristic, however. This condition may occur anywhere in the gastrointestinal tract; it must be considered as one form of partial obstruction. A diagnosis of partial obstruction may be made only after observing, on repeated examinations, retardation of the passage of barium at the same location. Special methods of examination are necessary for this investigation.

Small Intestinal Enema (Schatzki). If a barium mixture consisting of six parts barium to twenty parts of water by volume (500 to 1000 cc. is necessary for the examination) is introduced directly into the duodenum by a Rehfuss tube, the head of the advancing barium colon can be observed fluoroscopically during its advance in the small bowel. The flow must be continuous. It should reach the cecum in about fifteen to thirty minutes. Any variation in its normal appearance can at once be investigated with pressure manipulation and spot film examination. By this means it is possible to detect and evaluate small constrictions or defects in the bowel which do not completely obstruct. This is a most valuable method of examination in selected cases.

SMALL INTESTINAL EXAMINATION (Archer). If ice-cold physiological saline solution is used as the vehicle for barium mixture it usually is passed promptly from the stomach into the small bowel. The mixture traverses the small intestine rapidly; in 90% of all cases it should reach the cecum within an hour or less. Any prolongation of this time is indication of abnormality. Four ounces of barium sulphate in four ounces of ice-cold physiological saline is given and an initial 14 x 17 film is taken. A second glass of similar mixture is then administered and another 14 x 17 film is taken after a five minute interval. Similar films are taken at ten minute intervals thereafter until the head of the barium column reaches the cecum. Fluoroscopic examinations can be made at any time when the roentgenographic examinations show any indication of pathology, (Good and Fletcher). In deficiency states, sprue, and other intestinal conditions the motility is decreased. In enteritis it is delayed and the intestinal pattern may be segmented. In cases of sensitization there is hypermotility, (the head of the barium column reaching the cecum in fifteen to thirty minutes); reduction of the calibre of the intestines to one-half or less than its normal size, and segmentation of the bowel pattern. There is associated abdominal cramping. The usefulness of this method in detection of small bowel tumors, partial obstruction from intestinal bands or adhesion, constriction from terminal enteritis, etc., is self-evident, (Tennent).

REGIONAL ENTERITIS*—TERMINAL ILEITIS-ILIOJEJUNITIS (Fig. 254F). All of these probably represent similar pathological conditions. By re-

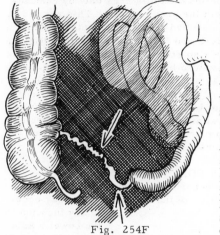

Fig. 254F

gional enteritis is meant a peculiar hyperplastic thickening of the intestinal wall of unknown etiology which occurs in an isolated segment of the bowel—usually near the terminal ileum, although it may have its inception at any location in the small intestine, or it may spread to adjacent large bowel involvement (Marshak and Wolf). Rare instances have been reported where it involved the stomach, (Martin and Carr), and duodenum, (Keats and Brady).

Two phases of development are recognized, (Marshak, et al.). The nonstenotic phase shows mucosal changes in the small intestine usually the jejunum, due to inflammatory thickening of the submucosal and mucosal layers.   As ulceration progresses a cobblestone appearance of the mucosa develops. The valvulae conniventes become thicker and more irregular encroaching upon the lumen of the intestine. This results in diminished mobility, straightening out of the intestinal loops and rigidity with wide spacing between the loops. As the condition progresses there is narrowing of the lumen and passage to the stenotic state.

In the stenotic stage the granulomatous lesion leads to encroachment upon the lumen of the intestinal canal until it permits only a fine stream of barium to pass, (known as Kantor's "string sign"). Occurring most commonly in the right lower quadrant the associated symptoms are often attributed to appendicitis. Clinically the following signs should lead to the suspicion of terminal ileitis.

1. Vaguely palpable mass in right lower quadrant
2. Tenderness on palpation in this area
3. Low grade fever 99° to 100.5° F.
4. Alternate attacks of diarrhoea and constipation; even signs of intestinal obstruction in advanced cases.
5. Anaemia due to varying amounts of blood lost in the stool. In atypical cases massive hemorrhage may be the only clinical sign.

Roentgenologically there is damming back of the barium meal so that at nine hours examination there will still be opaque material in the terminal ileum. The narrowed portion, giving the appearance of a "string sign," may be directly visualized, or it may be obscured by other loops of bowel. It is best detected by hourly examinations for five or six hours after administration of a barium meal. Kantor's "string sign" of the small bowel must not be confused with the "string sign" of the large bowel produced by mucus in the stool. By palpation at fluoroscopic examination the area of involvement may be connected up with the palpable mass. The condition gives rise to unusual intestinal forms in the right lower quadrant; this should always arouse suspicion and lead to a more detailed examination. There may be local spasm of the cecum similar to that seen in colitis or tuberculosis of the bowel. "Skip" areas of involvement along the bowel are frequent and both the roentgenologist and surgeon should bear this in mind during their examinations. Resection and by-passing of the involved area may completely eradicate the disease. About 20% recurrences are recorded. These may extend above or below the original site of involvement even onto the colon. Primary involvement of the colon is very rare. Fistula formation may occur either to the outside or between the loops of bowel. Enteroliths have been reported within the small bowel proximal to the constricted intestine, (Katz and Fischer).

SCLERODERMA (Hale and Schatski). The same lack of peristalsis and dilatation seen in the esophagus in scleroderma may be evident in the small bowel. The barium meal may remain in the jejunum for several hours and by eighteen hour examination there may still be considerable barium in the terminal ileum. Even the large bowel may show haustral pocketing and segmentation with barium enema. Stromme has pointed out that in the upright position fluid levels which may be present in diverticula of the small intestines may give the impression of intestinal obstruction.

DIVERTICULA OF SMALL BOWEL; MECKEL'S. Diverticula of the small bowel are frequently encountered. They may cause anorexia, crampy pains, vague distress an hour or two after meals should arouse suspicion and small bowel examination should be made. Inflammation may occur to the point of requiring resection, (Connolly). In this location they have no different characteristics than those found elsewhere in the gastrointestinal tract. They may not be easily demonstrated on direct examination and often go undetected until later when the barium mixture, after traversing the remainder of the small intestinal tract, leaves the diverticulum still filled with opaque material. Here also a bubble of gas may be entrapped above a fluid level if examination is made in the upright position, (Case). Being pseudo-diverticula without muscular coat they do not empty by direct muscular action. Meckel's diverticulum, on the contrary, is a true diverticulum with muscular structure in which peristalsis has been noted on fluoroscopic examination, (Lewitan). For the same reason they usually do not show a fluid level in the upright position, and are therefore more difficult to detect; this has, however, been accomplished in relatively few instances, (Poppel). A bubble of gas, constant in size and location should arouse suspicion, especially if associated with some barium retention. Bischoff and Stampfli have added to the barium filled or gas filled structure the presence of a "folded-ribbon-like (calcareous) shadow" within the gas bubble as a very helpful sign.

Moxon and Ollerenshaw point out that occasionally barium remaining as a residue in the diverticulum is the deciding factor which draws the pathology to one's attention. Before any conclusion can be drawn, the finding must be constant at repeated examinations. Mehth has reported a case on this basis.

Lerner, et al., have called attention to the presence of gas within the diverticulum on flat film examination of the abdomen as a presumptive sign, and confirmation by barium enema with reflux of opaque material into the terminal ileum and diverticular pouch. A case of intrauterine rupture of a Meckel's diverticulum has been reported by Rosza and Gross. Meckel's diverticulum may be the cause of intussusception, and is frequently the cause of hemorrhage.

TUMORS OF THE SMALL BOWEL.* Wherever melena is a symptom which cannot be adequately explained by the demonstration of a colonic lesion the small bowel should be carefully examined. While the small intestine will only be found to be the source in 5% of the cases the possibility of operative removal is great and the location of the lesion should be sought (Dedick and Collins). Improved methods of examination are bringing to light increasingly greater numbers of tumors of the small bowel. The small intestinal enema, fractional small bowel series with multiple examinations as the barium meal traverses the small intestine, and fluoroscopy with spot film examination of segmental loops under pressure have all led to more satisfactory examination, (Dundon).

Benign tumors which are encountered are:

Carcinoid
Adenomatous polyps
Lipoma
Lymphangioma
Leiomyoma
Hemangioma
Fibroma
Neurofibroma
Fibromyoma

The malignant tumors most frequently seen are:

Carcinoma
Lymphosarcoma
Fibrosarcoma
Leiomyosarcoma, and
Malignant carcinoid

Carcinoma of the small bowel, either primary or secondary, is very rare and produces no charac-

teristic appearance. Like carcinomatous involvement elsewhere the lumen is usually encroached upon by the growth (Fig. 255B). Regional dilatation of the small bowel from infiltration of the bowel wall with lymphoblastomatous lesions is the rule rather than the exception (Fig. 255C).

Infiltration of the muscular layer of the bowel wall is more likely to occur with lymphoblastomatous involvement. The sarcomatous infiltration renders the musculature ineffective and normal peristalsis does not progress thru the area of involvement: fecal material is propelled thru this area only by continuous pressure from the proximal end. This results in dilatation of the involved segment, smoothing out of the mucosal pattern and muscular inactivity. Richman, et al., have also stressed dilatation of the segment of bowel involved by lymphosarcoma. Extensive areas may be involved embracing almost entire jejunum and ileum. The walls are rigid and peristalsis absent in the involved area. In some instances infiltration of the muscular layer does not occur, the sarcomatous lesion merely obstructing the bowel as in carcinoma (Deeb and Stilson).

MULTIPLE POLYPI (Fig. 255A). Multiple polypoid masses occur most frequently in the colon and terminal portion of the ileum but they may occur in any location in the bowel. As a rule, when found in the distal portion of the ileum they are present as an extension from more pronounced involvement of the colon. Roentgenologically they appear as multiple rounded radiolucent areas within the barium-

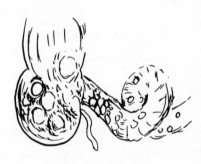

Fig. 255A

filled intestine. Such rounded defects, to be of significance must be constant at all examinations. Double contrast enema (injection of air after barium enema), is the most effectual method of demonstration in the colon, (see polyposis of colon). The association of melanum pigmentation of the lips and oral mucosa with intestinal polyps has been described.

NUTRITIONAL DISORDERS OF THE SMALL INTESTINE—AVITAMINOSIS—IDIOPOTHIC STEATORRHOEA—SPRUE—CELIAC-DISEASE—AMYLOIDOSIS and other deficiency states.

Although of widely varying etiology, all of these conditions give rise to unusual appearances of the intestinal pattern. The jejunum seems to be the site of greatest involvement.

SMALL INTESTINAL DYSFUNCTION IN AVITAMINOSIS. Avitaminosis, especially lack of vitamin B complex in the diet, may give rise to certain

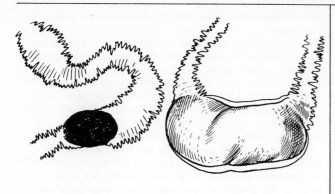

Fig. 255B   Fig. 255C

manifestations which are readily demonstrable roentgenographically. There is experimental evidence to
indicate that vitamins may influence gastro-intestinal
motility and absorption, (Learner, et al).

Roentgenologically the small intestinal pattern
produced by such deficiency states is characterized
in the early stages by hypermotility and hypertonicity,
and in the advanced stages by hypomotility and hypo-
tonicity. This is indicated roentgenographically by
irregular contraction of the bowel, abnormal segmentation of the small intestinal loops, interspersed with
widened loops of bowel showing coarsening and obliteration of the mucosal pattern, (Golden). The picture is not sufficiently distinctive to warrant an absolute diagnosis in all cases but where it is found it is
sufficient to justify a trial by vitamin therapy.

SPRUE AND PANCREATOGENOUS STEATOR-
RHEA. Sprue may give a similar picture. It may be
associated with pancreatic disease, such as stones
or carcinoma (Snell and Camp). The study of 3 cases
of amyloidosis has shown that its effect is the
marked slowing of the motility of the small intestine
and gas-distension occurring late in the disease. The
condition causes, 1) thickening of the mucosal folds
from infiltration of the mucosa, resulting in 2) narrowing and irregularity of the lumen, resembling regional ileitis, 3) gas distension due to replacement
of the tunica muscularis resembling ileus and 4)
4) slowing of the transit time. Gas distension appears
to be the most common finding. It may be accompanied by profuse bleeding. Marshak, et al., has
pointed out the continued roentgen picture of sprue
over 1 to 17 years followup. Three patients had
normal small intestinal pattern. The others showed
varying degrees if dilatation, segmentation, thickening of folds, scattering hypersecretion, fluid levels,
moulage sign and changes in motility. This is a
functional condition in which excessive amounts of
fat appear in the stool. Roentgenographically it is
characterized at first by coarsening of the mucosal
pattern which may pass on to complete loss of mucosal folds, the bowel segments assuming a smooth
waxy or moulage appearance, (Kantor). The process
is most pronounced in the jejunum and may not be
immediately demonstrable. A half-hour later, however, the mucosal pattern of the jejunum reveals a

peculiar appearance; it appears to have gathered in
curds, some small and irregular, others filling isolated dilated segments. Some coils have a coarse
serrated appearance while in others the barium
filled folds pass around the segments in ribbon-like
fashion (Brailsford). There is an associated failure
of normal calcium absorption and secondary manifestations in the bony structures. It is probably associated with pancreatic dysfunction (Marshak, et al.).

In celiac disease the mucosal pattern indicates
almost complete disintegration. This is associated
with serum protein deficiency, edema of the extremities and improper calcium absorption with secondary
manifestations in the bony structures. This is probably the infantile manifestation of the same condition
(Anderson, et al.).

Similar findings have been described, (Krause
and Crilly), in the presence of hookworms in the
small intestine. All of these conditions may be associated with vitamin deficiencies A, D, and E.

SCHONLEIN-HENOCH SYNDROME; (Henoch
Purpura). Handel and Schwartz have investigated the
gastrointestinal symptoms and signs of this condition
as manifested by areas of transient oedema of the
small bowel, demonstrable even before other skin
manifestations or purpura. They conclude that this
may be the gastrointestinal manifestation of polyarthritis nodosa.

Amyloidosis of Small Intestine (Golden).
"Amyloid is a protein material which exhibits certain
chemical reactions resembling starch." It may replace muscular tissue of the intestine giving rise to
various signs and symptoms resembling regional
enteritis. It may cause intestinal bleeding. Gas distention and disturbances in motility occur from infiltration of the muscular structure.

The present conception of the classifications
of steatorrhea may be divided into three types:
1) idiopathic, as seen in sprue and severe functional
disturbances, 2) pancreatogenous, from deficiency
of pancreatic enzyme, intrinsic inflammatory or
neoplastic ediseade, duct obstruction or extirpative
surgery and 3) symptomatic, the result of obstruction of small bowel lacteals by neoplastic or inflammatory processes. The general opinion is that
the two cannot be differentiated.

Hornsby and Bayling in a study of 19 cases of
sprue in comparison with 10 cases of pancreatogenous steatorrhea found in all cases of both types
steatorrhea was present.

In 3 cases of sprue sufficient gas-distended
loops of small intestine were present to resemble
paralytic ileus; this did not occur in any case of
pancreatogenous steatorrhea; the moulage sign was
frequently present in sprue, but not found in any case
of pancreatogenous steatorrhea; coarse folds and
flocculation were more frequent and pronounced in
sprue; neither group showed striking change in
transit time in about one-half of the pancreatogenous
steatorrhea patients, whereas only four of those with
sprue showed relatively normal intestinal patterns.

INTESTINAL PARASITES (Fig. 255D). Most intestinal parasites are small and cannot be recognized as such roentgenographically. They manifest themselves only by the irritability which they produce on the intestine. Hookworm infection manifests its presence roentgenographically by irregular segmentation of the small intestinal pattern; this is not specific, however, and may be caused by avitaminosis and other deficiency states. A similar intestinal disturbance has been reported in Giardia Lamblia infection, (Peterson). Henoch's Purpura has also been found to produce a similar picture (Whitmore and Peterson).

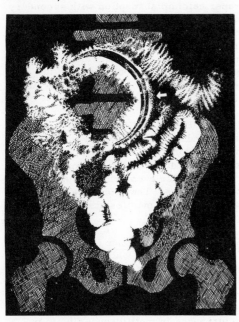

Fig. 255D

Round worms are 6 to 12 inches long, however, and produce a definite defect in the filling of the small intestine which permits indirect visualization of the worm itself. If the worm has been starved for a few days by the patient's fasting, and especially if a little chocolate flavor has been added to the barium, it may ingest the barium mixture. This shows in the roentgenogram as a fine line of increased density traversing the midportion of the worm throughout its entire length. At times round worms are very difficult to demonstrate roentgenographically and it may be necessary to make repeated roentgenographic examinations to determine the site at which the worm lies. Oftentimes, the intestine goes into spastic contraction and the worm cannot be seen from then on at that examination. Roentgen examination of 30, 60, and 90 minute intervals seems to be the best time for examination, (Minteer, et al.).

Free intraperitoneal air is almost always a sign of abdominal catastrophe. Perforated peptic ulcer is the most common cause. Other causes are perforation of the colon due to ulcerative colitis, volvulus or intussusception of the intestine due to a penetrating wound. Other means of introducing air should be excluded, such as by vaginal douche and by paracentesis or thoracentesis, before a diagnosis

of serious intraabdominal disease can be made, (Fischer).

Retroperitoneal air results from retroperitoneal perforation of the duodenum, secondary to peptic ulcer or severe crushing trauma. It may also occur from endoscopic instrumental perforation of the esophagus and stomach, or the rectum. The retroperitoneal structures, the kidney, the adrenals, are outlined by the dissecting air. When observed this sign likewise indicates abdominal catastrophe.

Foreign bodies usually pass through the entire small intestine without difficulty. If the object should be sharp or pointed, as an open safety pin or a needle, the passage may not occur. Roentgen examination is valuable to observe the progress of a radiopaque foreign body. If the foreign body remains strictly localized on the serial film examination, surgical removal is considered. If the foreign body continues to change position, making satisfactory progress down the alimentary canal, operation is not needed, and the object will eventually be passed per rectum.

CALCULI OF SMALL INTESTINE. A cluster of ring-like shadows in the right upper quadrant resembling gall stones, were found by exclusion to be calcified deposits in the wall of the colon. Similar lesions have been reported in the small intestine. It is usually associated with multiple strictures of the bowel.

PERITONEAL EXUDATION. A great deal more information may be obtained by closer attention to other details of the examination. The accumulation of abdominal fluid is manifested roentgenographically by the development of a homogeneous shadow in the flank, which displaces the intestines medialward. The subperitoneal layer as well as the fat spaces between the transversalis and internal and external oblique muscles show clearly as areas of greater radiolucency than the muscles themselves. These are known as the flank shadows. With the development of abdominal effusion the density of the medium surrounding the intestines is increased, the flanks bulge outward, but the clear subperitoneal areas are pushed ahead, but not invaded or obliterated by it. The invasion or obliteration of this space is indication of inflammation and exudation into the abdominal wall. This is a similar process to that seen in the obliteration of the shadow of the psoas muscles by infiltrating perinephritic abscess.

By applying these signs in cases of ileus, it is possible to determine whether or not there is associated fluid, either in the gas-distended intestine or in the peritoneal cavity, and whether this fluid is free or is a localized exudate. Since peritonitis with exudation is a common cause of paralytic ileus, its presence would be a factor in the differentiation between paralytic ileus and uncomplicated intestinal obstruction. By this method it is possible, under favorable conditions, to demonstrate appendiceal abscess and other localized exudates in the abdomen with or without ileus.

By transabdominal views—the patient lying on his back, the x-rays directed horizontally from side to side—marked variation in the picture can be shown in patients suffering from simple meteorism and those in which there is associated exudation. If there is no associated effusion, the coils of gas-filled intestine show well-defined thin walls and are close together; if exudation is present, it can be seen pushing its way between the intestinal coils and producing its impression upon them. By this means it has been possible to give the surgeon much more accurate information as to the condition present and to facilitate his approach to the pathological lesion.

THE APPENDIX

I. ANATOMY

Normal appendix

Variations of structure and position

ll. ROENTGEN EXAMINATION

Pathological manifestations

A. Chronic abnormalities of appendix

1. Normal findings

2. Criteria of pathology

B. Acute appendicitis

1. Methods of examination

2. Mucocele of appendix

3. Cecal spasm

4. Hyperplastic tuberculous appendicitis

The appendix varies greatly in its length, calibre, and position. Ordinarily it is about two and one-half to three inches long, extending downward from the cecum below the ileocecal junction, attached by a mesentery, yet freely movable. It may be represented by a stumplike rudimentary structure or it may be eight to ten inches in length, extending well over to the other side of the abdomen. Its lumen is ordinarily not more than two or three millimeters in diameter, but this may vary from a thin, threadlike structure when filled with barium to one well over a centimeter in width.

ROENTGEN EXAMINATION OF APPENDIX.* Normally, fecal material may enter the appendix in a large percentage of instances (Fig. 256A). The appendix may be visualized by the late films of a barium meal or on barium enema. Neither the filling or absence of filling of the appendix with barium can be considered of significance nor can retention of barium in the appendix for long periods after barium

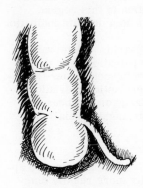

Fig. 256A

examination be considered as an indication of pathology.

Irregularity of filling (Fig. 256B), constrictions, kinking (Fig. 256C), inclusions, such as fecaliths, etc., are definitely abnormal conditions, but only in unusual instances are they associated with distinctive signs of disease.

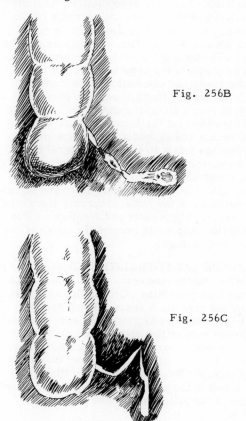

Fig. 256B

Fig. 256C

403

Malposition of the appendix may produce no definite indication of pathology. Instances have been observed where the cecum was inverted and the appendix was carried upward with it to a position near the gall bladder. If acute inflammation occurs in an appendix in this location, it would obviously become confused with gall-bladder pathology; mere change in position, however, produces no symptoms. Occasionally, an appendix which is closely restricted in the retrocecal position may give clinical indication of pathology. In instances where the lower end of the cecum presents an indented form (Fig. 256D), search for a retrocecal appendix, obscured by the intervening colon. Examine carefully with the patient lying on the left side on a stretcher, facing the examiner, before the vertical fluoroscope. The weight of the barium-filled colon will cause the cecum to rotate and gravitate toward the mid-line uncovering the appendix. It may be filled by double contrast method (Chrom and Gudbjerg).

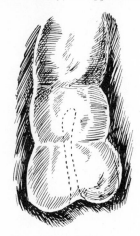

Fig. 256D

CHRONIC APPENDICITIS (Figs. 256A, B, C, and D). What sign or symptom is there of any value in determination of chronic appendicitis? Definite pain on palpation directly over the appendix region as indicated by fluoroscopic examination is suggestive but not conclusive. Other conditions may be associated with vague pains in the right lower quadrant such as ptosis of the hepatic flexure of the colon; close roentgen examination in such cases, however, will disclose that although the pain may be over McBurney's point, the underlying structure is not the appendix, but the hepatic flexure of the colon—the cecum and appendix having descended low down into the pelvis to a position lateral to the rectum. Sooner or later many of these patients have their appendices removed without relief of symptoms. Diverticula similar in nature and structure to diverticula of the bowel occurring elsewhere have been reported by Weiner and Jenkinson. It is conceivable that they might become the cause of infection or hemorrhage.

APPENDICEAL COPROLITHS. Calcareous deposits in fecal concretions occurring within the appendix are known as coproliths. Ordinarily, such structures would not give much concern but it has been found that when these exist associated with symptoms of appendicitis suppuration frequently follows even though the symptoms may subside. It is advisable, therefore, under such circumstances not to delay operation, (Thomas). Berg on the basis of his experience states that in the presence of a coprolith, when examination of the patient with acute abdominal

symptoms is performed, there is at least a 90% chance of the patient's having acute appendicitis, and a 48% chance that the appendix is perforated or gangrenous.

MUCOCELE OF THE APPENDIX. Mucocele of the appendix may present the appearance of a tubular or rounded distended mass even as large as the gall bladder. Norman, et al., have reported a case in which a rounded pressure defect produced on the cecum was constantly present. There may be calcium deposits in the wall resembling calcified gall bladder. Such conditions are very rare; they develop from stenosis of the cecal end of the appendix with continued mucous secretion in the absence of infection (Kalmoa and Winningham). Freedman has pointed out the frequent occurrence of cecal filling defects caused by granulomatous invaginated appendiceal stumps simulating neoplasm.

SPASM OF CECUM. Another very important sign of acute inflammation about the appendiceal region is spasm of the cecum and intestinal hypermotility. Roentgenologically this is observed as an irregular spastic contraction of the cecum and lower end of the ascending colon. It occurs with tuberculous infection of the cecum (Fig. 257), amebic dysentery, hyperplastic tuberculous appendicitis, actinomycosis, terminal ileitis and other types of acute inflammation in this region. When observed it may be taken as a definite indication of pathology.

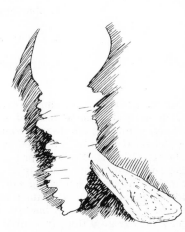

Fig. 257

It may be transitory, appearing at intervals during the examination. Deep palpation over the cecum usually stimulates its development under fluoroscopic observation. With hyperplastic tuberculous appendicitis, the appendix is large and bulbous, but spasm of the cecum may be lacking, especially if it is a subacute or chronic case.

ACUTE APPENDICITIS. Acute suppurative appendicitis is a condition usually more readily diagnosed clinically than by any roentgen sign. Since nothing is permitted by mouth in such instances, no barium meal examination may be made. Examination of the large bowel by barium enema must also be carried out with great care if undertaken at all, lest anything be done which might spread the infection.

Only very rarely is helpful information obtained; occasionally a large walled-off appendiceal abscess may cause a pressure defect on the cecum. If any roentgen examination is carried out at all, it is more advisable to make it without any manipulation and with the least disturbance to the patient. Frequently, a flat anteroposterior film of the abdomen, with patient lying on the back or on the left side, may render valuable information. The area of exudation causes displacement of the cecum and terminal ileum which frequently are outlined by gas from localized spastic ileus incident to the inflammation. Observance of the flank shadows will sometimes indicate whether an exudate is present and whether it has infiltrated the abdominal wall.

The subject of acute appendicitis cannot be passed over without calling attention to the close clinical resemblance of the disease to acute lobar pneumonia in children, especially when the pneumonic involvement is on the right side. This is so well recognized and so frequent that it would be hazardous to operate on any child for appendicitis without previous chest examination.

THE COLON (Chapter XXI)

I. ANATOMY

II. ROENTGEN EXAMINATION

III. PATHOLOGY

    A. Anomalies
        1. Of length
        2. Of position
            a. Nonrotation
            b. Descent
        3. Of fixation
            a. Mobile cecum (inverted)
            b. Volvulus of cecum on its long axis (Rotary ileus)
        4. Of size
            a. Megacolon (Hirschsprung's Disease)
        5. Malfusion of the omental layers
        6. Duplication of the entire colon

    B. Colitis
        1. Infections
            a. Acute colitis
            b. Ulcerative colitis
            c. Tuberculosis of colon
            d. Amebic dysentery
            e. Luetic involvement
            f. Lymphogranuloma inguinale
        2. Spasticity of colon
        3. Redundancy of colon
        4. Mucous colitis

    C. Obstruction of the colon
        1. From adhesive bands (postoperative)
        2. From peritoneal veils and membranes
        3. From strangulated hernia
        4. From pressure or invasion of extrinsic or metastatic growths
        5. From intrinsic growths
            a. Carcinoma
            b. Polypi (Multiple polyposis)

    D. Volvulus

    E. Intussusception

    F. Diverticula of colon
        1. Diverticulosis
        2. Diverticulitis

    G. Imperforate anus

    H. Foreign bodies in the rectum

Chapter XXI

COLON

ANATOMY. The colon skirts the outer margin of the abdomen from the cecum, through the ascending, transverse and descending portions, and sigmoid to the rectum. It is much larger in calibre than the small bowel, to permit the longer sojourn of intestinal material for absorption of fluids. The muscular coat has a longitudinal layer which, unlike that of the small bowel, is concentrated into three narrow elongated bands (taeniae coli). These muscular bundles are shorter than the colon itself which results in formation of numerous pouches in the bowel, (the haustra coli). Transverse rings of mucous membrane separate the haustra coli.

The ileocecal valve guards the small intestine from reflux of fecal material except under unusual conditions of colonic pressure and disease of the valve. This is accomplished largely by the valvelike action of its two lips which are firmly approximated by the pressure of colonic contents. Recent investigation would indicate that the ileocecal opening is further guarded by a sphincteric action of smooth muscle, (Lasser and Rigler).

ROENTGEN EXAMINATION. Roentgen examination of the colon may be carried out by two methods, barium meal and barium enema. The barium meal gives us an idea of the function of the colon but rarely completely fills the gut. Twenty-four hours after ingestion of a barium meal the colon should be filled. At forty-eight hour examination the bowel should be emptied except for small residues in the cecum and rectum—the reservoirs of the colon. The appearance of the large bowel by the two methods is very different, since with a barium meal the normal fluid absorption leaves the contents more concentrated and dry; the barium enema, however, is fluid and completely fills the gut, more clearly outlining its contour. The haustral markings are deeper and more distinct when the colon is filled by a barium meal. Normally the haustral markings are evenly spaced and balanced, the lumen is central and the sacculations on either side are about equal in size and symmetry.

Roentgenologically the two lips of the valve can often be demonstrated as they project longitudinally into the barium-filled cecum. Reflux of a barium enema into the terminal ileum is not attended with any untoward symptoms and is a matter of every day occurrence on administration of a barium enema.

Twelve to sixteen ounces of barium sulphate mixed with two quarts of warm water is introduced into the rectum by means of an ordinary enema apparatus. The roentgenologist observes the passage of the opaque mixture as it fills the colon, scrutinizing each successive segment of the bowel for constriction, obstruction or abnormal dilatation. After the colon is completely outlined, the contents are si-

phoned out by lowering the enema-can below the level of the patient's body, or the patient is allowed to evacuate, disclosing the appearance of the colon in its less distended form. For determination of mobility of the colon examination is made in the upright as well as the horizontal position.

After this, complete evacuation of the colon is permitted and further X-ray examination is made. If there is any question of polypoid growth, or any questionable lesion about the cecum or ileocecal valve, further examination by double contrast enema is advisable. To carry out this procedure, re-insert the nozzle and inflate colon with air by means of a rubber bulb; the barium clinging to the colonic wall makes any mucosal lesion clearly visible. Where barium enema is to be followed by air injection, rugar four tablespoonsful to one and one-half pints of water may be used as the initial injection. Powdered gum acacia added to ordinary barium sulphate is perfectly satisfactory. It may be found more satisfactory to inflate the colon with air first, and then follow by barium mixture. Many new types of adhering barium mixtures have recently been devised. For the best results this procedure requires an exact painstaking technique. Klami has recommended addition of hydrogen peroxide to the contrast medium for demonstration of ulcerative processes (see Manual of Roentgenological Technique).

ABNORMAL DEVELOPMENT. In the course of natural development the gastrointestinal tract originates as a longitudinal tube, extending through the abdominal cavity. The upper abdominal portion is expanded to form the stomach. A small pouch or diverticulum just behind the opening of the vitelline duct becomes the cecum. From this point distally the gut enlarges in calibre to form the colon. Up to this time both small and large bowel are attached by a common mesentery to the vertebral column, the small bowel is coiled up on the right side of the abdomen, and the colon is entirely on the left side. At this point, rotation of the colon occurs, the ascending portion rotating across the abdomen to take up its normal adult position.

NONROTATION OF COLON (Fig. 258). This anomalous position of the colon may persist into adult life with the cecum and appendix near the midline or even on the left side of the abdomen. Under such conditions the duodenum does not again ascend and extend to the left side of the spine but remains on the right side, passing directly into the jejunum. Normal rotation of the colon results in the adult position of this structure around the outskirts of the abdomen.

DESCENT OF CECUM (Fig. 259). Ordinarily after rotation, the cecum then descends into its normal position, but occasionally it remains high up in the right upper quadrant; the appendix remains with the

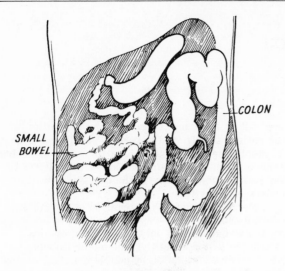

Fig. 258

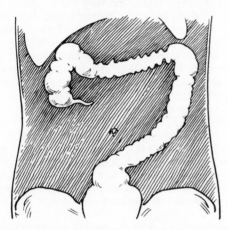

Fig. 259

cecum in a place high up in the right upper quadrant also.

Normally the cecum extends downwards to a position about one to one and one-half inches above the rim of the acetabulum; under certain developmental conditions, it may descend well below this point.

MOBILE CECUM (INVERTED) (Fig. 260). Ordinarily the ascending colon is relatively stable in position, descending perhaps an inch or so in the upright position. Occasionally, however, the ascending colon is so mobile that the cecum may become completely inverted, directed upward under the liver with the appendix in the gall bladder region. On assuming the upright posture it may revert to its normal position. Because of its wide range of mobility, it is very susceptible to volvulus (q.v.) and if inverted may even find its way into the lesser peritoneal cavity thru the foramen of Winslow (q.v.).

Rotary volvulus of the cecum (q.v.), a condition in which the cecum is twisted upon its longitudinal axis, has been described, (Jungmann). "At the junction between the barium-filled and air-filled parts of

the ascending colon it appeared to be turned upon its own axis." It gives rise to intermittent colicky pain. The terminal ileum may be involved in a similar type of rotary ileus, (Fig. 254C).

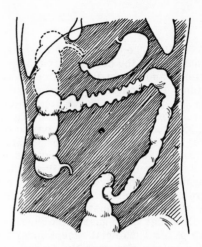

Fig. 260

MEGACOLON—(Hirschsprung's Disease) (Fig. 261A & B). Megacolon is a hereditary condition in which the colon is dilated to enormous size (Fig. 261A), many times the size of the normal, requiring gallons of fluid for complete filling by a barium enema. It is not advisable to fill completely the megacolon with barium because there is danger of excessive water absorption from the colon, and because it is difficult for the patient to expel the barium. It is probably due to faulty innervation of the colon, usually in the recto-sigmoid segment which develops separately and has separate innervation. Swenson has found by slow introduction of a barium enema that a constricted portion of the gut, usually in the recto-sigmoid region, can be demonstrated. An oblique view or lateral view is usually necessary to visualize this constricted segment, (Fig. 261B). In performance of the barium enema there should be no attempt to fill the entire colon, once the constricted, spastic distal segment is visualized. The patient will have difficulty evacuating the barium placed in the proximal colon. There is also danger of damage to the bowel from so much pressure.

Steinbach, et al., have called attention to the hazard of sudden death which may occur from administration of an enema, as a result of shock, presumably from "rapid absorption of water from the colon."

Careful study of the constricted area will show lack of normal ganglion cells in Auerbach's plexus, thereby eliminating or restricting peristalsis in this area and preventing normal propulsion of fecal material beyond this point. Strangely enough, surgical resection of the constricted portion of the sigmoid colon results in reestablishment of normal size and function of the rest of the bowel, (Swenson, et al.).

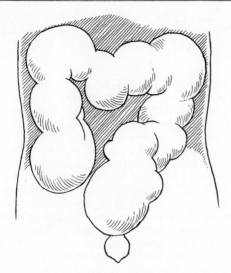

Fig. 261A

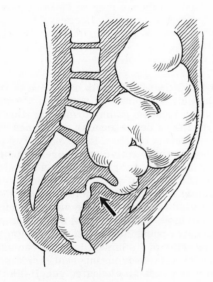

Fig. 261B

Keefer and Mokrohisky have shown that such aganglionic segments of bowel may be extremely elongated involving practically the entire colon and even the small bowel as well to the duodenojejunal junction.

MALFUSION OF OMENTAL LAYERS. During development of the greater omentum the posterior layer normally fuses with the transverse mesocolon so that the transverse colon is fixed in position beneath the stomach. If there is malfusion of these omental layers, the transverse colon may ascend higher than the stomach when the stomach and colon are examined simultaneously in the upright position.

DUPLICATION OF ENTIRE LARGE BOWEL. (Colon Duplex.) A very rare anomaly of development is seen in duplication of the colon. In a case reported

by Wever and Dixon, the upper end of the accessory colon did not communicate with the small bowel above nor the normal rectal pouch below.

Snodgras has described a case in which the reduplicated intestines passed through the diaphragm and were lodged in the thorax. Van Velzer, et al. have reported a case with duplication of the large bowel from congenital maldevelopment without symptoms.

ACUTE COLITIS. Acute colitis may not result in any organic pathology. The inflammatory process results in extreme hypermotility; large mass-movements of the colon can be seen under fluoroscopic examination sweeping the colon from cecum to rectum. Evacuation is so rapid that sufficient time does not elapse for fluid absorption and the bowel contents do not assume solid form. Such mass-movements may be seen in milder form in the normal colon, during expulsion of a barium enema; they are not necessarily an indication of inflammation. If the inflammation becomes very intense there may be hyperplasia of the lymph follicles giving rise to a feathered margin of the mucosal lining of the bowel. If the inflammation reaches this stage it must be considered as a very dangerous condition; the advent of antibiotic therapy has reduced the mortality to a minimum in these cases.

ULCERATIVE COLITIS* (Fig. 262A). Ulcerative colitis, in its acute stage, shows no different manifestations from that of acute colitis. When the disease becomes chronic it assumes certain distinctive characteristics. The gut loses its normal haustral markings and assumes a smooth appearance throughout the involved area, which has been likened to a sausage-skin appearance. The ulcerations themselves are very shallow mucosal ulcers which do not show at roentgenological examination. The ileocecal valve is held open by the thickening and edema of the gut, and the barium enema passes

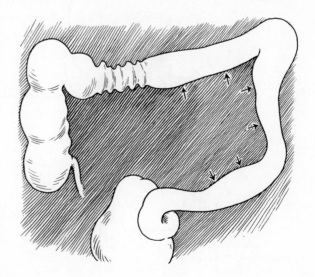

Fig. 262A

---

*An asterisk following any title indicates that roentgenographic reproductions illustrating this condition will be found in the pictorial supplement at the end of the chapter.

directly into the terminal ileum without hesitation, much more freely than normal. Sigmoidoscopic examination is the best method for detection of the ulcers. When ulcerative colitis becomes severe hypertrophy of the lymphoid tissue may produce the appearance of pseudo polypi; these may be very numerous throughout the colon. Pseudo polyps are also formed by ulceration leaving islands of mucosa, which appear to project into the bowel lumen.

TUBERCULOUS COLITIS (Fig. 262B). Tuberculous involvement of the colon is most likely to affect the cecum or rectum, the two points of stasis in the colon, but it may occur in any location. It is almost always found in individuals suffering with pulmonary tuberculosis. Tubercle bacilli, swallowed in sputum, lodge in the two points of stasis in the bowel and tuberculous lesions develop. Definite deformity of the colon can be seen at barium enema examination, frequently in several locations. While this is due in part to actual ulcerative or granulomatous lesions, the major portion of the defect is undoubtedly due to the extreme degree of hypersensitivity of the bowel causing local spasm.

As barium mixture is forced into the cecum either from the terminal ileum from a barium meal, or by enema, the cecum undergoes violent spastic contraction causing it to become narrowed down in calibre and irregular in outline. The contents are rapidly passed along into the colon, so that it is very difficult to obtain a roentgenographic examination of the cecum at any time.

Multiplicity of such areas in the colon speak for their tuberculous character. Likewise, the coexistence of pulmonary tuberculosis is an almost inseparable sign. Hyperplastic tuberculous appendicitis causes similar spasm of the cecum; in this case, however, the appendix itself can usually be visualized as a large hyperplastic structure. Solitary tubercu-

lous lesions of this sort may be difficult to distinguish from carcinomatous involvement. Roentgen examination offers the best method for diagnosis of this condition.

AMEBIC DYSENTERY. Hypersensitivity and spasm of the cecum are not confined to tuberculous lesions of the cecum and appendix. In amebic dysentery localized spasmodic contraction of the cecum and elsewhere is a very prominent feature and one which serves to direct attention to the inflammatory process present. Associated ulceration and induration probably contribute somewhat to the deformity. Since the cecum is a point of stasis the organisms probably therefore have greater opportunity for activity in this location. As treatment progresses these localized areas of spasm disappear. Chronic ulcerative colitis from amebic dysentery does not differ in appearance from chronic ulcerative colitis from other causes. The microscopic detection of the amebic in the stool is the only way in which an absolute diagnosis can be made. The localized inflammatory reaction to amebae may sometimes result in the formation of a large mass. Decrease in size of the mass in response to anti-amebic therapy helps in differentiating the mass from a true neoplasm of the right or transverse colon.

LUETIC COLITIS. With exception of the rectal region, luetic involvement of the colon is extremely rare. In this location gummatous ulceration of the rectum results in dense annular strictures which may almost completely obstruct the lumen. The ulcers themselves, in their active state, are not usually associated with great overgrowth of tissue and rarely stimulate carcinoma. By the time luetic involvement of the rectum reaches the stricture stage, the ulceration has healed and only a dense smooth stricture remains. Extrinsic pelvic lesions, such as tumors or pelvic exudates pressing against the rectum, may cause narrowing of its lumen, but this can usually be readily differentiated from inherent stricture. Pelvic cellulitis may cause an elongated pencil-like constriction of the rectum several inches long, from external pressure of the surrounding exudate. The early detection and treatment of syphilis has reduced the number of instances of rectal involvement.

LYMPHOGRANULOMA VENEREUM. Although primarily a veneral disease characterized by a small erosion or papule on the penis or vulva with enlarged inguinal lymph glands, the roentgenologist is more concerned with its secondary manifestations in the walls of the rectum and distal colon. The infection drains inward into the rectal wall causing a large infiltrating mass which has a tendency to produce extensive annular constriction of the rectum and sigmoid. There is destruction of the rectal mucosa, distention of the rectal pouch above the stricture and multiple sinuses and fistulous tracts (Klein).

In the active stage it produces large irregular filling defects of the colon especially in the rectal region with fistulous tracts which distinguish it from

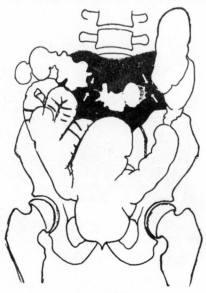

Fig. 262B

carcinoma. The Frei test for this condition indicates that this condition is more prevalent than formerly supposed especially in the colored race. It is possible that many of the cases of stricture of the rectum formerly thought to be luetic may be due to this cause.

SPASTICITY OF COLON (Fig. 263A). Spasticity of the colon is not considered as an inherent disease of the colon, but more likely as a local manifestation of a constitutional condition. High nervous tension in the routine of daily life, sedentary habits, constipation, etc., are contributory causes.

Roentgenographically the condition is manifested by accentuation and irregularity of the haustral markings of the colon. The condition is best seen at twenty-four hour examination after barium meal; it is not so well disclosed by enema.

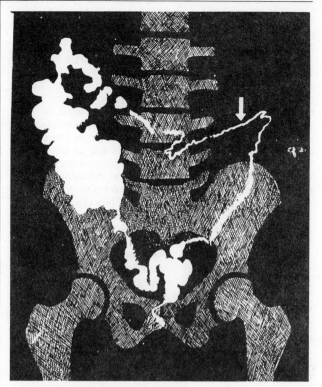

Fig. 263B

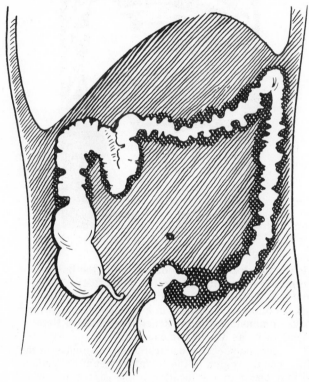

Fig. 263A

REDUNDANCY OF THE COLON likewise is rather a manifestation of a relaxed constitutional state than one of inherent defect unless it has reached the point of actual megacolon.

The most common site of redundancy in the colon is the sigmoid loop; this may become so long and dilated that it reaches a position well up under the left diaphragm. It is amazing how quickly this undergoes contraction and regains its tone after a cathartic or an enema.

MUCOUS COLITIS* (Fig. 263B). Mucous colitis is likewise a local manifestation of a constitution-

al condition. As a result of a highly nervous temperament large quantities of mucus are secreted into the bowel, encasing the normal stools at every bowel movement and sometimes even exceeding in quantity the amount of fecal matter passed.

Roentgenologically the presence of mucus can be detected by long opaque stringlike shadows remaining in the bowel after evacuation of barium meal or enema—the so-called "string-sign" of excessive mucus. This is much finer and more elongated than the "string-sign" of terminal ileitis with which it should not be confused.

OBSTRUCTION OF THE COLON. * The diagnosis of large bowel obstruction may be suspected from the plain film examination. Most colon obstructions occur on the left. The bowel proximal to the obstruction is dilated and retains fecal material and gas. Bowel distal to the obstruction, still being able to empty itself, contains no gas or fecal material. These generalizations apply to colon obstructions which are complete and have been present for more than a few hours. Incomplete obstructions will not show so decisive a difference in the x-ray appearance of the pre-obstruction segment compared to the post-obstruction segment. If the films are made very early in the course, even though the obstruction be complete, the distal bowel may not have had sufficient time to empty itself, and the proximal segments may not have begun to be greatly dilated as yet.

A careful appraisal of the gas-filled distended loops of bowel is necessary to differentiate large

bowel obstruction from small bowel obstruction and
paralytic ileus. With complete small bowel obstruction the loops have markings characteristic of jejunum or ileum. No gas is seen in the large bowel.
With ileus, gas is seen in both the more centrally
located small intestinal loops, and in the colon, although one or the other may disappear so dominant
on the films, that either small or large bowel obstruction is suspected. Large bowel obstruction
shows as a rule much greater distention of the colon
than is seen in ileus. The finding of gas in the
rectum excludes a complete colon obstruction (provided gas is not introduced by rectal examination or
enema). Gas in the distal colon and rectum is common in paralytic ileus. With large bowel obstruction,
distention of the small bowel is also observed, if the
ileocecal valve is incompetent and the obstruction
has been present for a time.

The diagnosis of large bowel obstruction should
always be confirmed by barium enema examination.
Rather than reliance on the impression obtained
from plain films, barium enema allows the diagnosis
to be made with certainty and enables the surgeon to
plan his operative procedure. The procedure carries
no risk to the patient and often prevents errors. Once
an obstructing lesion is detected, no attempt is made
to force barium beyond it to examine the remainder
of the colon. Attention to bowel care both before and
after surgery does away with the objection that barium may be long retained, and cause obstruction itself in the postoperative period.

Acute and complete obstruction of the colon is
commonly encountered in carcinoma of the left colon,
diverticulitis, and volvulus. The clinical history
must be correlated with the x-ray findings in every
case. Serious errors can be avoided by coordinating
the information obtained from roentgenologic examination with the bowel sounds, location of tenderness,
type of pain, and so forth. Unusual causes of colon
obstruction are postoperative adhesions, peritoneal
bands and membranes, strangulated herniae, pressure from extrinsic growths and intussusception.
Hewet and Ryan have reported a case of submucous
lipoma of the colon near the splenic flexure which
grew to such a size that it obstructed the colon.
There was a tendency to intussusception of the mass
but this was not complete.

INTUSSUSCEPTION* (Fig. 264A and B). Even
on the flat film of the abdomen a crescentic gas
shadow may mark the site of the advancing mass of
bowel leading to a suspicion of intussusception,
(Jackson). It produces a typical picture with barium
enema. The advancing head of the intussusception
forms a rounded impression upon the barium column
which is quite characteristic. The barium going
around the margin of the intussuscepted mass is
pressed out into a thin layer between the sheaths of
the intussusception giving rise to a "coiled spring"
appearance, Fig. 264B, (Ravitch). Intussusception
usually does not cause complete obstruction of the
bowel, so that there may not be any associated gaseous dilatation of proximal bowel; if there is sufficient pain or shock associated with the intussuscep-

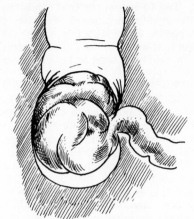

Fig. 264A

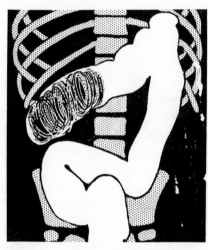

Fig. 264B

tion, some local gaseous dilatation of the bowel accompanies the intussusception, (Fig. 264). Figiel
and Figiel have pointed out that intussusception is
not uncommon in adults. In a number of cases they
have demonstrated a thickened, oedematous ileocecal valve as a possible cause.

Intussusception occurs most frequently in the
ileo-cecal region in the terminal ileum or cecum.
It may occur in any location in the gastro-intestinal
tract, even the stomach (q.v.) or duodenum. Tiscenco gives the percentage of occurrence in various
locations in the adult as follows:

1. Entero-colic:
   Ileocecal - 46%
   Ileocolic - 36%
   Cecal   - 2%
                 ────
                 84%
2. Colic (Colo-colic) 8%
3. Enteric (Ileo-ileal only) 8%

A few rare cases occur in the stomach and duodenum,
(Mauthe and Zwicky). Regardless of location their
roentgenological appearance is the same. Meckel's
diverticulum may be the cause in rare instances,
(Gay).

Reduction of the intussusception by hydrostatic pressure during barium enema is usually safe if carried out within the first 24 hours. As the barium solution enters it encounters the head of the intussusception shown under fluoroscopy as a rounded mass with multiple rings of distended intestine. As the enema proceeds the mass moves continually toward the cecum. With complete reduction, the barium solution passes well into the terminal portion of the ileum. To be sure that reinvagination does not occur, observe at intervals.

A great deal depends on the preparation of the patient for the successful reduction of the lesion. Girdany, et al., recommend washing out the stomach as a preliminary precaution to prevent aspiration if vomiting occurs. Insert child size BARDEX colon tube and wrap baby in restraining binder before proceeding; do not raise enema can more than 3 feet above body, to prevent application of excessive pressure.

Reduction of an intussusception of the colon by barium enema is usually safe early in the course of the lesion. This conservative method of reduction should be performed with the consultation of a surgeon. If there is any question of the viability of the bowel wall, or of the permanency of reduction of the intussusception, surgical exploration should not be delayed.

A very complete review of the subject is given by Hellmer.

CARCINOMA OF COLON* (Fig. 265A). In complete large bowel obstruction, postoperative adhesions, veils and membranes play a definite part; primary malignancy, however, is by far the most frequent lesion encountered (Samuel). Primary carcinoma may occur at any location in the bowel. The insensitive visceral peritoneum may permit the lesion to develop to enormous size before pain is produced. Not until it becomes of sufficient size to cause interference with function and partial obstruction is there any indication of abnormality.

The tumor, growing from the mucous membrane, encroaches upon the lumen of the bowel constricting the natural orifice. The natural fecal stream has difficulty passing this point so that the gut proximal to this point becomes dilated and often is impacted with fecal material. On barium enema examination the filling defect and constriction produced by the growth may be small, but the secondary manifestations of dilatation of the proximal portion with fecal impaction may direct the attention of the examiner to the site of the pathology (Fig. 265B).

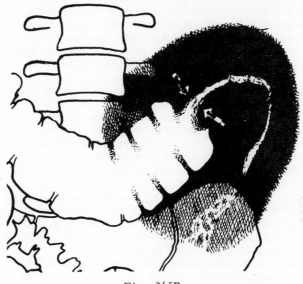

Fig. 265B

Pedunculated carcinomatous growths (Fig. 265C) which spring from one side of the gut and project into its lumen but do not necessarily obstruct, do not cause any change in calibre of the colon and may

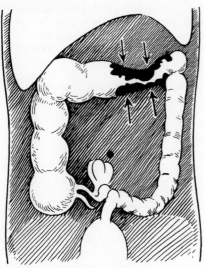

Fig. 265A

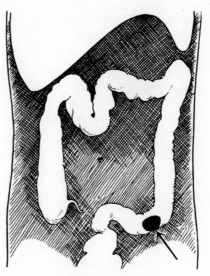

Fig. 265C

very easily be overlooked. The detection of carcinomatous lesions of the colon often taxes the utmost
skill of the roentgenologist.

The site of most frequent involvement is in the
recto-sigmoid area, a location in which the redundancy of the bowel may cause overlapping and obscuring of the lesion. Detailed examinations of this
area with the patient in the left posterior and right
anterior oblique views may be of advantage in
demonstrating the lesion. If it is obscured by an
over-distended rectum, drainage after filling the
upper segment may permit visualization of an otherwise obscured lesion. A Chassard-Lapine' view,
taken with the patient sitting on the Bucky diaphragm
table, with body fully flexed, may clearly demonstrate a lesion of this area which may have escaped
detection in the other views (Ettinger and Elkin).
Multiple primary carcinomas may occur simultaneously in various locations in the large bowel,
(Tondreau).

Destruction of the carcinomatous growth,
either from avascularity or infection, may occur resulting in fistula formation between the colon and
other surrounding hollow organs; the small bowel,
gall bladder or even the stomach, (Scott).

POLYPOSIS OF THE COLON*(Fig. 266A and B).
Multiple polypoid growths may be encountered springing from the mucosa of the colon. Such polypi may
be solitary or they may be so numerous as to almost
fill the lumen of the gut; no matter how extensive
they are, however, they never cause complete obstruction of the bowel since they are pedunculated
and are freely movable within the gut. They give
rise to periodic unexplainable attacks of diarrhea,
with bloody mucous stools and sometimes frank massive hemorrhages. They should be thought of as a
possibility in every obscure case having these symptoms where ordinary barium enema examination has
not disclosed the cause. Here, as in other hollow
organs, pedunculated growths projecting into the
lumen, unless large, may be completely obscured
by the opaque material filling the bowel, with an or-

dinary barium enema. To avoid this another method
of examination has been devised utilizing contrasting
mediums—barium sulphate solution to provide the
denser medium to coat the intestinal wall and the
surface of the polyps, and air to provide a medium
of lesser density than the soft tissues to throw the
polyp into relief. Such a double contrast enema is
carried out by first completely cleansing the bowel
of all extraneous material, with 2 oz. of castor oil
the evening before, and high cleansing enemas the
next morning on the day of examination.

First: using a viscid barium sulphate mixture,
introduce the solution to the region of the hepatic
flexure of the colon.

Then, drain the solution back into the enema
can by lowering the can to the floor.

Next, inflate the colon with air by means of a
pressure bulb until the entire colon is distended as
indicated fluoroscopically.

Finally, withdraw the nozzle and make examinations radiographically in the A-P, upright; right
and left lateral decubitus, and axial view with the
patient seated on x-ray table being well forward.
The latter view and a P-A view are of the pelvis
only and may be best accomplished immediately after
the patient has expelled the remaining fluid barium
solution from the rectum just before the air, (for detailed instructions of the technique the reader is referred to the Manual of Roentgenological Technique).
The tenacious barium sulphate, clinging to the mucosa and covering the surfaces of the polypi, is
thrown into bold relief by the air in the colon, .
(Douglas; Stevenson).

While this method produces beautiful roentgenograms it often presents pitfalls in diagnosis
which are very aggravating; small fragments of fecal
material remaining after cleansing preparation may
resemble or may hide polyps; bubbles of air from
the inflation procedure may resemble polyps; diverticula may be very difficult to differentiate from
polypi and overlapping of loops of the colon may obscure small lesions.

These, and other difficulties of double contrast
method of examination, have led to the recommendation of the use of a thinner barium mixture, 75 grams
of barium sulphate and 5 grams of powdered gum

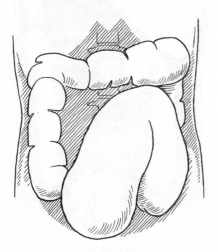

Fig. 266A

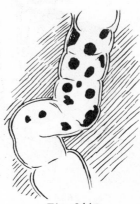

Fig. 266B

acacia to two quarts of water, has been recommended, (Doppel and Bercow; Potter), as a contrast medium. It is believed that by use of this thinner mixture small lesions such as polypi will not be so easily blotted out by the opaque mixture.

Carbon dioxide may be used in place of air. Comparative study was made by Levene of the use of carbon dioxide and air as mediums for double contrast study of the colon. Carbon dioxide was almost completely absorbed from the colon in 45 minutes; air showed little if any absorption in 2 hours. Moreover, the carbon dioxide injection caused no pain whereas the air caused cramping pains. This would indicate the superiority of carbon dioxide for this purpose.

The use of higher kilovoltage technique has also been advocated with regular barium mixture, (Gianturco and Miller). The higher kilovoltage penetrates the barium-filled colon more readily. Robinson has reviewed the advantages and disadvantages of the various methods of examination for this purpose and has suggested a judicious utilization of them all. He now relies on a single contrast barium enema study in which the barium column is made translucent by high kilovoltage exposure, controlled syphonage and extensive use of spot films made with compression. Fundamentally, the procedure is an elaboration of the technique developed by Gianturco and Miller. Andren and Frieberg have observed partial regression of polyps of the colon in children over a prolonged period by the double contrast method.

"BARIDOL," a finely divided barium sulphate, has tenacious qualities especially advantageous in double contrast colon examination, likewise it does not dry out as quickly as ordinary barium mixture and does not checker. It has one disadvantage in that it is thick and viscid requiring introduction with a syringe. (Manufactured by Pacific Chemical Co., 617 Montgomery Street, San Francisco, California.) We have found ordinary I-X barium meal satisfactory for this purpose, (Dick X-Ray Co., St. Louis, Missouri) utilizing both lateral decubitus position for examination. See Manual of Roentgenological Technique. With examination of 1,274 patients by this method using heavy barium, Andrén et al. succeeded in detecting polyps in 12.5%. Ninety per cent of these were under 1 cm. and 60% less than 1/2 cm. in size.

If the region of involvement is small and favorably located, surgical resection is possible; if, as occasionally happens, the growths are widespread throughout the colon and extend back beyond the ileocecal valve into the terminal ileum, then successful surgical intervention is impossible and reliance must be placed on medical measures, diet, enemas, etc.

VOLVULUS OF THE COLON (Fig. 266A). Certain portions of the colon, because of faulty embryological development, may be subject to a twisting deformity known as Volvulus, (Figiel and Figiel). Such twisting deformities may be either transverse, across the bowel or rotary along its axis, —axial torsion.

It is generally agreed that the development of volvulus of the colon is predicated upon some fault of embryological development of the intestinal attachment; hypermobility of one portion of the bowel due to unusually long mesentery, associated with close fixation of another from failure of mesenteric development. With such predisposing anatomical variations many conditions may provide the exciting cause for volvulus development, such as: unusual physical activity, overexertion, constipation, purgation, hypermobility, abdominal tumors, etc. The sites of most frequent involvement are those in which developmental variations of mesenteric attachment are most frequently encountered, the cecum and ascending colon, and the sigmoid.

Volvulus of the cecum and ascending colon is characterized roentgenologically by extreme gaseous distention of these structures showing, in the upright position, one or two elongated fluid levels within the dilated bowel, (Jakobsen, Frimann-Dahl). The gas-distended cecum can usually be identified without difficulty owing to its enormous size since small intestine could not possibly be distended to such a degree. Depending upon the degree of obstruction which may be associated with the volvulus of the cecum, there may be associated gaseous dilatation of the adjacent small bowel. Torsion of 180^0 or less may permit gas to pass thru the constricted loop so that it may be possible to have volvulus without associated complete obstruction. Displacement of the cecum and ascending colon into some other position in the abdomen, depending upon the degree of torsion and rotation, is one of the distinguishing features of volvulus. This may manifest itself as a larger oval or kidney-shaped gas balloon in the right hypochondrium, prevertebral or left subphrenic region, (Mondron, et al.). Failure to detect the cecum in its normal position in the right lower quadrant of the abdomen at once leads to suspicion of displacement from volvulus. Cecal volvulus may be secondary to a left colon obstructing lesion and such should be sought by a barium enema examination if there are no contraindications.

Detorsion of volvulus of the right colon is possible at times by barium enema and change in the position of the patient, lateral decubitus, knee, chest, etc. This is accompanied by immediate filling in of the deficient portion of the colon by the barium enema and relief of symptoms, (Figiel and Figiel). As with intussusception and volvulus of the sigmoid colon, there is danger that the bowel wall is nonviable, and that barium may perforate the damaged intestinal wall and enter the peritoneal cavity. The place of surgical treatment is obvious.

Volvulus of the Sigmoid.* This is another common location for the development of this condition, (Hall). The configuration of sigmoid renders it most susceptible to this type of involvement. Axial torsion or twisting of the bowel along its long axis may be demonstrated at times by roentgenographic methods. It may be accompanied by twisting of the mesentery and interference with the blood supply. It may give rise to severe symptoms or may be entirely symptomless, (Norgaard). Another unusual location for volvulus is the splenic flexure of the colon. This has been reported by Buenger. In 50% of the cases showing volvulus or torsion of the ascending colon and cecum at the Boston City Hospital, Ritvo, et al., have found some other associated lesion of the colon distal to the site of volvulus. Under such circumstances it is very easily possible to overlook such concomitant lesions. Barium enema may be helpful but this should not be performed in the presence of gangrene or perforation.

"The principal conditions which must be considered in differential diagnosis are paralytic ileus, mesenteric thrombosis, pancreatitis, peritonitis, strangulation of an internal hernia, Hirschsprung's disease, adhesions, neoplasm of the colon and a markedly dilated obstructed stomach."

A typical sigmoid volvulus is revealed by a long dilated gas-filled loop of colon appearing to rise out of the pelvis. The colon proximal to the twisted loop shows varying degrees of distention. Often both limbs of the twisted loop can be seen, but sometimes only a single but enormous gas-filled structure is readily visible. The diagnosis is confirmed by barium enema which shows a normal rectum and recto-sigmoid colon up to the point of obstruction, the twisted loop. The barium coming up against the twisted loop has a point shape, resembling the ace of spades. This appearance may be only fleeting, for reduction of the volvulus may be accomplished by the barium enema. Actually reduction by barium enema is preferred if feasible and the condition has not progressed to colon wall necrosis.

DIVERTICULOSIS OF THE COLON * (Fig. 267A).

Diverticula occur in the large bowel more commonly than in any other portions of the gastrointestinal tract. They occur most frequently in the sigmoid and descending colon but may be present in any location. They are more common in males than in females, and in the older age patient. Diverticulosis is probably the most frequently encountered lesion of the colon.

Small sacs of mucous membrane protrude outward between weak places in the muscular fibers of the gut to form blind pouches, connected with the lumen of the gut. They usually are much smaller and more numerous in the colon than at any other point in the gastrointestinal tract. They are usually patent, allowing bowel contents to pass into and fill them. The diverticula themselves are devoid of muscular structure and empty only because of contractions of the remainder of the colon.

Roentgenologically they appear as budlike projections extending outward from the lining of the gut at the tips of the pouch-like protrusion of the haustra coli, they are either completely filled with opaque mixture or show rings of opaque material about their fecal content. They may retain barium for several days after complete evacuation from the rest of the bowel. The mere presence of diverticula without evidence of local spasm or inflammation is known as diverticulosis of the colon.

DIVERTICULITIS OF THE COLON* (Fig. 267B).

Frequently, however, chronic retention of fecal material in these diverticula results in local inflamma-

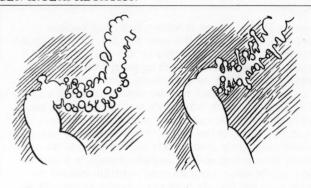

Fig. 267A   Fig. 267B

tion and infection which is manifested roentgenologically by local spasmodic contraction of the gut, and the formation of a tender palpable mass. As the inflammation subsides, the plica semilunares become thickened and the haustra become narrowed and deepened giving a saw-toothed appearance which is permanent evidence of previous diverticulitis not an indication of active inflammation (Goulard and Hampton).

By correlation of the clinical signs and symptoms, with the roentgen examination and the operative findings in a large number of cases, Wolf, et al., have come to certain valuable conclusions concerning the differentiation of these two conditions.

The mere presence of diverticula even with irregular sacculation of the haustral pattern and wide interhaustral plicae is not sufficient to indicate infection and is probably incident to the changes produced by the formation of the diverticula. Even "serration" of the bowel margin, if the segment of the bowel is pliable, does not necessarily indicate infection. Diverticulitis, on the other hand, is indicated by a failure to fill with barium the diverticulum which is the origin of the inflammatory process. The inflammation may subside and these may heal only to be repeated by the same process in others; when drainage does not take place infection supervenes and the process spreads to the surrounding tissues, even to the peritoneal covering and an inflammatory mass ensues.

A working classification of diverticulitis has been postulated by Wolf, et al.:

1. Acute diverticulitis with or without perforation.
2. Recurrent or multiple acute diverticulitis.
3. Healed or subsided diverticulitis, single or multiple.
4. Chronic diverticulitis with or without demonstrable fistula and sinus formation.

Carcinoma of the colon may develop on the basis of an old chronic inflammation from diverticulitis. At times it may be almost impossible to determine whether the palpable mass is inflammatory or actually carcinomatous. To add to the difficulty in diagnosis, such diverticula may rupture spontaneously with development of abscesses which may extend into the bladder or vagina, producing fistulous tracts (Stewart).

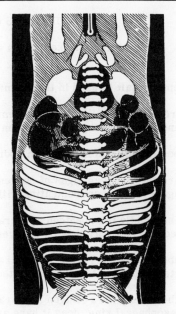

IMPERFORATE ANUS (Fig. 267C). Occasionally, at birth, it may be found that the rectum has not established proper connection with the anus (imperforate anus). Such a condition is of course incompatible with life and must be remedied surgically. The amount by which the gut fails to meet with the anal margin is the all-important consideration at surgical operation.

This information can be obtained in a very ingenious manner devised by Rigler. The bulb of a fever thermometer is placed at the anal margin to act as a marker for localization of this spot. Roentgenographic examination is made of the infant in an inverted position so that the rectal gas distends the distal end of the rectal pouch. The distance between the distal end of the gut and the thermometer marker is the distance over which continuity of the gut will have to be established. It is advisable to hold the child with buttocks elevated for five to ten minutes before x-ray examination to assure maximum filling of the rectum with gas, (Wilson). The rectum may be filled with meconium so that gas cannot enter; to be safe it is always advisable to take a lateral view of the rectum also.

GEOPHAGIA. Clayton and Goodman have called attention to the possibility of Geophagia or clay eating as an explanation of massive amounts of radio-opaque material inadvertently found in the colon. This is a practice extensively followed by adult negro women in some parts of the South.

Foreign Bodies in the Rectum. All manner of foreign bodies have been discovered in the rectum,

Fig. 267C

from fragments of a colon tube and enema nozzles to full-sized glass tumblers, electric light bulbs and crockery preserve jars. Prisoners frequently secrete bottles containing morphine in this manner. Perforation of the bowel wall by an ingested or inserted foreign body will result in abscess or fistula formation, with radiographic findings simulating tumor or localized inflammatory process.

QUESTIONS ON THE GASTROINTESTINAL TRACT

Questions marked with a dagger deal with rare and less-important conditions.

1. What opaque salt is used in the examination of the gastrointestinal tract?

2. Give procedure usually followed in making an examination of the gastrointestinal tract. What is a 5-hour meal and for what purpose is it given?

3. What position do disclike foreign bodies assume when lodged in the upper esophagus? Trachea? Why?

†4. What are the roentgen signs of congenital atresia of the esophagus? How may associated broncho-esophageal fistula communicating with the lower segment be demonstrated?

5. Describe briefly the roentgen appearance of benign stricture of the esophagus. How are such strictures acquired and how may they be differentiated from malignant conditions?

6. Describe briefly the roentgen appearance of cardiospasm and to what is it due? By what distinguishing characteristic may it be differentiated from other types of esophageal constriction?

7. Describe briefly the roentgen appearance of carcinoma of the esophagus and explain. What is meant by lower esophageal ring; does it have any relationship to carcinoma?

8. Describe briefly the roentgen appearance of diverticula of the esophagus and where do they most frequently occur? Name the different types and describe difference in their origin.

†9. How may esophageal varices be detected? What is meant by "curling" of the esophagus?

†10. What are the conditions known as "congenital short esophagus," eventration and diaphragmatic hernia? Is "short esophagus" always congenital? To what does it owe its origin?

11. Draw a stomach orthotonic for a sthenic individual and show all of the normal markings and label.

12. What is meant by: sthenic, hyposthenic, hypersthenic, asthenic individuals and what types of stomach are normal for these individuals?

13. Where should the head and tail of the barium column be five hours after the ingestion of a carbohydrate meal? twelve hours? twenty-four hours? forty-eight hours?

14. What are the signs of ulcer of the stomach and show by a diagram the typical appearance of a penetrating ulcer. What is the difference between perforating and penetrating ulcers?

15. Describe the roentgen appearance of gastric carcinoma of the adenomatous and scirrhous types.

†16. What is Linitis Plastica and what are its roentgen characteristics?

†17. What are the roentgen manifestations of syphilis of the stomach? Is it a rare or common lesion? What is appearance of emphysematous gastritis and to what is it due?

†18. Are benign tumors of the stomach rare? Name examples. How do they differ from malignant tumors?

19. What are the roentgen-ray indications of a hypertrophic gastritis and in what condition does it commonly occur? Is the roentgen diagnosis always accurate? What other method of examination of surface lesions is available?

20. To what are massive hemorrhages from the stomach due? What is meant by diapoedetic hemorrhage and under what circumstances does it occur? What is perigastric hematoma; to what is it due and how may it be recognized roentgenographically?

†21. What is multiple polyposis and explain its roentgen appearance.

†22. What are tricho- and phytobezoar and what are their roentgen characteristics? How frequently are they encountered?

†23. Do diverticula occur in the stomach? Frequently? Where are the sites of most frequent occurrence?

24. What is meant by marginal ulcer and under what circumstances does it occur?

25. What is meant by "cascade stomach" and how is this condition produced?

26. Upon what roentgen signs is the diagnosis of duodenal ulcer made? What is their incidence in relationship to gastric ulcer? Do they ever occur in children?

27. What are the criteria of diagnosis of duodenal diverticulum; carcinoma of head of pancreas? Aberrant pancreatic tissue?

28. What diagnostic points are observed in an roentgen examination of the stomach and what is their significance? How may ptosis be demonstrated and of what significance is it?

29. What are the usual causes of complete obstruction of the small intestine and to what are they due? What is the roentgen appearance and how may it be differentiated from paralytic ileus? What are causes of partial obstruction? Where does volvulus usually occur and how may it be recognized?

†30. What are the roentgen findings in mesenteric hernia?

31. Name at least three conditions in which there is associated hypermotility of the intestines and explain how you would differentiate.

†32. How may round worms be demonstrated roentgenographically?

†33. What is regional ileitis and how may it be detected? What other tumorous formations occur in the small bowel?

34. Can a diagnosis of appendicitis be made by roentgen-rays? Under what conditions would you say that an appendix was abnormal?

35. What types of deformity of the appendix would you consider as pathological? Of what significance is spasm of the cecum in diagnosis? Of what significance are fecaliths?

36. How may the large bowel be examined by roentgen examination and what diagnostic points should be especially considered? Name and explain several anomalies of development of the colon.

37. What are the roentgen characteristics of chronic ulcerative colitis? Amebic? Tuberculous?

38. In what respects does obstruction of colon differ from obstruction of small bowel?

†39. What are the roentgen characteristics of volvulus and what portions of the colon are most affected?

40. How does carcinoma of the large bowel appear and where does it most frequently occur?

41. What is meant by diverticulosis of the large bowel and where do diverticula most frequently occur? How may it be distinguished from diverticulitis?

42. What is polyposis of colon and how may it be demonstrated?

43. What is megacolon; how may it be diagnosed and to what is it due? How may it be cured?

44. How may the perineal defect in imperforate anus be demonstrated roentgenographically?

45. What are the characteristic signs of intussusception on barium enema examination? How may it be reduced?

REFERENCES FOR GASTROINTESTINAL TRACT

Esophagus:

Bockus, H. L., Gastroenterology, W. B. Saunders Co., 1943-46.

Saunders, J. B. de C., Davis, C., and Nuller, E. R., "Mechanism of Deglution (Second Stage) as Revealed by Cineradiography," Ann. Otol., Rhin. and Laryng., 60:897, 1951.

McLaren, J. W., Brit. J. Radiol., 16:270, 1943.

Middlemass, I. B. D., "Deformity of the Oesophagus in Bronchiogenic Carcinoma," J. Faculty Radiol., 5:121, 1953.

Freidenfelt, H., "A Double Contrast Method for the Roentgen Examination of Esophageal Structures," Acta Radiol., 46:499, 1956.

Leborgne, F., "Intubation in Carcinoma of the Oesophagus," Brit. J. Radiol., 29:344, 1956.

Palmer, E. D., "Achalasia: Anatomy of the Cardia as it Relates to the Regional Pathophysiology," Radiol., 67:79, 1956.

Kay, E. B., "Observations as to Etiology and Treatment of Achalasia of Esophagus," J. Thoracic Surg., 22:255, 1951.

D'Alessio, C. M., "Volvulus of the Esophagus," Am. J. Roentgenol., 70:425, 1953.

Baer, P., and Sicher, K., "The Association of Achalasia of the Cardia with Oesophageal Carcinoma," Brit. J. Radiol., 20:528, 1947.

Grossmann, M. E., "Non-malignant Conditions of the Oesophagus," Brit. J. Radiol., 19:114, 1946.

Kramer, P., and Ingelfinger, F. J., "Esophageal Sensitivity to Mecholyl in Cardiospasm," Gastroenterol., 19:242, 1951.

Conway-Hughes, J. H. L., "Oesophageal Reflux," Brit. J. Radiol., 29:343, 1956.

Lindsay, J. R., Templeton, F. E., and Rothman, S., "Lesions of the Esophagus in Generalized Progressive Scleroderma," J.A.M.A., 123:745, 1943.

Hale, C. H., and Schatzki, R., "The Roentgenological Appearance of the Gastrointestinal Tract in Scleroderma," Am. J. Roentgenol., 51:407, 1944.

Sennett, E. J., "Chordoma: Its Roentgen Diagnostic Aspects and Its Response to Roentgen Therapy," Am. J. Roentgenol., 69:613, 1954.

Schatzki, R., and Hawes, L. E., "Roentgenological Appearance of Extramucosal Tumors of Esophagus," Am. J. Roentgenol., 48:1, 1942.

Truchot, P., and Coutou, I., "Cystic Dysembryoma of Lower Esophagus," J. Radiol., et electrol., 32:512, 1951.

Antoine, Cayotte, Stehlin, and Sommelet, "Le retropneumoperitoine dans l'etude de la portion abdominale de l'oesophage," J. Radiol. et electrol., 32:446, 1951.

Melamed, A., and Walker, L. J., "Dissecting (Intramural) Pharyngoesophageal Diverticulum," Radiol., 49:712, 1947.

Nelson, S. W., "The Roentgenologic Diagnosis of Esophageal Varices," Am. J. Roentgenol., 77:599, 1957.

Brick, I. B., and Palmer, E. D., "Comparison of Esophagoscopic and Roentgenologic Diagnosis of Esophageal Varices in Cirrhosis of Liver," Am. J. Roentgenol., 73:387, 1955.

Waldenstrom, J., and Kjellberg, S. R., "The Roentgenological Diagnosis of Sideropenic Dysphagia (Plummer-Vinson's Syndrome)," Acta Radiol., 20:618, 1939.

Lindvall, N., "Hypopharyngeal Carcinoma in Sideropenic Dysphagia," Acta Radiol., 39:17, 1953.

Waldmann, H. K., and Turnbull, A., "Esophageal Webs," Am. J. Roentgenol., 78:567, 1957.

Spiro, M., "Oesophageal Atresia with a Review of Twelve Cases," Brit. J. Radiol., 29:345, 1956.

Hutton, C. F., "Plummer-Vinson Syndrome," Brit. J. Radiol., 29:338, 1956.

English, D. W., "Ectopic Stomach," Am. J. Roentgenol., 36:309, 1936.

Lust, F. J., "Herniation of Stomach into Scrotum," Am. J. Roentgenol., 37:666, 1937.

Johnstone, A. S., "Non-malignant Conditions of the Esophagus," Brit. J. Radiol., 19:101, 1946.

Wolf, B. S., Marshak, A. H., Som, M. L., and Winkelstein, A., "Peptic Esophagitis, Peptic Ulcer of Esophagus, and Marginal Esophagogastric Ulceration," Gastroenterol., 29:744, 1955.

Robinson, A. W., and Hennessy, J. D., "Reflux Oesophagitis of Unusual Aetiology," Brit. J. Radiol., 29:348, 1956.

Grossman, M. E., "Non-malignant Conditions of the Esophagus," Brit. J. Radiol., 19:114.

Wolf, B. S., Som, M., Marshak, R. H., "Short Esophagus with Esophagogastric or Marginal Ulceration," Radiol., 61:473, 1953.

Schatzki, R., and Gary, J. E., "Dysphagia due to a Diaphragm-like Localized Narrowing in the Lower Esophagus, (Lower Esophageal Ring)," Am. J. Roentgenol., 70:911, 1953.

Schatzki, R., and Gary, J. E., "The Lower Esophageal Ring," Am. J. Roentgenol., 75:246, 1956.

Inglefinger, F. J., and Kramer, P., "Dysphagia Produced by a Contractile Ring in the Lower Esophagus," Gastroenterol., 23:419, 1953.

Dawson, J., "Reflux Oesophagitis and Its Radiological Differential Diagnosis," Brit. J. Radiol., 26:310, 1953.

Andren, L., and Theander, G., "Roentgenographic Appearances of Esophageal Moniliasis," Acta Radiol., 46:571, 1956.

Gay, B. B., "Esophageal Perforations," Am. J. Roentgenol., 68:183, 1952.

Christoforidis, A., and Nelson, S. W., "Spontaneous Rupture of Esophagus," Am. J. Roentgenol., 78:574, 1957.

Migliaccio, A., Forsythe, T., and Cavanaugh, C., "Spontaneous Rupture of the Esophagus: Report of Case Occurring 5 Years after Gastric Resection," Surgery, 36:826, 1954.

Bodi, T., Fanger, H., and Forsythe, T., "Spontaneous Rupture of Esophagus," Ann. Int. Med., 41:553, 1954.

Madsen, E., "Dysphagia in Bulbar and Pseudobulbar Lesions Simulating Esophageal Carcinoma," Acta Radiol., 41:517, 1954.

Keates, P. G., and Magidson, D., "Dysphagia Associated with Sclerosis of Aorta," Brit. J. Radiol., 27:184, 1955.

Langton, L., and Laws, J. W., "Dysphagia Associated with Sclerosis of Aorta," Radiol., 6:134, 1954.

Stomach:

Jackson, C., and Jackson, L. J., Disease of the Nose, Throat, and Ear, W. B. Saunders Co., Philadelphia, 1946.

Almy, M. A., Volk, F. H., and Graney, C. M., "Situs Inversus of Stomach," Radiol., 61:376, 1953.

Mills, R. W., "Relation of Bodily Habitus to Visceral Form, Position and Motility."

Hodges, F., Snead, L. O., and Berger, R. A., "A Stellate Impression in the Cardiac End of the Stomach Simulating Tumor," Am. J. Roentgenol., 47:578, 1942.

Gross, K. E., and Durham, M. W., "Pyloric Antral Mucosal Diaphragm," Radiol., 61:368, 1953.

Ettman, I. K., Bouchillon, C. D., and Halford, H. H., "Gastrointestinal Roentgen Findings Due to Untoward Effects of Hexamethonium," Radiol., 68:673, 1957.

Campbell, R. J. C., "Gastric Ulcer of the Greater Curvature," Brit. J. Radiol., 21:146, 1948.

Feld, H., and Olivetti, R. G., "Benign Ulcer of the Greater Curvature of the Stomach," Radiol., 60:53, 1953.

Moutier, F., "Formation Cavitaire d'Origine Dynamique," Presse. Med., 34:681, 1932.

Lilja, B., "Gastric Block," Acta Radiol., 39:353, 1953.

Hinds, S. J., and Harper, R. A. K., "Shortening of the Lesser Curvature in Gastric Ulcer," Brit. J. Radiol., 25:451, 1952.

Wilson, J., and Wilson, B. J., "Pseudo-Ulceration of the Stomach and Duodenum Produced by Traction Diverticula," Am. J. Roentgenol., 75:297, 1956.

Carman, R. D., The Roentgen Diagnosis of Diseases of the Alimentary Canal, p. 421, Fig. 374, W. B. Saunders Co., Philadelphia, 1920.

Golden, R., and Stout, A. P., "Superficial Spreading Carcinoma of the Stomach," Am. J. Roentgenol., 59:157, 1948.

Kendig, T. A., Gaspar, M. R., Secrest, P. G., and Shackford, B. C., "Calcification in Gastric Carcinoma," Radiol., 68:30, 1957.

Livingston, E. M., and Pack, G. T., End Results in Treatment of Gastric Carcinoma, Paul Hoeber, Pub., 1939.

Meneghini, C., and de Marchi, R., "Pneumoperitoneum in Radiologic Diagnosis of Tumors in and Near the Cardia," Ardiol. Clin., 22:97, 1953.

Dragstedt, L. R., "A Concept of the Etiology of Gastric and Duodenal Ulcer," Am. J. Roentgenol., 75:219, 1956.

Kirklin, B. R., and Gilbertson, E. L., "Roentgenograms of Thorax that Suggest Carcinoma of Stomach," J.A.M.A., 134:1228, 1947.

Klein, M. M., and Bradley, R. L., "Gastric Ulcer in the Older Age Group," Am. J. Roentgenol., 77:25, 1957.

Elliott, G. V., Wald, S. M., and Benz, R. I., "Roentgenologic Study of Ulcerating Lesions of the Stomach," Am. J. Roentgenol., 77:612, 1957.

Katz, I., and Bierenbaum, M. C., "Multiple Chronic Gastric Ulcers," Am. J. Roentgenol., 77:623, 1957.

Evans, J. A., and Delany, F., "Gastric Varices," Radiol., 60:46, 1953.

Melenchini, M., and Roca, J., "Tumors of the Upper Third of the Stomach," Am. J. Roentgenol., 60:323, 1948.

Bell, H. G., "The Problems of Gastric Cancer in a University Hospital," Surg., 23:351, 1948.

Vickers, J. E., "Recurrent Gastric Ulcer Incident to Cortisone," Radiol., 69:412, 1957.

Camp, W. H., "Carcinoid of the Stomach," Radiol., 65:753, 1955.

Alexander, F. K., "The Prepyloric Suspect Lesion," Radiol., 61:523, 1953.

Sirak, H. D., "Boeck's Sarcoid of Stomach Simulating Linitis Plastica," Arch. Surg., 69:769, 1954.

Rubin, C. E., and Nelson, J. F., "Exfoliative Cytology as an Aid in the Differential Diagnosis of Gastric Lesions, Discovered Roentgenologically," Am. J. Roentgenol., 77:9, 1957.

Jenkinson, E. L., Epperson, K. D., and Pfesterer, W. H., "Primary Lymphosarcoma of the Stomach," Am. J. Roentgenol., 77:44, 1954.

Wang, C. C., and Petersen, J. A., "Malignant Lymphoma of the Gastrointestinal Tract," Acta Radiol., 46:523, 1956.

Mendl, K., Jenkins, R. T., and Hughes, J. R., "Congenital and Acquired Syphilis of the Stomach," Brit. J. Radiol., 29:48, 1956.

Thorgersen, J., "Anatomy of the Pyloric Canal," Am. J. Roentgenol., 71:76, 1954.

Rogers, J. V., and Adams, E. K., "Gastric Lipoma," Radiol., 67:84, 1956.

Roberts, R. I., "Benign Tumors of the Stomach," Brit. J. Radiol., 26:3, 1953.

Evans, J., and Weintraub, S., "Accessory Pancreatic Tissue in the Stomach Wall," Am. J. Roentgenol., 69:22, 1953.

Littner, M., and Kirsch, I., "Aberrant Pancreatic Tissue in the Gastric Antrum," Radiol., 59:201, 1952.

Davis, J. J., and Adams, D. B., "The Roentgen Findings in Gastric Leiomyomas and Leiomyosarcomas," Radiol., 67:67, 1956.

Gillespie, H. W., "Neuroepithelioma of the Stomach," Brit. J. Radiol., 20:433, 1947.

Cooley, R. N., "Primary Amyloidosis with Involvement of the Stomach," Am. J. Roentgenol., 70:428, 1953.

Grove, J. H., "Kaposi's Disease," Radiol., 65:236, 1955.

Flannery, M. G., and Caster, M. P., "Hemangioma of the Stomach with a Roentgenologic Diagnostic Point," Am. J. Roentgenol., 77:38, 1957.

Allen, E. H., Batten, J. C., and Jefferson, K., "Sarcoidosis of the Alimentary Tract," Brit. J. Radiol., 29:57, 1956.

Rappaport, E. M., Rappaport, E. O., and Alper, A., "Incidence and Clinical Significance of Transpyloric Prolapse of Gastric Mucosa," J.A.M.A., 150:182, 1952.

Rappaport, E. M., Rappaport, E. O., and Alper, A., Symposium, Radiol., 59:317, 1952.

New, P. F. J., "Prolapse of Prepyloric Mucosa," Brit. J. Radiol., 24:441, 1951.

deFeo, E., and Meigher, S. C., "Gallstones Impacted in the Stomach and Duodenal Bulb Demonstrated by Roentgenological Examination," Am. J. Roentgenol., 77:40, 1957.

Richards, H. G. H., "The Pathology of Benign Polypoid Gastric Tumours," Brit. J. Radiol., 26:121, 1953.

Rigler, L., Kaplan, H. S., and Fink, D. L., "Pernicious Anemia and The Early Diagnosis of Tumors of the Stomach," J.A.M.A., 128:426, 1945.

Melamed, M., and Pantone, A. M., "Hematoma of the Duodenum," Radiol., 66:874, 1956.

Rigler, L. G., Blank, L., and Hebbel, R., "Gastric Granuloma with Eosinophils," Radiol., 66:169, 1956.

Smith, M. J., "Gastric Granuloma with Eosinophilic Infiltration," Radiol., 66:177, 1956.

Vanek, J., "Gastric Submucosal Granuloma," Am. J. Roentgenol., 49:442, 1943.

Walk, L., "The Roentgen Signs of Gastritis," Am. J. Roentgenol., 60:77, 1948.

Miller, B., and Nushan, H., "Phlegmonous Gastritis," Am. J. Roentgenol., 67:791, 1952.

Lumsden, K., "Radiological Demonstration of Gas in the Stomach Wall," Brit. J. Radiol., 29:347, 1956.

Weens, H. S., "Emphysematous Gastritis," Am. J. Roentgenol., 55:588, 1946.

Henry, G. W., "Emphysematous Gastritis," Am. J. Roentgenol., 68:15, 1952.

Ostrum, H. W., and Serber, W., "Tuberculosis of the Stomach and Duodenum," Am. J. Roentgenol., 60:315, 1948.

Henry, G. W., "Detection of Gastrointestinal Bleeding with a Barium-Hydrogen Peroxide Mixture," Am. J. Roentgenol., 78:698, 1957.

Roberts, D. E., "Carbonated Soft Drinks in Roentgen Diagnosis of Foreign Bodies in the Stomach," Am. J. Roentgenol., 71:239, 1954.

Brizzola, A. J., "Magnet Extraction of Bobby Pins from Gastrointestinal Tract," Ann. Otol., Rhin., and Laryng., 61:237, 1955.

Canlas, E. M., and Fildes, C. E., "Radiopaque Phytobezoar," Radiol., 60:261, 1953.

Johnstone, A. S., Editorial: "Reflections on Hiatus Hernia and Related Problems," Radiol., 62:750, 1954.

Marchand, P., "An Aid to the Radiological Diagnosis of Oesophageal Disease," Brit. J. Radiol., 25:476, 1952.

Kleinfelter, E. W., "Invagination of the Esophagus in Hiatus Hernia," Radiol., 67:562, 1956.

Harrington, S. W., "Roentgenologic Considerations in the Diagnosis and Treatment of Diaphragmatic Hernia," Am. J. Roentgenol., 49:185, 1943.

Feldman, M., "Retrograde Extrusion or Prolapse of Gastric Mucosa into Esophagus," Am. J. Med. Sc., 222:54, 1951.

Marks, J. H., "Esophageal Hiatus Hernia with Inversion of the Stomach," Am. J. Roentgenol., 60:63, 1948.

Jenkinson, D. L., and Bate, L. C., "Volvulus of the Stomach," Am. J. Roentgenol., 69:54, 1953.

deLorimier, A. A., and Penn, L., "Acute Volvulus of the Stomach Emphasizing Management Hazards," Am. J. Roentgenol., 77:627, 1957.

Jungmann, H., and Venning, P., "Radiological Observations of Stomach Changes Accompanying the Threat of an Injection, and Further Data on the Normal Variation of Peristaltic Rate," Brit. J. Radiol., 26:93, 1953.

Davies, P. M., "Some Diagnostic Difficulties in Cases with Cascade Stomach and Chronic Gastric Volvulus," Brit. J. Radiol., 29:345, 1956.

Jungmann, H., "Gastro-duodenal Invagination," Brit. J. Radiol., 19:292, 1946.

Poppel, M. H., and Herstone, S. T., "Intussusception of the Stomach," Am. J. Roentgenol., 53:585, 1945.

Lands, E., "Pouch Formation after Gastroenterostomy," Am. J. Roentgenol., 60:69, 1948.

Palmer, E. D., "Retrograde Intussusception at Gastrojejunal Stoma," Am. J. Digest Dis., 21:309, 1954.

Golden, R., "Functional Obstruction of the Efferent Loop of Jejunum Following Partial Gastrectomy," J.A.M.A., 148:721, 1952.

Dragstedt, L. R., Clarke, J. S., Harper, P. V., and Woodward, E. R., "Supradiaphragmatic Section of the Vagus Nerves to the Stomach in Gastrojejunal Ulcer," J. Thoracic Surg., 16:226, 1947.

Wisoff, C. P., "Jejunogastric Intussusception," Radiol., 61:363, 1953.

Maisel, B., and Weintraub, S., "Prolapsing Gastric Mucosa Thru Gastro-Jejunostromy Simulating Cancer of the Stomach," Surg., 29:777, 1951.

Hajdu, N., Harris, M. A., and Ramsay, G. S., "Closed Loop Obstruction of the Afferent Limb, A Late Complication of Antecolic Partial Gastrectomy," Brit. J. Radiol., 29:344, 1956.

Solis-Cohen, L., and Levine, S., "Roentgen Diagnosis of Lacerated Spleen," Radiol., 39:707, 1942.

Schwarz, J., Silverman, F. N., Adriano, S. M., Straub, M., and Levine, S., "Relation of Splenic Calcifications to Histoplasmosis,"

Culver, G. J., and Pierson, H. S., "Splenic Artery Aneurysms," Radiol., 68:217, 1957.

Duodenum:

Aye, R. C., "Peptic Ulcers in Children," Radiol., 61:32, 1953.

Meyer, R. R., "Air Contrast Study of Duodenal Bulb," Radiol., 58:393, 1952.

Elkeles, A., "Penetrating Ulcer of the Descending Duodenum with Severe Secondary Anemia Caused by a Foreign Body," Brit. J. Radiol., 21:508, 1948.

Jacobs, E. A., Culver, G. J., and Koenig, E. C., "Roentgenologic Aspects of Retroperitoneal Perforations of the Duodenum," Radiol., 43:563, 1944.

Hayden, R. S., "Perforation of Duodenal Ulcer During Fluoroscopy," Radiol., 57:214, 1951.

Hampton, A. O, "A Safe Method for the Roentgen Demonstration of Duodenal Ulcers," Am. J. Roentgenol., 38:565, 1937.

Kirklin, B. R., "Duodenitis and Its Roentgenologic Characteristics," Am. J. Roentgenol., 31:581, 1934.

Whitmore, W. H., "Duodenal Diverticula with Ulceration," Am. J. Roentgenol., 59:343, 1948.

Mendl, K., and Tanner, C. H., "Carcinoma of the Duodenum," Brit. J. Radiol., 21:309, 1948.

Dodd, G. D., Fishler, J. S., and Park, O. K., "Hyperplasia of Brunner's Glands," Radiol., 60:814, 1953.

Brunschwig, A., and Templeton, F. E., "Roentgenographic Diagnosis of Neoplasms of the Peri-ampullary Region and Head of the Pancreas," Radiol., 41:438, 1943.

Frostberg, N. A., "Characteristic Duodenal Deformity in Cases of Different Kinds of Peri-Vaterial Enlargement of the Pancreas," Acta Radiol., 19:164, 1938.

Frostberg, N. A., "Pancreatic Ductal and Vaterian Neoplasms Thru Roentgen Manifestations," Radiol., 62:1, 1954.

Freedman, E., Rabwin, M. H., and Sava, M., "Benign and Malignant Tumors of the Duodenum," Radiol., 65:557, 1955.

Stiennon, O. A., "The Anatomical Basis for the Epsilon Sign of Frostberg," Am. J. Roentgenol., 75:282, 1956.

Hinkel, C. L., and Moller, G. A., "Routine Barium-Gas Examination of the Duodenal Bulb," Am. J. Roentgenol., 75:291, 1956.

Uncapher, R. P., and Holder, H. G., "Megaduodenum in an Adult," Am. J. Roentgenol., 77:634, 1957.

Goin, L. S., and Wilk, S. P., "Intermittent Arteriomesenteric Occlusion of the Duodenum," Radiol., 67:729, 1956.

McClenahan, J. E., and Fisher, B., "Idiopathic Megaduodenum," Am. J. Digest Dis., 15:414, 1948.

Sturtevant, M., "Megaduodenum and Duodenal Obstruction," Radiol., 33:185, 1939.

Barnett, Wm. O., and Wall, Lester, "Megaduodenum Resulting from Absence of the Parasympathetic Ganglion Cells in Auerbach's Plexus," Ann. Surg., 141:527, 1953.

Chamberlin, G. W., and Imber, I., "Pyelography for Diagnosis of Lesions of the Body and Tail of the Pancreas," Radiol., 63:722, 1954.

Felson, B., and Levin, E. J., "Intramural Hematoma of Duodenum," Radiol., 63:823, 1954.

Castigliano, S. G., "Pseudotumoral Syndrome; Syphiloma of Pancrease," Am. J. Roentgenol., 72:45, 1954.

Lehman, E. P., "Annular Pancreas as a Clinical Problem," Ann. Surg., 115:574, 1942.

Feldman, M., and Weinberg, T., "Aberrant Pancreas, a Cause of Duodenal Syndrome," J.A.M.A., 148:893, 1952.

Hope, J. W., and Gibbons, J. F., "Duodenal Obstruction Due to Annular Pancreas," Radiol., 63:473, 1954.

Keats, T. E., "Generalized Pulmonary Emphysema as an Isolated Manifestation of Early Cystic Fibrosis of the Pancreas," Radiol., 65:223, 1955.

McGeorge, C. K., and Widmann, B. P., Ostrum, H., and Miller, R. P., "Diffuse Calcification of the Pancreas," Am. J. Roentgenol., 78:599, 1957.

Farber, S., "Some Organic Digestive Disturbances in Early Life," J. Michigan Med. Soc., 44:587, 1945.

Sage, H. H., "Multiple Diffuse Pancreatic Lithiasis," Am. J. Roentgenol., 53:28, 1945.

McCort, J. J., "Roentgenographic Appearance of Metastases to the Central Lymph Nodes of the Superior Mesenteric Artery in Carcinoma of the Right Colon," Radiol., 60:641, 1953.

Clayton, R. S., and Thornton, W. L., "Benign Duodenocolic Fistula," Radiol., 60:832, 1953.

Doubilet, H., Poppel, M. H., and Mulholland, J. H., "Pancreatography: Technics Principles and Observations," Radiol., 64:325, 1955.

Figiel, L. S., and Figiel, S. J., "Gallstone Obturation of the Duodenal Bulb," Am. J. Roentgenol., 76:24, 1956.

Jejunum and Ileum:

Sloan, R. D., "The Mucosal Pattern of the Mesenteric Small Intestine - An Anatomic Study," Am. J. Roentgenol., 77:651, 1957.

Margulis, A. R., Conklin, F. P., Nice, C. M., and Rigler, L. G., "Deficiency of Intestinal Gas in Infants with Diarrhea," Radiol., 66:93, 1956.

Case, J. T., "Roentgenological Aids in the Diagnosis of Ileus," Am. J. Roentgenol., 19:413, 1928.

Frimann-Dahl, J., "Administration of Barium Orally in Acute Obstruction: Advantages and Risks," Acta Radiol., 42:285, 1954.

Bird, G. C., Fissel, G. E., and Young, B. R., "Pathognomonic Roentgen Sign of Retroperitoneal Abscess," Am. J. Roentgenol., 59:351, 1948.

Young, B., "Significance of Reginal or Reflex Ileus in the Roentgen Diagnosis of Cholecystitis, Perforated Ulcer, Pancreatitis and Appendiceal Abscess, as Determined by Survey Examination of the Acute Abdomen," Am. J. Roentgenol., 78:581, 1957.

Rendich, R. A., and Harrington, L. A., "Roentgenologic Observations in Mesenteric Thrombosis," Am. J. Roentgenol., 52:317, 1944.

Benjamin, D., "Mesenteric Thrombosis," Am. J. Surg., 76:338, 1948.

Mellnis, H. Z., and Rigler, L. G., "Roentgen Findings in Obstruction of the Small Intestine," Am. J. Roentgenol., 71:404, 1954.

Gannon, W. E., and Harrington, L. A., "Volvulus of the Entire Small Bowel in the Immediate Postoperative Period," Radiol., 67:569, 1956.

Tiscenco, E., "Subacute Volvulus of the Terminal Ileum (Case Report)," Brit. J. Radiol., 19:243, 1946.

Newman, H., and Frische, L. H., "Lesser Omental Bursa Abscess Simulating Gastric Neoplasm," Radiol., 69:567, 1957.

Cimmino, C. V., "Lesser Sac Hernia via the Foramen of Winslow," Radiol., 60:57, 1953.

St. John, E. G., "Herniation thru the Foramen of Winslow," Am. J. Roentgenol., 72:222, 1954.

Parsons, P. B., "Paraduodenal Hernia," Am. J. Roentgenol., 69:563, 1953.

Callander, C. L., Rusk, G. V., and Nemir, A., "Mechanism, Symptoms and Treatment of Hernia into the Descending Mesocolon," Surg. Gynec. and Obst., 60:1052, 1935.

Exner, F. B., "Roentgen Diagnosis of Right Paraduodenal Hernia," Am. J. Roentgenol., 29:585, 1933.

Gotlieb, G. G., "A Case of Intersigmoid Hernia with Illustrations of X-Ray Appearances," Brit. J. Radiol., 19:429, 1946.

Wallen, L., "Roentgen Examination of the Deep Rectogenital Pouch," Acta Radiol., 39:105, 1953.

Wolf, B. S., and Marshak, R. H., "Segmental Infarction of the Small Bowel," Radiol., 66:701, 1956.

Baggenstoss, A. H., Powers, M. H., and Grindlay, J. H., "Further Studies on Pathogenesis of Fibrocystic Disease of the Pancreas," Arch. Path., 51:510, 1951.

Bruwer, A., and Hodgson, J. R., "Intestinal Obstruction in Fibrocystic Disease of the Pancreas," Am. J. Roentgenol., 69:14, 1953.

White, H., "Meconium Ileus: A New Roentgen Sign," Radiol., 66:567, 1956.

Neuhauser, E. B., "The Roentgen Diagnosis of Fetal Meconium Peritonitis," Am. J. Roentgenol., 51:421, 1944.

Pratt, T. L. C., "Meconium Peritonitis," J. Faculty of Radiologists, 5:62, 1953.

Lester, J., "Meconium Peritonitis," Acta Radiol., 46:650, 1956.

Lerner, H. H., and Gazin, A. I., "Pneumatosis Intestinalis," Am. J. Roentgenol., 56:464, 1946.

Ramos, A. J., and Powers, W. E., "Pneumatosis Cystoides Intestinalis," Am. J. Roentgenol., 77:678, 1957.

Rosenbaum, H. D., "Pneumatosis Cystoides Intestinalis," Am. J. Roentgenol., 78:681, 1957.

McGee, A. R., Penny, S. F., and Williamson, N. L., "Pneumatosis Cystoides Intestinalis," Radiol., 66:88, 1956.

Good, A. C., and Fletcher, E. H., "The Roentgenologic Examination of the Small Intestine," J.M.A. Georgia, 37:67, 1948.

Tennent, W., "Recent Advances in Investigation of the Small Intestine," Brit. J. Radiol., 19:22, 1946.

Marshak, R. H., and Wolf, B. S., "Chronic Ulcerative Granulomatous Jejunitis and Ileojejunitis," Am. J. Roentgenol., 70:93, 1953.

Martin, F. R. R., and Carr, R. J., "Crohn's Disease Involving Stomach," Brit. Med. J., 1:700, 1953.

Keats, T. E., and Brady, R. M., "Duodenal Involvement in Regional Enteritis," Am. J. Roentgenol., 77:639, 1957.

Marshak, R. H., Friedman, A. I., Wolf, B., and Crohn, B. B., "Roentgen Findings in Ileojejunitis," Gastroenterol., 19:383, 1951.

Kantor, J. L., "Regional (Terminal) Ileitis: Its Roentgen Diagnosis," J.A.M.A., 103:2016, 1934.

Katz, I., and Fischer, R. M., "Enteroliths Complicating Regional Enteritis," Am. J. Roentgenol., 78:653, 1957.

Hale, C. H., and Schatzki, R., "The Roentgenological Appearance of the Gastrointestinal Tract in Scleroderma," Am. J. Roentgenol., 51:407, 1944.

Connolly, P. J., "Diverticula of Jejunum and Ileum," J. Michigan Med. Soc., 53:868, 1954.

Stromme, A., "Fluid Levels in Diverticula of the Small Intestine: A Radiological Sign, Simulating Obstruction," Brit. J. Radiol., 29:346, 1956.

Bischoff, M. E., and Stampfli, W. P., "Meckel's Diverticulum," Radiol., 65:572, 1955.

Poppel, M. H., "The Roentgen Demonstration of Meckel's Diverticulum," Am. J. Roentgenol., 51:205, 1944.

Lewitan, A., "Roentgenologic Study of Meckel's Diverticulum," Radiol., 61:796, 1953.

Moxon, C. P., and Ollerenshaw, T. D., "Meckel's Diverticulum," Brit. J. Radiol., 26:649, 1953.

Mehth, M. M., "Meckel's Diverticulum," Am. J. Roentgenol., 77:644, 1957.

Lerner, H. H., Levinson, S. S., and Kateman, A. E., "Meckel's Diverticulum; New Roentgen Diagnostic Sign," Am. J. Roentgenol., 69:268, 1953.

Dedick, A. P., and Collins, L. C., "The Roentgen Diagnosis of Bleeding Lesions of the Small Intestines," Am. J. Roentgenol., 69:926, 1953.

Dundon, C. C., "Primary Tumors of the Small Intestine," Am. J. Roentgenol., 59:492, 1948.

Richman, S., Goodman, H., and Russi, S., "Lymphosarcoma of Small Intestine and Its Mesentery," Gastroenterol., 28:623, 1955.

Deeb, P. H., Stilson, W. L., "Roentgenological Manifestations of Lymphosarcoma of the Small Bowel," Radiol., 63:235, 1954.

Learner, N., Stauffer, H. M., and Brown, C. L., "Small Intestinal Disorders in Avitaminosis," Ann. Int. Med., 20:675, 1944.

Golden, R., Radiologic Examination of the Small Intestines, J. B. Lippincott Co.

Kantor, J. L., "The Roentgen Diagnosis of Idiopathic Steatorrhoea and Allied Conditions. Practical Value of the Moulage Sign," Am. J. Roentgenol., 41:758, 1939.

Marshak, R. H., Wolf, B. S., and Adlersberg, D., "Roentgen Studies of the Small Intestine," Am. J. Roentgenol., 72:380, 1954.

Snell, A. M., and Camp, J. D., "Chronic Idiopathic Steatorrhea," Arch. Int. Med., 53:615, 1934.

Anderson, C. M., Astley, R., French, J. M., and Gerard, J. W., "Small Intestinal Pattern in Celiac Disease," Brit. J. Radiol., 25:526, 1952.

Krause, G., and Crilly, J., "Roentgenologic Changes in the Small Intestine with Presence of the Hook Worm," Am. J. Roentgenol., 49:719, 1944.

Handel, J., and Schwartz, S., "Gastrointestinal Manifestations of the Schonlein-Henoch Syndrome," Am. J. Roentgenol., 78:643, 1957.

Golden, R., "Amyloidosis of the Small Intestine," Am. J. Roentgenol., 72:401, 1954.

Hornsby, A. T., and Bayling, J., "Sprue vs Pancreatogenous Steatorrhea," Radiol., 63:491, 1954.

Peterson, G. M., "Intestinal Changes in Giardia Lamblia Infection," Am. J. Roentgenol., 77:670, 1957.

Fischer, H. W., "Free Intraperitoneal Air," Am. J. Roentgenol., 76:143, 1956.

Culver, G. J., and Concannon, J. P., "Retroperitoneal Emphysema," Radiol., 55:86, 1950.

Altaras, J., "Calculi of the Small Intestine," Brit. J. Radiol., 29:348, 1956.

Whitmore, W. H., and Peterson, G. M., "Henoch's Purpura: Small Intestinal Changes," Radiol., 46:373, 1946.

Minteer, D. W., Hayes, J. D., and Youngstrom, K. A., "Intestinal Ascariasis in Man," Am. J. Roentgenol., 71:416, 1954.

Herson, R. E., "Meconium Ileus," Radiol., 68:568, 1957.

Appendix:

Weiner, M. A., Jenkinson, E. L., "Diverticula of Appendix," Am. J. Roentgenol., 78:678, 1957.

Norman, A., Leider, S., and Carman, J., "Mucocele of the Appendix," Am. J. Roentgenol., 77:647, 1957.

Thomas, S. F., "Appendiceal Coproliths: Their Surgical Importance," Radiol., 49:39, 1947.

Berg, R. M., and Berg, H. M., "Coproliths," Radiol., 68:839, 1957.

Kalmoa, E. H., and Winningham, E. V., "Mucocele of the Appendix," Am. J. Roentgenol., 72:432, 1954.

Freedman, E., "Roentgen Simulation of Polypoid Neoplasms by Invaginated Appendiceal Stumps," Am. J. Roentgenol., 75:380, 1956.

Chrom, Sv. A., and Gudbjerg, C. E., "Studies in Contrast Filling of the Normal Appendix," Acta Radiol., 40:583, 1953.

Colon:

Lasser, E. C., and Rigler, L. G., "Observations in the Structure and Function of the Ileocecal Valve," Radiol., 63:176, 1954.

Klami, P., "On the Visualization of Ulcerative Processes Using Hydrogen Peroxide in the Contrast Medium," Acta Radiol., 39:98, 1953.

Jungmann, H., "Volvulus of the Coecum," Brit. J. Radiol., 21:346, 1948.

Swenson, O., Rhinlander, H. F., and Diamond, I., "Hirschsprung's Disease: A New Concept of the Etiology," New England J. Med., 241:551, 1949.

Swenson, O., Neuhauser, F. B. D., and Pickett, L. J., "New Concepts of the Etiology, Diagnosis and Treatment of Congenital Megacolon (Hirschsprung's Disease)," Pediat., 4:201, 1949.

Steinbach, H. L., Rosenberg, R. H., Grossman, M., and Nelson, T. L., "Potential Hazard of Enemas in Patients with Hirschsprung's Disease," Radiol., 64:45, 1954.

Keefer, G. P., and Mokrohisky, J. F., "Congenital Megacolon," Radiol., 63:157, 1954.

Weber, H., and Dixon, C. F., "Duplication of the Entire Large Intestine, (Colon Duplex)," Am. J. Roentgenol., 55:319, 1946.

Snodgras, J. J., "Transdiaphragmatic Duplication of the Alimentary Tract," Am. J. Roentgenol., 69:42, 1953.

Van Velzer, D. A., Barrick, C. M., and Jenkinson, E. L., "Duplication of the Colon," Am. J. Roentgenol., 75:349, 1956.

Klein, I., "Roentgen Study of Lymphogranuloma Venereum," Am. J. Roentgenol., 51:70, 1944.

Hewet, J., and Ryan, M. J., "Submucous Lipoma of Colon Causing Large Bowel Obstruction," Brit. J. Radiol., 29:343, 1956.

Norgaard, F., "Periodic, Spontaneously Remittent Volvulus and the Symptoms in Cases of Colon Elongation," Acta Radiol., 26:163, 1945.

Jackson, H., "A Sign of Intussusception," Brit. J. Radiol., 26:323, 1953.

Ravitch, M. M., "Consideration of Errors in Diagnosis of Intussusception," Am. J. Dis. Childhood, 84:17, 1952.

Tiscenco, E., "Subacute Ileo-ileal Intussusception in the Adult (Case Report)," Brit. J. Radiol., 19:374, 1946.

Andren, L., and Frieberg, S., "Spontaneous Regression of Polyps of the Colon in Children," Acta Radiol., 46:507, 1956.

Gay, B. B., "Roentgenologic Demonstration of an Invaginated Intussuscepted Meckel's Diverticulum," Radiol., 60:60, 1953.

Girdany, B. J., Bass, L. W., and Grier, G. W., "Reduction of Ileocecal Intussusception by Hydrostatic Pressure," Radiol., 60:518, 1953.

Greenwood, F., and Samuel, E., "Radiological Features of Jackson's Membrane," Brit. J. Radiol., 23:485, 1950.

Ettinger, A., and Elkin, M., "Study of the Sigmoid by Special Roentgenographic Views," Am. J. Roentgenol., 72:199, 1954.

Tondreau, R. L., "Multiple Primary Carcinomas of the Large Bowel," Am. J. Roentgenol., 71:794, 1954.

Scott, M. G., "Gastro-colic Fistula with Reflux into the Esophagus," Brit. J. Radiol., 26:268, 1953.

Douglas, J. B., "The Double Contrast Examination of the Colon," Radiol., 60:490, 1953.

Stevenson, C. A., "Indication for Double Contrast Colon Examination," Am. J. Roentgenol., 71:298, 1954.

Moreton, R. D., "Double Contrast Examination of the Colon," Radiol., 60:510, 1915.

Potter, R. M., "Dilute Contrast Media in the Diagnosis of Lesions of Colon," Radiol., 60:500, 1953.

Mauthe, H., and Zwicky, G., "Gastroduodenal Intussusception," Radiol., 65:86, 1955.

Levene, G., "Rates of Venous Absorption of Carbon Dioxide and Air Used in Double Contrast Examination of the Colon," Radiol., 69:571, 1957.

Gianturco, C., and Miller, G. A., "Routine Search for Colonic Polyps by High Voltage Radiography," Radiol., 60:496, 1953.

Andrén, L., Freiberg, S. and Welin, S., "Roentgen Diagnosis of Small Polyps in the Colon and Rectum," Acta Radiol., 43:201, 1955.

Robinson, J. M., "Polyps of the Colon: How to Find Them," Am. J. Roentgenol., 77:700, 1957.

Figiel, L. S., and Figiel, S. J., "Volvulus of the Cecum and Ascending Colon," Radiol., 61:496, 1953.

Jakobsen, A., "Volvulus Coeci," Acta Chir. Scandinav., 92:199, 1945.

Frimann-Dahl, J., "Volvulus of the Right Colon," Acta. Radiol., 41:141, 1954.

Mondor, H., Porcher, P., Olivier, C., and Simon, G. C., "Roentgenologic Diagnosis of Volvulus of Right Colon," Press. Med., 60:901, 1952.

Figiel, L. S., and Figiel, S. J., "Detorsion of Volvulus of the Right Colon," Am. J. Roentgenol., 72:192, 1954.

Hall, M. R., "Roentgenological Diagnosis of Volvulus of Sigmoid Megacolon," Am. J. Roentgenol., 39:925, 1938.

Ritvo, M., Farrell, G. E., and Stauffer, I. A., "The Association of Volvulus of the Cecum and Ascending Colon with Obstructive Colonic Lesions," Am. J. Roentgenol., 58:587, 1957.

Buenger, R. E., "Volvulus of the Splenic Flexure of the Colon," Am. J. Roentgenol., 71:81, 1954.

Goulard, A., and Hampton, A. O., "Correlation of Clinical, Pathological and Roentgenological Findings in Diverticulitis," Am. J. Roentgenol., 72:213, 1954.

Wolf, B. S., Khilnani, M., and Marshak, R. H., "Diverticulosis and Diverticulitis: Roentgen Findings and Their Interpretation," Am. J. Roentgenol., 77:726, 1957.

Stewart, J. W., "Diverticulitis of the Sigmoid Colon with Perforation," Surg. Clin. N. Am., 30:1491, 1950.

Wilson, A. K., "Roentgen Examination in Congenital Intestinal Obstructive Defects in Infants," Am. J. Roentgenol., 54:498.

Clayton, R. S., and Goodman, P. H., "Roentgenographic Diagnosis of Geophagia (Dirt or Clay Eating)," Am. J. Roentgenol., 73:0203, 1955.

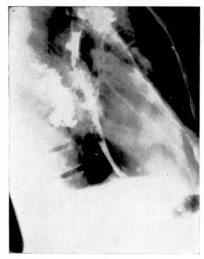

Carcinoma of esophagus showing irregular filling defect, with barium escaping into surrounding structures.

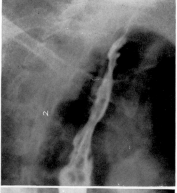

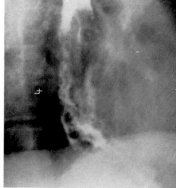

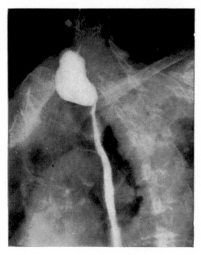

Diverticulum of the esophagus showing the rounded pouch-like sac springing from the upper portion of the esophagus.

←
Esophageal varices producing nodular appearance of mucosa.

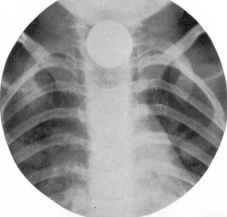

←
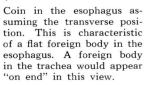
Coin in the esophagus assuming the transverse position. This is characteristic of a flat foreign body in the esophagus. A foreign body in the trachea would appear "on end" in this view.

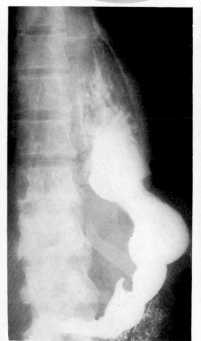

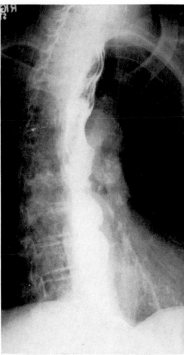

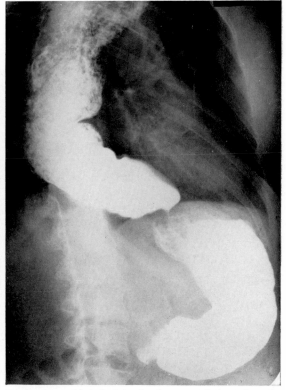

Operative resection of carcinoma of esophagus, anastomosis of resected end to stomach displaced high into mediastinum.

Tertiary contractions of the esophagus due to interference with normal nerve control of peristalsis.

Cardiospasm (Achalasia), showing constriction of esophagus at the cardia. Note enormous dilatation of esophagus; ten years duration. In no other condition is such extreme dilatation encountered.

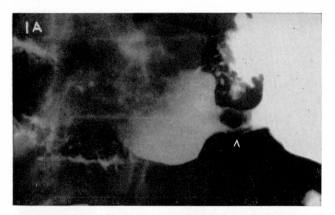

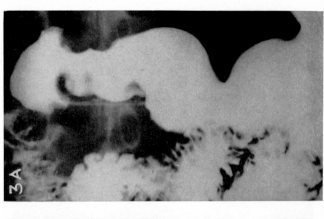

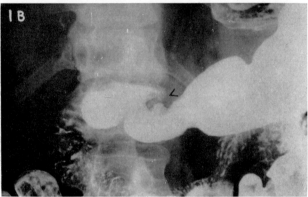

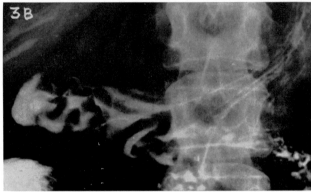

1A. Small polyp springing from the prepyloric mucosa, producing rounded filling defect. B. Small niche due to prepyloric ulcer.

3A. Irregularity of pylorus might easily be mistaken for carcinoma. B. Mucosal study shows plainly rounded niche of benign ulcer.

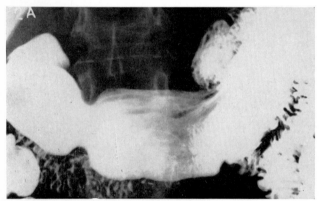

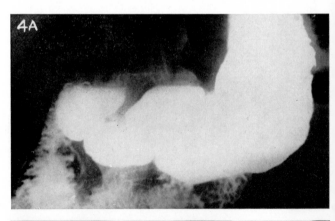

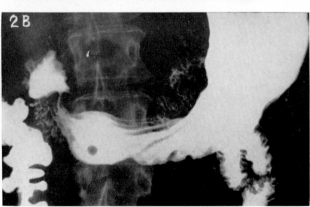

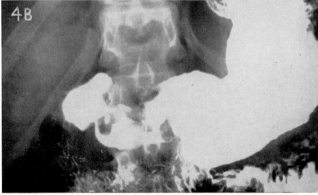

2A. Small polypoid growths may easily go undetected when overshadowed by barium. B. Same patient; small polypoid growth demonstrated with smaller quantity of barium.

4A. Pyloric end of stomach with complete filling. B. Mucosal relief showing giant rugae which might easily be mistaken for malignant growth.

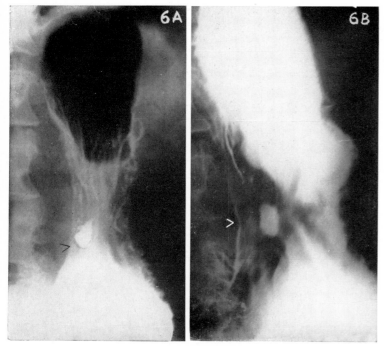

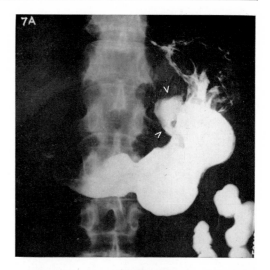

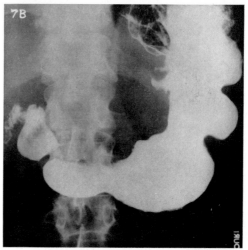

6A Benign ulcer of the stomach showing pouch-like niche on lesser curvature. B. pressure over niche shows clear-cut margins of ulcer crater and convergence of rugae in toward niche.

7A Large irregular niche on lesser curvature. B. Almost complete healing after 20 days bedrest indicating its benign character.

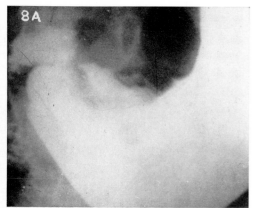

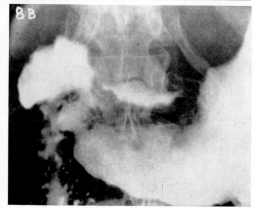

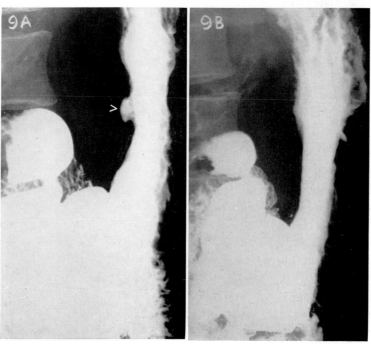

8A Meniscus sign produced by large ulcerating carcinoma. B. With pressure; a true meniscus sign must be entirely intrinsic.

9A Benign ulcer on lesser curvature of hypotonic stomach. B. Complete permanent healing after 20 days of complete bedrest without medication or special diet.

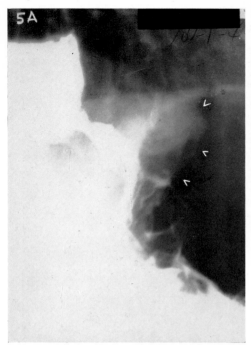

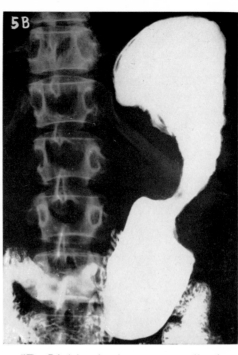

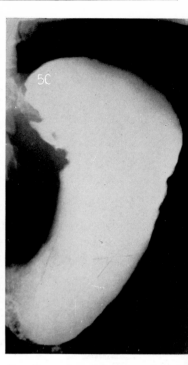

5A. Carcinomatous growth of fundus causing deflection of barium stream as it enters stomach. Mass outlined by gas in fundus.

5B. Linitis plastica or generalized infiltration of entire gastric wall, causing so-called "leather bottle" stomach.

Small undermining carcinoma of fundus lesser curvature just below esophageal orifice.

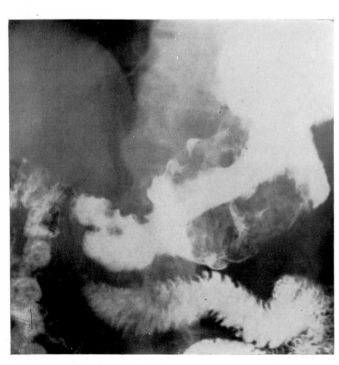

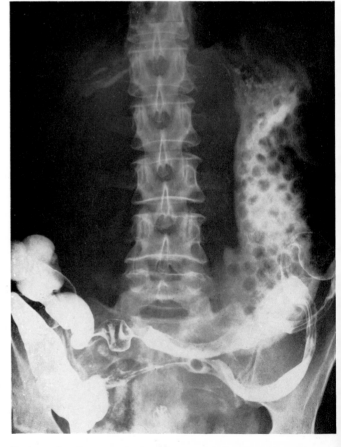

Large carcinoma of the stomach showing filling defect extending around the stomach in the pars media.

Polyposis of stomach showing multiple radiolucent areas throughout stomach. These may be benign but, like polyps elsewhere, may become malignant. Note polyp in transverse colon.

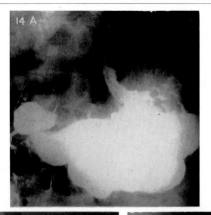

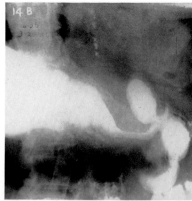

14A. Large gastric ulcer crater in pyloric region resembling duodenal bulb. B. Same patient in prone position with pressure showing complete filling of crater and indurated margin. In spite of these indications of malignancy the ulcer proved to be benign.

→

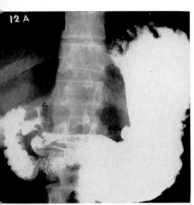

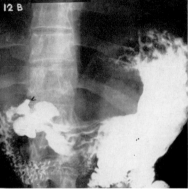

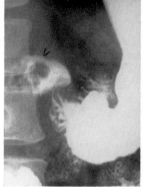

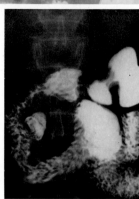

12A. Gastric and duodenal ulcer occurring in same patient—a not uncommon occurance. B. Gastric ulcer healed after bed rest only; duodenal ulcer deformity persistent.

Duodenal Polyp.

Duodenal Diverticulum.

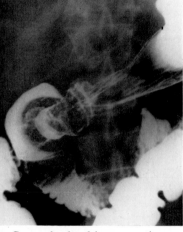

Deformity of the duodenal bulb, evidence of duodenal ulcer.

→

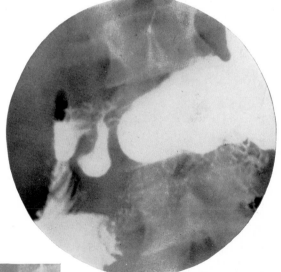

Gastro-duodenal intussuception.

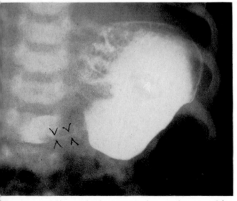

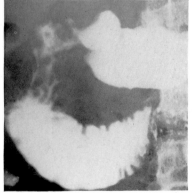

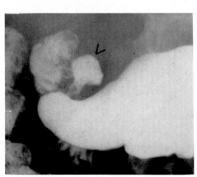

Hypertrophic pyloric stenosis; only a thin string-like stream of barium passes thru the canal.

Small areas of swelling in duodenal mucosa, due to hypertrophy of Brunner's glands.

Large prepyloric ulcer; in section a round worm was found in the base of the crater.

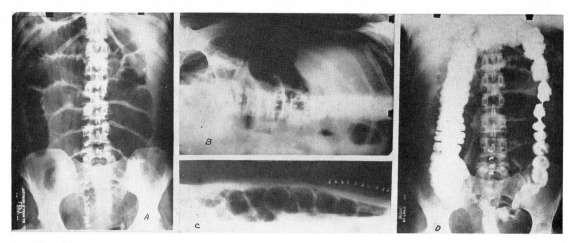

A. Flat film of abdomen showing complete small intestinal obstruction; gas distended loops of small bowel proximal to obstruction, showing "herring bone" design and "ladder pattern." The bowel distal to the obstruction is flaccid and the rectum is devoid of gas or fecal material.

B. Second position, with patient in lateral decubitus (right side uppermost) and the x-ray projected horizontally. This view serves best to show multiple fluid levels in the bowel and demonstrates any possibility of gas free in the abdomen.

C. Third position, with the patient on his back and the x-ray beam projected horizontally across abdomen from side to side. This transabdominal view serves well to show multiple fluid levels, but is the best position for demonstrating exudate between the intestinal walls.

D. Additional examination by barium enema serves to differentiate the small from the large bowel. In intestinal obstruction the distal portion of the bowel is flaccid and empty; barium enema should disclose relaxed, undistended character of colon.

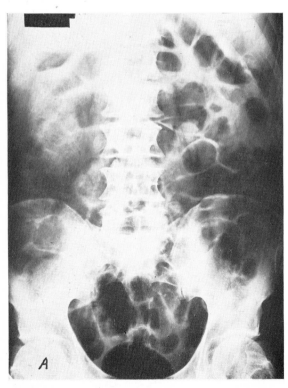

A. Paralytic ileus producing extreme gaseous distension of small and large bowel alike; multiple fluid levels are present in this condition also. Note that gas distended loops of bowel have a tendency to produce pressure upon each other, also that entire colon is distended and gas is present in the rectum.

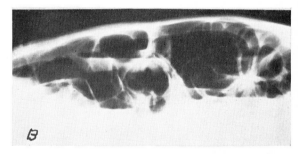

B. Transabdominal view showing multiple fluid levels in gas distended bowel.

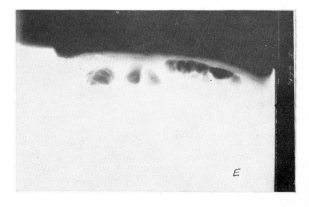

Exudate between loops of bowel is best seen in transabdominal position.

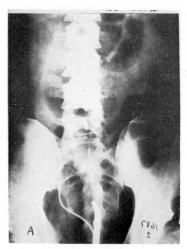
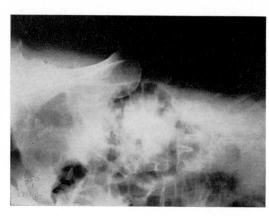
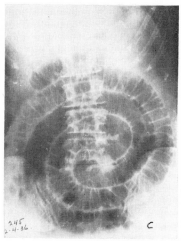

A. Localized spastic ileus from pain associated with passage of a urinary stone or catheter. Spastic ileus may be local or general; it is caused by reflex inhibition of intestinal movement often in isolated loops, always associated with pain with or without peritoneal infection.

B. Localized spastic ileus caused by inhibition in movements of the gut surrounding an appendiceal abscess. Patient is in left lateral decubitus.

C. Mesenteric (Richter's) hernia caused by a small knuckle of bowel herniating into a hole in the mesentery. Extreme pain results with production of a double loop of gas distended bowel forming circular intestinal patterns in the abdomen. Gaseous dilation is due to spastic ileus, not to intestinal obstruction.

Stomal ulcer at margin of gastro-enterostomy opening. Barium-filled crater remains after localized pressure with cone. →

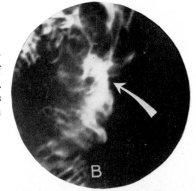

Paralytic ileus from injury to the spleen. Note the gas-filled loops of intestine throughout the entire abdomen involving even the rectum.

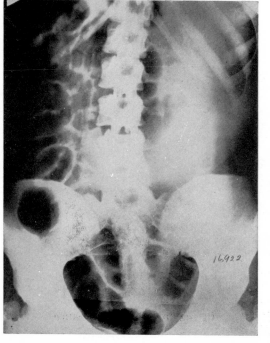

→

Paralytic ileus from traumatic laceration of liver. Large amount of blood in peritoneal cavity indicated by homogeneous density at periphery and clustering of gas-filled intestinal loops in center of abdomen. Such injuries are frequently followed by massive hemobilia even after the laceration has been repaired, due to autolysis.

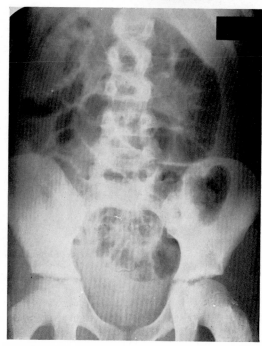

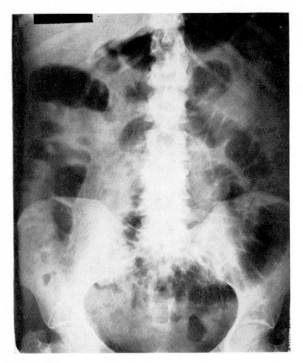

A. Mesenteric (arterial) thrombosis before it has become well established shows bizarre appearance of gas distribution. This in itself is suggestive of the condition.

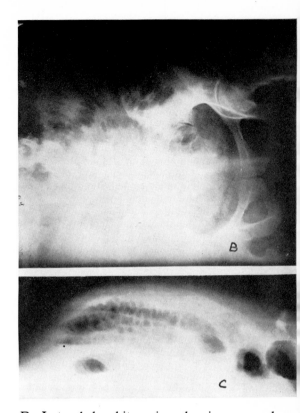

B. Lateral decubitus view showing unusual appearance of gas pattern.

C. In the transabdominal view, likewise, the gas pattern is unusual in appearance.

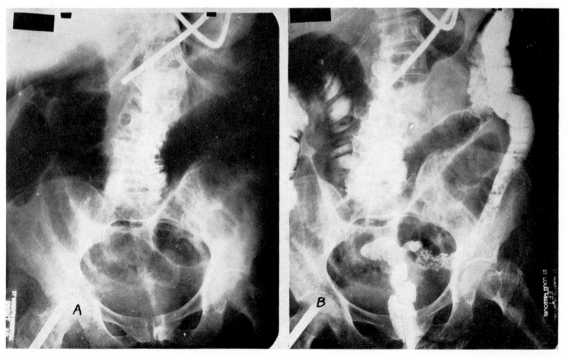

A. Mesenteric arterial thrombosis (advanced stage) producing gaseous distention of both small and large bowel up to the region of the splenic flexure of the colon, without gas in the descending colon or rectum, giving a picture similar to that of intestinal obstruction.

B. Barium enema failing to reveal any evidence of obstruction in region of splenic flexure, indicating that the condition is due to mesenteric (arterial) thrombosis.

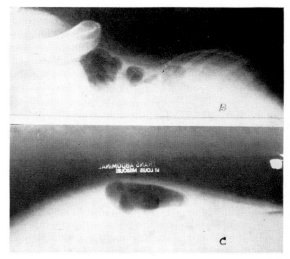

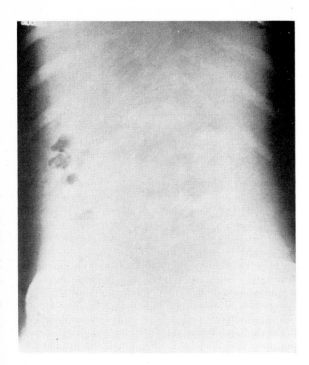

A. Venous mesenteric thrombosis showing almost complete lack of gas formation. Entire abdomen shows a homogenous appearance due to waterlogging edema.

B. In the lateral decubitus view only a small amount of gas is seen.

C. Also in the transabdominal view, there is almost complete absence of gas.

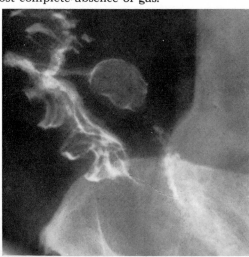

Coprolith in appendix, associated with suppurative appendicitis.

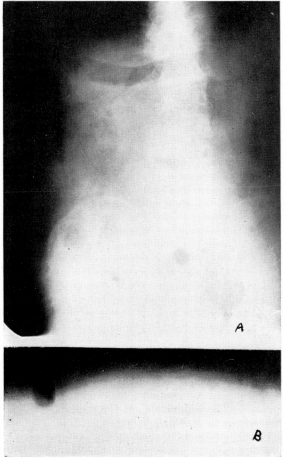

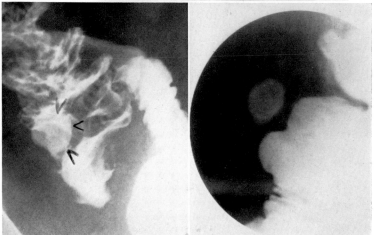

Tumor of the terminal ileum near ileocecal valve.

←   A. Venous mesenteric thrombosis showing almost complete lack of gas; only small amount is seen in the undistended transverse colon.

←   B. Lateral decubitus position also; only a small amount of gas was visible. (Courtesy of Dr. W. K. Mueller).

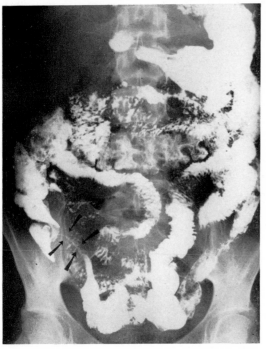

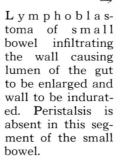
→ Lymphoblastoma of small bowel infiltrating the wall causing lumen of the gut to be enlarged and wall to be indurated. Peristalsis is absent in this segment of the small bowel.

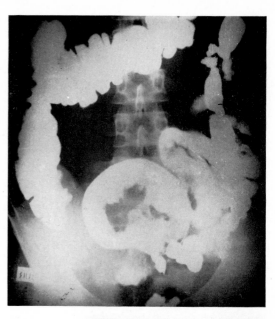

Regional enteritis or terminal ileitis showing extreme narrowing of terminal ileum producing so-called "string sign" of the small intestine.

→ Round worm high up in jejunum demonstrated by barium meal.

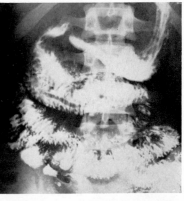

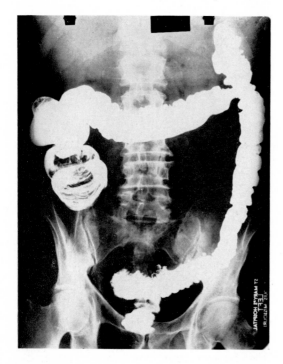

Barium enema in a case of intussusception showing the cap-like defect of the advancing head of the barium pressing the invaginated bowel. If intussusception does not obstruct, no gaseous-dilated loops of bowel result.

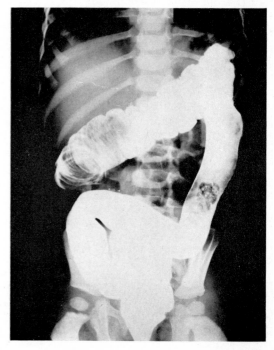

Intussusception of small bowel in colon; note ring-like appearance produced by pressure of advancing intussusception.

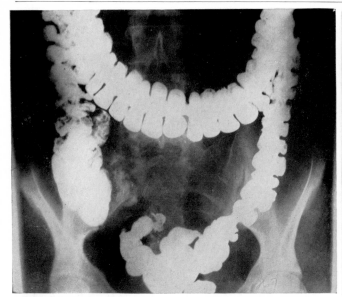

Normal colon after the injection of barium solution.

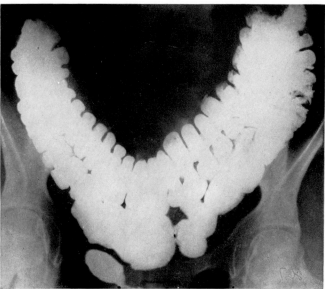

Ptosis of the colon showing the transverse colon descending almost to the symphysis pubis in the upright position.

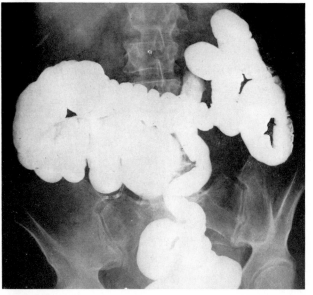

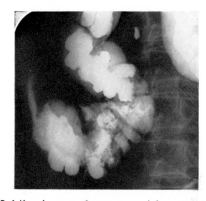

Mobile, inverted cecum with appendix in right upper quadrant.

Developmental anomaly. Incomplete rotation of colon; mobile cecum.

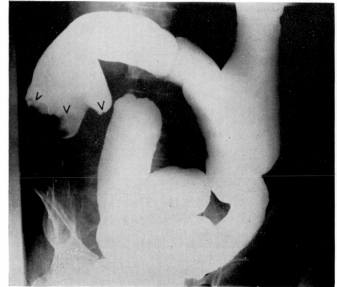

Large filling defect of the cecum due to carcinoma.

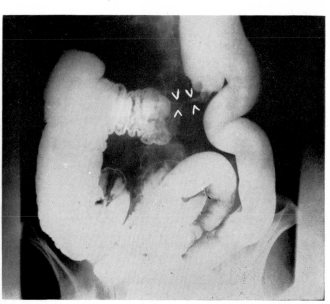

Carcinoma of the transverse colon causing pencil-like constriction of the bowel. Unless the bowel is completely obstructed toxic symptoms do not result.

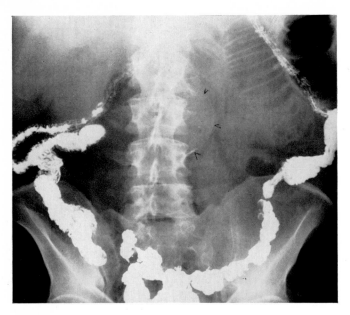

Localized spastic ileus from pain associated with dissecting aneurysm which is clearly visible because of calcium deposit in vessel wall. Note gas-distended loops of small bowel.

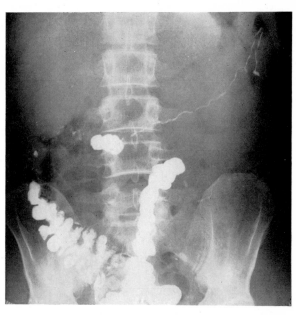

Mucous colitis, or excessive mucus in colon producing a "string-sign" in the colon after evacuation.

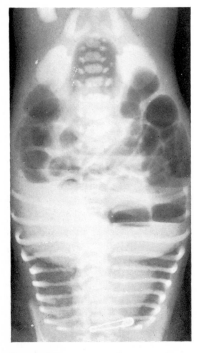

Imperforate anus in new born. Examination in inverted position shows failure of gas to completely fill rectum. Anus marked with bulb of a thermometer will disclose extent of defect.

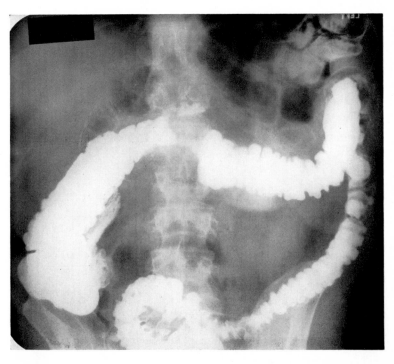

Herniation of greater portion of small intestine into lesser peritoneal cavity behind stomach causing intermittent obstruction. Malfusion of omental layers indicated by position of transverse colon above stomach.

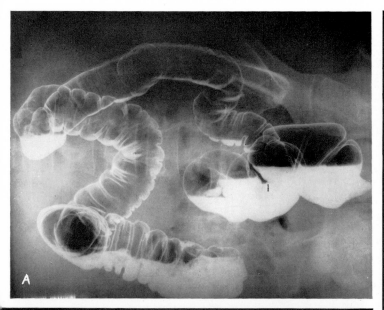

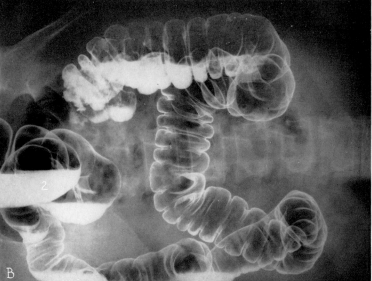

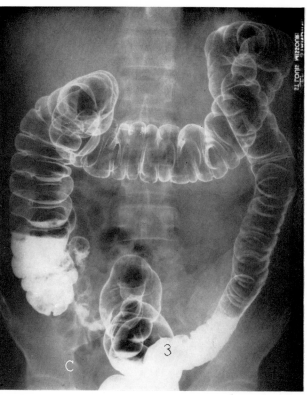

Double contrast enema especially useful for demonstration of polyps. Most successfully carried out by first administering a gelatinous barium mixture, partial evacuation, and then injecting air. **X**-ray examination with the patient in right, (**A**), and left, (**B**), decubitus and upright, (**C**), positions gives most satisfactory results.

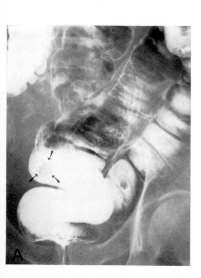

Multiple Polyposis of colon showing polyps in rectum and descending colon with double contrast enema.

A. Posterior view, rectal polyp surrounded by barium mixture. **B.** Anterior view, rectum filled with gas disclosing polyp.

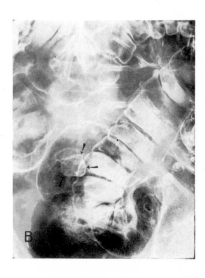

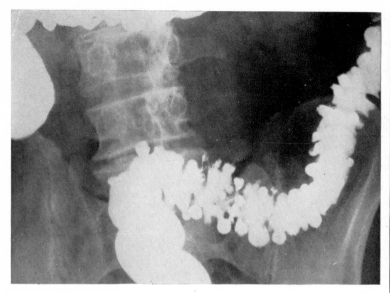

Diverticulosis of the colon showing large numbers of rounded pouch-like sacs coming off of the sigmoid portion of the colon.

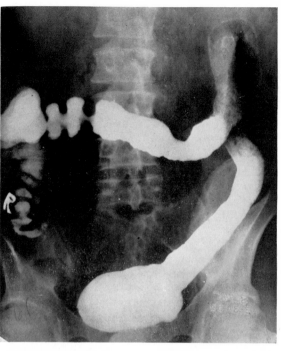

Chronic ulcerative colitis showing the loss of haustral markings in the transverse and descending colon. The bowel assumes a sausage-like appearance.

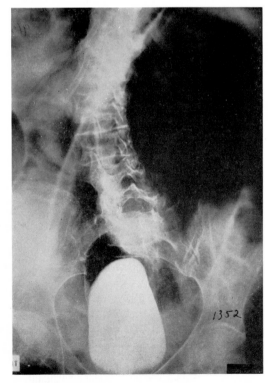

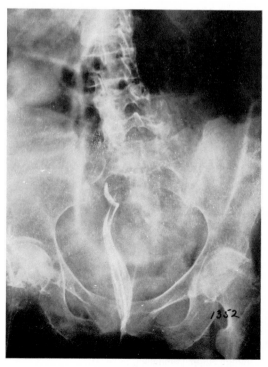

Volvulus of sigmoid portion of colon showing rectum distal to obstruction filled with barium; note enormous dilation of descending colon with gas. After evacuation rectum empties but colon still remains filled with gas.

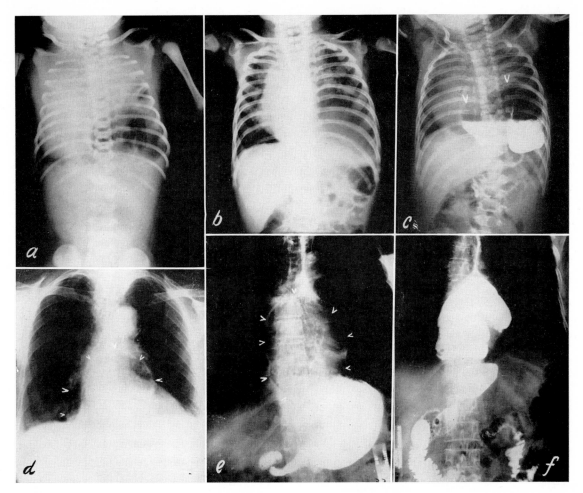

a. Diaphragmatic hernia in a newborn infant, with practically all intestinal structures in the chest. Note the narrowly constricted abdomen and bulging thorax.

b. When the left leaf of the diaphragm is poorly defined, especially in a newborn infant, a diaphragmatic hernia must be suspected.

c. A barium-filled stomach herniated through the posterior segment defect of the left leaf of the diaphragm with inversion of the stomach.

d. Large hiatus hernia showing a gastric air bubble through the cardiac shadow.

e. Results of a "soda pop" test in the case illustrated in d showing accentuation of the gas bubble after administration of a bottle of soda pop.

f. Another roentgenogram of the patient in d showing the barium-filled stomach extending well up into the retrocardiac position. The esophagus was of normal length.

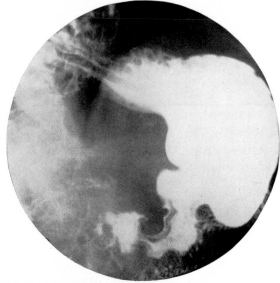

Diaphragmatic hernia of portion of stomach back through esophageal haitus.

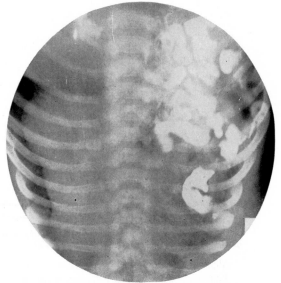

Congenital diaphragmatic hernia showing intestines in pleural cavity.

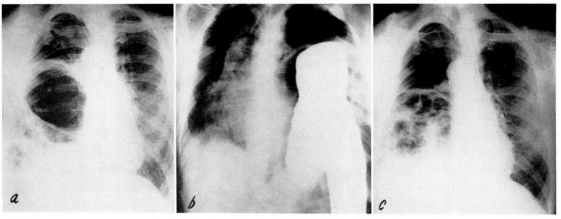

a. Congenital eventration of the diaphragm. The first manifestation of this eventration was in adult life when the patient experienced paralysis of a vocal cord as a result of pressure on the recurrent laryngeal nerve by a huge mass of intestines and other abdominal organs displaced upward into the thorax.

The gas-distended colon caused pressure upon the mediastinum.

b. A posterior roentgenogram of the patient showing the colon filled with barium extending into the thoracic cavity.

c. Another roentgenogram of the patient showing that at times the small bowel almost filled the pleural cavity.

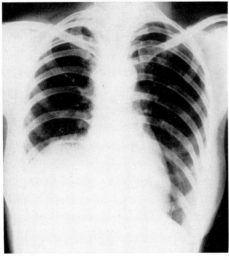

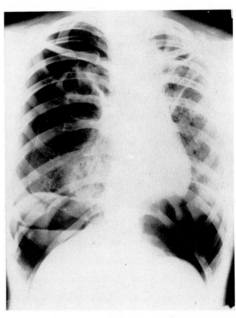

Roentgenogram showing paralysis of the right leaf of the diaphragm from phrenic nerve resection performed more than fifteen years before for the treatment of tuberculosis. With complete paralysis, the diaphragm atrophies rapidly and within a short time becomes a flail fibrous membrane. The extreme displacement of this diaphragm caused unusual traction on the stomach and duodenum with resulting profound digestive disturbances. Such disturbances have proved fatal.

Scalloped diaphragm still maintaining its appearance after the removal of any influence of adjacent structures by simultaneous induction of pneumothorax and pneumoperitoneum. indicating that the scalloping is due to irregular contraction of the diaphragm's muscular digitations from the ribs.

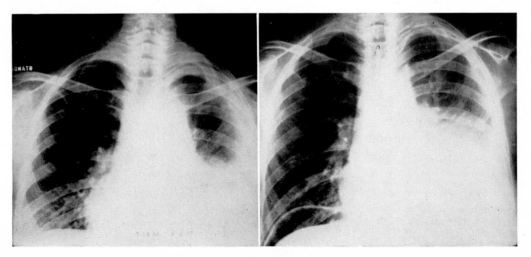

a. Subphrenic abscess may give rise to a "sympathetic" exudate in the base of the adjacent pleural cavity.

b. A small amount of air introduced into the peritoneal cavity will extend into the subphrenic regions if these areas are free from involvement. Failure of the air to extend into the subphrenic space indicates that it is involved by a subphrenic abscess.

PART IV

BILIARY TRACT

GALL BLADDER (Chapter XXII)

I. ANATOMY

II. PHYSIOLOGICAL FUNCTION

III. ROENTGEN EXAMINATION: CHOLECYSTOGRAPHY

    A. Direct

        1. Opaque and nonopaque stones

        2. Milk of calcium bile, (Limy Bile)

        3. Calcified gall bladder

    B. After administration of contrast medium

        a. Oral method

        b. Intravenous method

        1. Normally functioning gall bladder

          a. Stones in

        2. Pathology of the gall bladder

          a. Non-functioning

          b. Layering of nonopaque stones

          c. Polypoid growths

          d. Phrygian cap

          e. Diverticula
            (Rokitansky-Aschoff Sinus)

        3. In infants

BILE DUCTS

    1. RETROGRADE INJECTION OF, AFTER OPERATION: CHOLANGIOGRAPHY

        A. With lipiodol

        B. With water-soluble media

        C. Fistula

        D. Gas in hepatic ducts

    2. DEMONSTRATION BY INTRAVENOUS INJECTION

    3. DEMONSTRATION BY DOUBLE DOSE ORAL TELEPAQUE

Chapter XXII

BILIARY TRACT

Illustrations by Cesare Gianturco, M.D.

The gall bladder is a reservoir for the bile which is utilized for the emulsification of fats in preparation for digestion. It is composed of three portions: the distal end or fundus, the mid-portion or body and the proximal conical portion or infundibulum (Hartmann's Pouch) which connects with the cystic duct. A fine fibro-muscular layer is present in the fundal and infundibular regions, but the mid-portion is rich in elastic tissue. A sphincter-like mechanism appears to be present between the infundibulum and cystic duct, known as Lutken's Sphincter. No muscle fibers have ever been demonstrated in the bile ducts; the cystic duct is furnished with a spiral valvular arrangement known as Heister's valves and a smooth pars glabra portion which unites with the common hepatic duct to form the common bile duct which empties into the duodenum, (Sachs).

The gall bladder empties its contents into the duodenum as a result of the stimulation received from introduction of fatty material into the duodenum from the stomach. This expulsion of bile is probably produced by contraction of the fine muscular coat of the gall bladder as a result of stimulation produced by an enzyme or secretion formed in the small intestine, as a response to the presence of fatty material through direct absorption into the blood stream. Contraction and emptying of the gall bladder has been demonstrated following hypodermic injection into the blood stream of an extract of the duodenal mucosa, (Ivy and Oldberg).

ROENTGENOLOGICAL EXAMINATION OF THE GALL BLADDER. Roentgenologically, the bile-filled gall bladder is of similar density to the surrounding tissues; therefore, direct roentgenographic examination of the gall bladder for evidence of pathology can be successful in only a small percentage of cases. The chief pathological condition for which the gall bladder is examined is gallstones.

GALLSTONES * (Fig. 270A to D). Unfortunately, only a small percentage of gallstones contain sufficient calcium salts either throughout the stone or as the nucleus of the stone to render them detectable with x-ray examination (Figs. 270A to D); the majority are composed of cholesterin and other bile salts which have such slight difference in density from the surrounding soft tissues that they cannot be detected by ordinary roentgenographic examination. Such cholesterin stones may even be of lesser density than the bile in which they lie; when the bile is made radiopaque by cholecystography, these cholesterin

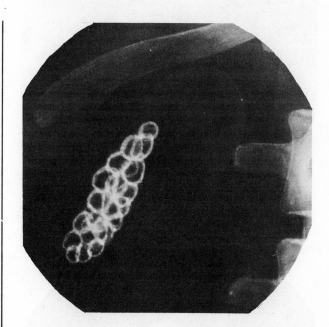

Fig. 270A. Calcium cholesterol stones

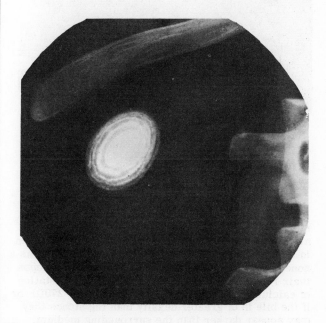

Fig. 270B. Single laminated calcium cholesterol stones

*An asterisk following any title indicates that roentgenographic reproductions illustrating this condition will be found in the pictorial supplement at the end of the chapter.

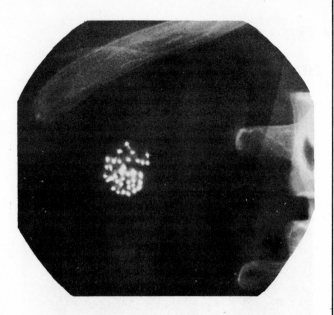

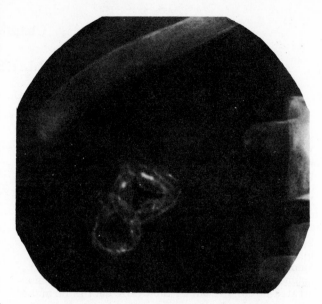

Fig. 270C. Multiple small calcium bilirubin stones.

Fig. 270D. Two calcium cholesterol stones with star formation.

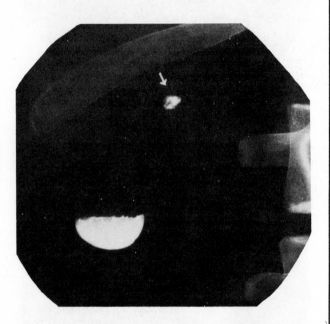

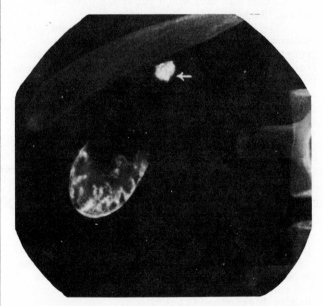

Fig. 271A. Milk of calcium bile with stone in cystic duct.

Fig. 271B. Calcified gall bladder with stone in cystic duct.

stones are visible as areas of lessened density, and are known as negative shadows.(Fig. 272D). If taken in the upright position such stones may layer out as a zone of decreased density in the bile depending upon their relative density. If covered by an incrustation of calcium salts they may be detected (Fig. 270D); or if the bile is of greater density than the stones they may appear darker than the surrounding medium. Small stones in the cystic duct, if calcified, can be demonstrated above the level of the 1st transverse process (Figs. 271A and B); stones in the common

duct lie near the 1st or 2nd transverse process. It has been reported that contrast media used in chole-cystography appears to have caused an opaque precipitation in the gall bladder in rare instances, (Theander).

Calcified omental fat deposits produce ring-like shadows in the abdomen, which, if they occur in the region of the gall bladder, might be mistaken for gall stones. They really represent infarction of a globule of omental fat which undergoes necrosis and calcification, (Holt and MacIntyre).

MILK OF CALCIUM BILE, (LIMY BILE) (Fig. 271A). Only in very rare instances does the bile content of the gall bladder become visible. In a condition known as Milk of Calcium bile, the heavy lime salt content of the bile renders the gall-bladder visible by ordinary roentgenographic methods. At operation the gall bladder contents is seen to be a greenish-yellow mass resembling putty or marshmallow. Stones may be imbedded in the mass, (Rose).

The formation of limy bile is basically part of stone formation. It is believed that the greater portion of bile calcium is secreted by the liver and the normal gall bladder acts to remove calcium from the bile. There is some discrepancy about the origin of the calcium in the bile. Phemister, Rewbridge and Rudisill found evidence that calcium carbonate is secreted by the gall bladder wall and is not derived from the bile. When a block of the cystic duct occurs in association with low grade chronic inflammation of the wall there is precipitation of calcium carbonate. The presence of unexplained increase in density of the bile should indicate some involvement of the gall bladder, (Cohen).

CALCIFIED GALL BLADDER (Fig. 271B). Calcareous deposits in the gall bladder wall is an occasional occurrence. It is usually the result of chronic gall bladder infection. It should not be confused with milk of calcium bile since the calcareous incrustations are irregular in outline and are in the gall bladder wall.

ORIGINAL GRAHAM TEST OF GALL BLADDER FUNCTION—USING TETRAIODOPHENOLPHTHALEIN (IODEIKON) (Figs. 272A, B, and C). Not until the evolution of the Graham-Cole-Copher-Moore test was very much definitely known about gall-bladder function. They conceived the idea that if the chlorine radical of tetrachlorphenolphthalein (a substance which had long been known to be secreted in the bile and which has been used as a test of liver function), could be replaced by a similar element (iodine) which was opaque to x-rays, it might be possible to render the bile radiopaque. This proved to be the case and the tetraiodophenolphthalein test was evolved.

The fundamental principle upon which this test is carried out should be briefly reviewed. (See detailed instructions in the Manual of Roentgenological Technique.) The examination was carried out by either the intravenous or the oral method.

At first the intravenous method was thought to be the most accurate means of performing the test; for the past several years, with the development of new chemical materials, the intravenous method has given place to the oral method as the preferred means of routine examination. The intravenous method is reserved for instances in which the oral method is found impossible. The drug originally used, Iodeikon (Tetraiodophenolphthalein), has likewise given place to a number of others which have been developed for this purpose. Detailed instructions for carrying out these various examinations

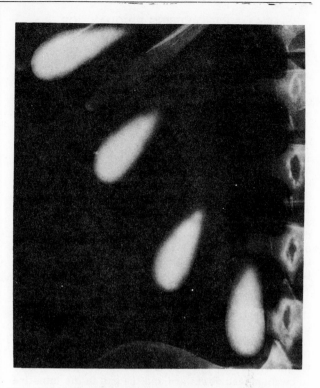

Fig. 272A. Position of gall bladder in individuals of different habitus: Hypersthenic type, above rib margin; sthenic type, just below rib margin; hyposthenic type, position lower down; asthenic type, hangs down into the abdomen.

will be found in the Manual of Roentgenological Technique.

The gall bladder may be found in widely varying locations on the right side of the abdomen. Rarely it may even be displaced into the left upper quadrant or be overshadowed by the spine. Since so much depends upon its visualization a thorough search should be made before a nonfunctioning gall bladder is diagnosed.

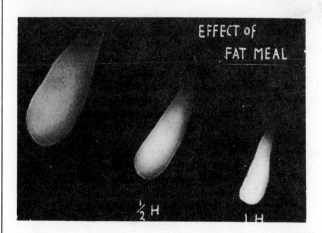

Fig. 272B. Effect of fat meal on size and density of gall bladder.

ORAL METHOD USING PRIODAX* OR TELEPAQUE.* Time has shown that the oral method is fully as reliable as the intravenous method. (A number of other drugs of similar composition seem to be very effective and are preferred by some.)

Six Priodax or Telepaque tablets or one per every twenty-five pounds of body weight if over 150 pounds, is administered the night before the examination after the evening meal. The meal should be fat-free or very sparing in fat content. A study of the gall bladder shadows obtained with Telepaque with and without a fat-free and a non-fat-free meal in preparation for the examination would indicate that the preparatory fat-free meal gives much the best gall bladder shadows, (Whitehouse). The tablets should be taken whole without chewing since this causes a burning sensation in the throat. They should be taken a few minutes apart. The patient then reports the next morning without breakfast twelve to fifteen hours after ingestion of the tablets for roentgen examination.

Since no cathartic is given by this method, at times intestinal gas may obscure the shadow of the gall bladder. To eliminate this, one view is taken in the right lateral decubitus with the patient lying on the right side, x-ray beam directed horizontally (Figs. 272C$_1$ and C$_2$).* This permits the gall bladder to be displaced downward and the gas in the intestine to rise giving a clear unobstructed view of the gall bladder shadow; it also permits "layering" of small inorganic stones if they happen to be in the gall bladder and thus favors their detection (Fig. 272)* (Kirklin). If visualization of the gall bladder is not successful at 12 hours, films should be repeated three hours later.

After the gall bladder is visualized a fat meal or synthetic fat meal, Neo-Cholex is then administered and re-examination is made at 8, 15 and 30 minute intervals to determine the degree of emptying, and to visualize the ducts.

Normal function of the gall bladder does not absolutely exclude organic lesion, however, such as gall stones or polyps. It must be quite obvious that a few small stones or a small polyp lying in a gall bladder filled with opaque material may be entirely overshadowed. This examination then must be thought of primarily as a test of function and secondarily as a method for detection of space occupying lesions. In many instances, gall stones, otherwise invisible, may be thrown into relief by the density of the bile and become detectable in this way. It is possible by careful examination made at half-hour intervals after fat meal until the gall bladder is almost entirely empty to detect even very small stones which could not otherwise be demonstrated, and thus to materially increase the number of cases in which a diagnosis of gallstones can be made in gall bladders showing normal function.

Roentgenographic examination made in the upright position may displace gallstones so that they float as a layer either in or on the bile; in this way they become more readily visible (Fig. 272D). A single rounded filling defect in the center of an otherwise normal gall bladder shadow may be due to a polypoid growth or to a single stone imbedded in the wall (Fig. 272E), (Greenwood and Samuel). Hilliard has reported a case of papiloma of the gall bladder. The 33-year-old male patient had suffered pain for 15 years; after food but no fixed interval which lasted two to three hours. Intervals free of pain had never been longer than a week. There were no other symptoms.

If no shadow of the gall bladder appears after administration of the contrast material at any examination, it is obvious that this means either that there may be some extensive disease of the liver preventing removal of the contrast material from the blood or that there is some obstruction to the cystic duct or pathology in the gall bladder itself, preventing entrance of bile. Delayed emptying of the stomach or other reason for failure of absorption from the intestines is another cause for failure of gall bladder visualization, (Loring and Herczeg). Where a shadow

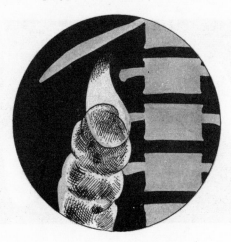

Fig. 272C$_1$. Gall bladder overshadowed by gas in colon.

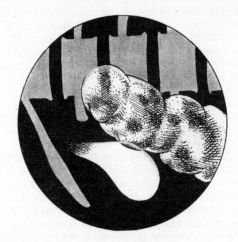

Fig. 272C$_2$. Same patient re-examined in the lateral decubitus (patient lying on left side, x-rays projected horizontally causes gall bladder to fall downward and gas-filled colon to rise).

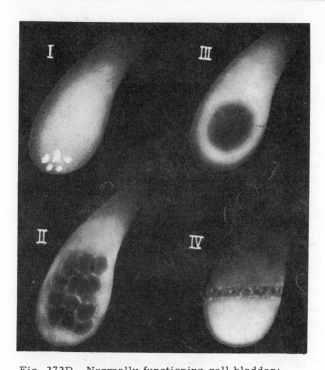

Fig. 272D. Normally functioning gall bladder:
 I. With multiple calcium bilirubin stones,
 II. with multiple cholesterol stones,
 III. with single large cholesterol stone,
 IV. with multiple cholesterol stones floating between layers of bile, (upright position).

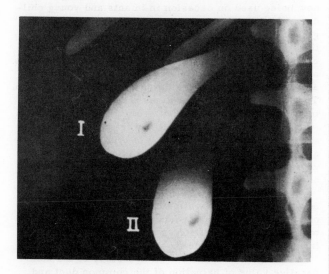

Fig. 272E. Normally functioning gall bladder with papilloma; position of defect is not changed in upright and prone positions. Papillomas can be demonstrated at the edge of the gall bladder on rotation of patient.

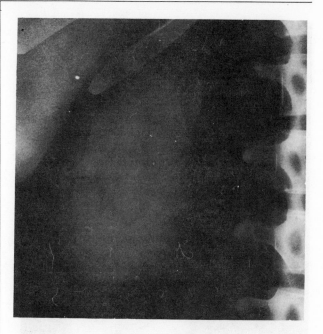

Fig. 272F. Non-functioning gall bladder with large hydrops.

of the gall bladder cannot be detected, this means pathology of the gall bladder in approximately 97% of all instances. The small remaining percentage of failures is usually due to technical difficulties or errors (Fig. 272F). Initial nonvisualization of the gall bladder cannot be considered an absolute indication for surgery. Because technical failures and errors do occur, the examination should be repeated, or repeated with a double dose of Telepaque or Priodax, and with medication to stimulate common duct sphincter spasm. (See Biliary ducts, p. 432.) With special attention, additional information can be obtained, either showing more definitely that the gall bladder is pathological or contains stones, or that normal function is after all present.

It should always be remembered that nonvisualization indicates pathology at the time of testing. Acute cholecystitis subsides, and if the gall bladder is not too badly damaged, later cholecystography will show normal function. Hepatitis prevents visualization because the diseased liver cells cannot excrete the contrast agent in high enough concentration. Cholecystography in the presence of jaundice gives no useful information about the gall bladder because of the accompanying liver impairment. In very rare instances the gall bladder may be congenitally absent.

The gall bladder may be deformed from pressure or adhesions or it may take on the appearance of a Phrygian Cap from tilting over of the fundus but this is of no pathological significance (Fig. 272G).

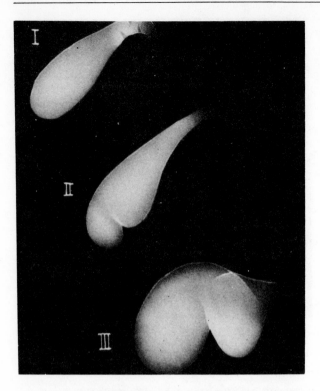

Fig. 272G. Various shapes of normal gall bladder:
   I. Appearance of valves in cystic duct,
   II. phrygian cap,
   III. convoluted gall bladder; this may be so
        pronounced as to give the impression of
        a double gall bladder.

Ross has reported a case of double gall bladder as
demonstrated by cholecystography.

Whitehouse advocated cholecystography with 2
gram doses of Telepaque in order to see stones and
other defects better. Faint shadow and nonvisualization he interpreted as cholecystitis with a large degree of confirmation. In his experience increase in
dose at subsequent examination of nonvisualizing gall
bladder is of little use.

Cimmino has found great satisfaction on upright fluoroscopic spot-film examination of the dye-
filled gall bladder utilizing compression when necessary in ridding the field of gas. The layering of
stones and the immovable character of polypoid
adenomas are valuable points.

Diverticula of Gall Bladder, (Rokitansky-
Aschoff Sinus). Deep, often irregular outpouchings
of the gall bladder mucosa extend into or through the
fine muscular coat of the gall bladder into the peri-
muscular layer. Such herniations are thought to be
due to chronic inflammation and over distention. The
condition is very rare, (Zinober). Moore has reported two additional cases of diverticula
(Rokitansky-Aschoff Sinuses) of the gall bladder
with findings indicating that this must be due to
chronic cholecystitis.

Acute gaseous cholecystitis is an infection of
the gall bladder characterized by the production of
gas within the gall bladder. The symptoms are not
essentially different from other patterns of acute
cholecystitis, so that differentiation is made radiologically. A plain film shows a radiolucent zone in
the shape and position of the gall bladder. Gas may
infiltrate into the gall bladder wall and pericholе-
cystic tissue. The gall bladder wall being subjected
to greater tension from the gaseous distention,
necrosis of the wall and perforation is frequent,
(Heifetz and Senturia). Recognition of this finding
makes surgery imperative.

Emphysema of the gall bladder is due to an
infection of the gall bladder wall usually by Bacillus Welchii or Coli. Roentgenographically the gas
can be seen in the gall bladder wall and within the
gall bladder itself forming a fluid level over the
bile in the upright position.

CHOLECYSTOGRAPHY IN INFANTS. Satis-
factory cholecystograms in children over three years
of age have been obtained with the adult dose of contrast agent, (Harris). With younger infants, their inability to concentrate bile in the gall bladder or lack
of sphincter control may prevent gall bladder visualization. Under age 3, about half of the attempts
are successful. Oral doses of Priodax and Telepaque
for infants is 0.15 gm. per kg. of body weight, but
double and triple doses have been given without
toxicity. Gall bladder studies are best timed four to
nine hours after giving of the oral contrast material.

Intravenous cholangiography (Cholegraphin) is
now being used on occasion in infants and young children. Moseley has reported a case in a 5-year-old
girl of choledocal "cyst" or idiopathic dilatation of
the common bile duct which was visualized by cholecystography and successfully operated upon. Success
of visualization was probably due to the fact that examination was done after the jaundice was cleared up.
The lesion appeared merely as a cyst-like enlargement of the common duct.

Investigation of the biliary tract in children
after the intravenous injection of biligrafin (Cholografin, single dose 0.1-0.3 gm/kg body weight) revealed good visualization of biliary system in all but
one in which there was congenital atresia of the duct.

The appearance of contrast medium in the
bowel without visualization of the bile ducts may be
of value in excluding atresia of the ducts; contrast
material in the renal pelves only may indicate liver
insufficiency, (Theander).

Borgstrom and Norman in a study of the comparative value of palpation of the common duct and
cholangiography for the detection of stones, came to
the conclusion that both methods are highly successful in detection of stones larger than 2 mm. in size;
below that size cholangiography has distinct advantages.

They felt that palpation against a probe and
cholangiography should both be used in combination
for greatest accuracy in diagnosis.

GALL BLADDER FUNCTION FOLLOWING TRAUMA. Howard studied the effect of nonspecific trauma on the secretory function of the liver in soldiers for 10 days following combat duty as well as many other cases of injury to the body exclusive of the gall bladder itself and found failure of secretion and concentration of the opaque media. Nonvisualization was practically the rule after injuries to the brain, chest, abdomen or extremities; after operative procedures such as herniorrhaphy for incarceration of the small bowel and one burned patient who had not received anaesthesia.

The author feels that there is reasonable evidence to support the hypothesis that the gall bladder participates in paralytic ileus following injury.

BILE DUCTS
(Figs. 273A & B)

Oral cholecystography as routinely performed only occasionally visualize the bile ducts, making the use of other technics necessary. Cholangiography may be accomplished by oral or intervenous injection of contrast material, or by direct introduction of the contrast substance into the bile ducts by surgical procedure.

Oral cholangiography: Using Telepaque, Sachs visualized the extrahepatic ducts in a fairly high percentage of instances, by roentgen examination at 8, 15, and 30 minutes following administration of a fatty meal (Neocholex) in the routine cholecystography. He suggests the simultaneous hypodermic injection of physostigmine to cause spasm of the sphincter of Oddi so as to retain the opaque material within the common duct under pressure.

Further refinement of oral cholangiography is described by Twiss and Gillette. They recommend a

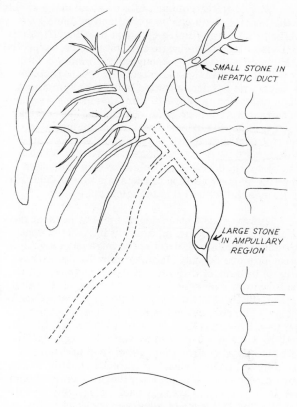

Fig. 273A₂

double dose of Telepaque on the evening preceding the examination, with an additional single dose of Telepaque on the morning of examination. Paregoric is given by mouth after ingestion of the doses of Telepaque to promote common duct sphincter spasm. The large dose of Telepaque combined with the withholding of fluids from the patient for 12 hours prior to filming allows maximal concentration of the opaque agent in the biliary ducts. If the gall bladder is visualized, a fatty meal is given, followed by films at 10 and 30 minutes, including upright films. In a series of cases examined by this method, visualization of the bile ducts was obtained in 72%.

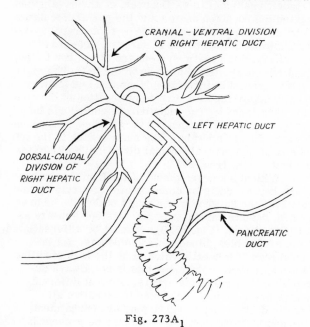

Fig. 273A₁

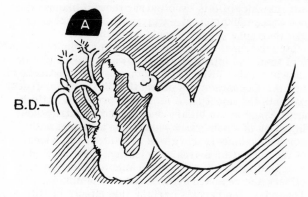

Fig. 273B. Ulceration of gall stone into the intestine.

Stones in the common bile duct, or more rarely, in the hepatic ducts can be visualized by the above methods. A large dilated common duct insufficiently well visualized to delineate a stone may be suspected of harboring a stone. Although the common duct normally dilates after cholecystectomy, such dilatation is slight and not accompanied by biliary symptoms. When dilatation is above 10 mm., symptoms are usually present and there is an obstructing lesion to account for the dilatation. The largest diameter to which a duct may dilate and still not be associated with symptoms is not yet known, however. Visualization of cystic duct and gall bladder remnants, and fibrosis or compression of the sphincter of Oddi may be successful with oral cholangiography.

Intravenous Cholangiography is at present dependent upon Cholografin, a newly introduced contrast material. When rapidly injected intravenously, this agent is more dependable in visualizing the extrahepatic bile ducts than oral cholangiography. Oral cholecystography remains the standard, most reliable and safest technic for roentgenologic investigation of the gall bladder, but in the post-cholecystectomy patient, and in the patient in whom neither gall bladder or bile ducts is visualized by routine or special oral technics, intravenous cholangiography is often extremely valuable. When the patient is unable to absorb oral medication, or when there is acute abdominal emergency, intravenous cholangiography is indicated. The incidence of adverse reactions to the injection is low. Films are made at intervals from 15 minutes to 2 hours after injection. Some use medication (Demerol, Morphine) to induce sphincter of Oddi spasm, thereby retaining the opaque material for a long time in the ducts.

Dyskinesia. Symptoms simulating biliary colic without actual obstruction from stone often following bile duct operation are thought to be due to a spastic condition of the musculature of the sphincter of Oddi. In 1928 Ivy demonstrated the occurrence of a hormone, cholecystokinin, secreted by the duodenal mucosa and acting specifically upon the musculature of the gall bladder. In 1934 Ivy and Sanblom reported that in experimental animals the sphincter of Oddi can resist a pressure of 800 mm. of H_2O_1; that the pressure at which bile is expelled into the gall bladder does not exceed 300 mm. of water and that the sphincter can therefore prevent expulsion of the bile. They injected duodenal extract into 19 healthy volunteers; in 3 of them the injection was followed by biliary colic indicating that biliary symptoms may be functional in origin. Gunnarson has shown that in symptom-free patients the injection of morphine produced little if any change in the biliary ducts filled by intravenous injection of Cholografin whereas in a patient with severe dyskinesia there was relaxation and widening of the duct after morphine injection. The method by which Biligrafin (Cholografin) acts and certain side effects are reported by Oeser and Frommhold, (Ref.). Theander also reports certain side effects of Biligrafin. Holmdahl has found that lactation does not interfere with Cholecystography and infants are not adversely affected by the iodine in the milk.

Intravenous cholangiography finds its greatest use in demonstrating a dilated common bile duct and the cause for its dilatation (in most cases a stone) in the patient suspected of having biliary tract disease. Other causes of duct dilatation which have been diagnosed are tumors, pancreatitis, and sphincter of Oddi fibrosis and spasm. Cystic duct and gall bladder remnants, gall bladder and cystic duct stones are other abnormal findings which give rise to biliary symptoms. As with oral cholecystography, jaundice and impaired liver function prevent the excretion of adequate amounts of Cholografin for diagnostic information. Body-section radiography about 40 minutes after Cholografin administration has a distinct advantage in visualization of the duct system according to Bell, et al., by eliminating disturbing shadows.

Mitchell has combined the use of Telepaque for oral cholecystography as well as Biligrafin (Cholografin) for intravenous cholangiography given 11 hours after administration of the oral administration. Combined use of both methods produces complete combined visualization of the entire biliary system, (Cholecystangiography).

Operative Cholangiography: Injection of water-soluble contrast material (Diodrast, Hypaque, Urokon, Neoiopax) into the bile ducts or gall bladder at time of surgery is of great value in helping the surgeon to ascertain the cause of biliary tract disease. The injection is made by syringe and needle or tubing, and a film which has previously been placed beneath the patient's upper abdomen is exposed by an x-ray tube temporarily placed over the operating table.

Knowledge of the roentgen anatomy of the hepatic ducts is essential to interpretation of operative and T-tube cholangiograms. Dochner, et al., have investigated the roentgen anatomy of the portal circulation 1) by injecting cadavers and 2) by photographing living subjects in the course of surgery. The main branches of the hepatic system are three, two to the right lobe of the liver, and one to the left. The right ventral cranial branch extends upward and forward, usually appearing as a direct continuation of the common hepatic duct. The right dorsal-caudal can be recognized by the distinct curve it makes as it bends downward and backward. The main branch to the left lobe runs in a ventral-cranial direction, and is often the last to fill, (Fig. 273A).

With quick development of the film a calculus in the hepatic ducts or common bile duct may be located for the surgeon which might otherwise be overlooked, despite careful probing. A stone appears as a filling defect, (Fig. 273B). It must be differentiated from air bubbles, blood clots and debris. An indirect sign of a hepatic calculus is the lack of filling of a major hepatic duct, but this is not always dependable. To minimize errors, films at different angles are recommended so as to visualize all hepatic ducts without overlapping or concealment, (Norman). More than one stone may be present in the biliary tree. Cholangiography can also be of assistance to the surgeon for detecting anomalies of the hepatic ducts, such as the drainage of a duct in abnormal manner into the cystic duct. An anomaly of some kind is present in 7.5% of cases, most of them not of clinical significance.

T-tube cholangiography is the injection of an organic iodide contrast material into the bile ducts through a chatheter left in place at previous surgical procedure. The surgeon desires to know that the sphincter of Oddi is unobstructed and the ducts free of overlooked or possibly newly formed calculi before he withdraws the biliary decompression tube from the bile ducts of the post-operative patient. Lipiodol, an oily substance, is no longer used for cholangiography. Its immiscibility with the bile gives appearances falsely suggestive of stones. See Fig. 273. Cholangiography is similarly performed by the injection of contrast material through a biliary fistula, should such occur spontaneously or following surgery.

Percutaneous cholangiography has been used in the diagnosis of obstructive jaundice, (Nurick). In this rarely indicated procedure, a long needle is inserted through the intact abdominal wall into the liver substance until a biliary radicle is encountered. Injection of water-soluble organic iodide contrast solution then outlines the biliary system and demonstrates the cause of obstruction. All other radiological non-operative diagnostic measures must be exhausted before this procedure is appropriate.

BILIARY FISTULA (Fig. 273C & D). Ulceration of a gall stone into the gastro-intestinal tract leaves an abnormal opening between the two systems. The observation of gas in the biliary tree indicates the presence of the fistula, for gas is not normally seen there (Fig. 273D). Each roentgenographic study of the patient with acute abdominal symptoms should include a search of the right upper quadrant of the abdomen for this abnormal distribution of air, which indicates serious gall bladder disease with calculi and the possibility of obstruction of the intestine from the gall stone.

Barium by mouth may escape through the fistulous opening into the bile ducts showing their outlines more clearly (Fig. 273C). Careful examination of the plain films will minimize this possibility. Air or barium may pass into the biliary ducts following surgical anastomosis of the gall bladder or common bile duct to the intestine, as in resections of the head of the pancreas. Fistulae between the biliary system and colon are more unusual than those of the intestine, and are demonstrated by barium enema.

Gas in the gall bladder may be present without a fistula between the biliary system and the gastrointestinal tract. In these instances, an acute cholecystitis due to gas-forming organisms is present.

Gall stone ileus may accompany the erosion of such a stone into the intestine and its passage by the alimentary tract. As the stone descends it may lodge at various locations in the bowel causing obstruction until gaseous dilatation of the bowel permits dislodgement and passage along to a new area of obstruction. At operation each area of intermittent obstruction may be detected by deposits of fibrinous exudate on the peritoneal coat of the intestine. This evidence of intermittent obstruction especially if accompanied by gas in the region of the biliary tract is evidence of gall stone ileus, (Bridenbaugh, et al.).

INTRAVENOUS CHOLOGRAFIN. Batt, after investigating the use of Cholografin in cholecystectomized patients has found it of great advantage in patients who have again developed symptoms. One-fourth of these patients have stones in the ducts, dilated ducts, gall bladder remnants, and long cystic duct stumps.

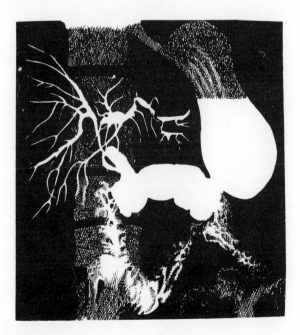

Fig. 273C. Spontaneous passage of barium into the biliary tract.

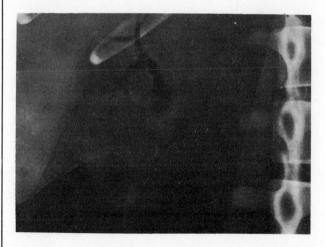

Fig. 273D. Spontaneous passage of gas into the biliary tract.

Intravenous Cholegraphin in Massive Hemobilia.
Traumatic lacerations of the liver (Sparkman), although meticulously sutured surgically, may become the site of subsequent biliary collections which prevent normal repair. Such collections of bile under pressure in a cavity may bring about autolysis of liver tissue lining the cavity and cause massive bleeding into the bile ducts which discharge into the gastro-intestinal tract. The triad of abdominal injury with subsequent gastro-intestinal hemorrhage and pain simulating biliary colic should lead one to suspect traumatic hemobilia.

Intravenous injection of Cholegraphin should prove an effective method for the detection of such an aberrant biliary collection and for the demonstration of derangement of the biliary radicals following liver damage, (Orloff, et al.). It is possible that injection of opaque material (Diodrast) into the portal vein might disclose any vascular damage to the liver.

Margulis, et al., found that the presumptive diagnosis of hepatoma could be made in children on the basis of relationship of a tumor mass in the upper abdomen to the other structures as indicated by the available methods of examination, such as gastro-intestinal, urological, etc., making use of a AP and lateral view.

The problem of portal hypertension and aids to its surgical attack has been undertaken by Doehner, et al. By surgical and autopsy procedures an attempt was made to evaluate the development of compensatory circulation in the portal venous system in order to aid the surgeon in selecting a vessel for anastomosis to relieve portal hypertension. After extensive investigation their conclusions were that:

1. When no natural shunts occur, except for gastro-esophageal varices (originating over the coronary vein) any type of portocaval surgery is permissible.

2. When there is already present an "effective" natural shunt (above 10 mm. in diameter) beside the coronary-gastro-esophageal varices, the choice of vessel for anastomosis should be limited to the "non-collateral portal tributaries".

From a technical standpoint, the surgeon will naturally choose the largest available vessel for anastomosis for shunting procedure. This may lead to unintentional sacrifice of a valuable natural collateral. As a means of evaluation of the situation present it is well to remember that normally the portal vein is larger than the splenic vein, which in turn is larger than the inferior mesenteric vein; a change in this relationship suggests that the disproportionately larger vessel carried collateral blood.

HEMOCHROMATOSIS. This is a condition in which heavy deposits of iron pigment in liver cells causes an increase in roentgenographic density of the liver. It is seldom diagnosed before death.

Zatzkin has reported a case with diabetes associated with cystitis emphysematosis, another rare condition in which gas bubbles accumulate in the bladder wall causing a radiolucent zone to appear about this structure. The simultaneous existence of these two rare conditions is unusual.

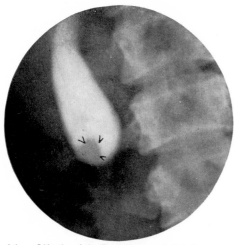

Gall bladder filled with Iodeikon eight hours after the intravenous administration. Note the shadow caused by negative stone.

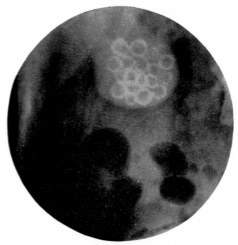

Gall bladder filled with Iodeikon showing a large number of calcium encrusted stones.

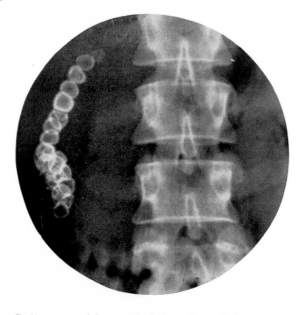

Gall stone without administration of dye.

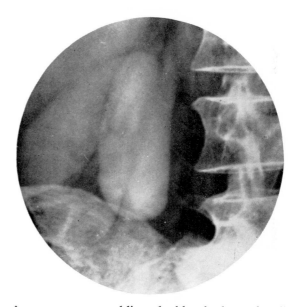

Appearance resembling double shadow of gall bladder caused by overlapping margins of liver and kidney.

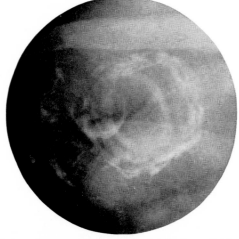

Large stone within pathological gall-bladder with calcium-encrusted wall.

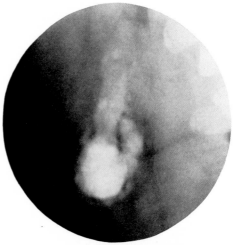

Numerous small diverticula-like extension into gall bladder wall,—Rokitansky-Aschoff Sinuses.

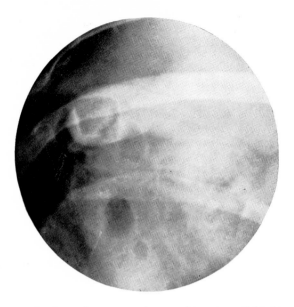
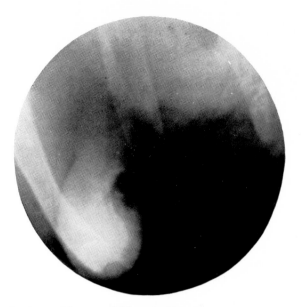

In the ordinary recumbent position the gall bladder shadow is obscured by gas which resembles stone; re-examination with the patient in the right lateral decubitus shows clear view of gall bladder without stone.

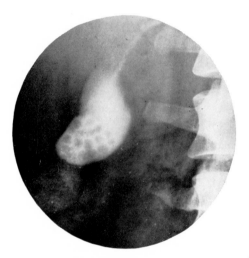
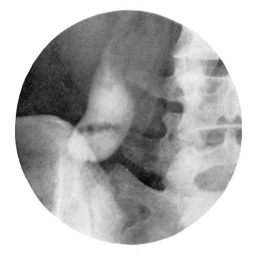

In the recumbent position gall stones spread out in the gall bladder and may even be overlooked; on assuming the upright position they float in a layer in the bile.

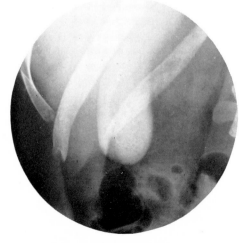
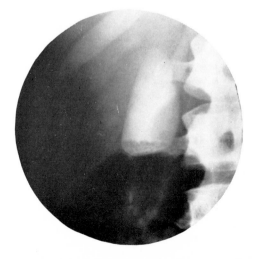

In recumbent position small stones may be invisible; in the upright position they may settle out and fall to the bottom.

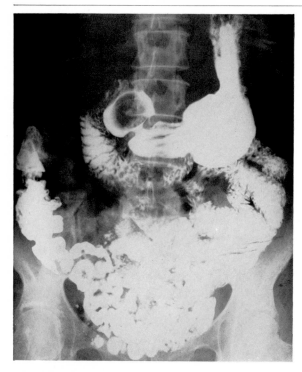

Gall Stone eroded through into duodenal bulb; small amount of barium in tract—Courtesy Dr. Frank Bihss.

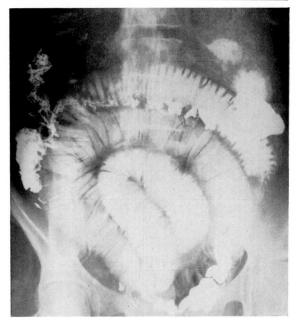

Intermittent obstruction and spastic ileus during passage of stone produces bizarre clinical symptoms.

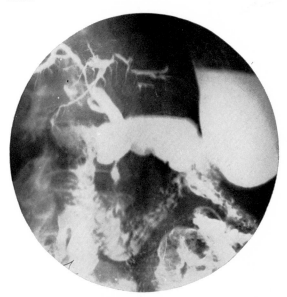

Barium meal extending out into bile ducts from destructive lesion of duodenum.

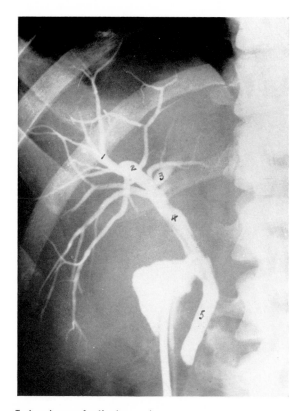

Injection of diodrast into common bile duct through a "T" tube. 1. Right ventral-cranial branch; 2. right dorsal-caudal branch curves and descends; 3. left lobe branch not completely filled; 4. common hepatic duct; 5. common bile duct.

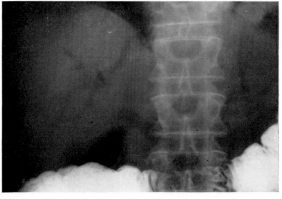

Gas outlining entire biliary tract after erosion of stone into duodenum.

CHOLECYSTOGRAM

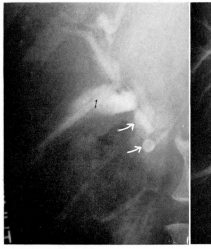
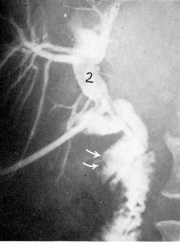

Two rounded stones in common duct definitely localized by injection of Diodrast thru a "T" tube.

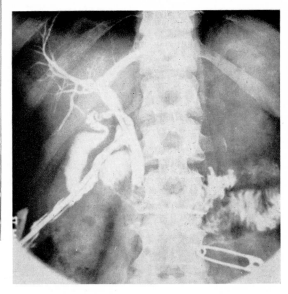

Injection through "T" tube into common duct; shows gall bladder, cystic duct, common and hepatic ducts and entire biliary tree.

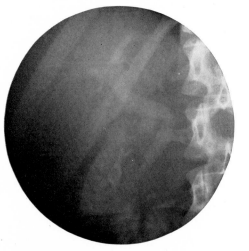

← Outline of biliary ducts after cholecystectomy by use of Cholografin.

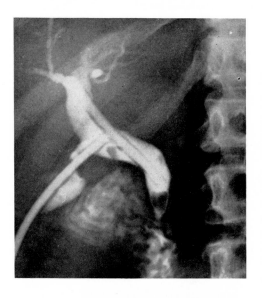

Two stones show by filling defects, one in common bile duct near the ampulla, the other as the "T" tube enters the common duct. →

Filling of biliary tree with regurgitation of opaque material backward into the pancreatic duct. →

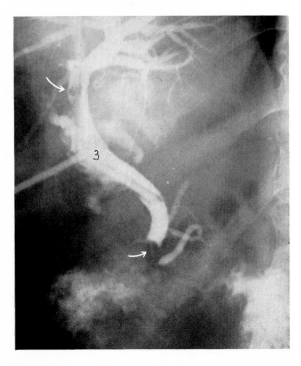

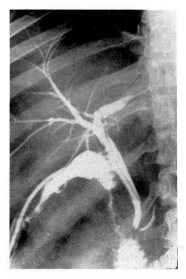

← Stones in hepatic and common ducts. Some extravasation about ducts. Regurgitation into finer radicals of pancreatic duct.

QUESTIONS ON BILIARY TRACT

1. Why is direct examination of the gall bladder not entirely satisfactory?

2. Approximately what percentage of gallstones can be visualized in flat films of the gall bladder area? Why?

3. How may the gall bladder be visualized?

4. Describe briefly the technique and procedure of the tetraiodophenolphthalein (Graham) test for gall-bladder function, using the intravenous and oral methods.

5. Upon what principle does the test depend?

6. What significance is attached to failure of a shadow of the gall bladder to appear after injection of the dye? In what percentage of cases is such a diagnosis found to be correct?

7. Is the visualization of the gall bladder an indication that it is free from organic pathology?

8. Is it possible for gall bladders showing normal function to be the site of other pathology? In what percentage of instances are stones found in such cases?

9. What x-ray findings are present in the case of a polypoid adenomatous growth? Might this appearance be simulated by any other pathology?

10. Would you depend upon failure to secure a gall-bladder shadow with the oral method as indication of pathology? Are present day oral methods considered as reliable as the intravenous methods?

11. What is milk of calcium bile like and how does it appear in the roentgenogram? Would it be detected by a preliminary examination of the gall bladder?

12. What method may be used to detect a stone remaining in the common bile duct?

13. What are the most common causes of biliary fistula and how may they be demonstrated roentgenographically?

14. How may the common bile duct be visualized in a patient in whom the gall bladder has been removed?

15. What is cholangiography and how is it carried out?

16. What information can be gained from cholangiographic examination after gall bladder removal?

17. What complications may develop after massive injuries to the liver?

REFERENCES FOR BILIARY TRACT

Sachs, M. D., "Visualization of the Common Duct during Cholecystography," Am. J. Roentgenol., 69:745, 1953.

Ivy, A. C., and Oldberg, E., "Gallbladder Function," Proc. Soc. Exper. Biol. and Med., 25:113, 1927.

Holt, J., and MacIntyre, R. S., "Calcified Omental Fat Deposits; Their Roentgenologic Significance," Am. J. Roentgenol., 60:612, 1948.

Theander, G., "Precipitation of Contrast Medium in the Gall Bladder," Acta Radiol., 44:467, 1957.

Rose, J. A. G. F., "Milk of Calcium" or "Limy" Bile. Brit. J. Radiol., 19:323, 1946.

Cohen, O. H., "Limy Ductus Choledochus," Radiol., 65:78, 1955.

Kirklin, B. R., "Cholecystographic Diagnosis of Neoplasms of the Gallbladder," Am. J. Roentgenol., 29:8, 1933.

Greenwood, F. Samuel, E., "Layering of Stones; the Pathological Gallbladder," Brit. J. Radiol., 21:438, 1948.

Whitehouse, W. M., "Re-evaluation of Fat-Free Preparatory Meal in Telepaque Cholecystography," Am. J. Roentgenol., 76:21, 1956.

Hilliard, C. H., "Papilloma of the Gall Bladder Diagnosed Radiologically," Brit. J. Radiol., 29:342, 1956.

Loring, P., and Herczeg, T., "Cholegraphic Demonstration of Cystic Duct Obstruction," Acta Radiol., 46:723, 1956.

Ross, J. A., "Double Gall Bladder with Report of a Case," Brit. J. Radiol., 29:339, 1956.

Whitehouse, W. M., "Correlation of Surgical Pathology with Telepaque Cholecystography in Doses of Two Grams," Surg., Gynec. and Obst., 100:211, 1955.

Cimmino, C. V., "Experience with the Upright Fluoroscopic Spot-Film Examination of the Gallbladder," Radiol., 67:74, 1956.

Zinober, M., "Rokitansky-Aschoff Sinuses of the Gallbladder," South African M. J., 26:35, 1952.

Moore, R. D., "Diverticula of the Gall Bladder," Am. J. Roentgenol., 75:360, 1956.

Stromme, A., "Emphysematous Cholecystitis," Acta Radiol., 44:39, 1955.

Harris, R. C., and Caffey, J., "Cholecystography in Infants," J.A.M.A., 153:1333, 1953.

Moseley, J. E., "Radiographic Demonstration of Choledochal Cyst by Oral Cholecystography," Radiol., 68:849, 1957.

Heifetz, C. J., and Senturia, H. R., "Acute Pneumocholecystitis," Surg., Gynec. and Obst., 86:424, 1948.

Sachs, M. D., "Visualization of the Common Duct during Cholecystography," Am. J. Roentgenol., 69:745, 1953.

Theander, G., "Cholegraphy in Children," Acta Radiol., 42:11, 1954.

Borgstrom, S., and Norman, O., "Palpation of Common Duct vs Preoperative Cholangiography in Diagnosis of Common Duct Stones," Acta Chir. Scandinav., 108:13, 1954.

Howard, J. M., "Gall Bladder Function (Cholecystographic Studies) Following Non-Specific Trauma," Surg., 36:1051, 1954.

Twiss, J. R., Gillette, L., Beranbaum, S. L., Poppel, M. B., and Hanssen, E. C., "Post Cholecystectomy Oral Cholangiography," Arch. Int. Med., 95:59, 1955.

Gunnarson, E., "The Bile Ducts of Cholecystectomised Patients with and without Dyskmesia Before and After Morphine Injection," Acta Radiol., 45:298, 1956.

Oeser, H., and Frommhold, W., "Cholegraphy," Acta Radiol., 43:355, 1955.

Theander, G., "Side Effects of Biligrafin," Acta Radiol., 43:369, 1955.

Holmdahl, K. H., "Cholecystography During Lactation," Acta Radiol., 45:305, 1956.

Mitchell, D. J., "Basic Combined Cholecystangiography," Brit. J. Radiol., 29:133, 1956.

Bell, A. L., Immerman, L. L., and Arcomano, J., "Body-Section Cholangiography with a New Intravenous Medium, (Cholografin)," Radiol., 66:84, 1956.

Dochner, G. A., Ruzicka, F. F., Hoffman, G., and Rousselot, L. M., "Portal Venous System: Its Roentgen Anatomy," Radiol., 64:675, 1955.

Dochner, G. A., Ruzicka, F. F., Rousselot, L. M., and Hoffman, G., "The Portal Venous System On Its Pathological Roentgen Anatomy," Radiol., 66:206, 1956.

Norman, O., "Studies on the Hepatic Ducts in Cholangiography," Acta Radiol. Suppl., 84, 1951.

Nurick, A. W., Patey, D. H., and Whiteside, C. G., "Percutaneous Transhepatic Cholangiography in the Diagnosis of Obstructive Jaundice," Brit. J. Surg., 41:27, 1953.

Bridenbaugh, R. B., Bridenbaugh, J. H., and Berg, H. M., "Gallstone Ileus," Am. J. Roentgenol., 77:684, 1957.

Shehadi, W. H., "Telepaque: New Cholecystographic Medium with Improved Visualization of Gall Bladder and Visualization of Bile Ducts," Am. J. Roentgenol., 68:360, 1952.

Ivy, A. C., "Hormone Mechanism for Gall Bladder Contraction and Evacuation," Am. J. Physiol., 86:599, 1928.

Sparkman, R. S., "Massive Hemobilia Following Traumatic Rupture of the Liver," Ann. of Surg., 138:899, 1953.

Batt, R., "Intravenous Cholecystography," Radiol., 65:926, 1955.

Margulis, A. R., Nice, C. M., and Rigler, L., "Roentgen Findings in Primary Hepatoma in Infants and Children," Radiol., 66:807, 1956.

Zatzkin, H. R., "Hemochromatosis with Diabetes Associated with Cystitis Emphysematosa," Radiol., 66:744, 1956.

Anderson, F. G., "Cholecystangiography Using Biligrafin Forte," Brit. J. Radiol., 29:504, 1956.

Orloff, T. L., Sklaroff, D. M., Cohn, E. M., and Gershon-Cohen, J., "Intravenous Choledochography with a New Contrast Medium, 'Cholegrafin'," Radiol., 62:868, 1954.

Boreadis, A. G., "Upright Cholangiography," Radiol., 63:227, 1954.

INDEX
TO
URINARY TRACT

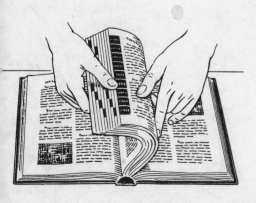

PART V

URINARY TRACT

I. ANATOMY—Roentgen (Chapter XXIII)
  A. Structures of roentgenological importance
    1. Normal position of urinary organs
    2. Urine collecting apparatus
    3. Points of natural ureteral constriction
    4. Psoas muscles

II. ROENTGEN EXAMINATION
  A. Methods of examination
    1. Ordinary x-ray examination—flat film; stereoscopic
    2. Injection methods
      a. Urography
        Retrograde
        Intravenous—excretory
          Advantages and disadvantages of each

III. PATHOLOGY—Roentgen evidence of,
  A. Kidney and ureter
    1. Urinary calculi
      a. Types
        Opaque
        Nonopaque
      b. Location
      c. Size
      d. Differentiation from,
        Gallstones
        Calcified costal cartilages
        Calcified mesenteric nodes
        Fecaliths
        Phleboliths
        Foreign bodies in intestinal tract
        Warts
        Artifacts
    2. Urography
      Pyelography and ureterography
      a. Normal pelvic and ureteral structure
      b. Pyelovenous, pyelolymphatic and pyelotubular backflow
      c. Dilatation of kidney pelvis and ureter
        Hydronephrosis
          Causes of dilatation and sequence of changes
          Influence of obstruction on renal function—nephrogram
        Infection—pyelonephritis
          Pyogenic
          Tuberculous
      d. Tumors of kidney
        Parenchyma
          Malignant
          Benign
          Cyst
          Polycystic kidney
        Kidney pelvis
          Papillary
          Malignant
          Benign
          Non papillary
          Malignant
          Benign
      e. Parenchymal (cortical) necrosis
        From tumor
        From pyogenic abscess; carbuncle of kidney

From tuberculous infection
f. Anomalies of kidney
    Agenesia
    Malposition
    Unilateral
    Rotated
    Fused
    Horseshoe
    Kidney pelvis and ureter
        Bifurcated kidney pelvis
        Branching ureter
        Double ureter
g. Injuries of kidney and ureter
    External
        Postoperative fistulae, urinary suppression from
    Internal
        From instrumentation and other causes

B. Psoas muscles
  1. Obliteration of psoas shadow from
    a. Hemorrhage
    b. Perinephritic abscess
    c. Infiltrating malignancy

C. Bladder
  1. Methods of examination
  2. Foreign bodies in
  3. Calculi
    a. Opaque
    b. Nonopaque
    c. Laminated
  4. Cystograms—opaque media
    Abnormalities of size and shape
    a. Contraction
    b. Dilatation
    c. Atony
    d. Pressure defects from extrinsic structures
    e. Diverticula
    f. Ureterocele
    g. Trabeculation—neurogenic bladder
    h. Congenital valves
    i. Tumors of bladder
    j. Ruptured bladder
  5. Pneumo—cystograms for,
    a. Small growths
    b. Polypi
  6. Cystitis
  7. Cystitis emphasematosa—air cysts of bladder

D. Prostate
  1. Calculi

E. Urethrography
  1. Method of examination
  2. Normal urethra
  3. Pathological changes
    a. Deep urethra
        In prostatic lesions
        From congenital constriction
        From neurogenic bladder
        From rupture
          Infection
          Trauma
    b. Pendulous urethra
        Stricture
        Diverticula

F. Seminal vesicles
G. Artificial pneumoperitoneum
H. Perirenal insufflation
I. Aortography

Chapter XXIII

URINARY TRACT

ANATOMY. Normally the kidneys lie on either side of the spine in the lower dorsal and upper lumbar regions between the levels of the upper margin of the eleventh dorsal and lower margin of the third lumbar vertebrae. They are tucked up well under the rib margin posteriorly, the right kidney extending slightly lower than the left. They are flattened from before backward and lie with their long axes verticle to the spine and their short diameter horizontally. Maintenance in this position is due in part to the perirenal structures but mainly to the intra-abdominal pressure produced by the tone of the abdominal muscles.

The urine is collected as it is excreted by numerous small cuplike structures, the minor calices; passed on into the larger branches or major calices which in turn empty into the main portion of the kidney pelvis and ureter. Ordinarily, there are three major calices, the superior (or cephalic), the middle, and the inferior (or caudal) calyx, each being formed by the union of varying numbers of minor calices, usually in clusters of two or three to each. Occasionally there may be only two, but rarely is there a greater number than three major calices. There may be wide variation in the structure of the pelvis in different individuals but regardless of the type they usually are similar on both sides.

The kidney pelvis joins with the ureter at the uretero-pelvic junction; with the exception of the lowest point of the inferior calyx, the ureter drains the pelvis at its lowest point. The ureters course downward parallel with the lumbar spine at about the outer margin of the transverse processes of the vertebrae. They cross the bony pelvis near the sacroiliac joints and empty into the bladder slightly lateral to the midline on either side low down in the bladder area. There are three points of natural narrowing of the ureter in its course:

1. At the uretero-pelvic junction,
2. As the ureter crosses the brim of the bony pelvis, and
3. At the uretero-vesicle junction.

The bladder itself forms a rounded hollow muscular structure lying low down in the bony pelvis, rising upward into the abdomen as it becomes distended with urine. The prostate lies immediately behind the symphysis pubis, surrounding the urethra at its attachment to the bladder. This portion of the urethra is known as the prostatic or deep urethra while the distal portion is known as the pendulous urethra.

The psoas muscles form strong heavy structures having attachment as high up as the last two dorsal vertebrae and extending obliquely downward on either side of the spine.

ROENTGENOLOGICAL EXAMINATION. None of these structures can be seen roentgenologically with a similar degree of clearness to the heart and great vessels in the chest; this is because there is not sufficient difference in density between the structures examined and the surrounding tissues. Usually, however, the size, shape, location and homogeneous structure of the kidneys, and their surrounding perirenal fatty deposits is sufficient to render the kidney outlines clearly visible. It is quite obvious that overshadowing fecal material in the intestines will hinder proper visualization of the kidney structures so that thorough cleansing of the gastrointestinal tract is essential. (See Manual of Roentgenological Technique, for preparation of patient.) Stereoscopic examination is ordinarily unnecessary, although some radiologists favor this method of examination. Before a roentgenogram may be considered as of proper quality for detection of stone, it should have the following qualities: it should include the last two ribs and the symphysis pubis; there should be detail in the transverse processes of the vertebrae; the psoas muscles should be clearly visible and there should be definite indication of the kidney outlines.

UROGRAPHY. The kidney pelves, ureters, and bladder usually cannot be seen in ordinary roentgenographic examination. Occasionally, the bladder, if well distended with urine, may be detected. To render these structures more clearly visible, the urine must be rendered radio-opaque by introduction of some suitable drug. This can be done by either intravenous, oral, or subcutaneous administration of a drug which will be excreted in the urine (the excretory method) or by retrograde injection of opaque material into the urinary tract (the retrograde method). In young infants the oral method using Hippuran, or the subcutaneous method using Urokon, although they often do not give pyelograms as dense as by other methods, are satisfactory (Friese-Christiansen). (See Manual of Roentgenological Technique for details of preparation and technique of examination.)

By reason of the increased density of this material the kidney pelves, with their major and minor calices, and the ureters are clearly outlined. For bladder visualization a similar procedure may be followed, injecting radiopaque solution into the bladder through an ordinary catheter.

In extremely small infants, an intraosseous method of injection has been used with reasonably satisfactory results. The intraosseous method of injection is mentioned only to be condemned since it is sometimes followed by osteomyelitic infection.

EXCRETORY UROGRAPHY. In recent years, a number of drugs have been made available, which, when injected intravenously, are excreted in the urine (Diodrast, Skiodan, Neo-Iopax, Hippuran, Hypaque, Diaginol, and Urokon). These solutions, being radiopaque, render the urinary tract clearly visible on roentgen examination. All produce satisfactory visualization; each has its advantages and disadvantages, so that a selection can be made which is suitable under almost any circumstances, (See Manual of Roentgenological Technique).

ADVANTAGES OF THE INTRAVENOUS METHOD.

1. It avoids disagreeable instrumentation and if successful under most circumstances is equally satisfactory to the retrograde method.

2. It utilizes the natural method of excretion and gives thereby, some indication of kidney function at the time of examination. It must be borne in mind that temporary suppression may occur after injury or in association with obstruction which may be relieved on subsequent examination; and that urography only to a certain degree affords a qualitative indication of renal function; when an exact measure of renal function is necessary, urography cannot replace quantitative tests upon the individual kidney, (Edling, et al.).

3. It can be used in cases where cystoscopy is impossible (as in cases of bladder neck obstruction) or where it is undesirable as in very young children or in the presence of infection).

4. It is often of advantage in detecting anomalies of the genito-urinary tract.

DISADVANTAGES OF THE INTRAVENOUS METHOD.

1. Often the diseased kidney, information concerning which is most desired, may be non-functioning and fail to excrete the drug in sufficient quantity for satisfactory visualization.

2. The pyelograms produced by the dye are often not as clear as those obtained by the retrograde method.

3. There are certain dangers, although remote, of shock and allergic reaction to the drugs.

4. It does not permit cystoscopic examination of the bladder, and thereby misses the possibility of detection of infection and its localization.

The use of the intravenous method is usually restricted to:

1. Patients in which bladder neck obstruction prevents cystoscopy.

2. Very young infants or other individuals on whom it is undesirable to do cystoscopic examination, and

3. Patients in whom anomalies of the urinary tract are suspected but cannot be demonstrated by the retrograde method.

RETROGRADE PYELOGRAMS. Since retrograde pyelograms present the clearest outline and greatest detail, this should be the method of choice wherever possible. It also affords a cystoscopic view of the bladder which at times gives valuable information.

The only valid objection to the retrograde method is the instrumentation which it requires for cystoscopy. The technique of this procedure has been so greatly improved as to minimize the disagreeable features of the examination and the danger of the procedure has been practically eliminated; even such accidents as false passage of the catheter and injection of the drug into the surrounding structures rarely if ever produce deleterious symptoms. In very rare instances where neither retrograde or intravenous urography is possible Wichbom has used direct puncture of the kidney pelvis for pyelography without deleterious effect; it is only recommended as a remote method where other less drastic methods are impossible.

ROENTGEN EVIDENCE OF PATHOLOGY

URINARY CALCULI.* Perhaps the most frequent examination of the urinary tract is for the detection of stones. Stones may have their origin, 1) in the parenchyma or, 2) within the kidney pelvis itself. Parenchymal stones develop usually in the papillae as the result of toxic action or infection. There seems to be an unusual attraction of calcium salts for regions of parenchymal destruction. Either pyogenic or tuberculous infection may be the cause of this destruction giving rise to stone formation. Depending upon the character of the urine at the time this occurs, these stones may be calcium oxalate, carbonate, phosphate, or whatever salt predominates in the urine at the time. Stones developed in this fashion pass down into the calices, pelvis and finally may descend into the ureter and bladder. Pelvis stones which have their origin within the kidney pelvis are usually due to retardation of urinary flow. Any slowing of the passage of urine favors precipitation of its salts and stone formation. Foreign or necrotic material, the products of infection, blood clot, etc., may serve as the nucleus of stone formation. Fortunately a large percentage (about 97%) of stones found in the urinary tract are inorganic and therefore are opaque to x-rays. Even stones of organic composition may, by indirect means, become visualized also. Calcium oxalate stones are especially dense having feathery edges. They cannot be dissolved or gotten rid of by any method other than removal. Uric acid stones are especially non-opaque; they are visualized by the filling defect they produce in opaque injected media.

Calcium deposits may occur in any location in the urinary tract, (Goldstein and Abeshouse). They may be found very rarely in the parenchyma of the kidney; when they occur in the region of the papillae they are usually calcareous deposits which have resulted from other pathological processes, such as tuberculosis or hyperparathyroidism. When they result from tuberculous infection they usually affect

*An asterisk following any title indicates that roentgenographic reproductions illustrating this condition will be found in the pictorial supplement at the end of the chapter.

the papillae of only a few of the calices; whereas in nephrocalcinosis from hyperparathyroidism (hypercalcemia) they are widespread involving usually the papillae for all caliceal structures in both sides. Similar calcium deposits have been reported in association with Sarcoidosis, (Davidson, et al.).

Calculi are most frequently found in the urinary passages: the kidney pelves, ureters, or bladder. Small calculi, passing down the ureter, are most likely to be held up at one of the three points of natural constriction; at the uretero-pelvic junction, as the ureter crosses the bony pelvis, or at the uretero-vesicle junction. Careful search should be made in these locations, although it is possible for a stone to be obstructed in its passage at any location.

For identification of a small structure such as a urinary stone it is necessary to localize it to the ureter or pelvic structure. In order to do this it is necessary either to pass a catheter into the ureter by cystoscopy or fill the urinary tract with opaque substance. Even though this shows a small shadow to lie directly over the catheter this is not sufficient for its absolute localization to the ureter. Double exposures on the same film, or on two successive films, with shift either of the x-ray tube or the patient is necessary. If the stone is in the ureter it should follow the ureteral catheter at both exposures maintaining its close relation. If it separates from the catheter in either exposure (Fig. 274) then this indicates that it is not within the ureter.

Stones in the urinary tract vary greatly in size; they may be tiny, hardly larger than a grain of sand—in fact, large quantities of such stones are referred

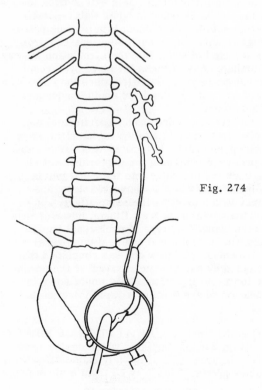

Fig. 274

to as urinary "sand." Sand of this type is rather rare since it usually is readily passed and does not have an opportunity to accumulate. It can occur in such amounts, however, as to completely pack the ureter. Small irregular stones forming in the calices or kidney pelvis give rise to typical symptoms of renal colic as they pass down the ureter; such stones even when they are scarcely more than a few millimeters in diameter are usually readily visible. Such stones, arising in the kidney pelvis may not pass but remain in situ, gradually enlarging by successive urinary deposits until they reach enormous size; they sometimes form complete casts of the kidney pelvis, known as "stag-horn calculi." Such large calculi cause few if any symptoms for many years, but finally they are usually followed by infection from local irritation. In such cases pyelography is of value in localizing the stone to the kidney pelvis and determining the extent of kidney damage which has resulted from the stone formation.

Numerous conditions occur in the abdomen which may be confused with urinary calculi. Chief among these are:
1. Gallstones
2. Calcifications in costal cartilages
3. Calcified mesenteric lymph nodes
4. Fecaliths
5. Phleboliths
6. Calcified necrotic fat nodules in the omentum
7. Foreign bodies in the intestinal tract
8. Warts and moles on skin
9. Artifacts of other types

Gallstones, of course, can only be confused with urinary stones when on the right side. Being nearer to the anterior abdominal wall, their shadows will be smaller in posteroanterior examination since they are nearer to the film in this position than in the anteroposterior view in which kidney examinations are ordinarily made. Lateral view examination may be helpful in differentiating.

Calcified deposits in the costal cartilages may fall over the kidney shadow giving the impression of stones. Re-examination by special technique, tucking the edge of the cone under the costal margin, eliminates all costal cartilages from the examination, permitting a definite diagnosis of stone.

Calcified mesenteric lymph nodes are usually quite movable; often they can be widely displaced under fluoroscopic examination by abdominal palpation. If fluoroscopic visualization is impossible, a second roentgenographic examination in the upright position will disclose any change in relationship between the kidney and the suspicious shadow.

Fecaliths, or concretions in the intestinal wall, appendix or diverticula; phleboliths, or rounded calcareous deposits in the walls of the veins or surrounding small areas of fat necrosis in the omentum and foreign material in the intestinal tract, such as fruit pits, etc., all can be differentiated from urinary calculi by their inconstancy of appearance in relationship to the urinary tract. On roentgenographic examination such a small calcareous deposit may lie directly over the shadow of the ureteral catheter. To

determine if the deposit lies in the ureter merely
make a second roentgenogram after shifting the position of the patient or x-ray tube and if the shadow is
a ureteral stone it will maintain its close relationship with the catheter.

Warts and moles on the skin of the back, when
closely pressed against the cassette, may cause very
suspicious shadows on the roentgenogram. Their
constancy in appearance in the same location at subsequent x-ray examination makes them even more
confusing. Examination in upright position, causing
some displacement of the kidney, reveals their change
in relationship with that organ. Close inspection of
the skin will detect the offending skin lesion.

Other artifacts, such as marks on the film or
intensifying screen, as small mouldy growths on
either, can be identified by their constant position on
the film even when the screen is turned around into
some other relationship with the part examined. A
roentgenogram taken with another screen will cause
such artifacts to disappear.

PYELOGRAPHY AND URETEROGRAPHY.*

The kidney pelvis, being of similar density to other
surrounding soft part structures is invisible under
ordinary roentgenographic examination. Injection of
opaque solution (10% skiodan) into the kidney pelvis
through catheters introduced into the ureters by
cystoscopic examination renders the outline of the
pelvic structure and ureter clearly visible. Kidney
pelves vary considerably in different individuals but
there are certain common characteristics seen in
practically all: there are usually three major
calices, superior (or cephalic), middle, and inferior
(or caudal), each of which drains clusters of two,
three, or even more minor calices; the cup-shaped
ends of the minor calices should show as sharp
points at the rim. The kidney pelvis should drain at
its lowest point, with perhaps the exception of the
lowermost point of the inferior calyx. The lower
border should be convex upward; occasionally an
anomalous renal vessel causes the lower border to
be at right angles to the ureter; this may or may not
be of pathological significance. The ureter courses
downward, parallel to the spine near the outer margins of the transverse processes; ordinarily it is not
more than half a centimeter in diameter.

At times where a more detailed examination of
the ureter is required or for some reason it cannot
be secured by ordinary means, the employment of a
conical-tipped Braasch-bulb ureteral catheter for
plugging the lower end of the ureter during injection
may be resorted to thus insuring a well-filled ureter
during roentgen examination (Fig. 274).

Ordinarily the kidney pelvis holds about 7.5 cc.;
injection of this quantity of material should completely fill the pelvis. Dilatation of the pelvis may be so
great that the retained urine will dilute 7.5 cc. of
opaque solution so much that scarcely any shadow
will be seen on the roentgenogram.

PYELORENAL BACKFLOW; (PYELOVENOUS,* PYELOLYMPHATIC AND PYELOTUBULAR) (Fig. 275 A, B, C).

Too great pressure on injection will result

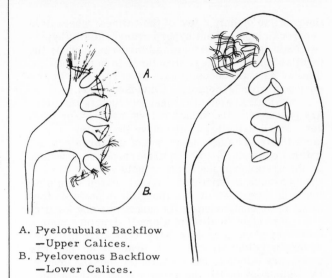

A. Pyelotubular Backflow
   —Upper Calices.
B. Pyelovenous Backflow
   —Lower Calices.

Fig. 275A and B   Fig. 275C

in expressing the opaque solution back into the tubules
and vascular and lymphatic structures of the kidney
known as pyelorenal backflow. Pyelotubular backflow gives rise to the appearance of numerous fine
opaque lines, radiating outward into the kidney substance from the centers of the minor calices toward
the periphery along the lines of the kidney tubules.
Such backflow may extend entirely to the subcapsular
region (A). If the opaque material is forced back into
the venous channels (pyelovenous backflow), fine radiating lines appear at the margins of the cups of the
minor calices (B); whereas in pyelolymphatic backflow (C) definite tortuous channels extend back toward
the midline. When Skiodan or other water-soluble
nonirritating solutions are used, this is of no pathological significance, since such solutions can ordinarily be injected directly into the circulation anyway
without mishap. Any of these forms of pyelorenal
backflow can be readily identified since they disappear
at once and are gone by the time another roentgenogram can be made.

Bauer has concluded from experimental and
clinical observations that pyelorenal backflow seen in
intravenous pyelography is the result of excess abdominal pressure retarding the ureteral flow thus
damming back the pressure into the renal pelvis producing similar conditions to those in retrograde
pyelography which produce the same effect, - increased intrapelvic pressure. Hinkel, however, has
observed the brush-like type of pyelorenal backflow
in patients who have not had ureteral compression
during intravenous backflow and has concluded that it
may be caused by use of concentration of the opaque
media or too rapid injection. This would seem to be
the explanation where it follows rapid injection in
aortography.

HYDRONEPHROSIS; DILATATION OF KIDNEY PELVIS* (Fig. 276A).

Anything which obstructs the
natural flow of urine will ultimately cause dilatation
of the kidney pelvis. This may be from a stone plug-

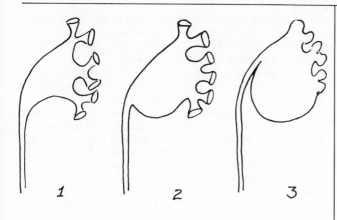

Fig. 276A

ging the ureter or stricture of the ureter from previous passage of a stone; it may be due to kinking of the ureter from pressure of an aberrant vessel, ptosis of the kidney or pressure of an extrinsic growth. The first roentgenographic indication of dilatation of the pelvis is usually seen in the lower border of the pelvis; it loses its natural upward curve, at first becoming flattened, and later, as dilatation continues, bulges downward. As the pressure increases and dilatation continues, the major calices become shorter and thicker and the minor calices become stubby and the margins of their cusps become rounded; dilatation may reach such a profound degree that the kidney pelvis merely appears as a rounded dilated sac with a few knoblike projections at the sites of the calices. The succession of events which take place with dilatation of the kidney pelvis from increase in pressure may be more clearly understood by observing the inflation of a toy animal balloon. With a normal degree of air pressure the balloon is distended to such a degree that the animal assumes its natural shape, rounded body, slender legs, and sharp clear-cut ears, snout and hoofs. Any increase in pressure is at first indicated by dilatation of the body and rounding of the belly of the animal; upon further inflation, the legs become shorter and thicker and finally on extreme inflation the snout, ears and hoofs lose their sharp, clear-cut outlines and assume the appearance of rounded bumps.

As the process of dilatation progresses, the lower border of the kidney pelvis sags more and more, and the uretero-pelvic junction creeps progressively upward in relationship to the kidney pelvis, so that the ureter no longer drains the pelvis at its lowest point but at a point much higher up, providing a water trap for the retention of the urine. Stagnation of urine always favors infection, and sooner or later this complication is bound to occur. Such dilation of the kidney pelvis is known as hydronephrosis; if infection has supervened, the condition is referred to as infected hydronephrosis or pyonephrosis. Dilatation of the terminal calices only is known as caliectasis.

Large saccular diverticula of the ureter have been reported which may resemble pelvic dilatation, (Culp).

Persistent hydronephrosis results in thinning of the kidney parenchyma. That this is an index of the damage which has been done by the pelvic dilatation would seem self-evident. Measurement of the parenchymal thickness whenever possible should be contained in the roentgenological interpretation, (Robins and Fischmann).

URETERAL OBSTRUCTION FROM OCCLUSION, CONSTRICTION OR KINKING. * Obstruction of the ureter from whatever cause, occlusion from stone, a new growth, cicatricial contraction or fibrous band, or kinking from pressure of an aberrant vessel or ptosis, may lead to enormous dilatation of the ureter. Even obstruction low down in the region of the neck of the bladder or posterior urethra from congenital valve formation, may cause ureteral dilatation which may even attain the calibre of the small intestine; as it dilates it becomes tortuous and may be thrown into folds.

Such obstruction may occur at any point along the urinary tract. Obstruction at the ureteropelvic junction is a very common site. It is most frequently due to:

1) occlusion from a stone, new growth or blood clot plugging the lumen,
2) constriction from pressure of an aberrant renal vessel or fibrous band,
3) kinking of the ureter due to ptosis of the kidney.

An opaque stone detected on flat film examination can easily be localized to the uretero-pelvic junction by pyelography (Fig. 276B$_1$). A nonopaque stone can usually be dislodged into another position in the kidney pelvis by introduction of a ureteral catheter. Blood clots are rarely so firm in consistency that they cannot be dislodged by lavage. Tumors, on the other hand, although they may present a somewhat different outline, usually remain undisturbed in the same location at subsequent examinations.

A very common cause of obstruction is con-

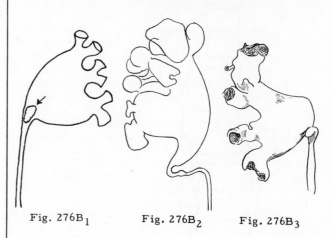

Fig. 276B$_1$ Fig. 276B$_2$ Fig. 276B$_3$

striction at the uretropelvic junction by pressure from an aberrant renal vessel (Fig. 276B$_2$). Any dilatation, confined to the kidney pelvis (unassociated with ureteral dilatation) must be assumed to be due to this cause. If the kidney pelvis is over distended the presence of an aberrant vessel defect may be readily over-shadowed; at some degree of filling however the characteristic appearance should be obtained. This may vary from an elongated cordlike defect from pressure of the vessel across the ureteropelvic junction, to merely a squaring of the lower margin of the kidney pelvis at its junction with the ureter. Fibrous bands may also give a similar appearance (Fig. 276B$_3$).

Kinking of the ureter from ptosis of the kidney is a very frequent cause of hydronephrosis and chronic septic infection (Fig. 276B$_4$). It can be demonstrated readily by examination in the upright position. Special urological x-ray tables are designed for elevating the patient into the upright position. Comparison of the films made in the horizontal and upright positions readily discloses the difference in position of the kidney with kinking of the ureter and pelvic dilatation. Prather has called attention to medial ptosis of the kidney as a cause of possible pathology.

Ptosis of the kidney in itself may not be of any pathological significance; it may however, cause urinary obstruction with subsequent infection and become a chronic source of septic infection. In searching for an obscure cause of septic infection it must always be borne in mind. At the time of obstruction the urine may be so completely blocked off from the diseased side that urinalysis will not show the presence of infection. In assuming the recumbent position, however, the infected side drains promptly and the temperature falls to normal. It must be considered that in any obscure case of prolonged temperature reaction, separate specimens of urine must be examined from each ureter and pyelograms must be made to exclude any anomalous development of the urinary tract, before the urinary tract can be completely eliminated as a source of possible infec-

tion. Ptosis implies descent of a kidney which was formerly in its normal high position; an ectopic kidney may have its normal position low down in the abdomen without abnormal function.

Obstruction of the ureter is most frequently caused by occlusion of stone, opaque or nonopaque, during its passage through the ureter.

Cicatrices produced by old scars from ureteral injury resulting from previous passage of urinary stones, may be single or multiple and may occur in any location in the ureter; the degree of dilatation of the ureter above the constriction depends upon the degree of obstruction produced. Obstruction at the ureterovesical junction leads to dilatation of the ureter often extending to the kidney pelvis (Fig. 276B$_5$).

URETERITIS CYSTICA. Ureteritis cystica, pyelitis cystica and cystitis cystica are similar conditions resulting from chronic inflammation. After the study and analysis of 57 cases, Loitman and Chiat are convinced that Von Brunn's widely accepted theory is the most plausible; cell nests develop from the downward proliferation of lining epithelium, separate and undergo central degeneration to become cysts. The typical roentgen appearance is that of multiple small round lucent defects producing a characteristic scalloping of the ureteral margins, when seen in profile. Such fibrocystic areas of thickening in the ureteral wall may so encroach upon the ureter that they cause obstruction.

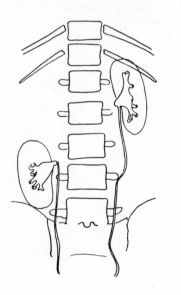

Fig. 276B$_4$

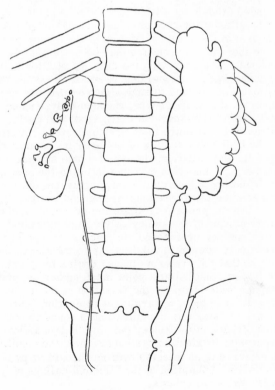

Fig. 276B$_5$

Occasionally such areas of thickening, although not obstructive in themselves, produce obstruction when combined with ptosis of the kidney.

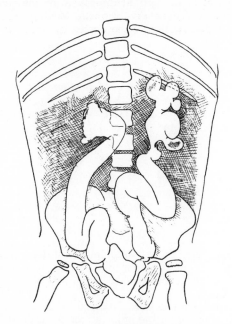

Fig. 276B₆

CONGENITAL VALVES. Congenital valves at the bladder neck in the posterior urethra produce the most extreme manifestation of ureteral dilatation. Transmission of the constant pressure from the bladder up through both ureters and kidney pelves results in enormous dilatation of the ureters so that they may attain fully the size of the small bowel and lie in folds upon themselves. This ultimately results in impaired renal function and death. Such stagnation of urine always favors infection.

Congenital ureteral valves (Fig. 276B₆) may produce a similar picture. These consist of redundant ureteral mucosa containing bands of smooth muscle. These are more common than are usually supposed (5% of new born infants) but do not obstruct and disappear in later life, (Wall and Wachter).

Bladder neck pathology can sometimes be demonstrated by micturating ureterograms taken during the act of urination, showing the neck of the bladder and urethra. Demonstration of congenital valves and other anomalous developments is possible (Williams).

INFLUENCE OF OBSTRUCTION ON RENAL FUNCTION (Fig. 277A and B). The excretory function of the kidney is influenced by delicately balanced pressures within the kidney and in the blood vessels. We have seen that excessive pressure exerted upon the pelvic structure by injection of opaque material

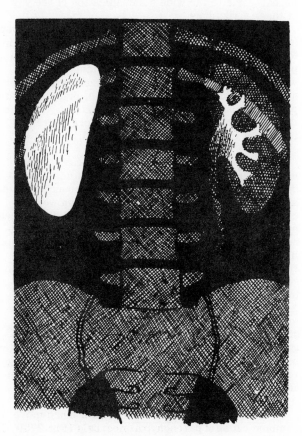

Fig. 277A

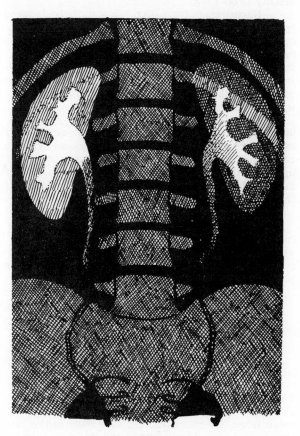

Fig. 277B

for pyelography results in forcing the contrast material back into the venous structures, resulting in pyelovenous backflow. Urinary excretion, then, depends upon a proper regulation of pressures between these structures; it would be expected that increased intrapelvic pressure might inhibit normal function.

This is found to be the case in excretory urography. Diodrast or Neo-Iopax injected intravenously should show excretion in the urine almost immediately and within a few minutes both kidney pelves should be well visualized on roentgenographic examination.

If there is excessive pressure in one kidney pelvis, excretion will be inhibited for a long period of time, even several hours. This may lead to an erroneous impression of a non-functioning kidney from parenchymal destruction. If the parenchymal tissue is unimpaired, the contrast medium will be stored up in the kidney tubules causing the kidney to assume a pronounced increase in roentgenographic density even though there is no evidence of excretion of the contrast medium. This we speak of as a "Nephrogram " (Fig. 277A).

If such a condition develops, roentgenograms should continue to be taken at hourly intervals and it will be found that from two to eight hours (or even longer) after injection the contrast material held up in the kidney substance, will be suddenly dumped into the kidney pelvis; the pelvic structures will become well outlined and the kidney will lose its abnormal density (Fig. 277B).

Nephrogram formation can usually be induced by either rapid injection of concentrated solution of opaque material, or by simultaneous intravenous and retrograde pyelograms (Herzan). The retrograde injection is made first and the catheter clamped; this is followed by intravenous injection. The increased pressure within the pelvis inhibits excretion of the intravenous material.

Nephrogram formation, intentionally induced, is utilized in examination of the kidney for certain types of parenchymal pathology, especially renal cysts and carcinoma. Defects of this sort will not contain the opaque material and will appear as less dense areas in the kidney. Tomography facilitates the demonstration of such pathology, (Evans, et al.).

INFECTION.* We have seen that infection is a frequent development in hydronephrosis secondary to urinary stasis. Active infection may occur without stasis however. Infection from direct blood stream inocculation may result in:
1) Pyelonephritis which primarily involves the kidney pelvis, or
2) Parenchymal infection of the kidney by direct blood stream inocculation.

PYELONEPHRITIS.* At the onset there is no perceptible difference in the pyelogram and at this stage diagnosis depends upon urine examination. The first indication of infection in the pyelogram is slight blunting of the calices. When infection is fully established, the minor calices lose their sharp cusps becoming rounded and clubbed and there is constric-

tion of the infundibula resulting in caliectasis (Fig. 278A). The kidney itself may show little involvement. Deformity of the pelvic structure may remain for life even after the patient improves, or the condition may become progressively worse leading to almost complete destruction of the cortex by pyogenic

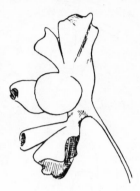

Fig. 278A

infection. Such an extreme degree of destruction of the kidney from infection is known as Pyonephrosis. It may be due to any type of organism, pyogenic or tuberculous.

Attention has been directed to the development of osteomyelitis of the spine as an occasional complication of urinary tract infection (Leigh, et al.), probably due to the wide communication of the veins of these structures.

That there is an important relationship between hypertension and chronic atrophic pyelonephritis, not found with other surgical renal lesions, has been amply demonstrated. The most important diseases which may be responsible for acquired renal atrophy are: atrophic chronic pyelonephritis, primary atrophy and pyonephrosis. Demonstration of a small unilateral contracted kidney may therefore be a very important finding, (Pendergrass, et al.).

Pyogenic infection,* gaining access to the kidney substance by way of the blood stream, may produce large abscesses or so-called "carbuncles of the kidney." Such infected areas may remain well encapsulated until the abscess ruptures and discharges by a fistulous tract into the kidney pelvis. The kidney itself undergoes enlargement presenting a tumor-like mass but rarely affects the kidney pelvis until rupture occurs when a fistulous tract results. Such abscesses are associated with constitutional symptoms of infection. Fortunately, they are very rare. A very unusual type of infection associated with numerous bubbles of gas throughout the kidney substance and pelvis is sometimes encountered due to gas bacillus infection. Kalmi has combined hydrogen peroxide with contrast media for retrograde pyelography for the detection of small areas of ulceration as indicated by formation of small bubbles.

Tuberculosis of the kidney* is a much more common cause of parenchymal necrosis (Fig. 278B, C, and D). Renal tuberculosis is always secondary to tuberculosis elsewhere in the body, usually pulmonary. Tubercle bacilli gain access to the kidney by way of the blood stream. In its early stage renal tuberculosis may not be recognized roentgenographically. The demonstration of tubercle bacilli in the urine is the only true method of diagnosis of the disease at this stage. The urine may be clear at this time but in its later stage albumin and leucocytes appear. Often the first clinical symptom is hematuria. Renal tuberculosis may attack the medulla or the cortex of the kidney. If the medulla is the site of involvement, it has a tendency to caseation and pelvic involvement; whereas, when cortical involvement predominates, caseous necrosis is less frequent and there is a tendency to fibrosis and calcification and healing with atrophy.

After the bacilli are found in the urine, pyelograms should

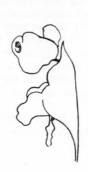

Fig. 278B

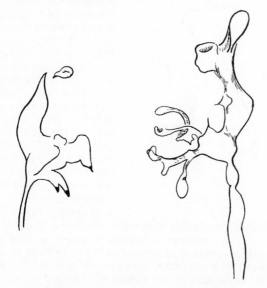

Fig. 278C   Fig. 278D

be made to determine the extent and location in the kidney. In a goodly number of cases, renal tuberculosis is bilateral; therefore, it is doubly essential to search carefully for evidence of involvement in the supposed "good" kidney before the removal of any diseased organ. Roentgenographically the pyelogram produced by leukoplakia is one of irregular cyst-like formations in the pelvis. This associated with passage of epithelial fragments is sufficient for the diagnosis. It is a precursor of squamous cell carcinoma and the kidney should be removed if possible, (Landes and Hamlin).

The earliest manifestation of renal involvement may be erosion of the minor calices, often of the upper pole. The lesion produced is essentially a pye-

lonephritis of tuberculous etiology. The tuberculous infection causes small areas of destruction in the papillary structures, resulting in a moth-eaten appearance in the minor calices. Continuous pouring of tuberculous infection into the calices, pelvis, ureter and bladder results in involvement of all of these structures. Tuberculous lesions of the pelvis result in strictures at the normal points of narrowing, especially the infundibula, with even complete pinching off of the minor calix, with formation of caliectasis or renal cysts. Such cysts may accumulate calcium (Holm). There may be stricture at the ureteropelvic junction and at numerous other regions in the ureter, giving the ureter a beaded appearance. Similar strictures may be produced by nontuberculous infections.

Calcium deposits may occur within caseous tuberculous areas in the medulla. Involvement may be so extensive that the kidney may become completely destroyed by caseous necrosis with calcification, giving rise to the so-called "putty kidney." Pyelonephrosis with complete destruction of the kidney may develop similar to that seen in infection from other causes.

Unusual complete calcification of the kidneys can also occur following vitamin D intoxication and from other conditions in which there is hypercalcemia with associated pyelonephrosis (Vaughn, et al.).

Complete saclike calcification may develop, encasing the entire kidney like a bag, from calcification of a subcortical hemorrhage from trauma.

TUMOR OF THE KIDNEY* (Fig. 279A, B, and C). Tumors may originate from any position or structure of the kidney. From the roentgenological standpoint those most frequently encountered may be roughly classified as to their location and physical characteristics as follows:

Tumors of the kidney:
I. Parenchyma
   A. Malignant
      1. Carcinoma
      2. Hypernephroma
      3. Sarcoma
      4. Wilm's tumor

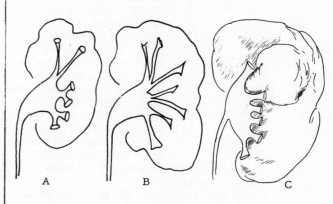

Fig. 279

B. Benign
  1. Solitary cysts
  2. Polycystic kidney
  3. Embryonic tumors—rare
    Other rarer tumors—adenoma,
    angioma, lipoma, fibroma, etc.
II. Pelvis
  A. Papillary tumors
    1. Benign papilloma
    2. Papillary carcinoma
  B. Nonpapillary tumors
    1. Squamous cell epithelioma (carcinoma)
    2. Transitional cell carcinoma
    3. Angiosarcoma

Parenchymal malignant tumors, unlike those arising in the pelvis, may attain considerable size before they give rise to symptoms. Depending upon their location, enlargement may be in either pole of the kidney (Fig. 279A) or it may be general. Tumors of the kidney, by their growth, may cause distortion and elongation of the kidney pelvis and calices due to enlargement of the tumor mass (Fig. 279B) or they may actually encroach upon and occlude any segment of the pelvic structures by pressure (Fig. 279C). If all of the calices are involved they may be drawn out and elongated giving the appearance of a "spider-leg" pelvis, (Fig. 279B). Such malignant tumors occurring in older individuals such as, carcinoma and hypernephroma, sarcoma, cannot be differentiated roentgenographically. They frequently form large rounded tumors with smooth margins similar to the benign solitary cyst. In children, Wilms' tumor produces enormous homogeneous enlargement of the kidney with pressure distortion of the kidney pelvis. They occur very rarely in adults, (Esersky, et al.).

SOLITARY CYST OF KIDNEY * (Fig. 280). Benign parenchymatous tumors of the kidney are

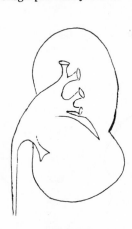

Fig. 280

much rarer in occurrence than malignant tumors. Of these solitary cysts of the kidney are least uncommon. Solitary cyst of the kidney cortex may, by pressure on the kidney pelvis, produce a rounded pressure defect which is evident in the roentgenogram. Such pressure may cause elongation of one or more calices, but they are never as slender and drawn out as those seen with new growth. Cysts of the lower pole displace the pelvis upward, those occurring in upper pole depress the pelvis. They are smooth and rounded and often appear denser than the kidney.

Cysts of this type may be due to simple serous cysts, hemorrhagic cysts, cysts associated with tumor, calcified cysts, hydatid, dermoid and tuberculous cysts, (Gutierrez). Such benign cysts are relatively rare; their appearance may be indistinguishable from hypernephroma.

Diagnostic Kidney Puncture. Diagnostic puncture of the kidney especially for differentiation between renal cysts, tumors and perirenal processes has been advocated by Lindblom. This is not done routinely but only where there is doubt. Injection of contrast medium is made if the diagnosis is questionable. In cysts the medium may sink to the bottom or become evenly mixed, with repeated withdrawals and injections. In tumors the contrast medium diffuses out into the growth in a characteristic manner.

POLYCYSTIC KIDNEY * (Fig. 281). Congenital polycystic kidney presents, first of all, an enlarged

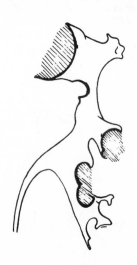

Fig. 281

kidney with a somewhat irregular nodular outline. The kidney pelvis is usually large in extent but often rather small in capacity. Pressure of numerous small cysts of the cortex on the calices and kidney pelvis produce an almost characteristic spindlelike narrowing of the major calices and flaring of the minor calices. When fully developed the diagnosis is simple, but in its early stages it may be quite difficult. Injection of the vasculature of the renal structures by aortography (q.v.) may produce conclusive diagnostic evidence, (Billing).

The condition is usually bilateral; in only a small percentage of instances (15 to 18%) is it observed as a unilateral involvement at autopsy. Almost invariably if one kidney is removed surgically for polycystic involvement, even if the other appears normal, the second kidney soon develops polycystic characteristics. It is, of course, congenital in origin but it may be dormant for many years and not give manifestations of its presence until well into adult life.

Polycystic disease in infants may be most difficult to recognize since they usually range from microscopic to a few millimeters in size. Collection of the opaque material in the tubules due to difficult excretion produces a tendency to nephrogram development which may be a clue to the examination. If the margin of the kidney is visualized through the stomach bubble the granular-like appearance of the tiny cysts may be visualized, (Hinkel and Saktini).

HEMANGIOMA OF KIDNEY. Hemangioma of the kidney is an unusual type of benign tumor. It usually occurs in the kidney parenchyma adjacent to the pelvic structures. It is associated with intermittent attacks of hematuria, a fact which may lead to a diagnosis of tuberculosis or carcinoma.

Roentgenologically the tumor produces rather suggestive manifestations; there is: compression of the fornix of a major calyx, with deformity of the infundibulum and filling defect throughout its major portion. A small amount of contrast material escapes from the edge of the calyx into the adjacent blood vessel tumor. The expanded club-shaped major calyx and its decrease in density are probably due to blood clots which it contains.

When such roentgen manifestations are present in a patient (usually under 40 years of age) having recurrent episodes of hematuria and renal colic, a diagnosis of renal hemangioma should be considered, (Friedman and Solis-Cohen).

Malignant tumors of the kidney frequently metastasize. In order of frequency the structures most often involved are: lungs, bones, liver, lymph nodes, and mediastinum.

Papillary Tumors (Fig. 282) arising in the pelvis rarely attain sufficient size to cause great enlargement of the kidney; because of their location they cause symptoms early in the disease. Pyelography cannot differentiate benign from malignant papillomata in the kidney pelvis. Papillomatous growths springing from the renal mucosa (A), project into the kidney pelvis. They may be single isolated lesions, in which case they must be differentiated from an air bubble, nonopaque stone, or blood clot. Air bubbles introduced by injection with the opaque material of course, will be easily displaced or eliminated by change in position of the patient. An unusual condition in which air bubbles appear in large numbers in the pelvis is in associated infection with gas bacillus, following septic infection from such causes as septic abortion. Nonopaque stones are usually small and may be displaced into new positions by position of the patient or may appear in different locations on subsequent examination. Polyps are attached to the surface and remain constant at all examinations projecting out into the kidney pelvis as rounded nonopaque filling defects. At times they extend down the ureter either as prolongations of pelvic growths or as implants in

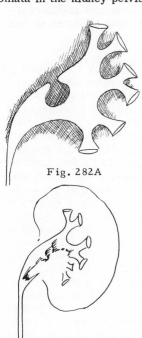

Fig. 282A

Fig. 282B

the ureter from the primary growths in the pelvis above. If multiple, they may completely fill the pelvis giving the appearance of polyposis. Such an appearance can be stimulated by ringlike gall stones superimposed on the kidney pelvis. Multiple gas bubbles, mentioned above, associated with gas bacillus infection may give this appearance; fortunately such infections are very rare. Small blood clots, if fresh, are usually rounded; but if organized, show an irregular margin and decomposition. Lavage of the pelvis changes their appearance on subsequent examination.

Nonpapillomatous tumors of the kidney pelvis (B) form filling-defects which project into and prevent complete filling of the pelvis the same as any other cavity. Their margins may be ragged and irregular or fairly smooth. They may be difficult to differentiate from blood clots but subsequent examination after lavage will show changes in appearance if they are due to a blood clot. Almost all tumors arising from the flat surface of the pelvis are malignant; their cell type cannot be differentiated roentgenologically. They may fill the pelvis and project down into the ureter causing complete occlusion. Squamous cell carcinoma of the renal pelvis is sometimes associated with longstanding kidney calculi.

PARENCHYMAL (CORTICAL) NECROSIS * (Fig. 283). The three conditions chiefly concerned in the production of parenchymal necrosis are: new growths, pyogenic abscess, and tuberculosis.

At times a large bulky tumor, by reason of deficient blood supply, becomes necrotic in the center of the growth, forming a large softened area. This finds its way to the kidney pelvis into which it discharges its necrotic infected material (A). Obviously, in such a case, opaque solution injected into the kidney pelvis will pass out beyond the normal confines of the pelvis into the ragged irregular cavity in the parenchyma. Any condition then, in which injected opaque solution escapes from the pelvis into the surrounding kidney cortex must be due to "parenchymal necrosis." The cause of necrosis cannot always be determined from the roentgenogram

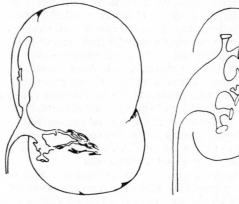

Fig. 283A   Fig. 283B

alone, but usually correlation with the other roentgen findings and clinical history is sufficient to come to a conclusion.

When necrosis occurs as a result of tumor formation, it rarely occurs until the tumor is large and bulky. By this time, during its growth, the tumor has left other unmistakable signs of its presence on the other pelvic structures, such as elongation of calices or pressure and destruction of the pelvis (Fig. 283A). The fistulous tract is relatively small.

Primary abscess of the kidney from direct blood stream inoculation causes local necrosis of the kidney substance, breaking through by a fistulous tract to discharge its pus into the kidney pelvis, intestine or through the diaphragm. The fistulous tract is relatively small. The pelvic structure itself may show no dilatation or other abnormality, or there may be distortion of the calices from pressure of the abscesses (Fig. 283B). The pinching off of calices from scar tissue retraction with caliectasis of the terminal calices is a very reliable sign in chronic tuberculous infection.

Hematuria, usually of an intermittent type, is a common accompaniment of both tuberculous infection of the kidney, and tumor; it may be difficult to differentiate between the two conditions. In tumor the effect of new growth on the kidney pelvis is the chief manifestation, necrosis is only secondary, whereas in tuberculous infections there are less manifestations of distortion of the pelvis from new growth. In tuberculosis likewise there are often multiple fine calcifications at the periphery. The detection of tubercle bacilli in the urine is, of course, an absolute indication of the true nature of the disease.

RENAL PAPILLARY NECROSIS; (NECROTIZING PAPILLITIS).

This is an unusual type of acute infection of the papillary structures of the kidney which usually occurs in diabetic patients; of 181 cases reported to 1956, only 10% did not have diabetes; Evans and Ross in a study of the subject point out that, "1) it is a suddenly developing and rapidly progressing necrotizing bacterial lesion that must be treated aggressively and without delay. 2) The selective necrosis involving the tips of the papillae impairs the urinary drainage of the associated nephrons, making definitely hazardous the use of sulfanamide drugs and related compounds with their known tendency to precipitate out in the renal tubules under conditions of urinary stasis or acid-base imbalance."

The infection starts with scattered abscesses located in the renal pyramids; these coalesce causing necrosis and sloughing of the pyramid structures which may be passed in the urine and recognized microscopically leading to the diagnosis. All pyramids of both kidneys may be involved in complete sequestration of these vital structures.

Roentgenologically the early diagnosis may be difficult or impossible. Since the infection does not immediately attack the calyceal structures (Ottoman, et al.), pyelograms may not disclose the destruction taking place in the renal papillae, and not until these are involved does haziness of the calyceal structures become evident. The findings bear a striking resemblance to renal tuberculosis.

Christoffersen and Andersen have concluded after the study of 8 cases of renal papillary necrosis that this rare condition is almost invariably fatal with its highest mortality in elderly patients with diabetes mellitus or other urologic pathology. It is always associated with pyelonephritis and its symptoms include those of any other profound infection, such as high fever, pain, chills, pyuria, even anuria, etc. The onset is severe and the symptoms pronounced; it is the severity of the symptoms in a known diabetic which gives the initial clue. Olson has found that neither diabetes nor obstruction is necessary for production of necrotizing papillitis but both are most frequent etiological factors in the presence of infection. Although many diabetics have both, in only a few does the condition develop. Either spontaneous renal or perirenal emphysema or necrotizing papillitis may occur with similar factors of obstruction and infection.

CALYCEAL DIVERTICULUM.

These are rounded cyst-like structures occurring in the parenchyma and connected by a narrow channel with the pelvis, therefore visible on pyelograph examination. They are thought to be congenital in origin. They may resemble the saccular lesions of papillary n-necrosis but are not attended with the same degree of profound illness.

ANOMALIES OF THE KIDNEY.*

Anomalies of development, size, position, form or outline, and structure give rise to many bizarre appearances which under most instances must be considered as normal for the individual. First of all, there may be a congenital failure of development of one kidney known as RENAL AGENESIA. Under such conditions the remaining kidney is larger than normal and is more apt to be the site of disease. Or an entirely separate extra kidney may be present known as a supernumerary kidney. Their structure may be in every respect similar to fully developed kidneys. The kidneys may be located in almost any position in the abdomen, or even in the thorax, (Weens and Johnston; Schwartz and Frankel). They may be low down, in the true pelvis (ectopic) (Fig. 284A), or they may both be on the same side of the abdomen (crossed ectopic). They may be rotated on their vertical or horizontal axes giving rise to a peculiar axial appearance of the calices as views "on end" (Fig. 284B). Both ureters may go to a single kidney structure or the two kidneys may be fused on one side of the abdomen (fused kidneys), (Fig. 284C). Small kidneys known as atrophic or infantile kidneys are occasionally encountered.

The two kidneys may be fused by their cortical portions across the spine, each retaining its own separate kidney pelvis and ureter producing a so-called "horseshoe" kidney (Fig. 285); in this event the cortical portions are directed inward near the

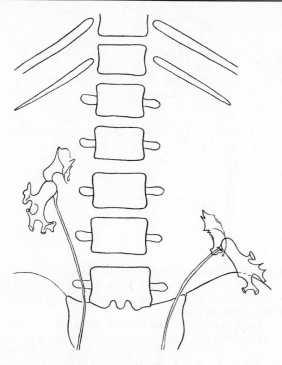

Fig. 284A

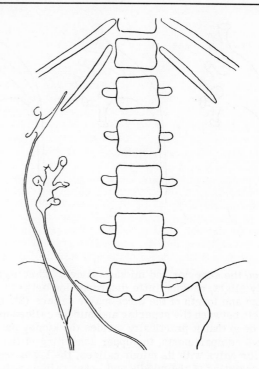

Fig. 284C

lower poles over the spine and the pelves are on either side with the calices of each directed inward. In horseshoe kidney the basal-pyelographic angle is often less than 20^0 as pointed out by Gutierrez, whereas in the normal individual it is usually 90^0. The apex of this angle is in the midline at the level of a line drawn across the iliac crests; the sides of the angle are formed by lines projected upward through the innermost calices. Petrovcic and Milic report an unusual case on asymmetrical "horseshoe" kidney in which the left ureter was situated both to the left and right of the midline of the body possessing two pelves connected together; a single ureter emerged from the right pelvis, crossed the body to enter the bladder on the left.

The various types of crossed ectopia with fusion have been very well illustrated by Abeshouse.

ANOMALIES OF KIDNEY PELVIS AND URETER (Fig. 286). *

The kidney pelvis and ureter are more commonly the site of anoma-

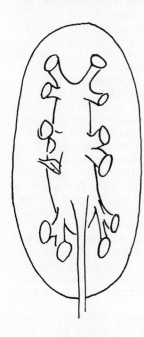

Fig. 284B

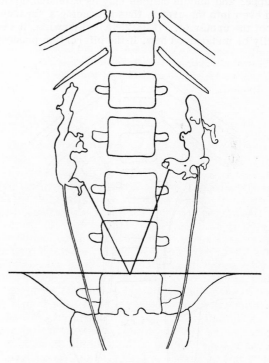

Fig. 285

lous development (1). The various configurations of the kidney pelves observed in different individuals may be most disconcerting unless the natural process of development is borne in mind. The chief variation in kidney pelves is seen in the degree of indenture

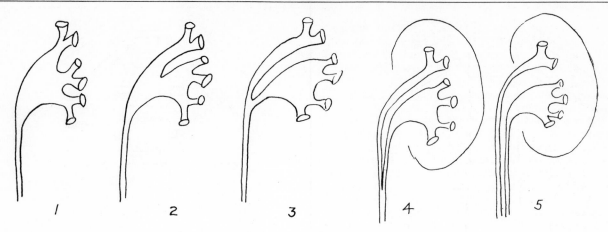

Fig. 286

between the superior and middle calices. This may be only slight, causing little disproportion between the size and length of the three major calices (2). Or the cleft between the superior and middle calices may be so deep that it practically divides the kidney pelvis into two compartments, the upper consisting of the superior calyx with its minor calices, the lower portion consisting of the middle and lower calices with their groups of minor calices, giving rise to a "bifurcated" kidney pelvis (3). This same cleft between the upper and middle calices may be extended downward even into the ureter, thus producing a "branching" of the ureter (4) (Fig. 286A). Likewise, it can readily be understood how, if the bifurcation process

extends far down the ureter to the bladder region, it will result in complete division and duplication of the ureter, "double ureter," both opening by separate orifices into the bladder (5).

Such anomalies are usually, at least in some degree, bilateral. They are normal for the individual and are in themselves of no pathological significance. It is necessary, however, to know of their existence and characteristics in order that they may not be falsely suspected as pathological phenomena. Very rarely caudal bifurcation of the ureter has been reported with two openings in the bladder, (Phokitis). There were no untoward symptoms and apparently no predisposition for disease.

INJURIES TO THE KIDNEY. In this day of mass construction and high speed transportation, the kidneys are frequently the site of accidental injury. The kidney substance may be damaged, with appearance of blood in the urine. Injection of opaque solution shortly after the accident may or may not reveal any escape from the pelvic structure into the parenchyma. If extravasation of the injected material is evident, there can be no doubt of injury, but if it is not present this does not exclude injury to the parenchyma. Intravenous urography would seem to be a safe method of procedure (Echternacht). Such fistulous tracts may not heal for many months. If injury to the cortex has been great and blood has escaped in great quantities into the surrounding perirenal tissues, there may be obliteration of the shadow of the psoas muscle. The psoas shadow may also be obliterated in fractures of the transverse processes of the spine as a result of hemorrhage and from a number of other conditions. The diagnosis may depend largely upon the clinical judgment of the urologist. Subcapsular hemorrhages from injury may ultimately result in a calcified, bag-like structure enveloping the entire kidney. This may remain as a permanent landmark for life.

Aneurysm of the renal artery may follow injury to the kidney region. Pulsation of a tumor mass in

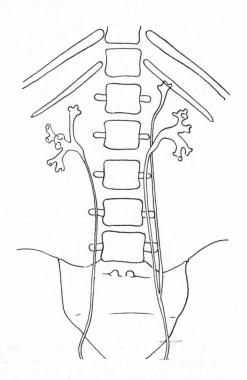

Fig. 286A

the kidney region is usually very difficult or impossible. Calcium deposit in the aneurysmal wall may lend a clue to the diagnosis. Abdominal aortography should establish the diagnosis. Previous trauma or infection are the usual etiological factors; syphilis does not seem to be a factor in its cause, (Solis-Cohen and Steinbach).

Foreign bodies of a wide variety have been found in the kidney and kidney pelvis. These may gain access from the outside, as shrapnel from a gun-shot wound or a tooth pick from the gastrointestinal tract or from insertion into the urinary tract, as for instance a blade of grass which, following insertion into the bladder by the urethra found its way up the ureter from its peristaltic action and finally reached the kidney pelvis where it became the center for a stone (Osmond).

Injury to the kidney from operative procedure may occur; fistula formation may even result if the pelvis or ureter is damaged; such false passages can easily be visualized after opaque injection.

Intravenous injection may show complete suppression of secretion after injury. This may be due merely to shock and is not in itself evidence of injury. After recovery from the immediate shock, function may again be resumed.

Spontaneous pneumopyelogram and perirenal emphysema may occur in diabetes. The writer has encountered a case in which perirenal emphysema occurred from gas bacillus infection following septic abortion.

Circumcaval Ureter. This is a condition of malposition of the ureter in which it swings to and beyond the midline in its lower portion passing posterior to the vena cava. Lateral view shows the ureter posterior,—not anterior normally located—to the vein. This is due to anomalous development and is ordinarily of no pathological significance. Operative correction has been successful.

Deviation of Ureter from Retroperitoneal Metastasis. Extension of testicular tumors to the retroperitoneal pre-aortic lymph nodes may result in deviation of the upper portion of the ureter and kidney away from the spine. If previous roentgenograms have shown normal relationship, and displacement subsequently develops, it may be considered as evidence of retroperitoneal metastasis.

PSOAS MUSCLE SHADOW

PERINEPHRITIC ABSCESS (Fig. 287). Positive roentgen findings are of value; lack of roentgen evidence does not exclude the condition. Roentgen manifestations are:
1. obliteration of the shadow of the psoas muscles; this sign is somewhat variable
2. kidney outline maintained, may be slightly enlarged—a very constant sign
3. scoliosis of the spine, concavity toward side of involvement. This is a sign which is most frequently present in chronic cases

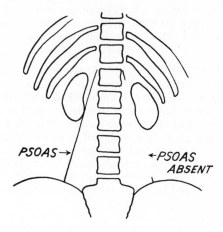

Fig. 287

4. decrease diaphragmatic movement on respiration; a rather constant sign but one which occurs with many types of infection or irritation, (Butts and Conley)
5. fixation of the kidney on inspiration-expiration pyelogram.

Normally the shadows of the psoas muscles are clearly defined running obliquely downward and outward along the lower two dorsal and lumbar vertebrae. We have seen how intramuscular and interstitial hemorrhage in this region may obliterate the shadow of the psoas muscle; pus collected in the perirenal region may produce a similar obliteration of the psoas muscle shadow; the kidney itself may remain clearly outlined in the midst of perinephritic infection. If the infection is not diffuse but remains localized the psoas shadow may not be obliterated. Similarly carcinomatous infiltration may obliterate the psoas muscle if the process is expensive.

The kidney itself is not involved and usually presents a clearly outlined border.

BLADDER

METHODS OF EXAMINATION OF THE BLADDER. Normally, the bladder filled with urine offers sufficient contrast with the surrounding structures to be faintly visible in the ordinary roentgenogram (Fig. 288A). It appears as a smooth, rounded, sharply defined structure extending upward just above the symphysis. Injection methods for demonstration of bladder pathology utilize media either of greater density than the body tissues, such as skiodan or potassium iodide solution or media of lesser density, such as air inflated through a catheter into the bladder. The

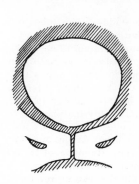

Fig. 288A

opaque injection is of advantage in outlining the mucosa for large growths, diverticula, etc.; the air injection is more satisfactory for detection of polypi and other small or pedunculated tumors.

FOREIGN BODIES IN BLADDER. The bladder is a large rounded hollow viscus, easily accessible from the outside through the urethra. All manner of foreign bodies have, therefore, been found in this organ from sticks of wood, straws, nails and fever thermometers, to beeswax, tallow and chewing gum. Fragments of catheters may be broken off or an entire catheter may be introduced into the bladder by the patient. The danger of such foreign bodies remaining in the bladder is from the fact that they become the nuclei for stones.

BLADDER CALCULI. Stones may, of course, occur in the bladder without the presence of a foreign body. A large percentage of urinary stones are calcareous and are therefore opaque to x-rays; but a small percent are organic. Many bladder stones are composed of a number of different chemicals which are deposited as the stone continues to form. Uric acid and urate stones are common in the bladder but rare in the kidney pelvis; they are nonopaque. Calcium oxalate stones can usually be identified by their shape. They may produce heavy starshaped radiations, the so-called "jack stone", or if more fully developed these radiations may be finer terminating in a small bumpy surface giving the appearance of a mulberry. Nonopaque stones may be visualized by injection of a small amount of opaque media. On cystoscopic examination calcium oxalate stones appear black.

Small stones, even of the opaque variety, may be very easily overlooked in the bladder, owing to the scattering of the x-rays produced by the large volume of urine in the bladder. The patient should therefore be instructed to clean out the rectum with an enema and to evacuate the bladder before examination.

Stones in the bladder may attain enormous size; a single stone even completely filling the bladder. They may be multiple and faceted; they may be smooth in outline and structure or they may be laminated from layer upon layer of deposits over long periods of time. Such stones may form within large diverticula.

CYSTOGRAPHY.* The bladder, like most other hollow organs, can be filled with opaque solution to obtain a silhouette of its mucosal lining. The tendency of any particle of foreign material remaining in the bladder to form the nucleus for stone deposits, however, makes it imperative that anything injected into the bladder be perfectly soluble and easily expelled. Barium sulphate solution, for instance, should never be used in the bladder.

Lipiodol likewise, although not dangerous, is not satisfactory for this purpose. Because of its oily consistency it is not freely miscible with water, breaking up into droplets within the watery medium.

In an emergency, if skiodan or other non-irritating preparation is not available, 5 to 10% sodium iodide solution from a radiological standpoint is just as satisfactory. It is much more irritating, however, and should be flushed out immediately after the examination is made.

CUNNINGHAM'S SOLUTION

Sodium Iodide	36.
Red Iodide of Mercury	0.1
Water q.s. ad	300.

has the added advantage of being an antiseptic.

If there is any possibility of rupture of the organ the non-irritating skiodan solution must be used.

This is especially useful where it is desirable to determine a rough estimate of residual amount of urine retained after voiding (Brailsford, et al.).

ABNORMALITIES OF SIZE AND SHAPE OF BLADDER. The normal bladder is rounded and smooth in outline, extending upward from behind the symphysis pubis in the midline. Following an extended period of tenesmus or inflammation from any cause, the bladder may become very small in size although it still maintains its rounded contour. The bladder may assume an oval shape in the anteroposterior diameter giving the appearance in the posterior view of a double superimposed ringlike shadow.

Atony of the bladder (Fig. 288B) occurs most frequently in women after repeated childbirth has resulted in relaxation of the pelvic floor; the bladder loses its rounded contour and becomes flattened in appearance. If cystocele occurs it may bulge outward under the symphysis. Occasionally tumor masses in the pelvis arising from the pelvic organs or the uterus itself may encroach upon the bladder so much that pressure defects are produced on the bladder from extrinsic pressure. In carcinoma of the sigmoid such defects occur. These may be the first indication of existence of the growth.

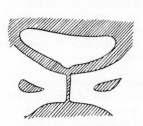

Fig. 288B

DIVERTICULA OF BLADDER* (Fig. 289). Diverticula of the bladder are not uncommonly found associated with bladder neck obstruction. They are most frequently of the pulsion variety, oval, pouchlike extension from the bladder. They are frequently multiple and vary in size from scarcely larger than a pea to greater capacity than the bladder itself. They may spring from any location in the bladder but are most commonly encountered on the posterior wall. They are frequently seen laterally on either side near the ureters. In this location they may cause pressure on the ureters. Very rarely the ureters may empty into them—under such conditions operative removal is a much more difficult and serious procedure. When they occur on the anterior surface or fundus they are most readily accessible for removal.

Diverticula springing from the anterior or posterior wall of the bladder would be obscured in

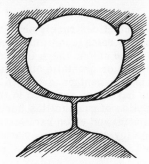

DIVERTICULA

Fig. 289

the roentgenogram when the bladder is filled with opaque material—for this reason other examinations should be made in the oblique views after evacuation in suspected cases; the diverticulum is smooth, the bladder wall roughened.

If the diverticular pouch exceeds the size of the bladder itself, it may be found difficult to identify the bladder structure itself from roentgen examination; post-evacuation examination will readily determine this point since the bladder will empty, leaving the diverticula partially filled.

Occasionally diverticula may be filled with debris and cannot be readily demonstrated without inserting a ureteral catheter by cystoscopic examination through the orifice of the diverticulum into its cavity, filling the cavity of the diverticulum directly.

Such diverticula may be filled with stones. They have frequently been observed packed with faceted stones resembling gall stones. Malignant growths may occasionally occur in diverticula.

A diverticulum-like pouch is occasionally encountered as a remnant of the urachus; it may be distinguished by its wide neck, located at the fundus of the bladder. Snow has reported a urachal cyst with round opaque calculi in the right lower quadrant of the abdomen with operative confirmation.

URETEROCELE. These are small rounded pouch-like projections of the ureters as they bulge into the bladder; usually a minute pin-point ureterovesicle orifice is the cause of the local dilatation. Urine, dammed back by the small opening, dilates the terminal end of the ureter until by its size it dilates the orifice sufficiently for urine to pass through the hole, when decompression rapidly results.

Roentgenologically these appear as rounded projections at the ends of the ureters, filled with opaque material during excretory urography, shown only immediately after micturation. If the bladder is filled with opaque solution, the rounded bulging ureteroceles, filled with non-opaque urine, show as negative shadows within the bladder; they remain constant within the same location. The cystogram

may assume a "cobra head" appearance due to pressure from the bilateral cystocele pouches, (Gottlieb, et al.).

TRABECULATION OF THE BLADDER. In chronic obstruction of the bladder neck by hypertrophy of the prostate or other cause, progressive enlargement of the bladder develops. At first the bladder retains its rounded outline but as distention progresses it loses its smooth border with the formation of cuplike projections through the muscular fibers into the bladder wall—this is known as trabeculation. As the condition progresses these pouches become larger forming multiple diverticula which may stud the entire surface of the bladder wall. Distention of the bladder may continue until it is enormous in size extending well up to the level of the umbilicus.

NEUROGENIC BLADDER. Interference with the normal innervation of the bladder may result in overdistention and paradoxical incontinence. As a result of chronic overdistention the bladder becomes trabeculated and irregular in outline with the formation of numerous cuplike projections. These may even go on to multiple diverticula formation. This condition commonly occurs in tabes dorsalis.

CONGENITAL VALVES. Congenital valves in the posterior urethra (q.v.) are occasionally encountered which cause chronic obstruction resulting in enormous dilatation of the entire urinary tract including the ureters and kidney pelves.

TUMORS OF BLADDER* (Fig. 290). Tumors most frequently encountered are:

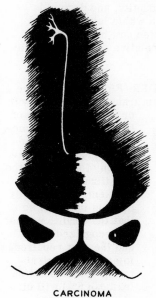

CARCINOMA

Fig. 290

A. Papillomata
  1. Benign
  2. Papillary carcinoma
B. Nonpapillary tumors
  1. Leiomyomata (benign) and leiomyosarcoma have been reported in the bladder wall
  2. Squamous cell epithelioma (carcinoma)
  3. Transitional cell carcinoma
  4. Adenocarcinoma (rare)

Differentiation between a benign and malignant papilloma is impossible. For demonstration of small pedunculated growths springing from the bladder wall and projecting into the bladder, air-cystography is essential. To obtain the best view for demonstration of the tumor, examination must be made in anterior, the posterior and both oblique views. The air rising to the top over any residual urine envelops the growth and renders it clearly visible. Opaque cystograms would obliterate the shadow.

Larger growths produce a definite filling defect in the bladder wall similar to filling defects produced by carcinomatous lesions in the gastrointestinal tract. Determination of the cellular type of the tumor from the roentgen appearance is not possible. Carcinomatous infiltration of the ureterovesical junction may either completely obstruct the orifice causing destruction of the ureter or may render the orifice widely patent so that opaque media will encounter no resistance but reflux up into the ureter and kidney pelvis. Occasionally cell implants from carcinoma of the kidney pelvis above form metastases in the bladder. Blood clots in the bladder may produce similar filling defects but lavage and reexamination will determine the inconstancy of the lesion.

Benign leiomyoma, and leiomyosarcoma (when it has undergone malignant degeneration), produce a rather destructive picture when they occur in the bladder. Like benign tumors of this sort, when they occur elsewhere in other hollow organs, they produce smooth rounded defects which clearly disturb the mucosal markings. When filled with opaque material, the rounded smooth defect produced by this type of tumor is very characteristic; the only other things which it might be confused with would be large nonopaque stone, or ureterocele at proper stage of distention, (Samuel).

Ovarian tumors and fibroids occurring in the female pelvis may have extensive calcium deposits readily establishing their identity, and dermoids may have rudimentary teeth within large rounded tumors. Cusmano has pointed out, however, that many dermoids show only relative radiolucency due to their fat content.

RUPTURE OF BLADDER (Fig. 291). Rupture of the distended bladder from trauma may occur with

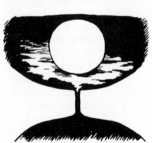

RUPTURED BLADDER

Fig. 291

or without fracture of the pubic bones immediately over the bladder region. Extravasation of urine into the soft tissues is very frequently followed by serious infection so that the condition must be recognized early and the rent repaired. Injection of nonirritating opaque solution (skiodan 5%) will disclose whether the bladder is intact or if there is a rupture of the organ permitting escape of opaque material into the surrounding tissues. If the rupture is into the retro-

peritoneal interstitial tissue there is irregular diffusion of the drug into the soft tissues; if it is into the peritoneal cavity, the outlines of intestinal loops of bowel can be seen impressed upon the opaque fluid. Fistulous tracts into perivesical abscesses or adjacent organs may also be demonstrated in this manner. For detection of a small rent in the posterior portion of the bladder which might be obscured by the media-filled organ another film should be taken after evacuation or a second film should be made laterally.

CYSTITIS. Bladder infections rarely show any demonstrable evidence on the roentgenogram. The mucosal outline is smooth and unless there is communication with a perivesicle or prostatic abscess no evidence can be seen in the roentgenogram. All manner of rare infections have been reported in the bladder but with the exception of gas bacillus infection (gas in interstitial tissue) and colon bacillus infection in diabetic patients (cystitis emphysematosa) these show no distinctive features.

CYSTITIS EMPHYSEMATOSA. Under rare unusual conditions, usually associated with diabetes, air cysts may develop beneath the bladder mucosa, giving rise in the roentgenogram to an appearance of a fine zone of air encircling the bladder (Lund, et al.; Boijsen and Lewis-Jonsson).

THE PROSTATE

PROSTATIC CALCULI. Prostatic calculi are not uncommon. Multiple minute stones form in the many prostatic ducts giving an appearance in the roentgenogram of a rosette or cluster of calcareous deposits immediately beneath the symphysis pubis.

Enlargement of the prostate causes elevation of the bladder which results in upward "hooking" of the ureters at their vesicular junctions, a condition which can frequently be suspected from the ordinary excretory urogram (Kretschmer).

Both air and opaque cystograms are of value in demonstrating enlargement of the prostate. Opaque cystograms may outline very clearly the prostatic enlargement if the bladder is not overfilled. Reexamination after micturition reveals the amount of residual urine. Air cystograms taken in the right oblique view reveal the enlarged prostate projecting upward into the air-filled bladder. Both lateral lobes and the posterior commissure can be visualized. The spherical projection caused by enlargement of the gland of Albarran can be identified. By far the greatest amount of information is obtained however from the combined use of air cystogram and urethral examination with opaque material. Prostatic enlargement and other prostatic pathology are best demonstrated by the secondary effects which they produce on the posterior urethra, (Middlemiss).

Injection of the prostatic and periprostatic veins may be of aid in diagnosis of thrombophlebitis of these and other pelvic structures, (Abeshouse and Ruben); (for teaching see Manual of Roentgenological Technique).

THE URETHRA

FOREIGN BODIES IN URETHRA. The urethra, being readily accessible also, is the site of many foreign bodies. These, of course, cause pain and discomfort and cannot remain for as long a time in place as they can in the bladder, but must be removed.

URETHRAL CALCULI. Urethral calculi are indeed very rare, usually a stone which will pass through the upper portion of the urinary tract will pass through the urethra readily; occasionally, however, they are temporarily delayed. Occasionally stones actually form in a dilated urethra behind a stricture. They may become as large as ordinary gallstones and form in clusters showing facets. Flat film examination is sufficient for detection of these conditions, since practically all stones occurring in this location contain some calcium salts and are therefore readily visualized. Calcium incrustation about a foreign body, such as a small segment of a catheter, is also readily detected.

URETHROGRAPHY

Examination. For the visualization of the urethra injection of opaque material is essential. For this purpose a viscous jellylike medium is more satisfactory than a thin aqueous solution. Skiodan Viscus Solution or Umbradil-Viscous-U Solution has proven most satisfactory for this purpose, (Coe and Arthur; Morales and Romanus). Examination must be made while the material is still being injected—otherwise the posterior urethra will not be properly filled. The combined use of air cystography and opaque urethrography taken in the right posterior oblique position, as suggested by Flocks, has been found most satisfactory. Urethrocystographic examination during micturation has yielded valuable information as to the condition of the bladder and urethra in demonstrating areas of induration, differentiation of true stricture from spasm, etc. This is a method which should be used more extensively, (Edling). Jensen has perfected an instrument for the ready performance of urethrography which is based upon the tube and cuff principle of intubation anaesthesia.

The instrument consists of a rubber catheter with a stopcock and air inflatable cuff located a short distance from the subterminal aperture connected to a rubber tube. The catheter is introduced only so far into the urethra that the cuff lies in the fossa navicularis. The cuff is then inflated by an ordinary hypodermic syringe so that the catheter is held firmly in the urethra. The air pressure in the cuff is maintained by the application of a clamp to the rubber tubing. After injection of opaque material the fluid is maintained in place by the stopcock.

Normal Urethra* (Fig. 292). The urethra consists of two portions, the deep or prostatic portion and the pendulous or cavernous part. The deep urethra extends from the inner sphincter at the bladder neck, to the external sphincter at its junction with the pendulous urethra. It is three to four centimeters in length and varies in calibre throughout. The anterior wall of the deep urethra makes a smooth sweep backwards, while the posterior wall shows a more acute backward angulation, with widening of the calibre just below the verumontanum, an impression of which can often be visualized on the urethral margin. Definite narrowing is seen at both the internal and external sphincters.

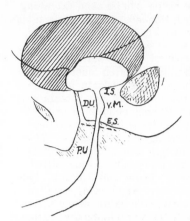

D.U. - Deep or Prostatic Urethra
P.U. - Pendulous Urethra
I.S. - Internal Sphincter
V.M. - Verumontanum

Fig. 292

During its course it extends through the prostate gland so that pathological changes in the gland are reflected in the impressions made upon the urethra.

Prostatic Enlargement.* Any type of prostatic enlargement will by its growth cause elongation of the posterior urethra.

Prostatic Carcinoma* (Fig. 293A) usually causes tense enlargement of the gland because of limitation by its capsule until late in the disease. This results in, 1) uniform annular constriction of the calibre of the posterior urethra and 2) straightening of its entire course.

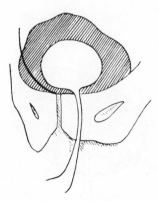

Fig. 293A

Prostatitis because of the edema and inflammatory reaction causes a similar effect which often simulates the findings of carcinomatous involvement.

Usually however, the clinical history serves to differentiate the conditions. If a prostatic or periurethral abscess exists which communicates with the urethra, the pouchlike cavity can be seen extending out into the periurethral tissues. Osteoblastic metastases may be demonstrated in the bony structures, (q.v.).

Benign Hypertrophy of the Prostate* (Fig. 293B) is the condition which so often must be differentiated from carcinoma. Here the pathological process is one of localized fibrous hyperplasia with gradual pressure of the fibrous nodules on the remaining normal prostatic tissue until it becomes thinned by pressure forming a false capsule. This pressure takes place in both lateral lobes flattening the membranous urethra from side to side called "spreading" of the urethra (Kerr and Gillies). This is one of the most distinctive signs of hyperplasia of the lateral lobes. Forward angulation of the upper end of the urethra above the verumontanum, called "tilting", is indication of hypertrophy of the posterior commissure.

In all of these conditions the air cystogram discloses the enlarged prostate projecting into the air-filled bladder (Fig. 293C). In the oblique view the two lateral lobes can be identified by two overlapping curves and the posterior commissure can be clearly identified, projecting upward posteriorly. A spherical defect is produced by an enlargement of the gland of Albarran. Correlation of these findings with those obtained from the opaque urethrogram

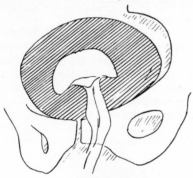

Fig. 293B

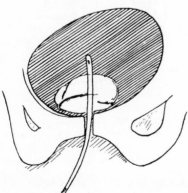

Fig. 293C

serve not only to determine the location but also the extent of the involvement. Obstruction of the posterior urethra without associated prostatic hypertrophy may be caused by a "median bar." This is due to a fold of tissue at the posterior surface of the neck of the bladder. The orifice between the urethra and bladder is so constricted that the viscus solution shows a "tooth-paste" like appearance which is quite characteristic (Kerr and Gillies).

Congenital Constriction of the Bladder Neck from fibrous bands may be clearly demonstrated. Opaque cystographic examination will show reflux into the ureters and kidney pelves with marked ureterectasis and hydronephrosis. Diverticula of the urethra have been found with greater frequency in women by this method; these show merely as pouches, (Higgins and Rambousek).

Neurogenic or "Cord" Bladder may result in similar trabeculation of bladder, ureterectasis and hydronephrosis. Urethrographic examination however in these instances reveals complete relaxation of the internal sphincter resulting in conical widening of the urethra at the vesicle neck; the external sphincter remains intact.

Rupture of the Posterior Urethra from external trauma, instrumentation and infection may result in fistulous tracts into the periurethral tissues, perineum or adjacent hollow viscera. These may be clearly outlined by the injected material.

The pendulous or cavernous portion of the urethra varies in length with the length of the organ; its shadow when distended with opaque material usually measures about two centimeters (Fig. 294). The pendulous portion of the urethra is the most frequent site of stricture from gonorrhoeal involvement. Chronic infection of this type results in extreme uniform constriction of the calibre throughout this entire portion of the urethra which apparently remains throughout life. The surface is smooth unless false passages occur resulting in periurethral involvement. Excessive pressure where such pouches exist may result in escape of the opaque material into the

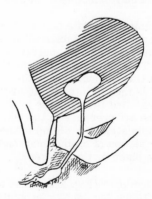

Fig. 294

corpus cavernosum or even into the vascular system. The material being nontoxic and nonirritating does not seem to produce any deleterious effect. Diverticula, single or multiple, have been noted involving the urethra.

Seminal Vesicles, (Fig. 295). The seminal vesicles are occasionally seen in the flat roentgenogram when calcified. They appear as two "wormlike" structures curling upward and outward from the midline just above the prostate. The ejaculatory ducts can be injected with opaque material through an endoscope for the demonstration of the seminal vesicles and ducti deferentia. Tucker, et al. have carried out direct injections into the vas deferens in its passage through the scrotum for filling these structures. Pereira has carried out a large number of such examinations and has been able to identify dysfunction in failure to empty, hypoplasia or lack of proper filling due to chronic inflammation and ectasia. The scrotal portion of the vas deferens is surgically exposed for the injection. The seminal vesicle may be the site of stones. Dull aching subpubic pain of 8 years duration was found by Cornwell to be due to stones in the seminal tract. Operative specimen showed stones to be present in right vas deferens.

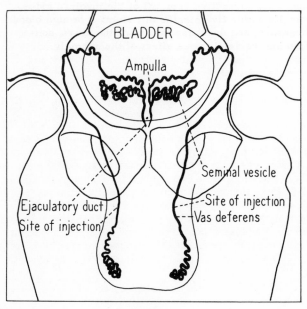

Fig. 295

PERINEAL OPERATIVE PROCEDURES COMPLICATIONS: OSTEITIS PUBIS AND ISCHII

Operative procedures in close relationship to the prostate, posterior urethra or other perineal structures, may be followed within a few days or weeks by a low grade infection of the pubic bones and ischii which is very painful and intractable in its course but ultimately usually heals without permanent disability (Lame and Chang). This infection may even spread to involve the hip joint or spine (deFeo; Lewitan and Nathanson). This is explained by injury to the deep venous plexus incident to operative procedure; hip or spine involvement, by spread along the adjacent venous plexuses (Batson). Roentgen therapy to the involved areas has been found very satisfactory as a therapeutic agent in many cases.

Phlebography of the prostatic and periprostatic region, (Abeshouse and Reben), may be helpful in diagnosis of prostatic lesions and in thrombophlebitis.

ARTIFICIAL PNEUMOPERITONEUM AS AN AID IN KIDNEY DIAGNOSIS (q.v.). Air introduced into the peritoneal cavity envelops the abdominal organs and renders them readily visible on roentgen examination. This method is particularly helpful in differentiating between tumors which arise in the abdominal cavity and those which are retroperitoneal (kidney tumors) in origin. For detection of perinephritic abscess, also, the method is of value. With regular urinary tract examination the kidney outline is still well preserved and the surrounding infection is not visible; the shadow of the psoas muscle may, or may not, be obliterated by the infiltrating infection. Pneumoperitoneum shows the homogeneous infiltration of the retroperitoneal space due to pus. Psoas abscess will show as homogeneous infiltration confined behind the psoas muscle bulging forward but not surrounding the kidney.

PERIRENAL INSUFFLATION (q.v.). This method, although not without danger, is in selected cases indispensable for demonstration of the perirenal tissues and adrenal glands. Tumors of the adrenal cannot be demonstrated in any other manner. For technique see Manual of Roentgenological Technique.

PRESACRAL AIR INJECTION. This method, also not without some danger, is considerably safer than perirenal insufflation. Guided by a rectal finger the needle is introduced around the spine to a position in the hollow of the sacrum. The outline of the kidneys and adrenals can frequently be clearly demonstrated by this method.

AORTOGRAPHY (q.v.). A procedure which has been found advantageous in differential diagnosis in selected cases is Aortography. Injection of contrast medium into the abdominal aorta at the origin of the renal vessels immediately preceding roentgen examination will show the renal circulation in brilliant contrast. This method can be resorted to in cases where it is desired to know the character of a kidney mass and its relationship to the circulation; for instance, to determine the character of the blood supply to a mass in differentiation of a neoplasm and a cyst of the kidney; a neoplasm would be very vascular throughout, whereas a cyst would have its blood vessels arranged about the periphery. For instance, Lofgren has reported a small rounded tumor present in the parenchyma of the upper pole of the kidney did

not show any deformity of the kidney pelvis on pyelographic examination, but on angiography was clearly
demonstrated by the worm-eaten appearance of excessive vascularity. It should be valuable in detecting
aneurysm of the renal artery. This method gives
promise of becoming very valuable means of differential diagnosis in selected cases (for detailed instructions of technique of the procedure see Manual
of Roentgenological Technique).

PERCUTANEOUS CATHETERIZATION OF THE
RENAL ARTERY. Selective catheterization of either
renal artery by means of a puncture needle introduced
into the femoral artery and a metal guide used to pass
a polyethylene catheter up the aorta to the renal artery, has been recommended by Edholm and Seldinger
as a method for the selective injection of either renal
artery. This has been successfully accomplished with
untoward hazard and affords the advantage of maintaining the dosage to the proper amount safe for the
kidney tissues, and avoids the mishap which sometimes occurs with aortography of overloading the
renal circulation by direct injection of the full aortic
dosage into the swollen renal vessels. Certain disadvantages were noted however: it was found that in
22% of the cases an additional apparent renal vessel
was present arising separately from the aorta which
was not filled by renal artery injection. This will
probably invalidate its use except in special cases.

Tillander has reported similar renal artery

catheterization, from the aorta using a magnetically
influenced metal-tipped catheter for guiding the end
of the catheter into the renal artery, which has been
quite successful. They feel that the smaller amounts
of less concentrated opaque media necessary is a
great advantage. The matter of aberrant vessels they
do not take as too serious an objection since when
these do occur they produce a sufficiently accurate
picture to recognize without difficulty.

ANEURYSM OF RENAL ARTERY. A rounded
calcareous deposit with the calcium deposit most
pronounced about the periphery, occurring in the region of the hilum of the kidney as verified by intravenous urography is the criterion for diagnosis of
aneurysm of the renal artery, (Provet, et al.). A
similar appearing lesion of the splenic artery may
be confused with this condition.

Isaac, et al. have demonstrated a cirsoid anomaly or network of vessels replacing the renal artery.
This has the effect of restriction of the renal circulation causing development of high blood pressure.
Translumbar aortography is essential to demonstrate
the network of smaller arteries which replace the
renal artery. A "scalloped" undulating deformity of
the ureters is suggestive of the presence of such an
anomaly. Operative removal of the involved kidney
results within five months in reduction of high blood
pressure, and decrease in size of the heart, confirming the deleterious effect of the anomaly.

QUESTIONS ON THE URINARY TRACT

Questions marked with a dagger deal with rare and less important conditions.

1. What qualities must an x-ray film show before it is considered satisfactory for the diagnosis of urinary stone? Name in order of frequency the positions in which calculi are found in the urinary tract.

2. What percentage of urinary calculi can be shown roentgenographically? How may a nonopaque stone be detected?

3. Name five conditions which may be confused radiographically with urinary stone.

4. How may a suspicious shadow in the region of the ureter be confirmed as a ureteral stone?

5. What is meant by pyelorenal "back flow" and to what is it due?

6. What is meant by pyelography, urethrography, cystography? What solutions are used and what procedure is followed in making such examinations? Explain retrograde and excretory methods for pyelography.

7. Show by diagram a normal kidney pelvis and explain the structure.

8. Show by diagram and explain how dilatation of the kidney pelvis results in interference with its drainage. What is the significance of constriction, obstruction or kinking of the ureter?

9. What is meant by ptosis of the kidney and how may it be demonstrated radiographically? What symptoms does it produce? What is meant by kinking of the ureter and by stricture of the ureter and to what are they due?

10. What structure does pyelitis first affect and how is it manifested in the pyelogram?

11. What conditions cause "filling defects" in the kidney pelvis?

12. What influence does new growth of the kidney have upon the pyelogram?

13. What effect does polycystic kidney have on the pyelogram? Solitary cysts?

14. To what may parenchymal necrosis of the kidney be due and explain its appearance in the roentgenogram. What are some other characteristics of tuberculous involvement?

15. Trace by diagrams the embryological development of double or divided kidney pelvis, branched ureter and double ureter.

16. What is the characteristic pyelographic appearance of "horseshoe" kidney? Of rotated kidney? Of fused kidneys?

17. Is there any conclusive roentgen evidence of injury to the kidney?

18. What roentgen sign is there indicative of perinephric abscess? Is it specific or does it occur from other conditions also?

19. By what two methods may the bladder be outlined, and what are they called?

20. What is the danger of foreign bodies remaining in the bladder?

21. How may diverticula of the bladder be shown?

22. What is the appearance of the cystogram in large carcinoma of the bladder? In trabeculation of the bladder?

23. How may rupture of the bladder be detected roentgenographically?

†24. Do stones occur in the urethra? How may they be detected?

25. What is meant by urethrography and how is it carried out? For what conditions is it of value?

26. How may rupture of the urethra be demonstrated?

†27. How may artificial pneumoperitoneum be of value in urinary tract diagnosis?

†28. Of what value is perirenal insufflation and what are its dangers?

†29. Describe the procedure for aortography and under what conditions is it of value in urinary tract diagnosis? Dangers?

†30. Of what value is Body-Section Roentgenography in kidney diagnosis and under what circumstances is it most effectively used?

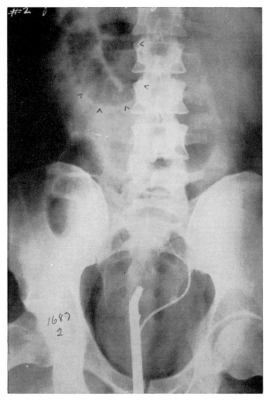

Stone in the ureter near the uretero-vesical junction. A cystoscope is seen in place and a urethral catheter passes the stone.

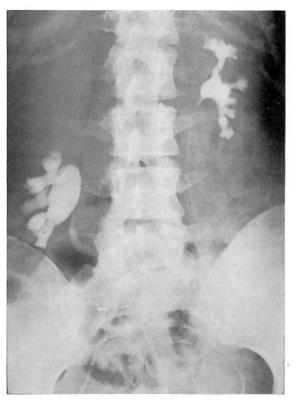

Ptosis of the right kidney with kinking of the ureter and dilatation of the kidney pelvis. The left kidney appears normal.

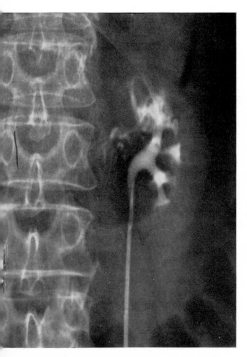

Pyelolymphatic back-flow showing the injected material extending back through the lymphatic pathways.

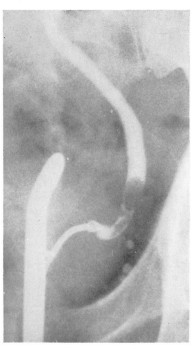

Non-opaque stone in lower ureter demonstrated by Braasch bulb technique.

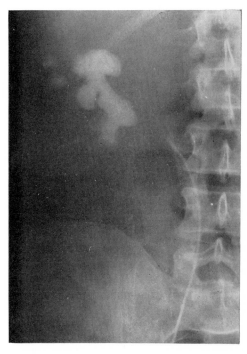

Large staghorn calculus in the kidney pelvis.

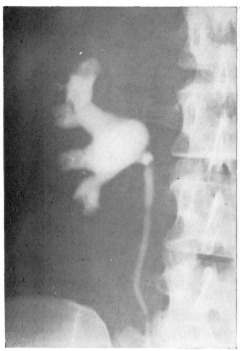

Aberrant vessel causing obstruction at uretero-pelvic junction.

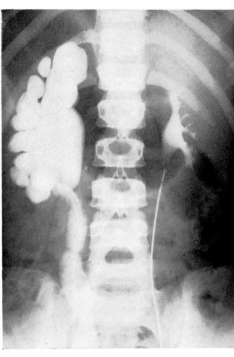

Dilatation of kidney pelvis and ureter from obstruction lower down.

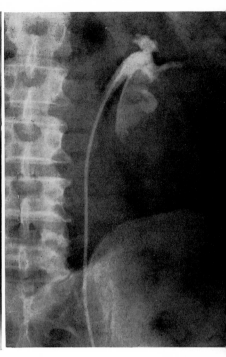

Round pressure-defect on the lowe portion of the kidney pelvis due a large hypernephroma. Such rounded growth could hardly be di tinguished from a solitary cyst of t kidney.

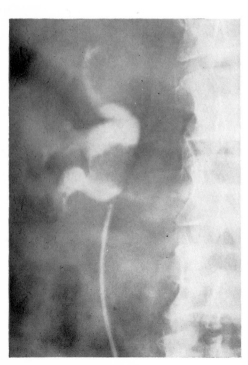

Pedunculated tumor of kidney pelvis causing filling defect.

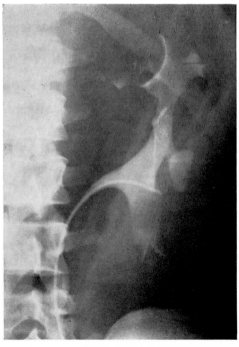

Large polycystic kidney showing an extreme degree of dilatation of the pelvis with rounded pressure defects of the cysts, upon the kidney pelvis, characteristic of the condition.

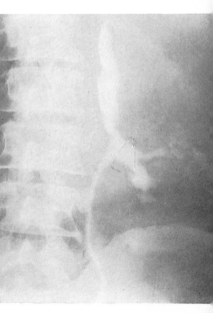

Parenchymal necrosis from lar tumor of kidney.

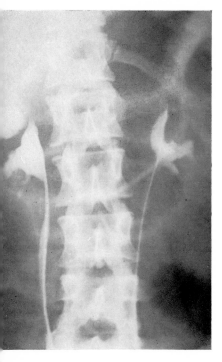

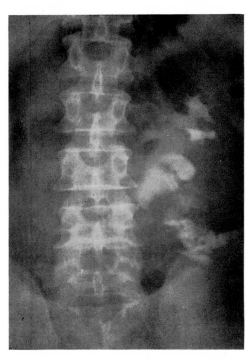

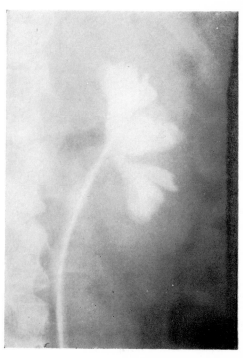

berculosis of kidney showing pinch-off of calices and caliectasis.

Extensive tuberculosis of the kidney, showing escape of the injected material into large area of parenchymal necrosis.

Pyelonephritis from pyogenic infection with constriction of infundibula and blunting of calices.

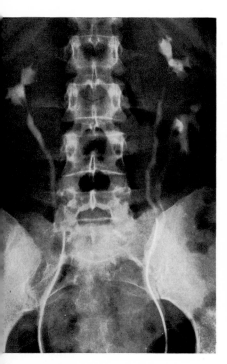

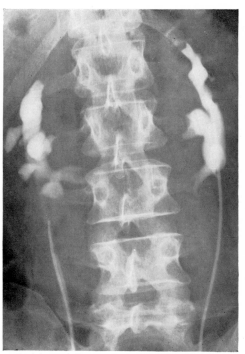

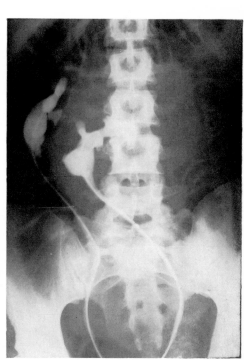

buble ureters and kidney pelves owing both sides injected.

Horseshoe kidney showing typical rotation of kidneys and inward inclination of lower calices.

Crossed fused kidneys.

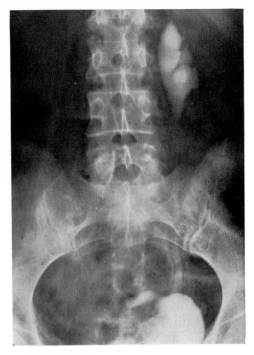

Large filling-defect of the bladder caused by carcinoma. The carcinomatous infiltration has a l l o w e d the injected material to extend directly up the ureter and into the pelvis of the kidney.

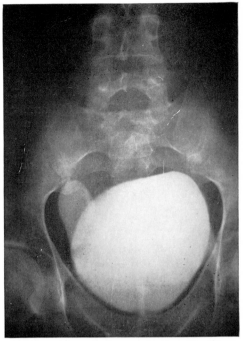

Large diverticulum of the bladder showing the pouch extending out from the bladder wall.

Calcification of the semi- →
nal vesicles.

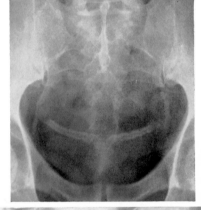

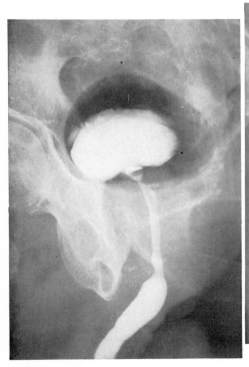

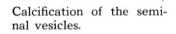
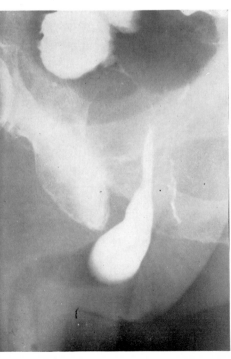

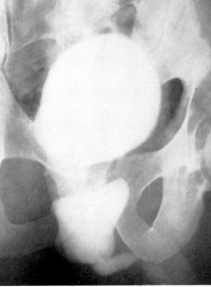

Normal urethrogram showing typical configuration of deep and pendulous urethra.

Carcinoma of prostate showing uniform tubular constriction of deep urethra and enlargement of prostatic lobes.

Large periurethral pouch from abscess of deep urethra.

Friese-Christiansen, A., "Urography on Children after Administration of Contrast Substance by Mouth," Acta Radiol., 27:197, 1946.

Edling, N. P. G., Edvall, C. A., Helander, C. G. and Pernow, B., "Comparison of Urography with Selective Clearance Tests of Renal Function," Acta Radiol., 45:85, 1956.

Wickbom, I., "Pyelography After Direct Puncture of Renal Pelvis," Acta Radiol., 41:505, 1954.

Goldstein, A. E., and Abeshouse, B. S., "Calcification and Ossification of the Kidney," Radiol., 30:544, 1938.

Davidson, C. N., Dennis, J. M., McNench, E. R., Wilson, K. V., and Brown, W. H., "Nephrocalcinosis Associated with Sarcoidosis," Radiol., 62:203, 1954.

Bauer, D., "Pyelorenal Backflow," Am. J. Roentgenol., 78:296, 1957.

Hinkel, C. L., "Opacification of the Renal Pyramids in Intravenous Urography," Am. J. Roentgenol., 78:317, 1957.

Culp, O. S., "Ureteral Diverticulum," J. Urol., 58:309, 1947.

Loitman, B. S., and Chiat, H., "Ureteritis Cystica and Pyelitis Cystica," Radiol., 68:345, 1957.

Williams, D. I., "Roentgenological Diagnosis of Lower Urinary Tract Obstruction," Brit. J. Radiol., 27:473, 1954.

Prather, G. C., "Medial Ptosis of the Kidney," New England J. Med., 238:253, 1948.

Wall, B., and Wachter, H. E., "Congenital Ureteral Valve," J. Urol., 68:684, 1952.

Herzan, F. A., "Artificial Nephrography by Combined Retrograde and Intravenous Urography," Am. J. Roentgenol., 71:228, 1954.

Evans, J. A., Dubilier, W. J., and Monteith, J. C., "Nephrotomography," Am. J. Roentgenol., 71:213, 1954.

Leigh, T. F., Kelly, R. P., and Weens, H. S., "Spinal Osteomyelitis Associated with Urinary Tract Infections," Radiol., 65:334, 1955.

Klami, P., "Retrograde Pyelography with Hydrogen Peroxide in Contrast Medium," Acta Radiol., 42:181, 1954.

Landes, R. R., and Hamlin, J. T., "Leukoplakia of Renal Pelvis," J.A.M.A., 155:1053, 1954.

Esersky, G. L., Saffer, S. H., Panoff, C. E., and Jacobi, M., "Wilm's Tumor in the Adult," J. Urol., 58:397, 1947.

Benzing, W., Jr., "Wilms' Tumor of Infancy and Childhood," Radiol., 58:674, 1952.

Friedman, P. S., and Solis-Cohen, L., "Hemangioma of the Kidney," Am. J. Roentgenol., 60:408, 1948.

Gutierrez, R., "Large Solitary Cysts of the Kidney," Arch. Surg., 44:279, 1942.

Lindblom, K., "Diagnostic Kidney Puncture in Cysts and Tumors," Am. J. Roentgenol., 68:209, 1952.

Billing, L., "The Roentgen Diagnosis of Polycystic Kidney," Acta Radiol., 41:305, 1954.

Hinkel, C. L., and Santini, L. C., "Polycystic Disease of the Kidney in Infants," Am. J. Roentgenol., 76:153, 1956.

Echternacht, A. P., "Injuries of the Urinary Tract," Urol. and Cutan. Rev., 49:357, 1945.

Solis-Cohen, L., and Steinbach, M., "A Case of True Aneurysm of the Right Renal Artery," Radiol., 31:173, 1938.

Osmond, J. D., "Foreign Bodies in the Kidney," Radiol., 60:375, 1953.

Evans, J., and Ross, W. D., "Renal Papillary Necrosis," Radiol., 66:502, 1956.

Ottoman, R. E., Woodruff, J. H., Wilk, S., and Isaac, F., "The Roentgen Aspects of Necrotizing Renal Papillitis," Radiol., 67:157, 1956.

Christoffersen, J. C., and Andersen, K., "Renal Papillary Necrosis," Acta Radiol., 45:27, 1956.

Olson, K. L., "Renal Escherichia Coli Infection Associated with Diabetes Mellitus," Am. J. Roentgenol., 78:719, 1957.

Yow, M., and Bunts, C. B., "Calyceal Diverticulum," J. Urol., 73:663, 1955.

Weens, S., and Johnston, M. H., "Thoracic Renal Ectopia," Am. J. Roentgenol., 70:793, 1953.

Schwartz, A., and Frankel, M., "High Renal Ectopy, Detection in Routine Chest Examination," Acta Radiol., 37:583, 1952.

Gutierrez, R., Clinical Management of Horseshoe Kidney, Paul Hoeber, Pub., 1934.

Petrovcic, F., and Milic, N., "Horseshoe Kidney with Crossed Ureter Condition After Right Nephrectomy," Brit. J. Radiol., 29:114, 1956.

Phokitis, P., "Caudal Bifid Ureter," J. Urol., Paris, 60:45, 1954.

Abeshouse, B. S., "Crossed Ectopia with Fusion," Am. J. Surg., 73:658, 1947.

Butts, J. B., and Conley, J. E., "Perinephric Abscess," U.S. Navy Med. Bull., 45:1081, 1945.

Brailsford, J. F., Donovan, H., and Mucklow, E. H., "A Simple Estimation of Residual Urine in Cases of Prostatic Disease Following the Ingestion of Hippuran by Mouth," Brit. J. Radiol., 27:183, 1954.

Snow, W. T., "Urachal Cyst with Calculi," Am. J. Roentgenol., 78:323, 1957.

Gottlieb, C., Beranbaum, S. L., and Hamilton, R., "Radiographic Features of Ureterocele," Radiol., 60:64, 1953.

Samuel, E., "The Radiological Features of Vesical Leiomyoma and Leiomyosarcoma," Brit. J. Radiol., 20:423, 1947.

Cusmano, J. V., "Dermoid Cysts of the Ovary," Radiol., 66:719, 1956.

Lund, H. G., Zingale, F. G., and O'Dowd, J. A., "Cystitis Emphysematosa," J. Urol., 42:684, 1939.

Boijsen, E., and Lewis-Johsson, J., "Emphysematous Cystitis," Acta Radiol., 41:269, 1954.

Kretschmer, H. L., "Solitary Cyst of the Kidney," J.A.M.A., 95:179, 1930.

Middlemiss, J. G., "Radiology in Diseases of the Prostate," J. Faculty Radiol., 4:115, 1952.

Abeshouse, B. S., and Ruben, M. E., "Prostatic and Periprostatic Phlebography," J. Urol., 68:640, 1952.

Coe, F. O., and Arthur, P. S., "A New Medium for Cystourethrography," Am. J. Roentgenol., 56:361, 1946.

Morales, O., and Romanus, R., "Urography in the Male with Highly Viscous Water-Soluble Contrast Medium, Umbradil-Viscous-U," Acta Radiol. Supp., 95, 1952.

Morales, O., and Romanus, R., "Urethrography in the Male," Acta Radiol., 39:453, 1953.

Flocks, R. H., "The Roentgen Visualization of the Posterior Urethra," J. Urol., 30:711, 1933.

Edling, N. P. G., "Urethrocystography in Male with Special Regard to Micturition," Acta Radiol., Supp., 58:1, 1945.

Jensen, V., "A Simple Device for Urethrocystography," Acta Radiol., 45:403, 1956.

Kerr, H. D., and Gillies, C. L., The Urinary Tract, Year Book Pub. Co., 1944.

Higgins, C. C., and Rambousek, E. S., "Diverticula of the Urethra in Women," J. Urol., 53:732, 1945.

Tucker, A. S., Yanagihara, H., and Pryde, A. W., "A Method of Roentgenography of the Male Genital Tract," Am. J. Roentgenol., 71:490, 1954.

Pereira, A., "Roentgen Interpretation of Vesiculograms," Am. J. Roentgenol., 69:361, 1953.

Cornwell, P. M., "Seminal Tract Calculi," J. Urol., 72:243, 1954.

Lame, E. L., and Chang, H. C., "Pubic and Ischial Necrosis Following Cystostomy and Prostatectomy," Am. J. Roentgenol., 71:193, 1954.

de Feo, E., "Osteomyelitis of the Spine Following Prostatic Surgery," Radiol., 62:396, 1954.

Lewitan, A., and Nathanson, L., "Osteitis Ischii and Pubis Following Abdominoperineal Resection of Carcinoma of Rectum," Radiol., 63:402, 1954.

Baston, O. V., "Role of Vertebral Veins in Metastatic Processes," Ann. Int. Med., 16:38, 1942.

Lofgren, F. O., "Renal Tumor not Demonstrable by Urography but Shown by Angiography," Acta Radiol., 42:300, 1954.

Edholm, P., and Seldinger, S. I., "Percutaneous Catheterization of the Renal Artery," Acta Radiol., 45:15, 1956.

Tillander, H., "Selective Angiography of the Abdominal Aorta with a Guided Catheter," Acta Radiol., 45:21, 1956.

Provet, H., Lord, J. W., and Lisa, J. R., "Aneurysm of the Renal Artery," Am. J. Roentgenol., 78:266, 1957.

Isaac, F., Brem, T. H., Temkin, E., and Movius, H. J., "Congenital Malformation of the Renal Artery, A Cause of Hypertension," Radiol., 68:679, 1957.

INDEX

TO

SPECIAL EXAMINATIONS

AND

PROCEDURES

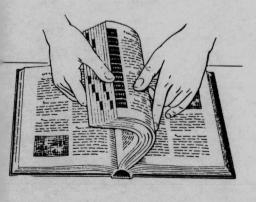

Nasal Sinuses

Mastoids

Teeth

Brain

Ventriculography

Encephalography
Angiography

Spinal Canal
Myelography

Artificial
Pneumoperitoneum

Perirenal
Insufflation

Aortography

Female Pelvic Organs:
Uterosalpingography

Fetal Development
Amniography

Radiation Therapy

PART VI

SPECIAL EXAMINATIONS AND PROCEDURES

I. ACCESSORY NASAL SINUSES
  A. Roentgen anatomy
  B. Pathology
    1. Sinusitis
      a. Catarrhal
        Acute
        Chronic
      b. Purulent
        Acute
        Chronic
      c. Hyperplastic
        Granulations
        Polypi
      d. Atrophic
      e. Allergic
      f. Aerosinusitis
    2. Malignant tumors
    3. Iodized oil injection
    4. Lung infection, associated

II. MASTOIDS
  A. Roentgen anatomy
    1. Types of mastoid development
      a. Infantile
      b. Diploetic
      c. Pneumatic
        Large cell
        Small cell
        Mixed cell
  B. Pathology
    1. Mastoiditis
      a. Acute catarrhal—edema of cells
      b. Purulent
      c. Destructive—necrosis of cell walls
      d. Perisinus abscess
      e. Epidural abscess
      f. Sclerotic—condensing osteitis
      g. Chronic
      h. Suppuration of petrous apex
      i. Cholesteatoma

III. TEETH
  A. Roentgen anatomy
    1. Structure of teeth
  B. Pathology
    1. Caries
    2. Apical infection
      a. Acute abscess
      b. Chronic abscess
      c. Granuloma
      d. Root cyst
      e. Osteomyelitis
    3. Pyorrhea
    4. Anomalies of eruption
    5. Tumors

IV. EXAMINATION OF BRAIN AND SPINAL CANAL
  Brain
  A. Without injection media
    1. Local evidence of pathology
      a. Erosion of bone

463

        b. Local pressure on,
           Sella turcica
           Auditory canal
           Optic canal
           Enlargement of skull
        c. Intracranial calcification in:
           Choroid plexus
           Falx cerebri
           Pacchionian bodies
           Blood vessels
           Tentorium
           Pituitary
           Pineal
        d. Abnormal blood vessel markings
           Deformities of skull in head injuries, "Stress coat" technique
    2. Intracranial neoplasms
        a. Gliomas
        b. Pituitary tumors
        c. Acoustic nerve tumors
        d. Angioma
        e. Meningioma
        f. Osteoma
        g. Hyperostosis internus cranialis
    3. Increased intracranial pressure
        a. Separation of sutures
           Enlargement of skull
        b. Convolutional atrophy
        c. Changes in the sella turcica
  B. With injection media
    1. Ventriculography and encephalography
    2. Cerebral angiography
Spinal Canal
A. Measurement of interpedicular spaces
B. Myelography
    1. Opaque oil
    2. Air
        a. Herniated disc
        b. Tumor
        c. Cysts
        d. Arachnoiditis
        e. Diastematomyelia
C. Discography
        a. Herniation
        b. Rupture

  V. SPECIAL EXAMINATION OF ABDOMINAL ORGANS
    A. Artificial pneumoperitoneum
      1. For outlining abdominal organs
      2. For detection and localization of masses
      3. For retroperitoneal tumors
      4. For subdiaphragmatic involvement
    B. Perirenal insufflation
      1. For examination of kidney and adrenal gland
    C. Intravenous thorium dioxide injection
      1. For demonstration of liver and spleen

  VI. AORTOGRAPHY
      1. For demonstration of abdominal circulation

  VII. FEMALE PELVIC ORGANS
    A. Uterosalpingography
    B. Pregnancy—Placenta
    C. Pelvimetry
    D. Amniography

Chapter XXIV

SPECIAL EXAMINATIONS AND PROCEDURES

ACCESSORY NASAL SINUSES

ROENTGEN ANATOMY. The accessory nasal sinuses, when fully developed, are large air spaces in the bones (Figs. 295A, B and C). Their air content furnishes a contrasting medium which renders them clearly visible roentgenographically. The maxillary sinuses or antra are evident within a short time after birth; the ethmoid cells are next to develop; the sphenoidal and frontal sinuses appear later. The frontals do not often attain their natural development until eight to ten years of age.

The antra (Figs. 295A and B) appear as two triangular-shaped air spaces on either side of the nose. In the anterior views the level of the floors of the antra in relationship to the floor of the nasal cavity can be noted; this is of importance if subsequent operative drainage is contemplated. At times the maxillary antra may extend downward and inward so as to almost meet in midline. They may also dip down into the alveolar process even surrounding the teeth in their sockets.

The ethmoidal cells lie just above the maxillary antra and are clustered on either side between the nasal cavity and the orbits. They usually extend outward over the superior rims of the orbits on either side—supraorbital cells. They are in close proximity to the orbits and are often separated only

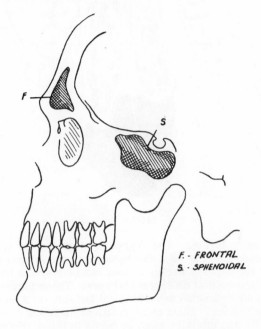

Fig. 295B. Lateral View Normal Sinus.

by a thin bony plate from the optic nerve in its course through the optic canal. This relationship is important since infection of the ethmoid cells can, by pressure on the optic nerve, cause blindness. Prompt detection of the infection and drainage may result in complete restoration of sight.

The full extent and development of the ethmoid cells is best demonstrated by oblique views (such as those obtained for showing the optic canals). However the "anterior" ethmoid cells cannot be distinguished from the "posterior" cells even in this view since by "anterior" or "posterior" the rhinologist refers to the location of the openings in the nose.

Camp's special localizer for the demonstration of the optic canal is useful for this purpose (See Manual of Roentgenological Technique).

The frontal sinuses lie above the ethmoidal cells, representing expanded air spaces in the frontal bone. They extend outward over both orbits from their bases at the glabella, usually forming symmetrical structures on either side. They are often crossed by bony septa which, if they do not interfere with natural drainage, are of no consequence. In the lateral view the depth of the frontal sinuses can be noted. A proper evaluation of the degree of aeration for sinuses of various sizes as indicated on the roentgenogram can be obtained only after considerable experience.

The sphenoidal (Fig. 295C) sinuses are paired air compartments in the sphenoid bone just beneath

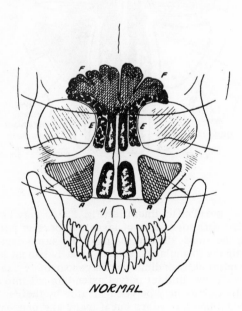

A - Antra
E - Ethmoids
F - Frontals

Fig. 295A. Anterior View Normal Sinuses.

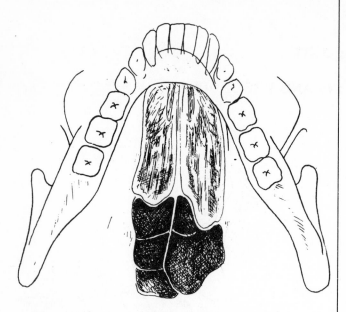

Fig. 295C. Normal.

the sella turcica. The degree to which the air space extends into the sella can be noted in the lateral view and the depth of the air spaces can be noted in the vertico-mental or sphenoidal view. These sinuses may be somewhat asymmetrical but this is of no significance. Their close relationship to the cranial cavity and pituitary must be borne in mind. If operative procedure is contemplated, preliminary roentgenographic examination with a probe in the sinus extending to its posterior wall may be found helpful in establishing the distance from the margin of the nose to the posterior sphenoidal wall. The air space may extend well up into the clinoid processes.

SINUSITIS.* Normally the accessory nasal sinuses are lined by mucous membrane closely applied to a periosteal layer; this is known as muco-periosteal membrane. In exceptionally clear roentgenograms this membrane may be seen as a thin translucent line running along the outer margin of the sinus, usually best seen in the maxillary antrum.

In acute catarrhal infections of the sinuses (Fig. 296, right side), there is congestion and edema of this membrane which results in definite thickening of this thin clear linear shadow along the sinus wall; at this stage little or no exudation is present and the sinus still remains well aerated. Catarrhal inflammation may become chronic, presenting much the same appearance as in the acute stage, lacking only the acute symptoms. Chronic infection produces rarefaction of the septa of the ethmoid cells. This is a matter of judgment and is often difficult to detect.

In acute purulent infection (Fig. 296, left side) of the accessory nasal sinuses the orifice by which the infected sinus drains into the nose may become closed up by edema and the products of infection dammed back and retained in the sinus. This causes a replacement of the normal air content with fluid

which can be readily recognized roentgenologically by a dense homogeneous opacity of the sinus. All of the sinuses on either or both sides may show such involvement—pansinusitis. After the acute stage of infection subsides and the orifice is opened, partial drainage to the outside becomes reestablished; products of the infection may still remain however, resulting in chronic thickening of the lining membrane—chronic purulent sinusitis.

Such pyogenic membrane may proliferate and appear as an irregular thick band extending around the outer borders of the sinus as if it had been cut in cross section. It is most frequently seen in the maxillary antra but does occur occasionally in the frontal and sphenoidal sinuses; the ethmoid cells are such small individual compartments that when chronically infected they are usually entirely filled with granulation tissue. Thin white lines produced by the dense bony septa resulting from condensing osteitis due to chronic infection serves to differentiate chronic from acute infection in the ethmoid cells. The antra may become so filled with granulation tissue that little, if any, air space remains. This is known as the hyperplastic type of chronic sinusitis.

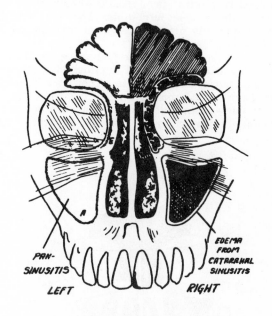

Fig. 296

Hyperplastic sinusitis (Fig. 297A) may be associated with formation of large numbers of polypi filling the sinus. These, being of the same density as ordinary granulation tissue, usually cannot be differentiated by ordinary roentgenographic examination. A few distinct polypi extending out into an air-filled sinus may be recognizable by their rounded smooth borders but if many are present they are crowded together and their individual rounded contour is lost.

*An asterisk following any title indicates that roentgenographic reproductions illustrating this condition will be found in the pictorial supplement at the end of the chapter.

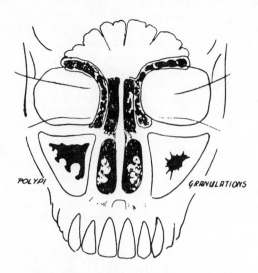

Fig. 297A. Hyperplastic Sinusitis.

Atrophic sinusitis (Fig. 297B) is recognized as a condition in which, as a result of long standing infection, condensing osteitis results in an irregular bony deposit about the walls of the sinuses, causing them to be reduced in size, even, in the case of the ethmoidal cells, to the point of obliteration.

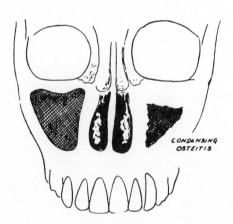

Fig. 297B. Atrophic Sinusitis.

ALLERGIC SINUSITIS (Fig. 298A). The mucous membrane of the accessory nasal sinuses responds readily and very characteristically to sensitization reactions. Oedema of the submucosal structures lifts the mucous membrane from the bony wall giving rise to a boggy swelling which is quite characteristic. The antra are most commonly affected.

AEROSINUSITIS (Fig. 298B) (Schneider; Cooke). The rapid descent from a high altitude in an airplane leaves the air within the nasal sinus at a much reduced pressure in comparison with the sur-

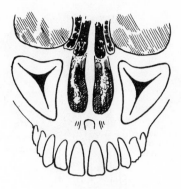

Fig. 298A

rounding atmospheric pressure. If the ostia connecting with the nasal passage are open and rapid exchange of air pressure is possible, nothing unusual happens; but, if they become partially obstructed or closed from any cause the pressure remains low and the mucous membrane lining the sinus becomes subjected to a negative pressure. This change is so rapid that it does not permit time for equalization of pressure but actually causes oedema and submucous hemorrhage. This is attended with sudden severe pain in the region of the affected sinuses.

Roentgenographically the bulging mucous membrane can be visualized protruding like a mucocele from the wall out into the sinus. Several days or weeks may be necessary for the condition to subside and for the roentgenogram to return to normal.

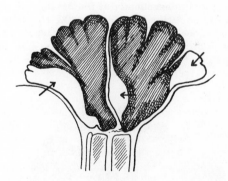

Fig. 298B

TUMORS OF SINUSES:

Mucocele and Pyocele* (Fig. 299) is a rounded, cystlike tumor containing mucus which springs from the mucous membrane gradually enlarging and causing pressure atrophy similar to any other soft tumor mass when it encroaches on bone. They may even cause bulging of the eye. It is recognized roentgenographically by its relatively large size and rounded outline when viewed against an aerated background. They may level out in the upright position. Mucoceles of this type are more common in the antra.

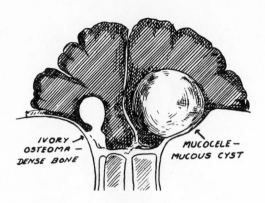

Fig. 299

Meningocele. This may have a similar appearance projecting downward into the frontal sinus.

Ivory osteoma* (Fig. 299). These are usually dense bony structures, rounded in outline and varying from the size of a pea to several centimeters in diameter. They are usually seen projecting into the frontal sinus. Unless by their size they involve surrounding structures or by their position they tend to obstruct the natural drainage of the sinus, they are of little pathological significance. They may remain quiescent or they may continue to grow slowly, enlarging over a period of years to sufficient size to cause expansion of the sinus and erosion of the bone.

Malignant tumors* (Fig. 300), carcinoma and sarcoma, have the same density as the products of infection, and consequently at the outstart they cannot usually be differentiated from the roentgen appearance alone. Correlation with clinical symptoms will aid in differentiation; if the process has advanced to the stage of expansion of the sinus or destruction

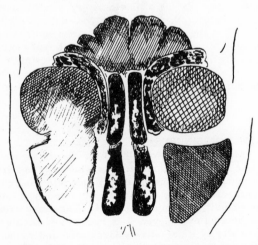

Fig. 300. Tumor of Maxillary Antrum.

of bone, then the diagnosis is readily made. Such tumors are very inaccessible to treatment; surgical exposure for the use of radium offers the only hope and this is none too encouraging.

IODIZED OIL INJECTION INTO NASAL SINUSES (Fig. 301). We have at our disposal, however, a method by which the contour of such polypoid growths can be mapped out and the remaining air space can be demonstrated. Introduction of iodized oil into the sinuses, either by direct injection or by the displacement method described by Proetz, fills the remaining air space with a medium of much greater density than the soft tissues and demonstrates both the size of remaining air space and the character of its contents. By this method anomalous septa and partitions in the sinuses may be demonstrated.

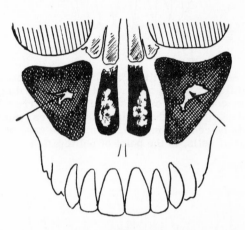

Fig. 301. Lipiodol in Antra.

CHRONIC LUNG INFECTION FROM SINUSITIS.* Chronic inflammation and infection of the lungs may result from chronic sinusitis as a result of the constant postnasal drip which always accompanies such infections. This is especially true in children who frequently give no subjective signs of the disease. Roentgenographic examination of the chest (q.v.) showing extensive increase of the peribronchial lung markings, especially in the cardiophrenic regions, must always be viewed with suspicion, and infection of the sinuses must be eliminated as a possible source of the infection. It is possible that, in many cases, such chronic sinus infection may be the direct cause of bronchiectasis.

Body section roentgenography (q.v.) may prove very valuable in examination of the accessory nasal sinuses. This is especially true for the demonstration of rounded tumor masses within the antra and for observation of the ethmoidal and sphenoidal cells. Erosion or destruction of the sinus walls may be shown in this way facilitating the diagnosis of malignant involvement. Accessory septa dividing the sinus and other anomalous structures may be shown by this method.

MASTOIDS

ROENTGEN ANATOMY. The mastoids, when fully developed, consist of multiple air cells in the bone. By reason of their air content they become readily detectable in the roentgenogram.

At birth (Fig. 302A) the mastoid process and the petrous portion of the temporal bone are represented by dense compact bony structure. Roentgen examination at this time will disclose the semicircular canals, cochlea, and other middle ear structures, but no evidence of air cells in the mastoid process. This is the infantile type which persists ordinarily

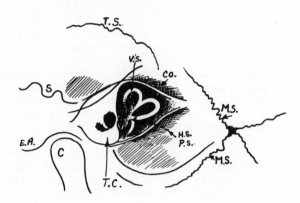

V.S.-Vertical Semicircular Canal
H.S.-Horizontal Semicircular Canal
P.S.-Posterior Semicircular Canal
T.C.-Tympanic Cavity
CO. -Cochlea

T.S. -Temporal Suture
M.S.-Mastoid Suture
C   -Condylar Process of Mandible
E.A.-Eminentia Articularis of Temperomandibular Joint
S   -Sella Turcica

Fig. 302A. Infantile Mastoid.

without much indication of cell formation for the first one or two years. As the individual grows, cellular development of the mastoid process progresses (Fig. 302B). In some individuals this cellular development is greater than in others, due to individual peculiarities of size and bony structure. This results in abundant, large, thin-walled cells in some individuals, and smaller, thicker-walled cells of scanty distribution in others. In some individuals scarcely any cell formation seems to take place and the structure of the mastoid process remains diploetic in character. For descriptive purposes, mastoids in which the air cells are well developed are referred to as of the large, small or mixed cell pneumatic type; those in which the diploetic character of the bone still predominates are referred to as of the diploetic type (Fig. 302C).

As a rule, however, regardless of the type, the mastoids on the two sides are similar in structure, unless normal cell development has been interfered with by disease in early childhood. Both mastoids should always be examined, therefore, for purposes

of comparison. Occasionally, however, cells may be well formed on one side and remain of the undeveloped diploetic type on the other. This is usually due to some ear infection of childhood which has resulted in destruction or inhibition of the normal cell-forming structures.

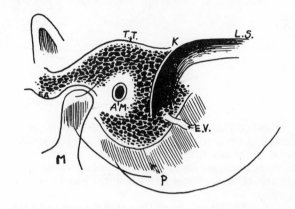

M.   -Mandible with its Condylar Process
E.A. -Eminencia Articularis of the Temperomandibular Joint
A.M. -Auditory Meatus; Internal and External Superimposed

T.T.-Tegmen Tympani
P. -Mastoid Process with Air Cells
L.S.-Lateral Sinus
K. -Knee of Lateral Sinus
E.V.-Emissary Vein

Fig. 302B. Mixed Cell Normal Mastoid.

Such cell development may be confined closely to the mastoid process, or it may extend forward into the zygomatic arch (zygomatic cells); upward into the squamous portion of the temporal bone (squamous cells) or backward into the occipital bone (occipital cells). It is important that such extension of the cell structure be recognized, since it may help to explain the development of certain clinical manifestations in the case. Likewise, if the surgeon is to remove all of the cell structure he must be advised of its extent.

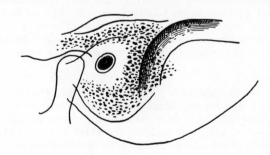

Fig. 302C. Diploetic Mastoid.

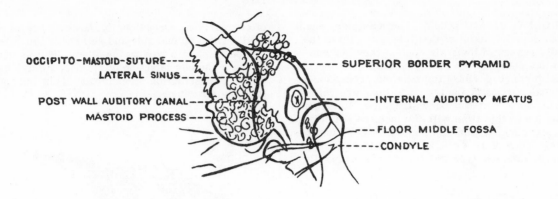

OCCIPITO-MASTOID-SUTURE

LATERAL SINUS

POST WALL AUDITORY CANAL

MASTOID PROCESS

SUPERIOR BORDER PYRAMID

INTERNAL AUDITORY MEATUS

FLOOR MIDDLE FOSSA

CONDYLE

Fig. 302D. Schüller Position.

ROENTGENOLOGICAL EXAMINATION. A number of projections have been devised for examination of the petrous bone and mastoid process for the more accurate detection of pathology of its intricate structures. These are essentially of three types:

1. The lateral views (in same direction as the petrous pyramid)
   Law Position
   "Swimming" Position
   Schüller Position
2. The antero-posterior or postero-anterior views (perpendicular to the long axis of the petrous bone)
   Stenver's Position (also Low-Beer modification)
   Arceline Position
3. The axial view (along the long axis of the petrous bone)
   Mayer Position

The positions in each group present similar roentgenographic appearances; the anatomical landmarks shown in these views should be studied carefully and correlated with each other.

NORMAL MASTOID. In examining a roentgenogram of the mastoid area first identify certain key structures such as the condyle of the mandible, temporomandibular joint and eminentia articularis, the tegmen tympani or roof, and mastoid process, in order to orient yourself. Next locate the auditory meati, internal and external, noting their relationship to each other in order to determine the angle of projection. Then examine the cellular structure, its type, location and extent; the lateral sinus and its relation to the mastoid process, any emissary veins, etc.

MASTOIDITIS.* The mastoids, like other air sinuses, are subject to infection. Infection usually spreads from the middle ear, although occasionally a patient is seen with mastoiditis which was not preceded by otitis media. Such cases must be due to blood- or lymph-borne infection. The first roentgenographic evidence of infection is haziness over the entire mastoid area. This is due to outpouring of cells and serum into the mastoid cells to combat the infection. Such a condition may clear up completely, leaving no evidence of damage to the cell structure; it is spoken of as catarrhal mastoiditis.

If the infection is prolonged, the process may become more intense and the haziness of the mastoid structures may become more pronounced, but still there may be no evidence of bone destruction and the cell walls remain clearly defined. The appearance of the limiting plate of the lateral sinus becomes more clearly defined than on the uninvolved side due to the presence of exudate in the cells producing a structure of more uniform density. Such a condition is referred to as purulent mastoiditis without cell destruction (Fig. 303).

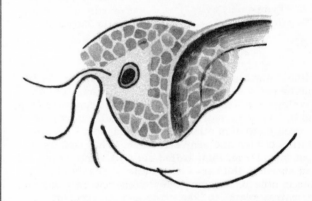

Fig. 303. Purulent Mastoiditis.

The next step in the progress of infection is softening and actual destruction of the bony walls of the cells—destructive mastoiditis. This is indicated in the roentgenogram by loss of the fine bony texture and by irregular areas of decreased density over the process. Destruction often begins in the region of the knee of the lateral sinus (Fig. 304A). If the knee of the lateral sinus is not sharply defined, this is indication that perisinus abscess is present with erosion of the adjacent bony plate (Fig. 304B).

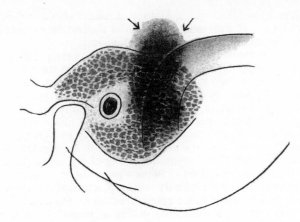

Fig. 304A. Destructive Mastoiditis.

It is obvious that large cells having thin bony walls will be more readily broken down and that surgical interference for control of infection is most urgent in this type of mastoid. Mastoids of this type, however, usually drain more readily. Mastoids of the smaller cell or diploetic type with thicker cell walls do not require such prompt operation for the control of infection, but this type is likewise more apt to become chronic, giving rise to thickening of the bony septa (condensing osteitis) and general increase in density of the bone structure, known as chronic sclerotic mastoiditis (Fig. 305).

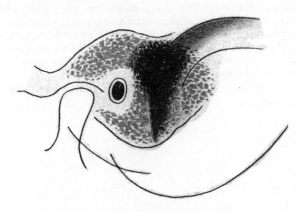

Fig. 304B. Perisinus Abscess.

CHRONIC MASTOIDITIS: APICAL PETROUSITIS; SUPPURATION OF THE PETROUS APEX. Failure to completely cure pyogenic discharge from the middle ear or mastoid by operation usually indicates failure to remove all cell structure from which such infection can arise. Zygomatic, squamous or occipital extension of cells may be overlooked at operation. One source of continued infection may be from extension of the suppurative process to the bony structures of the petrous apex.

Apical petrousitis (Fowler, et al.; Munk) may be considered as "an inflammation of the petrous bone, medial and anterior to the arcuate eminence (which marks the site of the upper vertical canal of the labyrinth). The clinical manifestations for the Gradenigo Syndrome is, if fully developed, a sixth

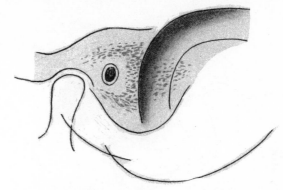

Fig. 305. Sclerotic Mastoid.

nerve paralysis (partial or complete paralysis of the external rectus) with fifth nerve involvement (radiating pain in the distribution of the nerve)." It may occur in cases of purulent otitis media or before or after mastoid operation.

Even if the petrous apex appears radiographically to be acellular there is still sufficient cell structure present to permit extension of infection. Depending upon the degree of infection there is first osteoporosis, then the formation of defects in the petrous apex and finally frank bone destruction. Abscess radiologically presents itself as "disappearance through absorption of the upper contour of the apex," (Mayer). Rupture of such an abscess into the cranial cavity is attended with serious complications.

In the basal view of the skull, and in Stenver's position (Fig. 306), actual extension of the air cells into the petrous bone and destruction of the apex can be demonstrated. Not until all sources of infection are removed will recovery take place.

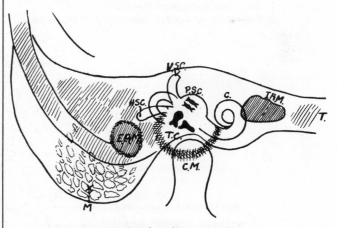

E.A.M.   external auditory meatus.
I.A.M.   internal auditory meatus.
M.   mastoid process.
C.M.   condylar process.
H.S.C.   horizontal semicircular canal.
V.S.C.   vertical semicircular canal.
P.S.C.   posterior semicircular canal.
C.   cochlea.
T.C.   tympanic cavity.
T.   apex of temporal bone.

Fig. 306

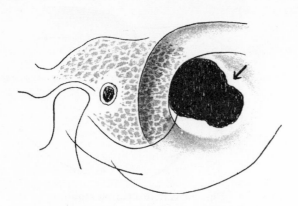

Fig. 307A. Cholesteatoma in Lateral Position.

CHOLESTEATOMA OF THE TEMPORAL
BONE, (Hodgson). The external auditory canal extends from the external auditory meatus to the tympanic membrane. This membrane separates the external canal from the middle ear, which connects by the eustachian tube to the nasopharynx. Practically all middle ear infections arise from the nasopharynx and travel through the eustachian tube to the middle ear cavity. From this point the infection extends to the attic through the aditus to the mastoid antrum and from this point to the mastoid cells.

The internal auditory canal is for passage of the auditory nerve; this occupies the upper edge of the petrous bone; it communicates with the cochlea and semicircular canals. Enlargement of the internal auditory meatus is significant in detection of acoustic nerve tumors.

Two conditions are necessary for the production of a cholesteatoma:

1. Low grade chronic infection,
2. Diploetic or poorly pneumatized mastoid.

It is associated with a history of long standing copious drainage of pus; demonstration of cholestrin crystals in the discharge clinches the diagnosis.

If the mastoid is of the cellular variety, infection spreads from the middle ear, through the aditus ad antrum into the mastoid antrum and from here into the mastoid cells. In a poorly pneumatized or diploetic mastoid, especially if the infection is of low grade and of a more insidious type, the process is slower. Normal mucosa is replaced by epidermal cells either from the external canal or by metaplasia. An infolding of the epithelial lining of the canal gives rise to this condition. Being squamous epithelium these cells are continually replaced, gradually collecting in the epitympanic recess, aditus or mastoid antrum forming a constantly enlarging mass. Pressure of this enlarging mass of epithelial cells causes erosion. A thin layer of sclerotic bone forms around the edge of the mass. Not until the mass erodes through the wall of the cavity will its presence be detectable. Perforation finally occurs; this is usually into the external auditory canal or it may be through the tegmen tympani into the middle fossa of the skull. Or the cholesteatoma may occur in the mastoid antrum or rupture into the labyrinth through the external canal where the latter projects into the mastoid antrum (Fig. 307A). Examination in Mayer's position (Fig. 307B) is of especial value where cholesteatoma is suspected, since it demonstrates very clearly the relation of the bony defect to the auditory canal.

Welin sums up the roentgen finding in cholesteatoma as follows: The sharp definition, angularity and polygonal shape of cholesteatoma cavities, their occurrence in the temporal bones with reduced pneumatization, and a linear calcareous zone between them and the surrounding bone tissue, have so far been held to the characteristic of these cavities.

Nothing short of surgical evacuation can cure the disease.

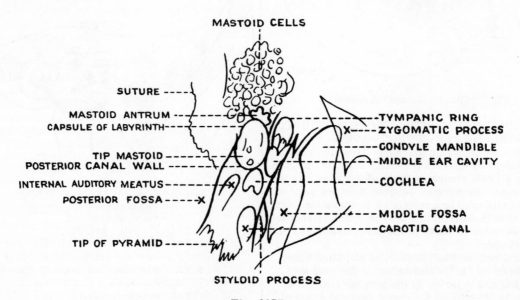

Fig. 307B

TEETH AND JAW

ROENTGEN ANATOMY (Figs. 308A and B). The teeth are dense structures, partly embedded in the cancellous bony tissue of the alveolar process and partly protruding above the aveolar margin. The portion which extends into the alveolar socket is called the root; that portion which protrudes above the gingival margin is called the crown. The tooth structure throughout is made up largely of dentine. The crown is covered by dense extremely hard enamel which can be distinguished in the roentgenogram as a denser covering. The root, covered with pericementum, fits snugly into the alveolar socket, which is lined by the peridental membrane. In the interior of the crown, the pulp chamber appears as a symmetrical cavity extending downward to the end, or apex, of the root; this harbors the nerve and blood supply of the tooth.

Normally there are 32 adult teeth; they are symmetrical and are similar in the upper and lower jaws. From the midline posteriorly they are: central incisor, lateral incisor, cuspid, 1st and 2nd bicuspid, 1st, 2nd and 3rd molar. They may be indicated roentgenographically before eruption as tooth buds forming below the deciduous teeth.

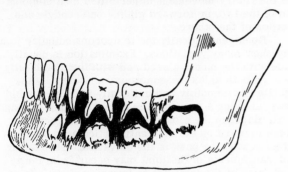

Fig. 308A. Deciduous Teeth.

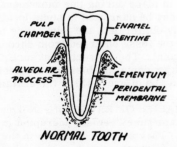

NORMAL TOOTH

Fig. 308B. Normal Tooth Structure.

DENTAL CARIES (Fig. 308C). Dental caries is indicated roentgenographically by radiolucent areas in the crown of the tooth. Such areas may become quite large, developing beneath the surface, before they are detected by roentgen examination. If they are encased deeply in the tooth structure they may cause pain to heat or cold; if open, they rarely cause pain unless they encroach on the pulp chamber.

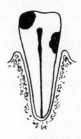

Fig. 308C

APICAL INFECTION (Figs. 309A, B, C and D). As physicians, our main concern in examination of the teeth is for detection of infection. The teeth are notorious as sources of focal infection. The most frequent location of such foci of infection in the teeth is at the apices of the roots; the nerve dies or is killed and is removed by the dentist; it is replaced by a root canal filling, sealing the canal. Infection entering by the open canal continues to persist at the apex of the tooth even for years after the tooth has been filled, thereby furnishing a constant source of infection for

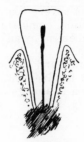

Fig. 309A
Acute
Abscess.

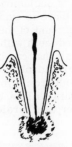

Fig. 309B
Chronic
Abscess.

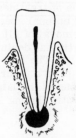

Fig. 309C
Apical
Granuloma.

absorption by the circulation. If the individual is in good health and has good resisting power, the body takes care of and neutralizes the effects of infection; just as soon, however, as this bodily defense breaks down from sickness or age, the effects of bacterial infection manifest themselves.

Roentgenographically these areas of apical infection are manifested by a break in the peridental membrane which surrounds the apex of the tooth and diffuse absorption of the periapical alveolar membrane

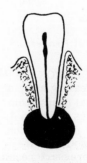

Fig. 309D
Root
Cyst.

which surrounds the apex. If the abscess is acute the area of absorption is more diffuse and irregular (Fig. 309A); if chronic it is more clearly defined (Fig. 309B). As the disease progresses the area of apical infection becomes rounded and smooth indicating the formation of an apical granuloma (Fig. 309C); such a condition is indicated roentgenographically as a rounded radiolucent area at the very apex of the root surrounded by a slight zone of sclerosis in the alveolar process. Inflammatory root cysts (Fig. 309D) of varying size may develop as the result of chronic infection. Roentgenologically they appear as large well-rounded radiolucent areas in the bone, one centimeter or more in diameter, usually with the root of a tooth projecting into the cyst. Infected teeth, when bordering on the antra, may be a factor in keeping up sinus infection. Diffuse infection of the bone, osteomyelitis, is similar to osteomyelitis occurring elsewhere.

PYORRHEA. Another very serious source of infection from the teeth is pyorrhea (Fig. 310). This is indicated on roentgenographic examination by alveolar absorption at the gingival margins about the teeth. This may be so severe that the alveolar process almost completely recedes. If it progresses to involve the interradial area (the portion between the roots of a tooth), then the infection can no longer be eradicated and the tooth must be sacrificed before a cure can be obtained. Extensive instrumentation and treatment of the periapical tissues followed by correction of errors of occlusion are the only methods of treatment. If there is evidence of severe constitutional upset on account of the infection, complete removal of all infected teeth with replacement by an artificial denture is all that can be done.

The loss of the periodontal membrane and lamina dura is a natural result from pyorrheal involvement. Loss of the lamina dura without infection is a diagnostic finding in hyperparathyroidism, (p. 129).

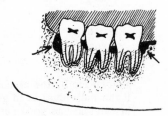

Fig. 310. Pyorrheal Absorption of Process.

INFLUENCE OF DENTAL OCCLUSION ON TEMPOROMANDIBULAR JOINT. Wearing away of the molar teeth and loss of the normal cusps from decay and filling with amalgam fillings causes a drop in the normal plane of the "bite" and malocclusion. This, in turn, may cause abnormal motion at the temporomandibular joint and nerve pressure resulting in neuralgia. Some feel also that this is a potent factor in the cause of pyorrhea. Raising the "bite" by building up the cusps with gold inlays reestablishes normal occlusion and does away with the abnormal pressure on the joint.

Examination of the temporomandibular joint may provide the diagnostic clue (Fig. 311), (Doub and Henny). Normally this is a very complicated joint, consisting of the condylar process of the mandible, the glenoid fossa of the temporal bone and an intervening meniscus of fibrocartilage which separates the joint into two compartments. The glenoid fossa projects anteriorly onto a rounded bony projection, the eminentia articularis. Movement at this joint is of the hinge, gliding, and rotary type. The hinge movement is between the condyle and the meniscus,

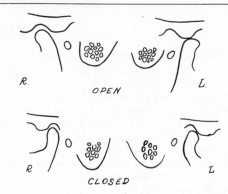

Fig. 311. Variations in function of temporomandibular joints due to malocclusion of teeth. Left joint shows excessive forward luxation of condyle over eminentia articularis with mouth open and failure to glide back into normal position with mouth closed showing relaxation of ligaments and flail joint. Right joint, on the other hand, never leaves the socket on opening mouth.

permitting opening of the mouth; the gliding movement is due to the movement of the meniscus in the glenoid, permitting forward protrusion of the jaw; and the rotary movement is permitted by a combination of the two, by forward gliding one condyle and rotation of the other.

Roentgenologically the temporomandibular joint may show many variations. Examination is usually made with the mouth closed and with the mouth fully open, on both sides for comparison. Normally the condyle fits smoothly and uniformly into the glenoid fossa, showing a narrow intervening radiolucent band of cartilage; in the closed mouth view, the condyle glides forward on the eminentia articularis but does not go beyond the peak of the elevation. All manner of derangements of the joint may occur from faulty mechanics of the joint due to lowering of the bite of the teeth. One condyle may glide forward, the other remaining in the socket on opening the mouth or both may remain in place during this movement. The joint space may be narrowed in some location or may be completely obliterated; the joint space may be widened and the fossa enlarged from chronic derangement of the joint. The correction of such defects may become a major dental problem. Body section examination may be of great aid in the examination.

ANOMALIES OF ERUPTION. Normal tooth structures sometimes remain unerupted in the alveolar process. They may lie obliquely in the process across the ends of other teeth or they may be free. Third molar teeth show some striking anomalies of eruption. Impaction of a third molar tooth against an adjacent second molar is very common; often the unerupted third molar lies horizontally in the process, the end of the crown being impacted against the side of the second molar. Upper third molar teeth may be reversed in direction, growing upward into the antrum or region of the eustachian tube giving rise to symptoms of trifacial neuralgia or ear infection. Such impactions and failures of normal eruption are potent causes of tic douloureux.

TUMORS OF THE MANDIBLE. Any of the soft part tumors common to other regions of the body may occur in the region of the jaw as well. They are of importance roentgenologically only in so far as they may encroach upon and invade the bony structure of the mandible. Tumors of the mandible itself may be benign or malignant. The benign tumors, owing to their close relationship to the teeth and dental development, have certain characteristics peculiar to this region; they are either of osseous or dental origin. The malignant tumors are more inclined to be similar to other osseous tumors occurring elsewhere in the body. The classification of tumors of the jaw in use in the Surgical Pathological Laboratory at Johns Hopkins Medical School (as quoted from Geschicter and Copeland) is as follows:

Dental and Benign Osseous Tumors
    Radicular or dental root cysts
    Follicular or dentigerous cysts
    Adamantinomas
    Odontomas
    Giant-Cell epulis (soft part tumor of
        alveolar margin)
    Central giant-cell tumors
    Osteomas and ossifying fibromas.

Malignant Osseous Tumors
    Osteogenic sarcomas
        Sclerosing
        Chondral
    Ewing's Sarcoma
    Tumors with skeletal and jaw involvement.

BENIGN. Any type of tumor occurring elsewhere in the body may arise in the mandible. There are, however, some tumors which occur peculiarly in this position.

RADICULAR OR DENTAL ROOT CYSTS are epithelial cysts of inflammatory origin occurring about the root of a chronically infected devitalized tooth. The apex of the root usually projects into the cyst cavity (Fig. 309D). It is circular in outline, with a well-defined border occasionally showing a sclerotic zone about its margin. These may cause few symptoms at the outstart but when they become larger they may, owing to pressure, produce neuralgic symptoms. These cysts have a fibrous wall and smooth epithelial lining. They may be filled with mucus or pus.

FOLLICULAR OR DENTIGEROUS CYSTS are cysts having a well-defined cyst cavity containing one or more usually well-formed teeth (Fig. 312A). They arise from the epithelium of the enamel organ during development. They are most frequently seen in the third molar region. They may occur without the presence of tooth structure; under these conditions they are known as simple cysts.

Simple cysts of the jaw are very common. They are often very extensive, involving almost the entire side of the jaw. The bony wall is thin and crackles easily on pressure; such cysts fill in with new bone and heal after curettement or fracture.

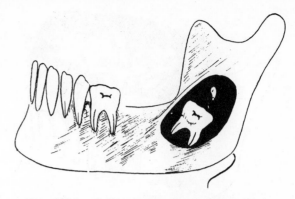

Fig. 312A. Follicular or Dentigerous Cyst.

ADAMANTINOMA, Fig. 312B, is a tumor arising within the alveolar border of the jaw from the paradental epithelial remains of the enamel organ. It usually contains irregular masses of various tissues which go to make up tooth structure but no definitely formed tooth. They show multiple cystic areas and patchy sclerosis at the border of the tumor; they are traversed by septa very similar to giant cell tumor and are often associated with dentigerous cyst. They do not have limiting membranes and tend to recur locally unless widely removed. They are slow growing (five years or more) and do not tend to metastasize. The lower molar region is the most frequent site of involvement.

One symptom which is frequently present and the significance of which is often overlooked is the loosening of a tooth. This is a condition frequently associated with malignant growths of all kinds.

Roentgenologically the adamantinoma is a clearly defined, centrally located solid or cystic tumor. It may be monocystic but is more frequently of polycystic type giving a honey-combed appearance which is quite characteristic of the condition. They may contain tooth remnants. Strangely enough, tumors of this type have also been described in the shafts of bones, especially the tibia. As pointed out by Sherman and Caumartin, they may in rare instances take on a low grade malignancy and metastasize to the cervical nodes or even lungs.

ODONTOMA is a solid mixed tumor composed of tooth elements, dentine, cementum, enamel, etc.,

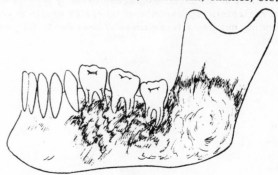

Fig. 312B. Adamantinoma.

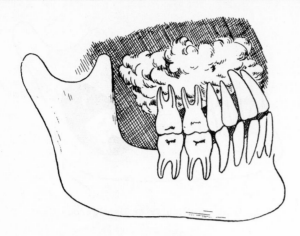

Fig. 312C. Ossifying Fibroma.

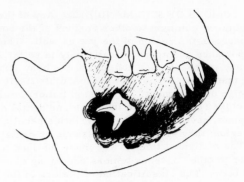

Fig. 313. Carcinoma of Mandible.

irregularly distributed without capsule or limiting membrane. It can be readily seen in the roentgenogram.

Roentgenographically they appear as irregular masses of calcification occurring in a rarefied area often in close relationship to a tooth. These calcareous deposits represent all manner of tooth remnants. They are benign and do not tend to recur after operative removal.

CENTRAL GIANT CELL TUMORS of the mandible resemble giant cell tumors occurring elsewhere. They have the same type of trabecular formation, with expansion of the bone. They occur at a much earlier age here than in the long bones (ten to twenty-five years) and respond to conservative treatment.

OSTEOMA may appear as an outgrowth of bone from any part of the mandible.

Heavy overgrowths of bone sometimes occur in the midline of the palate (torus palatinus) or at the alveolar ridge (torus lingulis); filmed in profile these show as projecting growths in no relation to the tooth structure. They are usually of no pathological significance.

OSSIFYING FIBROMA, Fig. 312C. These are slow-growing fibrous tissue tumors which slowly undergo ossification. The process is slow and painless, the first symptom noted being swelling and disfigurement of the face. Roentgenologically they give a characteristic appearance of irregular ossification extending out into a large mass of less dense fibrous tissue.

OSTEITIS FIBROSA. As part of the bony changes associated with generalized osteitis fibrosa (von Recklinghausen's Disease) the lamina dura of the teeth is not visible and loses its identity roentgenographically. This is a point in differential diagnosis from tumor. They present the appearance of an eggshell expanding, unilocular lesion, with flecks and strands of bone. They produce a rather unique appearance due to their tendency to the dissolution of the neighboring bone without pressure displacement.

CHERUBISM-FAMILIAL FIBROUS DISYPLASIA OF THE JAWS. A peculiar type of fibrous tissue growth invading the mandible causes loss of dental structure and enlargement of the bone imparting a characteristic cherub-like appearance to the individual. Roentgenographically the condition resembled that seen in fibroma. It affected only the jaws of these individuals. Operative procedures for correction of the deformity were well borne.

MALIGNANT TUMORS. Primary osteogenic sarcoma may occur in the mandible just as well as any other bone in the body. Malignant involvement of the mandible (sarcoma or carcinoma) is most frequently encountered as a secondary growth. Carcinoma most frequently occurs as an extension from carcinomatous involvement of the mouth (Fig. 313). It causes a ragged irregular destruction of bone from invasion of the malignant process.

INFANTILE CORTICAL HYPEROSTOSIS. The jaw is frequently involved in infantile cortical hyperostosis, (q.v.). Search should be made for other bone involvement if the diagnosis is in doubt, but usually this will not be necessary since the symptoms and signs are typical.

BRAIN

INTRACRANIAL PATHOLOGY. Where examination of the skull is made for fracture it is sufficient that various flat views should be taken with every portion of the bony structure in intimate contact with the film to insure the greatest detail. Where intracranial pathology is suspected, in addition to the five ordinary routine positions (right and left lateral, frontal, occipital, and basal), several other special positions to show the petrous bone, sella turcica, etc., should be taken. Stereoscopic exposures are also advisable, especially in the lateral positions.

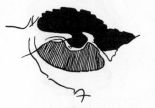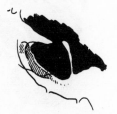

Normal Sella Turcica   Pituitary Tumor

Fig. 314

BONE EROSION PRODUCED BY TUMORS. If a tumor, in its growth, encroaches upon bony structure, it may cause destruction from pressure or invasion. Any such destruction within the skull is evidence of tumor or infection. The chief positions in which such pressure atrophy or erosion usually occurs are the sella turcica, the petrous bone, the optic and the auditory canals, and the sphenoidal fissure. Any portion of the bony structure may be involved, however. Tumors of the pituitary usually do not occur in children under fifteen years of age. Any enlargement of the pituitary or cystic involvement of the sellar or supra sellar region found in children, therefore, is probably due to craniopharyngioma. Such tumors have a very high incidence of calcification in and about the sella.

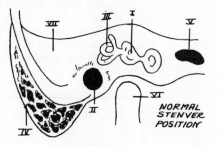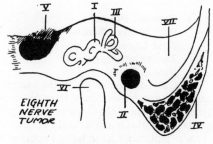

I. Cochlea   V. Internal Auditory Meatus
II. External Auditory Meatus   VI. Condyle of Mandible
III. Semicircular Canals   VII. Petrous Bone
IV. Mastoid Cells

Fig. 315

Tumors of the pituitary gland may, by their growth, so enlarge the sella turcica that pressure atrophy or destruction of the sella takes place (Fig. 314). The posterior clinoid processes, being the least stable of the bony structures composing the sella, are most frequently affected. Such involvement may be associated with headache and contraction of the visual fields or even blindness. In intrasellar tumors the dorsum sella may escape destruction but in extrasellar growths this is the first portion of the pituitary fossa to suffer. It is possible, however, by prolonged increased intracranial pressure, to have complete atrophy of the posterior clinoid processes without actual pathology of the pituitary. The processes may be pressed forward and decalcified in four months; on relief of pressure recalcification may occur in a like period.

Tumors of the middle and posterior fossa may encroach upon the petrous bone, causing rarefaction which is distinguishable in the roentgenogram. Cerebropontine angle tumors show destruction of the medial portion of the petrous ridge.

Hoelsh has found that about one-half of the tumors of the glomus jugulare arise in the adventitia of jugular bulb and then extend through the floor of the middle ear, into the tympanic cavity. Radiological findings are erosion of the petrous apex, sclerosis of the mastoid, destruction of the lower part of the petrous pyramid, enlargement of the jugular foramen. On arteriography a tortuous mass of new vessels were seen in the neck in the petrotemporal region.

In eighth nerve tumors, growth of the tumor caused expansion of the auditory canal and enlargement of the internal auditory meatus. This can often be detected by careful examination in Chamberlain-Towne or in Stenvers' position of the skull by comparison of the two sides (Fig. 315) (see Manual of Roentgenological Technique). Acoustic nerve tumors accounted for 8.7 percent of Cushings 2023 verified brain tumors.

Gliomas of the optic nerve may expand the optic canal. Comparison of the optic canals on both sides should show the abnormally enlarged canal on the affected side (Fig. 316).

INTRACRANIAL CALCIFICATIONS (Camp). Calcified deposits may be present in the cranial cavity as a result of many conditions, some of which are of no pathological significance, others of which are guide posts to various pathological lesions.

Calcareous deposits are found so consistently in certain locations in healthy individuals that they must be considered as physiological evidence of degeneration without pathological significance. These are:

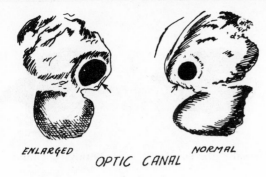

ENLARGED   OPTIC CANAL   NORMAL

Fig. 316

Choroid Plexus
Pacchionian Bodies
Falx Cerebri
Tentorium Cerebelli
Pineal Gland

Calcified deposits in the choroid plexes are readily recognized since they produce characteristic fine networklike shadows in the regions of the lateral ventricles which are usually bilateral, and usually fixed. Instances have been reported where the glomi were pedunculated permitting change in position of the calcareous deposits (Malbin). Calcifications in the Pacchionian bodies are represented by small irregular deposits along the superior longitudinal sinus under the vault of the skull. Calcifications elsewhere in the falx cerebri are commonly encountered in frontal examinations for nasal sinuses or in frontal views of the skull; such deposits may not be visible in the lateral roentgenogram since the calcified area presents itself as a thin layer in the lateral view. Calcification of the tentorium cerebelli is occasionally seen as a triangular-shaped structure in this region, seen on the lateral view. Calcification of the petroclinoid ligaments is not of significance.

Calcification of the pineal gland occurs in approximately 50% of all adults. Calcification is of itself not of pathological significance, but its presence allows determination of the pineal's position (Fig. 317A). Displacement of the pineal is seen in some, but by no means all, space-occupying intracranial

lesions. Shift of the pineal from its midline position as seen on antero-posterior view indicates an expanding lesion of the other hemisphere. Pineal displacement in the antero-posterior or superior-inferior direction as seen on lateral view is less frequently observed, but is an accurate indication of a mass lesion provided the displacement is beyond the known normal limits of pineal position.

Vastine and Kinney have charted the location of the pineal gland in a large number of normal individuals in order to establish a criterion for its normal location in the lateral view (Fig. 317B). The distance from the inner table of the frontal bone to the pineal was plotted against the distance of the antero-posterior diameter (chart 1); and the distance from the inner table of the vault to the pineal, against the distance of the inner table to the base (chart 2); as a result of charting the position of a large number of calcified pineal glands, a zone of normal locations was established.

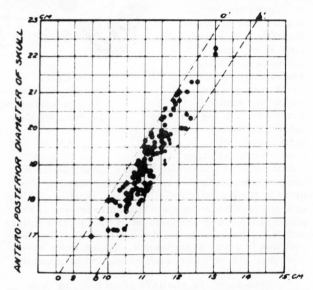

Chart 1. Distance, inner table of frontal bone to pineal.

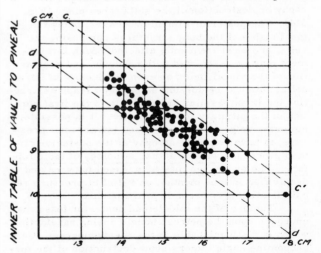

Chart 2. Distance, inner table of vault to base.

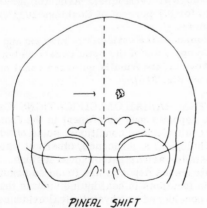

PINEAL SHIFT

Fig. 317A

Fig. 317B

Other intracranial calcareous deposits of pathological importance include calcifications in association with:

Vascular Structures -
Arteriosclerosis of cranial vessels
Aneurysms of cranial vessels
Hemangiomas associated with large vascular tumors of scalp and face
Angiomatous malformations
Hematomas—intracranial

Previous Destruction -
Encephalitis, multiple, fine, dense calcifications
Degenerated brain substance—calcified
Toxoplasma infection when healed—small calcareous deposits irregularly distributed

Degenerative Nerve Processes—
Calcification of basal nuclei
Tuberous sclerosis

Calcified deposits in the wall of an aneurysm of the carotid artery in the skull may show as a comma-like shadow within the orbit in the frontal view; in the lateral view the calcified walls show as parallel lines traversing the region of the sella. Ringlike periarterial calcifications about the vessels have been described but are very rare. Calcified deposits in the pituitary itself are much less frequent; they cannot be considered as of significance unless associated with symptoms. Cysts about the pituitary region often are the site of calcareous deposits; hematomas may show deposits at their margins; even chronic abscesses may have calcium deposits. Calcareous deposits other than these must be viewed with suspicion as evidence of intracranial new growth.

Encephalitis or any other type of degenerative or destructive brain lesion may be followed by calcium deposit.

Toxoplasmosis is the most frequent cause of multiple areas of intracranial calcification present at birth or in the first year of life.

Calcification of the basal nuclei usually occurs bilaterally in the regions of these structures.

Tuberous sclerosis (Ackermann; Dickerson) produces irregular areas of calcification in the brain within the tumorous masses. These may affect almost any structure of the brain, so that their location is not restricted; their symptomatology is variable depending upon the area involved. Tuberous sclerosis may also involve bony structures producing cyst-like areas in the cancellous structure simulating polyostotic fibrous dysplasia. When the lungs are involved fibrocystic changes occur which may be present throughout both lungs.

DEFORMITIES OF SKULL IN HEAD INJURY, "STRESS COAT" TECHNIQUE.
By a very technical method of "stress coating" the skull studies have been made of deformities of the skull following head injuries for the detection of resulting stress and strain. By this method it is possible to predict the likelihood of fractures occurring at various locations in the skull when subjected to certain trauma, (Gurdjian, Lissner, Webster).

INTRACRANIAL NEOPLASMS. The most common types of intracranial neoplasms are: (Percival Bailey):
Glioma
Pituitary Adenoma
Chromophobe
Chromophile
Eosinophilic
Basophilic
Mixed
Meningioma
Neurinoma-Acoustic Nerve Tumor.

Gliomas occur in many different forms, according to their cell derivation. From their x-ray standpoint they show no difference in characteristics; they may occur in any location. Localizing symptoms may be so few or confused that it may even be difficult to determine the side on which the lesion is located.

The presence of a brain neoplasm may be indicated by calcification seen on the skull films. In a series of 661 proven brain tumors, calcification was noted in 15%, (Gilbertson and Good). The most frequently occurring type of tumor, the glioblastoma multiforme, shows radiographic calcification infrequently. Other tumors of less common occurrence show calcification more often. Although oligodendrogliomas comprise about one-tenth of the total number of gliomas seen, half of these tumors calcify to some degree. Ependymomas, also not too common in general occurrence, calcify in one-fourth of instances. Astrocytomas calcify in a frequency of 13%. Medulloblastomas and ganglioneuromas rarely if ever show calcification.

Meningiomas of themselves show calcific densities appreciably often, but the detection of their presence is aided by the accompanying bone changes, erosion or hyperostosis. Craniopharyngiomas calcify very often, particularly in children. Tumors of hemangiomatous nature, metastatic carcinomas and sarcomas were not observed with calcium deposits. Calcification is thought to be of predominantly strand-like nature in oligodendrogliomas and astrocytomas. In spongioblastoma multiforme and ependymoma, punctate calcification is more to be expected.

Detection of calcification is a reliable roentgenographic sign of the presence and approximate location of a brain tumor. Films of excellent technic are required for often the calcification is highly localized and very faint. Differentiation must always be made from areas of physiological calcification, or areas of calcification which are not of pathological significance.

Another method by which this may be determined, if the pineal gland is calcified, is to observe any deflection of the pineal gland from its normal position in the midline. Tumors on one side of the brain, even when located in the frontal or occipital lobes far beyond the location of the pineal, may cause its shift to the opposite side; this is probably due to the edema from interference with circulation, caused by the tumor. Since approximately 50% of all adults have calcified pineal glands, it is obvious that this may be a very helpful sign (Fig. 317A). Tumors of this sort rarely produce bone erosion or production but may be associated with the manifestations of increased intracranial pressure. Of Cushing's 2023 verified brain tumors 42.6% were of this type, constituting by far the greatest percentage of neoplasm found in the brain. Displacement of the calcified pineal body in the antero-posterior or superior-inferior axis is less common, but does occur with some large tumors. Displacement beyond the normal range of position, known from measurement of normals, is significant. Vastine and Kinney have prepared charts for this purpose (Fig. 317B).

Pituitary adenomas* are of three general types: the chromophobe adenoma, in which the granules do not stain; the chromophile adenoma, in which the granules stain, with eosin (eosinophilic adenoma) or with hematoxylin (basophilic adenoma) or with both (mixed cell adenoma). Of Cushing's 2023 verified brain tumors pituitary adenomas accounted for the second highest percentage, 17.8%.

The chromophobic adenoma produces a large bulky tumor which expands the sella turcica, causing backward displacement of the posterior clinoid processes and erosion. It may attain considerable size before its presence is suspected. The sella has a "ballooned" appearance, suggesting the pathological process is enlarging the sella from within. This is to be distinguished from the decalcification and exclusion of the posterior clinoids as seen in generalized increased intracranial pressure. Disturbance of the visual field and headache is often the first manifestation of the condition. By far the greatest number of pituitary adenomas are of this type. This type is associated with pituitary insufficiency. The chromophobic type shows the greatest response to x-ray therapy; the tumor becomes checked in its growth or subsides enough to cause improved vision and remission of headaches but care must be exercised before any evaluation of treatment is made; long remissions are frequently encountered.

The eosinophilic adenoma produces some enlargement of the pituitary but never the large bulky tumor seen in the chromophobic type. About 90% show some enlargement of the sella turcica but in only one-third of these is the enlargement sufficient to cause disturbance of the vision. This type is associated with pituitary hyperfunction, producing gigantism in young individuals and acromegaly when the hyperfunction begins in adulthood. The osteochondrodystrophic changes in the bones of the hand and jaw of the acromegalic is due to secretion of excess growth hormone after the epiphyses have closed.

Basophilic adenoma, or pituitary basophilism never produces enlargement or deformity of the bony sella. A diffuse osteoporosis of all bones is seen in this (Cushing's) syndrome.

Meningioma. This is a bulbous encapsulated tumor arising from the meninges or arachnoid granules which often attains considerable size. Meningiomas may occur at any location but are most fre-

quently encountered in the parasagittal center region (one-fourth) in the cribriform, ophthalmic and sphenoidal regions, along the transverse sinus and near the foramina of the cranial nerves especially the olfactory groove. Of Cushing's 2023 verified brain tumors 13.4% were of this type.

This tumor gives rise to certain localized changes in the skull which may be characteristic when correlated with the slow progression of the clinical symptoms. These roentgen manifestations consist of local evidence of bone erosion and bone production. Erosion is indicated by irregular localized thinning of the bone. Bone production may occur however from invasion of the tumor into the Haversian canals stimulating new bone formation which may be so pronounced that it appears radiographically as spicules of bone radiating perpendicular to the cranial vault. Usually however the picture is one of both new bone production and destruction going on simultaneously. There is often associated dilatation of the diploetic veins in the region of the tumor. The tumor may become so large that it causes a palpable mass in the cranium. Endothelioma, originating in this region, may grow through the bony spaces of the skull to the outside, forming palpable tumors also. They may or may not be attended with demonstrable bone destruction on roentgen examination.

Somewhat similar areas of irregular bone production are encountered in healthy adult individuals without intracranial tumors (Fig. 318). This is known as hyperostosis internus cranialis, and may occur at any location of the skull. Such areas are most common in the frontal region (frontalis). They have been variously ascribed to endocrine disorders, atrophy of the brain with bony proliferation from the arachnoid, etc. Roentgenologically they can be differentiated from calcifications of meningeal tumors in that they do not occur in an isolated location but are bilateral showing a symmetrical pattern on both sides of the head most frequently encountered in the frontal region. Pedersen, following a correlated study of the roentgen findings in the skulls of 908 female patients and their endocrine manifestations, with

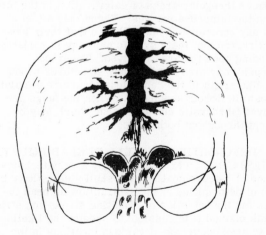

Fig. 318

special reference to adiposity and hypertrichosis, concluded that their coexistence cannot be considered of clinical significance; nor, was there any significant relationship between the instances of hyperostosis frontalis internus and epilepsy.

Neurinoma, (acoustic). Acoustic nerve tumors arise from the vestibular division of the eighth nerve within the auditory canal. By their slow growth they cause expansion and erosion of the internal auditory meatus. Here then is another instance in which x-ray examination may be of value; comparative examination of the two sides in the Stenvers and Chamberlain-Towne positions may disclose this characteristic expansion on the involved side.

Other rarer types of intracranial tumors are:
Congenital tumors
Sarcoma, primary
Papilloma of choroid plexus
Metastatic tumors
Granulomatous "tumors"
    Tuberculoma
    Syphiloma
Angioma
Osteoma
Craniopharyngioma
Chordoma

Of these the angioma and osteoma are of greatest roentgenological importance since they give roentgen manifestations of their presence.

Angiomata are frequently accompanied by excessive blood vessel markings of the cranial bones. Sometimes these markings are of unusual design and communicate directly with the intracranial neoplasm. Extensive angiomatosis of the retina and brain is known as Von Hipple's disease (See Tumors of Bone).

Osteomata are rarely seen as intracranial tumors; they do occur, however, and manifest themselves as dense well-defined bony growths. They are dense and hard and often are referred to as ivory osteomata. They frequently occur in the nasal sinuses (q.v.), especially the frontal, and have been encountered in the orbit and within the cranial cavity.

Other intracranial conditions not strictly of neoplastic origin, but of great importance, are cyst and subdural hematoma. Both of these may be of traumatic origin, and both by the pressure which they exert on the brain may cause serious symptoms. They may cause no roentgenological manifestations but may require ventriculography to demonstrate their presence and location. Occasionally the pineal may be shifted by these space-occupying lesions.

Craniopharyngiomas are seen appreciably often in children, less often in the adult. Hint of their presence is given by detection of calcification superior to the sella, and in some cases by enlargement of the sella itself. Chordomas are rare tumors. Erosion or calcification may be produced at the base of the skull.

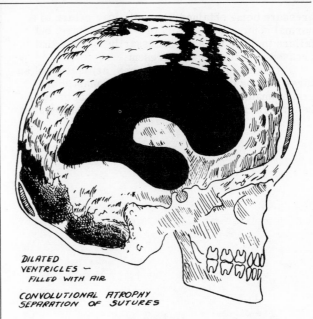

DILATED VENTRICLES — FILLED WITH AIR

CONVOLUTIONAL ATROPHY SEPARATION OF SUTURES

Fig. 319

INCREASED INTRACRANIAL PRESSURE:* The radiographic signs of increased intracranial pressure are three: separation of the cranial sutures, excessive convolutional markings of the skull and decalcification and erosion of the sella turcica. For separation of the sutures to occur, the increased intracranial pressure must begin in the infant or young child. Once the sutures have made progress toward closure, this finding is not often seen. It is rare over the age of ten, and practically non-existent over the age of 20, (Bull). In very young children this finding may be quite pronounced.

Increased convolutional markings of the skull, known as convolutional atrophy, increased digital markings, beaten silver appearance, as well as other terms, may at times indicate increased intracranial pressure. This finding is so often present without increased intracranial pressure, and is found in normals, particularly children, that it is felt not to be a reliable sign. It must always be correlated with other signs, both clinical and radiographic, of increased pressure.

Decalcification of the dorsum sellae and erosion of the dorsum are reliable signs of increased intracranial pressure. The changes in this portion of the base of the skull are thought to be secondary to pressure from the dilated, enlarged third ventricle in cases of internal hydrocephalus. These changes which affect the dorsum of the sella are in almost all cases distinct from the bony erosion occurring within the sella from a tumor arising in the sella itself. In cases of primary pituitary tumor, the sella is ballooned, that is enlarged, from within. The decalcification and erosion of the dorsum suggest that factors from outside the sella are at work. Any long-standing and significant cause of generalized increased intracranial pressure may give these alterations of the dorsum. With relief of the increase in pressure being obtained, the sella may return to a normal contour and density of bony structure, but failure to do so does not necessarily indicate that increased pressure is still present.

Under certain circumstances, separation of sutures may be due to infiltration of neoplastic or granulomatous tissue, as in xanthomatosis or leukemia. Decalcification of the dorsum sellae is seen to a certain degree in older age group without correlation of increased intracranial pressure. For this reason it is not quite as reliable a sign in the aged patient as in a young adult. In young children sella erosion and decalcification is not frequently seen, for with the separation of the sutures, the pressure is more or less relieved. Once the sutures have closed, sella changes are prominent.

VENTRICULOGRAPHY

VENTRICULAR SYSTEM. The ventricular system of the brain consists of a series of cavities, centrally located within the brain substance. They are four in number: right and left lateral which form the largest structures occupying the two hemispheres of the brain; the third ventricle, representing a small flat compartment located exactly in the midline just below and somewhat between the two lateral ventricles, and finally the fourth ventricle consisting of a triangular structure below the level of the other ventricles. They are filled with cerebrospinal fluid which is secreted by the choroid plexes, delicate vascular structures covering the posterior portions of the floors and lateral walls of the lateral ventricles. These ventricles communicate anteriorly with the third ventricle by the foramina of Monro, and the third ventricle, in turn, empties into the fourth ventricle by way of the Aqueduct of Sylvius, a slender canal which extends almost vertically downward between the two ventricles, when the head is held in the

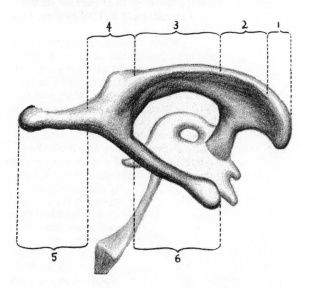

Fig. 320A. Lateral view; lateral ventricle divided into six parts.

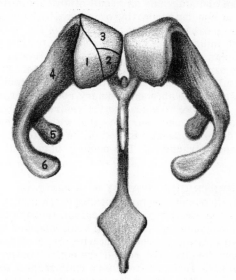

Fig. 320B. Anterior view of ventricles.

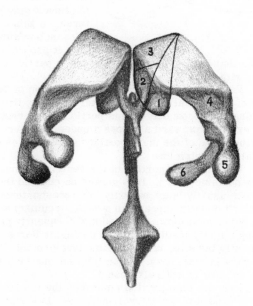

Fig. 320C. Posterior view of ventricles.

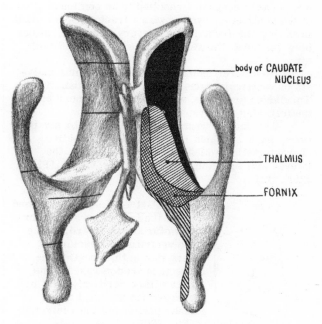

Fig. 320D. Ventral view of ventricles.

Fig. 320. Model of the ventricular system after A. Torkildsen and A. H. Pirie, (Am. J. R., and R. Th. 32:145, 1934).

upright position. From the fourth ventricle the cerebrospinal fluid not only finds its way into the spinal canal, but into the subarachnoid spaces of the brain also by way of the Foramina of Luschka and Magendie. It is excreted by the pacchionian bodies, which lie along the superior longitudinal sinus, into the blood stream. Any interference of hypersecretion or deficient elimination will result in generalized dilatation of the ventricular system or internal or communicating hydrocephalus. Excessive collection of fluid in the subdural space is known as external hydrocephalus. Occlusion of the foramina of Luschka and Magendie as result of arachnoiditis is known as noncommunicating or internal hydrocephalus.

A great majority of the tumors of the brain do not give indication of their presence by ordinary x-ray examination because they are similar in density to the brain tissue in which they lie. The ventricular system, because of its fluid content, likewise fails to show on ordinary roentgen examination. In order to visualize the ventricular system, therefore, it is necessary to fill it with some medium of different density to that of the surrounding soft tissue structures. The medium in general use is air.

VENTRICULOGRAPHY.* A needle is inserted, through a trephine opening in the skull, (usually in the occipitoparietal region), through the brain substance into the lateral ventricle, and the fluid withdrawn. Replacement with air, a medium of lesser density, will render the entire ventricular system clearly demonstrable on radiographic examination. This method for examination of the brain was first suggested to Dandy, its originator, by a roentgenogram taken by Wm. H. Stewart in which pneumocephalus resulted from communication of the ventricular system with a fracture of the skull involving the frontal sinus; every time the patient blew his nose the ventricular system filled with air.

No clearer method for the fundamental analysis of ventriculograms has been devised than that by Torkildsen and Pirie, which is briefly described in the following paragraphs.

The lateral ventricle is divided into six portions, each of which bears certain distinctive characteristics which can be identified in the lateral and also the anteroposterior views, (Fig. 320A, B, C).

Part 1. Anterior flattened tip of the frontal horn as it turns downward and outward. Since the ventricular structure is very thin in this location the roentgen shadow cast by this part will be relatively faint in comparison with that of the other portions of the ventricle, (Fig. 320E).

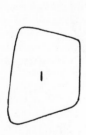

Fig. 320E

Part 2. The portion of the ventricle just posterior to the anterior horn and in front of the thalmus constitutes the second part. The shadow cast by this portion is more intense; it is more triangular and does not deviate from the midline as does the frontal horn, (Fig. 320F).

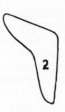

Fig. 320F

Part 3. Air filling the lateral ventricle posterior to part two produces a third shadow which extends across the upper portion of part two due to the narrowed portion of the lateral ventricle in this region, (Fig. 320G).

Fig. 320G

When all three shadows are superimposed they produce a composite representation of the body of the lateral ventricle as seen in the Ventriculogram, (Fig. 320H and J). "If the head is tipped backward when the film is taken, shadow three is seen to merge into one outline with shadow two because the latter becomes situated at a higher level than the thalmus. Because of the length of the air-filled space it throws a darker shadow than any other part of the ventriculogram," (Fig. 320I). If the head is tipped forward when the film is taken, shadow two is seen to extend upward almost overshadowing part three. If this occurs on one side only it probably means that the ventricle on this side is partially filled with fluid.

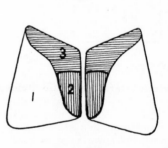

Fig. 320H

Part 4. This is the remaining portion of the body of the lateral ventricle posterior to the thalmus. The shadows produced by this portion of the ventricles extend downward as more slender structures on either side of the main portions of the bodies of the lateral ventricles.

Part 5. This portion of the ventricle consists of the posterior horn. It is viewed on end and therefore can usually be shown only in a foreshortened view. "It usually appears as a dark circumscribed area between shadows four and six, frequently projecting slightly medially." The posterior horns are frequently the sites of anomalous development; they may vary in size, form and outline on one or both sides or may be entirely absent.

Part 6. This portion embraces the inferior or temporal horn of the lateral ventricle. In the anteroposterior view this portion of the ventricle also appears somewhat foreshortened because of the projection of the rays along the long axis of the horn.

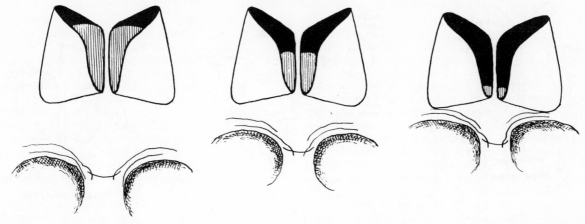

Fig. 320I   Fig. 320J   Fig. 320K

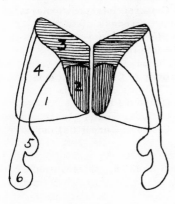

Fig. 320L

The tips deviate medially at their anterior ends. Figure 320L shows a composite view of all of the ventricular shadows.

In the postero-anterior position, if the ventricles are well filled with air, these same structures can usually be recognized; their appearance is similar with the exception that the structures closest to the film are smaller and more clearly outlined. The anterior ends of the temporal horns frequently do not show in this position due to gravitation of the cerebrospinal fluid remaining in the ventricles. Similarly, in the anteroposterior position, small amounts of air trapped in the tips of the temporal horns may appear as isolated globules of air.

In the lateral view, these structures can usually be well outlined. Brains fit the skulls which encase them and their ventricles conform to the size and shape of the brains which contain them. The third ventricle is flat in this position and therefore casts a very faint shadow but it can usually be detected with the aqueduct of Sylvius which extends almost vertically downward into the triangular fourth ventricle below. If it is desired to see the third ventricle in greater detail a lateral film with the patient's head hanging backward over the edge of the stretcher, vertex downward, will allow air to better fill this structure. For the temporal horns, Clark's position, projecting the rays from behind forward, patient in the upright position with head depressed forward, gives a very satisfactory auxiliary view.

From the fourth ventricle the cerebrospinal fluid passes into the spinal canal and by way of the foramina of Luschka and Magendie into the subarachnoid passageways which cover the brain. From these spaces the fluid is removed by the pacchionian bodies into the superior longitudinal sinus.

Roentgenologically by following these diagrammatic divisions (Fig. 321A to D) it is often possible to more accurately establish the location and extent of a lesion and to come to a clearer understanding of the pathology present.

Excessive secretion of cerebrospinal fluid by the choroid plexus or its defective elimination by the pacchionian bodies will result in increased fluid accumulation in and enlargement of the ventricular system (Fig. 321F). Any interference with its natural circulation as for instance closure of the foramina of Luschka and Magendie, from an inflammatory process such as meningitis, will have a similar result.

Blockage of the flow of fluid by invasion or pressure of a tumor mass will cause dilatation of the ventricular system proximal to the obstruction. Dilatation of the lateral ventricles without deviation or displacement would indicate a third ventricle tumor. Dilatation of the third ventricle as well as the lateral ventricle, either a lesion in the region of the Aqueduct of Silvius or in the fourth ventricle. Outlining of the tumor in the third or fourth ventricles by air ascertains the position of the obstructing lesion. Dilatation of the ventricular system then without displacement of ventricles to one side or the other, and without encroachment upon the ventricular wall from one side or the other, indicates a midline tumor. More often in addition to dilatation of the ventricular system there is displacement or encroachment on the ventricular structures, indicating that the space-occupying lesion is unilateral.

The types of lesions most commonly encountered in which ventriculography is of value are space occupying lesions such as brain tumors, cysts or hematomas. Since the density of all such lesions is ordinarily the same as that of the brain they cannot be differentiated roentgenographically from the surrounding tissue, unless, as occasionally happens, they may show fine calcium deposits. They all take

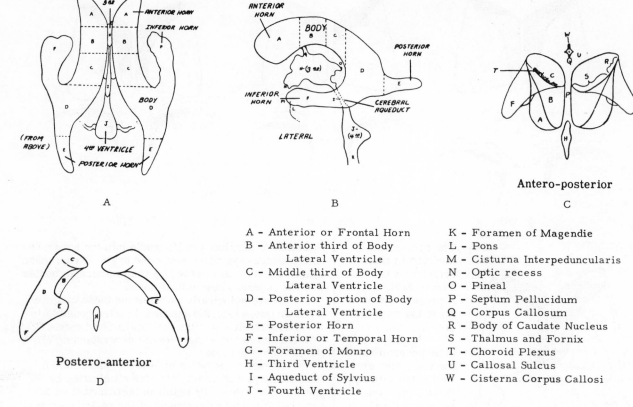

A

B

Antero-posterior

C

Postero-anterior

D

A - Anterior or Frontal Horn
B - Anterior third of Body
    Lateral Ventricle
C - Middle third of Body
    Lateral Ventricle
D - Posterior portion of Body
    Lateral Ventricle
E - Posterior Horn
F - Inferior or Temporal Horn
G - Foramen of Monro
H - Third Ventricle
I - Aqueduct of Sylvius
J - Fourth Ventricle

K - Foramen of Magendie
L - Pons
M - Cisturna Interpeduncularis
N - Optic recess
O - Pineal
P - Septum Pellucidum
Q - Corpus Callosum
R - Body of Caudate Nucleus
S - Thalmus and Fornix
T - Choroid Plexus
U - Callosal Sulcus
W - Cisterna Corpus Callosi

After A. Torkildsen and A. H. Pirie. Am. J. Roentg. and Rad. Th., 32:145, Aug. 1934.

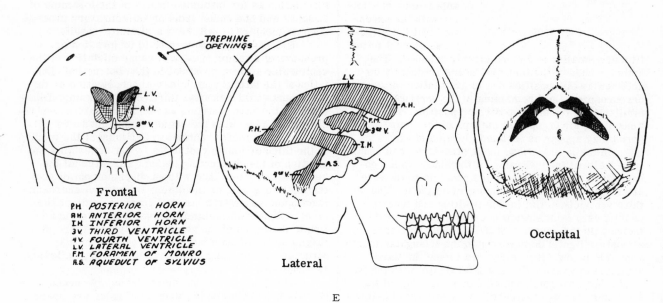

Frontal

PH POSTERIOR HORN
AH ANTERIOR HORN
IH INFERIOR HORN
3V THIRD VENTRICLE
4V FOURTH VENTRICLE
LV LATERAL VENTRICLE
FM FORAMEN OF MONRO
AS AQUEDUCT OF SYLVIUS

Lateral

Occipital

E

Fig. 321

up space within the cranium, however, and cause displacement of the normal structures. In this way it may be possible, from a study of the displacement of the air-filled ventricular structures, to determine the location and approximate size of abnormal space-occupying lesions. Correlation of such findings with

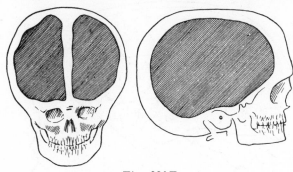

Fig. 321F

the clinical history and neurological findings may serve to determine the type of lesion and even the location of the involvement.

A knowledge of the structures in immediate contact with the ventricles in certain locations may be of value in determining the structure involved in any lesion of this specific location. For instance: the body of the caudate nucleus is in contact with the floor of the lateral ventricle throughout its anterior half and along its lateral margin farther back; the fornix lies on its inner side with the thalmus in between, (Fig. 320D). The third ventricle is in close relation anteriorly to the optic recess, below to the infundibulum (of pituitary) and posteriorly to the pineal body so that tumors of these structures may be indicated by encroachment on this structure.

Cortical lesions of the parietal region have a tendency to depress the lateral ventricle on the side involved. Temporal lobe lesions displace the ventricular system to the opposite side, compressing the lateral ventricle on the affected side and swinging the upper portion of the third ventricle to the opposite side without disturbing its lower midline attachment, (Fig. 321G). This is because of the firm unyielding position of the falx cerebri. Subtentorial tumors almost always block the flow of cerebrospinal fluid, causing dilatation of the third and lateral ventricles.

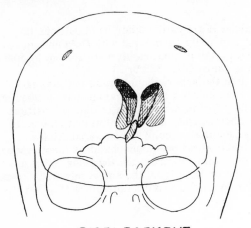

DISPLACEMENT

Fig. 321G

Areas of cortical necrosis frequently rupture into the ventricular system forming fistulous tracts, thereby permitting air to escape into the destroyed area in the brain on ventriculographic examination. Such areas may be congenital or may be acquired from injury; the condition is referred to as Porencephalus.

Cortical atrophy from trauma, hemorrhage, degenerative disease, or other cause, results in dilatation and displacement of the ventricular structures also. Here a different mechanism is at work. The ventricle on the side of atrophy enlarges, occupying the space which was formerly brain tissue.

In addition to acquired pathological lesions there are many due to congenital developmental defects, (Lowman, et al.). Anomalies of the septum pellucidum may be encountered. Normally the septum pellucidum is the membranous structure which separates the two lateral ventricles. Ordinarily it is only a few millimeters in thickness but in agenesis of the corpus callosum it becomes very broad, widely separating the two lateral ventricles causing them to project upward as sharp horn-like structures. Tumors of the septum pellucidum may cause similar widening.

Or the septum pellucidum may itself house a cavernous space which is spoken of as the fifth ventricle, or if it is dilated, as a cyst of the septum pellucidum.

Strand-like structures have been encountered crossing the lateral ventricles—probably due to remains of blood vessel structures from the developmental period.

Herniation of small portions of various ventricular structures have been observed and identified. They are of importance only in so far as they help to explain certain symptoms present in the case.

The complexity of symptoms and signs sometimes encountered is almost beyond understanding. It is only by astute correlation of these with the ventriculographic findings that a diagnosis can be made.

A glomus of vascular structures presents a rounded or ovoid structure within the choroid plexus in the lateral ventricle near its junction with the inferior horn. It is a normal structure which may frequently be seen in the lateral view of the ventricles. Situated in this position it is under unusual conditions subject to injury during ventricular puncture. Hemorrhage or oedema of the glomus may cause it to swell up to considerable size giving the appearance of a tumefaction from neoplastic cause. Reexamination after a week or so in any suspicious case will see the "glomus tumor" completely regressed.

THORIUM DIOXIDE FOR VENTRICULOGRAPHY (Fig. 321H). Thorium dioxide solutions have been utilized for outlining the ventricular system. There is no doubt about the advantage of the fine opacity obtained. Thorium dioxide, although used in small quantity for this purpose, is of restricted value because of its radioactivity.

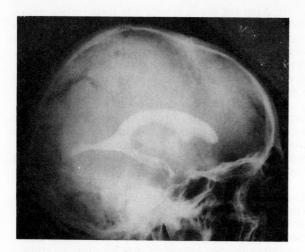

Fig. 321H

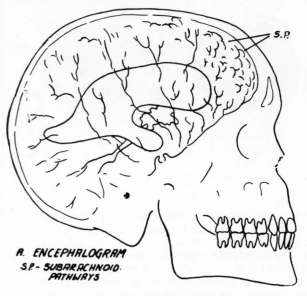

A. ENCEPHALOGRAM
S.P.- SUBARACHNOID.
PATHWAYS

Fig. 322A₁

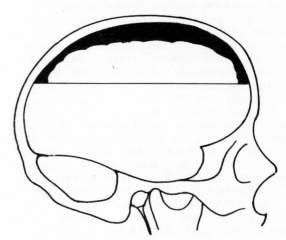

Fig. 322A₂. Air in Subdural Space.

ENCEPHALOGRAPHY* (Fig. 322A). Small amounts of cerebrospinal fluid may be drained at a time and air substituted by means of lumbar puncture. This may be done only if there is no evidence of increased intracranial pressure; otherwise the brain stem may be jammed down into the foramen magnum and death may occur from respiratory paralysis. Air introduced in this fashion in suitable cases finds its way not only into the ventricles but into the subarachnoid cisterns (Fig. 322A₁) and smaller subarachnoid pathways as well. The ventricles themselves, when completely filled with air by this method, appear exactly the same as when filled by the direct ventriculography. The subarachnoid passageways appear as fine tortuous, irregular channels at the periphery of the brain often showing especially pronounced in the anterior portion over the frontal area, due to the fact that the patient usually lies on his back and the air collects anteriorly. Laceration and hematoma from injury often cause obliteration of these markings over the involved area. Subtentorial tumors may obstruct the access of air to these spaces when introduced by lumbar puncture. Brain atrophy may be indicated by ventricular dilatation on the affected side, or by enlargement of the subarachnoid pathways.

Pneumocephalus (pneumocranium) is an abnormal collection of air within the skull, (Eagleshaw).

Intracranial pneumocephalus is usually due to trauma such as fracture involving the accessory nasal sinuses or mastoid air cells. It may, however, be non-traumatic due to erosion into these structures.

It may be extradural in which case it is usually small in amount remaining fixed in position, limited to the site of trauma.

Subdural air on the other hand outlines the brain; it is usually associated with fluid and moves freely within the cranial cavity with change in position of the skull, (Fig. 322A₂).

Air in the subarachnoid space outlines the passageways as seen in encephalography; it does not move freely within the skull on change of position, but may show variations of its distribution due to prolonged maintainance of the same position.

Intracerebral pneumocephalus is most frequently seen extending upward from the floor of the anterior fossa or back from the anterior wall in close apposition to frontal and ethmoid sinus fluid level.

CEREBRAL ANGIOGRAPHY

CEREBRAL ANGIOGRAPHY * (Fig. 322B, C and D). Roentgenographic examination of the skull after injection of opaque material (Diodrast, Urokon, Hypaque) into the cerebral circulation will disclose the vascular structures clearly. Injection is made into the carotid artery on the side examination is primarily desired. The injection of the contrast material is made rapidly, so as to provide sufficient concentration of opaque material in the vessels to be visualized. Films are taken in arterial phase, venous phase, or both arterial and venous phase, or films are taken in rapid succession with the aid of a cassette changer. Bilateral carotid angiography is performed when indicated. Vertebral artery injection of contrast material is similarly performed when primary visualization of the posterior contrast material, particularly when used in too large amount or too frequently within a short time, may damage the blood-brain barrier, causing convulsions and other disabilities.

Cerebral angiography is a valuable diagnostic procedure for many types of intracranial lesions. Foremost in importance are the lesions of the blood aneurysms, a few millimeters in diameter may be visualized. Some prefer stereoscopic films for greater accuracy. Aneurysms are most frequently seen arising from the anterior basilar vessels, and the anterior communicating artery. Arterio-venous malformations, thought to be congenital in origin, may simulate brain tumors or aneurysms in their symptomatology, but can be differentiated by their appearance on the angiogram. Blockage of a vessel by a thrombus, or by arteriosclerotic disease may also be recognized.

Displacement of the vascular pattern by space-occupying lesions leads to the recognition of intracranial abnormalities. Familiarity with the normal vascular pattern and its variations is of course required, before the minor distortions and displacements can be recognized, and a diagnosis is made. The finding of vessel displacement without other abnormality is a non-specific observation, for tumors, cysts, hematomas, both intracerebral and over the surface of the brain, and abscess may all exert pressure. Vascular tumors, regardless of their cell type, however, may be detected by the observation of a localized area of abnormal blood vessels. This visualization of the blood vessels within the neoplasm itself, is referred to as "tumor stain", especially when contrast material is seen in the tumor vessels at a different time, than in the surrounding normal vessels.

As with any other area of diagnostic radiology, familiarity must be obtained with normal findings, and then with typical pathological findings before proficiency can be approached. Cooperation between the neurosurgeon and radiologist is essential for accurate diagnosis. Diagrams of the normal vascular pattern, arterial phase, are shown in Figs. 322C and D. A complete examination requires films to be made in lateral and anterior-posterior projections. Fig. 322B illustrates subarachnoid cisterns.

Examination in both lateral views is of advantage for comparison. Reversal of one of the films gives similar images which are more readily compared. Colored pencils may be used to map out the distribution of each arterial structure.

The procedure is not without danger since replacement of the blood with a high percentage of contrast medium deprives the brain cells of proper oxygenation which cannot be prolonged for more than a few minutes without dire consequences. Danger from reaction from iodine sensitization can be averted by previous testing with small quantities of the drug before the full injection is made.

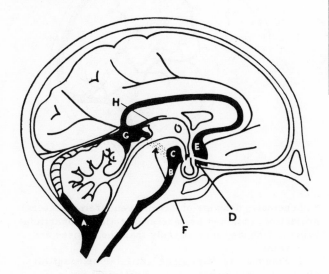

Fig. 322B. Diagrammatic sagittal section to show the subarachnoid cisterns (black). A. cisterna magna; B. cisterna pontis; C. cisterna interpeduncularis; D. cisterna chiasmatis; E. cisterna laminae terminalis; F. cisterna ambiens; G. cisterna venae magnae cerebri; H. central part of choroid fissure (usually obliterated). Joining E and G is the cisterna corporis callosi. Extending backwards over the cerebellum from cisterna magna cerebri is the superior cerebellar cistern. (After Graeme Robertson.)

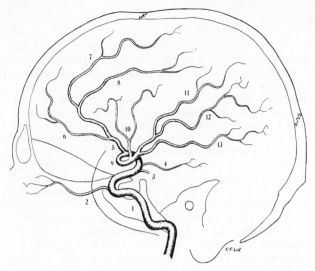

C. Lateral projection   D. Anteroposterior projection

Schematic drawings of normal arteriograms of the
internal carotid artery.

1. Internal carotid artery. 2. Ophthalmic artery. 3. Posterior communicating artery. 4. Anterior choroidal artery. 5. Anterior cerebral artery. 6. Frontopolar artery. 7. Callosomarginal artery. 8. Pericallosal artery. 9. Middle cerebral artery. 10. Ascending frontoparietal artery. 11. Posterior parietal artery. 12. Angular artery. 13. Posterior temporal artery.

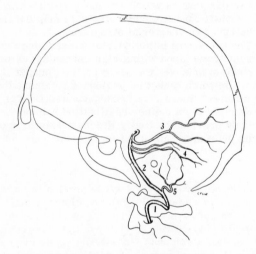

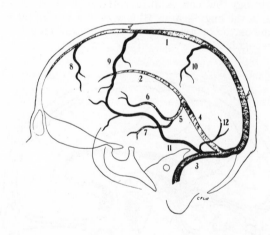

E. Schematic drawing of a normal vertebral arteriogram in lateral projection.

1. Vertebral artery. 2. Basilar artery. 3. Posterior cerebral artery. 4. Superior cerebellar artery. 5. Posterior inferior cerebellar artery.

(The schematic drawings on this page are used by courtesy of List, Burge and F. Hodges, Radiol., 45:1, 1945.)

F. Schematic drawing of normal venogram in lateral projection, obtained by carotid injection. Superficial veins are shaded more darkly than the sinuses and deep veins.

1. Superior sagittal sinus. 2. Inferior sagittal sinus. 3. Transverse sinus. 4. Straight sinus. 5. Great cerebral vein of Galen. 6. Internal cerebral vein. 7. Basal vein of Rosenthal. 8. Frontal ascending vein. 9. Rolandic vein of Trolard. 10. Parietal ascending vein. 11. Communicating temporal vein of Labbé. 12. Descending temporo-occiptal vein.

Fig. 322

MYELOGRAPHY

MYELOGRAPHY. * Tumors arising within the spinal canal often do not give evidence of their presence on ordinary roentgenographic examination. Tumors here, however, as elsewhere, may, by their gradual growth, cause pressure on the adjacent walls of the bony canal, causing pressure defects and widening of the interpediculate spaces. If these spaces are measured and chartered for the various levels of the spine and are compared to curves showing the maximum variation of normal, any unusual localized widening of the canal can be detected. In some instances, by this means, tumors of the spinal cord not otherwise evident can be diagnosed (Fig. 323A). Interpediculate space measurements in children do not show the sudden change at T9 or T10 shown in adults; a difference of 1 cm. between T12 and L5 is indication of possible intraspinal pathology requiring myelography. By age of 12 the curve assumes its normal adult appearance (Landmesser).

Even where neurological signs give unmistakable evidence of the presence of a lesion (tumor) of the cord it is important to determine the exact location of the pathology before surgical exploration. The lowest extent of the lesion is usually very well demonstrated by the neurological findings, but the upper level is most important to the surgeon.

Roentgenographic examination after the introduction of contrast medium, either of greater density (Lipiodol or Pantopaque) or lesser density (air) than the surrounding bony structures is known as Myelography.

Where there is a question of a block from a spinal cord tumor, 6 cc. of Pantopaque may be injected into the cisterna magna and its descent observed as the patient is tilted into the upright position on a fluoroscopic table. The oil being heavier than the spinal fluid should descend rapidly and smoothly to the sacrum. For this examination the patient lies upon his back on the tilt table since in this position the oil flows more freely over the natural curves of the spine. If there is any block-

age of the oil in its descent roentgenograms are made using the overhead radiographic tube with the cassette in the Bucky holder under the patient (Fig. 323B). The patient should be tilted up and down several times to make sure of the constancy of the level; care should be taken not to allow the head to become too low since in this position the contrast material may run into the ventricles of the brain. Injection of contrast material by lumbar puncture allows determination of the lower border of a completely obstructing lesion. When the level of a block is established care must be taken to observe the surrounding bony structure carefully, lest disease of the bone may be the cause of the obstruction.

Where the lesion to be investigated is probably due to herniation of an intervertebral disc in the lower lumbar and upper sacral regions, the opaque oil may be injected into the lumbar region with a No. 18 gauge lumbar puncture needle. The space between the third and fourth or fourth and fifth lumbar vertebrae may be used. The lower space facilitates removal of the oil after the examination is completed. For this purpose 6 cc. of oil is usually used.

The patient lies upon a fluoroscopic tilt table for this procedure. During the insertion of the lumbar puncture needle the patient lies on his side, spine in extreme flexion with head down and knees drawn up as far as possible. It is important that the body be straight and that the needle be inserted perpendicularly precisely in the midline. With the needle in place the patient then raises the dependent arm well above the head, straightens out the legs, and rolls over onto the abdomen taking care not to make any unusual movement of the extremity. The patient must lie flat before the oil is injected. The oil should be warmed to body temperature by placing the bottle in hot water to lessen its viscosity. To guard against slipping of the needle during injection a small piece of rubber tubing with suitable connectors interposed between the syringe and the needle

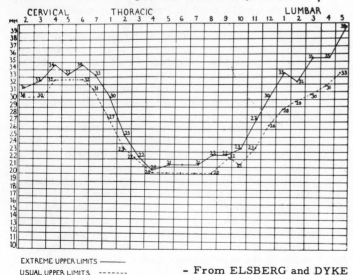

EXTREME UPPER LIMITS ———
USUAL UPPER LIMITS - - - - - -

- From ELSBERG and DYKE

Fig. 323A

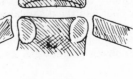

Fig. 323B

may be found useful. A dry syringe must be used to inject the Pantopaque and once started the injection must be completed without any withdrawal of spinal fluid. After injection the needle is left in place and a guard on the fluoroscopic screen set so that the undersurface of the fluoroscopic screen cannot descend to touch the needle during the examination.

For exploration of the lower lumbar and sacral segments, sufficient downward tilt of the head of the table is supplied by most fluoroscopic units. By slowly tilting the table the column of oil may be observed passing up and down in the lumbosacral region. Care should be taken to avoid sudden movements since this may cause segmentation of the oil column. Spot film examination should be made in the antero-posterior, right and left oblique segment of the lumbar spine.

It has been our practice to confirm the findings of the conventional antero-posterior exposures, with lateral transdorsal views directed horizontally from side to side with the patient still lying in the prone position.

After the examination is completed the opaque oil may be removed by tilting the table until the column of oil is immediately beneath the tip of the needle, with the patient lying on abdomen. A fenestrated needle with a small additional hole on the side of the needle above the point will facilitate removal (Klemme).

The opaque oil may be removed by gentle suction with a small syringe or by forcibly exhaling against pressure (Valsalva Exercise). The increased abdominal pressure produced by this method will cause the opaque oil in the canal to bubble up through the needle. With care and patience the oil can be almost completely evacuated, although Pantopaque left in the canal is slowly absorbed.

In case of inadvertent injection of oil into the extra arachnoid space, the opaque material is seen to break up into irregular deposits and extend outward along the nerve sheaths. This usually invalidates the examination and makes it necessary to postpone examination until a future time after the oil has been sufficiently absorbed.

Air myelography has been advocated by some (Camp and Chamberlain) in order to avoid introduction of foreign material into the spinal canal. In such cases with the lower spinal segment filled with air, the head must be lowered considerably and the patient maintained in this position throughout the examination. The roentgenographic images produced are not so precise and now that less viscid Pantopaque is usually readily removed or absorbed, there would seem little reason for continuing the use of air myelography as a diagnostic agent. For a detailed account of the development of this procedure, the reader is referred to Camp. Myelography with water soluble organic iodides (Diodrast) is advocated by some, but has the disadvantage of requiring anaesthesia because of the pain production when these solutions are injected into the spinal canal.

Jacobsen prefers gas as a contrast medium in

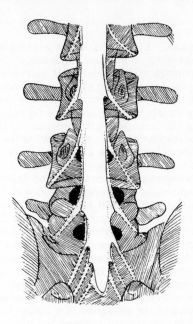

Fig. 323C

the cervical and suboccipital region in association with body section examination. By this method it is possible to demonstrate herniated disc or tumors with cord compression.

Roentgen Manifestations

Both tumors of the cord* and herniation of an intervertebral disc* may occur at any level; any defect present above the upper lumbar segments is most apt to be due to a tumor of the cord, whereas herniation of an intervertebral disc is most likely to occur between the third lumbar and first sacral segments. Tumors do occur in the lower lumbar segments, and disc displacements do occur in the upper spine (even in cervical region) but in these locations they are relatively rare (Fig. 323J) (Bucy and Chenault). Hematoma subdural of the cord is a rare occurrence after injury, (Rader).

Normally 6 cc. of Pantopaque should fill the lower subarachnoid space from the fourth lumbar to the second sacral segment with the patient in the upright position. The nerve root sheaths and axillary pouches should be indicated. From many roentgenographic examinations a composite diagram showing the location and course of the various spinal nerves has been constructed by Hampton and Robinson, (Fig. 323C).

The spinal nerves take origin from the cord several segments above their vertebral level. They course downward with the cord and emerge about opposite the intervertebral space of the vertebra below, extending obliquely downward and outward beneath the pedicles of the vertebrae on either side, to the lower outer margin of the vertebral body. The opaque material may actually extend down the nerve root sheaths and fill the small axillary pouches. Careful examination will disclose the location of these in the myelogram. Great importance is attached to the proper filling of these sheaths. With less viscid Pantopaque these spaces should fill more readily; failure of the nerve sheaths to fill with Pantopaque constitutes evidence of pathology.

Defects produced by herniation of the intervertebral disc vary widely depending upon the extent and location of the displacement, (Soule, et al.). Defects caused by various displacements are as follows:

1. Backward midline protrusion of the disc, if large, produces
   a. Complete "block" of the canal—this is rare except at the fifth lumbar vertebra and usually cannot be distinguished from that produced by tumor of the cord (Fig. 323D).
   b. If the backward protrusion is not so great it may produce a "gap" between the upper and lower segments of the opaque medium (Fig. 323E).
   c. Or it may be that the backward protrusion of the disc is just sufficient to press out some of the opaque material leaving a thin

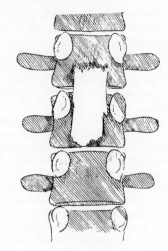

Fig. 323D

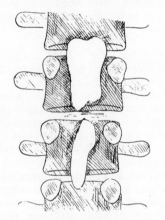

Fig. 323E

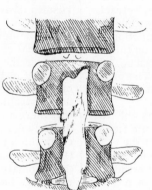

Fig. 323F

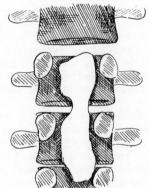

Fig. 323G

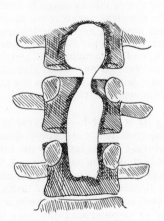

Fig. 323H

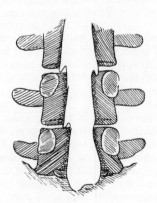

Fig. 323I

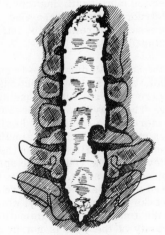

Fig. 323J

layer over the top of the projection producing a "veil-like" defect over this area (Fig. 323F).

2. Lateral herniation of a disc produces
   a. A lateral "pressure defect" or notch on either side in the region of the disc. This is the most common type of defect (Fig. 323G).
   b. If such notch defects are bilateral they produce an "hour glass" deformity (Fig. 323H), a condition which must be carefully differentiated from pressure sometimes caused by exostosis.
   c. If the lateral herniation of a disc compresses the nerve root sheath without encroaching upon the subarachnoid space it may produce a "root" defect or obliteration ("amputation") of the root shadow (Fig. 323I).

Estimates of 90% or more of correct diagnosis by this method have been made (Camp and Chamberlain).

Failure to find a defect where a loose disc is present probably is due primarily to the fact that it may, under bedrest and flexion of the spine, retract. Likewise, meningoceles and other tumors within the sacrum have been reported below the termination of the spinal canal. These can be recognized on the flat film by the sacral deformity which they produce, but may not show a defect on the myelogram. The myelogram merely shows the extent of the canal into the sacrum.

Taylor has demonstrated that it is possible to injure the cord in the cervical region by acute flexion without fracture of the spine. Thickening of the ligamentum flavum can be demonstrated from this cause. Under such conditions symptoms of herniation may be present without demonstration of a herniated disc. Tumors are more apt to occur in the cervical region (Fig. 323J).

In scarcely any other field are the results of operative correction more gratifying; complete removal of the protruding portion of the disc removes the abnormal pressure and relieves the intractable pain, (Woolsey and Tsang).

Cysts of the Spinal Membranes;—Perineurial Cysts* (Fig. 323K) are cyst-like projections from the subarachnoid space which fill with opaque material on myelography. They may be single or multiple and may attain more than a centimeter in size; they may produce symptoms which closely simulate those of herniated disc. They usually occur in the sacral roots but may develop in the roots of the spinal nerves at any place in the spine. Cyst-like diverticular structures may develop at the nerve roots, some days or weeks after myelography, which are not evident at the time of first examination. If, however, the cavity of the cyst is not in communication with the subarachnoid space as occurs frequently in the sacral region, myelography may be of no diagnostic value. Extradural meningeal cysts may be congenital; they may occur at any location in

the spine but are prone to occur in the thoracic region. They usually do not fill with opaque medium on myelography and ultimately result in a partial or complete block.

Roentgenologically they cannot ordinarily be differentiated from any other type of spinal cord tumor causing similar involvement. Occasionally they communicate with the subarachnoid space and fill with myelographic fluid, (Jacobs, et al.).

Cyst-like lesions of these types may be equally disabling as protrusion of a disc and operative removal may be equally satisfactory. Holman, et al., have demonstrated a diamond-shaped defect in the myelogram due to bifurcation of the spinal cord.

They may cause pressure erosion of the bone seen only in the lateral view of the sacrum, (Seaman and Furlow).

Arachnoiditis* (Fig. 323L). This condition is characterized by inflammatory deposits involving the arachnoid which prevent free movement of the spinal fluid up and down the canal producing irregular deposits of opaque material in the myelogram. Operative freeing of the space and the administration of cortisone therapy have shown some beneficial results (Seaman, et al.; Wood, et al.).

Diastematomyelia* (Fig. 323M) is a condition of the spinal cord in which there is a division or duplication of the cord. This is usually associated with widening of the vertebrae and an expanded condition of the spinal canal; a bony ridge or septum is usually demonstrable dividing the canal (Cowie). Some feel that there is merely spinal dysraphism and that diplomyelia never occurs, that there is merely one cord which is split at an early stage of development, (Lichtenstein). Herren and Edwards merely consider this anomaly as an incipient form of twinning. Tomography has been found of great diagnostic value in the demonstration of the bony septum (Cowie; Holman, et al.).

AVULSION OF BRACHIAL PLEXUS. The principal feature of myelographic findings in avulsion or high rupture of the cervical nerve roots is extravasation of the contrast medium into diverticulum-like pouches beyond the level of the root pouches. This is indication of rupture of the arachnoidal and dural investments of the nerves. It serves to give an estimate of the damage done. Surgical repair in the face of such a picture is impossible, (Rayle, et al.).

Discography* (Fig. 323N). Discography consists of radiographic examination of the spine after injection of opaque material (Diodrast) into the intervertebral disc. (For technique of injection see Manual of Roentgenological Technique.) For a normal disc .5 to 1 cc. of 35% Diodrast will usually be found to be sufficient to satisfactorily outline the disc structures. A ruptured or degenerated disc may require from 2 to 5 cc. to fully outline this structure. The normal nucleus pulposis will be found contained in a homogeneous compartment, centrally located well within the vertebral margins. Herniation of the disc

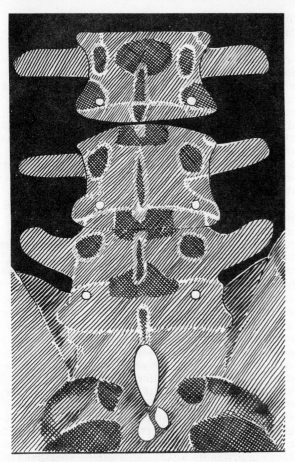

Fig. 323K. Perineurial cysts of spinal membranes often cause signs of herniated disc.

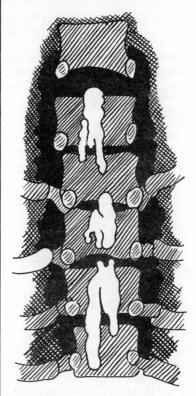

Fig. 323L. Arachnoiditis. Adhesions and inflammatory tissue are present in the subarachnoid space. On myelography, there is fragmentation of the contrast column.

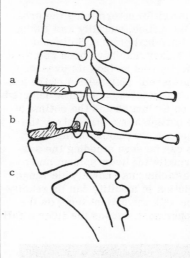

Fig. 323N. Discography; examination of spine after direct injection of opaque material directly into the nucleus pulposus itself, in order to show rupture or herniation. a) Normal disc; b) Herniation into vertebral body; c) Herniation posteriorly.

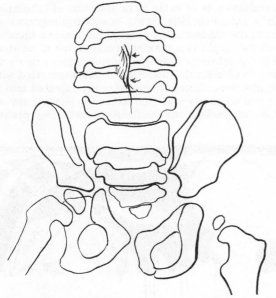

Fig. 323M. Diastematomyelia, a condition in which there is division or duplication of the spinal cord. A thin bony plate is seen dividing the canal.

either forward or backward into the spinal canal is readily demonstrated. Schmorl's nodes are seen to correspond directly with herniations of the disc through the cartilaginous and bony plates of the vertebra.

While the procedure of discography is very exact in depicting the extent and character of the pathology present it is by no means without pain and some surgeons do not approve of the procedure in view of the damage inflicted upon the disc structure by insertion of a needle for contrast injection. At any rate it is a very accurate method for detection of a herniated disc if other methods (myelography) have been found of no avail, (Cloward and Buzaid; Walk). Friedman and Goldner have added their endorsement to the accuracy of discography as a diagnostic agent; they agree however that it may be a painful procedure.

SPECIAL EXAMINATION OF THE ABDOMINAL ORGANS
BY ARTIFICIAL PNEUMOPERITONEUM*

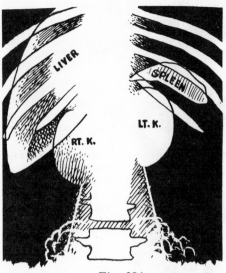

Fig. 324

Owing to the fact that the abdominal viscera are of so nearly the same density as their surrounding media, they do not lend themselves readily to roentgen-ray examination. Induction of artificial pneumoperitoneum by the introduction of air or other gas into the abdominal cavity provides a medium of lesser density surrounding the abdominal viscera which renders them clearly visible. (See technique in "Manual of Roentgenological Technique".)

This method is useful for determining the presence, location, size, and outline, mobility and attachments of the various abdominal organs (Stein and Stewart) (Fig. 324). A kidney may have been removed or destroyed by disease; by this method its presence or absence can be established. Malposition of the kidney, spleen, or other abdominal organs can be detected. The relative size can be estimated and the outline of the organs noted. The outline alone may betray the character of the disease; in carcinoma of the liver, large nodular growths can be seen studding the surface of the organ. Normally the liver, spleen, and organs with mesenteric attachments show a wide range of mobility; any restriction in mobility can be readily observed. Examination with the patient lying on the left side, right side uppermost, causes the liver to fall far over toward the midline leaving a clear unobstructed view of the right kidney (Fig. 325A). When viewed with the patient lying on a stretcher on his right side (right lateral decubitus), the spleen and left kidney become visible as well as the peritoneal attachment of the splenic flexure and descending colon (Fig. 325B).* This is the only means by which adhesions between the anterior abdominal wall and underlying viscera can be demonstrated (Fig. 326); the patient lies on his back on a stretcher and examination is made with the transabdominal projection of the ray.

The attachments of abdominal masses may be visualized and their origin determined. One of the most useful phases of this method of examination is the determination of the retroperitoneal character of a mass (Fig. 327). With the abdomen previously somewhat overinflated with air, the patient is rolled over, face downward on a hospital cart. Lying in this position, supported on two blocks, one under the chest and the other under the thighs, allowing the abdomen to sag freely between these two supports, a lateral transabdominal roentgen-ray examination is made.* In this position the air rises to envelop the retroperitoneal structures, the abdominal wall sags forward, the stomach, intestines and all organs with mesenteric attachment fall forward producing a prevertebral clear space. The kidney is overshadowed by the retroperitoneal structures and may not be detectible unless it is the site of tumor formation or is enlarged from other causes. If a mass is retroperitoneal in origin its attachments can be visualized directly by this method and it can be seen encroaching on the prevertebral clear space.*

Another condition in which pneumoperitoneum examination is of value is in detection of subdiaphragmatic pathology (Fig. 328). In subdiaphragmatic abscess the shadow of the underlying viscera blends with the diaphragm making visualization of an abscess in the subphrenic space impossible unless there happens to be a small collection of gas associated with the abscess. A small amount of air injected into the abdominal cavity will rise to the top beneath the dome of the diaphragm and disclose any pathology present.

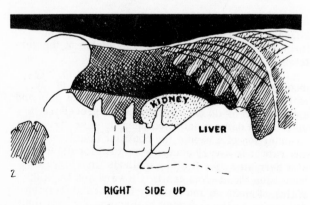

RIGHT SIDE UP

Fig. 325A

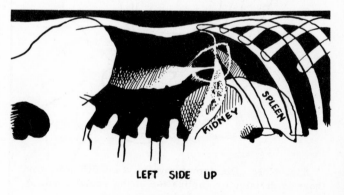

LEFT SIDE UP

Fig. 325B

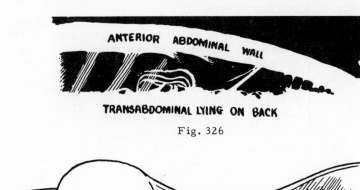

TRANSABDOMINAL LYING ON BACK

Fig. 326

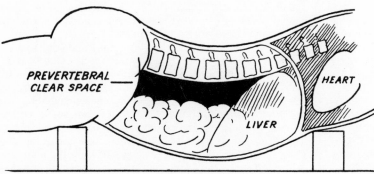

Fig. 327

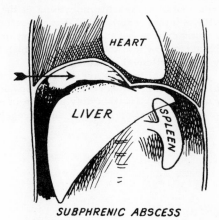

SUBPHRENIC ABSCESS

Fig. 328

Such small quantities of air have no tendency to interfere with the most delicate inflammatory adhesions and we have never seen any evidence of spread of infection. Subdiaphragmatic abscess cannot be definitely demonstrated in any other way. The patient must be rolled well over toward the abdomen to avoid missing a collection of pus far toward the back between the liver and the diaphragm.

Examination of the female pelvic organs by pneumoperitoneum has met with considerable success (Jacho), (Fig. 329). The uterus, tubes and ovaries can be visualized and their relationship can be noted. Tumors of the various organs can be detected and their size and location determined. Early pregnancy can, under favorable conditions, be diagnosed from the changes which occur in the uterus, long before the fetus is visible. Other more exact biological tests give more trustworthy information with regard to very early pregnancy, however.

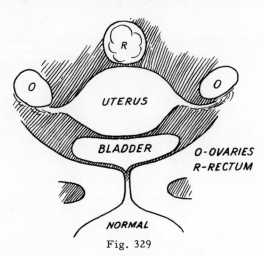

Fig. 329

INTRAVENOUS THORIUM DIOXIDE. The liver and spleen can be visualized by the intravenous injection of Thorotrast (thorium dioxide). The deposit of this opaque material in the liver and spleen, (see "Manual of Roentgenological Technique") results from the reticuloendothelial cells of liver and spleen phagocytizing the colloidal particles from the blood. Any carcinomatous nodules present will therefore stand out in clear contrast by their lack of opaque deposit. About 1 cc. per kilogram of body weight is used. This substance is radioactive; it remains in the tissues permanently. Taft has demonstrated that the amount of radiation coming from such a quantity of thorium dioxide is equivalent to doses of radium which have caused symptoms of poisoning. For this reason it is inadvisable to use any method involving injection of this quantity of radioactive material except under very exceptional circumstances. It may be combined with pneumoperitoneum. Smaller quantities of thorium dioxide are used for angiography but this too results in retention of radioactive material in the body.

PERIRENAL INSUFFLATION*; (PRESACRAL PNEUMATOGRAPHY). Perirenal insufflation is carried out by insertion of a long needle into the perirenal connective tissue spaces and insufflating air. The introduction of air (or other gas) into the retroperitoneal tissues is more safely accomplished by presacral injection, (Joelson, et al.). By either method (see "Manual of Roentgenological Technique" for details) the outline of the kidneys, adrenals, and psoas muscles can be visualized with clearness of detail. The size and shape of the adrenal gland can most accurately be demonstrated by this technic. Changes in size and contour of the kidneys are similarly detectable, but because of the good visualization of renal structures afforded by intravenous and retrograde pyelography, one need not be so dependent on this technic as for visualization of the adrenals. Presence of a pheochromocytoma of the adrenal medulla, a tumor which simulates essential hypertension to some degree because of its paroxysmal release of ephinephrines into the circulation, may be confirmed by retroperitoneal pneumography.

Adrenal tumors are occasionally detected by calcification in the adrenal area. Speckled and poorly defined calcification may be seen in neuroblastomas; calcification is heavy and irregular in adeno-

carcinoma, (Samuel).

For maximum precision in routine stratigraphy the exposure time must be brief in the order of 1/10 second. Axial transverse stratigraphy may be of value to the surgeon in localizing pulmonary lesions such as cavities, tumors, etc. It has been found very useful in interpretation of retroperitoneal air insufflation, (perirenal insufflation) especially for renal and pancreatic examination, (Vallebonna).

AORTOGRAPHY

AORTOGRAPHY.* To render the abdominal aorta and its tributary vessels opaque to x-rays, 70% Diodrast or Neo-Iopax is injected directly into the upper portion of this vessel. A 12 to 15 inch long 8 to 9 gauge needle is used with a suitable 50 cc. syringe; the needle is inserted in the lower thoracic aorta in the back and the opaque material must be "dumped" into the circulation with great rapidity in order to secure a sufficient concentrated mixture to render the vessels opaque, (for details of technique see "Manual of Roentgenological Technique"). The same dangers are attendant with this procedure as are met with wherever large amounts of foreign matter are injected into the circulation (Pendergrass, et al.).

If a satisfactory injection is made, the abdominal aorta and all of its tributary vessels should be well visualized, (Fig. 330A). Since the examination

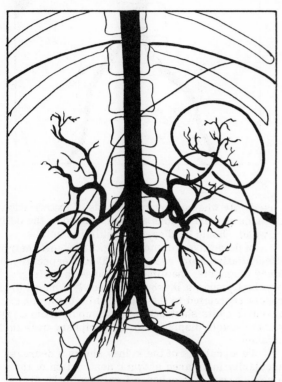

Fig. 330A

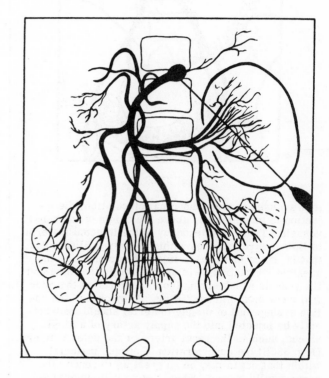

Fig. 330C

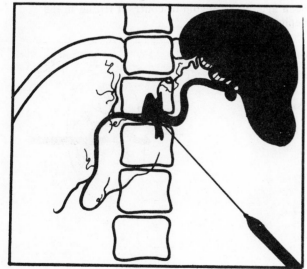

Fig. 330B

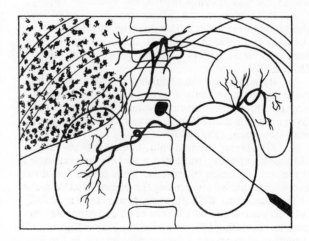

Fig. 330D

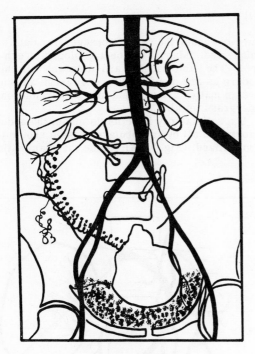

Fig. 330E

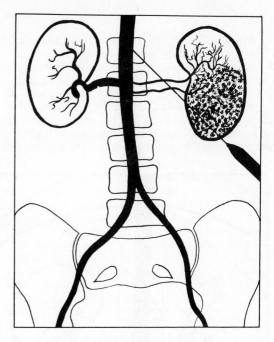

Fig. 330F

is often used to study the renal circulation, the injection is made high up above the origin of the renal vessels. There is a tendency of the injected material to flow in streams even within the blood-filled aorta; that is, if the material is injected into one side the greatest concentration is maintained in that side and the vessels which spring from the aorta on that side will show most intense filling. If by chance the entire syringe full of opaque material should inadvertently be injected into the supply artery of a single viscus, such as the renal artery or the splenic artery, (Fig. 330B) the concentration of opaque material within that organ may be so great as to render the organ totally opaque. This is of no pathological significance but it does blot out any information as to the extent and arrangement of the vascular supply.

If, by chance, the full amount is injected into the mesenteric artery, this may be disastrous since the anoxemia which results to the intestinal structure may be sufficient to cause gangrene of the bowel, (Fig. 330C).

By and large the abdominal organs show distinct channels as their source of vascular supply; organs which have vascular sinusoids such as the liver show a mottled appearance of their parenchymal structure, (Fig. 330D).

Similarly, the placenta, because of its large sinusoidal spaces, produces a blotchy appearance in the roentgenogram (Hartnett). This method is of value in determining with certainty the exact location and size of the placenta. With placenta praevia, (Fig. 330E) this structure can be clearly seen over the uterine outlet, covering the foetal head. Placentography by injection of contrast solution retrograde in the femoral artery appears to be less traumatic. This method

is used only when ordinary methods of examination fail since it merely adds another hazard to the delivery which should be dispensed with if possible.

In detection of tumors (Fig. 330F) and their differentiation from cysts (Fig. 330G), especially in kidney diagnosis, the tumors because of their great vascularity show a meshwork of newly-formed blood vessels restricted to the tumor while the almost avascular cysts show scant blood supply from a few sparse vessels displaced to the periphery over their surfaces.

Tuberculosis of the kidney shows a decrease in vascularity in an area showing destruction of the kidney. Areas of pinched-off calices in the pyelogram show decreased vascularity in the aortogram. Such areas are devoid of contrast filling in the nephrogram.

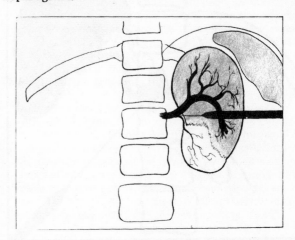

Fig. 330G

Farinas has devised a technique for the selective injection of the vascular supply of any specific organ by retrograde catheterization of the artery using a ureteral catheter inserted into an inguinal vessel.

It would seem that the greatest usefulness of this method of examination will be in determining the character of blood supply to the abdominal organs, especially the kidney for differentiation between a cyst and tumor of that organ and when evidence of an aberrant vessel is sought. This method of vascular catheterization has been successfully utilized to catheterize the renal artery for restriction of the injection to one renal blood vessel in order to preserve the function of the other kidney from possible harm of injection (see Urinary Tract). Virtually every vascular part of the body has been injected. The pelvis has been subjected to this type of examination; the vertebral vessels and spine; the extremities especially for the evaluation of peripheral circulation in varicosities; the portal (q.v.); even the foetal circulation.

In a similar manner by catheterization of the femoral vein the venous structures may be demonstrated for occlusion from the clots and often by the use of heparin these may be dissolved.

Angiography of the azygos vein and anterior venous plexus of the spine has been demonstrated in dogs by transitory occlusion of the inferior vena cava by a tube bearing an inflatable balloon with injection of contrast medium below the obstruction. The injected material is directed between the azygos vein and the inferior vena cava to fill the azygos system and internal venous plexus of the spine.

Transitory occlusion of the inferior vena cava above the opening of the hepatic vein causes a "catastrophic" fall of arterial pressure whereas temporary occlusion below the renal vein gives only moderate reduction.

Nordenstrom has carried on extensive animal research to determine the least harmful place for occlusion. The porto-canal vessels may be visualized in a similar manner by catheterizing the venous structures and injecting opaque material into the inferior vena cava. Or, a similar result may be obtained by direct injection into the spleen. Details of technique involved may be obtained from the "Manual of Roentgenological Technique".

SPLENO-(LIENO)-PORTAL VENOGRAPHY

Visualization of the portal system for the detection of portal hypertension may be accomplished by percutaneous injection of opaque material into the spleen.

Technique

The technique utilized by Gvozdanovic and Hauptmann is as follows: Under local anaesthesia (1% Novocain) the 8th, 9th and 10th interspaces in the axillary line on the left side a needle is inserted through the chest wall over the spleen; contact with the spleen is detected by a scratchy sensation; insert 2 to 3 cm. farther into the spleen and inject 20 cc. of non-irritating opaque material in 2 or 3 seconds, (Joduron or other aqueous organic iodine solution). Expose up to 4 films in rapid succession using an automatic film changer at the rate of 2 films per second for 7 to 10 seconds. Use 70-80 K.V., 400 M.A., 95 cm. distance and 1/10 sec. time.

Spalteholz describes the normal portal circulation (Fig. 330H), as follows:

The portal vein collects blood from the entire digestive system and abdominal viscera by union of the superior and inferior mesenteric veins, the splenic vein and the v. coronaria ventriculi (from along the lesser curvature of the stomach where it anastomoses at the pylorus with the v. pylorica and the cardia with the esophageal veins) where it opens into the v. portae or v. lienalis.

The regular anastomoses of the portal vein with the vv. cavae are:

1. At the cardia of the stomach between the v. coronaria ventriculi and the esophageal veins;

2. At the rectum through the hemorrhoidal vessels between the v. hemorrhoidalis superior (branch of v. inferior mesenteric), and the inferior and medial hemorrhoidal veins, which are in turn branches of the vv. hypogastric.

3. Paraumbillical veins forming an anastomosis about the umbillicus, the so-called caput meduci, between the superficial veins and the vv. epigastric inferior and extending near the ligamentum teres into the liver substance.

It would seem that from the radiological standpoint that the anastomosis of greatest importance would be that producing esophageal varices since the umbillical anastomosis should be readily recognized as the caput meduci characteristic of this region, and that produced by hemorrhoidal vessels is so commonly encountered from ordinary increase in pressure without relationship to portal hypertension.

Esophageal varices may be readily demonstrable by ordinary x-ray examination with barium swallow.

This method of splenic injection would seem to be most useful where operative procedure is contemplated for relief of portal hypertension.

Gvozdanovic and Hauptmann feel that the question of portal hypertension should be separated into two groups, certain and probable.

The first or certain group: Strong reflux into tributaries of the lienoportal venous system, development of the collateral circulation through the pre-existing anastomosis—including widened paraumbillical veins, and a marked slowing down of the circulation in the liver;

The second or probable group: The probable

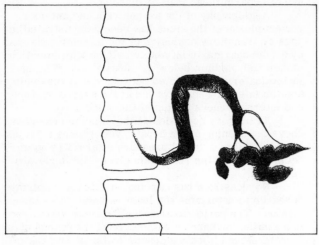

a

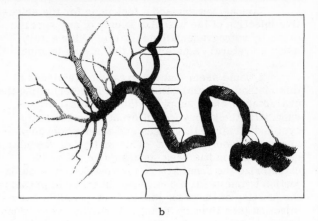

b

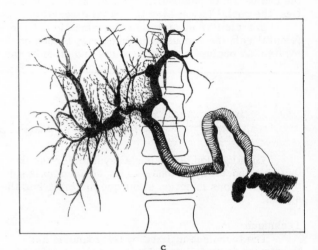

c

Fig. 330H. Normal splenic injection: a) 1.5 seconds after injection, opaque material fills the splenic vein up to the spine; b) at 3 seconds examination the entire course of the v. lienalis, v. portae and its intrahepatic branches is well demonstrated without dilatation or indication of collateral reflux into its tributaries; c) at 4 seconds exposure the terminal branches of the v. portae are also well demonstrated. Catalano, et al. have called attention to the opacification of the liver which is attendant with this method, which may be of value in detection of accessory lobes, etc.

Using the Elema film changing apparatus, as many as four films per second were exposed during the injection by Gvozdanovic and Hauptmann making it possible to follow the injection of the opaque material during its entire passage. They stress the importance of serial film exposure.

Bergstrand and Ekman discuss the complications attendant with this procedure in 31 cases.

Figures 330H to K redrawn by courtesy of authors and publishers Gvozdanovic, V., and Hauptmann, E., "Further Experience with Percutaneous Lieno-Portal Venography," Acta Radiol., 43:177, 1955.

signs embrace widening of the vv. lienalis and portae and the marked tortuous course of these veins. These signs in themselves are insufficient for a diagnosis of portal hypertension but only if combined with individual signs of the first group. The scantness of branches in the liver, although present in cirrhosis may be due merely to premature taking of film in a slowed down circulation in the liver. In cirrhosis of liver the circulation time is increased almost double (see Figs. 330H to L).

Giuseffi and Largen have devised a method for determining the status of anastomosis following shunt procedures. For details of this procedure the reader is referred to the original article.

Demonstration of tributary veins of the portal system, specifically the coronary vein of the stomach, and the inferior mesenteric vein, indicates a reverse flow in the portal system, secondary to portal block. The actual filling of gastric and esophageal varices may be seen (Fig. 330L). Slow disappearance of contrast medium from the portal circulation is another indication of portal block. Of great value is the making clear of the portal venous anatomy for the surgeon to plan his operative attack on portal hypertension, (Bruwer).

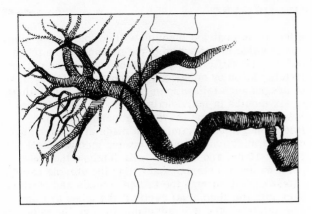

Fig. 330 I. Unusually long branch of the left portal vein (arrow).
- Courtesy of Gvozdanovic and Hauptmann

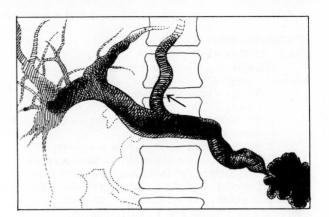

Fig. 330K. Collateral circulation is carried out through the dilated v. coronaria ventriculi in this instance of portal hypertension (hepatic cirrhosis). The course of both the splenic and portal veins is almost linear.
- Courtesy of Gvozdanovic and Hauptmann

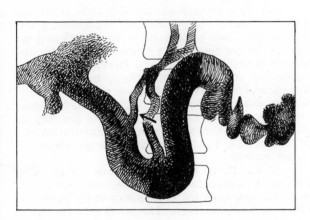

Fig. 330J. Extremely wide splenic and portal veins in portal cirrhosis. The collateral circulation is accomplished through vv. gastricae breves (arrow) and v. coronaria ventriculi. The finer radicals of the portal vein are not well outlined probably due to premature exposure of the radiograph.
- Courtesy of Gvozdanovic and Hauptmann

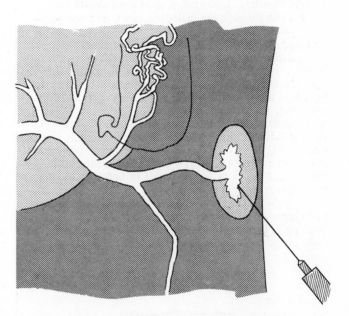

Fig. 330L. Collateral circulation through the gastric and coronary veins forming esophageal varices. This is probably one of the most important sites of varicosities.

FEMALE PELVIC ORGANS

UTERO-SALPINOGRAPHY (HYSTERO-SALPINOGRAPHY) *

Intrauterine injection of contrast medium is used as a diagnostic procedure:

1. To determine the patency of the Fallopian tubes,
2. To detect pathology in the uterine cavity and other pelvic organs,
3. To determine extrauterine pregnancy.

Opaque materials available for this purpose are of two varieties: a) those having an oily base such as Lipiodol, Lipiodine, and Pantopaque, and b) those in aqueous solution such as Skiodan (Viscous) Acacia Solution and Visco-Rayopake.

The disadvantages of lipiodol and other oil-based media is the danger of oil embolism if the oily material inadvertently is injected into the circulation. Under such conditions multiple miliary droplets of opaque oil may be readily recognized uniformly distributed throughout the lung fields, resembling somewhat the appearance of miliary tuberculosis. Even where this does occur it rarely causes severe or lasting results. Likewise if oil-based media is spilled out through the fallopian tubes into the peritoneal cavity, the material absorbs only very slowly and may leave an encysted mass for a long time.

Aqueous solutions then, such as Skiodan (Viscous) Acacia Solution or Medopaque-H, are preferable for injection media on account of their non-irritating qualities and their ready absorbability, (15 to 20 minutes), (Roland, et al.).

Details of the technique of examination are discussed fully in the Manual of Roentgenological Technique. About 10 cc. of medium is used for injection. It is best to make roentgen examination after injection of 2, 3 and 5 cc. of material in order to be able to properly interpret the findings.

This method finds one of its greatest fields of usefulness in examination of the fallopian tubes for patency (Fig. 331A). Occlusion of the fimbriated ends of the tubes is a common cause of sterility.

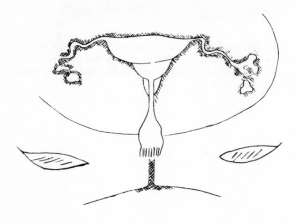

Fig. 331A

Injection of contrast medium will not only be of diagnostic value in determining the patency of the tubes but may be sufficient to open tubes which are not too firmly closed by adhesions. Reports as high as 35% of pregnancies following such procedure within three to six months in individuals previously sterile for long periods of time have been made (Martin). Roentgenographic examination made after each successive injection of 2 cc. of opaque medium until a total of 10 cc. are injected will disclose the contrast medium, entering and filling the uterine cavity, extending out through the fallopian tubes and spilling over into the abdominal cavity if the tubes are open. For safety's sake it is advisable to have the injection tube connected with a manometer so that the degree of pressure can be accurately gauged. Ordinarily 60 mm. Hg. pressure will be sufficient; if there is occlusion, gradual increase in pressure up to 100 mm. or even 150 mm. Hg. is considered permissible, but any pressure higher than this must be carried out with great caution. I. C. Rubin has devised an instrument properly equipped with a manometer for this purpose.

Gas such as oxygen, carbon dioxide or air may be used instead of opaque medium. Auscultation with a stethescope over the adnexal regions will elicit the sound of the gas escaping from the tubes into the abdominal cavity if they are open. Roentgenographic examination of the abdomen in the upright position after such procedures will disclose gas free in the abdomen under the diaphragm; this is definite indication of patency of the tubes. Sufficient gas may be introduced in this manner to permit examination of the abdominal and pelvic organs by the pneumoperitoneum method.

Both artificial pneumoperitoneum and injection of contrast medium into the uterine cavity can be used simultaneously for examination of the pelvic organs to good advantage. The gas free in the abdominal cavity serves to outline the pelvic organs (see section on artificial pneumoperitoneum) and the injected contrast medium serves to identify the structures outlined by the pneumoperitoneum and to demonstrate their inner cavities.

Uterosalpinography either alone or in combination with pelvic pneumoperitoneum is of value in many pelvic conditions.

1. It will indicate the location, size and structure of the uterus disclosing any dislocation of position or anomaly of development, such as double uterus (Fig. 331B).
2. Where several masses are palpated in the pelvis it will identify the uterus.
3. It will show the relationship of tumors, especially fibroids, or interligamentous cysts (Fig. 332A) to the uterus by pressure defects on the uterus or uterine cavity.
4. Carcinoma of the uterus can be demonstrated in this manner; its location and size may be determined thus guiding biopsy forceps for

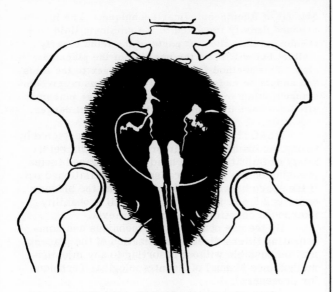

Fig. 331B

obtaining a specimen of the growth (Fig. 332B).

5. It has been used by some for diagnosis of early pregnancy without producing abortion. It would seem that with our present accurate tests for early pregnancy such methods should be abandoned.

6. In unusual cases it may be essential to utilize uterine injection to determine extra-uterine pregnancy.

7. In addition to disclosing the patency of the fallopian tubes, it will show their position, length and tortuosity. Occlusion and distention of the tube with hydrosalpinx will be indicated. Where oily media is used it may separate into clusters of spherical droplets within the fluid-filled dilated tube (Fig. 333).

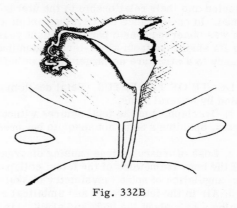

Fig. 332B

COLLOIDAL THORIUM DIOXIDE. Colloidal thorium dioxide has been recommended as an injection medium to outline the mucosal relief. This material is injected, retained for a few minutes, and then allowed to completely run out; this forms an insoluble albuminate with the mucous secretion and adheres to the walls of the uterine cavity outlining the mucosal pattern.

PREGNANCY.* As soon as the fetus shows calcium deposits in its skeleton x-ray demonstration is possible. Ordinarily, pregnancy cannot be diagnosed by this means with any degree of consistency earlier than four to four and one-half months gestation. Under favorable conditions a fetus eleven to twelve weeks old can occasionally be demonstrated. (Other biological tests for pregnancy are more accurate in the early months.)

Examination of full-term fetus for position and size, however, is at times very helpful. With present-day roentgenographic methods the bones of the fetus can be readily outlined in practically all cases during the latter half of pregnancy.

ANOMALIES OF FETAL DEVELOPMENT. Anomalies of development of the fetus, anencephaly, acrania, hydrocephalus, monsters of any sort can readily be diagnosed, (Thomson). Lithopedions can

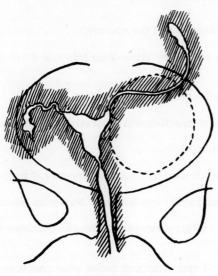

Fig. 332A

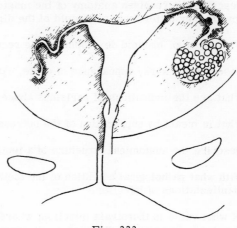

Fig. 333

be detected and their relationship to the uterus determined. In one instance the development of a lithopedion was observed over a period of eight years during its shrinkage from a full-term abdominal pregnancy to a structure no larger than one's fist.

DEATH OF THE FETUS. Fetal death may be indicated by several signs:

    1. Overlapping of the fetal sutures without engagement, Spalding's Sign, not absolute but presumptive.

    2. Loss of muscular tone causing disorganization of the bony framework of the fetus; collapsed thorax, angulation of spine, asymmetry of skull.

    3. Air in the fetal tissues and umbilical region producing a halo about the body and skull. Air may be in the fetal blood vessels.

PELVIMETRY. The relationship of the size of the fetal head to the size of the pelvic inlet of the mother can be accurately measured by present methods of pelvimetry. (See Manual of Roentgenological Technique.)

AMNIOGRAPHY. In cases of suspected placenta praevia, amniography may be carried out. This is a method by which strontium iodide, in concentrated solution, is injected directly through the abdominal uterine wall into the amnionic cavity. (See Manual of Roentgenological Technique.) The increased density imparted to the amnionic fluid will render not only the soft parts of the fetus clearly visible, but will show the position of the placenta also. This method is not without danger to the fetus and should be undertaken only under unusual circumstances; other methods of determining the placental site have been developed which are without danger.

PLACENTA PRAEVIA can often be detected by filling the bladder with air or opaque media before x-ray examination. The head of the engaged foetus pressing on the bladder causes it to be flattened out. If the space between the fetal head and the bladder exceeds 2.5 cm. the placenta is in all probability interposed constituting placenta praevia.

By the use of soft tissue technique and compensating filters direct visualization of the placenta may be possible without resorting to any injection method (see Manual of Roentgenological Technique for procedure).

Aortography (q.v.) may produce accurate and immediate information on placenta praevia. Diodrast (70%) injected directly into the abdominal aorta will disclose the circulation of the abdominal organs, as well as that of the placenta. The blood, pooling in the placental sinuses gives a mottled effect which is characteristic. The placenta located in the lower segment can be readily recognized. (For technique of Aortography see Manual of Roentgenological Technique.)

QUESTIONS ON SPECIAL EXAMINATIONS AND PROCEDURES

1. Why is x-ray examination of the accessory nasal sinuses possible?

2. What are the roentgen manifestations of catarrhal, purulent, hyperplastic and atrophic sinusitis and how may they be differentiated?

3. What x-ray manifestation is characteristic of neoplastic involvement of the sinuses?

4. Describe the roentgen anatomy of the mastoid. What are the characteristics of an infantile mastoid and how do they differ from a mastoid of the diploetic type?

5. What types of mastoid development are recognized and describe their characteristics.

6. Describe the x-ray appearance of acute, catarrhal, purulent, destructive and sclerotic mastoiditis.

7. What are the indications of perisinus abscess? Of cholesteotoma?

8. What is meant by suppuration of the petrous apex? When does it usually occur? How may it be detected?

9. Describe the anatomical structure of a tooth and its roentgenographic appearance. Name the adult teeth.

10. With what pathological condition of the teeth is the physician chiefly concerned? Why? Describe the manifestations of infection.

11. Of what value is thorotrast injection; where is the thorium salt deposited and under what conditions is it of value? Dangers from radioactivity from large quantities? Use in Ventriculography?

12. Describe the methods of introduction of air into the ventricles of the brain. Discuss briefly the principle involved in this type of examination for intracranial pathology.

13. What is meant by (a) ventriculography; (b) encephalography? How do they differ and what are their respective values in diagnosis of intracranial lesions?

14. Show by diagram the normal markings of the ventricular system of the brain.

15. What is meant by subarachnoid pathways and of what significance is their obliteration?

16. How may the presence of a calcified pineal gland be utilized in the detection of an intracranial tumor?

17. What other roentgenographic findings are present in: (1) Increased intracranial pressure? (2) Tumor of the pituitary? (3) Tumor elsewhere in the cranial cavity? (4) Suprasellar cysts?

18. Of what significance are calcified intracranial deposits?

19. What are the x-ray characteristics of meningiomata and where do they most frequently occur? How does it differ roentgenographically from hyperostosis internus cranialis?

20. What is meant by cerebral angiography and how is it carried out? In what condition is it of value? Danger?

21. How may the interpretation of cerebral angiograms be examined to the best advantage? Is this of importance?

22. Describe briefly the method used in detection of a tumor of the spinal cord and determination of its location.

23. Describe briefly the technique of producing artificial pneumoperitoneum and discuss the principle of its use in association with the x-ray examination of the abdominal viscera.

24. In what particular type of cases is pneumoperitoneum examination of greatest value?

25. How may pneumoperitoneum be produced in the female without abdominal puncture? Advantages? Dangers?

26. What is aortography and how is it carried out? What are the dangers of the procedure?

27. Of what value is aortography in abdominal diagnosis? Kidney diagnosis?

28. Of what value is the intrauterine injection of contrast media?

29. What is meant by amniography and in what particular condition is it of value? Dangers?

30. How may placenta praevia be detected? Is it a safe procedure?

31. Of what value is roentgenographic examination in pregnancy? How early may pregnancy be detected?

32. What roentgen signs are indication of fetal death in utero?

REFERENCES FOR SPECIAL EXAMINATIONS AND PROCEDURES

Schneider, M., "Aerosinusitis," Am. J. Roentgenol., 53:563, 1945.

Cocke, J. A., "Aerosinusitis," Am. J. Roentgenol., 57:298, 1947.

Proetz, A., "Displacement Method of Sinus Diagnosis and Treatment," Annals Pub. Co., St. Louis, 1939.

Fower, P. E., and Swanson, P. C., "Petrositis," Am. J. Roentgenol., 41:317, 1939.

Mayer, E. G., "Roentgenological Analysis of an Unusual Deformity of the Temporal Bone and the Technique of Its Examination," Acta Radiol., 5:135, 1926.

Hodgson, H. K. G., "Cholesteatoma of the Temporal Bone," Brit. J. Radiol., 20:202, 1947.

Welin, S., "On Roentgen Diagnosis of Cholesteatoma in Temporal Bone," Acta Radiol., 25:227, 1944.

Doub, H. P., and Henny, F. A., "Roentgenological Study of the Temporomandibular Joints," Radiol., 60:666, 1953.

Geschicter, C. F., and Copeland, M. M., "Classification of Bone Tumors," Bull. Hosp. Joint Dis., 12:498-513, Oct. 1951.

Sherman, R. S., and Caumartin, H., "The Roentgen Appearance of Adamantinoma of the Mandible," Radiol., 65:361, 1955.

Hoelsh, S., "Diagnosis of Tumors of the Glomus Jugulare," Lancet, 1:169, 1955.

Camp, J. D., "Pathologic Non-Neoplastic Intracranial Calcification," J.A.M.A., 137:1023, 1948.

Malbin, M., "Mobile Calcified Choroid Plexuses," Radiol., 51:383, 1948.

Vastine, J. H., and Kinney, K. K., "The Pineal Shadow as an Aid in the Localization of Brain Tumors," Am. J. Roentgenol., 17:320, 1927.

Ackermann, A. J., "Tuberous Sclerosis," Am. J. Roentgenol., 51:315, 1944.

Dickerson, W. W., "Roentgenographic Changes with Tuberous Sclerosis," Arch. Neurol. and Psychiatry, 53:199, 1948.

Gurdjian, E. S., and Lissner, H. R., "Deformations of Skull in Head Injury Studied by 'Stress Coat' Technique, Quantitative Determinations," Surg., Gynec., and Obst., 83:219-233, Aug. 1946.

Gurdjian, E. S., Lissner, H. R., and Webster, J. E., "Mechanism of Production of Linear Skull Fracture; Further Studies on Deformation of Skull by 'Stress Coat' Technique," Surg., Gynec., and Obst., 85:195-210, Aug. 1947.

Gurdjian, E. S., Webster, J. E., and Lissner, H. R., "Mechanism of Skull Fracture," J. Neurosurg., 7:106-114, March, 1950; Radiol., 54:313-338, March, 1950.

Gurdjian, E. S., Webster, J. E., and Lissner, H. R., "Observations on Predictions of Site of Head Injury," Radiol., 60:226-235, February 1953.

Bailey, Percival, "Intracranial Tumors," Chas. S. Thomas, Pub., Springfield, 1933.

Gilbertson, E. L., and Good, C. A., "Roentgenographic Signs of Tumors of the Brain," Am. J. Roentgenol., 76:266, 1956.

Torkildsen, A., and Pirie, A. H., "Interpretation of Ventriculograms," Am. J. Roentgenol., 32:145, 1934.

Eagleshaw, D. C., "Radiological Aspects of Intracranial Pneumocephalus," Brit. J. Radiol., 18:335, 1945.

Pedersen, J., "Hyperostosis Cranialis Interna. Morgagni and Stewart-Morel Syndromes. Examination of Females Suffering from Diabetes Mellitus and Other Endocrine Disorders as Well as Female Epileptics. (Studies on Hypertrichosis)," Acta Med. Scandinav., 128:71-102, 1947.

Bull, J., "The Radiological Diagnosis of Intracranial Tumors in Children," J. Faculty Radiol., 4:149, 1953.

Robertson, E. G., Encephalography, MacMillan Co., London, 1941.

Lindblom, K., "Roentgenographic Study of the Vascular Channels of the Skull," Acta Radiol., Supp. 30.

Elsberg, C. A., and Dyke, C. E., "The Diagnosis and Localization of Tumors of the Spinal Cord by Means of Measurement Made on the X-Ray Films of the Vertebrae, and the Correlation of Clinical and X-Ray Findings," Bull. Neurol. Institute of New York, 3:359-394, 1933-34.

Landmesser, W. E., Jr., and Heublein, G. W., "Measurement of Normal Interpedicular Spaces in Children," Connecticut M. J., 17:310, 1953.

Klemme, R., Scott, W., and Woolsey, R. D., "Special Needle for Injection and Removal of Lipiodol," Missouri State Med. J., 39:131, 1942.

Camp, L. D., "Contrast Myelography," 54:477, 1950.

Jacobsen, H. H., "Suboccipital Gas Myelography in the Diagnosis of Herniated Disc in the Cervical Segment," Acta Radiol., 46:28-30, 1956.

Rader, J. P., "Chronic Subdural Hematoma of the Spinal Cord," New England J. Med., 253:374, 1955.

Hampton, A. O., and Robinson, J. M., "The Roentgenographic Demonstration of Rupture of the Intervertebral Disc into the Spinal Canal after Injection of Lipiodol," Am. J. Roentgenol., 36:782, 1936.

Soule, A. B., Jr., Gross, S. W., and Irving, J. J., "Myelography by the Use of Pantopaque in the Diagnosis of Herniations of the Intervertebral Discs," Am. J. Roentgenol., 53:319, 1945.

Woolsey, R. D., and Tsang, J. L. K., "A Review of Three Hundred Cases of Protruded Intervertebral Disc Treated Surgically," J. International Coll. Surg., 18:456, 1952.

Taylor, A. R., "Mechanism of Injury to Spinal Cord in Neck without Damage to Vertebral Column," J. Bone and Joint Surg., 33B:543, 1951.

Seaman, W., Marder, S. N., and Rosenbaum, H. E., "Myelographic Appearance of Adhesive Spinal Arachnoiditis," J. Neurosurg., 10:145, 1953.

Wood, E. H., Taveras, J. M., and Pool, J. H., "Myelographic Demonstration of Spinal Cord Metastasis from Primary Brain Tumor," Am. J. Roentgenol., 69:221, 1953.

Cowie, T. N., "Diastematomyelia with Vertebral Column Defect," Brit. J. Radiol., 24:156, 1951.

Cowie, T. N., "Diastematomyelia, Tomography in Diagnosis," Brit. J. Radiol., 25:263, 1952.

Rayle, A. A., Gay, B. B., Jr., and Meadors, J. S., "The Myelogram in Avulsion of the Brachial Plexus," Radiol., 65:65, 1955.

Lichtenstein, B. W., "Diastematomyelia," Arch. Neurol. and Psychiat., 44:792, 1940.

Herren, R. Y., and Edwards, J. E., "Diastematomyelia," Arch. Path., 30:1203, 1940.

Holman, C. B., Svien, H. J., Bickel, W. H., and Keith, H. M., "Diastematomyelia," Pediatrics, 15:191, 1955.

Seaman, W. B., and Furlow, L. T., "The Myelographic Appearance of Sacral Cysts," J. Neurosurg., 13:88, 1956.

Cloward, R. B., and Buzaid, L. L., "Discography: Technic, Indications and Evaluation of Normal and Abnormal Intervertebral Disk," Am. J. Roentgenol., 68:552, 1952.

Walk, L., "Diagnostic Lumbar Disk Puncture: Clinical Review and Analysis of 67 Cases," A.M.A. Arch. Surg., 66:232, 1953.

Friedman, J., and Goldner, M. Z., "Discography in Evaluation of Lumbar Disk Lesions," Radiol., 65:653, 1955.

Jacobs, L. G., Smith, J. K., and VanHorn, P. S., "Myelographic Demonstration of Cysts of Spinal Membranes," Radiol., 62:215, 1954.

Stein, A., and Stewart, W. H., Pneumoperitoneal X-Ray Diagnosis, Southworth Co., Troy, N. Y., 1921.

Jarcho, J., Gynecological Roentgenology, Paul B. Hoeber, Inc., New York, 1931.

Joelson, J. J., Persky, L., and Rose, F. A., "Radiographic Diagnosis of Tumors of the Adrenal Gland," Radiol., 62:488, 1954.

Samuel, E., "Calcification in Suprarenal Neoplasms," Brit. J. Radiol., 21:139, 1948.

Vallebonna, A., "Recent Progress in Field of Stratigraphy," Acta Radiol., Supp., 116:175, 1954.

Cadman, E. F. B., and Tinkler, L. F., "Localization of Pheochromocytoma," J. Faculty Radiol., 4:211, 1953.

Melick, W. F., and Vitt, A. E., "Present Status of Aortography," J. Urol., 60:321, 1948.

Pendergrass, E. P., Chamberlain, G. W., Godfrey, E. W., and Burdick, E. D., "A Survey of the Deaths and Unfavorable Sequelae Following Administration of Contrast Media," Am. J. Roentgenol., 48:741, 1942.

Sante, L. R., "Evaluation of Aortography in Abdominal Diagnosis," Radiol., 56:183, 1950.

Hartnett, L. J., "Possible Significance of Arterial Visualization in the Diagnosis of Placenta Previa," Am. J. Roentgenol., 55:940, 1948.

Weyde, R., "Abdominal Aortography in Renal Disease," Brit. J. Radiol., 25:353, 1952.

Roland, M., Carpenter, F., and Rich, J., "New Water-Soluble Opaque Medium in the Study of Hysterograms and Hysterosalpingograms," Am. J. Obst. and Gynec., 65:81, 1953.

Farinas, P. L., "A New Technique for the Arteriographic Examination of the Abdominal Aorta and Its Branches," Am. J. Roentgenol., 46:641, 1941.

Figley, M. M., Fry, W. J., Orebaugh, J. E., and Pollard, H. M., "Percutaneous Splenoportography," Gastroenterol., 28:153, 1955.

Gvozdanovic, V., and Hauptmann, E., "Further Experience with Percutaneous Lienportal Venography," Acta Radiol., 43:177, 1955.

Giuseffi, J., and Largen, T., "A Method of Determining Patency of the Portocaval and Splenorenal Shunts," Arch. Surg., 70:707, 1955.

Bruwer, A. J., and Hallenbeck, G. A., "Roentgenologic Findings in Splenic Portography," Am. J. Roentgenol., 77:324, 1957.

Nordenstrom, B., "A Method of Angiography of the Azygos Vein and the Anterior Internal Venous Plexus of the Spine," Acta Radiol., 44:201, 1955.

Spolteholz, W., "Hand Atlas of Human Anatomy," 2nd Ed., 2:259, J. B. Lippincott Co., Philadelphia, Pennsylvania.

Catalano, D., Giardiello, A., and Ruggiero, A., "Hepatography after Percutaneous Lieno-Portal Venography," Acta Radiol., 43:285, 1955.

Bergstrand, I., and Ekman, C. A., "Percutaneous Lieno-Portal Venography," Acta Radiol., 43:377, 1955.

Thomason, J. L. G., "The Differential Diagnosis of Spalding's Sign," Brit. J. Radiol., 23:122, 1950.

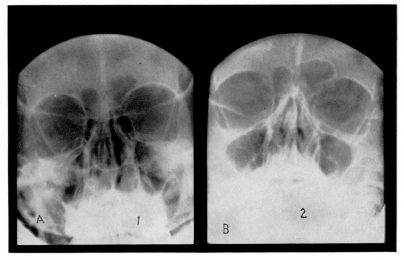

Normal accessory nasal sinuses, A., 23° angle position, and B. Waters' position, giving clear antral view.

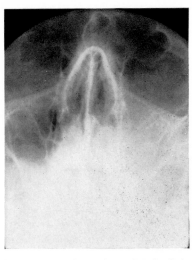

Dense opacity of patient's left antrum from pronounced infection.

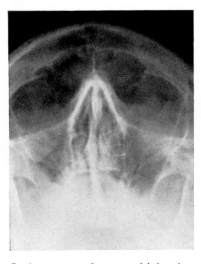

Oedematous boggy thickening of the patient's right antrum from allergy.

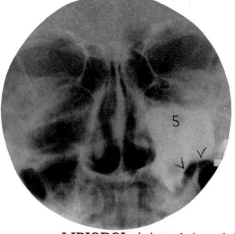

LIPIODOL injected into left antrum reveals large rounded filling defect caused by polyp, (arrows).

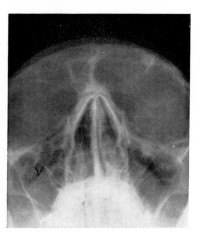

Rounded polyp in the patient's right antrum.

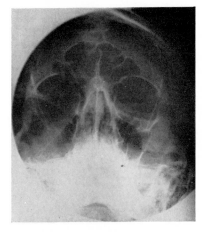

Sarcoma involving the patient's left antrum. Note bone destruction of roof of antrum and zygomatic process with extension into orbit.

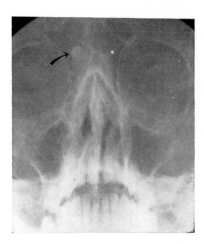

Small ivory osteoma of the frontal sinus.

MASTOIDS

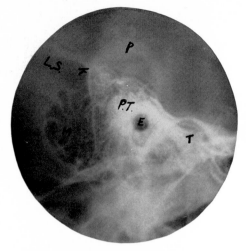

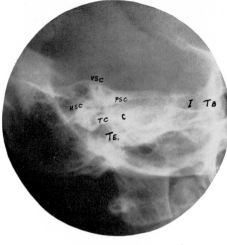

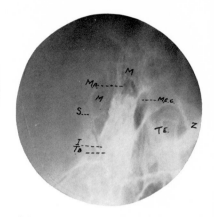

Left: Normal Mastoid; Law position; T, temporomandibular joint; E, external auditory canal viewed on end as it traverses petrous bone, P.; L-S, lateral sinus as it extends downward behind petrous bone; M, mastoid cells; K, knee of lateral sinus.

Middle: Arceline position; I, internal auditory meatus; T.B., temporal bone; T.C., tympanic cavity; T.E., temporal fossa; C, cochlea; V.S.C., vertical semicircular canal; H.S.C., horizontal semicircular canal; P.S.C., posterior semicircular canal.

Right: Mayer position; M, mastoid cells; Ma, mastoid antrum; M.E.C., middle ear cavity; I, internal auditory meatus; T.B., temporal bone; T.E., temporal fossa; M.E.C., middle ear cavity; Z, zygoma.

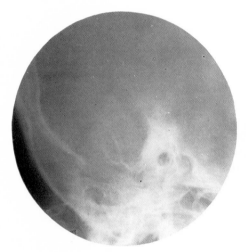

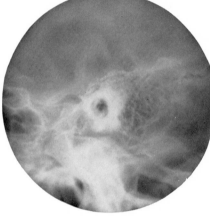

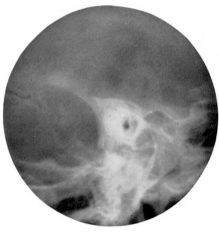

Left: Destructive mastoiditis with destruction of cells and sinus plate with perisinus abscess. Middle: Normal side for comparison. Right: Bony defect following operation.

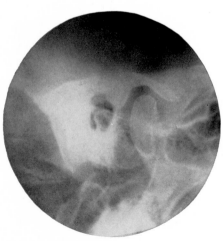

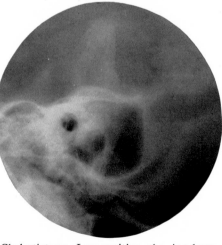

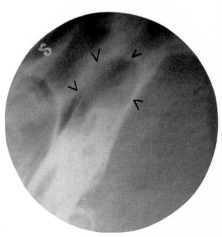

Selerotic mastoiditis showing dense sclerosis of the bone and lack of cell formation from chronic infection.

Cholestiatoma, Law position, showing large area of cell destruction with sclerotic margin.

Cholestiatoma, Mayer position, showing large destroyed area eroding thru auditory canal and communicating with inner ear.

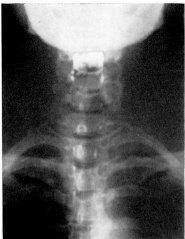

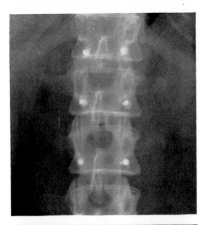

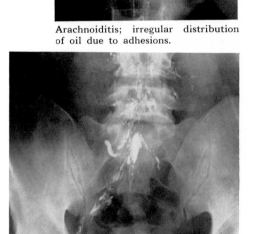

Lipiodol injected into the cisterna magna is blocked in its descent by a tumor of the cord in the lower cervical region.

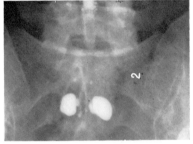

Arachnoiditis; irregular distribution of oil due to adhesions.

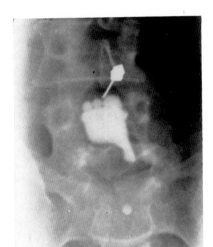

Multiple tiny cyst-like collections of opaque oil in sacral region and at each nerve root appearing several months after myelography, detected on subsequent gastrointestinal examination.

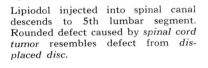

⟶

Opaque media in extraarachnoid space extending along nerve sheaths.

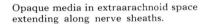

◄⟶

Lipiodol injected into spinal canal descends to 5th lumbar segment. Rounded defect caused by *spinal cord tumor* resembles defect from *displaced disc.*

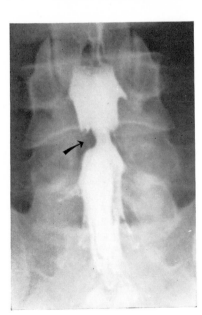

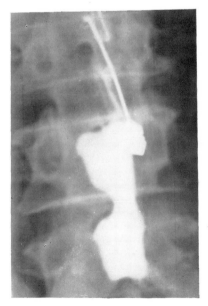

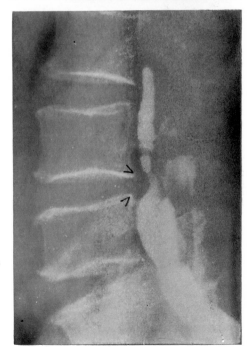

Antero-posterior and lateral views of lumbar spine after lipiodol injection showing protrusion of disc between 4th and 5th lumbar vertebrae.

Backward protrusion of the interarticular disc as outlined by lipiodol injected into the spinal canal (Myelography).

PNEUMOPERITONEUM—PERIRENAL INSUFFLATION

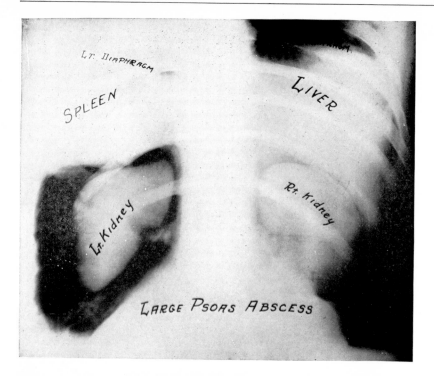

← Pneumoperitoneum examination with the patient in the prone position showing both kidneys well outlined and showing a large psoas abscess springing from the spine and bulging outward on either side.

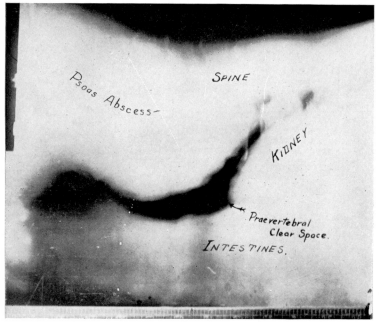

← Retroperitoneal position, same patient as above, showing the psoas abscess bulging forward from the retroperitoneal region into the prevertebral space.

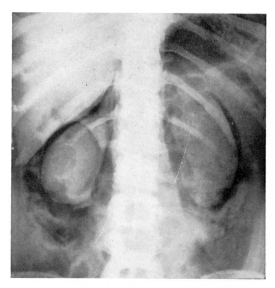

↑ Perirenal insufflation showing air in the connective tissue about the kidneys. Note diffuse calcification throughout the adrenal gland.

← Pneumoperitoneum examination with the patient in the retroperitoneal position showing diffuse infiltration of the entire retroperitoneal space with pus forming perinephritic abscess.

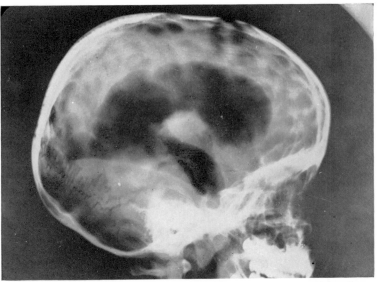

Ventriculogram showing enormous enlargement of the ventricles from pressure. Note the accentuation of the convolutional markings (convolutional atrophy) and the separation of the sutures due to chronic increase in intracranial pressure.

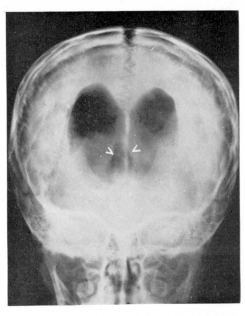

Antero-posterior view of the same patient showing dilatation of the third ventricle as well as the lateral ventricles. The condition was due to a diffuse glioma.

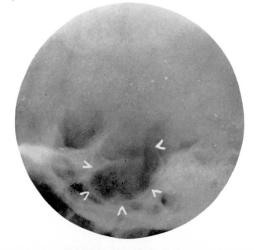

← Bulky tumor of the pituitary gland due to a pituitary adenoma. Note the enlargement of the sella turcica and the erosion of the posterior clinoid processes.

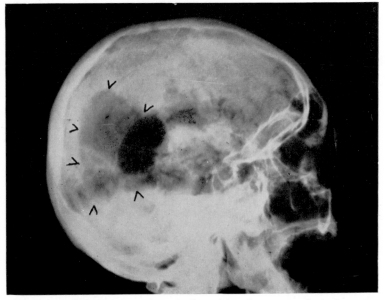

Large area of cortical necrosis as indicated by the escape of air from the ventricle into the necrotic area.

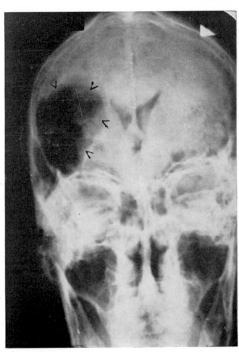

Anterior view of the same patient showing an extensive area of cortical necrosis. The ventricles are not dilated and appear normal.

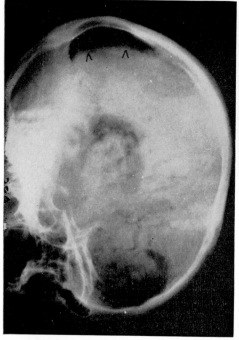

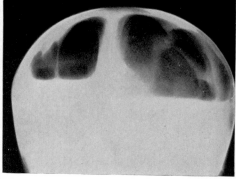

Extreme dilatation of the ventricles due to internal hydrocephalus. Very little cortical substance remains.

← Air in the subdural space after encephalography. Air may escape into the subdural space during injection; this is not necessarily an indication of cortical necrosis.

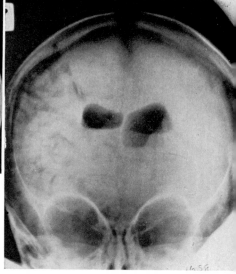

Encephalogram showing air in the ventricles and in the subarachnoid spaces on one side but a lack of filling of the subarachnoid pathways on the other side. This is sometimes associated with epilepsy.

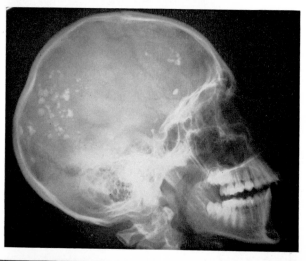

← Calcified areas in brain due to healed lesions of Toxoplasmosis acquired in infancy. Courtesy Dr. C. Zoller.

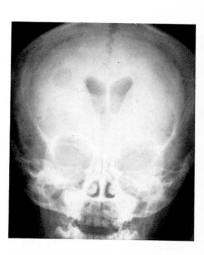

Same patient showing ventricular system in postero-anterior position. →

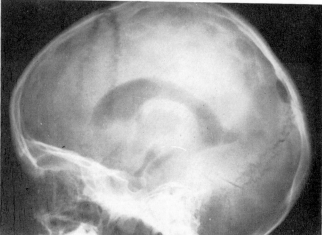

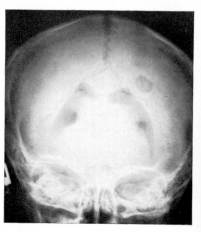

Same patient showing ventricular system in antero-posterior position. →

Lateral view of skull showing ventricular structures well filled with air from cerebellar tumor. Note separation of sutures. For details of structures compare diagrams in text.

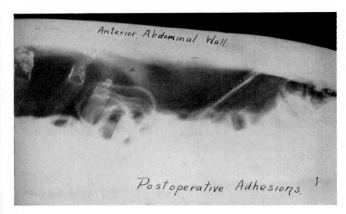

Transabdominal view with pneumoperitoneum showing post operative adhesions to anterior abdominal wall.

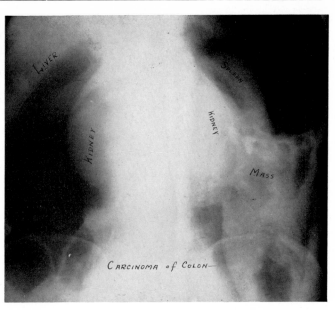

Prone view with artificial pneumoperitoneum, showing extension of carcinomatous growth of descending colon to lateral abdominal wall.

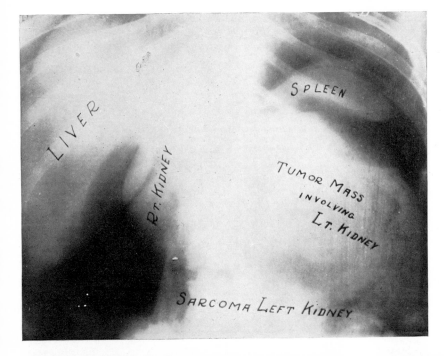

← Large tumor (sarcoma) left kidney, differentiated from spleen, which appears as a flattened structure beneath the dome of the diaphragm. Both kidneys and liver normal.

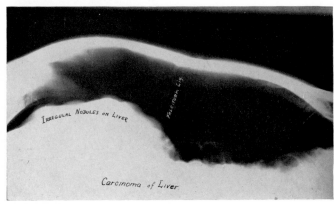

Transabdominal view, patient lying on his back, x-rays directed horizontally across abdomen; liver studded with carcinomatous nodules.

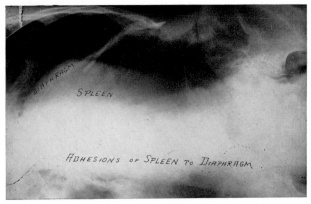

Right lateral decubitus; patient lying on right side, x-rays directed horizontally; spleen adherant to dome of diaphragm.

FEMALE PELVIC ORGANS

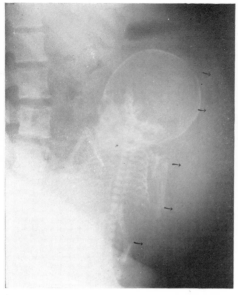

Lateral view, breech presentation showing placenta attached to anterior uterine wall.

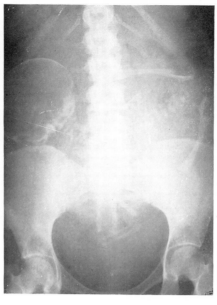

Transverse position of foetus with arm presentation.

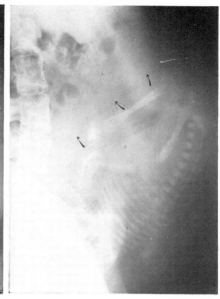

Lateral view, cephalic presentation; placenta in fundus of uterus.

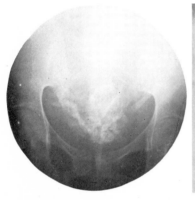

Anencephaly; characteristic deformity of head.

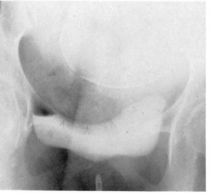

Opaque material injected into bladder in pregnancy to determine the presence of placenta-previa. More than 3 cm. between head and base of bladder is indication of placenta-previa.

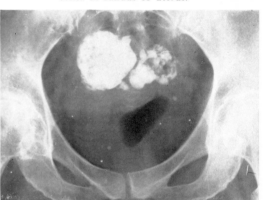

Irregular calcareus deposit in uterine fibroid.

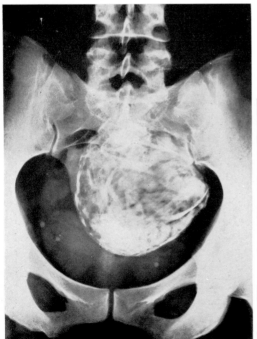

Lithopedion 8 years after full term abdominal pregnancy.

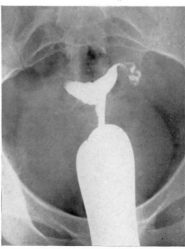

Lipiodol injection into uterus showing one tube occluded.

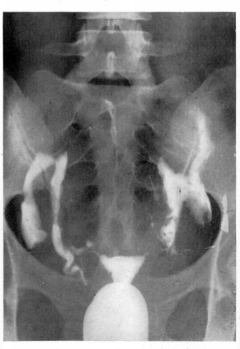

Lipiodol injected into the uterine canal filling the uterine cavity, extending through tubes into abdominal cavity indicating patency of tubes.

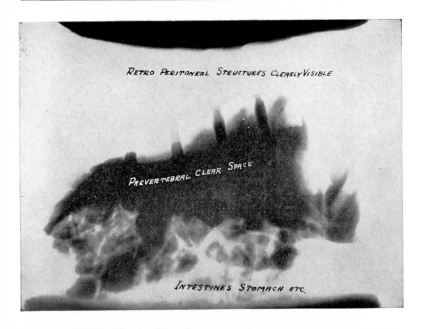

← Pneumoperitoneum examination of the patient in the retroperitoneal position (lying face downward, x-rays directed horizontally from side to side), showing the bodies of the vertebrae in the lateral view, the prevertebral clear space and the intestines and other organs with mesenteric attachment sagging forward with the anterior abdominal wall.

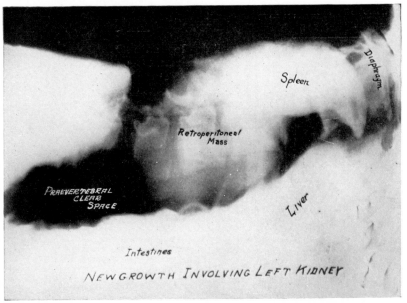

← New growth involving the left kidney clearly shown bulging forward into the prevertebral clear space. The spleen is still held in position by the growth. The patient is in a similar position to that shown above.

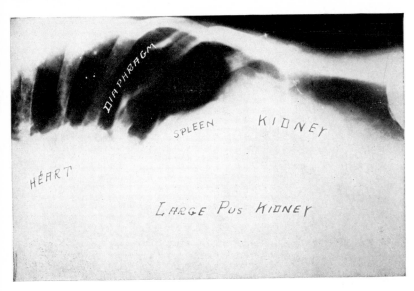

← Pneumoperitoneum examination with the patient in the lateral decubitus position (lying on right side) showing a large pus kidney.

PNEUMOPERITONEUM

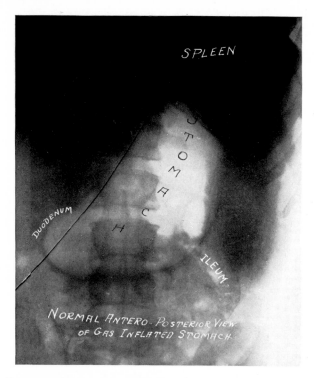

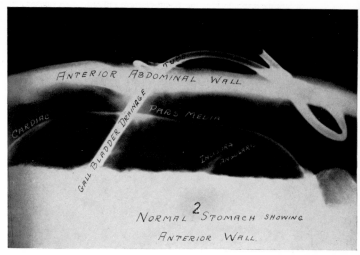

Normal Stomach: Transabdominal position; full thickness of anterior wall of entire stomach visible in its descending portion.

Pneumoperitoneum and gas-filled normal stomach by separate administration of the two packages of a sedlitz powder or soda-pop; supine position; peristalsis visible.

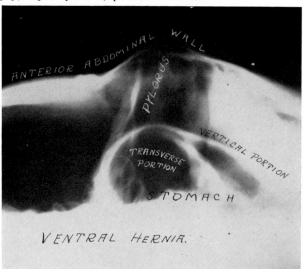

Ventral herniation with pylorus extending into hernial sac.

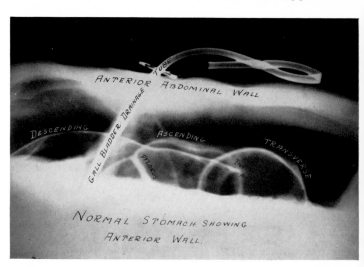

Same as above with patient slightly rotated to show transverse and ascending portions.

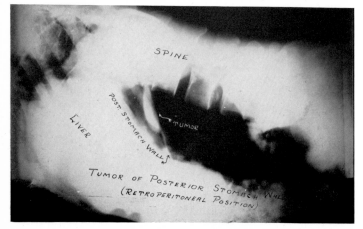

Tumor of posterior stomach wall shown by pneumoperitoneum and gas-filled stomach.

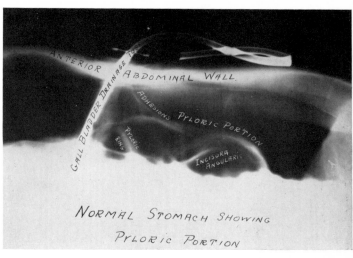

Same as above with patient rotated so as to show more clearly pyloric portion and pyloric ring. Peristalsis clearly visible.

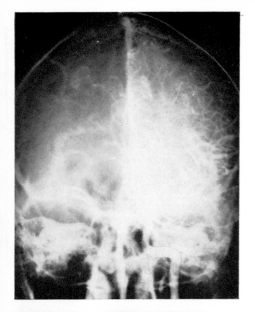

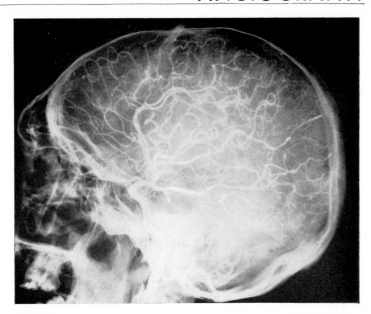

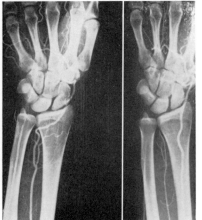

CEREBRAL ANGIOGRAPHY. Diodrast (70%) injected into internal carotid artery outlines cerebral circulation on one side.

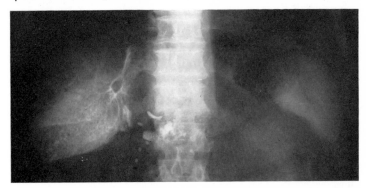

Thorotrast remaining in liver and spleen 11 years after injection.

Arteriograms of wrists of two different patients indicating variations in arterial structures.

Angiography of Extremities. A. Arteriography of leg. B. Venography of deep circulation of leg. C. Venography of superficial circulation of leg. D. Venography; varicose veins of leg. E. Retrograde venography showing valve structures.

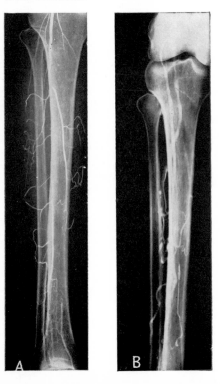

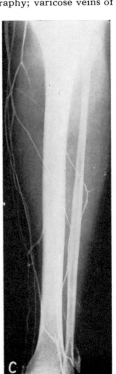

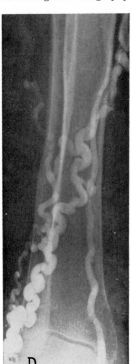

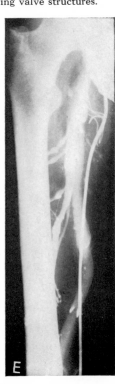

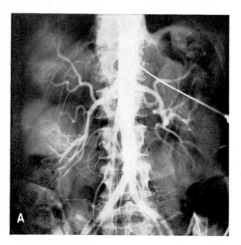

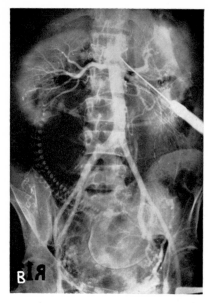

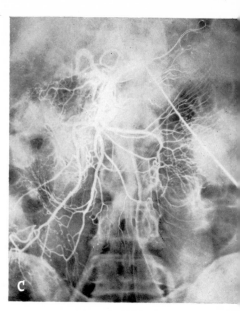

A. Normal aortogram showing circulation of all abdominal organs. B. Aortogram showing placenta previa; "puddling" of blood in sinusoids gives an irregular density to placental structure. C. Aortogram showing direct injection into mesenteric artery; this mishap may be followed by gangrene of the bowel.

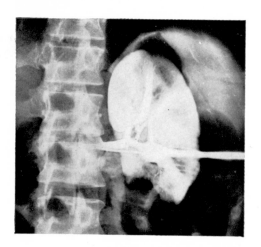

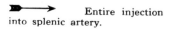 Entire injection into left renal artery; failure lower pole to fill could be from cyst or aberrant blood supply. May cause some damage to kidney.

Entire injection into splenic artery.

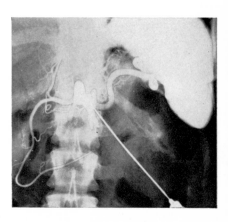

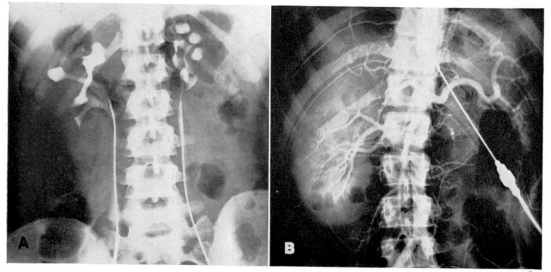

A. Double kidney pelves, with or without associated complete duplication of the ureters, often receive their blood supply from two separate arteries. B. Aortography discloses readily the presence and distribution of such vascular structures.

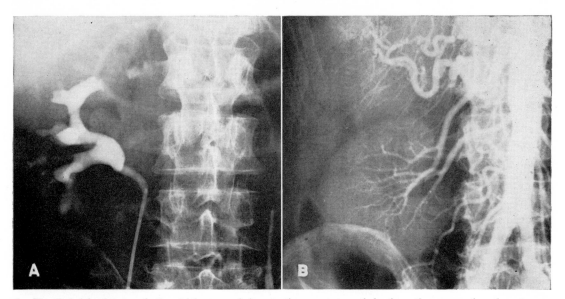

A. Partial blockage of the kidney pelvis at the ureteropelvic junction may be due to an aberrant renal vessel.

B. Aortography discloses readily the origin, size and distribution of such an aberrant vessel.

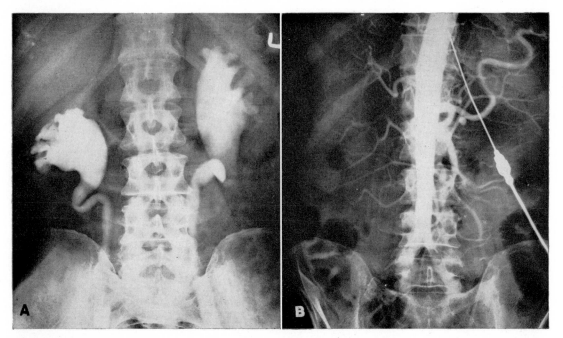

A. Bilateral hydronephrotic kidneys showing enlargement of pelves and ureters, with pressure from pelvic dilatation.

B. Aortogram showing scant blood supply to kidneys, almost to the point of ischemia.

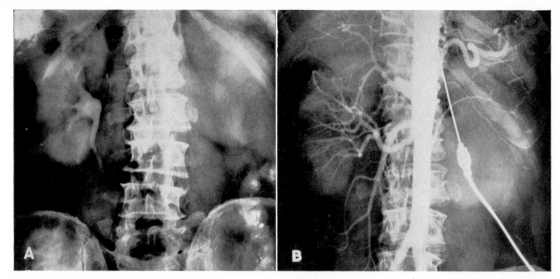

A. Intravenous pyelogram of non-functioning left kidney, with large hydronephrosis.   Right side normal.
B. Aortogram of same patient, showing good blood supply to right kidney but almost complete avascularization of left kidney, indicating that conservative measures will be of no avail in salvaging the diseased kidney.

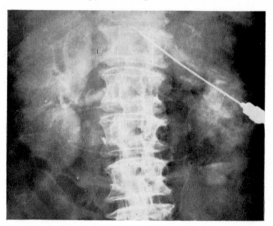

Neoplasm of left kidney, indicated by "puddling" seen within the mass in lower pole.

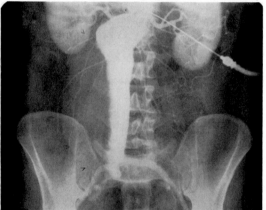

Large aneurysm abdominal aorta, bulging to left; recanalization thru old clot. Successfully removed and replaced with aortic graft.

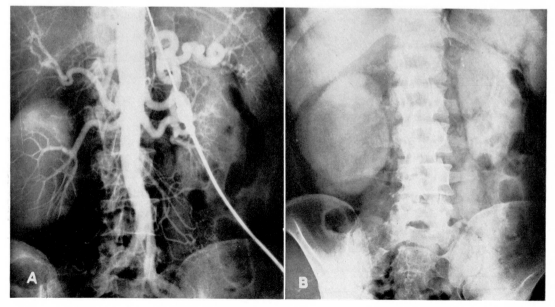

A. Large rounded mass in right kidney; fine slender arterial branches indicate that it probably is a cyst.
B. Aortogram made a few seconds later, showing arterial circulation swept clear, some retention in kidneys, but no "puddling" in the mass.   "Puddling" would have indicated a neoplasm.

Chapter XXV

RADIATION THERAPY

It is obviously impossible in such a short communication to present more than the essential facts concerning radiation therapy. Technical details of application and dosage are beyond the province of this article and will not be attempted. Radiation therapy has become so extensively employed as a means of combating malignant disease however that a knowledge of the fundamental principles governing its use have become essential to all practitioners. It will be considered under the following headings:

1. The nature and method of application of radiation therapy.
2. The effect of radiation on living tissues.
3. Results which can be expected from this method of treatment.

THE NATURE AND METHOD OF APPLICATION OF RADIATION THERAPY

While the term radiation therapy, strictly speaking, includes all types of radiation, common usage has restricted its meaning to the use of the penetrating types of radiation, x-rays and the gamma rays of radium. These two agents are similar in character and should always be used to supplement each other; both are forms of radiant energy which will penetrate solid substances.

X-RAY THERAPY. High voltage x-rays, although not as penetrating as gamma rays of radium, may be generated in great quantities; gamma rays being of much shorter wave length are more penetrating in character but are very small in quantity. By and large, therefore, it may be assumed that deep x-ray therapy is most efficient in delivering a greater quantity of radiant energy into a tumor in the depth, whereas, radium may be very effectively used to produce an intense local dosage for an isolated surface lesion.

The student is not concerned with the technical details of x-ray dosage, suffice it to say that long usage has proven that for all practical purposes x-rays generated at 200 K. V., using suitable filter and other factors, have proved most satisfactory for deep x-ray therapy and are universally used. The novice might expect that x-rays generated at higher voltages, 400 K. V., 600 K. V., or even 1.000.000 volts, might be proportionately "better" for the treatment of malignant disease, but this is not the case. X-Rays generated at these higher voltages not only fail to produce more than slight increase in dosage at 10 cm. depth over those generated by 200 K.V. but also introduce other adverse factors which tend to offset any advantage this may afford. After all, the cure of cancer is not to be found in any such small increase in depth dose such as 10 or 15% or even in dosage increases many times as high. Two hundred thousand volt x-rays have proved most efficient by a long period of experience. Great things have been accomplished by this means both for palliation as well as for cure of malignant tumors.

In order to formulate an orderly method of procedure, some method of measurement of the "strength" of the x-ray beam had to be devised. This was done by utilizing the ionization effect of x-rays upon gases. Further, it was found that the ionization effect upon the air closely paralleled, if it was not identical with, the biological effect upon the body tissues so that this method was found to be especially well suited to this purpose and became the means adopted by the U. S. Bureau of Standards and other standardization bodies throughout the world.

The unit of measurement is called the "roentgen" or "r-unit" in honor of Wm. Roentgen, the discoverer of x-rays. An international "roentgen" (unit of radiation) as revised by the Fifth International Congress of Radiology may be defined as follows: The roentgen shall be the quantity of x or Gamma Radiation such that the associated corpuscular emission per 0.001293 gram of air produces, in air, ions carrying 1. E.S.U., (Elecrostatic Unit), of quantity of electricity of "either" sign. This permits the application of the "r" unit to gamma as well as x-rays. This definition sounds very complicated but need not be remembered except by physicists engaged in checking instruments used in measuring x-radiation. One does not attempt to remember the origin of the standard measurements of a "foot" or a "meter" and yet these units of measurement are in continuous use. The r-unit however has one vital difference; its actual value varies with every wave length. The biological effect produced by an "r" unit of radiation varies widely depending upon the quality (wave length and filter) of the x-ray beam producing it. In other words, a mere statement of the number of "r" delivered to a tumor is meaningless unless the quality of the beam is also mentioned. Likewise, the number of "r" delivered to a tumor by x-rays of differing wave lengths or by the gamma rays of radium cannot be added together as an expression of the total biological dosage delivered. One might think that this would invalidate the use of such a unit for measurement but this is not the case; if a beam of the same quality, suitable for the purpose in question, is adhered to throughout the course of treatment, the dosage can be determined quite accurately both on the skin and in the depth. The number of "r" utilized in the treatment of any patient remains the province of the radiologist; it is not a commodity which can be directed in an order without a complete and detailed description of all other factors.

We must not suppose that, since we have found an accurate method of measurement and agreed upon a standard unit, the problem has become simple. A review of the physical properties of x-rays will recall the fact that when x-rays strike other substances they cause them to give off secondary radiations; in the case of the body tissues this radiation is of heterogeneous character depending upon the nature of the primary beam which gives rise to it. One can see therefore that the number of r-units recorded by an ionization chamber placed in the path of an x-ray beam in air will vary materially from the values obtained if the chamber is in contact with the skin, since in the latter case there is not only the effect of the primary beam but also the added effect of the scattered radiation from the tissues. The r-unit measurement therefore must be further qualified as to whether the reading was taken in air or with back scatter (tissue dose). The picture is still further complicated by the fact that the percentage of scattered radiation occurring in the tissues varies with the quality of the beam (kilovoltage and filter), with the size of the x-ray field, with the thickness of the part treated and with the homogeneity of the tissues irradiated. All of these points are cited merely to point out to the student the complexity of the problems connected with radiation therapy.

Modern apparatus for administration of deep x-ray therapy has been so perfected that the accuracy and constancy of the x-ray beam which it emits can be definitely relied upon thus reducing radiation therapy to a much more scientific basis. Integrating ionization measuring instruments incorporated in the machine may be set for the number of r-units desired. Shock proof tubes and cables make it possible to carry out treatments which would be otherwise impossible such as intracavity treatments of malignant tumors of the mouth or throat and cancer of the uterine cervix and female pelvis through small cones introduced into the cavities directed to the area of involvement.

Apparatus for the generation of x-rays up to many million electron volts has been perfected, so that their wave lengths approach that of the gamma rays of radium, yet their biological effect on cancer cells does not show any material advantage over 200 K. V. x-rays; many factors enter into this which cannot be discussed here.

One type of apparatus, revolutionary in design, which holds some promise of a different approach to the problem is the Betatron. The principle upon which it works is the setting into rapid revolving movement of a stream of electrons within the intense magnetic field produced by two large, rounded, flat-faced, doughnut-shaped electromagnets; the process is similar to the current induced within a coil of wire when placed in an alternating magnetic field except that in this case the electron stream itself comprises the induced circuit. Thus freed from the impediment of a metallic circuit the electron stream gains high velocity as it revolves around and around in the magnetic field; as it continues to gain speed it approaches the outer edge of the flat-faced magnets attaining a speed comparable to that of light. This stream of high speed electrons is then permitted to strike a thin metallic target and x-rays of shortest wave length yet known are produced. X-ray therapy

with these rays has not resulted in any spectacular advantage.

In recent years however, means have been devised for the transmission of the high speed electron stream itself, outside of the tube; this has shown physical properties which may be described as almost revolutionary in our conception of penetration of solid structures and may well be applied to radiation therapy, (Leucutia). When such a beam of electrons is applied to a block of paper for sufficient time, several sheets of paper may be charred from the effects of the beam at several centimeters depth and yet no effect will be noted either on the surface or in the tissues beyond the zone of destruction. This zone of destruction can be restricted to any desired depth, depending upon the degree of acceleration of the electron stream. One can conceive how such a beam of high speed electrons might be used in radiation therapy, provided a tumor mass was closely constricted to a given area and was not located within or near a vital organ (the normal tissues would of course be subjected to the destructive effect of the beam as well as the tumor mass). Still, some means might be perfected of widening the effective zone and of applying the electron stream in such a manner that it would have a greater differential effect upon the tumor cells than on the normal tissue, a condition which makes x-ray and radium therapy possible.

RADIUM THERAPY. The rays emitted by radium are of essentially the same character as x-rays; their method of application is similar and they must always be considered as complementary agents. The method by which these radiations are produced however is somewhat different.

Radium is a metal; contrary to popular opinion it is not radioactive in the sense of giving off rays. By the spontaneous emission of an alpha particle (the nucleus of a helium atom, bearing 2 positive charges) it loses two from its atomic weight and becomes a new element, Radon. This element differs in its physical properties in that it is a colorless odorless gas. Radon in the true sense of the word is likewise without radioactivity. With spontaneous emission of a positively charged alpha particle radon likewise loses two from its atomic weight and changes into another new element, Radium A. By the further rapid emission of alpha particles Radium A changes in succession to Radium B, C, D, E, F-Polomium and finally ends up as Uranium-lead. Radium B and C, known as Radium Active Deposit, are solids; they constitute the potent part of the radium series giving off gamma rays which are utilized in radium therapy. It will be noted that the immediate degeneration product of radium is radon, a gas, which is not radioactive in itself but is none the less the parent substance of Radium A, B, and C, the active deposit of radium which gives off the rays which are utilized in radium therapy. Now this gas is so inactive immediately after it has been withdrawn from the radium that it can be handled without danger and sealed into small glass or gold tubes for use in treatment. These small 2 to 4 mm. long capillary gold tubes are called gold radon "seeds" and are used for "planting" deep into tumors so that their radiation effect may be expended in intimate contact with the growth.

Since the radon gas is separated from the radium which gave rise to it, the continuous decay of the radon will result in a reduction of its quantity of radiation by 1/6 every twenty-four hours until it becomes inert. (See Radium Emanation Plant, Manual of Roentgenological Technique.)

The amount of radon gas which is found to be exactly in equilibrium with 1 milligram (mg) of radium element is designated as 1 millicurie (mc) (in honor of the discoverers of Radium, M. and Mme. Curie). 1 mghr. of dosage therefore is exactly equal to 1 mchr.

It has been determined by mathematical calculation that each millicurie of radon gas by the time it completely disintegrates exposes the surrounding tissues to 133 mchrs. of radiation. Such dosage is referred to as "millicuries destroyed." The dosage of radiation received by a tumor into which radon seeds have been planted would be expressed as number of gold radon seeds x the amount in mc. of each seed x 133 = number of mc. hours.

The radiations given off by Radium Active Deposit (Radium B and C) are of three types:
Alpha particles, (positive charges)
Beta particles, (negative electrons)
Gamma rays, (true wave motions in the ether)

Alpha particles have very little penetration; ordinarily they will be blocked by a single piece of paper and they never have sufficient penetration to pass outside of the wall of the glass tube in which they are contained so that under ordinary circumstances we do not need to consider them in treatment.

Beta particles, on the other hand, have much greater penetrating power and their effect must always be considered in radium therapy. Their effect is expanded almost entirely in the first few millimeter of tissue. All beta rays are eliminated by 1/2 mm. platinum or gold, 1 mm. lead or silver, or 2 mm. brass.

Gamma Rays are the most penetrating of all radiations, requiring two to three inches of lead for complete protection.

The penetrating power of these various types of radiation is: Alpha: Beta: Gamma as 1:100: 10:000; however the biological effect is in reverse proportion, alpha: beta: gamma as 10:000: 100:1.

This means that beta particles have a low penetration but a very caustic effect, whereas gamma rays are more penetrating and spread their effect over a longer pathway without being so intense in any one area.

It is possible by interposing various metallic filters (monel metal, brass, silver, gold, platinum, etc.) to produce, by a selective absorption of the corpuscular emissions, a beam composed entirely of gamma radiations. Most radiation therapy is carried out at the present time by the use of gamma rays only.

There is one great advantage in the treatment with radium, namely, the constancy of its emission; the rate of spontaneous change continues regardless of any outside influence which is brought to bear; no change of temperature or pressure causes any variation. It is therefore possible to determine with accuracy the number of milligrams of radium present from the amount of ionization which it produces in an ionization chamber, regardless of whether it is in the form of a salt of radium or is mixed with other substances. The radiation coming from a milligram of radium is constant therefore, the world over, under any circumstances. It is possible therefore to express dosage satisfactorily by designating the number of milligrams of radium times the number of hours of application in "milligram-hours." When coupled with a detailed description of the method of application, filter, distance, length of tube or arrangement and size of applicator, this may be considered as a satisfactory method of expressing dosage; however it expresses only the dosage applied to the part to be treated, it does not give any indication of the amount of radiation received by the tumor.

The adoption of the gamma roentgen (γ r) as a standard unit of measurement has made it possible to formulate a more accurate method of tissue dosage. Using 1/2 mm. of platinum as a filter to exclude all other gamma rays, at a 1 cm. distance, from a theoretical point source it has been found that 8.4 gamma-ray roentgens are delivered per milligram-hour. Since it has been determined that a Threshold Erythema Dose to the skin (a very faint erythematous reaction) is equivalent to 1000 gamma r, it is obvious that under such conditions 120 mg. hrs. should produce such a reaction. Of course, this figure varies with every form and length of applicator; single radium tube applicators vary for every length and position, applicators of varying size and construction differ depending upon the size of the lesion to be treated and the distance at which it must be treated. All of these have been worked out in great detail by physicists; Patterson and Parker charts have been constructed for this purpose; they are based on continuous or divided dose treatments over an eight day period. The entire process may be very complicated. Since 1000 gamma ray r is equivalent to a threshold erythema dose (T. E. D.), if it were known how many T. E. D. were necessary to kill tumor cells of various types, it would be possible to administer radium therapy with greater accuracy.

THE EFFECT OF RADIATION ON LIVING TISSUES. The effect which radiation has upon living tissues may be considered as:
1. Physical
2. Chemical
3. Physiological
The beam of radiation may be considered as a stream of projectiles directed against an army of living cancer cells which by their relentless growth

are constantly advancing. The relative size of the atomic structure of the cellular elements and the rays which go to make up the beam of radiation may be likened to machine gun fire directed against an army in wide open formation; some may be killed outright by direct hits, others may escape injury entirely unless intensive fire is kept up for considerable time; a great many will be injured but not killed outright, some of these may ultimately die, others may recover and again march forward. So it is with radiation of a malignant growth—many cells may be injured so badly that they die almost immediately, others may be wounded so that their growth is temporarily inhibited, but later on they may recover and start in growing again producing a recurrence of the tumor.

The physical impact of the quanta of radiation upon the atomic structures causes displacement of their orbital electrons into other orbits or ejects them entirely. If the impact has not been severe and the change produced not too radical, immediate recovery may take place by rearrangement of the orbital electrons from surrounding structures; if however the change produced has become so great that recovery of the normal status cannot take place, then a permanent charge results in the atom.

Chemical changes always accompany rearrangement of the atomic structure of the atom. Some of these chemical changes wrought in the protein substances of the cells are foreign to its normal function thus leading to the next phase.

Physiological action in the presence of such foreign chemical material may not be possible so that the cell disintegrates and dies finishing the cycle of the destructive process.

All cell structure is not affected to the same degree by radiation but certain cells are more vulnerable than others. Adult body tissue cells are more resistant than those of newly growing tumor cells so that it may be possible to destroy the more sensitive tumor cells without affecting (beyond recovery) the normal body tissue cells in which it lies. It is this differential effect of irradiation upon tumor cells that makes the entire process of radiation therapy possible.

The administration of sufficient radiation may leave definite evidence of the effect of the radiation on normal tissue bed in which it lies. This may be indicated by intense fibrosis of the tissue; in the lung this may be evident as fibrosis of the lung tissue, pleural thickening and the results of scar tissue contraction, (see Bate and Guttman).

Almost from the beginning of radiation therapy it was realized that, by and large, cells were more resistant to the effects of irradiation depending upon their degree of differentiation; the higher in the scale of differentiation, that is, the more specialized their function, the more resistant to radiation they become. The ovum and spermatids being fundamentally sex cells were found to be most profoundly affected, whereas highly differentiated cells like muscle cells and glandular structure were more resistant; nerve tissue, being the most highly differentiated of all, showed greatest resistance.

Furthermore, it has also been found that the sensitivity of cells varied greatly depending upon the phase of their activity; during the stage of cell division all cells are found to be more sensitive to irradiation. The life cycle of tumor cells varies greatly; some tumors are slow in their growth, others are extremely rapidly growing. It would seem logical therefore to time the irradiation so that the greatest number of cells would be irradiated during mitosis.

The life cycle of epidermal cells of the skin is relatively long compared to most neoplasms; it is possible therefore to deliver to the tumor such intense irradiation that it cannot survive whereas the skin which is less sensitive may be able to recover promptly without apparent injury. This is the basis for the divided dose therapy formulated by Regaud and Coutard, which is universally used today.

C. Regaud, utilizing the testicle of a ram, demonstrated the increased effect of radium exposure during the process of cell division and advocated the use of small intensities over a longer period of time in order to expose more cells during mitosis. On microscopic examination it was found that in the case of the single massive dose of interstitial radiation, the immediate surrounding tissues were necrosed but that the spermatids and other primitive cells were still viable at a short distance from the radium needle, whereas with surface application and divided dose method the spermatids were destroyed without evidence of necrosis.

H. Coutard soon followed by extending the divided dose technique to x-ray therapy. Under this plan daily doses of high voltage heavily filtered radiation were applied for periods of one to four weeks or even more. This was done in the early 1930's; up to that time there were relatively few instances of malignant neoplasm cured by irradiation; since that time the entire field of radiation therapy has been lifted to a new level. In certain instances the response of tumor tissue to this method of treatment has been almost phenomenal; in others the effects have been very disheartening. Success or failure in radiation therapy depends upon two factors: 1) the sensitivity of the tumor cell to radiation, and 2) the bed in which the tumor lies.

For instance, a primary tumor of the skin may be readily affected by radiation not only because of the effect of the radiation on the tumor cells themselves but also because of the effect of radiation on the newly-formed blood vessels which nourish the tumor in its rapid growth. A metastatic focus from the same tumor into the regional lymph nodes requires many times the amount of radiation to kill the tumor cells. This is probably because of the fact that in this new location the tumor cells derive their nutrition from the lymph spaces in which they lie, and any radiation effect produced must be attributed to the direct effect upon the tumor cells themselves.

RESULTS WHICH CAN BE EXPECTED FROM RADIATION THERAPY. The success or failure of radiation therapy depends largely upon these two factors. The vulnerability of the body tissue cells will always remain the limiting factor in radiation therapy. Obviously a vital organ cannot be destroyed in an effort to kill the tumor. No matter how "powerful" an x-ray machine may be, the vulnerability of the normal tissues will always limit the amount of radiation which can be applied to a tumor.

Broder has endeavored to grade tumors as to the degree of anaplasia of their cellular structure as a general rule into grades 1, 2, 3 and 4. Tumors of adult cell type (least anaplastic) are designated as grade 1, whereas those of embryonal type (most anaplastic) are designated as grade 4. Obviously this graduation should also express the degree of radiosensitivity, since the more anaplastic a tumor the greater the degree of radiosensitivity. While such an analysis of the cell structure gives valuable information as to the cellular composition of a tumor, in actual practice it cannot be depended upon to furnish a definite index for the response of the tumor to radiation. The actual "test of radiation," or exposure of the tumor-bearing area to a tolerance dose of radiation, (a dose which the normal tissue will stand without destruction), and observing the result three weeks later, is the only practical means of determining the sensitivity of the tumor. It will often be found that the tumors having relatively little cellular structure and large amounts of stroma, which would seem to be of the least favorable variety for radiation therapy, may show the best response. If the tumor shows, by its favorable regression, that it is amenable to treatment, radiation should be continued to its maximum effect; if on the other hand, the tumor does not show satisfactory response to the test dosage, then no matter how much further radiation is applied, favorable response cannot be expected. If there is any chance for cure, one is justified in subjecting the patient to the most drastic methods, but if palliation is all that can be expected, there is no point in making the patient more miserable by the continuous drastic application of radiation.

Three types of reaction of tumors to radiation may be considered clinically:
1) Autolytic
2) Necrotic
3) Growth restraining

By autolytic type of reaction is meant the rapid regression and resolution of the tumor by autolysis, without pain, toxic reaction or other local or constitutional manifestation. The tumor literally seems to melt and disappear; there is no evidence of toxic manifestation and the patient feels well. This may be considered as the most favorable type of radiation reaction as far as the local tumor is concerned; however, it does not always prove most favorable for the patient, since it often happens that tumors which respond locally in this favorable fashion are most apt to show early metastases to remote locations.

A necrotic reaction on the other hand, is one in which the radiation reaction must be carried to the point of necrosis before the death of the cancer cells can be affected; any point short of destruction of normal tissue will still leave viable cancer cells. Obviously the normal tissues cannot be carried to any such degree of necrotic reaction except where the tumor is very small, is readily accessible and is located in a non-vital organ.

Between these two extremes of great radiosensitivity and radioresistance are many tumors, which although they cannot be totally destroyed, may have their growth restrained by repeated sublethal doses of radiation applied over a prolonged period. By this method the growth of the tumor cells is inhibited long enough to permit the surrounding fibrous tissue to proliferate and restrain the growth of the tumor. Such a reaction is known as a growth restraining reaction. This form of reaction, although never curative, may prolong the life of the individual and relieve his discomfort for many years.

After all, the success or failure of a procedure is determined by the results obtained. The statistics quoted concerning the various types of growth are all approximate; obviously these vary greatly from different clinics and depend a great deal upon the extent and characteristics of the growth. For this reason most clinics determine upon certain factors for different stages of a growth.

Consideration of criteria for staging of tumors, gleaned from many sources (especially those used in the Tumor Clinic of Stanford University School of Medicine; Pack and Livingston, Pfahler, League of Nations, etc.) and from our own experience, has lead us to adapt those which seem particularly applicable in each instance for use in the Radiology Departments of the St. Louis University School of Medicine and Associated Hospitals and the St. Louis City Hospital.

Another factor in the success or failure of radiation therapy is the accessibility of the growth. Skin cancers because of their location are readily accessible, aiding the application of radiation and giving almost universally good results. Tumors of this sort are of either basal or squamous cell type. Basal cell epitheliomata have one characteristic which is highly favorable—they do not tend to metastasize, whereas squamous cell epithelioma tends to metastasize early to the regional lymph nodes. The primary growth is readily killed by irradiation but the metastases in the regional lymph nodes require many times the radiation needed to kill the primary growth before the cells in this new location succumb. It is very important therefore to distinguish between basal cell and squamous cell carcinoma. This is especially difficult at times since in large skin tumors about the face microscopic sections taken at different locations give a conflicting appearance; some resemble basal cell while others appear as squamous cell epitheliomas. Under such conditions it is better to assume that the growth is of the epidermoid or squamous cell type even though no metastases are present. As a matter of practical observation it may be well to remember that if a line is drawn across the side of the face from the corner of the mouth to the lobe of the ear, approximately 90% of skin tumors of the face occurring above this line are of basal cell type whereas approximately 90% occurring below this line are squamous cell epitheliomata.

In carcinoma of the lip, the primary lesion can usually be very readily destroyed by radiation therapy (x-rays or radium); it matters not how the primary growth is destroyed whether it be by radiation, surgery or actual cautery; radiation therapy usually produces less scar but the other methods are none the less effective. The question which is of grave importance is how to take care of the regional lymph nodes. There are those who advocate prophylactic neck dissection before any glands appear, thus subjecting a large number of patients (90%) to a useless operative procedure since many never develop glandular metastases at all. Likewise, in a considerable number of instances cervical metastases develop later even after lymph node dissection has been carried out. Others wait for lymph node dissection until metastatic glands appear, but when this occurs few are ever saved by surgical procedure; recurrence is usually prompt and tragic. Many radiologists feel that the patient's welfare can best be served by radiological treatment to the metastatic glands if and as they appear. Surface application of radiation from the outside is not sufficient in most instances to kill metastatic lesions in lymph nodes; this usually requires the supplemental use of interstitial radiation using gold radon seeds implanted directly into the metastatic mass.

In this type of epithelioma statistics show the following results:

Lesions 1 cm. or less, 90%, five year arrests

Lesions 1 cm. to 2.5 cm. in size without extensive infiltration into the deeper structures about 50%, five year arrests

Lesions larger than 2.5 cm. in size with evidence of infiltration into the deeper structures, muscle, cartilage or bone, or with metastatic regional lymph node involvement, approximately 10 to 20%, five year arrests.

In other words, as long as a lesion remains small, 1 cm. or less in size, without lymph gland metastases or extension in other structures, the possibility of cure is in the order of 90%; if lymph node metastases occurs, at once the possibility of cure drops the figure below 20 %.

Other epithelial tumors in certain locations of the head and neck require special consideration.

Epitheliomas involving the eyelids are probably best treated with x-ray therapy with small cones to direct and limit the x-ray beam closely to the area involved, since the gamma rays of radium if given in large amounts may have effect on the eye especially on the lens. If radium is used, it may be found best to treat with beta radiation since this will produce an intense local dose in a short time thereby preventing exposure of the eye to prolonged irradiation with gamma rays. In any event in addition to the eye, the eyebrows and lashes should be well protected with lead to prevent epilation.

Epitheliomatous growths in the region of the naso-labial fold are notoriously radioresistant and require heavy dosage.

Epitheliomas of the ear even if they involve the cartilage may be treated by radiation therapy. We have never hesitated to apply full adequate doses of radiation even if the cartilage is involved; treatment should be made by topical (surface) application however not by interstitial implantation of gold radon seeds into the cartilage. If a cartilage infection or slough should follow, this can best be treated after the acute reaction has subsided by administration of ultra violet light using a quartz applicator. Attempts to clear up infection by using ultra violet applicator before radiation therapy should never be carried out since this may tend to spread or augment the growth.

Cystic adenomatous (malignant) growths of the skin are notoriously radioresistant and should be completely removed by actual cautery.

Melanoepithelioma (malignant pigmented mole) is very resistant to any form of treatment. Wherever they occur they should be removed completely surgically or with actual cautery.

Epitheliomas of the upper extremity usually occur on the back of the hand or extensor surfaces of the forearm; they are usually of the squamous cell type and frequently metastasize to the supracondylar and axillary lymph nodes. The procedure for treatment is the same as for epidermoid epithelioma elsewhere.

Epidermoid growths of the lower extremities especially occurring on or about the ankle or dorsum of the foot are very frequently due to melanoepithelioma; they should be treated similarly to those elsewhere in the body, by wide surgical extirpation or actual cautery. The regional glands, if involved, are deeply pigmented, even black in appearance.

Tumors of the oral cavity are a group in which radiation therapy may be of distinct palliative or curative value. Malignant tumors occur in the tongue and floor of the mouth, alveolar process, tonsil, palate and buccal mucous membrane. Of these the tongue and floor of the mouth present the vast majority of cases. The method of treatment in these locations is essentially similar. Intense local irradiation is necessary, using interstitial radiation with gold radon seeds or radium element needles implanted directly into the tumor. Any regional lymph node metastases are treated like similar metastases elsewhere. In the oral cavity such treatment can be supplemented by further x-ray therapy using an intracavity cone to limit the radiation to a small selected field. Here again the size of the primary lesion, its metastases location and the possibility of lymph node are the all important factors in prognoses. Early lesions, 1 cm. or less in size without lymph node metastases, 25 to 50% may show 5 year arrests whereas as soon as extension occurs into lymph nodes this falls to 10% or even less.

Carcinoma of the pharynx and larynx are best treated by external application of x-radiation, by Coutard's divided dose method over a prolonged period of weeks. By this method an appreciable percentage of patients may be cured and palliation can be effected in most instances for long periods of time. Early cases of carcinoma of the larynx, where the growth is confined to a small portion of the vocal cords and has not infiltrated the surrounding tissues, are suitable for operative extirpation. The difficulty arises in the inability to determine whether the growth is still localized.

Carcinoma of the breast forms a large percentage of the malignant growths which present themselves for treatment. Most are of the adeno-carcinomatous type which is very resistant to radiation therapy. Carcinoma of the breast therefore is primarily a surgical disease. No amount of radiation therapy can compare with complete surgical removal. Many patients however are beyond the surgical stage when they first report for treatment.

The breast is a pendulous structure which can be radiated from both sides producing a cross-fire effect on the tumor, which is often very effective in causing complete resolution of the growth. Metastatic lesions in the lymph glands are so much more resistant than the primary growth, however, that their destruction usually cannot be effected from surface radiation; they require the intensive doses supplied by gold radon seeds directly implanted into the tumor tissue. It is difficult if not impossible to do this with any degree of accuracy in a great number of widely scattered nodes so that such therapy must be considered as palliative only. When adeno-carcinoma metastasize to the bony structure however it is amazing to observe its radiosensitivity. This is one incidence in which the metastatic lesions are more sensitive than the primary growth. Relatively small doses of radiation applied to large metastatic areas of bone destruction cause almost immediate regression of the tumor and relief of pain with filling in of the destroyed area by dense new bone formation. Batson has shown how distant metastases can occur without passage through the heart by venous extension which may explain some of these bone lesions.

It is difficult to formulate a classification of breast tumors. The qualifying factors, such as movability of breast, fixation of metastatic nodes etc., by which various stages are designated is based so much on the judgment of the individual examiner that uniformity of staging can hardly be expected.

As a general rule all attempts at staging are built upon the following criteria: Stage 1. Small growths localized to the breast, freely movable and without evidence of axillary metastases, purely operable lesions; approximately 75% five year surgical survivals. Stage 2. Those in which such an operable primary lesion is associated with involvement of axillary nodes, not fixed, still operable; approximately 25% five year survivals. Stage 3. All cases in which the disease has advanced beyond this stage, very small (less than 10%) five year survivals.

It will be noted that with surgical resection alone (stage 1 cases) there is approximately 75%

five year survivals. The overall statistics of operable cases however where there is some axillary node involvement show a much lower survival rate, in the neighborhood of 25%. These figures vary, depending upon the relative numbers of localized and axillary involved cases in the series. Pfahler has shown that by operation only there are 28% average alive and well in 5 years; using preoperative irradiation, operation, plus postoperative irradiation, 57% alive and well in five years. This would indicate that operable cases with axillary involvement is the field in which radiation therapy has a real beneficial effect. In reality this increase in percentage is probably due to the average percentage of radiosensitive tumors found among breast carcinomas.

Haagensen and Stout have formulated from statistics certain criteria which will aid the physician in deciding whether a patient with carcinoma of the breast should be operated on or be subjected only to palliative therapy.

"Women of all age groups who are in good enough general condition to run the risk of major surgery should be treated by radical mastectomy except as follows: (1) when the carcinoma is one which developed during pregnancy or lactation (now no longer included as a contraindication); (2) when extensive edema of the skin over the breast is present; (3) when satellite nodules are present in the skin over the breast; (4) when intercostal or parasternal tumor nodules are present; (5) when there is edema of the arm; (6) when proved supra-clavicular metastases are present; (7) when the carcinoma is the inflammatory type; (8) when distant metastases are demonstrated; (9) when any two or more of the following signs of locally advanced carcinoma are present; (a) ulceration of the skin; (b) edema of the skin of limited extent (less than one-third of the skin over the breast involved); (c) fixation of the tumor to the chest wall; (d) axillary lymph nodes measuring 2.5 cm. or more in transverse diameter and proved to contain metastases by biopsy; (e) fixation of axillary lymph nodes to the skin or the deep structures of the axilla and proved to contain metastases by biopsy."

Roentgen castration has been widely advocated as a supplementary method of treatment in the immediate pre-menopausal patients. The influence of endocrine secretion on malignant growths is well recognized so that the elimination of ovarian secretion should have a tendency to restrain growth and lessen the chance of metastases. Each case should be examined individually; if a woman is in the immediate pre-menopausal period (42 to 45 years of age) and other circumstances make it improbable that she will have further increase in her family, roentgen castration is permissible. Observations of the beneficial effect of removal of the effects of female ovarian secretion would suggest the inadvisability of the use of Theelin in any patient having carcinoma. In fact, the use of testosterone has been advocated as a deterrent in such cases.

CARCINOMA OF THE UTERINE CERVIX

The uterine cervix is one of the most frequent sites of carcinomatous involvement. This is primarily a radiological disease. The cervical growth is in an ideal situation for radiation therapy; the cervical canal permits the introduction of a radium tube deep into the center of the growth and the vaginal fornix permits the application of other radium tubes on either side, thus developing a system of cross fire radiation. In addition to this, x-radiation applied from the outside through the abdominal wall augments the local application of radium to the adjacent adnexal areas. Furthermore, the cervix and uterus itself are insensitive organs which will stand large quantities of irradiation without destruction.

Carcinoma of the cervix has been classified by the League of Nations into four stages, according to its extent and involvement. A summary of the classification is as follows:

Stage I. The cancer is limited strictly to the cervix uteri and the uterus is mobile.

Stage II. Extension of the cancer into one or more fornices with or without infiltration of the parametrium, the uterus retaining some degree of mobility.

Stage III. a) Nodular infiltration of the parametrium on one or both sides extending to the wall of the pelvis with limited mobility of the uterus or massive infiltration of one parametrium with fixation of the uterus.

b) More or less superficial infiltration of a large part of the vagina, although the uterus may be movable.

c) Isolated metastases in the pelvic lymph nodes with a relatively small primary tumor.

d) Isolated metastases in the lower part of the vagina.

Stage IV. a) Massive infiltration of both parametria extending to the walls of the pelvis.

b) Carcinoma involving the bladder or rectum.

c) Entire vagina infiltrated (rigid vaginal passage) or one vaginal wall infiltrated along its whole length with fixation of the primary cancer.

d) Remote metastases.

e) "Frozen pelvis"

The percentage of five year arrests in carcinoma of the uterine cervix after radiation therapy is approximately:

Stage I.   - 80%
Stage II.   - 40%
Stage III. - 10%
Stage IV.   - 0%

Overall percentage for all cases average about 22%.

Of course the highest percentage of cures is in the stage I and II cases; in stage III cases, the percentage of cures falls off materially, in stage IV cases there are practically no survivals. Surgical removal is occasionally performed in stage I cases but the recovery statistics with this method cannot compare with those of radiation therapy. Nor is there any advantage in surgical removal after radiation therapy since surgery is apt to open up nests of quiescent cells which are being choked off by fibrous tissue and allow them free unrestrained growth.

CARCINOMA OF THE UTERINE FUNDUS

Carcinoma of the fundus of the uterus on the other hand must be considered as a disease treated most effectively by a combination of radiation and surgery. The uterus is a thick muscular organ which offers a barrier to the spread of malignancy; it is not so abundantly supplied with lymphatics and it can be readily extirpated without detriment to the patient. Radiation therapy can not be applied to fundus carcinoma with the same degree of precision as it can to carcinoma of the cervix since the location and extent of the growth cannot be visualized. On this account carcinomas in this location are treated with multiple radium tubes introduced into the uterine cavity, combined with x-ray therapy from outside. Radiation therapy followed by surgical removal offers the best chance for survival in fundus carcinoma.

Clinical classification:
Stage I.   Small localized growth.
Stage II.   Infiltration of uterus with possible extension beyond uterine wall but without evidence of fixation.

It is almost impossible to differentiate with any degree of accuracy between these two stages, I and II.

Stage III. Invasion of growth into parametria with limited mobility.
Stage IV.   Frozen pelvis, or distant metastases.

The differentiation between these two stages III and IV may also be very difficult.

Where the disease is limited to the uterus (stage I cases) a large percentage of five year arrests fully 80% can be expected from hysterectomy —this is much better than can be hoped for from radiation therapy alone. Carcinoma of the fundus is clearly a surgical disease.

Where extension has occurred beyond the uterine wall the five year arrests drop off to 20 to 25%.

If the growth has extended into the parametria the percentage of five year arrests is very small, less than 10% and in frozen pelvis it is practically 0%.

CARCINOMA OF THE OVARY

The ovary is a frequent site for the development of carcinoma. Early surgical removal is of course the method of choice; only too often, however, the disease goes unrecognized until there are large cysts and metastatic nodules covering the peritoneal surface of the pelvis and abdomen.

An appreciable percentage of such tumors, even after they have metastasized to the peritoneum, are found to be very amenable to x-ray therapy; many cases of five year survivals have occurred even after peritoneal metastases and ascites have been present for a long period of time.

Carcinoma of Ovary (Schmitz) (from Cancer Handbook, Liljencrantz).

Stage I. Growth limited to one ovary. Capsule intact. No fixation; no demonstrable glandular or peritoneal involvement.

Stage II. Invasion of opposite ovary. Normal mobility of pelvic organs. No demonstrable metastasis.

Stage III. Tumor adherent to surrounding viscera. Loss of mobility of pelvic organs. Involvement of pelvic nodes, which remain discrete.

Stage IV. Advanced, fixed growths and widespread implants.

Radical operative removal of tumor both ovaries and panhysterectomy is the procedure of choice wherever possible. Postoperative x-ray therapy enhances the five year arrests; these are approximately 20 to 25%. Even in stage III and IV where there is widespread metastatic implants x-ray therapy may give lasting palliation even for periods of three to four years.

Carcinoma of the vulva is primarily a surgical disease. The vulva does not take well to radiation therapy; this, taken with the fact that carcinomatous growths of this region are usually very resistant, makes a poor combination for radiation therapy. Actual cautery has been found the most satisfactory method of treatment.

Carcinoma of the vagina is usually squamous cell in type; it can often be effectively treated with local application of radium and pelvic irradiation with x-rays.

The urethral orifice may be the site of carcinomatous involvement. Local treatment with radium therapy or if very small, the destruction of the growth by fulguration has been the best method of attack in our experience.

Prostatic carcinoma is slow-growing often extending over a period of five years even without any therapy. Interstitial radiation with gold radon seeds evenly inserted into the prostate has been tried with some success but ordinarily surgical extirpation gives best palliative results. It is ultimately a fatal disease.

Carcinoma of the bladder is best treated by interstitial radiation with gold radon seeds inserted directly into the base of the growth with the bladder open under direct observation, combined with external pelvic irradiation. Papillomatous growths may be cured in 75% of the cases. The percentage of ultimate recovery is relatively low even with small growths, however, if there is any infiltration at the base of the lesion.

Carcinoma of the gastro-intestinal tract offers a very poor prognosis regardless of the method of treatment.

Complete regression of esophageal carcinoma has been produced by external application of x-radiation, likewise esophageal carcinoma has been successfully resected surgically but these are isolated cases. In general, no effective method has been found to cope with carcinoma in this location.

Carcinoma of the stomach, likewise, presents very unfavorable prospects. Surgical resection, even in selected cases, yields only 5% over-all five-year cures in the hands of able surgeons; 18% in carcinoma of the pylorus; radiation therapy offers nothing at all.

The small bowel fortunately is seldom affected by malignant growths.

The colon and rectum are common sites of carcinoma; of all of the sites, it is the one in which surgical resection offers the greatest hope for success. Radiation therapy may be used postoperatively only as a palliative measure for pain.

Carcinoma of the anus is usually of the squamous cell type and is more accessible to treatment by radiation.

Primary malignant tumors of bone do not ordinarily respond well to radiation; in certain instances they may show regression and quiescence after irradiation as a preparatory procedure for operation. Operation during this period nets a greater percentage of cures. Ewing's endothelial myeloma is the only type of primary malignant bone tumor which responds with any degree of consistency to radiation therapy; a few instances of cure have been recorded by this method alone.

Metastatic malignant tumors to bone, on the other hand, often show surprising sensitivity. Areas of destruction fill in with new bone and the patient may go even as much as ten years.

The xanthomatous lesions involving bone usually respond to small doses of radiation with ultimate cure.

BENIGN CONDITIONS

Many benign conditions are favorably affected by radiation therapy. Small divided doses of low voltage x-radiation are used for the treatment of many varieties of skin lesions. Eczema, contact dermatitis, fungus infections such as epidermophytosis are prominent examples.

Warts of various types such as verruca vulgaris, verruca plantaris and even veneral warts are destroyed by irradiation. A wart is one of the few tumors known to be caused by a virus; if warts are excised, macerated, extracted with saline solution and then passed through a Berkefeld filter to exclude bacteria, the filtrate injected intradermally will produce warts in another individual. This is what makes excision of plantar warts so difficult and unsuccessful; if any of the virus contained in the wart is squeezed into the wound, more warts will appear in or near the operative scar. Radiation therapy, either x-ray or radium, is the most satisfactory means for complete cure.

Small skin tabs, mulluscum fibrosum, and horny growths of epidermis may be removed in a similar way.

Nevi of many varieties may be completely destroyed by application of small quantities of radiation. Even when of large size covering a great portion of the face, it is remarkable what favorable results can be obtained in suitable cases. Port wine stains and Spider nevi usually do not respond favorably nor do blood vessel tumors composed of adult fully developed blood vessels such as those produced by venous varicosities. Tiny spider nevi often require fulguration.

Moles can be removed by radiation therapy but this represents a chemical agent and if destruction is not complete it may cause irritation of the growth. It is better to remove such growths by wide surgical excision or by thorough cauterization.

Pyogenic infections of the skin and subcutaneous tissues such as furuncles and carbuncles usually react very promptly to superficial radiation therapy. It seems that the greater the involvement of the skin itself, the more profound is the effect of radiation on the infectious agent. In carbuncles x-ray therapy usually has a profound effect causing their reduction in size and ameliorating the symptoms within 24 to 48 hours and often aborting the course of infection to a seven to ten day period. If the carbuncle is associated with diabetes care must be exercised in application of x-ray therapy because sometimes they "freeze" forming a hard cake which becomes chronic neither breaking down nor resolving. Surgical removal under such circumstances is the only solution. Furuncles also respond readily but usually not as rapidly as carbuncles.

Where the pyogenic infection involves the hair follicles, (folliculitis), of the axilla or other hairy parts, radiation therapy to the point of epilation will be very effective in curing the infection.

In Psychosis Barbae or Tenea Barbae, forms of infection of the bearded areas of the face, (Barber's Itch) complete epilation of the entire bearded area is practically the only effective method of treatment. For complete epilation four weeks must elapse; the amount of radiation necessary for epilation in this area is much greater than elsewhere in the body.

Ring worm infection of the scalp or favus both require complete epilation of the entire scalp for effective cure. This is a very technical procedure but it has been worked out with great exactness so that it can be readily performed. The hair begins to fall out in three weeks and by four weeks complete epilation should have taken place. The x-radiation does not have any effect upon the fungus itself but merely removes the hair thereby eliminating the site in which the infection grows. Regrowth of the hair should occur within 3 or 4 months.

In other types of infection it has also been advocated. In nasal sinusitis and mastoiditis the effects may be gratifying but this is usually due to the influence of the radiation on chronic granulation tissue and chronically infected hyperplastic lymphoid tissue which is usually associated in infections of this type. It has never given spectacular results in acute cases of this type in our experience. Radium applied to the nasopharynx in cases of chronic infection and deafness may, by its influence on the chronic hyperplastic lymphoid material, result in cure of the infection and restoration of hearing.

Extremely small doses of surface radiation administered with a radium plaque to the cornea may clear up interstitial keratitis and corneal opacities and may even have a favorable influence on pannus.

Radiation therapy for hyperthyroidism. (Refer to Isotopes.)

In acute thyroiditis, the infection can be controlled with very small doses of radiation, producing prompt and lasting results.

X-Ray therapy for "enlarged thymus" is another field in which there is much dispute. In the first place it is difficult to evaluate any effect of therapy on this structure since it varies in size with every phase of respiration; it becomes large on crying and small on regaining composure. Perhaps the only condition in which it should be used is when lateral roentgenographic examination shows compression of the trachea by the thymus. Even then, only very small doses of radiation should be given, always being mindful of the harmful effect which thymic irradiation may have on testicular development and bone growth as shown experimentally on animals.

It is questionable whether x-ray therapy has ever been shown to have beneficial effect on lung infections. Its use in the treatment of pneumonia has been advocated but results of such cases are always hard to evaluate. In lung abscess it has not had demonstrable benefit; surely with present day chemotherapy we have a more scientific and effective means of combating these diseases.

There are few if any benign lesions of the gastro-intestinal tract in which it is of any value. Regional enteritis produces a granulomatous lesion which one might think would be amenable to radiation therapy but repeated attempts have never led to any beneficial effect.

Certain benign conditions of the female generative organs may be very successfully treated by radiation. Pre-menopausal bleeding from endometritis or submucous fibroid may be cured in practically all instances by a sterilizing course of x-ray therapy.

This should of course never be done except in

patients in the early forties in the pre-menopausal period. The influence which radiation therapy has on fibroids is probably due in large part to its effect on the ovarian function; with cessation of this function fibroids regress naturally under any condition.

Lymphomata

Malignant disease of the lymphoid system can be well treated by external radiation therapy. Symptoms can be alleviated, tumorous masses made to decrease in size or disappear and life prolonged. Hodgkins disease is treated by irradiation of the involved node masses. Good palliation is obtained, the results of treatment being better in less advanced disease. Lymphosarcoma is almost always palliated by roentgen therapy and cures have been reported when the disease is limited to a localized area or organ. Leukemia patients are benefitted by radiation therapy when the disease is chronic. The elevated white count is lowered by irradiation over the spleen or by total body irradiation. The well being of the patient is furthered and life is prolonged. Radiation therapy is contraindicated in acute leukemia.

Kidney

Radiation therapy is of value only in palliation of carcinoma in the adult. In the child, embryonal carcinoma, Wilms tumor, should be treated by surgery primarily followed by radiation of the area. Five year survivals are increased thereby. Neuroblastoma, originating in the adrenal, is radiosensitive but not necessarily radiocurable. Radiation therapy is of value as palliation and cures may be obtained in a small percentage of cases. Certain tumors of the testis namely the seminoma group are very radiosensitive. Up to 80% of five year survivals are experienced if the lymph node areas of the testis are irradiated after the primary tumor is excised. Other tumors of the testis are highly malignant and x-ray therapy is ineffectual.

Lung Carcinoma can be palliated in some instances by deep x-ray therapy, but on the whole the results are not very satisfactory.

Central Nervous System

Radiation has a definite place in the treatment of pituitary tumors. Surgery for pituitary tumors also has a definite place, depending upon the symptoms, rapidity of growth, and other factors, but results from radiation therapy alone are as good or better than surgery in larger series of cases. Medulloblastomas have as the treatment of choice radiation since surgery can offer only confirmation of diagnosis and decompression of increased intracranial pressure. The cerebellar region and the spinal cord are treated with relatively high doses because of the tendency of these tumors to metastasize down the spinal cord. Hemangioblastomas are radiosensitive. The more rapidly growing tumors of other types are more radiosensitive than the less rapid growing, more differentiated neoplasms, but radiation offers only temporary improvement.

Bursitis is helped by x-ray therapy, alleviating pain and shortening the course of disability. Most often occurring in the shoulder, but also in the elbow and hip, the condition is common and deserves treatment. Symptoms of rheumatoidspondylitis are often alleviated by a short course of deep-x-ray therapy.

Radioactive Isotopes as Therapeutic Agents, (H. W. Fischer). New as the subject of atomic medicine may be to the general physician, the basic principle of alteration of cell function by ionizing radiation is the same which has formed the foundation of traditional radiation therapy with x-rays and radium. The cyclotron and uranium pile produce radioactive isotopes of many elements, only a few of the total number having known therapeutic application at this time. Like radium and other naturally occurring radioactive elements, the artificially produced radioactive isotopes may give off alpha, beta, or gamma rays or combinations of these. (See pp. 508-509 for discussion of radium disintegration.) Although their action on tissues is essentially the same, it is their deliverance to the tissue which is new and different in many instances. The roentgen as defined applies only to x and gamma rays. In attempting to measure the radiation delivered by an isotope emitting beta rays, the "roentgen equivalent physical," (rep), is the corresponding unit. It is the amount of beta radiation which releases 93 ergs of energy per gram of tissue. When the isotope is deposited in certain tissues or is distributed throughout the entire body, the dosage received cannot be measured. Calculations must be made for each isotope, depending upon the physical characteristics of that isotope, and physiological factors concerned in deposition and excretion of the isotope. The suitability of an isotope will depend upon the type of radiation emitted, whether alpha, beta, or gamma rays. The period of effective action will determine the practicality of usage; elements having a very short half-life (12 hours or less) are uneconomical to deliver to the patient from the production source. Elements with too long a half life have excessively prolonged activity when internally administered, with the potential danger of carcinogenesis, and too slow deliverance of the major portion of their radiation to allow practical evaluation of results. Biological and chemical behavior of the isotopes must be well understood, such as toxicity, differential organ uptake, absorption, storage, and excretion. Technical efficiency in production of an isotope is also important, as is the ease of handling, and the protection required for patient and operator in its usage.

Cobalt 60 as Therapeutic Agent. Radioisotopes may be used in the same manner as radium. Large quantities of isotopes are used for external radiation at a distance, as with teleradium therapy. Cobalt 60 with a half life of five years is the most suitable radioisotope available for this purpose, with iridium and cesium 137 also considered for this role. A 1100 curie cobalt 60 unit supplies a depth dose equivalent to that produced by a three million volt peak x-ray machine. The emitted gamma rays give a greatly increased depth dose as compared to a 200 kv x-ray machine. Advantages of telecobalt therapy are the constant output of a relatively homogeneous beam of high energy gamma rays which does not require filtration. The initial cost and upkeep is stated to be less than for a million volt x-ray machine.* Disadvantages are that the cobalt must be replaced at intervals, that the output of the unit is less than of a million volt machine. The physical characteristics are essentially the same as those emitted by radium, and no essential difference in results in treatment is to be expected. The value lies in that now many curies of radioactive substance are now available, where formerly only a limited number of curies of radium were assembled at any one place for tele-radium therapy.

Strontium 90 as a Therapeutic Agent. Cobalt 60 and other isotopes (Tantalum 182, Gold 198) when properly sheathed may be used for external, interstitial and intracavitary therapy in the same fashion as radium plaques, needles, and capsules. Dependent upon the half lives and the activity of the isotope, new tables of exposure are necessary to give radiation effects comparable to well observed radium technics, but the biological effect is no different.

Radioactive strontium, Sr 90, is used in the same manner as a radium plaque for irradiation of external eye lesions. It has the advantage of having a very energetic pure beta spectrum, whereas beta ray therapy with radium (or radon) is complicated by the simultaneously emitted gamma rays.

INTERNAL ADMINISTRATION OF ISOTOPES

Internal administration of radioactive isotopes is relatively recent in its usage. Isotopes are administered internally for uptake by specific cells or tissues, or are deposited into local areas to remain there. Radioactive phosphorous, P 32, and radioactive iodine, I 131, typify the novel internal deliverance of ionizing radiation to specific tissues in the body or to all body tissues, and radioactive colloidal gold, Au 198, typifies the deposition of particles of radioactive material into local areas.

Phosphorus 32 as a Therapeutic Agent. Tissues which normally take up phosphorus and tissues which have a high rate of mitotic division have also a high uptake of radioactive phosphorus. Bone, bone marrow, liver and spleen, and neoplastic tissue therefore have a high uptake of P 32 and this fact is utilized in the treatment of polycythemia and leukemia. The ionizing radiation is delivered to the cells more specifically and more effectively than any form of externally administered radiation. Polycythemia vera is effectively treated by one or more appropriately sized doses of P 32 in 90% of cases. Relief of symptoms and disappearance of hematological abnormalities is obtained far more consistently by this treatment than

by external x-ray therapy or chemical inhibitors of the bone marrow. The treatment is simple to give, and has no particular disadvantages. Except for partial lack of absorption of orally ingested P 32, oral and intravenous therapy are equally effective. Radiophosphorus can be used effectively in the treatment of chronic granulocytic leukemia. Small, repeated doses of oral or intravenous P 32 result in clinical remissions accompanied by lowered white blood cells count, and improvement in anemia. The response in chronic lymphatic leukemia is more variable and less successful. The remissions obtained are essentially comparable to those obtained with external roentgen therapy such as total body spray and irradiation of the spleen or bone marrow. The advantage is ease of administration.

Iodine 131 as Therapeutic Agent. Radioactive isotopes of iodine have opened up an entire new field of therapy of thyroid diseases. Orally or intravenously administered I 131 is taken up by the thyroid gland proportional to its activity. When thyrotoxicosis exists, the uptake is high, and the proper sized dose of radioiodine will destroy the major portion of functioning thyroid tissue. Radioiodine is a very efficient form of therapy, low in cost, and accompanied by few risks. It is recommended particularly for poor surgical risk, and patients refusing surgery, for patients in whom medical therapy has not been successful, for recurrent hyperthyroidism after thyroidectomy, for uncomplicated hyperthyroidism in older patients, and for patients with malignant exophthalmos. Natural caution has held back the use in younger patients not because of less good results to be obtained, but for fear that there may be a late tendency to neoplasia of thyroid or other tissue following internal use of a radioactive material. Results of treatment are better in diffuse thyroid hyperplasia than in nodular toxic goitre.

The large nodular goitre may contain a neoplastic area which would not be adequately treated by the size of the dose directed at hyperthyroidism. Dosage is not yet precise, being dependent on the size of the gland and the percentage uptake of a tractor dose of radioactive iodine. Some patients require two or more doses at intervals to obtain remission of symptoms. The percentage of good results is very high, above 90%. Ill effects are hypothyroidism in a minority of patients, and rarely definite myxedema, due to too vigorous attack upon the gland. Adverse generalized reaction to radiation is nil, and local symptoms are not of importance. No deaths, tetany, or vocal cord paralyses are associated with this treatment as may happen with surgery. Radioiodine is a new weapon in the attack on thyroid cancer, but early hopes for wide success have not been realized. A high index of malignancy is associated with proportionate loss of function. The more malignant the tumor, the less tendency to take up iodine or radioactive iodine. Consequently the iodine cannot be effectively delivered to the neoplastic cell,

---

*A true estimate of the cost of cobalt 60 and other isotopes must take into consideration the huge cost of the governmental atomic energy programs, and not just the present cost charged for production and delivery of each order.

except when its function and structure approaches the normal. Uptake of iodine by the thyroid neoplasm can be increased by prior defunctionalization of the normal thyroid tissue, by feeding of antithyroid drugs, or the administration of thyroid stimulating hormone, but even with these aids, results are good in only a few cases.

The normal functioning gland may be reduced to hypofunction when the occasion so demands by radio-iodine. In cardiac failure and angina pectoris, intractable to other forms of therapy, the administration of radioiodine brings relief in a substantial number of patients by reducing their general level of metabolism. Relatively large and repeated doses are required since the gland's uptake of iodine is not elevated. Myxedema will be produced in some cases and if the symptoms are not tolerated, thyroid extract may be given. Failure of such treatment occurs when a balance of relief of cardiac symptoms and those of hyperthyroidism cannot be achieved. Surgical thyroidectomy formerly used for this type of patient can now be eliminated from consideration because radio-iodine therapy carried no inherent risk.

Gold 198 as a Therapeutic Agent. Radioactive colloidal gold has found use in the treatment of pleural and peritoneal effusions due to malignant disease, in which the rapid and excessive formation of fluid causes more distress than other aspects of the neoplasm's growth. Au 198 when injected intracavitarily is rapidly removed from the free fluid and is fixed on or near the surface of the cavity lining, the effective radiation penetrating only to a depth of 2 or 3 mm. In about one half of the patients treated in this manner, the formation of fluid is successfully inhibited. Better results are obtained in pleural effusions than in ascites. The mechanism of action is not clear, but production of fibrosis on the affected surfaces by the ionizing radiations is thought to inhibit fluid formation. The radioactive gold has no special affinity for tumor tissue and the serosal surfaces are not rid of tumor. A small amount of radioactive material enters the blood stream, and is deposited in bone marrow, liver and spleen, as well as excreted in the urine. This has not been of clinical consequence. Radioactive colloidal chromic phosphate has been used for intracavitary injections and behaves similarly to Au 198, but because some of the material becomes ionized a somewhat higher deposition in neoplastic tissue is observed.

Gold 198 has been used successfully in the treatment of prostatic carcinoma. Its greatest use is in the moderately advanced cases in which neoplasm has spread beyond the gland, but has not yet become widely and distantly spread. For more localized tumors, surgery is the procedure of choice. Other forms of palliative therapy are more appropriate for the patient with distant metastases.

Adequate deliverance of ionizing radiation to neoplastic tissue is best accomplished by the visualization afforded by the open suprapubic operation, and direct injection into tumor masses in and around the gland and the regional lymphatics. Perineal and transrectal injection have a definite place in certain patients.

The fascial planes and compartments of the area allow the injected radioactive colloid to remain essentially localized or to spread along the course of the lymphatic drainage. Absorption of radioactive material into the general circulation for ultimate retention in the reticuloendothelial system has not been a problem when injections are performed skillfully and with experience. Injection of too little or too poorly distributed gold does not control the tumor. Injection of too much or too poorly distributed gold results in irradiation complication, sloughing of the prostatic tissue or rectal ulceration. Excision of as much obviously neoplastic tissue as possible is advised at time of injection to minimize complications.

Injection of Au 198 into parametrial tissue in cases of carcinoma of the cervix is a logical approach to delivering of a cancerocidal amount of radiation to the local extension of neoplasm and its regional lymph node metastases, without causing necrosis of normal tissue. The colloidal radioactive gold is injected into the parametrium alongside the uterus. Some of the gold enters the local lymphatics and travels to the regional lymph nodes along the lateral pelvic wall, where often insufficient irradiation is obtained with the conventional radiation techniques. The method shows promise in the early evaluation. So far, it has been used along with intracavitary radium, and Wertheim hysterectomy and lymphadenectomy, with omission of external radiation therapy.

The use of solutions of radioactive colloidal gold for injection into other tumor masses whether superficial or deep is being investigated. Intravenous administration of Au 198 for chronic leukemia cases has been used but the preference is for radioactive phosphorus.

The possibilities of therapeutic usage of radioactive isotopes can be suggested by the consideration of a recent experimental work. Boron becomes a source of alpha radiation by virtue of slow neutron capture. The boron injected intravenously into the patient with a cerebral glioblastoma multiforme reaches a maximum concentration in the tumor tissue in about 15 minutes. The patient is then exposed to a nuclear reactor which produces the slow neutrons. The resulting alpha particles produced in the tissues penetrate only to a depth of nine microns from their source. By this means highly selective local irradiation of great biological effectiveness is delivered to tumor cells, since their boron content is several times that of normal brain. This is but an example to indicate the fields in which development of technics may lead to better tumor therapy.

Table I

I-131 UPTAKES OF NORMAL AND
HYPERFUNCTIONING GLANDS

Normal:
   Anterior neck   4004
   Posterior neck 1893
   Right neck   2624
   Left neck   2941

Average 2866 counts per minute

Standard   12790 cpm.
Background   337 cpm.

$$\% \text{ Uptake} = \frac{\text{Average neck counts} - \text{background count}}{\text{Standard} - \text{background count}}$$

$$= \frac{2529}{12453} = 20.3\%$$

Hyperthyroidism:
   Anterior neck   9801
   Posterior neck 4295
   Right neck   8440
   Left neck   7108

Average 7411

Standard   12790
Background   337

$$\% \text{ Uptake} = \frac{\text{Average neck counts} - \text{background}}{\text{Standard} - \text{background}}$$

$$= \frac{7074}{12453} = 56.9\%$$

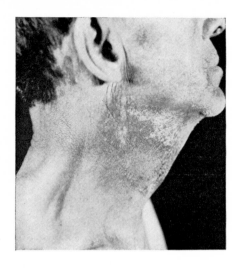

← Desquamating x-ray reaction; the skin becomes erythematous followed by fine scaling and pigmentation. For completely denuding (epidermite) reaction see pelvic irradiation.

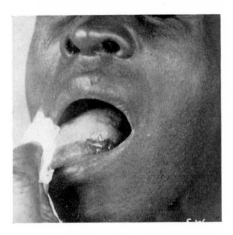

Heavy pseudomembranous reaction on mucous membrane (epithelite), following radium or intense x-ray therapy, subsides and returns to normal in a few weeks.

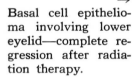

Basal cell epithelioma involving lower eyelid—complete regression after radiation therapy.

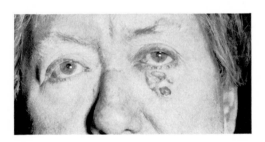

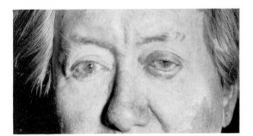

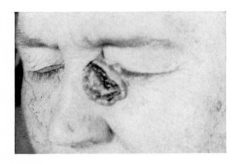

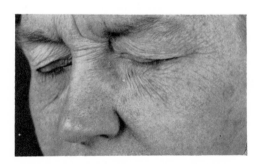

← Basal cell epithelioma near inner canthus of eye overlying the extremely thin lacrymal bone. Complete regression after radiation therapy without damage to bone structure.

Basal cell epithelioma encroaching upon cartilage of ear. Complete regression without damage to cartilage after radium therapy. →

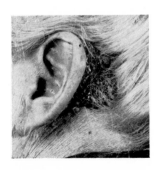

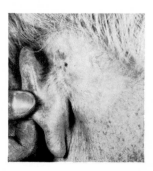

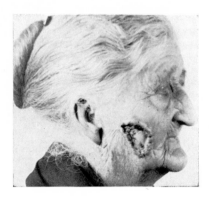 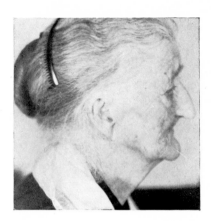

Basal cell epithelioma before and after radium therapy. Radiosensitive growth; does not tend to metastasize.

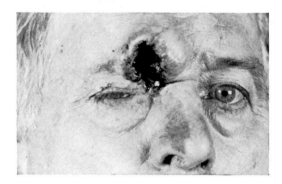 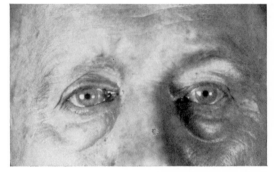

Basal cell epithelioma; deep ulceration denuding bone. Radiosensitive growth readily destroyed by either x-rays or radium.

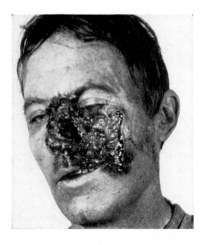 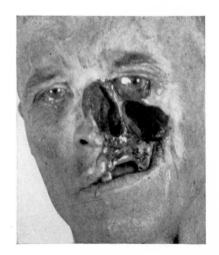

Large basal cell lesion destroying cartilage of nose, eyelid, bone forming antral wall and alveolar process. Alive and well without recurrence, more than 20 years after radiation therapy. An obturator of plastic material can be constructed to fill in the remaining defect.

Small squamous cell epithelioma of lower lip. These lesions are usually readily destroyed by radiation; when confined to the lip there is better than 90% chance of recovery. →

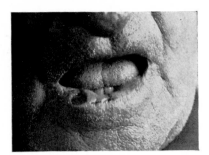
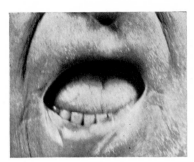

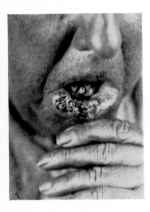
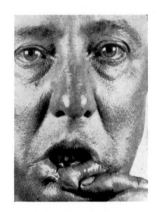

← Extensive squamous cell epithelioma of lower lip showing complete regression after radiation therapy. No metastases. If lymph node metastases occur, 5 year recovery rate drops to less than 20%.

Basal cell epithelioma of upper lip; complete regression. These do not tend to metastasize to local lymph nodes. →

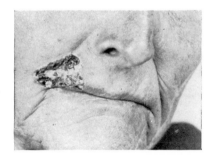
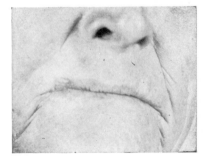

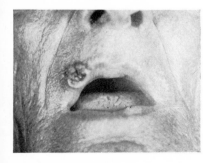
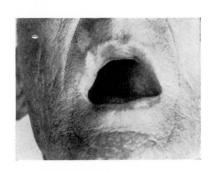

← Epitheliomata of the upper lip are more apt to be of the basal cell type and therefore have a better prognosis.

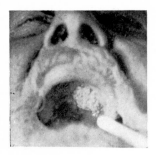
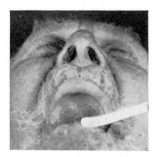

← Squamous cell carcinoma of palate; bone not involved. Complete regression after topical application of radiation. Such tumors are readily accessible to intracavity treatment with x-rays.

Squamous cell carcinoma of the buccal mucous membrane. Complete regression after irradiation. Often spoken of as "tobacco chewer's cancer." →

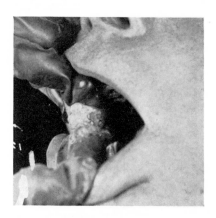
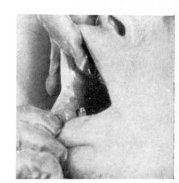

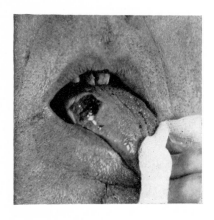
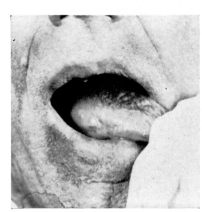

← Carcinoma of the tongue treated with interstitial implantation of gold radon seeds with complete regression. Radiation finds a large place in treatment of carcinoma of the tongue since surgical removal usually implies extensive mutilation.

Carcinoma of the tip of the tongue treated with local application of radiation. Tumors of the tongue in this location can just as well be treated with surgical removal or cautery. →

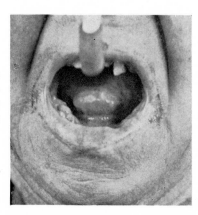
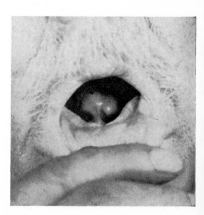

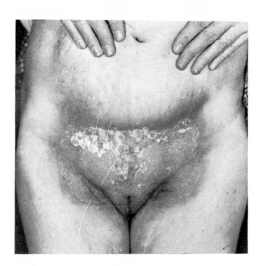
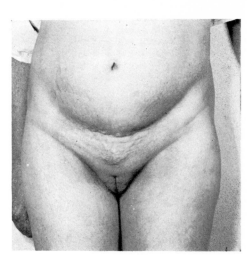

"Epidermite" reaction or complete desquamation of outer layer of skin following irradiation of female pelvis for carcinoma of cervix uteri. The weeping skin surface soon heals. →

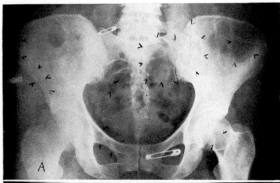

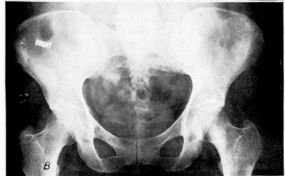

← Metastatic bone lesions from Scirrhus carcinoma of breast. Large areas of destruction in pelvic bones, both femurs and the vertebral structures. A, before; B, after treatment.

Note healing of destroyed areas with replacement by dense new bone after x-ray therapy. Such paliation can often be continued for periods of 5 to 10 years, or even longer.

↓ Vertebral Destruction, left; after treatment, right.

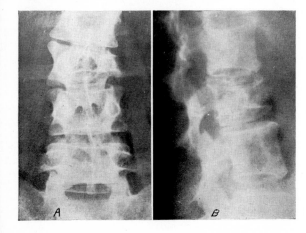
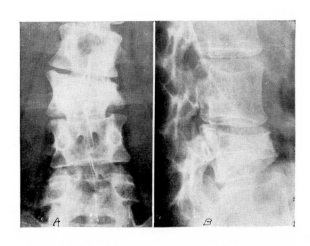

BENIGN LESIONS—INFECTION

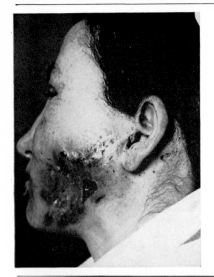

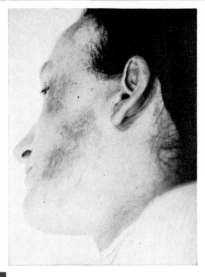

← Actinomycosis of the jaw; bone was not involved. Complete healing after superficial x-radiation.

Epidermophytosis and other fungus infections of the feet and hands are usually very amenable to x-ray therapy, healing after about 2 weeks.
↓

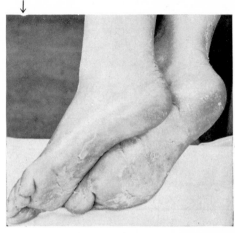

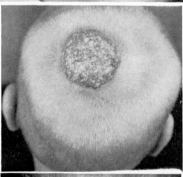

← Onychimycosis or fungus infection of the nails may also be successfully treated. When the disease is destroyed the new nail pushes the old nail off.

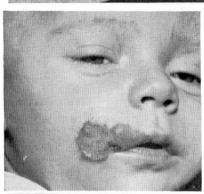

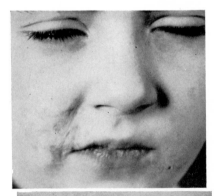

← Hemangioma involving vermilion border of lip. Note how, after a period of years, the normal vermilion characteristics have returned to the lip.

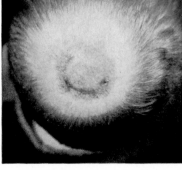

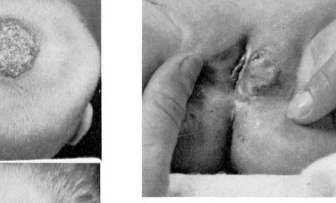

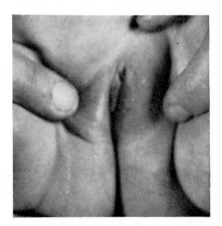

↑ Angioma of vulva in infant treated by radiation therapy with complete recovery.

← Microsporon infection of the scalp. Epilation of entire scalp has been carried out with x-ray; remaining granulations caused by fungus can be seen. Complete regrowth of hair after 3 months. Fungus is healed. Epilation is used for treatment of ringworm and favus of the scalp.

Chapter XXVI

RADIOACTIVE ISOTOPES AS DIAGNOSTIC AGENTS

Harry W. Fischer, M.D.

(Radioactive isotopes as therapeutic agents are discussed on p. 517.)

With the growth and development of nuclear physics in recent years, radioactive isotopes were produced by the cyclotron. It was inevitable that some of these isotopes should find a use in medicine. At first, limited quantities of a few isotopes were made available, and research and clinical experience was likewise limited. With the advent of the chain reacting uranium pile, the availability of radioactive materials has increased prodigiously. The firm establishment of isotope diagnostic and therapeutic technics has followed.

Atoms with different atomic weights but identical atomic numbers and chemical properties are called isotopes. Radioactive isotopes, either natural occurring or artificially produced, are unstable in their nuclear combination of protons and neutrons. With the spontaneous breakdown of the unstable nuclear arrangement, an energetic particle is emitted. By this single or repeated activity, a stable configuration is reached, the resultant atomic number and weight of the element depending upon the number and nature of the emissions. Emission of a beta ray, that is, an electron from the atom, results in an increase in atomic number of one without change in the atomic weight. Emission of an alpha ray, identical with the helium atom, results in a decrease of two in the atomic number and four in the atomic weight. Gamma radiation are emitted in the course of nuclear transformations but such activity is not characterized by change in atomic number or weight per se. Since the chemical properties of radioactive isotopes are identical with the stable atoms of an element, they are handled identically by the body in absorption, excretion, anabolism, catabolism, circulation and so forth. During their participation in metabolic processes, radioisotopes may be detected by suitable equipment at any time by the emission of their characteristic rays. Far smaller amounts of radioactive materials than non-radioactive materials may be measured because of this characteristic. The rate of emission of rays from any one radioisotope is constant, and specific, and uninfluenced by any physical or chemical factors. The number of radioactive atoms partaking in any process may therefore be indicated by measuring the number of emissions per unit time. The diagnostic application of radioactive isotopes rests then on their use as indicators in "tagged" or labelled substances utilized by the body. Significant physiological and pathological information is furnished by study of uptake, distribution, or excretion of radioisotopes. The counting of beta or gamma rays in certain body locations gives valuable information, as does analysis of body fluids, and excretory products. The histological locations of metabolized radioisotopes are recorded by placing thin tissue sections in contact with a photosensitive emulsion, a process called autoradiography.

Certain general principles must characterize the isotope to be used in biology and medicine. The half life, or the time in which half of any given number of atoms undergoes disintegration, should be neither too long nor too short. It is not practical or convenient to prepare and deliver an isotope and make use of it in a very brief interval, as with isotopes of half lives of hours or minutes. Isotopes with long half lives may remain radioactive in the body for a longer time than desired, or their effect may be so delayed as to be unsuitable for clinical use. For counting on the external body surface, a radioisotope need emit a gamma ray, which will penetrate many centimeters of tissue. In all but a very few special instances beta rays will not be measurable outside the body because they travel only a few millimeters in water or tissue. Alpha particle emission measurement is not practical since alpha particles cannot penetrate a fraction of a millimeter of tissue. Positron emitters are utilizable since the positron is annihilated with resultant production of two coincident gamma rays, which are detected without difficulty. The suitable radioisotope must be one which is not retained unduly long by the body, nor have undesirable selective concentration in certain tissues. Concentrations of elements not tolerated in non-radioactive isotopic form must also be avoided with radioisotopes. This implies knowledge of the chemical and biological behavior of the element. Measurement of either beta or gamma rays is feasible when body fluids, tissues or excretory products are examined separate from the body. The specimen may be concentrated or dried for counting of the entire specimen, or an aliquot may be counted.

Counting Instruments

With the interest in radioactive materials in biology, improved equipment has been developed for measurement of radioactivity. The Geiger-Muller counter works on the principle of ionization of a gas enclosed in a tube by the entering particle or photon. The ionization produced is measured by a potential applied between two electrodes in the chamber. When amplified, this discharge may be recorded in one of several ways. The design, size, and shape of the Geiger Muller tube depends upon the type of radiation to be detected and the nature of the specimen to be examined. Scintillation counters work on the principle of conversion of energy of photons or emitted particles into light. The energetic particle or photon striking certain crystals called phosphors (sodium iodide; anthracene) produces extremely brief minute flashes of light which are detected and greatly amplified by a photomultiplier tube, so that the pulses of current may be counted and recorded. The efficiency of counting is greater with the scintillation counter because of quicker response to impulses rapidly following one another. The scintillation counter is coming to be the preferred instrument, except when increased sensitivity could be considered a disadvantage. The actual recording of impulses is carried out by electronic devices since the GM tube or scintillation apparatus counts too fast for mechanical recording. A scaler is the electronic instrument which stores pulses, releasing only a definite proportion of the counts received to a mechanical counter. The electronic recording equipment may be devised to give simultaneous readings of counts per second or minute, as the subject is being examined, or the total number of counts in a selected period. Regardless of type of counter, counts must always be corrected for the radiation detected from other than the subject being examined. The natural radioactivity of the earth, radioactivity of cosmic rays, and any other possible radioactive substances near the counter make up "background" radiation. Background count is increased with the sensitivity of the counter, being higher with scintillation counters than with GM counters. It may be reduced somewhat by shielding of the counter with lead, and excluding contamination from other radioactive sources, but cannot be entirely eliminated. The background radiation count must always be subtracted from the recorded count to obtain the true count. Weak radioactive specimens cannot be counted accurately when their counting rate is little different from that of the background count, which fluctuates within a certain range. The lower the background count in relation to the true count, the more accurate the determination. Accuracy can be increased in the counting of weakly radioactive specimens by counting a very large number of impulses.

Radiological Safety

Protection of the patient and the physician and his assistants is a vital aspect of the use of any radioactivity. The problem assumes added importance with new, untried materials, particularly when they are internally administered and retained in the body. Outside of the body protection must be afforded during transportation, preparation and administration of the full strength isotope, and during disposal of the radioactive residue. Shielding with lead and utilization of a safe distance is satisfactory for these purposes. Inside the body, the local and general harmful effects of excessive radiation present problems which cannot be solved by shielding with heavy metals or protection by distance. Local effects may be acute or chronic, temporary or permanent. Obtaining dosage within limits considered

to be safe is the only means of protection. The possible harmful effects of even small amounts of radioactive isotopes as used in tracer studies must be taken into consideration.

USEFUL ISOTOPES

Iodine 131 in Thyroid Disease

The most useful of the radioisotopes from a clinical diagnostic aspect is Iodine 131. The thyroid takes up ingested iodine, brought to it by the circulation after absorption from the intestine. In the gland, the inorganic iodine is converted into thyroid hormone, and is then discharged into the blood in organic form or stored within the gland. The individual body cells are stimulated metabolically by the circulating hormone, Thyroxine. Radio iodine I-131 undergoes all steps in the process as does ordinary non-radioactive iodine, and can therefore be utilized in assessing thyroid function. When the gland is hyperactive, the rate and amount of iodine taken up is increased and the conversion of the inorganic ion to the organic hormone is likewise speeded up. The reverse holds true for underactivity. Iodine not metabolized by the thyroid gland is excreted by the kidney, whether this be ordinary iodine or radioactive iodine, (Schilling, et al.).

A small dose, 10 to 50 microcuries, when administered by mouth or by vein is rapidly and progressively concentrated by the gland. Since the gamma rays emitted from the I 131 within the thyroid cell penetrate the surrounding tissue without difficulty, they can be counted externally by a Geiger or scintillation counter positioned over the neck. The counter is suitably shielded by a lead collimator to count mainly the gamma rays from the thyroid area (Fig. 1) and to exclude those from the remainder of the body. An estimation of the uptake of I 131 by the gland is obtained by comparing the counts per minute over the gland at 24 hours with the counts per minute from a standard solution of I 131 at the same time. The standard was originally calibrated to be of the same number of microcuries as the tracer dose. For accuracy, the standard is placed in a water phantom to simulate the actual geometrical conditions of counting the patient's neck. The uptake of the gland is expressed as a percentage of the standard. The hyperfunctioning gland concentrates more I 131 than the normal gland. Studies by various laboratories using different counting equipment and technics of counting give slightly different figures for the per

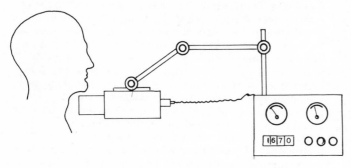

Fig. 1. Wide angle counter being used to measure the total uptake of radioactive iodine in the thyroid gland. Counting is recorded by a scaler.

cent uptake by normal glands. About a 35-40% up-take is assumed as the upper limit of normal. Almost all hyperthyroid patients have a higher uptake than this level and almost all normal patients have an up-take lower than this level (Table I, p. 520). As in other physiological tests, there is an overlap zone between the normal and pathological. The hypofunc-tioning gland concentrates less I 131 than the normal gland. The overlap zone between euthyroidism and hypothyroidism is large, decreasing the usefulness of this measurement.

Another method of assessing the thyroid func-tion is the measurement of radioactivity of the urine following the administration of a tracer dose of I 131. The portion of the test dose not taken up by the thyroid is excreted in the urine, except for an un-accounted for fraction which is not dependent upon the thyroid activity. The amount of I 131 detected in the urine varies inversely with the thyroid activity. A high urine radioactivity indicates a hypofunctioning gland, a low urine radioactivity indicates a hyper-functioning gland. To obtain the per cent of the dose excreted, comparison of the urine specimen in counts per minute and a standard tracer dose in counts per minute at the same time, usually 24 hours, and under identical conditions must be made. A urinary excre-tion below 40% is considered evidence of hyper-thyroidism. Due to large overlap zones between hy-perthyroid, euthyroid, and hypothyroid patients and since complete collection of iodine is often imprac-tical, this test is no longer in favor.

The rate of uptake of I 131 as well as the total amount has also been used for a test of thyroid func-tion. High uptake rates generally indicate hyper-thyroidism; lower rates of uptake, normal function. Measurement of rate of uptake of I 131 is not as practical as total uptake measurements or urinary excretion analysis.

Without certain qualifying conditions, I 131 up-take studies are invalid. Ingestion of organic or in-organic iodine up to seven weeks prior to the test reduces the uptake of I 131 to very low levels, with a falsely low uptake value resulting. Organic iodine retained in the body from previous radiographic pro-cedure, such as myelography, bronchography, cholecystography, pyelography, or angiography, have a similar effect in producing false low uptake values or high urinary excretion values. Thyroid extract ingested by the patient will also depress the I 131 up-take for as many as two weeks, even though the medication is stopped. Antithyroid compounds, propyl thiouracil and others, lower the radioactive iodine uptake. Within four days of ingestion of these com-pounds, the test is not valid. Sulfa derivatives have some antithyroid effect. Dietary iodine, iodized salt or iodine rich foods cannot be ingested in sufficiently large amounts in the normal diet to influence the test. Uptake of I 131 into the thyroid may be slowed by circulatory failure, and a false low 24 hour value be obtained. Repeat uptake determination at 48 hours in these cases will show a more accurate value. Similarly in poor kidney function, falsely low urinary outputs appear due to retention of the I 131 in the blood.

If the limitations of the method are realized, the advantages are apparent. The tracer study is easy to perform, takes a minimum of time and ex-pense, and is not subject to the vagaries of the emo-tional state of the patient as is the basal metabolism test. Comparatively, the accuracy of this method compared to other methods is high. The previous utilized tests of thyroid function are still used in the investigation of thyroid disease, and all have definite value. The I 131 uptake like any biological test is subject to error, and all factors must be considered in the diagnosis of the thyroid patient.

With the aid of a radiation counter, not only the percentage uptake of I 131 by the entire gland can be determined but local areas of the gland can be in-vestigated. A special collimator of lead placed over the counter allows the gamma rays from only one square centimeter of surface to be counted at one time. In this way, a nodule or lobe may be found to be hyperfunctioning by virtue of many counts per minute, while the remainder of the gland has a nor-mal uptake, as expressed by fewer counts per minute. The size of the gland may be mapped by counting of multiple coordinates over the neck surface (Fig. 4) and plotting the results on graph paper. A line drawn around the border of the high activity coordinates outlines the gland. The method is valuable in esti-mating the gland size and therefore its weight, since the weight of the hyperfunctioning gland determines in part the size of the therapeutic dose of I 131. Sub-sternal components of the thyroid either hyper or normal functioning have been detected and presence of functioning thyroid tissue in the neck following thyroidectomy is ascertained similarly. The pro-cedure could be likened to a "mine detector" as used in modern warfare, although the principle upon which detection is based differs. Location of metastases of thyroid carcinoma when the tumor concentrates sig-nificant amounts of I 131 can be detected almost any place in the body. As a rule, thyroid carcinoma does not concentrate iodine very well and the procedure is of limited value.

The I 131 tracer study can be further utilized to measure thyroid function by determination of the radioactive protein-bound iodine, (Fig. 2). The con-version of inorganic iodine into protein-bound, or hormonal, iodine is an essential gland function, and the measurement of such activity is obviously of value. Seventy-two hours after the ingestion of the test dose (it may be the same tracer dose used for a gland uptake or urinary excretion study), a blood

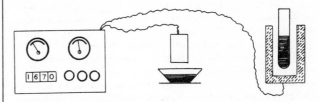

Fig. 2. Counter and scaler measuring the radio-activity of a urine or body fluid sample as used in thyroid function, blood volume studies, and cobalt 60-vitamin B.

sample of specified amount is withdrawn and counted. In euthyroids, the radioactive iodine being returned to the circulation as hormonal iodine is not sufficient to give a radioactive count above a certain level. The inorganic iodine has been removed from the circulation by the thyroid gland or by kidney excretion and does not participate in the blood sample radioactivity. In hyperthyroidism, high values of radioactivity are noted in the blood sample due to the large amounts of I 131 converted into protein-bound iodine of the plasma. False positives may be obtained when renal retention of inorganic I 131 results in high blood radioactivity. These cases may be differentiated by precipitating the plasma proteins, and taking separate counts on the two fractions. This test of thyroid function appears even more accurate than in vivo counting of the neck or urinary excretion studies. An overlap zone is present between normal and hyperthyroids, but it is very small. Drugs, like iodine, thyroid extract, and thiourea derivatives, which pervert the mechanism and rate of formation and liberation of protein-bound iodine, make invalid this test, as they do the I 131 uptake and urinary excretion studies. The radioactive protein-bound iodine test is far simpler in performance than the chemical protein bound iodine determination.

CARDIOVASCULAR STUDIES

The study of the circulation by tagged substances offers much useful clinical information. Cardiac output is measured by the dilution method, using iodinated human serum albumen, (IHSA). If a small volume of highly concentrated material, in this instance 150 microcuries of IHSA, is injected into the venous system, the average dilution of the material coming out of the heart will be a direct indication of the volume passing through the heart and causing the dilution. If the change in dilution is measured for a definite period of time, the output can be expressed as volume of flow per unit of time. The dilution curve is obtained by counting the blood led from the femoral artery with a scintillation counter, and then calibrating the flow system in terms of microcuries per cc. by comparing the final record at final dilution with the in vitro assay of blood withdrawn at the same time. As for many other procedures, the values of IHSA depend upon its non-diffusability out of the vascular system for a relatively long period of time. The method compares favorably with the older, more standard methods of cardiac output determination such as the Fick method.

Utilizing any one of several tagged substances or radioactive electrolytes, peripheral vascular flow and circulation time may be measured. After the injection of the radioactive material into an arm vein, a counter placed over the extremity begins to record radioactivity, the curve of counts per second rising to a plateau. The initial detection of impulses indicates the arm to foot circulation time. The slope of the curve and the height of the plateau indicate the peripheral circulatory status. The tagged material mixes with the patient's blood, and achieves equilibrium. The faster the rate of mixing of the radioactive material with the blood, the faster the counting curve will rise. An ample circulation through the extremity is indicated by a fast rising curve, a poor circulation by a slowly rising curve. The height of the curve's plateau indicates the volume of the vascular bed measured by counts per second. This may be decreased in diseased extremities (arteriosclerosis). Since the radioactivity being measured is primarily within the capillaries this indicates a decreased capillary volume. When radioactive sodium, Na 24, is used in the study of the peripheral circulation, it diffuses out into the extracellular space, where it contributes to the radioactivity count of the extremity. The counts per second are a measurement then of this diffusion rate as well as the capillary circulation, whereas with IHSA, which remains in the vascular system well beyond the measurement period, the counts per second indicate only the flow within the vessels.

Blood volume has been studied by several different radioactive isotopes. All methods are based on the dilution of an injected substance by the total amount of blood, a method which has been extensively used with non-radioactive materials such as Evans blue dye. The essential difference is that the analysis of dilution is based on counts of radioactivity rather than on a chemical or colorimetric analysis. The radioactivity per milliliter of blood after dilution is compared with the total injected activity, and the total blood volume thereby calculated. Either red cells may be tagged by radioactive P 32, Fe 55, Fe 59, Cr 51, or K 42, or IHSA may be used. The erythrocyte tagging methods are most accurate for measurement of plasma volume. Either can be used to calculate whole blood volumes in conjunction with the hematocrit determination, but total blood volume measurements by tagged red cell methods are lower than IHSA methods. This is because the average body hematocrit is lower than the peripheral vessel hematocrit. For accurate evaluation of the whole blood independent determinations of plasma and red cell volumes should be done. The extracellular field volume may be obtained by measurement of the dilution of radioactive sodium, which like the non-radioactive sodium does not enter blood or tissue cells. Total body water is likewise measured by the dilution of a sample of deuterium.

TUMOR DETECTION

Diiodofluorescein and human serum albumen, "tagged" with radioactive iodine, are used in the detection of brain tumors. The presence of these substances in any location in the body is made known by detecting the emitted gamma rays. The relative quantity of the tagged substance is measured by the number of impulses per unit time. After the giving of an intravenous injection of the tagged compound to the patient with a suspected intracranial lesion, a directional counter is placed on the patient's head, and the number of impulses at each of many positions is counted on the skull surface and compared with readings at symmetrical positions on the opposite side (Fig. 3). A significant difference between a

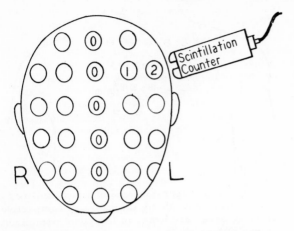

Fig. 3. Diagram of scintillation counter being used in a brain tumor tracer study. Multiple specific areas are counted following the intravenous injection of radioactive human serum albumen and compared with exactly symmetrical areas of the contralateral side. Increased uptake of the isotopic compound may be noted in tumor tissue.

focus and its adjacent area or a significant difference between identical right and left sided positions suggests a pathological area. Neoplastic tissue by virtue of its increased vascularity and its altered blood vessel permeability relationships contains more radioactive labelled material in a specific volume than does normal tissue. While neoplastic tissue produces a higher counting rate than normal tissue, an inflammatory lesion may also show a high counting rate for the same reasons. Some neoplasms are cystic, some are necrotic or have little vascularity and therefore show little distinguishing differences from normal tissue. Other neoplasms are deep seated and cannot be localized. The technic using radioactive diiodofluorescein and a Geiger counter consumes much time, 2-1/2 to 4 hours, and has been criticized for its lack of accuracy. The fluorescein rapidly leaves the circulation and the counts must be made within a limited period following injection. Using radioactive iodinated human serum albumen and scintillation counter, the counting procedure takes only 20 to 40 minutes and is considered more accurate. The initial count need not be hurried and repeated counts are permitted, since the albumen is retained in the circulation in sufficient quantity for 24 to 72 hours. Serial uptake studies have led in some cases to the detection of a focal lesion where a single set of counts had given doubtful values. P 32 and K 42 have also been used for brain tumor localization. K 42 is not very practical because of its short half life. P 32, a pure beta emitter whose rays cannot penetrate the skull can only be used for identification and delimitation of neoplasm from normal tissue at time of craniotomy with a special counter probe. Standard radiographic procedures of encephalography and ventriculography, whose accuracy approaches 100%, will not be replaced by the present tracer technics with radioactive materials. When the standard procedures are not yet indicated or give equivocal information, tracer studies

are indicated and valuable. They may help in diagnosing an intracranial metastasis from a lung neoplasm or in investigating a postoperative recurrence of a brain tumor.

The same principle of differential concentration of a radioisotope in tumor and adjacent normal tissue is utilized in the detection of intraocular tumors. A definite increased concentration of P 32 in tumor tissue over that found in normal tissue has been previously known. In addition to the postulated increased vascularity of a tumor, a rapid nucleic acid turnover and breakdown of the blood-tissue barrier account for the increased phosphorus content of the tumor. One half hour or more following an intravenous injection of a P 32 solution counts are made on the suspected eye and the normal eye. The pure beta emitter P 32 was purposely selected so that only the radioactivity within a few millimeters of a special probe-like Geiger counter would be counted. With a gamma emitter, the radioactivity for a more general area would be detected, rather than the radioactivity of a localized area. The procedure is valuable in determining whether retinal separation is due to tumor. When the cause of retinal separation is obvious, or the presence of a tumor can be diagnosed with certainty by other means, the radioactive phosphorus determination is not indicated.

The differential concentration of human serum albumen tagged with radioactive iodine in tumor and normal tissue is utilized in the diagnosis of liver metastases. Postmortem analysis of tumor and adjacent normal liver tissue bears out this higher concentration of IHSA in tumor tissue. Following an intravenous injection of the radioactive material, counts are taken by scintillation counter at coordinated points over the lower thorax and upper abdomen overlying the liver. The counting values are compared with control values obtained from a large series of normal patients. Abnormally high values are suggestive of liver metastases. A high accuracy is claimed for the method, but errors have occurred when ascites is present, and when there are inflammatory processes in the liver or adjacent organs.

VITAMIN B 12 - COBALT 60

Radioactive cobalt (Co 60) labelled vitamin B 12 is very useful in the laboratory diagnosis of pernicious anemia. The procedure has a specific use for patients who are suspected to have pernicious anemia, or who have already been treated with vitamin B 12 or folic acid, yet the diannosis is not certain. Symptoms of typical nature may not appear for long intervals, nevertheless it is not desirable to withhold treatment awaiting the development of hematological or neurological symptoms and signs which would make make the diagnosis clinically certain. In the typical case, this test confirms the clinical diagnosis.

Several different tests have been proposed, all based on the pernicious anemia patient's inability to properly absorb vitamin B 12 from the gastrointestinal tract, due to a deficiency of intrinsic factor provided by the stomach. Quantitation of the absorption and excretion of an orally administered dose of B 12 in which cobalt 60 is an integral part of the vitamin molecule can be made in different ways. One method is to measure the excretion in the stool. Another is to measure by external counting the amount retained in the liver, this being feasible since Co 60 emits gamma rays which penetrate the liver substance and abdominal wall. Or the minute amounts of Co 60 appearing in blood may be measured. The most acceptable method is that devised for measuring the Co 60 in the urine, after its original absorption from the intestine, circulation in the blood, and excretion via the kidney. One or two micrograms of cobalt 60 labelled vitamin B 12 are given to the fasting patient. Two hours later, 1000 micrograms of non-radioactive vitamin B 12 are given intramuscularly, to saturate the vitamin B 12 binding capacity of the plasma, and allow the absorbed radioactive B 12 to be excreted by the kidney in sufficient amount for accurate counting. It is termed a "flushing" dose. Commencing at this time, a 24 hours urine specimen is collected. An aliquot is counted for activity in a well type scintillation counter (Fig. 2), and the total amount excreted is expressed as a percentage of the previously administered radioactivity. Normal subjects excrete from 7 to 22%; pernicious anemia patients excrete from 0 to 2.3%. With the addition of intrinsic factor by mouth, and repeating of the test, pernicious anemia patients increase their excretion per cent into the normal range.

Total gastrectomized patients, who also do not have intrinsic factor, have greatly impaired absorption of B 12. Test results with radioactive B 12 are essentially the same as with pernicious anemia patients. Sprue and pancreatic insufficiency show im-

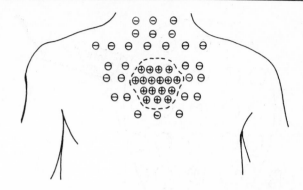

Fig. 4. Small operature chamber has outlined an intrathoraic thyroid by its uptake of radioactive iodine. ⊖ areas are areas of low count per minute, ⊕ areas of high count per minute.

paired B 12 absorption, which will not respond to the giving of intrinsic factor, thus indicating the primary disturbance to one of intestinal absorption, not of underproduction of intrinsic factor by the stomach.

Technics devised for study of pancreatic insufficiency based on the absorption of isotope labelled fat and protein would seem worthwhile provided they are simpler than chemical determination which is sometimes laborious. Isotope procedures to replace standard cholecystography and myelography to analyze cardiac function (radiocardiology) and liver function (radioactive rose bengal) have not been widely used.

QUESTIONS ON ISOTOPES

1. What general properties of radioactive isotopes make them useful in "tracer" studies?

2. Why is P 32 useful in some diseases of the blood forming tissues?

3. What is the place of isotope studies and what is their reliability in the diagnosis of thyroid disorders?

4. Thyroid function testing is dependent upon what properties of I 131? Therapy of hyperthyroidism is based upon what properties of I 131?

5. What is the value of an isotope study in brain lesions? How is it carried out?

6. What is a background count? Geiger counter? Scintillation counter? How do they differ from recording by a scaler?

7. List the ways in which radioactive colloidal gold has been used and describe the method of its action.

REFERENCES FOR ISOTOPES

Yuhl, E. T., and Stirrett, L. A., "Clinical Evaluation of the Hepatic Radioactive Survey," Ann. Surg., 138:857, 1953.

MacIntyre, W. J., Storaasli, J. P., Kruger, H., Pritchard, W., and Friedell, H. L., "I-131 Labelled Serum Albumin: Its Use in the Study of Cardiac Output and Peripheral Vascular Flow," Radiology, 59:849, 1952.

Brady, L. W., Cooper, D. Y., Colodzin, M., McClenathan, J. E., King, E. R., and Williams, R., "Blood Volume Studies in Normal Humans," S.G.O., 97:25, 1953.

Thomas, C. I., Krohmer, J. S., and Storaasli, J. P., "Detection of Intraocular Tumors with Radioactive Phosphorus," Arch. Ophthalmd., 47:276, 1952.

Ashkenazy, M., and Crawley, J. W., "The Value of Serial Studies of Cerebrovascular Permeability with Radioactive Iodinated Serum Albumin and the Scintillation Counter, Particularly in the Detection of Neurosurgical Lesions," American Surgeon, 19:155, 1953.

Hahn, Paul F., Editor, Therapeutic Use of Artificial Radioisotopes, New York, John Wiley and Sons, 1956.

Silver, S., Fieber, M. H., and Yohalem, S. B., "Blood Levels After Tracer Doses of Radioactive Iodine in the Diagnosis of Thyroid Disorders," Am. J. Med., 13:725, 1952.

Moore, G. E., et al., "Biophysical Studies of Methods Utilizing Fluorescein and Its Derivatives to Diagnose Brain Tumors," Radiology, 55:334, 1950.

Bate, D., and Guttman, R. J., "Changes in Lung and Pleura Following Two-Million-Volt Therapy for Carcinoma of the Breast," Radiol., 69:372, 1957.

Schilling, R. F., Clatanoff, D. V., and Korst, D. R., "Intrinsic Factor Studies. III. Further Observations Utilizing the Urinary Radioactivity Test in Subjects with Achlorhydria, Pernicious Anemia, or a Total Gastrectomy," J. Lab. and Clin. Med., 45:926, 1955.

Beierwaltes, W. H., Johnson, P. C., and Solari, A. J., "Clinical Use of Radioisotopes," W. B. Saunders, Philadelphia, 1957.

SUGGESTIONS FOR COLLATERAL READING*

General books on the subject of diagnostic roentgenology:
Small concise works:

Appleton, A. B., Hamilton, W. J., Tchaperoff, I. C., Surface and Radiological Anatomy, Williams and Wilkins, Baltimore, 1946.

Holmes, G. W., and Ruggles, H. E., Roentgen Interpretation, Lea and Febiger, Phil., 1941.

Rigler, L. G., Outline of Roentgen Diagnosis, J. B. Lippincott, Phil., 1943.

McLaren, J. W., Modern Trends in Diagnostic Radiology, Paul Hoeber, N. Y., 1948.

Hodges, F. J., Lampe, I., Holt, J. F., Radiology for Medical Students, Year Book Pub. Co., Chicago, Ill., 1954.

Markovits, E., Visceral Radiology, McMillan Company, Chicago, 1951.

More comprehensive volumes:

Appleton, A. B., Hamilton, W. J., and Tchaperoff, I. C. C., Surface and Radiological Anatomy, Wm. Wood and Co., Phil., 1938.

Friedman, L. J., Textbook of Diagnostic Roentgenology, D. Appleton-Century Co., N. Y., 1937.

Kohler, A., Roentgenology, Wm. Wood and Co., Baltimore, 1935.

Shanks, S. C., Kerley, P., and Twining, E. W., A Textbook of X-ray Diagnosis, H. K. Lewis and Co., London, 1938.

Harrison, B. J. M., Textbook of Roentgenology, Wm. Wood and Co., Baltimore, 1936.

Golden, Ross, et al., Diagnostic Roentgenology, Thos. Nelson and Son, N. Y., 1941.

Pillmore, G. U., Clinical Radiology, 2 vols., F. A. Davis Co., Phil., 1946.

Schinz, Baensch, Friedl, and Uehlinger, Ed. by J. T. Case, Grune and Stratton, N. Y., 1954.

For a review of latest developments in the field of roentgenology:

Hodges, F., and Kaplan, Ira, Yearbook of Radiology, Yearbook Publishing Co., Chicago, published annually since 1933.

On Bones and Joints:

Fairbank, Sir Thos., An Atlas of General Affections of the Skeleton, E. and S. Livingston, LTD., Edinburgh, 1951.

Cohn, I., Normal Bones and Joints, Paul Hoeber, N. Y., 1924.

Stewart, Wm. H., The Skull, Paul Hoeber, N. Y., 1925.

Bradford, F. K. and Spurling, R. G., Chas. Thomas, Springfield, Ill., 1945.

Brailsford, J. F., Radiology of Bones and Joints, Wm. Wood and Co., Baltimore, 1948.

American Committee for the Control of Rheumatism, Rheumatism Primer, A.M.A., Chicago.

Geschickter, C. F., and Copeland, M., Am. J. of Cancer, N. Y., 1936.

Kolodny, A., Bone Sarcoma (supplement of Nov. 1927 number Surg. Gyn. and Obst., Vol. 44) Surgical Pub. Co., Chicago, Ill., 1927.

Ferguson, A. B., Roentgen Diagnosis of Extremities and Spine, Paul Hoeber, N. Y., 1941.

deLorimier, Alfred, The Arthropathies, Year Book Pub. Inc., Chicago, 1943.

Archer, V. W., The Osseous System, Year Book Pub. Inc., Chicago, 1945.

Snapper, I., Medical Clinics on Bone Diseases, Interscience Pub. Inc., N.Y.

Weinmann, J. P. and Sicher, H., Bone and Bones, C. V. Mosby, St. Louis.

Todd, T. W., Atlas of Skeletal Maturation, C. V. Mosby, St. Louis, 1937.

Moselely, H. F., Shoulder Lesion - 1st edition - Chas. C. Thomas Publisher, Springfield, Illinois, 1947

Steindler, A., Post Graduate Lectures on Orthopedic Diagnosis and Indication, Vol. I, Chas. C. Thomas Publisher, Springfield, Illinois, 1950.

Hass, J., Congenital Dislocations of the Hip, Chas. C. Thomas Publisher, Springfield, Illinois, 1951.

Hollander, J. L., Editor, Comroe's Arthritis and Allied Condition, Lea and Febiger, Philadelphia, 1953.

Pugh, D. A., Bones and Joints, Williams and Wilkins, Baltimore, 1954.

On Respiratory System:

Wessler, H., and Jaches, L., Clinical Roentgenology of Diseases of the Chest, Southworth Co., Troy, N. Y., 1923.

Sante, L. R., The Chest, Paul Hoeber, N. Y., 1931.

Stoloff, E. G., The Chest in Children, Paul Hoeber, N. Y., 1930.

Jackson, Chevalier, and Jackson, Chevalier L., Foreign Bodies in the Air and Food Passages, Paul Hoeber, N. Y., 1934.

Miller, Wm. Snow, The Lung, Chas. C. Thomas, Springfield, Ill., 1937.

Pancoast, H. K., and Pendergrass, E. P., Pneumoconiosis, Paul Hoeber, N. Y., 1926.

*All references are to volumes which deal with the various subjects in a general way; no references have been made to specific articles appearing in medical journals.

Reimann, H. A., The Pneumonias, W. B. Saunders Co., Phil., 1938.

Cole, L. G., Lung Dust Lesions Versus Tuberculosis, Am. Med. Films, Inc., White Plains, N. Y., 1948.

Cole, L. G. and Cole, W. G., Pneumoconiosis, John B. Pierce Foundation, N. Y., 1940.

Pinner, M., Pulmonary Tuberculosis in the Adult, Chas. C. Thomas, Springfield, Ill., 1946.

Rubin, E. H. and Rubin, M., Diseases of the Chest, W. B. Saunders Co., Phil., 1947.

Drinker, C. K., Pulmonary Edema and Inflammation, Harvard Univ. Press, 1945.

Brock, R. C., Anatomy of the Lung, Oxford Univ. Press, London, 1946.

Lisa, J. R., Bronchiectasis, Oxford Univ. Press, 1943.

Snow, W., Roentgen Study of the Chest, Chas. C. Thomas, Springfield, Ill., 1946.

Rigler, L. G., The Chest, Year Book Pub., Chicago, 1946.

Westermark, N., Roentgen Studies of the Lungs and Heart, Univ. Minn. Press, 1948.

Myers, J. A. and McKinlay, C. A., The Chest and Heart, 2 vols., Chas. C. Thomas, Springfield, Ill., 1948.

Amor, A. J., An X-Ray Atlas of Silicosis, Williams and Wilkins, Baltimore, 1941.

Lisa, J. R., Rosenblatt, M. D., Bronchiectasis, Oxford University Press, 1943.

Neuhof, H., Jemerin, E. A., Acute Infections of the Mediastinum, Williams and Wilkins, Baltimore, 1943.

Norris, G. W. and Landis, H. R. M., Diseases of the Chest and Principles of Physical Diagnosis, W. B. Saunders, Philadelphia, Pa., 1940.

Ritvo, M., Chest X-Ray Diagnosis, Lea and Febiger, Philadelphia, Pa., 1951.

On the Circulatory System:

Master, A. M., Electrocardiogram and X-ray Configuration of the Heart, Lea and Febiger, Phil., 1939.

Trueta, J., Barclay, A. E., Franklin, K. J., Daniel, P. M. and Prichard, M., Studies of the Renal Circulation, Chas. C. Thomas, Springfield, Ill., 1948.

Schnitker, M. A., Congenital Anomalies of the Heart and Great Vessels, Oxford Univ. Press, New York, 1952.

Mayo Clinic Group, Congenital Anomalies of the Heart and Great Vessels, Chas. C. Thomas, Springfield, Ill., 1948.

Ungerleider, H. E. and Gubner, R., Roentgenology of the Heart and Great Vessels, 3rd edition, 1950, F. A. Davis Pub., Philadelphia, Pa., 1950.

Polevski, J., The Heart Visible, F. A. Davis, Phil., 1934.

Roesler, Hugo, Atlas of Cardiorentgenology, Chas. C. Thomas, Springfield, 1940.

Roesler, Hugo, Clinical Roentgenology of the Cardiovascular System, Chas. C. Thomas, Springfield, Ill., 1943.

Barclay, A. E., Franklin, K. J. and Prichard, M. L., The Foetal Circulation, Blackwell Scientific Publications, Ltd., Oxford, Eng., 1945.

Gross, R. E., Surgical Treatment for Anomalies of the Heart and Great Vessels, Chas. C. Thomas, Springfield, Ill.

New York Heart Assoc., Diseases of the Heart, N. Y. Heart Assoc., 50 West 50th St., N. Y.

Schwedel, J. B., Clinical Roentgenology of the Heart, Paul Hoeber, N. Y., 1946.

Stroud, W. D., Cardiovascular Disease, F. A. Davis, Co., Phil., 1945.

Taussig, H. B., Congenital Malformations of the Heart, Commonwealth Fund, N. Y., 1947.

Treiger, I. J., Atlas of Cardiovascular Disease, C. V. Mosby Co., St. Louis.

New York Heart Ass'n., Diseases of the Heart, N. Y. Heart Ass'n., N. Y., 1943.

On the Gastrointestinal Tract:

Carman, Russel, and Miller, Albert, Roentgen Diagnoses of Diseases of the Alimentary Tract, W. B. Saunders, 1917.

Buckstein, J., Peptic Ulcer, Paul Hoeber, N. Y., 1930.

Cole, L. G., et al., Radiologic Exploration of the Mucosa of the Gastrointestinal Tract, Bruce Pub., St. Paul, 1934.

Barclay, A. E., Digestive Tract, Macmillan, Chicago, 1933.

Alvarez, W. C., Mechanics of the Digestive Tract, Paul Hoeber, N. Y., 1928.

Kerley, C. G., and Lewald, L. T., Digestive Disturbances in Infants and Children, Paul Hoeber, N. Y., 1923.

Feldman, M., Clinical Roentgenology of the Digestive Tract, William Wood, Baltimore, 1945.

Templeton, X-ray Examination of the Stomach, Univ. of Chicago Press, Chicago, Ill., 1944.

Golden, Ross, Radiological Examination of the Small Intestine, J. B. Lippincott Co., Phil., Pa., 1945.

Hodges, F. J., The Gastro-Intestinal Tract, Year Book Pub. Inc., Chicago, 1944.

Bockus, H. L., Gastro-Enterology - 3 vols., W. B. Saunders Co., Phil., 1944.

Farrell, J. T. Jr., Roentgen Diagnosis of Diseases of the Gastrointestinal Tract, Chas. C. Thomas, Springfield, Ill., 1946.

Alvarez, W. C., Introduction to Gastro-Enterology, Paul Hoeber, New York, 1940.

Buckstein, J., Digestive Tract in Roentgenology, J. B. Lippincott, Philadelphia, 1948.

Ritvo, M., and Shauffer, I. A., Gastro-Intestinal X-Ray Diagnosis, Lea and Febiger, Phil., 1952.

On the Biliary Tract:

Graham, E. A., Cole, W. H., Copher, G. and Moore, S., Diseases of the Gall Bladder and Bile Ducts, Lea and Febiger, Phil., 1928.

On the Urinary Tract:

Young, H. H., and Waters, C. A., Urological Roentgenology, Paul Hoeber, N. Y., 1928.

Lower, Wm. E., and Nichols, B. H., Roentgenographic Studies of the Urinary System, Mosby Co., St. Louis, 1933.

Wesson, M. B., and Ruggles, H. E., Urological Roentgenology, Lea and Febiger, Phil., 1936.

Kerr, H. D., and Gillies, C. L., Urinary Tract, Year Book Pub. Co., Chicago, Ill., 1944.

Braasch, W. F., Emmett, J. L., Clinical Urography, W. B. Saunders, Philadelphia, 1951.

Lossley, O. S., Kirkwin, P. J., Clinical Urology, Williams and Wilkins Co., Baltimore, 1940.

On the Head and Neck:

Pancoast, H., Pendergrass, E., and Schaeffer, J. P., Head and Neck in Roentgen Diagnosis, Chas. C. Thomas, 1940.

Ritvo, M., Roentgen Diagnosis of Diseases of the Skull, Paul Hoeber, New York, 1949.

On the Nasal Sinuses and Mastoids:

Law, F. M., Nasal Accessory Sinuses, Paul Hoeber, N. Y., 1933.

Law, F. M., Mastoids, Paul Hoeber, N. Y., 1929.

Granger, A., Para-Nasal Sinuses and Mastoids, Lea and Febiger, Phil., 1932.

Proetz, A., Displacement Method of Sinus Diagnosis and Treatment, Annals Publ. Co., St. Louis, 1939.

Jackson, C. and Jackson, C. L., Diseases of the Nose, Throat and Ear, W. B. Saunders Co., Phil., 1946.

Young, B. R., The Skull, Sinuses and Mastoids, Year Book Pub. Co., Chicago, Ill., 1948.

Samuel, E., Clinical Radiology of Ear, Nose and Throat, Hoeber, N. Y., 1952.

On the Teeth:

Thompson, W. S., Operative and Interpretive Radiodontia, Lea and Febiger, Phil., 1936.

Simpson, C. O., Technic of Oral Radiography, C. V. Mosby, St. Louis, 1926; Advanced Radiodontic Interpretation, University Press, St. Louis, 1931.

Osgood, H. A., Teeth and Jaws, Paul Hoeber, N. Y., 1929.

Ennis, L. M., Dental Roentgenology, Lea and Febiger, Phil., 1936.

Main, L. R., Oral and Dental Roentgenography, C. V. Mosby, St. Louis, 1945.

On Artificial Pneumoperitoneum:

Stein, A., and Stewart, Wm. H., Pneumoperitoneal Roentgen-ray Diagnosis, Southworth Co., Troy, N. Y., 1921.

On Ventriculography and Encephalography:

Davis, Loyal, Intracranial Tumors, Paul Hoeber, N. Y., 1933.

Dandy, W. E., Section on Ventriculography in Dean Lewis' Practice of Surgery, W. F. Prior, Hagerstown, Md., 1936.

Davidoff, L. M., and Dyke, C., Normal Encephalogram, Lea and Febiger, Phil., 1937.

Bailey, P., Intracranial Tumors, Chas. Thomas, Springfield, 1933.

On Female Pelvic Organs:

Jacho, J., Gynecological Roentgenology, Paul Hoeber, N. Y., 1931.

Snow, W., Clinical Roentgenology of Pregnancy, Chas. C. Thomas, Springfield, Ill., 1942.

On Neuroradiology:

Orley, A., Neuroradiology, Chas. C. Thomas, Springfield, Ill., 1949.

Bing, R., Haymaker, W., Compendium of Regional Diagnosis and Lesions of the Brain and Spinal Cord, Mosley Publisher, St. Louis, 1940.

Ecker, A., Normal Cerebral Angiogram, Chas. C. Thomas, Publisher, Springfield, Illinois, 1951.

On Pediatrics:

Caffey, J., Pediatric Roentgenology, Year Book Publishers, Chicago.

INDEX